OKU 11

Orthopaedic Knowledge Update

AAOS

AMERICAN ACADEMY OF
ORTHOPAEDIC SURGEONS

OKU 11

Orthopaedic Knowledge Update

EDITOR:

Lisa K. Cannada, MD
Associate Professor
Department of Orthopaedic Surgery
Saint Louis University
St. Louis, Missouri

AAOS
AMERICAN ACADEMY OF
ORTHOPAEDIC SURGEONS

AAOS

AMERICAN ACADEMY OF ORTHOPAEDIC SURGEONS

The material presented in *Orthopaedic Knowledge Update 11* has been made available by the American Academy of Orthopaedic Surgeons for educational purposes only. This material is not intended to present the only, or necessarily best, methods or procedures for the medical situations discussed, but rather is intended to represent an approach, view, statement, or opinion of the author(s) or producer(s), which may be helpful to others who face similar situations.

Some drugs or medical devices demonstrated in Academy courses or described in Academy print or electronic publications have not been cleared by the Food and Drug Administration (FDA) or have been cleared for specific uses only. The FDA has stated that it is the responsibility of the physician to determine the FDA clearance status of each drug or device he or she wishes to use in clinical practice.

Furthermore, any statements about commercial products are solely the opinion(s) of the author(s) and do not represent an Academy endorsement or evaluation of these products. These statements may not be used in advertising or for any commercial purpose.

Published 2014 by the
American Academy of Orthopaedic Surgeons
6300 North River Road
Rosemont, IL 60018

Copyright 2014
by the American Academy of Orthopaedic Surgeons

ISBN 978-0-89203-865-7

Library of Congress Control Number: 2013955807

Printed in the USA

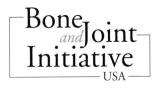

Acknowledgments

Contributors

WILLIAM A. ABDU, MD, MS
Associate Professor of Orthopaedic Surgery
Dartmouth-Hitchcock Medical Center
Lebanon, New Hampshire

JOHN A. ABRAHAM, MD
Chief of Orthopedic Oncology
Rothman Institute
Thomas Jefferson University
Philadelphia, Pennsylvania

ANIMESH AGARWAL, MD
Professor
Department of Orthopaedic Surgery
University of Texas Health Science Center
San Antonio, Texas

VINAY AGGARWAL, BA
Research Fellow
Department of Adult Joint Reconstruction
Rothman Institute at Thomas Jefferson
 University
Philadelphia, Pennsylvania

CHRISTOPHER S. AHMAD, MD
Associate Professor
Department of Orthopaedic Surgery
Columbia University Medical Center
New York, New York

JAIMO AHN, MD, PhD
Assistant Professor and Co-Director
Department of Orthopaedic Trauma and
 Fracture Service
University of Pennsylvania
Philadelphia, Pennsylvania

TAMARA ALLISTON, PhD
Associate Professor
Department of Orthopaedic Surgery
University of California, San Francisco
San Francisco, California

DONALD D. ANDERSON, PhD
Associate Professor
Department of Orthopaedics and Rehabilitation
The University of Iowa
Iowa City, Iowa

APRIL D. ARMSTRONG, MD
Associate Professor
Department of Orthopaedics
Penn State Milton S. Hershey Medical Center
Hershey, Pennsylvania

WILLIAM V. ARNOLD, MD, PhD
Instructor
Department of Orthopaedic Surgery
The Rothman Institute at Thomas Jefferson
 University
Philadelphia, Pennsylvania

GEORGE S. ATHWAL, MD, FRCSC
Associate Professor
Hand and Upper Limb Centre
Western University
London, Ontario, Canada

GEORGE C. BABIS, MD, PhD
Professor and Chairman
2nd Department of Orthopaedic Surgery
University of Athens, Medical School
Athens, Greece

DONALD BAE, MD
Assistant Professor of Orthopaedic Surgery
Department of Orthopaedic Surgery
Harvard Medical School
Boston Children's Hospital
Boston, Massachusetts

TESSA BALACH, MD
Assistant Professor
Department of Orthopaedic Surgery
New England Musculoskeletal Institute
University of Connecticut Health Center
Farmington, Connecticut

JAMIE BARATTA, MD
Instructor
Department of Anesthesiology
Jefferson Medical College
Philadelphia, Pennsylvania

SARINA BEHERA, MD
Clinical Instructor, Pediatric Cardiology
Department of Pediatrics
California Pacific Medical Center
San Francisco, California

JOHN-ERIK BELL, MD, MS
Assistant Professor
Department of Orthopaedic Surgery
Dartmouth-Hitchcock Medical Center
Lebanon, New Hampshire

KARL A. BERGMANN, MD
Assistant Professor
Division of Orthopaedics
Creighton University
Omaha, Nebraska

GREG BERRY, MDCM, FRCSC
Staff Surgeon
Department of Orthopaedic Surgery
McGill University Health Centre
Montreal, Quebec, Canada

MOHIT BHANDARI, MD, PhD, FRCSC
Professor and Academic Head
Division of Orthopaedic Surgery
McMaster University
Hamilton, Ontario, Canada

LOUIS U. BIGLIANI, MD
Frank E. Stinchfield Professor and Chairman
Department of Orthopaedic Surgery
Columbia University Medical Center
New York, New York

MICHAEL V. BIRMAN, MD
Hand Surgeon, Private Practice
Hand Surgery Associates, S.C.
Arlington Heights, Illinois

CHRISTOPHER M. BONO, MD
Chief, Orthopaedic Spine Service
Associate Professor
Harvard Medical School
Brigham and Women's Hospital
Boston, Massachusetts

PATRICK BOSCH, MD
Associate Professor
Department of Orthopaedic Surgery
University of Pittsburgh Medical Center
Children's Hospital of Pittsburgh
Pittsburgh, Pennsylvania

RICHARD E. BOWEN, MD
Associate Clinical Professor
Geffen School of Medicine at University of
*   California Los Angeles*
Los Angeles Orthopaedic Hospital
Los Angeles, California

RONALD C. BURGESS, MD
Clinical Associate Professor
Orthopaedic Department
University of Kentucky
Lexington, Kentucky

EDWIN R. CADET, MD
Assistant Professor
Department of Orthopaedic Surgery
Columbia University
New York, New York

MICHELLE S. CAIRD, MD
Assistant Professor of Orthopaedic Surgery
Department of Orthopaedics
University of Michigan
Ann Arbor, Michigan

JOHN T. CAPO, MD
Professor, Department of Orthopaedics
New York University Hospital for Joint
*   Diseases*
New York, New York

EUGENE J. CARRAGEE, MD
Professor and Vice Chairman
Department of Orthopaedic Surgery
Stanford University School of Medicine
Redwood City, California

CORDELIA W. CARTER, MD
Assistant Professor
Department of Orthopaedics and Rehabilitation
Yale University
New Haven, Connecticut

ANTONIA CHEN, MD, MBA
Junior Faculty
Rothman Institute
Jefferson University
Philadelphia, Pennsylvania

JOHN S. CLAPP, MD
Orthopaedic Surgeon
Department of Orthopaedic Surgery
University Hospital
Augusta, Georgia

RACHEL M. DEERING, MPH
Clinical Research Coordinator
Orthopaedic Spine Department
Brigham and Women's Hospital
Boston, Massachusetts

DANIEL R. DZIADOSZ, MD
Orthopaedic Trauma Surgeon
Department of Orthopaedics
Inova Fairfax Hospital
Falls Church, Virginia

SARA EDWARDS, MD
Assistant Professor
Department of Orthopaedic Surgery
Northwestern University Feinberg School
  of Medicine
Chicago, Illinois

KENNETH A. EGOL, MD
Professor and Vice Chair
Department of Orthopaedic Surgery
New York University Hospital for
  Joint Diseases
New York, New York

BRIAN T. FEELEY, MD
Assistant Professor
Department of Orthopaedic Surgery
University of California, San Francisco
San Francisco, California

MARCO FERRONE, MD
Department of Orthopaedic Surgery
Brigham and Women's Hospital
Dana Farber Cancer Insitute
Boston, Massachusetts

ANDRZEJ FERTALA, PhD
Professor
Department of Orthopaedic Surgery
Division of Orthopaedic Research
Thomas Jefferson University
Philadelphia, Pennsylvania

CHARLES FISCHER, MD, MHSc, FRCSC
Associate Professor
Department of Orthopaedic Surgery
University of British Columbia
Vancouver, British Columbia, Canada

CYRIL B. FRANK, MD
Professor
Department of Surgery
University of Calgary
Calgary, Alberta, Canada

LEESA M. GALATZ, MD
Associate Professor
Washington University Orthopedics
Barnes-Jewish Hospital
St. Louis, Missouri

KISHOR GANDHI, MD, MPH
Assistant Professor
Department of Anesthesiology
Jefferson Medical College
Philadelphia, Pennsylvania

ROBIN M. GEHRMANN, MD
Chief of Sports Medicine
Department of Orthopaedics
University of Medicine and Dentistry of
  New Jersey
New Jersey Medical School
Newark, New Jersey

ERIC GIZA, MD
Chief, Foot and Ankle Surgery
Department of Orthopaedics
University of California Davis Medical Center
Sacramento, California

JESSICA GOETZ, PhD
Research Assistant Professor
Department of Orthopaedics and Rehabilitation
University of Iowa
Iowa City, Iowa

GUILLEM GONZALEZ-LOMAS, MD
Assistant Professor
Department of Orthopaedic Surgery
Division of Sports Medicine
New York University Hospital for
  Joint Diseases
New York, New York

MELISSA M. GUANCHE, MD
Department of Rehabilitation Medicine
Thomas Jefferson University Hospital
Philadelphia, Pennsylvania

GEORGE J. HAIDUKEWYCH, MD
Academic Chairman, Orlando Health
Professor, University of Central Florida
Orlando, Florida

KURT D. HANKENSON, DVM, MS, PhD
Associate Professor
Department of Clinical Studies-New Bolton
    Center
University of Pennsylvania
Philadelphia, Pennsylvania

CHRISTOPHER CHAMBLISS HARROD, MD
Attending Orthopaedic Spine Surgeon
Baton Rouge Bone and Joint Clinic
The Spine Center
Baton Rouge, Louisiana

EDWARD J. HARVEY, MD, MSc
Professor of Surgery
McGill University
McGill University Health Center
Montreal, Quebec, Canada

THERESA A. HENNESSEY, MD
Assistant Professor
Department of Orthopaedics
University of Utah
Shriner's Hospital for Children
Salt Lake City, Utah

CHRISTINE ANN HO, MD
Assistant Professor
Department of Orthopaedic Surgery
University of Texas Southwestern Medical
    Center
Children's Medical Center
Texas Scottish Rite Hospital for Children
Dallas, Texas

XIAOBANG HU, MD, PhD
Clinical Research Assistant
Scoliosis and Spine Tumor Center
Texas Back Institute
Texas Health Presbyterian Hospital
Plano, Texas

JOSHUA J. JACOBS, MD
Professor and Chairman
Department of Orthopedic Surgery
Rush University Medical Center
Chicago, Illinois

CHARLES M. JOBIN, MD
Assistant Professor of Clinical Orthopaedic
    Surgery
Department of Orthopaedics
Columbia University
New York, New York

JOSEPH A. KARAM, MD
Post-Doctoral Research Fellow
Department of Orthopaedic Research
The Rothman Institute at Thomas Jefferson
    University
Philadelphia, Pennsylvania

DAVID B. KARGES, DO
Professor
Department of Orthopaedic Surgery
Saint Louis University
St. Louis, Missouri

DEREK M. KELLY, MD
Pediatric Orthopedic Surgeon
Campbell Clinic Orthopedics
University of Tennessee and Le Bonheur
    Children's Hospital
Memphis, Tennessee

GRAHAM J.W. KING, MD, MSc, FRCSC
Professor
Department of Surgery
University of Western Ontario
London, Ontario, Canada

BRIAN A. KLATT, MD
Assistant Professor
Department of Orthopaedic Surgery
University of Pittsburgh
Pittsburgh, Pennsylvania

GREGG KLEIN, MD
Vice-Chairman
Department of Orthopaedic Surgery
Hackensack University Medical Center
Hackensack, New Jersey

CDR Kevin M. Kuhn, MD, MC, USN
Director of Orthopaedic Trauma
Department of Orthopaedic Surgery
Naval Medical Center San Diego
San Diego, California

Stefanie Peggy Kuhnel, MD
Clinical Fellow
Department of Surgery
Hand and Upper Limb Centre
University of Western Ontario
London, Ontario, Canada

Alfred C. Kuo, MD, PhD
Assistant Professor
Department of Orthopaedic Surgery
University of California, San Francisco
San Francisco, California

Joshua Langford, MD
Director, Limb Deformity Service
Orlando Health Orthopedic Residency
    Program
Orlando Health
Orlando, Florida

Joseph M. Lane, MD
Chief, Metabolic Bone Disease Service
Professor
Department of Orthopaedic Surgery
Hospital for Special Surgery
New York, New York

Steve K. Lee, MD
Associate Professor of Orthopaedic Surgery
Hand and Upper Extremity Service
Hospital for Special Surgery
New York, New York

Paul E. Levin, MD
Associate Professor
Vice-Chairperson
Department of Orthopaedic Surgery
Montefiore Medical Center/Albert Einstein
    College of Medicine
Bronx, New York

Brett R. Levine, MD, MS
Assistant Professor and Residency Director
Department of Orthopaedics
Rush University Medical Center
Chicago, Illinois

William N. Levine, MD
Professor of Orthopaedic Surgery
Department of Orthopaedics
Columbia University
New York, New York

Richard L. Lieber, PhD
Professor of Orthopaedics and Bioengineering
Department of Orthopaedic Surgery
UC San Diego School of Medicine
San Diego, California

Isador H. Lieberman, MD, MBA, FRCSC
Medical Director
Scoliosis and Spine Tumor Center
Texas Back Institute
Texas Health Presbyterian Hospital
Plano, Texas

Jay R. Lieberman, MD
Director, New England Musculoskeletal
    Institute
Professor and Chairman
Department of Orthopaedic Surgery
University of Connecticut Health Center
Farmington, Connecticut

Frank A. Liporace, MD
Associate Professor
Director of Orthopaedic Research
New York University Hospital for Joint
    Diseases
New York, New York

Luke Lopas, BS
Research Fellow
Department of Orthopaedic Surgery
University of Pennsylvania
Philadelphia, Pennsylvania

Jeffrey Lotz, PhD
Professor and Vice Chair
Department of Orthopaedic Surgery
University of California, San Francisco
San Francisco, California

Anthony C. Luke, MD, MPH
Professor of Clinical Orthopedics
Director, Primary Care Sports Medicine
Department of Orthopedics
University of California, San Francisco
San Francisco, California

Terry C.P. Lynch, MD
Professor of Clinical Radiology
University of California, San Francisco
  Department of Radiology
San Francisco General Hospital
San Francisco, California

C. Benjamin Ma, MD
Associate Professor
Chief, Sports Medicine and Shoulder Surgery
Department of Orthopaedic Surgery
University of California, San Francisco
San Francisco, California

William G. MacKenzie, MD
Chairman, Department of Orthopaedic Surgery
Nemours/Alfred I. DuPont Hospital
  for Children
Wilmington, Delaware

Peter J. Mandell, MD
Assistant Clinical Professor
Department of Orthopaedic Surgery
University of California, San Francisco
San Francisco, California

Iain McFayden, MBChB, FRCS (Tr&Orth)
Chief of Trauma
Department of Trauma and Orthopaedics
Brighton and Sussex University Hospitals
Brighton, Sussex, United Kingdom

Amy L. McIntosh, MD
Assistant Professor
Department of Orthopedics
Mayo Clinic
Rochester, Minnesota

Simon C. Mears, MD, PhD
Associate Professor
Department of Orthopaedic Surgery
Johns Hopkins Bayview Medical Center
Baltimore, Maryland

Samir Mehta, MD
Chief, Orthopaedic Trauma and Fracture
  Service
Department of Orthopaedic Surgery
Hospital of the University of Pennsylvania
Philadelphia, Pennsylvania

Joshua Meier, MD
Pediatric Orthopaedic Surgeon
Children and Orthopedics of Louisville
Clinical Professor
Department of Orthopaedic Surgery
University of Louisville
Louisville, Kentucky

Eric Meinberg, MD
Assistant Clinical Professor
Department of Orthopaedic Surgery
University of California, San Francisco
San Francisco, California

Justin W. Miller, MD
Spine Surgeon
Indiana Spine Group
Indianapolis, Indiana

Hassan R. Mir, MD
Assistant Professor
Department of Orthopaedic Surgery
Vanderbilt University
Nashville, Tennessee

Berton R. Moed, MD
Professor and Chairman
Department of Orthopaedic Surgery
Saint Louis University School of Medicine
St. Louis, Missouri

Saam Morshed, MD, PhD, MPH
Assistant Professor
Department of Orthopedic Surgery
Orthopedic Trauma Institute
University of California, San Francisco
San Francisco, California

M. Lucas Murnaghan, MD, MEd, FRCSC
Assistant Professor
Department of Surgery
University of Toronto
Toronto, Ontario, Canada

Anand Murthi, MD
Attending Orthopaedic Surgeon
Chief, Shoulder and Elbow Surgery
Department of Orthopaedics
MedStar Union Memorial Hospital
Baltimore, Maryland

Unni G. Narayanan, MBBS, MSc, FRCSC
Associate Professor
Department of Orthopaedic Surgery
The Hospital for Sick Children
University of Toronto
Toronto, Ontario, Canada

Javad Parvizi, MD, FRCS
Professor of Orthopaedics
Department of Orthopaedic Surgery
The Rothman Institute at Thomas Jefferson
    University
Philadelphia, Pennsylvania

Adam Pearson, MD, MS
Assistant Professor
Department of Orthopaedic Surgery
Dartmouth-Hitchcock Medical Center
The Geisel School of Medicine at Dartmouth
Lebanon, New Hampshire

Brad Petrisor, MSC, MD, FRCSC
Associate Professor
Division of Orthopaedics
McMaster University
Hamilton, Ontario, Canada

David A. Podeszwa, MD
Associate Professor
University of Texas Southwestern Medical
    Center
Attending Surgeon
Texas Scottish Rite Hospital for Children
Dallas, Texas

Debra Popejoy, MD
Pediatric Orthopedic Surgeon
University of California, Davis
Sacramento, California

Anish Potty, MD
Fellow
Department of Orthopaedics
Hospital for Special Surgery
New York, New York

Raj D. Rao, MD
Professor of Orthopaedic Surgery and
    Neurosurgery
Department of Orthopaedic Surgery
Medical College of Wisconsin
Milwaukee, Wisconsin

Mark C. Reilly, MD
Associate Professor and Chief Orthopaedic
    Trauma Service
Department of Orthopaedics
New Jersey Medical School
Newark, New Jersey

William M. Ricci, MD
Professor, Chief Orthopaedic Trauma Service
Department of Orthopaedic Surgery
Washington University School of Medicine
St. Louis, Missouri

Jeffrey A. Rihn, MD
Associate Professor
Department of Orthopaedic Surgery
The Rothman Institute at Thomas Jefferson
    University
Philadelphia, Pennsylvania

Scott A. Riley, MD
Chief, Hand Surgery Service
Shriners Hospital of Lexington
Lexington, Kentucky

Vasileios I. Sakellariou, MD, PhD
Stavros Niarchos – Thomas Sculco
    International Fellow
Department of Orthopedic Surgery
Hospital for Special Surgery
New York, New York

JONATHON K. SALAVA, MD
OrthoCarolina Hip and Knee Center
Charlotte, North Carolina

RICK C. SASSO, MD
Spine Surgeon
Indiana Spine Group
Indianapolis, Indiana

ADAM SASSOON, MD
Orthopedic Fellow
Department of Orthopedic Traumatology
    and Reconstruction
Orlando Regional Medical Center
Orlando, Florida

JEFFREY R. SAWYER, MD
Orthopaedic Surgeon
Department of Pediatric Orthopaedics and
    Spinal Deformity
University of Tennessee, Campbell Clinic
Memphis, Tennessee

MARA L. SCHENKER, MD
Department of Orthopaedic Surgery
University of Pennsylvania
Philadelphia, Pennsylvania

JONATHAN G. SCHOENECKER, MD, PhD
Assistant Professor
Department of Orthopaedics
Vanderbilt University
Nashville, Tennessee

ANDREW J. SCHOENFELD, MD
Assistant Professor
Department of Orthopaedic Surgery
Texas Tech University Health Sciences Center
El Paso, Texas

ROWAN SCHOUTEN, MBChB, FRACS
Orthopaedic Surgeon
Orthopaedic Department
Christchurch Hospital
Christchurch, New Zealand

JOE SCHWAB, MD, MS
Instructor of Orthopaedic Surgery
Department of Orthopaedic Surgery
Massachusetts General Hospital
Boston, Massachusetts

ERIC SCHWENK, MD
Instructor
Department of Anesthesiology
Jefferson Medical College
Philadelphia, Pennsylvania

JESSE SLADE SHANTZ, MD, MBA
Clinical Research Fellow
Department of Orthopaedic Surgery
University of California, San Francisco
San Francisco, California

JODI SIEGEL, MD
Assistant Professor
Department of Orthopaedics
University of Massachusetts Memorial
    Medical Center
Worcester, Massachusetts

JEREMY SIMON, MD
Clinical Instructor
Physical Medicine and Rehabilitation
    Department
Thomas Jefferson University Hospital
Philadelphia, Pennsylvania

KERN SINGH, MD
Assistant Professor
Department of Orthopaedic Surgery
Rush University Medical Center
Chicago, Illinois

MICHAEL SIRKIN, MD
Vice Chairman
Department of Orthopaedics
New Jersey Medical School
Newark, New Jersey

GILLIAN SOLES, MD
Fellow, Orthopaedic Trauma
Department of Orthopaedic Surgery
Unversity of California Davis Medical Center
Sacramento, California

BRYAN D. SPRINGER, MD
OrthoCarolina Hip and Knee Center
Charlotte, North Carolina

JASON W. STONEBACK, MD
Assistant Professor
Director of Orthopaedic Trauma
Department of Orthopaedics
University of Colorado Hospital
University of Colorado Health Science Center
Denver, Colorado

ROBERT J. STRAUCH, MD
Professor of Clinical Orthopaedic Surgery
Department of Orthopaedic Surgery
Columbia University
New York, New York

MICHAEL P. STAUFF, MD
Assistant Professor and Spine Surgeon
Spine Center
Department of Orthopaedics and Physical
    Rehabilitation
University of Massachusetts Medical Center
Worcester, Massachusetts

MAX TALBOT, MD, FRCSC
1 Canadian Field Hospital
Canadian Armed Forces
Montreal, Quebec, Canada

VISHWAS R. TALWALKAR, MD
Associate Professor
Department of Orthopaedic Surgery and
    Pediatrics
Shriners Hospital for Children
Lexington, Kentucky

PETER TANG, MD, MPH
Assistant Professor
Department of Orthopaedic Surgery
New York Presbyterian Hospital
    Columbia Orthopaedics
New York, New York

PAUL TORNETTA III, MD
Director, Orthopaedic Trauma
Department of Orthopaedic Surgery
Boston Medical Center
Boston, Massachusetts

ROCKY S. TUAN, PhD
Professor
Department of Orthopaedic Surgery
University of Pittsburgh
Pittsburgh, Pennsylvania

EJOVI UGHWANOGHO, MD
Spine Surgery Fellow
Texas Back Institute
Plano, Texas

ALEXANDER R. VACCARO, MD, PhD
Orthopaedic Surgeon
Department of Orthopaedic Surgery
Rothman Institute
Philadelphia, Pennsylvania

BENJAMIN VAGHARI, MD
Instructor
Department of Anesthesiology
Jefferson Medical College
Philadelphia, Pennsylvania

EUGENE VISCUSI, MD
Director, Acute Pain Management
Department of Anesthesiology
Jefferson Medical College
Philadelphia, Pennsylvania

PARTH A. VYAS, MD
Fellow
Department of Orthopedic Surgery
Hospital for Special Surgery
New York, New York

J. TRACY WATSON, MD
Professor, Orthopaedic Surgery
Chief, Orthopaedic Trauma Service
Department of Orthopaedic Surgery
Saint Louis University School of Medicine
St. Louis, Missouri

JENNIFER WEISS, MD
Physician/Orthopedic Surgeon
Department of Pediatric Orthopedics and
    Sports Medicine
Southern California Permanente Medical Group
Los Angeles, California

Nathan A. Wigner, MD, PhD
Resident
Department of Orthopaedic Surgery
University of Pennsylvania
Philadelphia, Pennsylvania

Klane K. White, MD
Orthopedic Surgeon
Department of Orthopedics and Sports
  Medicine
Seattle Children's Hospital
Seattle, Washington

Philip Wolinsky, MD
Chief, Orthopaedic Trauma Surgery
Professor and Vice Chair
Department of Orthopaedic Surgery
University of California Davis Medical Center
Sacramento, California

Kirkham B. Wood, MD
Associate Professor
Chief, Orthopaedic Spine Service
Department of Orthopaedic Surgery
Massachusetts General Hospital
Harvard Medical School
Boston, Massachusetts

Brad Yoo, MD
Assistant Professor
Department of Orthopaedics
University of California Davis Medical Center
Sacramento, California

Bruce H. Ziran, MD, FACS
Director, Orthopedic Trauma
Orthopedic Surgery Residency Program
Atlanta Medical Center
Atlanta, Georgia

Preface

I would like to welcome you to *Orthopaedic Knowledge Update* 11 (OKU 11).

It is with great honor that I accepted the duties of editor of this incredible book. I fondly remember reading earlier editions to help provide an overview for residency rotations, prepare for my boards, and as a constant source of up-to-date knowledge. Fast-forward to OKU 11. My goal was to make this edition of OKU 11 the go-to guide for the most current information on a variety of orthopaedic topics. Almost immediately after OKU 10 was published, work on the 11th edition began with the assembly of an all-star team of section editors, who then enlisted their colleagues to write chapters. The section editors dedicated an extensive amount of time to this project, including traveling to Chicago, along with an author from each chapter, to review chapters published in this edition. In the age of social media and multiple venues for education, including webinars, lectures, and even You Tube videos, it is with great pride that we present this edition as an educational tool designed to be used regularly.

OKU 11 is different from previous editions in that several chapters have video references, including original videos from the authors. The high-quality surgical images throughout the book will enhance the reader's understanding of the material presented. In addition, each chapter ends with a summary and three key points. The other goal of this update was to ensure that at least 30% of the references in each chapter were published within the past 3 years. In this way, we are highlighting what is new and important since the last edition was published.

I would like to mention some of the new topics included in OKU 11. Discussions of American Academy of Orthopaedic Surgeons (AAOS) clinical practice guidelines and the Appropriate Use Criteria for distal radius fractures have been added to this edition. In Section 1, Principles of Orthopaedics, there are new chapters on professionalism and ethics, and the care of geriatric patients. The chapter on geriatric patient care is especially important because of the increasing number of older individuals and the rising rate of hip fractures that all orthopaedic surgeons must address, regardless of their specialty. In Section 2, Systemic Disorders, we have included a chapter discussing genomics, proteomics, and metabolomics. As a result of reader comments and feedback, the orthopaedic oncology section is now a separate chapter instead of being divided among the subspecialties. Section 3, Upper Extremity, is enhanced by several videos and interesting discussions of topics involving the shoulder, elbow, hand, and wrist. Section 4, Lower Extremity, has exciting educational videos and new topics, including soft-tissue coverage options and segmental bone loss. Section 5, Spine, highlights the latest and most up-to-date information on spine trauma and diseases, including vertebral compression fractures and osteoporosis. Section 6, Pediatrics, provides the most up-to-date information on a variety of pediatric subjects.

Some may ask why I accepted the challenge of being the editor of OKU 11. It is only because of the great support that I knew I would receive from the section editors, the authors, and the top-notch AAOS staff. I would like to acknowledge Lisa Claxton Moore for her tireless efforts and continued work, along with Michelle Wild, Kathleen Anderson, and Courtney Astle. The marketing department, particularly Tricia Arnold, has assisted with the promotion of this book. I would also like to thank the following individuals who provided editing assistance without expecting acknowledgment: Albert J. Aboulafia (Baltimore, MD), who helped with the tumor section; David J. Anderson (St. Louis, MO), who helped review pediatrics chapters; and Michael Delcore (St. Louis, MO), who helped assemble figures and reference charts for some of the chapters.

I appeal to residents and young practitioners to get involved in orthopaedic education— I started with writing chapters, became a section editor, and, ultimately, this honor! I encourage young orthopaedic surgeons who are reading this book to use this text and subsequent editions throughout their career, but also to remember to give back to the Academy through future contributions.

I would like to acknowledge my husband Jeff and my daughter Annalise; without them, nothing would be accomplished. I also would like to thank my parents, John and Theresa Metcalf, and my family for their continued support and encouragement of my career. The duties of being editor of OKU 11 would not have been completed without the support of my entire department at Saint Louis University, particularly J. Tracy Watson and David Karges, and my chairman, Berton R. Moed.

I hope that you refer to this edition often and look forward to your feedback.

Lisa K. Cannada, MD
Editor

Table of Contents

Section 6: Pediatrics

Section 1

Principles of Orthopaedics

SECTION EDITORS:

Theodore Miclau, MD

Saam Morshed, MD, PhD, MPH

Kristy L. Weber, MD

Chapter 1

Professionalism and Ethics

Paul E. Levin, MD

Medical Professionalism

A profession is an occupation or trade that is defined by a body of information and specific technical skills that are unique to each particular profession and its members. In an expansion of this definition, a medical professional must demonstrate additional personal traits and qualities beyond those of a nonmedical professional. Medical professionals also have an inherent ethical obligation to his or her patients and society.[1,2]

Society recognizes the unique nature of the different professions and expects every professional organization to ensure that its members maintain their education and skills to be able to safely and effectively function in their area of professional expertise. Governmental agencies also acknowledge the importance of individual professional societies and require these organizations to promote activities to ensure the professional expertise of their members. The federal government and state governments have created independent agencies that establish standards for professional licensure, oversee professional organizations, and set guidelines for professional responsibilities to society.

Medical professionalism is a dynamic and abstract concept. The American Academy of Orthopaedic Surgeons (AAOS), the Accreditation Council for Graduate Medical Education (ACGME), the American Medical Association (AMA), medical schools, and several specialty societies have each defined their vision of professionalism. They have identified a variety of personal characteristics, qualities, and professional activities consistent with each organization's concept of professionalism. The AAOS has adapted the guidelines proposed by the American Board of Internal Medicine (2002) in their position statement "Medical Professionalism in the New Millennium: A Physician Charter."[3,4] The charter includes overlying fundamental principles consistent with modern medical ethics, including the primacy of patient welfare, patient autonomy, and social justice. In addition to respecting the principles of medical ethics, medical professionalism requires that a

physician be altruistic, advocate for patients, be honest with patients, respect patient confidentiality, and maintain appropriate relationships with patients. Beyond responsibilities to patients, professionalism obligates physicians to strive to improve the quality of care and access to care for all citizens, help create a just distribution of finite healthcare resources, and further scientific knowledge.[3]

The authors of a classic text describe the cornerstone of medical professionalism as establishing "fidelity to trust."[5] A similar philosophy recommends that physicians develop a fiduciary relationship with their patients.[6] In a fiduciary relationship, the interests of the patient are paramount. Any recommendations made or treatment rendered should solely be for the benefit of the patient. Potential conflicts of interest need to be recognized, acknowledged, and, as much as is humanly possible, eliminated in the planning of patient care.

Several necessary personal characteristics have been proposed, including excellence, humanism, accountability, and altruism, which are supported by the professional skills of clinical competence, communication skills, and an ethical and legal understanding. "Professionalism is demonstrated through a foundation of clinical competence, communication skills, and ethical and legal understanding, upon which is built the aspiration to and wise application of the principles of professionalism—clinical competence, ethical understanding, and communication."[7]

Two intersecting attributes—healer and professional— have been described as exemplifying medical professionalism. Many common individual characteristics also are frequently cited by numerous ethicists, sociologists, and professional organizations[8] (Figure 1). The Association of American Medical Colleges and the National Board of Medical Examiners convened a conference in 2002 with the charge of defining medical professionalism and to develop strategies to teach medical professionalism in medical school. Their comprehensive report, "Embedding Professionalism in Medical Education: Assessment as a Tool for Implementation" challenges medical schools and professional societies to recognize professionalism as an integral trait of a successful physician.[9] They specifically identified altruism, honor and integrity, caring and compassion, respect, responsibility and accountability, excellence and scholarship, and leadership as necessary behaviors and characteristics consistent with medical professionalism (Table 1).

Dr. Levin or an immediate family member serves as a board member, owner, officer, or committee member of the American Academy of Orthopaedic Surgeons Committee on Ethics and the American Academy of Orthopaedic Surgeons Trauma Program Subcommittee.

The basic concepts of professionalism remain consistent among most ethicists and professional societies. Earning a professional degree is not synonymous with demonstrating professionalism. Professionalism requires that a physician respect and fulfill the basic principles of medical ethics as well as adhere to the aforementioned multifaceted personal characteristics and responsibilities. In addition, physicians must acknowledge the economic stresses faced by health care in the United States and abide by a commitment to social justice and a just distribution of finite resources.

Medical schools and residency programs have recognized the importance of teaching professionalism and are creating programs to teach and evaluate a student's professionalism. The ACGME has established six core competencies as necessary skills for a resident to successfully learn during his or her training. The required competencies include medical knowledge, patient care skills, professionalism, interpersonal and communication skills, practice-based learning and improvement, and systems-based practice. These six competencies are included in most definitions of professionalism.[10] These competencies also have been included in the new milestone project of the ACGME. The milestone project identifies a core of orthopaedic procedures in which the orthopaedic resident needs to demonstrate an appropriate level of medical knowledge and clinical competence, incorporating many of the components of professionalism in the evaluation process. According to a recent study, it is recommended that orthopaedic training programs develop formal and informal programs in the teaching of medical professionalism.[11]

Balancing Personal and Professional Life

Physicians have historically demonstrated professionalism by always being available for their patients. This availability was often associated with significant personal and family sacrifice and was accompanied by many unintended costs. A national survey of orthopaedic residents, resident spouses, attending physicians, and attending spouses uncovered an alarming rate of job dissatisfaction, burnout, and personal stress.[12] A high level of burnout, depression, and alcohol abuse is described in a report from the Governors' Committee on Physician Competency and Health of the American College of Surgeons, recounting the results of national surveys in 2008 and 2010. Common stressors were the number of hours worked per week, nights on call, having children younger than 21 years, and work-home conflict.[13] In a study of orthopaedic leaders, only 15% reported satisfaction with their personal/professional balance.[14] A secondary analysis of the Physician Worklife Survey attempted to identify the "difficult doctor."[15] The authors of this study found an association of a higher frustration level in physicians younger than 40 years and in those working more than 55 hours per week. Commonly reported symptoms among these physicians were stress, anxiety, and depression.[16]

Unnecessary personal sacrifice and loss of personal/

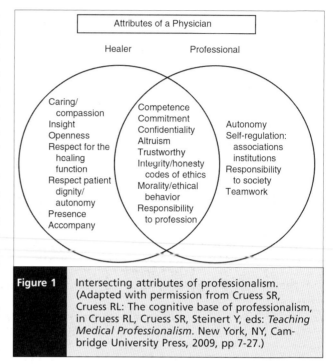

Figure 1 Intersecting attributes of professionalism. (Adapted with permission from Cruess SR, Cruess RL: The cognitive base of professionalism, in Cruess RL, Cruess SR, Steinert Y, eds: *Teaching Medical Professionalism*. New York, NY, Cambridge University Press, 2009, pp 7-27.)

professional balance creates excessive stress and premature burnout.[17,18] Stress affects physician interactions with patients and interpersonal relationships and increases the risk for substance abuse, depression, and suicide. Stress decreases professional satisfaction, increases frustration, and compromises the ability to demonstrate professionalism and care for patients. Balance allows physicians to be more successful in their personal and professional lives.

Professionalism, altruism, and trustworthiness can be maintained through a careful reassessment of how physicians care for patients in modern society. This will require a better understanding and a reevaluation of the skills necessary to create an effective doctor-patient relationship. An essential component necessary to achieve personal/professional balance is effective communication with patients and colleagues.[19,20] Patients understand that everyone has a personal life separate from one's professional life. Patients who are active participants in their health care, achieved through the process of shared decision making, gain a full understanding of their health-related issues and the strategy to address these problems. Patients' understanding of their active medical conditions will more successfully allow the patient to assist a covering physician if a problem arises (expanded discussion in Orthopaedic Knowledge Update 11, chapter 8, Patient-Centered Care: Communication Skills and Cultural Competence). In addition, physicians who have comprehensively advised their covering physicians of potential issues arising with their active patients can safely take time off and feel comfortable that their patients will be appropriately cared for.

Medical students and practicing physicians are recognizing the importance of personal balance and are

Table 1

Behaviors Reflecting Professionalism

Altruism
- Offers to help team members who are busy.
- Contributes to the profession; is active in local and national organizations, such as the Association of American Medical Colleges and the Organization of Student Representatives.
- Does not use altruism as an excuse to misprioritize or rationalize certain behaviors. ("I can't be with my family because my patients need me.")

Honor and Integrity
- Is forthcoming with information; does not withhold and/or use information for power.
- Admits errors.
- Deals with confidential information discreetly and appropriately.
- Does not misuse resources (for example, school computers and patients' food).

Caring and Compassion
- Treats the patient as an individual, taking into account lifestyle, beliefs, personal idiosyncrasies, and support system.
- Communicates bad news with sincerity and compassion.
- Deals with sickness, death, and dying in a professional manner with patient and family members.
- Supports a balance in personal and professional activities for peers and subordinates.

Respect
- Respects institutional staff and representatives; respects faculty during teaching sessions.
- Respects patient rights/dignity (privacy/confidentiality, consent); knocks on door, introduces self, drapes patients appropriately, and shows respect for patient privacy needs.
- Demonstrates tolerance to a range of behaviors and beliefs.
- Does not disturb small group sessions.

Responsibility and Accountability
- Demonstrates awareness of own limitations, and identifies developmental needs and approaches for improvements.
- Cares for self appropriately and presents self in a professional manner (demeanor, dress, hygiene).
- Recognizes and reports errors/poor behavior in peers.
- Informs others when not available to fulfill responsibilities and secures replacement.
- Takes responsibility for appropriate share of teamwork.
- Arrives on time.
- Accountable for deadlines; completes assignments and responsibilities on time.
- Answers letters, pages, e-mail, and phone calls in a timely manner.

Excellence and Scholarship
- Masters techniques and technologies of learning.
- Is self-critical and able to identify own areas for learning/practice improvement.
- Has internal focus and direction; setting own goals.
- Takes initiative in organizing, participating, and collaborating in peer study groups.

Leadership
- Teaches others.
- Helps build and maintain a culture that facilitates professionalism.
- Does not provide disruptive leadership (organizing pranks, inappropriately confronting authority).

(Adapted from an Invitational Conference Cosponsored by the Association of American Medical Colleges and the National Board of Medical Examiners: *Embedding Professionalism in Medical Education: Assessment as a Tool for Implementation.* National Board of Medical Examiners, Philadelphia, PA, 2002.)

choosing specialties and practice settings by giving strong consideration to personal lifestyle and quality of life. Working hour restrictions for medical students and residents, originally implemented to improve patient safety and physician education, have also put a focus on personal and professional balance. Physicians are choosing positions that allow for guaranteed free time, and more physicians are electing to become salaried employees with specific guarantees of free time.[21]

The Impaired Physician

An impaired physician, as defined by the AMA, "has any physical, mental or behavioral disorder that inter-feres with the ability to engage safely in professional activities."[22] Physician impairment deleteriously affects an individual's cognitive abilities, motor skills, and the ability to uphold his or her commitment to professionalism. Although impairment frequently infers chemical dependence/substance abuse (prescription and illicit drugs), many physicians are impaired by common psychological conditions such as anxiety and depression. Impairment is considered to be a disease and, if left untreated, will likely not resolve. Depression is estimated to affect 16% of the general population, and it is widely believed that a greater number of practicing physicians are affected. The rates of suicide among physicians are higher than in the general population and are often related to depression. Female physicians are affected at greater numbers than male physicians.[23]

Substance abuse among physicians is believed to have a lifetime incidence of 8% to 12% and includes alcohol, illicit drugs, and prescription drugs. The precise statistics are difficult to ascertain because of difficulty identifying and reporting physicians affected.[24,25] National anonymous, self-reporting surveys among physicians find a significant incidence of self-treatment with benzodiazepines and narcotics.[26] According to the results of a 2010 national survey of surgeons in the United States, 15.4% of the respondents had findings consistent with either alcohol abuse or other chemical dependencies. Female surgeons had nearly twice the prevalence for drug abuse or chemical dependence (25.6% versus 13.9%).[27] Anesthesiologists, emergency physicians, and psychiatrists have the highest incidence of prescription drug abuse.[28]

The medical profession has a long history of institutional and individual failures to identify and assist physicians who are burdened with the common personal problems encountered throughout life. Physicians often fail to recognize, acknowledge, or accept their own personal challenges and need a friend or a colleague to help them identify and acknowledge that assistance is needed.[29] Individual physicians, physician colleagues, and organizations delivering health care need to be proactive in identifying and assisting impaired physicians, and if problems are suspected they should be addressed immediately. Personality changes, mood changes, irritability, lateness, and falling asleep during the daytime are all potential signs of impairment.[30] Recognition of impairment is the first step in the treatment process. If a physician is not able to voluntarily accept the advice of a colleague and recognize that he or she requires help, that physician should be reported to the appropriate governmental agency to ensure that he or she receives help and that patients are not harmed. All health professionals have an ethical, professional, and legal responsibility to report an impaired physician.

The medical profession, as with so many other professions, has been guilty of underreporting and failure to appropriately assist impaired physicians. In an attempt to protect colleagues and help them avoid professional sanctions, physicians place these colleagues and their patients at risk. Because some physicians are often fearful of the legal implications associated with their impairment, admitting and confronting these problems is often avoided. Surveys demonstrate that physician colleagues are more likely to report a physician dealing with chemical dependence as opposed to a psychological disorder.[31]

All 50 states have agencies and programs to address the issues of impaired physicians and substance abuse, and all recognize impairment as an illness. The goals of these programs are successful treatment of the underlying medical condition and safely allowing the physician to return to practice in a setting that best suits the need of the individual practitioner. These programs protect patients, physician colleagues, and the medical profession. The success of these programs has been difficult to gauge. Success rates have been reported to be in the range of 27% to 92%, with abstinence rates of 70% to 90%.[25,32,33] A review of 904 physicians enrolled in 16 different state programs in 2008 described encouraging results: 78% of physicians had no positive drug tests over 5 years, and 72% continued to practice medicine.[32]

Disruptive Behavior

Disruptive behavior is unprofessional personal conduct that compromises patient safety and negatively affects the work environment. Approximately 5% of physicians demonstrate disruptive behavior, and orthopaedic surgeons are the fourth most common group of disruptive physicians after general surgeons, neurosurgeons, and cardiothoracic surgeons.[34] Common disruptive behaviors include a disregard for hospital regulations, such as an operating room "time-out"(a pause before an incision is made to ensure correct patient, correct procedure, correct site, and verification that all implants are available); sarcastic comments; offensive comments of a sexual nature; shouting and throwing instruments; and belittling or ignoring suggestions from associates, students, and residents. Surgeons can be particularly prone to disruptive behavior as a result of a long tradition of operating room hierarchy and culture. Disruptive behavior can have a significant effect on operating room morale and staff satisfaction, leads to high levels of staff turnover, and can have a deleterious effect on patient safety. In a disruptive environment, operating room personnel, students, and residents are discouraged from speaking up when they believe an alternative clinical management may be indicated or when they identify a patient safety concern.[35] Surgical residents report personal conflict and ethical dilemmas when they disagree with the management of a patient by a surgical attending physician. A disruptive surgeon fails to create a working environment of mutual respect, and, as a result, the residents are not given an opportunity to address their concerns, so patient safety is compromised.[35]

A variety of programs have been developed to address the issue of disruptive behavior, including educational forums; strategies for prevention, support, and counseling; and, when necessary, the removal of physicians from the medical staff. Maimonides Medical Center has developed a highly successful program "Code of Mutual Respect" that can be accessed online.[36,37] The comprehensive program at Vanderbilt University addresses disruptive and unprofessional behaviors and teaches professionalism.[38]

Medical Ethics

Morality

Morality is an individual's deep-seated beliefs and internal compass of right and wrong. Individuals develop their own personal morality as a result of upbringing, education, religion, culture, society, and personal experiences. A common morality is described as universally accepted "standards of action and moral character traits," and it has been proposed that all moral individuals would follow these standards[39] (exemplified by the following directives: do not kill, do not cause pain or suffering to others, prevent evil or harm from occurring, rescue persons in danger, tell the truth, nurture the young and dependent, keep promises, do not steal, do not punish the innocent, and obey the law). Character traits that reflect a strong moral code include "nonmalevolence, honesty, integrity, conscientiousness, fidelity, gratitude, truthfulness, lovingness and kindness."[39] These character traits are commonly identified as building blocks of professionalism.

Beyond the concept of a common morality, individuals in a multicultural society each develop their own personal moralities and will interpret some clinical presentations with very different moral "authority." Individuals view personal morality as clear, unwavering principles that are so obvious that explanations or justifications are not needed. However, in a multicultural society, and certainly when physicians act as professionals, they may be called on and should be able to explain the moral reasoning that underlies their specific recommendations and actions. Undoubtedly, an individual's morality will affect his or her personal ethical behavior.

Clinical Ethics and Bioethics

Ethics is a branch of philosophy that evaluates and examines people's moral actions in an attempt to understand the underlying moral reasoning behind those actions. Clinical ethics examines the justifications for a particular behavior in a specific clinical situation by evaluating common morality, sociologic norms, and societal needs; the psychological understanding of human actions; and a careful analysis of the facts associated with a particular presentation and action. Ultimately, these deliberations are designed to determine what is right and what is wrong, what is acceptable and what is not acceptable, and what is morally acceptable in the context of society.[40] Bioethics considers ethical dilemmas that encompass more global issues in health care, including research with human subjects, utilization of new technologies (such as stem cell research), animal research, and public health decisions.

The study of bioethical principles allows the development of a structure and a framework to resolve ethical conflicts. Bioethical deliberations can also guide the challenging economic and public health decisions currently at hand. Ethics consultation services can help give physicians guidance when addressing ethical dilemmas in the care of their patients. Ultimately, no physician is obligated to violate his or her own morality. However, when an institution's or a physician's moral views are irreconcilably different from those of the patient, the physician may need to honor the patient's autonomy and respect the patient's morality by referring him or her to another institution or to a physician whose personal morality is better suited to that patient's care.[41]

Basic Principles of Bioethics

The modern study of bioethics is based on four basic principles: respect for autonomy, beneficence, nonmaleficence, and distributive justice. These four principles integrate to form the foundation of the ethical practice of health care in the United States and many other countries throughout the world and are used to analyze individual actions, organizational decisions, and public health policies. Frequently conflicts will arise in balancing these principles in the implementation of sound ethical care of patients.[39,40,42]

Respect of Autonomy

Among the most cherished principles in a free society is an individual's right to live his or her life consistent with personal needs, desires, and morality. Respect of a patient's autonomy and individuality protects this freedom, is a core principle in the current practice of medicine, and should be the underlying principle in all healthcare decisions. This philosophy is diametrically opposed to older practices of paternalism, in which the physician identified the "best" treatment of his or her patient and simply advised patients on what needed to be done. The successful implementation of respecting patient autonomy requires that the patient have a full understanding of his or her medical condition and its implications, the various options for treatment, and the expected outcomes of each treatment option. Having all of this information available allows patients to determine which treatment is consistent with their own personal needs and morality. The principle of autonomy does not imply that patients should receive any care that they believe is indicated (see discussion on beneficence and nonmaleficence). Respecting autonomy does require the physician to acknowledge and address his or her differing opinion with the patient and, if necessary, refer the patient for an additional evaluation. This concept should be included in all medical evaluations, not just in situations in which an intervention is indicated (see chapter 8, Patient-Centered Care: Communication Skills and Cultural Competence, in *Orthopaedic Knowledge Update 11*).

Beneficence

The bioethical principle of beneficence obligates the physician to help his or her patient do well, that is, benefit his or her patient. Beneficence requires that the physician be much more than a neutral source of information that is respecting a patient's autonomy by simply explaining the problem and listing the treatments. To fulfill the principle of beneficence, the physician needs to develop an understanding of the patient's individuality (such as lifestyle or economic/moral factors) and help patients achieve the best individual outcome. A beneficent physician will be a strong advocate for his or her patient (see discussion on professionalism). Advocating for orthopaedic patients may include assisting the patient in obtaining necessary healthcare services to help treat both musculoskeletal and non-musculoskeletal conditions.

Nonmaleficence

Nonmaleficence simply states that physicians should not harm their patients. This concept is consistent with the commonly quoted Latin phrase *primum non nocere,* which means first do no harm. This principle implies that any treatment undertaken by the physician is expected to help not harm the patient. It is a principle with a very delicate balance. At times, nonmaleficence may seem to conflict with the principles of patient autonomy and beneficence. A physician may decline a patient's request for a diagnostic test or intervention, theoretically violating the patient's autonomy, because the physician does not believe that the request is necessary or beneficial and could be potentially harmful. This conflict is illustrated in the case of a scholarship-level high school athlete who requested a meniscectomy rather than a meniscal repair to allow him to more rapidly return to the field and be evaluated by college scouts.[43] Nonmaleficence may conflict with the principle of beneficence because physicians may initially "harm" their patients when treating musculoskeletal pathology. In this instance, although a meniscal repair is thought to achieve the best long-term prognosis, the athlete is potentially harmed as an individual by not being allowed to play football and gain a college scholarship.

Nonmaleficence also may conflict with an individual physician's personal morality. This conflict may potentially interfere with an individual's autonomy. For example, an orthopaedic surgeon may feel morally obligated to save a patient's life by performing an emergency amputation to resolve hemodynamic instability secondary to an uncontrollable foot infection. Performing the amputation to preserve life, against the patient's wishes, has potentially "harmed" the patient. The physician may view the failure to perform an amputation as a direct violation of his or her own morality and the principle of nonmaleficence. Other physicians, although not necessarily comfortable with the patient's choice, would be able to accept the patient's choice and attempt to care for the patient in a manner acceptable to the patient. (See discussion on informed consent.)

Distributive Justice

Living in a just society implies that all members are entitled to a basic set of rights and freedoms. Clearly, these rights and freedoms are vigorously debated. The principle of distributive justice requires the equitable delivery of healthcare services. Modern bioethicists contend that basic health care should be a guaranteed right of all members of society. The American Board of Internal Medicine and the AAOS in their policy statement on professionalism include social justice as one of the primary responsibilities of a medical professional.[3,4] This principle obligates the physician to treat all patients who present for care irrespective of a patient's sex, sexual orientation, religion, ethnicity, race, or ability to pay for care.

This is the only one of the four basic principles of bioethics that examines the needs of all the members of a society and not just the needs of each individual member of a society. Healthcare resources are limited, and the amount of money in which an economically successful society can spend for health care is also limited. Ethical utilization of these resources requires that guidelines be established to distribute these resources to most effectively care for all members of society. Orthopaedic surgeons should be actively involved in policy-making decisions to ensure appropriate, cost-effective musculoskeletal care for their patients. Value-based medicine has been discussed as a standard that potentially will improve outcomes and save healthcare resources.[44]

Current Ethical Challenges and Dilemmas

Decision-Making Capacity

Patients need to have the ability to understand their personal medical situation to be able to participate in discussions related to their healthcare needs. The patient's ability to understand his or her medical condition and assist in determining the best treatment is called decision-making capacity. The term decision-making capacity is normally used in medical settings and the term competence is used in legal forums. In practice, they are often used interchangeably. Capacity is not an all-or-none phenomenon. Patients may be able to demonstrate complete capacity in some aspects of their lives but have a complete inability to develop an objective understanding in other aspects of their lives.[45] A refusal to consent to a procedure with obvious indications does not indicate a lack of capacity. In addition, the presence of psychiatric illness does not automatically negate a person's autonomy and his or her ability to make decisions related to their health care.[45]

All physicians are ethically and legally permitted to make determinations of a patient's decision-making capacity. A basic guideline in this determination is the ability of a patient to demonstrate an understanding of his or her condition as well as an understanding of the different treatments and why a specific treatment is recommended. Having a patient explain what he or she has learned in discussions with the physician and being able to explain the choice of treatment that he or she has selected is an accepted minimal standard for determining capacity.[46] Whenever a question arises about a patient's capacity, a consultation with a psychiatry liaison service is recommended. In addition, it is recommended that the orthopaedic surgeon discuss the indications for the surgical procedure and describe his or her specific concerns about a patient's capacity with the liaison psychiatrist before the psychiatrist's evaluation.[47] Some institutions and legal jurisdictions require a psychiatry consultation for a patient with a history of psychiatric illness.

Failure to determine if a patient has decision-making capacity violates the principles of autonomy, beneficence, and nonmaleficence. Obtaining consent for a procedure from a patient who lacks capacity will rob that individual of his or her ethical and legal right to have a designated guardian or healthcare proxy make his or her autonomous decisions. Obtaining consent for a procedure from a family member without determining a patient's decision-making capacity also violates the principle of respecting a patient's autonomy. Using a family member to sign a consent because of language barriers or other medical comorbidities (such as paralysis or hearing loss) are common errors made in determining decision-making capacity and obtaining informed consent.

The AAOS has created a web-based ethics syllabus based on common patient presentations to assist orthopaedic residents and practicing physicians in learning about and understanding these challenging issues.[48]

Informed Consent

The practice of obtaining informed consent for any medical intervention is both an ethical imperative and a legal requirement. Of paramount importance is ensuring that the patient understands all pertinent issues involved in making a decision. Developing appropriate communication skills is critical for the physician to be able to successfully engage in a comprehensive discussion related to a recommended intervention. Obtaining informed consent fulfills the three basic tenets of biomedical ethics: respecting patient autonomy, beneficence, and nonmaleficence. Failure to successfully communicate with patients and obtain appropriate informed consent has been found to be associated with some malpractice claims.[49-52]

The consent process requires the orthopaedic surgeon to discuss all available information and options of management of the presenting musculoskeletal pathology that he or she is evaluating and treating. All medical interventions have alternatives, although at times the alternative treatment is an extremely poor option. Alternative treatments include an option of no intervention, even if this could result in the loss of a limb or death. Individuals with decision-making capacity have the moral and legal right to decline treatment.

Beneficence requires the physician to develop an understanding of his or her patient's individual desires and goals, along with an understanding of a patient's medical comorbidities, activity level, lifestyle, and personal morality to help the patient identify the most appropriate method of treatment. Nonmaleficence obligates the orthopaedic surgeon to arrive at a treatment that does not violate the patient's personal choices or his or her moral or religious beliefs. For example, administering a blood transfusion and violating an individual's religious beliefs may save a person's life but leave him or her permanently harmed.

Ethicists debate how much information is appropriate to communicate to a patient.[53] The goal of informed consent is to ensure that an individual understands the proposed intervention. Ideally, the process will inform the patient, provide assurance that the procedure will help resolve/improve his or her condition, and not deter a person from undergoing a procedure that could significantly improve his or her quality of life. Purposefully withholding information with the goal of ensuring that a patient consents to a recommended procedure is paternalist and not ethically acceptable.

Two common standards of the informed consent process are frequently used in both the medical and legal communities. The community standard obligates the physician to perform the consent process in a fashion similar to that of other members of the medical community. The reasonable person standard requires that information be discussed and an understanding established for any information of which a "reasonable person" would want to be aware. Obviously, determining what information a reasonable person would require is an area of significant debate.

A third approach, the subjective standard, believed to be more ethically sound,[39] recognizes that different individuals require/request different levels of information. Care must be taken in using the subjective standard. Clearly, different individuals are interested in different degrees of comprehension of their medical condition. Most patients are interested in gaining a reasonable level of understanding of their condition and treatment options. Some individuals require a far greater level of information and understanding prior to consenting to a surgical intervention. Some patients prefer not to be involved in comprehensive discussions. Patient preferences will usually become evident as the informed consent discussion evolves.[39] Insisting that an individual who is not interested in a comprehensive discussion participate in an overly comprehensive and technical discussion can violate the basic biomedical principle of autonomy.

Caution must be used in applying the subjective standard. A physician may assume that a patient does not need to be informed of an unusual but significant complication because of the belief that a person should not be burdened with too much information. Unfortunately, this approach would be paternalistic and not even meet the needs of a subjective standard. Six critical components need to be achieved to obtain a successful informed consent:[54,55] clinical issues, alternatives and options, pros and cons, uncertainties of the decision, assessment of understanding, and patient preference.

The patient's full understanding of the proposed intervention is paramount. Studies demonstrate that, in general, physicians believe that a full disclosure of a planned intervention meets the needs of informed consent. A common failure is not establishing that the patient understands the implications of the complications disclosed.[54] A reasonable guideline for the informed consent process is to discuss all common complications associated with the planned procedure, as well as less common complications, which may have significant long-term or permanent consequences.

Example of Informed Consent, Incomplete Discussion

Dr. Clarke is having an informed consent discussion

with Ms. Swanson regarding her upcoming total hip arthroplasty. He has listed all of the commonly encountered problems, including injury to the sciatic nerve. The patient develops a complete peroneal nerve palsy after surgery and ultimately requires an ankle-foot orthosis for ambulation. She is angry and complains to Dr. Clarke that she was never told this injury could happen.

Example of Informed Consent, Complete Discussion

Dr. Clarke has advised Ms. Swanson that if her sciatic nerve is injured, recovery may or not occur. He explains that if the nerve problem does not improve, a plastic leg brace may be required to prevent Ms. Swanson from tripping. Dr. Clarke pauses for a moment, and Ms. Swanson then inquires about the brace and the likelihood of that problem occurring.

These two discussions demonstrate the difference between a disclosure and helping the patient develop a full understanding of the complication. This explanation would meet the requirements of a reasonable person standard in that one could assume that an individual consenting to an elective surgical procedure would want to know how a possible complication could have a permanent functional implication.

Summary

The four basic principles of modern medical ethics are integral components of medical professionalism. Patients are all unique individuals, with their own morality and personal needs who require an appropriate understanding of pathology and treatment options. A successful medical professional will strive to meet the individual needs of each patient, develop a fiduciary relationship with his or her patients, and, as a result, practice and exemplify professionalism in the care of his or her patients.

Key Study Points

- Medical professionalism requires a physician to develop a trusting (fiduciary) relationship with a patient. Professionalism obligates the physician to be altruistic, caring, compassionate, and humanistic and to maintain a current level of excellence in his or her medical practice.

- The four basic biomedical principles of respecting a patient's autonomy, beneficence, nonmaleficence, and justice are the foundation of successful patient care. Adhering to these principles will allow physicians to embrace medical professionalism and be successful medical professionals.

- The practice of orthopaedic surgery is often stressful and time consuming. These stresses can lead to chemical dependence, psychological impairment, and early professional burnout. Establishing an appropriate professional and personal balance in life is consistent with modern medical professionalism and helps physicians be professionally and personally successful.

Annotated References

1. Cruess SR, Johnston S, Cruess RL: "Profession": A working definition for medical educators. *Teach Learn Med* 2004;16(1):74-76.

2. *Oxford English Dictionary*, ed 2. Oxford, United Kingdom, Clarendon Press, 1989.

3. ABIM Foundation, American Board of Internal Medicine, ACP-ASIM Foundation, American College of Physicians-American Society of Internal Medicine, European Federation of Internal Medicine: Medical professionalism in the new millennium: A physician charter. *Ann Intern Med* 2002;136(3):243-246.

4. American Academy of Orthopaedic Surgeons: Principles of medical ethics and professionalism in orthopaedic surgery. *Guide to Professionalism and Ethics in the Practice of Orthopaedic Surgery*. Rosemont, IL, American Academy of Orthopaedic Surgeons January 2012. http://www.aaos.org/about/papers/ethics/ethicalpractguide.pdf. Accessed September 12, 2013.

   Regularly updated AAOS guidelines of professionalism and current topics are presented.

5. Pellegrino ED, Thomasma DC: *The Virtues in Medical Practice*. New York, NY, Oxford University Press, 1993.

6. Lo B: *Resolving Ethical Dilemmas: A Guide for Clinicians*, ed 4. Philadelphia, PA, Lippincott Williams & Wilkins, 2009, pp 32-33.

7. Stern DT: *Measuring Medical Professionalism*. New York, NY, Oxford University Press, 2006, pp 11-20.

8. Cruess RL, Cruess SR: *Teaching Medical Professionalism.* New York, NY, Cambridge University Press, 2009.

9. Embedding professionalism in medical education: Assessment as a tool for implementation. Report from an Invitational Conference Cosponsored by the Association of American Medical Colleges and the National Board of Medical Examiners. Baltimore, MD, May 2002.

10. Accreditation Council for Graduate Medical Education Outcome Project: Common program requirements: General competencies. 2007. http://www.acgme.org. Accessed March 24, 2011.

11. Zuckerman JD, Holder JP, Mercuri JJ, Phillips DP, Egol KA: Teaching professionalism in orthopaedic surgery residency programs. *J Bone Joint Surg Am* 2012; 94(8):e51.

The authors describe a variety of forums for teaching professionalism to orthopaedic residents.

12. Sargent MC, Sotile W, Sotile MO, et al: Managing stress in the orthopaedic family: Avoiding burnout, achieving resilience. *J Bone Joint Surg Am* 2011;93(8): e40.

A sobering survey of the personal health and satisfaction of orthoapedic residents, faculty, and spouses is presented.

13. Kaups KL: Governors' Committee on Physician Competency and Health: An update. *Bull Am Coll Surg* 2011; 96(10):22-25.

The author presents comprehensive results of a national survey of general surgeon's job satisfaction, stress, and chemical dependence.

14. Saleh KJ, Quick JC, Conaway M, et al: The prevalence and severity of burnout among academic orthopaedic departmental leaders. *J Bone Joint Surg Am* 2007;89(4): 896-903.

15. Williams ES, Konrad TR, Linzer M, et al: Refining the measurement of physician job satisfaction: Results from the Physician Worklife Survey. *Med Care* 1999;37(11): 1140-1154.

16. Krebs EE, Garrett JM, Konrad TR: The difficult doctor? Characteristics of physicians who report frustration with patients: An analysis of survey data. *BMC Health Serv Res* 2006;6:128.

17. Dunbar RP Jr: The realities of relationship failure. *J Orthop Trauma* 2012;26(suppl 1):S32-S33.

A review of the professional stresses that threaten personal and family relationships is presented.

18. Marsh JL: Avoiding burnout in an orthopaedic trauma practice. *J Orthop Trauma* 2012;26(suppl 1):S34-S36.

Orthopaedic trauma practices can be extremely time consuming, threaten personal relationships, and lead to early burnout. This article reviews the prevalence of burnout and describes strategies to achieve balance.

19. Tongue JR, Epps HR, Forese LL: Communication skills. *Instr Course Lect* 2005;54:3-9.

20. American Academy of Orthopaedic Surgeons: Communication skills mentoring program. http://www3.aaos.org/education/csmp/index.cfm. Accessed September 18, 2013.

21. Bozic KJ, Roche M, Agnew SG: Hospital-based employment of orthopaedic surgeons—passing trend or new paradigm? AOA critical issues. *J Bone Joint Surg Am* 2012;94(9):e59.

A higher percentage of orthopaedic physicians are opting for salaried positions. This trend is multifactorial. Healthcare institutions are striving to maintain market share, control costs, and remain profitable, and this strategy includes employee physicians. Physicians are examining the economic changes and challenges in maintaining a private practice and reassessing professional and personal balance.

22. American Medical Association: Policies related to physician health: H-95.955 Substance abuse among physicians. Chicago, IL, Department of Physician Health & Health Care Disparities, February 2011. http://www.ama-assn.org/resources/doc/physician-health/policies-physicain-health.pdf. Accessed September 18, 2013.

This AMA policy statement recognizes that physician impairment secondary to substance abuse and psychological disorders affects a physician to safely practice medicine. They encourage research to be able to identify causes and possibly address practice issues that lead to impairment. State programs are encouraged to establish programs to successfully treat physicians with impairment issues.

23. Schernhammer ES, Colditz GA: Suicide rates among physicians: A quantitative and gender assessment (meta-analysis). *Am J Psychiatry* 2004;161(12):2295-2302.

24. Peterson RN: Background paper on physicians with substance abuse issues. Report to *AAOS Ethics Committee.* Rosemont, IL, American Academy of Orthopaedic Surgeons, June 15, 2012.

A comprehensive review of substance abuse among physicians, elaboration of physician responsibilities for reporting colleagues, discussions of programs available for treatment, and review of current AAOS positions is presented.

25. Baldisseri MR: Impaired healthcare professional. *Crit Care Med* 2007;35(2, suppl):S106-S116.

26. Hughes PH, Brandenburg N, Baldwin DC Jr, et al: Prevalence of substance use among US physicians. *JAMA* 1992;267(17):2333-2339.

27. Oreskovich MR, Kaups KL, Balch CM, et al: Prevalence of alcohol use disorders among American surgeons. *Arch Surg* 2012;147(2):168-174.

The authors report the result of a survey with 7197 respondents (28.7% of survey population) revealing a prevalence of alcohol abuse/dependence among male surgeons of 13.9% and female surgeons of 25.6%. Surgeons reporting depression and being burned out were more at risk for alcohol problems.

28. Garcia-Guasch R, Roigé J, Padrós J: Substance abuse in anaesthetists. *Curr Opin Anaesthesiol* 2012;25(2): 204-209.

Anesthesiologists have an approximately 2.7 times likelihood of substance abuse compared with other medical specialties. Among the commonly abused medications were opioids, induction agents, and benzodiazapines.

29. Center C, Davis M, Detre T, et al: Confronting depression and suicide in physicians: A consensus statement. *JAMA* 2003;289(23):3161-3166.

30. Boisaubin EV, Levine RE: Identifying and assisting the impaired physician. *Am J Med Sci* 2001;322(1):31-36.

31. Farber NJ, Gilibert SG, Aboff BM, Collier VU, Weiner J, Boyer EG: Physicians' willingness to report impaired colleagues. *Soc Sci Med* 2005;61(8):1772-1775.

32. Carinci AJ, Christo PJ: Physician impairment: Is recovery feasible? *Pain Physician* 2009;12(3):487-491.

33. Brewster JM, Kaufmann IM, Hutchison S, MacWilliam C: Characteristics and outcomes of doctors in a substance dependence monitoring programme in Canada: Prospective descriptive study. *BMJ* 2008;337:a2098.

34. Patel P, Robinson BS, Novicoff WM, Dunnington GL, Brenner MJ, Saleh KJ: The disruptive orthopaedic surgeon: Implications for patient safety and malpractice liability. *J Bone Joint Surg Am* 2011;93(21):e1261-e1266.

Disruptive behavior in the operating room affects patient safety. Orthopaedic surgeons are the fourth most frequently reported physicians to demonstrate disruptive behavior.

35. Knifed E, Goyal A, Bernstein M: Moral angst for surgical residents: A qualitative study. *Am J Surg* 2010; 199(4):571-576.

The authors describe interviewing 28 surgical residents to discuss the ethical challenges of surgical training. Among the issues reported were the belief that patients were not well informed of the resident's role, the desire to report intraoperative errors to patients, and concern that they were placed in ethically challenging situations during their training because of the existing models of training or in disagreeing with the attending surgeon's management plan.

36. Kaplan K, Mestel P, Feldman DL: Creating a culture of mutual respect. *AORN J* 2010;91(4):495-510.

The authors report on an initiative to create a "Code of Mutual Respect." This was designed to address the issues of disruptive and inappropriate behavior by physicians and establish a framework for successfully addressing this behavior in the author's institution.

37. Maimonides Medical Center: Code of Mutual Respect. Adopted November 2008, revised July 2009. http:// www.maimonidesmed.org/ Resource.ashx?sn=codeofmutualrespectrev709.

38. Hickson GB, Pichert JW, Webb LE, Gabbe SG: A complementary approach to promoting professionalism: Identifying, measuring, and addressing unprofessional behaviors. *Acad Med* 2007;82(11):1040-1048.

39. Beauchamp TL, Childress JF: Moral status, in *Principles of Biomedical Ethics*, ed 6. New York, NY, Oxford University Press, 2009, pp 122-124.

40. English DC: *Bioethics: A Clinical Guide for Medical Students*. New York, NY, Norton & Company, 2009, pp 16-28.

41. Curlin FA, Lawrence RE, Chin MH, Lantos JD: Religion, conscience, and controversial clinical practices. *N Engl J Med* 2007;356(6):593-600.

42. Lo B: *Resolving Ethical Dilemmas: A Guide for Clinicians*, ed 4. Philadelphia, PA, Lippincott Williams & Wilkins, 2009.

43. Ross JR, Capozzi JD, Matava MJ: Discussing treatment options with a minor: The conflicts related to autonomy, beneficence, and paternalism. *J Bone Joint Surg Am* 2012;94(1):e3, 1-4.

"Ethics in Orthopaedics" discussion in JBJS describing the conflict of menisectomy versus meniscal repair in a 17-year-old scholarship-level high school football player. The patient is a minor, and consent needs to be obtained from his mother or father with participation of the patient.

44. Bozic KJ, Chiu V: Emerging ideas: Shared decision making in patients with osteoarthritis of the hip and knee. *Clin Orthop Relat Res* 2011;469(7):2081-2085.

Large regional, racial, and socioeconomic disparities exist in the utilization of total joint replacement for the management of osteoarthritis. The authors propose a framework for an investigation to assess the benefit of shared decision making in resolving these differences in the management of patients with osteoarthritis of the hip and knee.

45. Ganzini L, Volicer L, Nelson WA, Fox E, Derse AR: Ten myths about decision-making capacity. *J Am Med Dir Assoc* 2005;6(3, suppl):S100-S104.

46. Appelbaum PS: Clinical practice: Assessment of patients' competence to consent to treatment. *N Engl J Med* 2007;357(18):1834-1840.

47. Capozzi JD, Rhodes R: Assessing a patient's capacity to refuse treatment. *J Bone Joint Surg Am* 2002;84-A(4): 691-693.

48. American Academy of Orthopaedic Surgeons Ethics Committee: Resident ethics series: Issues and scenarios for discussion and guidance. Rosemont, IL, American

Academy of Orthopaedic Surgeons. http://www. aaos.org/ethics. Accessed September 12, 2013.

49. Bhattacharyya T, Yeon H, Harris MB: The medical-legal aspects of informed consent in orthopaedic surgery. *J Bone Joint Surg Am* 2005;87(11):2395-2400.

50. Ambady N, Laplante D, Nguyen T, Rosenthal R, Chaumeton N, Levinson W: Surgeons' tone of voice: A clue to malpractice history. *Surgery* 2002;132(1):5-9.

51. Beckman HB, Markakis KM, Suchman AL, Frankel RM: The doctor-patient relationship and malpractice: Lessons from plaintiff depositions. *Arch Intern Med* 1994;154(12):1365-1370.

52. Levinson W, Roter DL, Mullooly JP, Dull VT, Frankel RM: Physician-patient communication: The relationship with malpractice claims among primary care physicians and surgeons. *JAMA* 1997;277(7):553-559.

53. Schwartz PH: Questioning the quantitative imperative: Decision aids, prevention, and the ethics of disclosure. *Hastings Cent Rep* 2011;41(2):30-39.

   A discussion on how much information to share with a patient, including debate over outcome statistics, is presented.

54. Braddock CH III, Fihn SD, Levinson W, Jonsen AR, Pearlman RA: How doctors and patients discuss routine clinical decisions: Informed decision making in the outpatient setting. *J Gen Intern Med* 1997;12(6):339-345.

55. Braddock CH III, Edwards KA, Hasenberg NM, Laidley TL, Levinson W: Informed decision making in outpatient practice: Time to get back to basics. *JAMA* 1999; 282(24):2313-2320.

1: Principles of Orthopaedics

Chapter 2

Fracture Repair and Bone Grafting

Mara L. Schenker, MD   Nathan A. Wigner, MD, PhD   Luke Lopas, BS
Kurt D. Hankenson, DVM, MS, PhD   Jaimo Ahn, MD, PhD

Introduction

Approximately 7.9 million fractures occur each year in the United States, and 5% to 20% of patients experience some degree of impaired healing.[1] Consequently, physicians need to understand the complex mechanisms of bone repair, with the ultimate goal to promote and accelerate proper fracture healing in patients. This chapter reviews the biology of bone repair and the possible failure of bone healing (that is, nonunion and delayed union), as well as recent technologic advances in the augmentation of fracture repair using grafts, biologic, and mechanobiologic materials.

Biology of Bone Repair

The vertebrate skeleton forms as a result of two processes: intramembranous ossification and endochondral ossification. Intramembranous ossification is the process by which flat bones, such as the cranium, the scapula, innominate pelvic bones, and the clavicle, develop. During intramembranous ossification, progenitor cells

Dr. Hankenson serves as a paid consultant to or is an employee of Venenum; has received research or institutional support from Synthes; and serves as a board member, owner, officer, or committee member of the Orthopaedic Research Society, American College of Laboratory Animal Medicine, and American Association for Laboratory Animal Science. Dr. Ahn or an immediate family member serves as a paid consultant to or is an employee of Merck and serves as a board member, owner, officer, or committee member of the American Academy of Orthopaedic Surgeons Basic Science Evaluation Subcommittee, the Foundation for Orthopaedic Trauma Research Committee, the American Physician Scientists Association Board of Directors, and the National Board of Medical Examiners Committee for United States Medical Licensing Examination surgery test material development. None of the following authors nor any immediate family member has received anything of value from or has stock or stock options held in a commercial company or institution related directly or indirectly to the subject of this chapter: Dr. Schenker, Dr. Wigner, and Mr. Lopas.

differentiate directly into bone-forming osteoblasts. Other bones of the vertebrate skeleton form by endochondral ossification, a biphasic process of chondrogenesis followed by osteogenesis. Endochondral ossification occurs via the replacement of cartilaginous anlage with bone. Endochondral bones derive from mesenchymal progenitors often termed mesenchymal stem cells (MSCs) that differentiate into chondrocytes. During endochondral ossification, chondroprogenitor MSCs condense and differentiate into chondrocytes that deposit cartilage matrix, principally collagen type II and aggrecan, a large chondroitin sulfate proteoglycan. In the growth plate, chondrocytes continually secrete extracellular matrix (ECM) proteins and undergo unidirectional proliferation, forming parallel columns of dividing cells that result in longitudinal bone growth. Chondrocyte differentiation culminates with terminal hypertrophy, apoptosis, and mineralization of the ECM. As the chondrocytes undergo apoptosis, blood vessels, osteoblasts, and osteoclasts penetrate this zone of hypertrophic chondrocytes. Although osteoclasts are responsible for resorbing ECM, osteoblasts use the devitalized cartilaginous anlage as a functional scaffolding to lay down new osteoid. Thus, the pathways of chondrogenic and osteogenic lineage progression are fundamentally linked during endochondral bone formation.

Fracture healing represents a unique postnatal process that recapitulates many of the developmental processes seen during embryogenesis and during periods of postnatal skeletal growth. Therefore, the same processes that occur during endochondral ossification also occur during fracture healing. During the initial phases of fracture repair, the skeletal defect is stabilized via the formation of a cartilaginous callus; the callus size often is inversely related to the mechanical competency across the bony defect. Thus, the callus not only provides immediate mechanical stability at the fracture site but also functions as a template on which new bone is formed.

Fracture healing may be characterized by its progression through a series of different biologic processes that comprise four temporally defined but overlapping phases of repair: the inflammatory phase, characterized by an inflammatory and marrow response; the early callus phase, predominated by mesenchymal and vascular infiltration and chondrogenesis; the mature callus phase, marked by endochondral ossification and

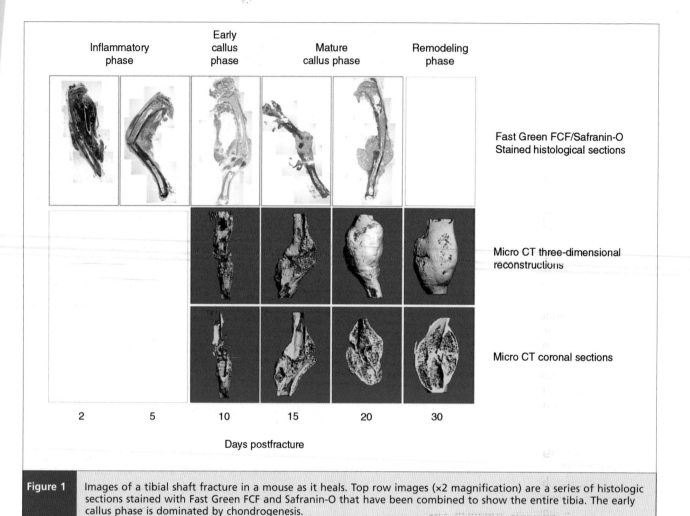

Inflammatory phase	Early callus phase	Mature callus phase	Remodeling phase	

Fast Green FCF/Safranin-O Stained histological sections

Micro CT three-dimensional reconstructions

Micro CT coronal sections

| 2 | 5 | 10 | 15 | 20 | 30 |

Days postfracture

Figure 1 Images of a tibial shaft fracture in a mouse as it heals. Top row images (×2 magnification) are a series of histologic sections stained with Fast Green FCF and Safranin-O that have been combined to show the entire tibia. The early callus phase is dominated by chondrogenesis.

primary bone (also called immature or woven bone) formation; and the remodeling phase, defined by secondary bone (also called mature or lamellar bone) formation[2] (Figure 1).

The Inflammatory Phase

The initial inflammatory stage of fracture healing in patients begins immediately following the fracture to typically 3 to 4 days postfracture. A hematoma forms that encompasses the fracture site and a systemic proinflammatory response is initiated.[3] Similar to other wound healing processes, this stage is characterized by the release of proinflammatory mediators, such as interleukin 1 (IL-1), IL-6, and tumor necrosis factor alpha (TNF-α) produced by T cells, macrophages, neutrophils, platelets, and injured bone cells. These inflammatory mediators play a critical role in initiating the repair process.[4] Proinflammatory molecules reach peak expression 24 hours following injury and subsequently decline to baseline levels by 72 hours following fracture. In addition to inflammatory mediators, numerous growth factors and critical signaling molecules are expressed in the immediate local environment, resulting in an influx of MSCs from the surrounding marrow cavity and the periosteal surface followed by proliferation.[3]

The Early Callus Phase

The second stage, which may begin within a few days postfracture and last up to several weeks, is characterized by vascularization, the proliferation of chondroprogenitor MSCs and differentiation into chondrocytes, and the expression of cartilage-specific matrix proteins. Chondrogenesis is a multistage process that functionally can be divided into six phases: MSC proliferation, MSC condensation, chondrocyte formation, chondrocyte maturation, hypertrophic differentiation, and apoptosis. The formation of a cartilage callus not only provides immediate mechanical stability to the fracture site but also establishes the spatial geometry on which new bone forms.[5] The cartilage callus is composed of many different ECM proteins, such as collagens and hyaluronic acid, and sulfated proteoglycans, such as aggrecan. During endochondral fracture healing, discrete phases of chondrogenic differentiation can be identified by monitoring the differential expression of stage-specific genes, which parallel associated phenotypic changes. For example, proliferating and mature chondrocytes predominantly synthesize collagen type II and aggrecan, whereas hypertrophic chondrocytes express collagen type X and alkaline phosphatase. Only the most terminally differentiated chondrocytes express proteases, such as matrix metallopeptidase 13 (MMP13), which degrade the cartilaginous ECM.[6]

The Mature Callus Phase

The final two stages of primary and secondary bone formation occur as the cartilaginous matrix is mineralized and primary bone is laid down on these surfaces. Prior to the onset of ossification, chondrocytes in these regions undergo apoptosis, the matrix becomes vascularized, and osteoblasts infiltrate the callus.[7]

The Remodeling Phase

Subsequently, the formation of more organized secondary bone begins. During this stage, the original long bone structure begins to reestablish as the newly formed woven bone remodels to reform the mature lamellar bone, restoring the original cortical structure.[2] In the clinical setting, fractures are typically considered healed during the late mature callus phase and early remodeling phase (several months postfracture). It is important to keep in mind, however, that late remodeling can continue beyond 1 year and can extend into many years.

Fracture Healing in Stable Mechanical Environments

The spontaneous healing of fractures typically occurs as mentioned previously, via secondary bone healing, in the presence of unstable fragment ends. However, in stable mechanical environments, bone has the potential to heal without significant callus formation. In 1949, rigid fixation without callus formation was first described as "primary bone healing."[8] A later study showed that healing occurs under these conditions via direct osteonal proliferation[9] (Figure 2). Stable abutment of the fracture ends is achieved by the application of rigid implants, such as compression plates and lag screws, and is used to precisely align the fracture ends, as routinely performed for stabilization of intra-articular fractures and simple fracture patterns.

Failure of Bone Repair: Delayed Unions and Nonunions

In the United States, the delayed healing of fractures has been reported in approximately 600,000 patients per year, with 100,000 progressing to nonunion.[10] Currently, no standard criteria exist to define nonunion, although the FDA defines nonunion as a fractured bone that has not completely healed within 9 months and shows no progression toward healing on serial radiographs over 3 consecutive months. The three types of nonunion are hypertrophic, oligotrophic, and atrophic.[10] Hypertrophic nonunions have a biologic capacity for healing, have inadequate mechanical stability,

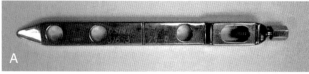

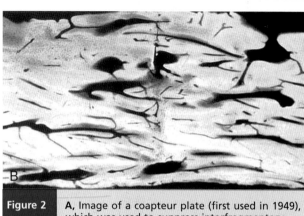

Figure 2 **A,** Image of a coapteur plate (first used in 1949), which was used to suppress interfragmentary motion and increase the stability of fixation through interfragmentary compression achieved by tightening the side screw. **B,** Direct osteonal proliferation in primary bone healing. (Reproduced with permission from Uhthoff HK, Poitras P, Backman DS: Internal plate fixation of fractures: Short history and recent developments. *J Orthop Sci* 2006;11[2]:118-126.)

and are characterized by abundant callus formation with a lack of bony bridging. Oligotrophic nonunions have the biologic capacity for healing, have no ability to initiate healing, and are characterized by little to no callus formation. Atrophic nonunions have little to no capacity for healing and are characterized by sclerotic bone ends with no callus formation and pseudarthrosis.

The risk factors for impaired bone healing in fractures can be classified as modifiable or nonmodifiable. Intervention in modifiable risk factors offers an opportunity to enhance bone healing in compromised patients.

Modifiable Risk Factors for Impaired Bone Healing

The potential risk factors for impaired bone healing that can be modified to improve bone healing are outlined in Table 1. Basic science studies have shown that smoking reduces local blood flow and decreases osteoblast formation and bone metabolism, thus impairing fracture healing.[11] Prospective and retrospective cohort studies have corroborated this basic science evidence and show trends toward higher rates of nonunion and longer mean healing times for fractures in patients who smoke.[12,13]

Diabetes mellitus, in addition to its associated risk of peripheral neuropathy and peripheral vascular disease, directly affects fracture healing. In a study of diabetic rats, fracture calluses were shown to have 29% less tensile strength and 50% less stiffness compared with those in the control group.[14] This disadvantage can be

1: Principles of Orthopaedics

Table 1

Risk Factors for Fracture Nonunion

Modifiable Risk Factors	Nonmodifiable Risk Factors
Substance abuse (alcohol, smoking)	Injury characteristics (pattern of bone injury, location of fracture, status of the soft tissues, severe bone loss)
Medication use (NSAIDs, steroids)	Patient disease (peripheral vascular disease, genetic disorders)
Infection	Advanced age
Diabetes mellitus	Sex
Metabolic deficiencies (vitamin D, calcium, parathyroid hormone, testosterone, thyroid, nutritional)	
Inadequate surgical fixation (for example, insufficient mechanical stability or high strain)	

normalized with improved glycemic control.[15] Clinical studies have shown a higher incidence of delayed union, nonunion, and prolonged healing times in patients with diabetes when compared with healthy patients.[16]

Nutritional deficiencies, particularly in dietary calcium and vitamin D, have long been associated with impaired fracture healing. One study noted that 84% of patients referred for treatment of a fracture nonunion were found to have a metabolic or an endocrine abnormality, and 68% were found to have a vitamin D deficiency.[17] Additionally, hyperparathyroidism and low growth hormone levels have been associated with higher rates of nonunion.[18] Based on the high rate of association between metabolic and endocrine abnormalities and nonunion, some authors have recommended referral to an endocrinologist for a complete workup in cases of nonunion.[17]

Certain medications have also been shown to limit the capacity for fracture healing. NSAIDs effectively reduce acute pain and swelling and decrease the requirement for concurrent narcotic therapy in the management of musculoskeletal injuries, including fractures. However, basic science evidence has raised concerns about the use of NSAIDs in routine management following a fracture, with the potential of slowing the intrinsic fracture healing process and increasing the risk of nonunion or delayed union.[19] A recent systematic review of the literature did not show a substantial detrimental role of clinical NSAID use in fracture healing; the authors concluded that clinical evidence is insufficient to deny patients with simple fracture patterns the benefits of these drugs.[20] Systemic administration of corticosteroids also has been shown to inhibit fracture healing and reduce callus strength in animal models[21] and increase the rate of nonunion in patients with intertrochanteric hip fractures.[22] Bisphosphonates are widely used for the treatment of osteoporosis and the prevention of fragility fractures. Systemically administered bisphosphonates bind to the hydroxyapatite in bone and inhibit bony resorption by osteoclasts, thereby decreasing the rate of bone remodeling. Several

animal models have shown increased callus volume, trabecular bone volume, and bone mineral content with bisphosphonate treatment but also have shown delayed maturation and remodeling of the callus.[23] Similarly, clinical studies have shown varied and uncertain effects on bone repair, making their role in fracture healing unclear.[24]

Nonmodifiable Risk Factors for Impaired Bone Healing

Nonmodifiable risk factors for impaired bone healing[10] are presented in Table 1. Fractures in several anatomic areas, including the fifth metatarsal metaphysis[25] and the proximal pole of the scaphoid,[26] are more prone to nonunion given the tenuous blood supply. Severe bone loss is also a risk factor for nonunion. Although the absolute critical size for a bone defect beyond which healing cannot occur in patients is not known, it represents a deficiency that is not expected to heal without secondary intervention.[10] Other proposed nonmodifiable risk factors for impaired healing may become modifiable in the future via improved mechanistic understanding of these factors.

Modulation of Fracture Healing

Several approaches to enhance fracture healing are widely used clinically, including optimization of patient risk factors for poor healing, direct augmentation of the fracture site with biologic materials (for example, bone morphogenetic proteins [BMPs]) and grafts (for example, autografts and allografts) and indirect augmentation of the fracture site with external stimulation (for example, electric stimulation, ultrasound, shock, and vibration). Much research has been dedicated to the enhancement of fracture healing, although most data have a low level of evidence.

Optimization of Patient Risk Factors for Poor Healing Capacity

Numerous modifiable risk factors predispose patients to a poor capacity for healing. Although cessation of substance abuse, discontinuation of specific medications, and optimization of symptoms for a patient's disease are presumed to enhance bone healing, little high-level clinical evidence exists to support this claim in patients who have sustained a fracture. Two randomized controlled trials have evaluated the effects of optimizing patient metabolic deficiencies during acute fracture healing.[1,27]

Parathyroid hormone (PTH) is released by the parathyroid glands and increases the blood levels of calcium by indirectly stimulating bone resorption, increasing renal reabsorption of calcium, and increasing intestinal calcium absorption. Low-dose intermittent administration of PTH has anabolic effects on bone metabolism, although high-dose continuous administration has catabolic effects. PTH 1-34 is the active form of PTH; a commercially available form is FDA approved for the treatment of osteoporosis in postmenopausal women who are at high risk of fracture or who have a history of osteoporotic fracture. Animal models have shown enhanced callus formation and mechanical strength of fractures with the administration of PTH.[28] In 2010, a prospective, randomized, double-blind study was conducted on 102 postmenopausal women with nonsurgically treated distal radius fractures who received 8 weeks of daily systemic administration of low-dose recombinant PTH (20 µg), high-dose recombinant PTH (40 µg), or a placebo. The time to cortical bridging was accelerated in the patients treated with low-dose recombinant PTH, but no difference was noted between patients treated with high-dose recombinant PTH and those treated with placebo.[1]

Dietary supplementation with calcium and vitamin D, long recommended for improving bone health, is thought to help reduce fracture risk in patients with osteoporosis and enhance fracture healing. Animal models have shown the benefit of systemic administration of calcium and vitamin D on bone healing after fracture.[29] In 2004, a double-blind prospective trial evaluated the effects of the daily administration of vitamin D (800 IU) and calcium (1 g) on patients with nonsurgically treated proximal humeral fractures compared with placebo. The results of the study showed increased callus formation (as measured by enhanced bone density) at 6 weeks in the treatment group when compared with the control group.[27] In 2012, the US Preventive Services Task Force published a recommendation against vitamin D supplementation for the prevention of osteoporotic fractures, citing insufficient current evidence to assess the benefits.[30]

Bone Grafting
Autogenous Bone Grafts
Autogenous bone grafting is the gold standard for the treatment of bone defects and the stimulation of new bone formation. Autograft can be harvested from the iliac crest or from local metaphyseal areas. Autograft is osteogenic (contains viable donor osteoblasts and their precursors in the tissue that promote bone formation), osteoinductive (recruits pluripotent MSCs that differentiate into osteoblasts and chondroblasts), and osteocon-

ductive (provides scaffolding and an environment for new bone formation by supporting vascular ingrowth, perivascular tissue, and osteoprogenitor cells). Autograft is also histocompatible and nonimmunogenic. The potential drawbacks of using autograft include donor site morbidity (deep infection, pain, and nerve injury), increased surgical time and blood loss, and limited quantity availability. Because of the potential drawbacks, significant research efforts have been dedicated to the development of bone graft substitutes.[31]

Allografts
Allografts are harvested from cadaver tissue, thereby avoiding all of the donor site morbidities associated with autografts. Allograft types include nonstructural grafts (cancellous or corticocancellous chips), structural grafts (cortical struts), and demineralized bone matrix (DBM). DBM is a highly processed allograft subtype prepared by demineralization of the allograft using an organic solvent, allowing the retention of both collagenous and noncollagenous proteins (for example, BMPs). More than 25 DBM products are commercially available in multiple forms (powder, putty, chips, crushed granules, or gel-filled syringes).[32] Although allograft has both osteoconductive and osteoinductive capacities, its osteoinductive capacity is less than that of autograft. It has been suggested that the process of demineralization for DBM may result in improved osteoinductive properties compared with traditional allograft.[32] DMB also has comparable capacity for bone formation compared with autograft, as reported in a subset of patients with humeral nonunions.[33] Allografts are not inherently osteogenic because they do not have viable cells. Allografts are typically processed via mechanical débridement of all soft tissues, washing with ethanol to remove blood and live cells, and gamma irradiation to sterilize the tissues. Although high-dose irradiation kills bacteria and viruses, it may also decrease the biomechanical properties of the allografts and affect the osteoconductive and osteoinductive properties in a dose-dependent fashion.[34] A potential drawback of allograft is the risk of disease transmission. A strict donor screening protocol, such as that implemented by the American Association of Tissue Banks, is critical to ensure the safety of bone allografts. According to donor screening recommendations, it has been reported that the chance of obtaining a bone graft from an HIV-infected donor is 1 in 1.67 million,[35] and the risk of obtaining DBM that contains HIV is 1 in 2.8 billion.[36] Other drawbacks of allograft include a risk of immunogenic response, longer healing times, and decreased osteoinductive capacity when compared with autograft.

Synthetic Bone Substitutes
Synthetic bone substitutes are an alternative to allograft and autograft and include calcium sulfate, calcium phosphate, tricalcium phosphate, and bioglass. Synthetic bone substitutes are available in multiple forms, including powder, pellets, and putty. They are osteoconductive but not osteoinductive or osteogenic.

Several clinical studies have evaluated the use of synthetic bone substitutes for bone defect filling in fractures of the tibial plateau, hip, distal radius, proximal humerus, and calcaneus.[37] One randomized controlled study evaluated the treatment of femoral neck fractures with closed reduction and percutaneous pinning.[38] No difference was found between the reoperation rates of patients whose treatment did include augmentation with calcium phosphate cement and those whose treatment did not. Another randomized controlled study evaluated the use of calcium phosphate for the treatment of depressed tibial plateau fractures.[39] Fewer complications and decreased articular subsidence were found in patients whose treatment was augmented with calcium phosphate cement compared with autograft,[39] although the effect on clinical outcomes remains unclear.

Platelet-Rich Plasma

Platelets are a key component of the inflammatory phase of bone healing, and activated platelets release many growth factors, including platelet-derived growth factor, transforming growth factor-beta (TGF-β), and vascular endothelial growth factor. These growth factors influence the proliferation and the differentiation of cells, including bone cells, and promote healing. The goal of platelet-rich plasma (PRP) therapy is to deliver supraphysiologic concentrations of platelets and growth factors to sites of injury to enhance healing; however, good-quality data that support the use of PRP for clinical applications in general are sparse. Studies of animal models using PRP therapy for the treatment of fractures have demonstrated enhanced early cellular proliferation and chondrogenesis as well as subsequent improved callus formation and mechanical strength.[40] A recent review identified 61 studies on PRP therapies for long bone healing in adults, but only 1 study fully met the inclusion criteria.[41] That study evaluated patients who had undergone corrective tibial osteotomies who were prospectively randomized to allograft alone or allograft and PRP therapy. No differences were found in functional scores at 1 year; however, enhanced radiographic integration of the graft was noted at the osteotomy site in the PRP group compared with the allograft-only group.[42] One additional study, which was excluded, was a randomized clinical trial that compared two different treatment types (BMP-7 versus PRP) without including a true-negative control group. This group included patients with long bone nonunions and showed enhanced healing in the BMP-7 group compared with the PRP group.[43]

Bone Marrow Aspirate and Stem Cell Therapies

Bone marrow aspirate and stem cell therapies are topics of considerable current research for the enhancement of fracture healing. Bone marrow is a source of circulating endothelial progenitors that can participate in bone healing either directly by differentiating into osteoblasts or indirectly by secreting various growth factors that enhance the differentiation of local stem cells and/or lead to enhanced vascular ingrowth. Several stem cell–based approaches have shown improved bone regeneration in animal models[44,45]; however, one study proposed that skeletal repair requires the structural and mechanical support provided by a scaffold to be successful.[46] Several products of bone marrow aspirate/allograft scaffold are currently clinically available.[47,48] A reamer-irrigator-aspirator system[49] is also available that provides continuous irrigation and suction during long bone reaming. The bone is collected in a suction bag and can be used as graft material. Despite the intense research interest in this field, considerable oversight by regulatory committees exists for regenerative sciences in general, which may slow the approval for stem cell based therapy in fracture healing in the near future.[50]

Bone Morphogenetic Proteins

BMPs are part of the TGF-β superfamily and are potent inducers of bone formation. BMPs are synthesized by skeletal cells and are critical for embryogenesis, skeletogenesis, and maintaining bone mass in the mature skeleton.[51] More than 30 BMPs have been identified, and murine studies of tibial fracture healing have shown temporal expression of BMP-2, -3, -4, -5, -6, and -7 at different stages of the fracture healing process, which suggests these proteins play a role in bone healing.[52] The biologic importance of BMPs in bone formation is exemplified in bone overgrowth disorders that result from genetic inactivation of an antagonist[53] or overactivation of a receptor.[54]

BMPs promote bone formation using several mechanisms.[55] The BMPs recruit MSCs from the surrounding muscle, bone marrow, and vessels and induce these cells to become osteoblasts to generate bone directly. In addition, BMPs induce chondrocytes to initiate the process of endochondral ossification and can promote vascularization.[55]

Two clinically available BMPs are FDA approved: recombinant human BMP-2 (rhBMP-2) and rhBMP-7. rhBMP-2 is currently approved for the treatment of acute open tibial fractures and for use in spine fusion surgery. rhBMP-7 is approved for the treatment of recalcitrant long bone nonunions for which autograft is unfeasible and alternative treatment options have failed, as well as in patients at high risk for fusion failure who require revision posterolateral lumbar spinal fusion. Several randomized prospective controlled studies have evaluated fracture healing augmented with rhBMP-2 and rhBMP-7.[55] Three studies evaluated the use of rhBMP-2 (1.5 mg/mL) in open tibial fractures delivered directly to the fracture site in an absorbable collagen sponge. Two of the studies showed accelerated fracture and wound healing times in severe open fracture injuries, a decreased need for secondary procedures (bone grafting, invasive procedures, procedures for delayed union), and lower rates of infection in severe open fractures.[56,57] The third study did not identify any differences in healing rate, infection rate, or the need for secondary surgeries in open tibial fractures treated by reaming with intramedullary nails.[58] A 2006 study evaluated the effects of treating patients who sustained tibial fractures with severe bone loss using rhBMP-2 and allograft versus autograft. The study noted decreased blood loss in the group treated with rhBMP-2 and allograft but no difference in healing rates or functional outcome scores.[59] Four studies evaluated the clinical use of rhBMP-7 for nonunions,[43,60] malunions,[61] and large fibular defects following high tibial osteotomies[62] in randomized controlled trials. rhBMP-7 (3.5 mg/mL) was shown to be equivalent to autograft for the treatment of tibial nonunion[60] and superior to PRP therapy for long bone nonunion.[43] The results of a 1999 study showed increased formation of bone and bridging of the segmental defect in fibular defects using rhBMP-7 compared with a control group.[62] However, a 2008 study found slower healing time in patients with distal radius fracture malunion treated with corrective osteotomies and augmented with rhBMP-7 compared with patients treated using autograft.[61]

External Stimulation: Electrical Stimulation, Ultrasound, and Vibration Therapy

Biophysical treatments, such as electrical stimulation, ultrasound, shock, and vibration therapy have the potential to improve fracture healing. In 1953, the first work on the effects of electric forces on bone healing was published.[63] In 1970, early evidence showed that electrical stimulation can lead to bone formation.[64] Since then, there has been considerable interest in the manipulation of electric forces in bone healing; however, clinical data in support of electrical stimulation, ultrasound, shock, and vibration for enhanced fracture healing are relatively sparse.

In a 2011 review, four randomized placebo-controlled studies were identified that evaluated the effects of electrical stimulation for treating delayed union or nonunion of long bone fractures in adults.[65] The data demonstrated that electrical stimulation was safe, with only two minor skin irritations reported. Further, the results favored electrical stimulation compared with placebo, but the overall pooled estimate was not significant (relative risk, 1.96; 95% confidence interval, 0.86-4.48).[65]

Ultrasound is high-frequency sound waves and is a form of mechanical stimulation. For the augmentation of fracture healing, the ultrasound probe is typically placed directly over the fracture site for 20 minutes per day. Three types of ultrasound therapy have been described: low-intensity pulsed ultrasound, high-intensity focused ultrasound, and extracorporeal shock wave therapy. Another recent review evaluated the effects of ultrasound and shock wave therapy for acute fractures in adults.[66] The authors identified 11 randomized controlled trials that evaluated low-intensity pulsed ultrasound and found that ultrasound therapy was favored in acute fractures, but no difference was found in delayed unions and nonunions. One randomized controlled trial that evaluated extracorporeal shock wave therapy for acute tibial and femoral fractures was identified and found no improvement in achieving union at 12 months, but small differences in the visual analog scale for pain at 3, 6, and 12 months in favor of extracorporeal shock wave therapy.[66]

Vibration therapy is based on Wolff's law, which states that bone adapts to its mechanical environment. The osteogenic effect of vibration therapy on intact bone and the stimulating effect on limb blood flow have been documented in animal and human studies[67] and is typically administered in a low-magnitude, high-frequency mode. Whole-body vibration therapy has been proposed for the treatment of osteoporosis.[68] Some animal models have demonstrated a marginal or beneficial effect of vibration therapy on fracture healing.[69] Well-designed clinical studies are needed to better assess the effects of biophysical stimulation on bone healing.

Summary

There is considerable interest in unraveling the complex regulation of bone repair to devise new strategies for the enhancement of fracture healing, both in acute fractures and in delayed unions and nonunions. Recent advances in augmented fracture repair through bone grafting, biologics, and biophysical stimulation have made significant progress toward enhancing bone repair, but substantial research is needed to further enhance the processes of fracture healing, particularly in the compromised patient. Given the high societal burden of delayed unions, nonunions, and routine fracture healing, additional strategies, including cell-based and scaffold-based therapies, are needed to enhance the fracture healing process.

Key Study Points

- The two ways in which fracture healing occurs mirrors endochondral (indirect bone formation through cartilage phase) and intramembranous (direct bone formation from progenitor cells) bone formation during development.

- Absolute stability with direct apposition of bone favors direct bone healing, and relative stability favors indirect healing through a fracture callus. Various treatments rendered by physicians and surgeons can alter the degree of stability and affect the mode of healing.

- The enhancement of problematic fracture healing (nonunion, delayed union, gap defect) can be treated by improving the mechanical environment; altering modifiable biologic factors systemically; or applying local therapies such as bone grafts, biologic factors, or cell-based enhancements.

1: Principles of Orthopaedics

Annotated References

1. Aspenberg P, Genant HK, Johansson T, et al: Teriparatide for acceleration of fracture repair in humans: A prospective, randomized, double-blind study of 102 postmenopausal women with distal radial fractures. *J Bone Miner Res* 2010;25(2):404-414.

   Although the clinically approved dose of recombinant PTH (teriparatide [20 µg]) reduced the time to cortical bridging in distal radius fractures when compared with placebo, the authors were unable show that recombinant PTH enhances healing in a dose-dependent manner. Level of evidence: I.

2. Gerstenfeld LC, Cullinane DM, Barnes GL, Graves DT, Einhorn TA: Fracture healing as a post-natal developmental process: Molecular, spatial, and temporal aspects of its regulation. *J Cell Biochem* 2003;88(5):873-884.

3. Barnes GL, Kostenuik PJ, Gerstenfeld LC, Einhorn TA: Growth factor regulation of fracture repair. *J Bone Miner Res* 1999;14(11):1805-1815.

4. Kon T, Cho TJ, Aizawa T, et al: Expression of osteoprotegerin, receptor activator of NF-kappaB ligand (osteoprotegerin ligand) and related proinflammatory cytokines during fracture healing. *J Bone Miner Res* 2001;16(6):1004-1014.

5. Hankemeier S, Grässel S, Plenz G, Spiegel HU, Bruckner P, Probst A: Alteration of fracture stability influences chondrogenesis, osteogenesis and immigration of macrophages. *J Orthop Res* 2001;19(4):531-538.

6. Gerstenfeld LC, Alkhiary YM, Krall EA, et al: Three-dimensional reconstruction of fracture callus morphogenesis. *J Histochem Cytochem* 2006;54(11):1215-1228.

7. Goldring MB, Tsuchimochi K, Ijiri K: The control of chondrogenesis. *J Cell Biochem* 2006;97(1):33-44.

8. Danis R: *Théorie et pratique de l'ostéosynthèse.* Paris, France, Masson, 1949.

9. Schenk R, Willenegger H: [On the histological picture of so-called primary healing of pressure osteosynthesis in experimental osteotomies in the dog]. *Experientia* 1963; 19:593-595.

10. Bishop JA, Palanca AA, Bellino MJ, Lowenberg DW: Assessment of compromised fracture healing. *J Am Acad Orthop Surg* 2012;20(5):273-282.

    The authors present a comprehensive review on fracture nonunions, including epidemiology, risk factors, clinical evaluation, and classification. Level of evidence: IV.

11. Rothem DE, Rothem L, Dahan A, Eliakim R, Soudry M: Nicotinic modulation of gene expression in osteoblast cells, MG-63. *Bone* 2011;48(4):903-909.

    Using MG-63 osteoblast-like cells, this study identified 842 genes whose expression was altered after exposure to nicotine. Gene ontologic analysis showed that many of the identified genes play key roles in cellular proliferation and/or apoptosis.

12. Castillo RC, Bosse MJ, MacKenzie EJ, Patterson BM; LEAP Study Group: Impact of smoking on fracture healing and risk of complications in limb-threatening open tibia fractures. *J Orthop Trauma* 2005;19(3):151-157.

13. Schmitz MA, Finnegan M, Natarajan R, Champine J: Effect of smoking on tibial shaft fracture healing. *Clin Orthop Relat Res* 1999;365:184-200.

14. Macey LR, Kana SM, Jingushi S, Terek RM, Borretos J, Bolander ME: Defects of early fracture-healing in experimental diabetes. *J Bone Joint Surg Am* 1989;71(5):722-733.

15. Kayal RA, Alblowi J, McKenzie E, et al: Diabetes causes the accelerated loss of cartilage during fracture repair which is reversed by insulin treatment. *Bone* 2009;44(2):357-363.

16. Loder RT: The influence of diabetes mellitus on the healing of closed fractures. *Clin Orthop Relat Res* 1988;232:210-216.

17. Brinker MR, O'Connor DP, Monla YT, Earthman TP: Metabolic and endocrine abnormalities in patients with nonunions. *J Orthop Trauma* 2007;21(8):557-570.

18. Lancourt JE, Hochberg F: Delayed fracture healing in primary hyperparathyroidism. *Clin Orthop Relat Res* 1977;124:214-218.

19. Brown KM, Saunders MM, Kirsch T, Donahue HJ, Reid JS: Effect of COX-2-specific inhibition on fracture-healing in the rat femur. *J Bone Joint Surg Am* 2004;86(1):116-123.

20. Kurmis AP, Kurmis TP, O'Brien JX, Dalén T: The effect of nonsteroidal anti-inflammatory drug administration on acute phase fracture-healing: A review. *J Bone Joint Surg Am* 2012;94(9):815-823.

    The authors present a review on the controversial topic of NSAID use during the acute postfracture period. Despite preclinical animal models suggesting COX-2 inhibition impairs early fracture healing, there was insufficient evidence to withhold NSAID use clinically. Level of evidence: IV.

21. Waters RV, Gamradt SC, Asnis P, et al: Systemic corticosteroids inhibit bone healing in a rabbit ulnar osteotomy model. *Acta Orthop Scand* 2000;71(3):316-321.

22. Bogoch ER, Ouellette G, Hastings DE: Intertrochanteric fractures of the femur in rheumatoid arthritis patients. *Clin Orthop Relat Res* 1993;294:181-186.

23. McDonald MM, Dulai S, Godfrey C, Amanat N, Sztynda T, Little DG: Bolus or weekly zoledronic acid administration does not delay endochondral fracture re-

© 2014 American Academy of Orthopaedic Surgeons

pair but weekly dosing enhances delays in hard callus remodeling. *Bone* 2008;43(4):653-662.

24. Goldhahn J, Féron JM, Kanis J, et al: Implications for fracture healing of current and new osteoporosis treatments: An ESCEO consensus paper. *Calcif Tissue Int* 2012;90(5):343-353.

    The authors present a review on current treatment options for osteoporosis, and they conclude that there is no evidence that osteoporosis treatments are detrimental to bone healing, and they may have some positive effects on bone healing. Level of evidence: IV.

25. Rosenberg GA, Sferra JJ: Treatment strategies for acute fractures and nonunions of the proximal fifth metatarsal. *J Am Acad Orthop Surg* 2000;8(5):332-338.

26. Kozin SH: Incidence, mechanism, and natural history of scaphoid fractures. *Hand Clin* 2001;17(4):515-524.

27. Doetsch AM, Faber J, Lynnerup N, Wätjen I, Bliddal H, Danneskiold-Samsøe B: The effect of calcium and vitamin D3 supplementation on the healing of the proximal humerus fracture: A randomized placebo-controlled study. *Calcif Tissue Int* 2004;75(3):183-188.

28. Andreassen TT, Fledelius C, Ejersted C, Oxlund H: Increases in callus formation and mechanical strength of healing fractures in old rats treated with parathyroid hormone. *Acta Orthop Scand* 2001;72(3):304-307.

29. Delgado-Martínez AD, Martínez ME, Carrascal MT, Rodríguez-Avial M, Munuera L: Effect of 25-OH-vitamin D on fracture healing in elderly rats. *J Orthop Res* 1998;16(6):650-653.

30. US Preventive Services Task Force: Vitamin D and calcium supplementation to prevent cancer and osteoporotic fractures in adults: US Preventive Services Task Force recommendation statement. DRAFT. June 12, 2012. http://www.uspreventiveservicestaskforce.org/uspstf12/vitamind/draftrecvitd.htm. Accessed February 14, 2012.

    Sixteen randomized controlled trials with considerable heterogeneity in populations and interventions were examined by the US Preventive Services Task Force. They concluded that the current evidence was insufficient to determine if vitamin D and calcium supplementation prevents fractures in premenopausal and postmenopausal women. Level of evidence: II.

31. Myeroff C, Archdeacon M: Autogenous bone graft: Donor sites and techniques. *J Bone Joint Surg Am* 2011;93(23):2227-2236.

    This review provides a comprehensive overview of autogenous bone grafts, primarily focusing on autogenous cancellous bone grafting, donor site techniques, associated complications, and relevant clinical data to inform clinical decision making. Level of evidence: IV.

32. Drosos GI, Kazakos KI, Kouzoumpasis P, Verettas DA: Safety and efficacy of commercially available demineralised bone matrix preparations: A critical review of clinical studies. *Injury* 2007;38(suppl 4):S13-S21.

33. Hierholzer C, Sama D, Toro JB, Peterson M, Helfet DL: Plate fixation of ununited humeral shaft fractures: Effect of type of bone graft on healing. *J Bone Joint Surg Am* 2006;88(7):1442-1447.

34. Nguyen H, Morgan DA, Forwood MR: Sterilization of allograft bone: Effects of gamma irradiation on allograft biology and biomechanics. *Cell Tissue Bank* 2007;8(2):93-105.

35. Buck BE, Malinin TI: Human bone and tissue allografts: Preparation and safety. *Clin Orthop Relat Res* 1994;303:8-17.

36. Russo R, Scarborough N: Inactivation of viruses in demineralized bone matrix. *FDA Workshop on Tissue Transplantation and Reproductive Tissue*. Bethesda, MD, 1995.

37. Larsson S, Hannink G: Injectable bone-graft substitutes: Current products, their characteristics and indications, and new developments. *Injury* 2011;42(suppl 2):S30-S34.

    This article describes the biomechanical properties of the most common injectable bone graft substitutes currently commercially available and their use in specific clinical situations. Level of evidence: IV.

38. Mattsson P, Larsson S: Calcium phosphate cement for augmentation did not improve results after internal fixation of displaced femoral neck fractures: A randomized study of 118 patients. *Acta Orthop* 2006;77(2):251-256.

39. Russell TA, Leighton RK; Alpha-BSM Tibial Plateau Fracture Study Group: Comparison of autogenous bone graft and endothermic calcium phosphate cement for defect augmentation in tibial plateau fractures: A multicenter, prospective, randomized study. *J Bone Joint Surg Am* 2008;90(10):2057-2061.

40. Kasten P, Vogel J, Geiger F, Niemeyer P, Luginbühl R, Szalay K: The effect of platelet-rich plasma on healing in critical-size long-bone defects. *Biomaterials* 2008;29(29):3983-3992.

41. Griffin XL, Wallace D, Parsons N, Costa ML: Platelet rich therapies for long bone healing in adults. *Cochrane Database Syst Rev* 2012;7:CD009496.

    One randomized controlled trial of 21 participants was included in this systematic literature review. Given the paucity of eligible studies, the authors determined that insufficient evidence exists to assess the efficacy of PRP therapies in long bone healing. Level of evidence: I.

42. Dallari D, Savarino L, Stagni C, et al: Enhanced tibial osteotomy healing with use of bone grafts supplemented with platelet gel or platelet gel and bone marrow stromal cells. *J Bone Joint Surg Am* 2007;89(11):2413-2420.

43. Calori GM, Tagliabue L, Gala L, d'Imporzano M, Peretti G, Albisetti W: Application of rhBMP-7 and

Chapter 3

Articular Cartilage and Intervertebral Disk

Alfred C. Kuo, MD, PhD   Tamara Alliston, PhD   Jeffrey Lotz, PhD

Introduction

Articular cartilage and the intervertebral disk are connective tissues that function in load transmission and motion. Extracellular matrix (ECM) accounts for most of the volume in both of these tissues and allows for their specialized functions. Proteoglycans and collagens are the major macromolecules in both cartilage and disk ECM. The glycosaminoglycan (GAG) side chains of proteoglycans carry a high negative charge density, which attracts cations and water and leads to hydrostatic tissue pressurization. These actions, in turn, support the compressive properties of cartilage and disk. Collagens form a fibrous network that encases the charged proteoglycans and contributes to tensile properties. In adults, cartilage and the nucleus pulposus of the disk lack a blood supply. Diffusion and convection (bulk fluid flow) account for the transport of nutrients and wastes. Because of these factors, as well as low cell density, both tissues have an extremely limited intrinsic healing response. Current and developing treatments of cartilage and disk disorders attempt to overcome these limitations.

Dr. Kuo or an immediate family member has received research or institutional support from the Musculoskeletal Transplant Foundation and StemRD. Dr. Alliston or an immediate family member serves as a board member, owner, officer, or committee member of the American Academy of Orthopaedic Surgeons and the Orthopaedic Research Society. Dr. Lotz or an immediate family member serves as a paid consultant to or is an employee of ISTO Technologies and Nocimed; serves as an unpaid consultant to Spinal Motion, Simperica Spinal Restoration, Relievant, and SMC Biotech; has stock or stock options held in ISTO Technologies, Spinal Motion, Relievant, Nocimed, Simperica Spinal Restoration, Orthofix, and Relievant; has received research or institutional support from Orthofix and Relievant; and has received nonincome support (such as equipment or services), commercially derived honoraria, or other non–research-related funding (such as paid travel) from ISTO Technologies.

Articular Cartilage

Structure/Composition/Function

Articular cartilage has a highly structured organization, with cellular characteristics and matrix composition varying throughout the depth of the tissue (Figure 1, A). From the joint surface to subchondral bone, cartilage is subdivided into the superficial zone, the intermediate (transitional) zone, the deep (radial) zone, and the calcified zone. The lamina splendens is a cell-free layer of matrix at the surface of the superficial zone. The superficial zone has the highest content of collagen and the lowest content of proteoglycan. Chondrocytes (cartilage cells) in this zone produce lubricin and have a flat shape, in contrast to round chondrocytes in the deeper zones. The superficial zone contains a population of cells with characteristics of progenitor cells; however, their role is unclear.[1] Collagen fibers in the superficial zone are aligned parallel to the joint surface and resist shear. Collagen content decreases and proteoglycan content increases from the superficial zone to the deep zone. Collagen fibers transition to an orientation perpendicular to the joint surface in the deep zone. The tidemark represents the junction between the deep zone and the zone of calcified cartilage. The zone of calcified cartilage contains high levels of type X collagen as well as a mineralized extracellular matrix. Calcified cartilage is permeable to small molecules; however, diffusion is diminished relative to uncalcified cartilage. Analysis of the three-dimensional structure of cartilage with electron microscopy shows that collagen is arranged not only as fibers but as layered, leaf-like structures that account for the fiber orientations discussed previously[2] (Figure 1, B).

Articular cartilage lines the ends of bones at synovial joints, functioning in load distribution and allowing almost frictionless movement. Chondrocytes comprise 10% or less of the volume of cartilage. Water makes up 60% to 80% of the wet weight of cartilage, with collagens comprising 10% to 30%, and proteoglycans comprising 5% to 15%. Type II collagen is the most abundant collagen in cartilage, which also contains smaller amounts of types VI, IX, X, and XI collagen. Aggrecan is the predominant proteoglycan in cartilage and contains large numbers of the negatively charged GAGs

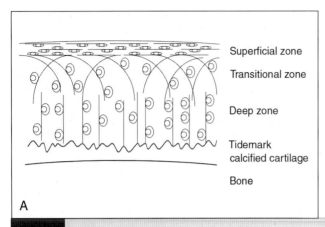

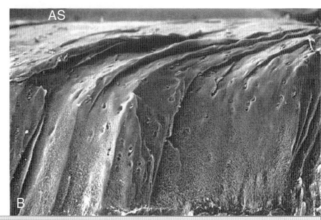

Figure 1 **A,** Articular cartilage cross-sectional architecture. The chondrocytes in the superficial zone are small and flattened; in the transitional and deep zones, they are rounded and reside in larger lacunae. **B,** Scanning electron microscopy image of bovine articular cartilage showing the arrangement of collagen leaflets. These leaflets are in a horizontal orientation at the articular surface (AS). (Panel A reproduced from Kim HT, Yoon ST, Jarrett C: Articular cartilage and intervertebral disk, in Fischgrund JS, ed: *Orthopaedic Knowledge Update*, ed 9. Rosemont, IL, American Academy of Orthopaedic Surgeons, 2008, pp 23-33. Panel B reproduced with permission from Jeffery AK, Blunn GW, Archer CW, Bentley G: Three-dimensional collagen architecture in bovine articular cartilage. *J Bone Joint Surg Br* 1991;73[5]:795-801.)

chondroitin and keratan sulfate. Most of the aggrecan is found in high-molecular-weight aggregates that also include hyaluronic acid and link protein. Additional proteoglycans include biglycan, decorin, fibromodulin, lumican, perlecan, and versican.

Although water, proteoglycans, and collagen contribute to cartilage's weight-bearing properties, several molecules contribute to cartilage lubrication. Lubricin/PRG4/superficial zone protein is a glycoprotein secreted by surface chondrocytes and synovial cells. Mutations in PRG4 lead to camptodactyly-arthropathy-coxa vara-pericarditis syndrome, an autosomal recessive condition that leads to early progressive arthropathy as well as perturbations of other organ systems. Hyaluronic acid and surface active phospholipids also reduce joint friction.

Metabolism/Nutrition/Homeostasis

In adults, cartilage has low metabolic activity. Cartilage matrix turnover is extremely slow: the half-life of collagen in normal cartilage is estimated to be more than 100 years,[3] whereas the half-life of aggrecan is estimated to be approximately 20 years.[4] Adult chondrocytes are sparsely distributed and undergo little or no cell division. Because cartilage lacks blood vessels, the transport of nutrients and wastes depends on diffusion and fluid flow through the tissue. Cartilage is hypoxic, and thus adenosine triphosphate (ATP) production occurs through glycolysis. Synovial fluid at the joint surface provides much of the nutrition for cartilage; however, transport can also occur across subchondral bone and calcified cartilage.

Given the low metabolic activity of cartilage, alterations in either matrix synthesis or degradation by chondrocytes can disrupt tissue function. Cartilage homeostasis—the maintenance of steady state—requires the careful calibration of cellular activity to physical and biochemical stimuli. Chondrocytes sense and respond to a diversity of cues: mechanical forces such as tension, compression, fluid flow, hydrostatic pressure, and shear stress; intrinsic physical cues such as ECM stiffness and topography; chemical cues such as oxygen tension and pH; and biochemical cues such as growth factors and inflammatory cytokines.[5] For example, compressive loads that mimic the frequency and the intensity of walking stimulate new cartilage matrix synthesis.[6] Cyclic compressive loads also contribute to fluid flow and therefore the transport of nutrients and waste through cartilage. Deformation of cartilage by compression leads to the migration of water from the tissue—akin to squeezing a sponge—whereas the release of load allows restoration of shape and return of water. Dynamic shear forces on articular cartilage, as might be encountered during joint movement and synovial fluid flow, increase the synthesis of lubricin.[7] In this way, the physical demands on cartilage are accommodated by a corresponding change in cellular activity.

Chondrocyte Integration of Physical and Biochemical Cues

Chondrocytes integrate cues from multiple sources to exert the appropriate response. This integration is critical in cartilage development as stem cells differentiate into chondrocytes, in mature cartilage as cells synthesize ECM, and in tissue engineering techniques to turn stem cells into cartilage. In cartilage development, mesenchymal cells condense into high-density aggregates that subsequently form cartilage in response to biochemical factors. Similarly, chondrogenesis (differentiation into cartilage) of mesenchymal stem cells (MSCs) is performed in high-density pellet cultures that mimic the mesenchymal condensations in cartilage development. The physical cues provided by pellet culture prime MSCs to more potently respond to differentiation factors, such as transforming factor-β (TGF-β). Furthermore, the TGF-β-mediated stimulation of chondrocyte differentiation is enhanced when cells are grown on materials that mimic the physical properties of articular cartilage.[8] This critical ability to integrate these diverse signals helps chondrocytes maintain homeostasis even within the challenging avascular, mechanically loaded tissue. Consequently, small changes in either the physical or the biochemical environment, as a result of the injury or genetic variation, can significantly affect chondrocyte homeostasis and cartilage integrity.

Although the mechanisms by which chondrocytes integrate these cues remain unclear, integrin signaling and primary cilia have been identified as critical components of this process. Integrins are cell surface proteins that bind ECM molecules such as type II and VI collagen.[9] This binding of ECM molecules can lead to intracellular signaling that can activate SOX9,[10] a transcription factor that is a key regulator of cartilage differentiation. Because SOX9 is regulated by many stimuli, it helps chondrocytes integrate cues from multiple sources. Chondrocytes also possess primary cilia, an organelle that acts as a cellular antenna. Cilia movement, in response to fluid flow, for example, couples physical stimuli to biochemical signaling cascades. Primary cilia are important for signaling that is induced by hedgehog, which is a molecule that plays key roles in cartilage development and has emerging roles in osteoarthritis.[11] Therefore, understanding the ability of primary cilia to couple physical and biochemical signaling in chondrocytes is clearly important for cartilage biology and disease.

Focal Chondral Injuries

Because of the lack of blood supply, cartilage has a limited capacity for self-repair. Despite the presence of progenitor-like cells, focal injuries that are confined to cartilage do not heal. In contrast, deeper injuries that extend into the subchondral plate allow reparative cells from the marrow cavity to migrate into damaged regions and generate fibrocartilaginous repair tissue. Surgical treatments of chondral injuries either directly introduce cells into injured areas or allow the migration of local reparative cells. Like full-thickness injuries, marrow stimulation techniques such as microfracture provide paths from the marrow cavity to chondral injuries. The advantages of marrow stimulation include low cost and ease, whereas a disadvantage is the formation of fibrocartilage, which may not match the longevity and the mechanical properties of native tissue. Autologous chondrocyte implantation (ACI) involves the direct surgical implantation of cartilage cells grown in tissue culture to sites of cartilage injury. ACI is limited by cost, the need for two procedures (harvest and subsequent implantation), technical difficulty, and frequent formation of fibrocartilage rather than hyaline cartilage. Osteochondral grafting fills osteochondral defects with cartilage and bone from an autologous or an allogeneic donor site. In contrast to other techniques, de-

fects are filled with native tissue with appropriate structure and mechanical properties. However, donor tissue availability is limited, and mismatches can exist in cartilage depth and contour between donor and recipient sites. These three categories of treatments all can lead to short-term clinical improvement, with defect and patient-specific factors affecting outcomes.[12]

Exciting new data suggest that the mobilization of endogenous stem cell populations may be a promising strategy for repairing articular cartilage defects. The administration of TGF-β3 to cartilage defects in rabbits was sufficient to fill critical-size lesions with repair tissue.[13] TGF-β3 is thought to act as a stem cell homing signal, inducing migration of this cell population to an injured site. Although the anabolic activity of the endogenous stem cell population declines with age, this discovery may be particularly valuable for younger individuals with sports injuries if the metabolically active stem cells can localize to the site and initiate repair of the cartilage injury. The source of the mobilizing stem cells is an area of intense investigation. Soft-tissue injuries about the knee, including chondral injuries, are discussed in detail in chapter 38, Soft-Tissue Injuries About the Knee, *Orthopaedic Knowledge Update 11*.

Osteoarthritis

Osteoarthritis (OA) is a degenerative process that affects all tissues of a joint. OA can be triggered by either genetic mutations or traumatic injury and mechanical factors. Whether the initiating events are the result of physical or biochemical factors, the progression of the disease is remarkably similar, ultimately leading to the loss of chondrocyte homeostasis and progressive articular cartilage degradation. Initially, osteoarthritic chondrocytes secrete high levels of key cartilage ECM constituents, including type II collagen and aggrecan, to compensate for the diminished ability of articular cartilage to withstand mechanical forces.[5] However, after this anabolic burst, matrix synthesis declines and osteoarthritic chondrocytes and synovial cells often secrete inflammatory cytokines, such as tumor necrosis factor-α (TNF-α) and interleukin-1β (IL-1β). This leads to the production of collagenases such as matrix metalloproteinase-13 (MMP-13) and aggrecanases such as a disintegrin and metalloproteinase thrombospondin motifs 4 (ADAMTS4) and ADAMTS5 that degrade ECM.[14] Between the reduced synthesis and the increased proteolysis of cartilage ECM, changes in the physical properties of cartilage ECM are among the earliest detectable signs of OA, which are apparent even in grade 1 lesions.[15] This matrix catabolism therefore impairs the ability of the tissue to support mechanical loads while corrupting key physical cues that help to maintain chondrocyte homeostasis. Collectively, these factors help explain the progressive nature of OA with the ongoing loss of cellular homeostasis and matrix degradation.

Some human mutations implicated in OA directly compromise the quality or the quantity of cartilage matrix synthesis. Others interfere with the ability of chon-

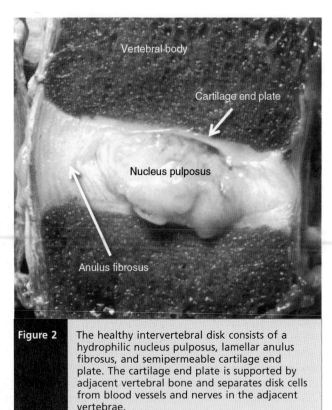

Figure 2 The healthy intervertebral disk consists of a hydrophilic nucleus pulposus, lamellar anulus fibrosus, and semipermeable cartilage end plate. The cartilage end plate is supported by adjacent vertebral bone and separates disk cells from blood vessels and nerves in the adjacent vertebrae.

drocytes to integrate their response to diverse physical and biochemical stimuli to maintain cartilage homeostasis, such as mutations in SMAD3—a key effector of TGF-β signaling.[16] Although several mutations that predispose individuals to OA have been identified, these do not account for most OA cases. Most likely, a predisposition for OA results from multiple factors that are not yet defined.

Factors such as traumatic injury or the increased mechanical loading of joints caused by obesity also reflect the complex interplay between physical and biochemical factors. Even in obesity, the increased mechanical loading on joints is unable to account for the increased risk of developing OA. Chondrocytes are also affected by changes in energy metabolism associated with obesity and by the increased levels of adipose-derived cytokines (adipokines), which are contributors to inflammation.[17]

Therapies Under Development

With more than 21 million Americans having OA, the demand for therapies to prevent or reverse cartilage degeneration is increasing.[18] Although many agents show promise in animal models, no therapy currently in clinical use modifies the natural history of the disease. Strategies that target individual aspects of the complex pathophysiology of OA are under development.[19] For example, intra-articular injection of recombinant lubricin may decrease friction and disease progression in osteoarthritic joints.[20] As indicated, OA involves disrupted cartilage homeostasis with increased catabolism and decreased anabolism. Bone morphogenetic protein-7 (BMP-7) is an anabolic growth factor that stimulates chondrocytes to synthesize aggrecan, collagen, and hyaluronic acid. BMP-7 has been well tolerated with a trend toward superior efficacy to placebo in patients with knee OA in a phase I trial.[21] Inhibition of catabolic cytokines is also being evaluated. For example, diacerein, recombinant IL-1 receptor antagonist (IL-1Ra), and autologous blood products are intended to decrease the activity of IL-1. However, clinical trials of these agents have not yet conclusively demonstrated clinical efficacy.[22-24]

Arthritis, including the use of platelet-rich plasma as a therapy, is further discussed in chapter 18, Arthritis and Other Cartilage Disorders, *Orthopaedic Knowledge Update 11*.

Intervertebral Disk

Structure/Composition/Function

Loads on the spine are shared between the intervertebral disk anteriorly and the two facet joints posteriorly. The intervertebral disk is a pliant, heterogeneous structure that separates spinal vertebrae. The disk functions to work synergistically with the facets and the interspinous ligaments to support spinal loads and constrain multiaxial flexibility. Disk/facet interactions vary between different spinal regions as a result of changes in facet orientation and biomechanical forces: from high rotation and low compression in the cervical spine to low rotation and high compression in the lumbar spine.

The healthy disk is composed of three distinct tissues: the nucleus pulposus, the anulus fibrosus, and the vertebral end plate (**Figure 2**). The nucleus pulposus consists largely of aggrecan, other proteoglycans, and small amounts of type II collagen. GAG side chains are negatively charged, bind mobile ions (mostly sodium), and thereby generate an osmotic pressure that attracts water, which makes up approximately 80% of the disk nucleus by volume. The nucleus is supported laterally by the anulus fibrosus, which is composed of approximately 50 layered, type I collagen sheets. The outer anulus layers have collagen fibers that are anchored via Sharpey fibers to the adjacent vertebral rims. Toward the inner portions of the anulus fibrosus, the fibers coalesce with the hyaline cartilage end plate.

The disk end plate is a sandwich composite of cartilage and bone. The cartilage end plate separates the nucleus pulposus from the adjacent vertebral bodies and is composed mostly of type II and type IX collagen. It has a low permeability and serves three principal functions: (1) to work with the inner anulus fibrosus to constrain nuclear swelling; (2) to act as a semipermeable membrane to control transport across the disk/vertebra boundary; and (3) to shield the subchondral bone from tensile loading that can cause end plate cracks.

The disk's overall biomechanical properties are determined by the combined actions of nuclear swelling and, in reaction, annular fiber tension. Together, these actions support axial compression and provide resistance to spine bending, torsion, and shear. Because the end plate is semipermeable, water moves out of the disk when spinal stress exceeds its swelling pressure, and vice versa. This time-dependent behavior leads to diurnal variations in disk water content, disk height, and spinal flexibility.

Development

During development, the intervertebral disks are formed at repeated, perinotochordal condensations of mesenchyme that are separated by the early cartilage of developing vertebrae. At birth, the nucleus pulposus contains notochordal cells that are remnants of this spinal development. In humans, notochordal cells are gradually replaced over the first two decades of life by chondrocyte-like cells. This loss of notochordal cells may be the result of a combination of increased pressure from gravity loading, plus decreases in nutrition secondary to changes in adjacent vertebral perfusion. Adult nucleus pulposus chondrocytes arise from either the cartilage end plate or the inner anulus fibrosus. Nucleus pulposus cells are considered analogous to articular chondrocytes because they express typical chondrocyte markers such as SOX9 (a master transcription factor for cartilage), aggrecan, and type II collagen. However, there are clear morphologic differences, and recently several genes unique to nucleus pulposus cells have been identified.[25]

Anulus fibrosus cells secrete several matrix proteins, including types I, II, III, and VI collagen. Outer anulus fibrosus cells do not express chondrogenic markers, whereas those in the transition zone express SOX9. Under certain circumstances, these inner anulus fibrosus cells can take on a chondrocyte phenotype and reversibly express aggrecan and type II collagen.

Metabolism/Nutrition/Homeostasis

Disk cells rely on diffusion from vertebral capillaries for the transport of nutrients and wastes. Competition for nutrients limits cell density to approximately 1,600 cells/mm^3. Because the disk tissue oxygen levels are low (0.5% to 5%), disk cells create energy via glycolysis, which uses glucose and generates lactic acid. Accumulation of lactic acid decreases disk pH to almost 6.3 and is detrimental to matrix because it decreases GAG production and cell viability. The dependence on anaerobic glycolysis for cell production of ATP makes glucose a critical nutrient. Other factors in serum are also important because serum deprivation results in decreased cell proliferation and increased cell senescence.[26]

In addition to nutrient availability and the accumulation of metabolic waste products, disk cell function is influenced by spinal load and consequent matrix deformations. Nucleus pulposus cells can rapidly detect and respond to fluctuations in hydrostatic pressure. Similarly, annular cells are exquisitely sensitive to stretch. Matrix loading also indirectly stimulates cells by compacting matrix, which decreases tissue permeability, water content, oxygen tension, and pH. These changes alter proteoglycan and collagen synthesis via changes in cell volume and the cytoskeleton. Time-dependent disk biomechanics and frequency-dependent cell responsiveness may underlie the U-shaped relationship between physical exposure and back pain, where both low and high exposures are observed to be detrimental.[27]

Degeneration

Disk degeneration is a normal, age-related process that begins in the second decade of life coincident with the disappearance of nucleus pulposus notochordal cells. Degeneration typically progresses at 3% to 4% per year, being fastest at the lowest level, L5/S1, where biomechanical demands are the greatest. Degeneration of at least one level is apparent in approximately 35% of individuals younger than 40 years and in almost all individuals older than 60 years.

Several factors may accelerate the rate or the severity of degeneration and include excessive mechanical load, smoking, and high body mass index. Studies of identical twins show that heritable factors explain most individual variability in disk degeneration (45% to 70%) versus more traditional risk factors such as occupational loading (2% to 7%).[28] Clarification of the mechanistic basis for genetic factors that implicate irregularities in ECM, inflammation, and pain signaling is in the early stages.[29]

The earliest and most conspicuous feature of disk degeneration is the loss of nuclear water as a result of reductions in the osmotic pressure of the nucleus pulposus. Because the disk is part of an integrated biomechanical system, the inability of the nucleus pulposus to attract sufficient water triggers a cascade of effects both intrinsic and extrinsic to the disk. Nuclear dehydration causes reductions of disk height, stress shielding of the inner anulus fibrosus, redistribution of vertebral end plate stress, motion segment hypermobility, and facet overloading. Over time, the nucleus pulposus and the inner anulus fibrosus become indistinct as the nucleus pulposus becomes fibrotic while the annular lamellae denature. Annular weakening leads to internal disk disruption that includes radial and circumferential fissures plus end plate cartilage disruptions. As the disk continues to deteriorate, progressive height loss and hypermobility can cause facet arthritis and spinal ligament hypertrophy. Ultimately, dehydration, tissue crosslinking, and disk height loss lead to stiffening and restabilization.

Fundamentally, degeneration happens because the rate of matrix damage exceeds the disk cell's ability to repair. Disk mechanical loading can damage the matrix and trigger a wound-healing response analogous to that reported for other tissues. Trauma can activate the release and the formation of prostaglandins, leukotrienes, and chemokines (for example, monocyte chemoattractant protein-1) that regulate early events. These chemoattractants recruit polymorphonuclear cells that migrate from postcapillary venules. Upregulation of proinflammatory cytokines, such as IL-1, IL-6, IL-8, and TNF-α, influence subsequent cell proliferation, chemotaxis, and connective tissue formation. These cytokines also induce matrix remodeling (or degeneration in the case of the disk) by triggering the production of enzymes such as MMP-2, MMP-9, and MMP-13.

Nuclear cells progressively lose their capacity to secrete aggrecan and collagen and begin to produce matrix-degrading enzymes and cytokines, ultimately becoming senescent and apoptotic. The root of these problems may be poor disk perfusion as the vertebral capillary network deteriorates with age. Deficient end plate perfusion not only limits disk cell nutrition but also causes the accumulation of degraded matrix fragments that interact with cells to trigger further catabolic behaviors. Paradoxically, there is no decrease in disk cell density with degeneration, which may be the result of shortened diffusion distances accompanying losses in disk height.[30]

The diagnosis and treatment of disk herniations are further discussed in chapter 51, Lumbar and Thoracic Disk Herniations, *Orthopaedic Knowledge Update, 11.*

Summary

Articular cartilage and intervertebral disk play crucial structural and functional roles in the musculoskeletal system. These tissues are composed chiefly of ECM, have a very low cell content, and have little or no blood supply. Because of these factors, cartilage and disk injuries and degeneration have limited ability to heal. Many approaches to improve healing are under development, including the use of cell-based therapies and anti-inflammatory treatments.

Key Study Points

- Articular cartilage and intervertebral disk have low rates of metabolism and low healing rates.
- Tissue degeneration occurs when the rate of matrix damage exceeds the rate of tissue repair.
- No current therapies reliably slow or prevent cartilage and disk degeneration.

Annotated References

1. Hattori S, Oxford C, Reddi AH: Identification of superficial zone articular chondrocyte stem/progenitor cells. *Biochem Biophys Res Commun* 2007;358(1):99-103.

2. Jeffery AK, Blunn GW, Archer CW, Bentley G: Three-dimensional collagen architecture in bovine articular cartilage. *J Bone Joint Surg Br* 1991;73(5):795-801.

3. Verzijl N, DeGroot J, Thorpe SR, et al: Effect of collagen turnover on the accumulation of advanced glycation end products. *J Biol Chem* 2000;275(50):39027-39031.

4. Verzijl N, DeGroot J, Bank RA, et al: Age-related accumulation of the advanced glycation endproduct pentosidine in human articular cartilage aggrecan: The use of pentosidine levels as a quantitative measure of protein turnover. *Matrix Biol* 2001;20(7):409-417.

5. Goldring MB, Marcu KB: Cartilage homeostasis in health and rheumatic diseases. *Arthritis Res Ther* 2009;11(3):224.

6. Guilak F, Fermor B, Keefe FJ, et al: The role of biomechanics and inflammation in cartilage injury and repair. *Clin Orthop Relat Res* 2004;423:17-26.

7. Nugent GE, Aneloski NM, Schmidt TA, Schumacher BL, Voegtline MS, Sah RL: Dynamic shear stimulation of bovine cartilage biosynthesis of proteoglycan 4. *Arthritis Rheum* 2006;54(6):1888-1896.

8. Allen JL, Cooke ME, Alliston T: ECM stiffness primes the TGFβ pathway to promote chondrocyte differentiation. *Mol Biol Cell* 2012;23(18):3731-3742.

   Chondrocytes grown on a substrate with the stiffness of articular cartilage produce more proteoglycan and exhibit more cartilage-specific gene expression than cells grown on other substrates. The combination of optimal stiffness and TGF-β further enhances cartilage gene expression.

9. Loeser RF: Chondrocyte integrin expression and function. *Biorheology* 2000;37(1-2):109-116.

10. Haudenschild DR, Chen J, Pang N, Lotz MK, D'Lima DD: Rho kinase-dependent activation of SOX9 in chondrocytes. *Arthritis Rheum* 2010;62(1):191-200.

    The authors studied Rho kinase activity and interactions related to increased cartilage matrix production via activation of SOX9.

11. Chang CF, Ramaswamy G, Serra R: Depletion of primary cilia in articular chondrocytes results in reduced Gli3 repressor to activator ratio, increased Hedgehog signaling, and symptoms of early osteoarthritis. *Osteoarthritis Cartilage* 2012;20(2):152-161.

    The effects of the loss of primary cilia on articular cartilage are discussed.

12. Harris JD, Siston RA, Pan X, Flanigan DC: Autologous chondrocyte implantation: A systematic review. *J Bone Joint Surg Am* 2010;92(12):2220-2233.

    The authors evaluated level I and II studies comparing ACI with cartilage repair or restoration methods. Level of evidence: I.

13. Lee CH, Cook JL, Mendelson A, Moioli EK, Yao H, Mao JJ: Regeneration of the articular surface of the rabbit synovial joint by cell homing: A proof of concept study. *Lancet* 2010;376(9739):440-448.

Replacement of the articular surface of rabbit humeral heads with bioscaffolds that contained TGF-β3 but no cells led to coverage with hyaline cartilage. These results suggest that targeted homing of endogenous cells can stimulate tissue regeneration.

14. Goldring MB, Otero M: Inflammation in osteoarthritis. *Curr Opin Rheumatol* 2011;23(5):471-478.

    This review article discusses novel stress-induced and proinflammatory mechanisms underlying the pathogenesis of OA.

15. Kleemann RU, Krocker D, Cedraro A, Tuischer J, Duda GN: Altered cartilage mechanics and histology in knee osteoarthritis: Relation to clinical assessment (ICRS Grade). *Osteoarthritis Cartilage* 2005;13(11):958-963.

16. van de Laar IM, Oldenburg RA, Pals G, et al: Mutations in SMAD3 cause a syndromic form of aortic aneurysms and dissections with early-onset osteoarthritis. *Nat Genet* 2011;43(2):121-126.

    Mutations in SMAD3, a key molecule in TGF-β signaling, are responsible for a connective tissue syndrome associated with early-onset OA as well as aortic aneurysms and dissections.

17. McNulty AL, Miller MR, O'Connor SK, Guilak F: The effects of adipokines on cartilage and meniscus catabolism. *Connect Tissue Res* 2011;52(6):523-533.

    The authors discuss the role of adipokines in increasing catabolism and the production of proinflammatory mediators in cartilage and meniscus.

18. Lawrence RC, Felson DT, Helmick CG, et al: Estimates of the prevalence of arthritis and other rheumatic conditions in the United States: Part II. *Arthritis Rheum* 2008;58(1):26-35.

19. Singh JA: Stem cells and other innovative intra-articular therapies for osteoarthritis: What does the future hold? *BMC Med* 2012;10:44.

    A review of promising but unproven therapies for osteoarthritis, including bone marrow stem cells, IL-1 receptor antagonists, BMP-7, and botulinum toxin, is presented.

20. Bao JP, Chen WP, Wu LD: Lubricin: A novel potential biotherapeutic approaches for the treatment of osteoarthritis. *Mol Biol Rep* 2011;38(5):2879-2885.

    A review describing the function of lubricin, animal studies of lubricin as a treatment of OA, and the possible role of lubricin as a therapy for human OA is presented.

21. Hunter DJ, Pike MC, Jonas BL, Kissin E, Krop J, McAlindon T: Phase 1 safety and tolerability study of BMP-7 in symptomatic knee osteoarthritis. *BMC Musculoskelet Disord* 2010;11:232.

    The authors describe a phase I, double-blind, randomized, multicenter, placebo-controlled trial of intra-articular BMP-7 for knee OA, which showed no dose-limiting toxicity and a trend toward more symptom relief than placebo. Level of evidence: I.

22. Bartels EM, Bliddal H, Schøndorff PK, Altman RD, Zhang W, Christensen R: Symptomatic efficacy and safety of diacerein in the treatment of osteoarthritis: A meta-analysis of randomized placebo-controlled trials. *Osteoarthritis Cartilage* 2010;18(3):289-296.

    The authors studied diacerein as an alternative treatment for OA; its symptomatic benefit after 6 months is unknown. Level of evidence: I.

23. Chevalier X, Goupille P, Beaulieu AD, et al: Intraarticular injection of anakinra in osteoarthritis of the knee: A multicenter, randomized, double-blind, placebo-controlled study. *Arthritis Rheum* 2009;61(3):344-352.

24. Yang KG, Raijmakers NJ, van Arkel ER, et al: Autologous interleukin-1 receptor antagonist improves function and symptoms in osteoarthritis when compared to placebo in a prospective randomized controlled trial. *Osteoarthritis Cartilage* 2008;16(4):498-505.

25. Minogue BM, Richardson SM, Zeef LA, Freemont AJ, Hoyland JA: Characterization of the human nucleus pulposus cell phenotype and evaluation of novel marker gene expression to define adult stem cell differentiation. *Arthritis Rheum* 2010;62(12):3695-3705.

    The authors discuss gene expression profiling to identify the human nucleus pulposus cell phenotype.

26. Johnson WE, Stephan S, Roberts S: The influence of serum, glucose and oxygen on intervertebral disc cell growth in vitro: Implications for degenerative disc disease. *Arthritis Res Ther* 2008;10(2):R46.

27. Heneweer H, Vanhees L, Picavet HS: Physical activity and low back pain: A U-shaped relation? *Pain* 2009;143(1-2):21-25.

28. Battié MC, Videman T, Gibbons LE, Fisher LD, Manninen H, Gill K: 1995 Volvo Award in clinical sciences: Determinants of lumbar disc degeneration. A study relating lifetime exposures and magnetic resonance imaging findings in identical twins. *Spine (Phila Pa 1976)* 1995;20(24):2601-2612.

29. Tegeder I, Lötsch J: Current evidence for a modulation of low back pain by human genetic variants. *J Cell Mol Med* 2009;13(8B):1605-1619.

30. Liebscher T, Haefeli M, Wuertz K, Nerlich AG, Boos N: Age-related variation in cell density of human lumbar intervertebral disc. *Spine (Phila Pa 1976)* 2011;36(2):153-159.

    The authors studied changes in cell density in defined regions of interest in complete human motion segments.

Chapter 4

Muscle, Tendon, and Ligament

Richard L. Lieber, PhD   Cyril B. Frank, MD

Skeletal Muscle

Functional Anatomy

Surgeons should be cognizant of the fact that a fundamental property of skeletal muscle is that the amount of force it generates depends on its length. This is because muscles are composed of sarcomeres, so-called molecular machines that are themselves length sensitive. Sarcomeres are composed of contractile filaments termed myofilaments. Two major sets of contractile filaments (one relatively thick, the other relatively thin) exist in the sarcomere. These thick and thin filaments represent large polymers of the proteins myosin and actin, respectively. The myosin-containing filaments and the actin-containing filaments interdigitate to form the muscle contractile machine. It is also this interdigitated pattern that gives muscle its familiar striated or striped appearance and is observable under a light microscope (Figure 1).

Sarcomere Properties

Various sarcomere regions are named based on their appearance so that they can be easily referenced (Figure 1). For example, the sarcomere region containing the myosin filaments is known as the A-band (for anisotropic, an optical term describing what this band does to incoming light). The region containing the actin filament is known as the I-band (for isotropic). The region of the A-band in which there is no actin-myosin overlap is called the H-zone (for *heller*, which is German for "light"). The dark narrow line that bisects the I-band is the Z-band (for *zwischen*, which is German for "between"). Most investigators who quantify sarcomere dimensions use the distance from one Z-band to the next as the definition of sarcomere length, which

is one of the most important variables for understanding muscle force generation. A device has been developed to measure sarcomere length in human muscles during orthopaedic surgery procedures.[1]

Muscle force generated is highly dependent on sarcomere length. The rigorous demonstration of this fact was provided at the level of the single muscle cell in a classic study.[2] In this relationship, skeletal muscle fiber force production is defined in terms of myofilament overlap, that is, in terms of sarcomere length (Figure 2). At optimal length, where actin-myosin interactions are maximal, muscle generates maximum force (region 2 in Figure 2). As sarcomere length increases (region 3 in Figure 2), force decreases because of the decreasing number of interactions between actin and myosin myofilaments. At lengths shorter than the optimum length (region 1 in Figure 2), force decreases because of double interdigitation of actin filaments with both myosin and actin filaments from opposite sides of the sarcomere. Additional information about sarcomere length changes in wrist muscles and back muscles and

Dr. Lieber or an immediate family member serves as a paid consultant to or is an employee of Allergan, Halozyme, and Mainstay Medical; has received research or institutional support from Allergan; and has received nonincome support (such as equipment or services), commercially derived honoraria, or other non–research-related funding (such as paid travel) from Allergan. Dr. Frank or an immediate family member has received research or institutional support from Pfizer and serves as a board member, owner, officer, or committee member of the Canadian Orthopaedic Association.

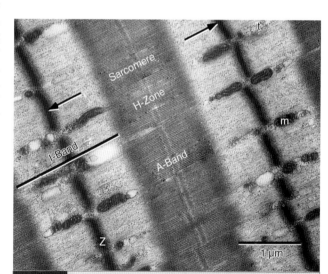

Figure 1	Longitudinal electron micrograph of a human vastus lateralis muscle that was fixed in glutaraldehyde, embedded in plastic, sectioned at approximately 60-nm thickness, and stained with heavy metal. This severe processing is necessary to view the tissue with an electron microscope. The calibration bar corresponds to a distance of 1 µm. m = mitochondrion, Z = Z-band, and t = transverse tubular system.

1: Principles of Orthopaedics

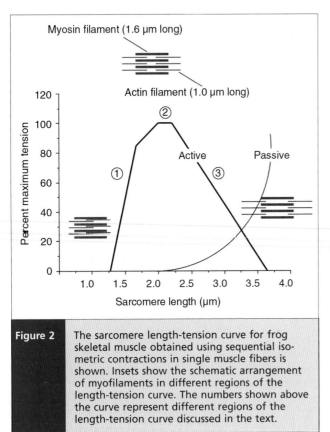

Myosin filament (1.6 μm long)

Actin filament (1.0 μm long)

Figure 2 The sarcomere length-tension curve for frog skeletal muscle obtained using sequential isometric contractions in single muscle fibers is shown. Insets show the schematic arrangement of myofilaments in different regions of the length-tension curve. The numbers shown above the curve represent different regions of the length-tension curve discussed in the text.

their functional significance is available.[3,4] The length-tension relationships of muscles are beginning to be measured intraoperatively[5] based on classic experiments.[6]

The total number of sarcomeres within a fiber depends on the muscle fiber length and diameter and is the most important determinant of muscle fiber function. Because of the series arrangement of sarcomeres within a myofibril, the total distance of myofibrillar shortening is equal to the sum of the shortening distances of individual sarcomeres. This is why an entire muscle may shorten several centimeters even though each sarcomere can shorten only about 1 μm. It should also be stated that the number of sarcomeres in a mature muscle can change given the appropriate stimulus. This means that muscle fibers have a great capacity to adapt after surgery, a finding that has been demonstrated in human muscle undergoing lengthening.[7]

Architecture

Skeletal muscle function is based on what is known as its fiber architecture. Architecture, or the orientation and the number of muscle fibers within a muscle, determines that muscle's force and excursion—not its mass or volume.[8] This is critical because most surgeons' impressions of muscles are based on intraoperative appearance, anatomic dissection, or view on MRI, all of which are dominated by size or volume. Rigorous experimental studies have since demonstrated that muscle function depends on the number and the orientation of muscle fibers, not on the size or the shape of the mus-

cle,[9,10] and thus the only way to accurately define muscle architecture is through direct anatomic microdissection.[11]

Although variability in muscle architecture exists among muscles within an individual, there is extremely consistent architectural design within muscles among individuals. Muscle architecture types are referred to by their arrangement of muscle fibers relative to the axis of force generation. Muscles with fibers that extend parallel to the muscle force-generating axis and extend most of the muscle length are termed parallel or longitudinally arranged muscles. Muscles with fibers that are oriented at a single angle relative to the force-generating axis are termed pennate muscles. (The angle between the fiber and the force-generating axis generally varies from 0° to 30°.) It is obvious when viewing actual human muscles that most muscles fall into the final and most general category, multipennate muscles—muscles composed of fibers that are oriented at several angles relative to the axis of force generation.

In terms of function, the sarcomere length-tension curve described previously can simply be scaled to the whole muscle once muscle fiber length and overall muscle architecture are known.[10] For example, the length-tension curve gets wider with increasing fiber length. The explanation for the relationship between muscle fiber length and excursion is based on the concept that a greater serial sarcomere number (greater fiber length) leads directly to a greater muscle excursion because the excursions of the individual sarcomeres in series are additive.

In terms of force production, a muscle's maximum force generated is based on the total number of muscle fibers within the muscle. Unfortunately, it is very difficult to quantify either muscle fiber number or the precise fiber arrangement within a muscle and therefore predict peak force. As a result, the total cross-sectional area of the muscle fibers is approximated mathematically, by physiologic cross-sectional area (PCSA). One excellent study performed in guinea pig hindlimb muscles[9] showed that PCSA is proportional to isometric force capacity, with a conversion factor of 22.5 N/cm² (approximately 250 kPa). Thus, it is possible to estimate the maximum isometric force a muscle can generate by multiplying its PCSA by 22.5 N/cm². This value can be used to predict force generation by a muscle after orthopaedic surgery.

Examples of Human Arm Architecture

The architectural properties of 25 upper extremity muscles have been defined and their fiber length and PCSA are plotted[12] in Figure 3. Upper extremity muscles possess a wide range of strengths and excursions that can be exploited to restore function. For example, in the forearm, the longest and largest muscles are the flexor digitorum profundus to the middle finger, (FDP M mass = 16.3 g, length = 200 mm) and the brachioradialis (BR mass = 16.6 g, length = 175 mm). The BR also contains the longest fibers (121 mm) and the highest relative fiber length (as quantified by the fiber

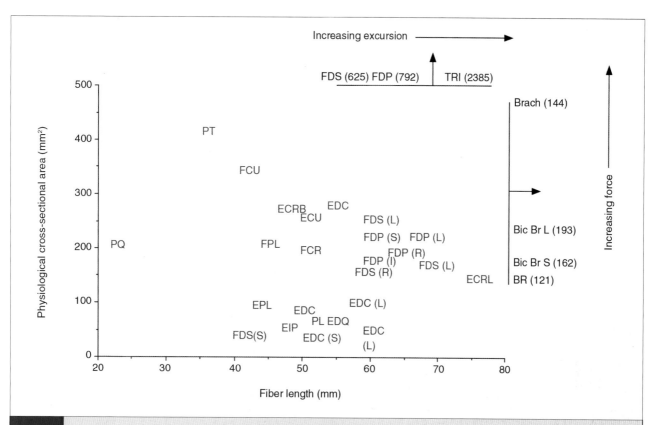

Figure 3 Scattergraph of the fiber length and physiologic cross-sectional areas of muscles in the human arm. Fiber length is proportional to muscle excursion, whereas physiologic cross-sectional area is proportional to maximum muscle force. Thus, this graph can be used to compare the relative forces and excursions of arm and forearm muscles. Muscles placed at extremes of the graph (FDS, FDP, TRI, BRACH, BR, and Bic Br) would be plotted off this scale at the position shown. BIC Br L = biceps brachii, long head; Bic Br S = biceps brachii, short head; BR = brachioradialis; ECRB = extensor carpi radialis brevis; ECRL = extensor carpi radialis longus; ECU = extensor carpi ulnaris; EDC = extensor digitorum communis; EDQ = extensor digiti quinti; FCU = flexor carpi ulnaris; FDP = flexor digitorum pollicis; FDS = flexor digitorum superficialis; I = index; L = long; PL = pronator longus; PQ = pronator quadratus; PT = pronator teres; R = ring; S = short. (Data from Lieber RL, Fazeli BM, Botte MJ: Architecture of selected wrist flexor and extensor muscles. *J Hand Surg Am* 1990;15A:244-250; and Lieber RL, Jacobson MD, Fazeli BM, Abrams RA, Botte MJ: Architecture of selected muscles of the arm and forearm: Anatomy and implications for tendon transfer. *J Hand Surg Am* 1992;17A:787-798.)

length/muscle length ratio—0.69). Even though the BR has the greatest mass in the forearm, it is not the strongest; the pronator teres (PT) has the greatest PCSA, which is more than three times that of the BR (4.1 versus 1.3 cm², Figure 3) and thus would generate more force. These types of comparisons highlight the dominance of architecture over raw muscle mass. If force generation were based on mass alone, the BR would be much stronger than the PT. An understanding of muscle architecture can be useful when selecting skeletal muscles for surgical tendon transfer. The idea here is that muscles of similar architecture will have similar functions. Thus, when choosing a particular donor muscle to substitute function, architectural properties should be matched.[13] A specific example is shown graphically in Figure 3, in the surgical restoration of digital extension following high radial nerve palsy, where potential donor muscles (which are transferred to the extensor digitorum communis [EDC]) include the flexor carpi radialis (FCR), the flexor carpi ulnaris

(FCU), the flexor digitorum superficialis (FDS) to the middle finger, and the FDS to the ring finger. From the standpoint of architecture alone, the FDS M most closely resembles the EDC in terms of force generation (cross sectional area) and excursion (fiber length) and would be the preferred donor.

Examples of Human Leg Architecture

Leg muscles also demonstrate unique architectural properties. For example, in the entire lower extremity, the three strongest muscles (based on PCSA) are the soleus, the vastus lateralis, and the gluteus medius. This is not surprising because they are all antigravity muscles, but it may be surprising that the single strongest muscle is observed distally in the leg where muscle volumes tend to be smallest. The muscles with the longest fiber lengths (implying the greatest excursion) are the sartorius, the gracilis, and the semitendinosus. Although they all cross the hip and the knee, the feature they share in common is knee flexion. The semitendinosus ranks high in fiber length only when the proximal and distal heads of the muscle are added in series, which is likely to reflect the actual function of the muscle based on its dual innervation.[14] In terms of fundamental design features, large mass and short fiber length both contribute to large PCSA when the lower extremity is considered as a whole. For example, the soleus has modest mass but very short fibers, which result in its exceptionally large PCSA. This is in contrast to the vastus lateralis, which has a much larger mass but modest fiber length. These types of comparisons are critical for surgeons to be able to make because the proper choice of muscles to be used in transfers, the length of muscles set during surgical procedures, and the prediction of muscle function after the insertion of prostheses all rely heavily on an understanding of architectural properties.

Fiber Types

The current view of muscle fiber types is that skeletal muscle fibers possess a wide and nearly continuous spectrum of morphologic, contractile, and metabolic properties. The appropriate view of any classification scheme, therefore, is that it is an artificial system superimposed on a continuum for convenience. Most modern muscle fiber classification schemes are based on some type of measurement of the myosin molecule. It is important to note that, in terms of functional importance, an understanding of muscle architecture, especially for the orthopaedic surgeon, is much more important than knowledge of the muscle fiber types.

Mammalian Fiber Types Are Based on Myosin Heavy Chain Isoforms

Using modern immunohistochemical methodology, a collection of antibodies was created that demonstrated selective reactivity between fiber types, and the pattern of reactivity was correlated with the traditional fiber typing scheme.[15,16] The result of these studies was to generate a set of monoclonal antibodies that could identify four major fiber types in adult rat skeletal muscle tissue. Of these four fiber types, one was clearly a slow fiber type, and three fiber types corresponded to fast isoforms. The slow fiber type is termed type 1, and the three fast fiber types are types 2A, 2X, and 2B. It is now known that these fast fibers vary slightly in speed and power in the order 2A < 2X < 2B.[17]

Like all mammals, humans have four myosin heavy chain (MyHC) genes in their genome: type 1, type 2A, type 2X, and type 2B.[18,19] However, despite the presence of these four MyHC genes, humans do not express the type 2B MyHC gene.[20] This appears to be an issue of scaling with size. For example, very small mammals have a relatively fast stride frequency, and analysis of their muscles reveals a high percentage of type 2B muscle fibers, even in what would be considered slow muscles such as the soleus.[21,22]

Functional Differences Among Fiber Types

The force-velocity relationship provides a convenient tool for muscle fiber type-specific characterization of speed. The muscle's maximum contraction velocity is termed V_{max} and can be compared among muscles that have large differences in fiber type distribution. This provides a fiber type-specific value for V_{max}. It is possible to perform contractile experiments on pieces of rat muscle fibers. Using this approach, one study has shown that V_{max} was found to be in the order type 2B > type 2X > type 2A > type 1.[17] The situation was actually even more interesting because the study demonstrated that even in a single cell, multiple MyHC isoforms can be expressed along the fiber's length.

In a manner similar to that used for measuring V_{max}, maximum tetanic tension (P_o) can be measured in muscles of different fiber type distributions. This value is then normalized to the PCSA of the muscle studied to yield the value known as specific tension, or the force of contraction per unit of cross-sectional area of muscle. In measuring the specific tension of whole skeletal muscle, most investigators find that muscles composed mainly of fast fibers have a greater specific tension than muscles composed mainly of slow fibers. The typical value for specific tension of fast muscle is approximately 22 N/cm² (250 kPa), whereas that for slow muscle is 10-15 N/cm² (125 kPa). The common interpretation of these whole-muscle experiments has been that fast muscle fibers have a greater specific tension than slow muscle fibers.

The endurance (or its opposite, fatigue) of muscle fibers is even more difficult to precisely define than speed or strength. This is because endurance depends on the type of work the muscle is required to perform. Because force generation involves a chain of events, it is possible to produce fatigue by interrupting any point in the chain. Thus, a danger exists in simply ascribing a drop in force to muscle fiber fatigue without understanding the basis for the drop.[23] Generally, type 1 fibers have the greatest endurance, followed by type 2A and type 2X fibers, and then type 2B fibers. This is not surprising because type 2B fibers have a very low oxidative capacity.

Passive Biomechanical Properties

The previous functional discussion refers to a muscle's active mechanical properties, but because muscles are soft tissues as are tendons and ligaments, they also have a passive stress-strain relationship—that is, a relationship obtained when the muscle is relaxed but passively stretched. This passive relationship is probably the single most common mechanical property that surgeons experience in the operating room.

In contrast to the active contractile properties of muscle that were described previously as being predicted accurately by sarcomere length, passive muscle tension is poorly understood. Increasing muscle length increases its passive tension (passive in Figure 2), but there is not a clear relationship between passive tension and active muscle force produced.[10] This idea has been discussed extensively with respect to hand surgery.[24,25] Experimental studies demonstrate that intracellular cytoskeletal proteins[26] in combination with extracellular matrix (ECM) material[27,28] combine to create a muscle's passive properties. Near optimal muscle length (the length at which active tension is maximum), passive tension is almost zero. However, as a muscle is stretched to longer lengths, passive tension increases dramatically (Figure 2).

Regeneration

Unlike tendons and ligaments, skeletal muscle as a tissue has a tremendous ability to regenerate. This is mostly because skeletal muscles have resident stem cells within the tissue known as satellite cells, so named because they were first identified at the fiber periphery more than 50 years ago—the only stem cell to be identified based on anatomic location.[29] Although satellite cells are normally quiescent, when the muscle cell is injured and the natural inhibitory influence of the basal lamina released, they enter the cell cycle, proliferate, and can repair injured muscle or create new muscle. It is thus no wonder that muscle satellite cells are widely used therapeutically in attempts to replace defective muscle[30] or even deliver specific factors to sick muscle.[31] This is a fantastic area of study, which promises both therapeutic and scientific insights.

Tendons

In simple terms, tendons form the anatomic connections between muscles and bones. All tendons are connected to muscles at one end, and these fusion points are referred to as myotendinous junctions. The connection point between the other end of the tendon and the bone is called an osteotendinous junction or what is better known clinically as the tendon insertion site. Tendons vary in breadth and length from very small diameters and very long to very large diameters and very short. Their shapes are also surprisingly diverse and range from flat to cylindrical, fan shaped, or ribbon shaped. Tendons' lack of vasculature and their composition creates a relatively dense white coloration.

Functional Anatomy

Tendons belong to a family of dense connective tissues, composed of mostly parallel collagen fiber bundles (Figure 4). They are primarily composed of type 1 collagen, with a smaller percentage of minor collagens, proteoglycans, elastin, and water.[32] At the finest level, collagen molecules assemble into fibrils that intertwine into fibril bundles, fascicles, and fiber bundles, forming a highly organized multihierarchical structure. At a more gross level, longitudinal fibers also do not run perfectly parallel to one another, but they do cross each other to some extent, actually forming spirals. At a slightly more macroscopic level (light microscopy), the collagen fibers in tendons exhibit regular undulations called crimp. During tendon elongation, this crimp disappears but returns after tensile forces are removed. This finding suggests some intrinsic resistance to tensile

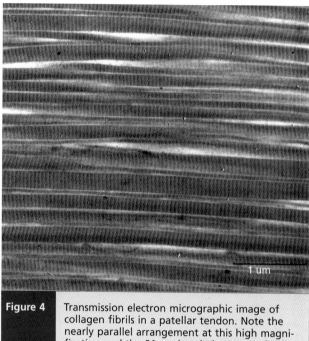

Figure 4 Transmission electron micrographic image of collagen fibrils in a patellar tendon. Note the nearly parallel arrangement at this high magnification and the 64-nm banded pattern of collagen fibrils as a result of quarter-stagger overlap of collagen molecules.

elongation that is conferred in part by whatever is maintaining the crimp pattern.

Tendons also display interesting biologic variations and are categorized as intrasynovial if they are covered by a synovial sheath or extrasynovial if they are not encapsulated by synovium. Some of these anatomic differences lead to relatively high gliding resistance for the extrasynovial tendon compared with an intrasynovial tendon.[33]

In contrast, intrasynovial tendons have only a single cell layer of epitenon with a relatively smooth surface; it is a fine connective sheath covering the tendon a level below the paratenon. As a sandwich layer, epitenon is contiguous with the paratenon on the outer surface and with the endotenon on its inner surface. The endotenon is a thin, loose, connective tissue layer that envelops the collagen fiber bundles or fascicles and is the tissue that carries neurovascular elements along the tendon.[34]

Tendon grafts can be used to replace an injured segment of tendon. The outcome is suboptimal when an extrasynovial tendon is used as a graft to replace a damaged intrasynovial tendon as a result of intrinsic biologic and biomechanical differences between the two tendon types. Although extrasynovial tendons generally have superior tensile properties, they exhibit elevated adhesion formation and inferior compressive properties when compared with intrasynovial tendons.[34]

Biomechanical Properties

Tendons primarily function by transmitting tensile loads from muscle to bone, thereby permitting locomotion along with supplementing the stability of the joints that they cross. The hierarchical structural unit for tendons described previously makes a tendon ideal for carrying and transmitting large tensile mechanical loads.[35] As demonstrated with increasing sophistication for the past 3 decades, tendons and tendon cells exhibit mechanosensitive properties, and, in response to mechanical loads, undergo adaptation by altering their structure, composition, and mechanical properties.

The stiffness and cross-sectional area of tendons increases in response to loading during development[36,37] and is attributed partly to increasing body and muscle mass and increasing muscular forces. Adult tendons exhibit greater stiffness compared with tendons from children, but there are apparently no major sex differences in their intrinsic material properties.[37] Although aging generally leads to a decrease in tensile strength, the mechanical properties of tendons also deteriorate because of low levels of resistive functional loading, especially in elderly patients.[35]

Different tendons in the body are subjected to different mechanical loads, which is roughly proportional to the PCSA (see previous discussion) of the associated muscle. In general, the greater the muscle or muscle group PCSA, the higher the force that it will produce, leading to a greater force on its tendon (for example, the quadriceps muscles loading the quadriceps and patellar tendons). Moreover, because of a combination of extrinsic forces and intrinsic muscle loads, different activities clearly induce quite different levels of forces on the same tendon.[38] Although tendon is regarded as a distinct force-transmitting structure, it remains to be determined whether forces are transmitted evenly throughout each structure and whether stresses experienced by collagen subunits within a tendon are uniform or not.[31]

Viscoelasticity is a biomechanical behavior of all connective tissues, meaning, as the word implies, that tissue properties are a combination of viscosity (velocity dependent) and elasticity (time independent). Tendons are viscoelastic because of complex interactions within and among collagen fibers, proteoglycans, and water. Recent studies have examined the molecular origin of viscoelastic behavior and concluded that the viscosity of individual collagen molecules is several orders of magnitude lower than the viscosity of single collagen fibrils, suggesting that additional molecular mechanisms, such as the movement of collagen molecules within collagen fibrils, must be contributing to gross tissue viscoelastic behavior in tendons.[39]

Functional Significance of Muscle-Tendon Interactions

As noted previously, muscles often shorten as they exert tensile loads on tendons. The affected tendon stretches and can subsequently recoil as the muscle relaxes, which essentially makes the tendon an elastic strain energy storage material. The capacity of tendons to store and recover energy is one mechanism that enables individual muscle-tendon units to customize their function to a particular need, such as high-efficiency (where compliant tendons store a great deal of energy) or high-

power productions (where stiff tendons transmit force directly to bones with little deformation).

Based on their functions, tendons are categorized as either energy-storing or positional tendons[40-43] (Table 1). Examples of energy-storing tendons include the Achilles tendon and the equine superficial digital flexor tendon, both of which sustain high strain during normal physiologic loads and are designed to stretch and recoil to ensure the efficient return of stored energy.[40] Positional tendons such as equine common digital extensor tendon or human anterior tibialis tendon are relatively inextensible. Because of the low strain, positional tendons are rarely injured.[32]

Biomechanical Alterations of Tendons With Aging and After Tendon Injury

Tendons can be damaged either because of acute injury or as a result of overuse and degeneration. Repeated occasional loading with abnormal load cycles can lead to overuse damage of tendons by progressively breaking individual collagen fibrils. Broken fibrils likely decrease loads on individual cells, causing them to initiate catabolic responses and degrade local matrix (a normal response to unloading that can eventually lead to gross tendon rupture.[44] Different animal models investigating the overuse of tendon (such as rotator cuff and Achilles) have demonstrated that increased repetitive activity can lead to local tendon matrix damage, with a catabolic cascade of degradative cellular events that can lead to decreased material properties in tendon. During these events, tendons can undergo gross thickening either in their midsubstance, at their insertions into bone, or near their muscle-tendon junctions.

Aging also increases the risk of tendon injury in both humans and animals.[45] Human tendon collagen content decreases with age, suggesting either a reduction in the synthesis of collagen, increased degradation, or a combination of the two. Furthermore, this decline in collagen synthesis may be caused by either a decrease in the number of tendon fibroblasts or a decline in their intrinsic ability to produce collagen.[45]

In general, injured tendons heal by the typical wound-healing processes of inflammation, proliferation, and remodeling, but there are functional differences in the way different tendons heal, which is an important factor to be considered during postoperative treatment.[44] For example, because flexor tendons of the hand are encased in synovial sheaths and their functional repair requires both tissue strength and intrasynovial gliding properties, the prevention of adhesion tissue formation between the tendon surface and its sheath is critical. The possibility of optimal periods of immobilization and subsequent loading regimens for different injured tendons are controversial topics.

Immobilization leads to the development of fibrous adhesions between the tendon and its synovial sheath during the repair of an injured flexor tendon, which can severely limit range of motion. Long-term removal of load from a healing tendon also weakens the repair tis-

Table 1

Summary of Functional, Material, and Biomechanical Differences Between the Positional and Energy-Storing Tendons

Tendons		
Energy Storing	**Positional**	**References**
Function		
Store and release of elastic strain energy	Transmit forces generated in muscles to bones	Birch[41]
Material Properties		
Bimodal with smaller fibril diameter	Unimodal with larger fibril diameter	Birch[41]
Greater glycosaminoglycan and water content: less stiff matrix	Lower glycosaminoglycan and water content rigid matrix	Batson et al[42]
Increased interfascicular gliding because of lower intrafascicular stiffness	Tightly packed fascicles lead to less interfascicular sliding at low loads	Thorpe et al[43]
Biomechanical Properties		
Extensible under physiologic loads	Inextensible under physiologic loads	Thorpe et al[43]
Higher failure strain	Lower failure strain	Thorpe et al[43]
Lower modulus and failure strain	Higher modulus and failure strain	Thorpe et al[43]
Rate of Injury		
More	Less	Thorpe et al[43]
Examples		
Human Achilles tendon Equine superficial digital flexor tendon	Human anterior tibialis tendon Equine common digital extensor tendon	Thorpe et al[43]

sue because of decreased production of extracellular matrix.

Biologic Alterations Following Tendon Injury

Degeneration in tendons is apparently not routinely accompanied by evidence of inflammation. Tendinosis has been reported to occur in the patellar, Achilles, posterior tibialis, rotator cuff, long head of the biceps brachii, and wrist extensor tendons. Histologically, tendinosis is characterized by the lack of inflammatory cells with disordered patterns of collagen fibrils, increased cellularity and vascularization (early), apoptosis or programmed cell death (later), and abnormal ECM resulting from degradative cell processes.

As noted in previous paragraphs, tendon healing after a rupture where there is local bleeding is similar to wound healing, including its cellular events. The infiltration of mast cells and macrophages in the injury site leads to the secretion of transforming growth factor-β (TGF-β), which in turn stimulates excessive production of ECM, resulting in the formation of scar. It has been shown that a neutralizing antibody of TGF-β can diminish excessive production of ECM and improve the postoperative range of motion in a rabbit model of flexor tendon transection.[46]

Nitric oxide (NO) is a small free radical that is generated by nitric oxide synthase (NOS). Normal, uninjured tendons have very little NOS activity, but chronic tendon overloading upregulates NOS isoforms, demonstrating NO responses to mechanical stress. Extraneous addition of NO can apparently improve some tendon healing by increasing collagen synthesis, whereas competitive inhibition of NOS activity inhibits tendon healing.[47]

Current Concepts in Tendon Repair

The common goal of the various reparative strategies used after tendon injury is to facilitate early return to preinjury activity levels by promoting early and strong repair. Improved suture repair techniques are the gold standard for repairing completely torn tendons, with minimal durations of immobilization and early (low load) loading being used to restore tendon function. In addition, several tendon augmentation techniques are still being evaluated.

Although tissue-engineered application of matrices loaded with growth factors, cells, and other regulators has been tested in an attempt to augment normal tendon repair, only transitory improvement has been noted without significant biomechanical improvements thus far.[48] Platelet-rich plasma (PRP) harvested from whole blood has an array of growth factors that are found in normal tissue repair. As of 2012, however, convincing clinical evidence for the success of PRP based on randomized trials remains limited.

Adult mesenchymal stem cells retain their ability to differentiate into various tissue types and thus are a potentially useful tool for repairing injured tendons, which do not heal intrinsically. The mesenchymal stem cells from tendon tissue, referred to as tendon stem/progenitor cells, possess multipotent differentiation capacity along with inducing cellular proliferation and angiogenesis as well as reducing apoptosis of endogenous cells.[49] As of 2012, tendon stem/progenitor cells are not yet in use clinically because they require further investigation for both safety and efficacy.

Ligaments

Ligaments are dense, fibrous, connective tissues that form the connecting link between two articulating bones.[50] Ligaments come in various shapes and sizes and are named based on their shapes (for example, deltoid), their relationships to a joint (for example, collateral) or to each other (for example, cruciate), or to the bones that they connect (for example, coracoacromial).

Functional Anatomy

Ligaments have many subcomponents that are known as major functional bands that tighten or loosen in different positions of the joint that they are guiding. The anterior cruciate ligament (ACL) is described as having two main functional bundles or bands—the anteromedial band (that tightens in knee joint flexion) and the posteromedial band (that tightens more in knee joint extension). Each functional band contains a much larger number of fibrous subcomponents that carry loads in slightly different three-dimensional positions of the bones and thus help guide the bones through these normal motions. This has significance to how ligaments are injured (for example, the tight parts fail first, and the parts that are tight are a function of joint position), why joints need to be examined in the position in which they were injured (which is why a Lachman test is effective in detecting unstable knee joints from ACL tears; most ACLs are likely injured by sudden tibial rotation at 15-30° of knee flexion), and how joints need to be positioned to minimize pulling torn ligament ends farther apart (the joint position will determine whether or not there is load on the healing part).

Adult ligaments typically attach to bones through specialized insertions.[51] Each direct insertion has a specialized gradation of cells and tissue matrix that merges from ligament matrix through fibrocartilage into mineralized fibrocartilage and then into bone. These insertions anchor ligaments firmly into bone because the ends of the collagen fibers that make up the body of the ligament are literally embedded in bone. Those embedded fibers are known as Sharpey fibers and are analogous to similar fibers seen at tendon insertions. A second type of ligament insertion is more typically seen in an immature ligament (for example, the tibial insertion of the medial collateral ligament [MCL] during growth) in which a ligament attaches into periosteum and is not yet embedded into bone. Those periosteal attachments are much weaker but do convert to the adult form (embedded into bone) at maturity.

In terms of histologic architecture and matrix composition, the exterior surfaces of extra-articular ligaments are enveloped by a very thin cellular and vascular layer known as the epiligament. The epiligament merges into the periosteum and shares the rich cellularity, vascularity, and sheet-like architecture of the periosteum. It likely contributes to healing in a way that is analogous to periosteal healing of bone. The cruciate ligaments are unique among all ligaments in having a synovial sheath that covers them, and they have some healing issues in common with synovial tendons.

Collagen fibers and fiber bundles in the main body of ligaments are configured grossly in a parallel arrangement along the long axis of the ligament with a crimp pattern similar to that seen in tendons (but with unique periodicity). This crimp has been shown to allow a ligament to elongate (slightly) under tensile loads without sustaining matrix damage.[52] Also similar to tendons, collagen bundles in a ligament exhibit a hierarchical structure, with intertwined collagen fibrils forming fibers, and fibers forming fiber bundles. Type I collagen is the primary structural constituent of a ligament, but ligaments also contain collagen types III, V, VI, XI, and XIV; proteoglycans; elastin; and other glycoproteins.[51]

Biomechanical Properties

The mechanical properties of ligaments are dictated mainly by the hierarchical organization of their collagen fibers. Ligaments are likely not loaded homogeneously and function normally at less than 20% of their tensile loading capacity, suggesting that they are somewhat overdesigned biomechanically.

Collagen content, which dictates the mechanical properties, varies among ligaments. For example, the concentration of collagen is higher in the MCL than in the ACL, making the MCL materially stronger.[53] The magnitudes of these differences can be quite large: the tangent modulus and the tensile strength of a human MCL are approximately 300 MPa and 40 MPa, respectively, whereas comparable modulus values for glenohumeral ligaments range from 5 to 42 MPa with tensile strengths of only 1-6 MPa.

The mechanical properties of ligaments change with age. An asynchronous maturation process has been noted between the bone-ligament-bone complex and the ligament midsubstance.[54] Both stress and motion are necessary for remodeling of normal ligament tissue, and even a few weeks of immobilization can affect joint stiffness and its structural properties. Load deprivation leads to increased osteoclastic activity, resorption of bone, and disruption of the normal attachment of the ligament to bone.

Like all connective tissues, ligaments exhibit interesting viscoelastic behaviors. Type III collagen and elastin contribute to the elastic behavior of ligaments,[55] whereas many factors appear to contribute to their viscoelastic properties, including the collagen fibers themselves,[56] the interaction of collagen fibers with other extracellular constituents,[57] water movement through the

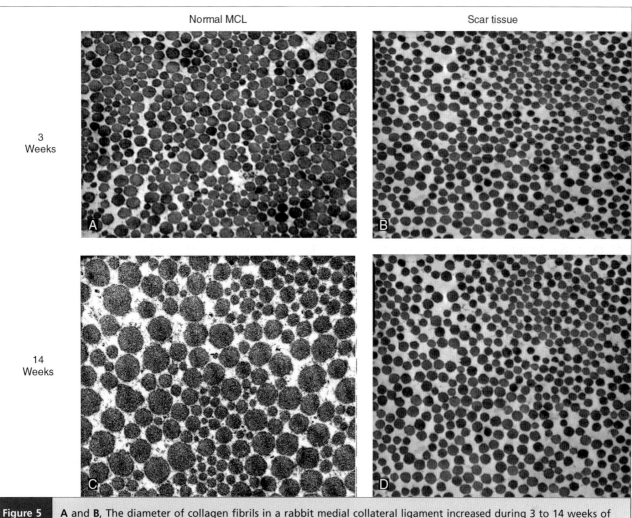

| Normal MCL | Scar tissue |

3 Weeks

14 Weeks

Figure 5   **A** and **B**, The diameter of collagen fibrils in a rabbit medial collateral ligament increased during 3 to 14 weeks of development. The collagen fibers changed from a relatively unimodal distribution of small diameter fibrils at 3 weeks to a bimodal distribution of small and large diameter fibrils at 14 weeks. **C** and **D**, The maturation of scar tissue from 3 to 14 weeks after injury displayed only small unimodal collagen fibrils, indicating that MCL remodeling may never reach the original levels following injury. (Adapted with permission from Achari Y, Chin JW, Heard BJ, et al: Molecular events surrounding collagen fibril assembly in the early healing rabbit medial collateral ligament—failure to recapitulate normal ligament development. *Connect Tissue Res* 2011;52:301-312)

matrix, and molecular bridges among collagen fibrils by sulfated glycosaminoglycans.[58] Ligaments apparently can accumulate damage with repetitive loading and fail at stresses below their normal ultimate tensile strength.[59]

Biomechanical Alterations Following Ligament Injury

The MCL of the knee has the capability of relatively good functional healing by scar formation and remodeling.[51] However, this remodeling process takes years, and the original levels of material strength are never fully restored (Figure 5). In contrast, because of the relative lack of a robust or functionally effective response within a joint, ACLs do not enjoy the same functional recovery. ACL fibroblasts have limited capacity for cellular proliferation and ECM production. Further, the ACL is ensheathed by a synovial membrane that, when disrupted, likely exposes the torn ACL to a relatively unfavorable synovial environment for healing.

Biologic Alterations Following Ligament Injury

A recent report evaluated cytokine levels over time in an ACL-deficient knee and found high levels of select interleukins—namely IL-1β, IL-6 and IL-8 immediately after injury.[60] The levels of tumor necrosis factor-alpha and interleukin 1 receptor agonist (IL-1Ra) were significantly lower following ACL injury and did not return to normal reported levels.[60] In a recent clinical trial, inflammation was blocked with a single intra-articular injection of IL-1Ra (anakinra 150 mg) in patients with an acute ACL tear. No decrease was noted in levels of IL-1β, although these patients experienced a reduction in knee pain and improved joint function over a 2-week interval.[60]

Current Concepts in Ligament Repair

Injury to the ACL is a major area of study to test ligament repairs. Several strategies for ACL repair or replacement have evolved. Anatomic placement of grafts within tibial and femoral footprints is now considered to be essential for optimal anatomic reconstruction.

Engineered ACL replacements or augmentations have been evaluated extensively. Such replacements have included sources of reparative cells with a capacity for proliferation and matrix synthesis; structural scaffold that facilitates growth of these cells; and an environment that provides sufficient nutrients. Recently, in an attempt to rejoin the torn ends of a ruptured ACL, a novel suture technique using a scaffold with a combination of collagen with PRP was applied.[61] Adding PRP may improve graft maturation and remodeling but not consistently. This composite scaffold also apparently improved the biomechanical properties of an ACL reconstruction.[61] Thus, as of 2012, there is no reliable augmentation for either ACL healing after suture repair and no reliable augment of tendon grafts for ACL reconstruction.

Summary

Skeletal muscles, tendons, and ligaments are all mechanosensitive connective tissues that alter their structure, function, and biology to alterations in loading and use conditions. Recent advances in muscle stem cell biology promise increased biologic understanding and therapeutic applications. Tissue engineering of ligaments and tendons promises similar advances and application.

Key Study Points

- Understanding muscle structural hierarchy is key to understanding its function, and can help with surgical decision making regarding changes in muscle length that occur during surgical tendon transfers and total joint replacement.

- Skeletal muscle performance depends on metabolic factors as well as structural factors. An understanding of muscle fiber types will help surgeons prescribe rational therapeutic regimens to increase muscle strength and endurance after injury.

- Ligament and tendon biomechanical properties serve as the prototype for almost all soft-tissue mechanics. Understanding this nonlinearity is key for making decisions that involve surgical tendon repair or joint replacement where ligaments must be transposed or displaced.

- Novel new treatments involving tissue engineering of artificial ligaments and tendons may provide a new source of tissue and offer new approaches to treatment.

Annotated References

1. Lieber RL, Loren GJ, Fridén J: In vivo measurement of human wrist extensor muscle sarcomere length changes. *J Neurophysiol* 1994;71(3):874-881.

2. Gordon AM, Huxley AF, Julian FJ: The variation in isometric tension with sarcomere length in vertebrate muscle fibres. *J Physiol* 1966;184(1):170-192.

3. Loren GJ, Shoemaker SD, Burkholder TJ, Jacobson MD, Fridén J, Lieber RL: Human wrist motors: Biomechanical design and application to tendon transfers. *J Biomech* 1996;29(3):331-342.

4. Ward SR, Kim CW, Eng CM, et al: Architectural analysis and intraoperative measurements demonstrate the unique design of the multifidus muscle for lumbar spine stability. *J Bone Joint Surg Am* 2009;91(1):176-185.

5. Smeulders MJ, Kreulen M, Hage JJ, Huijing PA, van der Horst CM: Overstretching of sarcomeres may not cause cerebral palsy muscle contracture. *J Orthop Res* 2004;22(6):1331-1335.

6. Freehafer AA, Peckham PH, Keith MW: Determination of muscle-tendon unit properties during tendon transfer. *J Hand Surg Am* 1979;4(4):331-339.

7. Boakes JL, Foran J, Ward SR, Lieber RL: Muscle adaptation by serial sarcomere addition 1 year after femoral lengthening. *Clin Orthop Relat Res* 2007;456: 250-253.

8. Brand PW, Hollister A: *Clinical Mechanics of the Hand,* ed 2. St. Louis, MO, Mosby, 1993.

9. Powell PL, Roy RR, Kanim P, Bello MA, Edgerton VR: Predictability of skeletal muscle tension from architectural determinations in guinea pig hindlimbs. *J Appl Physiol* 1984;57(6):1715-1721.

10. Winters TM, Takahashi M, Lieber RL, Ward SR: Whole muscle length-tension relationships are accurately modeled as scaled sarcomeres in rabbit hindlimb muscles. *J Biomech* 2011;44(1):109-115.

    The important contribution of this article is that it demonstrates experimentally that the three-dimensional model of a whole muscle as numerous sarcomeres in series and in parallel works for large rabbit muscles.

11. Lieber RL, Ward SR: Skeletal muscle design to meet functional demands. *Philos Trans R Soc Lond B Biol Sci* 2011;366(1570):1466-1476.

    This is an excellent review of the architectural design of skeletal muscle as well as the skeletal system to which it attaches.

12. Lieber RL, Jacobson MD, Fazeli BM, Abrams RA, Botte MJ: Architecture of selected muscles of the arm and forearm: Anatomy and implications for tendon transfer. *J Hand Surg Am* 1992;17(5):787-798.

13. Zajac FE: How musculotendon architecture and joint geometry affect the capacity of muscles to move and exert force on objects: A review with application to arm and forearm tendon transfer design. *J Hand Surg Am* 1992;17(5):799-804.

14. Bodine SC, Roy RR, Meadows DA, et al: Architectural, histochemical, and contractile characteristics of a unique biarticular muscle: The cat semitendinosus. *J Neurophysiol* 1982;48(1):192-201.

15. Schiaffino S, Reggiani C: Molecular diversity of myofibrillar proteins: Gene regulation and functional significance. *Physiol Rev* 1996;76(2):371-423.

16. Schiaffino S, Gorza L, Sartore S, et al: Three myosin heavy chain isoforms in type 2 skeletal muscle fibres. *J Muscle Res Cell Motil* 1989;10(3):197-205.

17. Bottinelli R, Canepari M, Pellegrino MA, Reggiani C: Force-velocity properties of human skeletal muscle fibres: Myosin heavy chain isoform and temperature dependence. *J Physiol* 1996;495(pt 2):573-586.

18. Yoon S-J, Seiler SH, Kucherlapati R, Leinwand L: Organization of the human skeletal myosin heavy chain gene cluster. *Proc Natl Acad Sci USA* 1992;89(24):12078-12082.

19. Weiss A, Schiaffino S, Leinwand LA: Comparative sequence analysis of the complete human sarcomeric myosin heavy chain family: Implications for functional diversity. *J Mol Biol* 1999;290(1):61-75.

20. Smerdu V, Karsch-Mizrachi I, Campione M, Leinwand L, Schiaffino S: Type IIx myosin heavy chain transcripts are expressed in type IIb fibers of human skeletal muscle. *Am J Physiol* 1994;267(6, pt 1):C1723-C1728.

21. Burkholder TJ, Fingado B, Baron S, Lieber RL: Relationship between muscle fiber types and sizes and muscle architectural properties in the mouse hindlimb. *J Morphol* 1994;221(2):177-190.

22. Eng CM, Smallwood LH, Rainiero MP, Lahey M, Ward SR, Lieber RL: Scaling of muscle architecture and fiber types in the rat hindlimb. *J Exp Biol* 2008;211(pt 14):2336-2345.

23. Fitts RH: Cellular mechanisms of muscle fatigue. *Physiol Rev* 1994;74(1):49-94.

24. Fridén J, Lieber RL: Evidence for muscle attachment at relatively long lengths in tendon transfer surgery. *J Hand Surg Am* 1998;23(1):105-110.

25. Lieber RL, Murray WM, Clark DL, Hentz VR, Fridén J: Biomechanical properties of the brachioradialis muscle: Implications for surgical tendon transfer. *J Hand Surg Am* 2005;30(2):273-282.

26. Labeit S, Kolmerer B: Titins: Giant proteins in charge of muscle ultrastructure and elasticity. *Science* 1995;270(5234):293-296.

27. Ward SR, Tomiya A, Regev GJ, et al: Passive mechanical properties of the lumbar multifidus muscle support its role as a stabilizer. *J Biomech* 2009;42(10):1384-1389.

28. Prado LG, Makarenko I, Andresen C, Krüger M, Opitz CA, Linke WA: Isoform diversity of giant proteins in relation to passive and active contractile properties of rabbit skeletal muscles. *J Gen Physiol* 2005;126(5):461-480.

29. Brack AS, Rando TA: Tissue-specific stem cells: Lessons from the skeletal muscle satellite cell. *Cell Stem Cell* 2012;10(5):504-514.

   These authors provide an authoritative and thoughtful review of the various stem cells present in muscle and the control of their development and differentiation.

30. Sampaolesi M, Blot S, D'Antona G, et al: Mesoangioblast stem cells ameliorate muscle function in dystrophic dogs. *Nature* 2006;444(7119):574-579.

31. Huard J, Fu FH: *Gene Therapy and Tissue Engineering in Orthopaedic and Sports Medicine (Methods in Bioengineering)*. Boston, MA, Birkhäuser, 2000, pp xvi, 286.

32. Franchi M, Ottani V, Stagni R, Ruggeri A: Tendon and ligament fibrillar crimps give rise to left-handed helices of collagen fibrils in both planar and helical crimps. *J Anat* 2010;216(3):301-309.

   This study examines the three-dimensional morphology of fibrillar crimp in tendons and ligaments and demonstrates that each fibril in the fibrillar region always twists leftward, changing the plane of running, and sharply bends, modifying the course on a new plane. Level of evidence: III.

33. Gott M, Ast M, Lane LB, et al: Tendon phenotype should dictate tissue engineering modality in tendon repair: A review. *Discov Med* 2011;12(62):75-84.

   The authors present a detailed discussion on intrasynovial and extrasynovial tendon morphology. Level of evidence: III.

34. Wang JH, Guo Q, Li B: Tendon biomechanics and mechanobiology—a minireview of basic concepts and recent advancements. *J Hand Ther* 2012;25(2):133-140, quiz 141.

   The biomechanical characteristics of tendons are discussed in relation to their unique hierarchical structure and composition, which enable them to carry and transmit muscular forces effectively. Level of evidence: III.

35. Arnoczky SP, Lavagnino M, Egerbacher M: The mechanobiological aetiopathogenesis of tendinopathy: Is it the over-stimulation or the under-stimulation of tendon cells? *Int J Exp Pathol* 2007;88(4):217-226.

36. O'Brien TD, Reeves ND, Baltzopoulos V, Jones DA, Maganaris CN: Muscle-tendon structure and dimensions in adults and children. *J Anat* 2010;216(5):631-642.

   In this article, the changes associated with fascicles, muscles, and tendons with maturation are discussed.

1: Principles of Orthopaedics

The study concludes that adult muscles are better designed for force production than children's muscles. Level of evidence: II-1.

37. Wang JH: Mechanobiology of tendon. *J Biomech* 2006; 39(9):1563-1582.

38. Magnusson SP, Langberg H, Kjaer M: The pathogenesis of tendinopathy: Balancing the response to loading. *Nat Rev Rheumatol* 2010;6(5):262-268.

    This article discusses the microstructure of tendons and suggests that one or more weak links are present in the structure. A deeper understanding of how tendon tissue adapts to mechanical loading will help in understanding tendinopathy. Level of evidence: III.

39. Duenwald SE, Vanderby R Jr, Lakes RS: Stress relaxation and recovery in tendon and ligament: Experiment and modeling. *Biorheology* 2010;47(1):1-14.

    As tendons and ligaments are considered interchangeable in surgical applications, this study evaluates the ability to predict the nonlinear and viscoelastic behavior of tendon and ligament during stress relaxation testing in a porcine model. Level of evidence: III.

40. Killian ML, Cavinatto L, Galatz LM, Thomopoulos S: The role of mechanobiology in tendon healing. *J Shoulder Elbow Surg* 2012;21(2):228-237.

    This article discusses how adhesion formation impairs the healing of tendons and the effect of loading and motion to improve tendon healing.

41. Birch HL: Tendon matrix composition and turnover in relation to functional requirements. *Int J Exp Pathol* 2007;88(4):241-248.

42. Batson EL, Paramour RJ, Smith TJ, Birch HL, Patterson-Kane JC, Goodship AE: Are the material properties and matrix composition of equine flexor and extensor tendons determined by their functions? *Equine Vet J* 2003;35(3):314-318.

43. Thorpe CT, Udeze CP, Birch HL, Clegg PD, Screen HR: Specialization of tendon mechanical properties results from interfascicular differences. *J R Soc Interface* 2012; 9(76):3108-3117.

    This article discusses the differences in the movement of fascicles in the energy storing and positional tendons. Level of evidence: III.

44. Galatz LM, Charlton N, Das R, Kim HM, Havlioglu N, Thomopoulos S: Complete removal of load is detrimental to rotator cuff healing. *J Shoulder Elbow Surg* 2009; 18(5):669-675.

45. Thornton GM, Hart DA: The interface of mechanical loading and biological variables as they pertain to the development of tendinosis. *J Musculoskelet Neuronal Interact* 2011;11(2):94-105.

    This article evaluates how tendon overuse injury is related to abnormal mechanical loading that deviates from normal mechanical loading in magnitude, frequency, duration, and/or direction. Level of evidence: III.

46. Chang J, Thunder R, Most D, Longaker MT, Lineaweaver WC: Studies in flexor tendon wound healing: Neutralizing antibody to TGF-beta1 increases postoperative range of motion. *Plast Reconstr Surg* 2000;105(1): 148-155.

47. Bokhari AR, Murrell GA: The role of nitric oxide in tendon healing. *J Shoulder Elbow Surg* 2012;21(2): 238-244.

    A detailed review that addresses the role of NO in relation to tendon injury and healing is presented. Level of evidence: III.

48. Visser LC, Arnoczky SP, Caballero O, Kern A, Ratcliffe A, Gardner KL: Growth factor-rich plasma increases tendon cell proliferation and matrix synthesis on a synthetic scaffold: An in vitro study. *Tissue Eng Part A* 2010;16(3):1021-1029.

    This article discusses the use of a bioactive scaffold created by a combination of growth factor-rich plasma and a synthetic scaffold that enhanced the deposition of a collagen-rich extracellular matrix. Level of evidence: III.

49. Cao Y, Liu Y, Liu W, Shan Q, Buonocore SD, Cui L: Bridging tendon defects using autologous tenocyte engineered tendon in a hen model. *Plast Reconstr Surg* 2002;110(5):1280-1289.

50. Frank CB: Ligament structure, physiology and function. *J Musculoskelet Neuronal Interact* 2004;4(2):199-201.

51. Frank CB, Hart DA, Shrive NG: Molecular biology and biomechanics of normal and healing ligaments—a review. *Osteoarthritis Cartilage* 1999;7(1):130-140.

52. Woo SL, Newton PO, MacKenna DA, Lyon RM: A comparative evaluation of the mechanical properties of the rabbit medial collateral and anterior cruciate ligaments. *J Biomech* 1992;25(4):377-386.

53. Quapp KM, Weiss JA: Material characterization of human medial collateral ligament. *J Biomech Eng* 1998; 120(6):757-763.

54. Jung HJ, Fisher MB, Woo SL: Role of biomechanics in the understanding of normal, injured, and healing ligaments and tendons. *Sports Med Arthrosc Rehabil Ther Technol* 2009;1(1):9.

55. Puxkandl R, Zizak I, Paris O, et al: Viscoelastic properties of collagen: Synchrotron radiation investigations and structural model. *Philos Trans R Soc Lond B Biol Sci* 2002;357(1418):191-197.

56. Scott JE: Elasticity in extracellular matrix "shape modules" of tendon, cartilage, etc.: A sliding proteoglycan-filament model. *J Physiol* 2003;553(pt 2):335-343.

57. Chimich D, Shrive N, Frank C, Marchuk L, Bray R: Water content alters viscoelastic behaviour of the normal adolescent rabbit medial collateral ligament. *J Biomech* 1992;25(8):831-837.

58. Ciarletta P, Micera S, Accoto D, Dario P: A novel microstructural approach in tendon viscoelastic modelling at the fibrillar level. *J Biomech* 2006;39(11):2034-2042.

59. Georgoulis AD, Papadonikolakis A, Papageorgiou CD, Mitsou A, Stergiou N: Three-dimensional tibiofemoral kinematics of the anterior cruciate ligament-deficient and reconstructed knee during walking. *Am J Sports Med* 2003;31(1):75-79.

60. Kraus VB, Birmingham J, Stabler TV, et al: Effects of intraarticular IL1-Ra for acute anterior cruciate ligament knee injury: A randomized controlled pilot trial (NCT00332254). *Osteoarthritis Cartilage* 2012;20(4):271-278.

    This study evaluates the clinical effectiveness of IL-1Ra for ACL tears. Level of evidence: I

61. Vavken P, Fleming BC, Mastrangelo AN, Machan JT, Murray MM: Biomechanical outcomes after bioenhanced anterior cruciate ligament repair and anterior cruciate ligament reconstruction are equal in a porcine model. *Arthroscopy* 2012;28(5):672-680.

    This article has evaluated that bioenhanced ACL repair produced biomechanical results that were not different from ACL reconstruction in a skeletally immature, large animal model, although both procedures produced significantly improved results over ACL transection. Level of evidence: III.

1: Principles of Orthopaedics

Chapter 5
Musculoskeletal Biomechanics

Donald D. Anderson, PhD   Jessica E. Goetz, PhD

1: Principles of Orthopaedics

Introduction

The scientific field of musculoskeletal biomechanics has matured considerably over the past three decades. Many educational resources are available to aid in understanding this engineering science in the context of orthopaedics.[1,2] A summary of the basic terminology of biomechanics is provided in Table 1. This chapter focuses on the evolving role that biomechanics is playing in orthopaedic practice, with background information presented as needed to support this focus. The chapter begins with a brief review of musculoskeletal tissue mechanics (bone, cartilage, tendon, and ligament), describes evolving biomechanical focus areas, and concludes with a discussion of specific areas in which biomechanical principles are being translated into clinical application.

Musculoskeletal Tissue Mechanics

Bone Mechanics

The macroscopic mechanical properties of bone have been extensively studied, and much is known in this area.[3] Bone is a highly mineralized tissue whose properties are largely dictated by its density (mass) and structure (global and local architecture). Because of the primary weight-bearing role of the skeleton, bone is subjected to a highly complex loading environment during the normal activities of daily living. The nature of these dynamic (time-varying) loads subjects bone to the risk of failure. At a macroscopic level, bone is weakest in shear, next weakest in tension, and strongest in compression. It is anisotropic, with a preferred directionality well suited to resisting routinely encountered loads.

Bone usually exists in a neutral homeostatic biologic state, with an even balance between mineral deposition and resorption. However, bone is commonly subjected to a more net-osteogenic or net-osteoresorptive state,[4,5]

such as in instances when fractures occur or as physical activity levels increase or decrease. The associated fluctuations in bone constitution involve changes in density and architecture, which can impart considerable change in the mechanical properties of the tissue.

Recent research in the area of bone mechanics has focused on methods for noninvasively assessing bone properties in live individuals, better understanding how pathologies (for example, osteoporosis) negatively influence the mechanical integrity of bone, and the development of new (often pharmacologic) approaches to maintaining or restoring more favorable mechanical properties. In this latter respect, bisphosphonates have played a primary pharmacologic role in treating osteoporosis. Physical interventions (such as certain types of exercise) also have been studied for this purpose, with targeted development of protocols to optimize the osteogenic signal provided by exercise.[6]

Cartilage Mechanics

Articular cartilage is generally well suited to the demands of joint motion. The tissue supports predominantly compressive loading and affords low-friction motion between opposing joint surfaces. Articular cartilage tissue has a unique biphasic (mixed solid/fluid) character, with corresponding mechanical implications. When loaded slowly, the fluid phase of cartilage (water) is able to flow through the porous solid matrix, and the apparent cartilage modulus is relatively low. The permeability of cartilage dictates how slowly the load must be applied to allow this fluid flow. When loaded more abruptly, there is inadequate time for the fluid to flow through the matrix, and the apparent modulus is on the order of 10 to 20 times higher than that associated with slow loading. Although there has been much debate in this area over the years, it is now widely accepted that for most functional activities, cartilage is loaded sufficiently fast to limit fluid flow.

Defects in cartilage can be focal or global, with focal defects tending to be more traumatic in origin and global defects reflecting a chronic pathologic state. Both types of defects influence tissue material properties and joint mechanics and are the focus of continuing research.[7] The repair of focal defects is associated with a need to restore local congruity and mechanical integrity in a stable, long-lasting manner. The challenges imposed by these twin necessities have made progress in this area difficult, but most efforts have focused on physical replacement with some type of graft. More

1: Principles of Orthopaedics

Table 1

Basic Terminology of Biomechanics

Term	Definition
Stiffness	The ratio of force to displacement (stiffness = force ÷ displacement). Units of measure are most commonly N/mm or N/m.
Load to failure	The force that is measured at the time that a specimen breaks in a test involving a continuous application of force.
Fatigue failure	Cyclical subfailure loading may result in failure caused by fatigue. Load-to-failure testing data are most often reported in the orthopaedic literature; however, clinical failure of fracture fixation constructs or implants is often caused by fatigue failure.
Strain	The amount of deformation per given length of an object. The units for strain are dimensionless, but they are often referenced as mm/mm or % strain.
Stress	The amount of internal forces acting over a given area of an object. The units of measure for stress are thus N/m^2 (Pascal [Pa]), but for most orthopaedic applications are more on the order of MPa (N/mm^2).
Elastic modulus	The ratio of the stress to strain over a region for which the deformation is elastic, which is analogous to stiffness for force displacement. The units are the same as for stress.
Yield point	The point on the stress-strain curve where deformation goes from elastic (fully recoverable on unloading) to plastic (unrecoverable).
Strength	The highest stress on a stress-strain curve to failure. Strength and stiffness are not the same thing, and the difference is important.
Anisotropy	The concept that properties vary along different directions. Isotropy (in contrast) implies that the properties are invariant with direction.
Brittle	A material that experiences little plastic deformation (strain) before it fails is said to be brittle (for example, glass or cortical bone).
Ductile	If a material has a large plastic deformation region before it fails, it is said to be ductile (for example, copper).
Toughness	A material that can absorb more energy before failure (large area under the stress-strain curve) is said to be tougher. Units for toughness are $(N/m^2)(m/m)$ or $joules/m^3$.

global defects in cartilage properties continue to be the purview of total joint arthroplasty, but mechanical joint-sparing procedures are also under development.

Soft-Tissue Mechanics: Tendon and Ligament

Tendons and ligaments are highly specialized to bear the predominantly tensile loads that occur from joining bones together into a joint and joining active contractile muscle tissue to bony insertions to facilitate skeletal movement. At a microscopic level, this function is accommodated by long, thin, collagen fibers, which exist in a partially crimped state. These crimped bundles are generally aligned along a single primary direction between bony (or muscular and bony) insertions, with some variability in the degree of alignment of the collagen fibers along that primary direction. This variability is frequently called the fiber dispersion and is expressed as a percentage of fibers aligned along the primary direction. This microstructure causes tendons and ligaments to be highly anisotropic. When tension is applied along the main fiber direction, the tissue demonstrates its stiffest behavior; however, when tension is applied perpendicular to the main fiber direction, the load is carried by the cross-links between fiber bundles and the

remaining disorganized matrix material, causing the tissue to appear more compliant. The more highly aligned the fibers are in the primary direction (that is, the lower the dispersion), the more dramatic is the anisotropic behavior of the tissue.

Tendons and ligaments are substantially more compliant than bone or cartilage and exhibit highly nonlinear stress-strain behavior, with relatively rapid extension under low loads and progressively stiffer behavior under higher loads. In the low-load, high-extension part of the stress-strain curve (frequently referred to as the toe region), the applied load is acting to align and straighten the crimps in the collagen fibers. The less crimped fibers will straighten sooner and begin taking up load, while other neighboring fibers continue to straighten. This tissue behavior causes an upward inflection in the shape of the stress-strain curve. After all of the collagen fibers have been pulled straight, they will take up load in a more uniform manner, and the stress-strain curve will become more linear and much steeper than in the toe region. Although a single elastic modulus can be calculated in this region of the stress-strain curve, it is only descriptive of the behavior of that tendon or ligament after it has been moderately loaded.

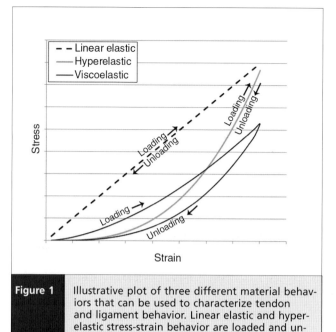

Figure 1 Illustrative plot of three different material behaviors that can be used to characterize tendon and ligament behavior. Linear elastic and hyperelastic stress-strain behavior are loaded and unloaded in the same manner. Viscoelastic material unloads in a different manner than it was loaded because of the time-dependent behavior of the material.

To fully describe the range of mechanical behavior of tendons or ligaments, more complex material property models must be used. Two common models appropriate for describing tendon and ligament behavior are hyperelastic or viscoelastic models (**Figure 1**). Rather than a direct stress versus strain relationship, hyperelastic models rely instead on equations describing the relationship between the strain energy density and tissue stretch ratios. The coefficients in the hyperelastic model equation are optimized to fit experimentally measured tissue behavior. Hyperelastic coefficients typically do not have any direct physical meaning, which is in contrast to Young's modulus. Hyperelastic material models used to describe tendon and ligament behavior range in complexity from the single coefficient neo-Hookean model, which results in a relatively linear stress-strain curve, to the more complex Ogden model, which can be of a first, second, or third order (with two, four, or six coefficients, respectively). Generally, hyperelastic models with more coefficients can more accurately describe highly nonlinear stress-strain behavior, although fitting large numbers of model coefficients requires extensive experimental testing.

Similarly, viscoelastic material models use equations describing changes in material behavior associated with time. When tendons or ligaments are loaded for extended periods of time, the solid tissue microstructure can deform and slightly rearrange under a constant strain or a constant load. Typically, viscoelastic models are fit to experimental data captured over an extended period of time, and these models are especially useful for modeling tendon and ligament behavior because these tissues are loaded over very different time scales

depending on the activity being performed (for example, jumping versus standing).

New and Developing Focus Areas in Musculoskeletal Biomechanics

The study of biomechanics has progressed substantially beyond macroscopic measurements of bulk tissue behavior. Advances in experimental testing equipment, imaging technology, and computing power have spurred new developments in musculoskeletal biomechanics. Such advances have driven the application of patient-specific (personalized) medicine, which has changed the way in which clinical treatment decisions are made. For example, rapid or real-time analysis of the mechanics of a given patient's joint, fracture, or gait pattern can be used to provide specific rehabilitation or surgical care. Continuing advancements in and experience with benchtop imaging tools (microscopy) and noninvasive clinical imaging modalities (such as ultrasound and MRI) have presented new ways to assess the mechanical properties of musculoskeletal tissues.

Patient-Specific Treatment Considerations
Macroscopic: Kinematic Modeling
Musculoskeletal modeling provides a comprehensive approach to joint and tissue mechanics. This type of modeling uses kinematic (relative positions and joint angles) and kinetic (forces and moments) data in conjunction with an engineering approach known as inverse dynamics to calculate forces acting in a series of joints, most frequently the arm (shoulder-elbow-wrist-finger) or the leg (hip-knee-ankle; **Figure 2**). Kinematic data are usually collected using an optoelectronic motion capture system, in which a series of cameras track markers placed directly on an individual while he or she performs a physical activity. Kinetic data are collected using a force platform or pressure sensors.[8,9] These two types of data can be used to calculate the effects of a load applied at the hand or the foot on the forces that develop in more proximal joints.

Because this type of modeling uses an individual's movement and loading patterns, it is inherently patient specific. If a pathologic condition is associated with a particular movement abnormality, movement retraining can be prescribed.[10,11] A key advantage to this type of intervention is that it is a conservative treatment specifically tailored to the needs of an individual patient. Although commonly used after neurologic problems such as trauma or stroke, gait retraining or modification in patients without neurologic damage is slowly becoming more popular. Typically, a patient is given detailed instructions on how to change one or more aspects of his or her normal walking motion to achieve a specific change in a movement pattern. The new motion is practiced while the individual receives biofeedback ranging in sophistication from verbal feedback to audio feedback to visual feedback based on motion capture systems.[12,13]

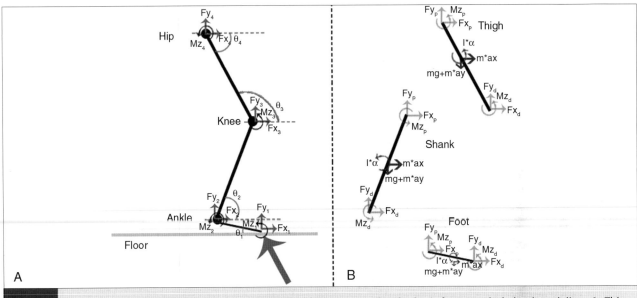

Figure 2 An example of a two-dimensional free-body diagram that provides the basis for musculoskeletal modeling. **A,** This basic model incorporates the joint angles and the applied forces (floor). **B,** The decomposed model allows for equation development. In each segment, the forces and the moments at the proximal (p) and distal (d) locations must balance. In addition to joint angles and externally applied forces, the equations also incorporate the weight of the limb segment (mg), the acceleration of the segment at the instant of the time being modeled (m*ax and m*ay), and the rotational acceleration (α) of the segment center of mass (I).

It has been suggested that an individual who has modified his or her gait to compensate for chronic joint pain or injured soft tissues may benefit from gait retraining. It is believed that such treatment would prevent any abnormal kinematics from stretching a surgical repair or increasing the load on implant hardware that could cause premature arthroplasty failure.[14,15] An example of a specific gait modification is intentionally increasing lateral trunk lean to decrease the adduction moment in the knee.[16] Because a decreased knee adduction moment would theoretically decrease medial compartment stress, such a modification may be useful in patients with arthritis. Similarly, a patient who reduces his or her hip adduction angle by 5° (23%) while running reduces the pressure on the lateral side of the patella and decreases patellofemoral pain.[17] As motion capture and computer modeling become more widely available and patient-specific treatment becomes the norm, it will become more common for the required modifications to be optimized to a patient's particular movement rather than the patient receiving generic instructions about a movement modification needed to achieve a particular mechanical goal.[18]

Localized: Numerical Modeling

Patient-specific analysis on a joint and tissue level is becoming much more common. Numerical modeling approaches, primarily computational stress analysis methods such as finite element analysis, have played a critical role in the engineering design of implants and devices used throughout orthopaedics. In that context, much of the focus has been on establishing a general inventory of products engineered to accommodate a range of patient sizes and requirements. In the simplest of cases, this could involve decision making regarding the placement and the diameter of a hole in a given plate so that it does not prematurely fail from stress concentration near the hole. In a more complex scenario, analyses might involve determining the sizes of polyethylene acetabular cups that are generally more prone to wear.

Recently, increased computational capabilities and the ubiquity of digital medical imaging have made patient-specific stress analysis tractable. As a result, treatment considerations are beginning to be analyzed on a patient- and case-specific basis. These methods begin with the ability of an analyst to proceed fairly directly from CT or MRI information to computational models of a patient's anatomy. In one example, incorporating bone density information can allow the assessment of the risks of vertebral fracture in one patient versus another.[19] Patient-specific analysis also could be applicable to planning a complex pelvic osteotomy aimed at improving femoral head coverage and thereby decreasing contact stress to reduce the risk of osteoarthritis. The degree of surface incongruity remaining after surgical repair of a fractured joint can be directly related to the expected levels of chronic contact stress exposure that the joint will experience[20] (Figure 3). This information could be helpful in guiding later treatment decisions.

Apart from finite element analysis, CT data obtained after an articular fracture can provide information to objectively assess the severity of a fracture, stratify the risk associated with the initial trauma, and guide treatment decision making.[21] Such methodology is based on

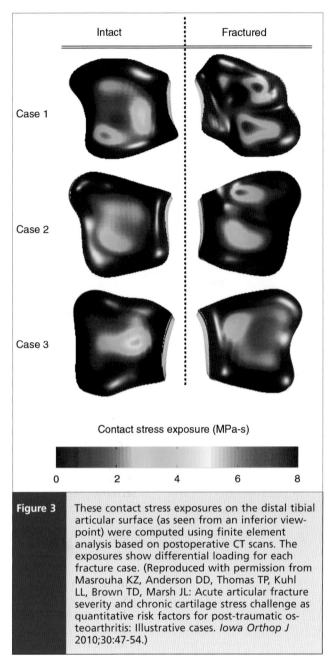

Intact | Fractured

Case 1

Case 2

Case 3

Contact stress exposure (MPa-s)

0   2   4   6   8

Figure 3 These contact stress exposures on the distal tibial articular surface (as seen from an inferior viewpoint) were computed using finite element analysis based on postoperative CT scans. The exposures show differential loading for each fracture case. (Reproduced with permission from Masrouha KZ, Anderson DD, Thomas TP, Kuhl LL, Brown TD, Marsh JL: Acute articular fracture severity and chronic cartilage stress challenge as quantitative risk factors for post-traumatic osteoarthritis: Illustrative cases. *Iowa Orthop J* 2010;30:47-54.)

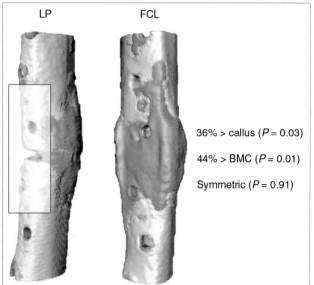

LP   FCL

36% > callus (*P* = 0.03)

44% > BMC (*P* = 0.01)

Symmetric (*P* = 0.91)

Figure 4 Differential callus formation associated with conventional locking plate (LP) and far cortical locking (FCL) techniques are shown in a volumetric rendering of callus from quantitative CT data obtained at 9 weeks after surgical treatment in an osteotomy gap fracture model. A 36% greater callus volume was observed in the FCL group compared with the LP group (*P* = 0.03). The bone mineral content (BMC) was 44% greater in the FCL constructs than in the LP constructs (*P* = 0.01). The box to the left (plate side) of the fracture highlights an area in which callus formation was retarded by preferential construct stiffness in the LP group. In FCL constructs, the medial half of the callus, termed near callus, had the same bone mineral content as the far callus (*P* = 0.91). In other words, callus formation was symmetric. (Reproduced with permission from Bottlang M, Lesser M, Koerber J, et al: Far cortical locking can improve healing of fractures stabilized with locking plates. *J Bone Joint Surg Am* 2010;92[7]:1652-1660.)

theories of fracture mechanics that allow the calculation of the amount of physical energy involved in fracturing a bone by calculating the amount of surface area liberated in the fracture.

Locked Plating and Related Concepts

Locked plating describes fixation systems that couple a plate possessing threaded holes and screws with corresponding terminal threads that allow the screw to lock into the plate when fully advanced. This construct has been mechanically likened to an "internal" external fixator when taken to the extreme of having the fixator itself in exceedingly close proximity to the periosteal surface of the bone. Some of the mechanical benefits imparted by locked plating are better stability in less

dense bone and less allowance of screw toggling within the plate holes, which limits the risk of screw pullout.

Important mechanical considerations arise, however, because the stiffness that can be obtained with locking plates far exceeds that attainable with conventional plate and screw combinations. This potential has led to several loading experiments using cadaver and bone surrogate specimens to better understand the mechanical influence of locking screw placement within a given plate. Plate designs that allow hybrid fixation in which certain holes may be locked and others left free further complicate the mechanics of the fixation construct. Researchers are attempting to fill this gap in knowledge.[22,23]

Recent research in locking plate fixation has begun to question whether such constructs can be made so stiff that they actually impede bone healing[22] (Figure 4). Novel designs and techniques, such as overdrilling the near cortex and using partially threaded screws to produce a far cortical locking construct, have arisen to further manipulate the mechanics of a locking plate construct.[23] Under axial loading, the initial stiffness of far cortical locking constructs has been shown to induce comparable amounts of interfragmentary motion at the near and the far cortex. This fracture-site motion was one order of magnitude greater than that of standard locking plate constructs.

The relative mechanical merits of one locking plate construct over another have not been determined, but there are an exceedingly large number of permutations associated with variations in plate design and surgical technique. This is another area in which biomechanical modeling, including patient-specific modeling, may provide a sensible method to select the best construct to stabilize a fracture and optimize the potential for healing.

Noninvasive Assessment of Mechanical Properties

It is reasonably well known that the mechanical properties of biologic tissues in different disease states often deviate from normal, which frequently leads to screening tests based on physical palpation of the tissue. When performed by a clinician, the tissue of interest is subjected to a manually applied force, and the difference in tissue stiffness is evaluated by subjective touch. Although this practice is reasonably effective, objectively quantifying differences in tissue stiffness (for example, tissue modulus) is highly desirable. In most biomechanical studies, quantitative measurement requires isolating (either excising or surgically exposing) the tissue of interest and physically deforming it in a controlled manner while measuring the applied loads and the actual tissue displacement. In some instances, tissues can be tested in situ using techniques such as mounting strain gauges onto the tissue of interest and directly measuring strain when the tissue is physiologically loaded. Tissue strain also can be measured without direct contact by using videos or photographs of the deformation of a pattern applied to the surface of the tissue in conjunction with image analysis routines to calculate strain. All of these methods require direct access to and visualization of the tissue.

The main advantage of direct physical testing is that measurements are made on the specific tissue of interest in a well-controlled environment and, therefore, provide more repeatable and reliable results. All of these direct physical measurement techniques are highly invasive, meaning that they cannot be routinely made on living patients. The main drawback of these direct measurement techniques is that the tissue is removed from its normal physiologic environment. Because the experimentally applied loads may not perfectly replicate those that occur in vivo, the mechanical data collected are less useful than measurements made under normal physiologic conditions.

Ideally, physical measurements of the mechanical behavior of a tissue would be conducted without altering it in any way (such as removing it from its normal lo-

cation within the body, attaching it to external instrumentation, or by exposing it to the outside environment for direct visualization). The goal of noninvasive mechanical testing has prompted the search for methods of measuring the mechanical behavior of tissues that do not disrupt the native system. One such technique, which is rapidly gaining in popularity, is elastography. This technique has been called "an imaging-based counterpart to palpation."[24]

In elastography, a mechanical stimulus is applied to the tissue of interest. The method of force application can vary in sophistication from a clinician manually pressing on the tissue to ultrasonically applied force or other external loading stimuli. While the tissue is mechanically loaded, images are collected using a noninvasive imaging modality, such as ultrasound, MRI, or optical coherence tomography. The mechanical properties are then calculated using the measured displacements from the imaging and the applied force data.

Micromechanics

It is well recognized that the musculoskeletal system adapts and responds to mechanical stimuli. These adaptive responses take place not at the whole-patient or the tissue levels but at a cellular level by prompting cell differentiation, changing membrane potentials, or activating signaling molecules. In situ, cells are attached to their surrounding matrix material by complex microstructures that alter load transmission from the tissue as a whole and can constrain the possible mechanical response of the cell itself. For example, in cartilage, chondrocytes are attached to cartilage via a complex of pericellular collagen fibrils that are oriented differently from the normal zonal distribution of collagen fibrils in the different layers of cartilage.[25] Macroscopic tissue mechanical behavior is not necessarily indicative of the mechanical environment that develops inside or immediately adjacent to cells.

Mechanical study at the microscopic level requires alternative tools and methodologies. Whereas the mechanical stiffness of a tendon or a piece of cartilage can be directly measured in simple benchtop studies using the assumption that the tissue acts as a continuum (it is continuously distributed and fills the region of space it occupies), accurate microscopic mechanical analysis requires incorporating information about the detailed microscopic structure of the tissue. A continuum assumption is no longer valid, and characteristics such as cell density, collagen fiber orientation, fluid permeability, and electrical charge density must be included in the mechanical evaluation. Advances in imaging methods and computer and materials science technology have made it possible to study the specific mechanical changes that cause adaptive tissue response at the microscopic and/or single-cell level.

Like any other material, cell membranes, cytoskeletal filaments, mitochondria, nuclei, and collagen fibers will mechanically deform under load. The mechanical study of these tissue and cellular components requires substantially different techniques than those traditionally applied to whole bones and tissues. The three main methods for evaluating microscopic mechanics are (1) analysis of microscope images, (2) computational modeling and submodeling, and (3) direct physical testing at or below the microscale. In imaging-based methods, displacements and deformations of cells or tissue components under load are recorded using a microscope. Strain behavior is calculated from microscopic measurements of deformation.[26,27] Microscopic computational modeling uses traditional mechanical evaluation techniques, such as finite element analysis; however, the mechanical history of output from a macroscopic finite element tissue model serves only as input for a submodel of one or more cells or tissue regions, with highly detailed mechanical property definitions and features such as aligned collagen fiber reinforcement. Direct measurement methods use microscopic testing methods such as nanoindentation, micropipetting plus mathematical modeling, or atomic force microscopy.[28,29]

These types of methods have made it possible to measure mechanical behavior at the level of a single cell. For example, chondrocyte deformation appears to be time dependent, with an initial rapid deformation under applied loading followed by a prolonged recovery period to the initial state after removal of the load.[26,28] Static load application causes a decrease in proteoglycan production, whereas dynamic compression causes increased proteoglycan production.[30] Chondrocytes appear to be more tolerant of compressive strain and are likely to be damaged by high tangential strains.[31] With the confluence of mechanics and biology that is so critical to orthopaedics, it is likely that these types of micromechanical studies will become more common and begin to explain tissue response to load on a more mechanistic level.

Translating Biomechanics Into Clinical Applications

Developments in biomechanics are being translated into new clinical applications in orthopaedics through various methods. A direct example of incorporating these new developments occurs when mechanical modeling and knowledge gained from physical testing provide insights into the likelihood of clinical success. In other instances, the risks for surgical complications are reduced based on biomechanical studies of optimal implant positioning, or mechanical unloading from joint distraction is proposed for the treatment of end-stage osteoarthritis. Patient-specific treatment and planning is beginning to reshape the way in which orthopaedics is practiced.

Mechanical Testing to Gain Insight in Fracture Treatment

Over the years, physical testing has provided a valuable tool to help surgeons differentiate between the performances of fracture fixation constructs. When done

well, this approach provides understanding about new fixation devices and application scenarios in relation to familiar clinical situations and promotes the adoption of new technologies with minimal risk to the patient. Laboratory mechanical assessment uses tight experimental control to answer specific mechanical questions, whereas there is little control in clinical assessments. For example, using laboratory testing, a given screw-plate construct can be definitively shown to be more or less stiff than another construct. However, mechanical testing is limited by its inability to predict the ideal mechanical environment for a given fracture and patient.

By more tightly connecting mechanical testing with animal testing and noninvasive imaging, researchers have achieved greater success in providing clinical understanding and mechanical insights. These advances often rely on the creation of new, objective measurement strategies, which can replace former subjective and categorical scoring methods. In a study involving locking plate fixation, the use of new methods to characterize callus formation over time after an experimental fracture in a sheep model clearly showed that far cortical locking enhanced symmetric callus formation.[23]

Optimal Implant Positioning to Reduce Complications

Proper positioning of total joint arthroplasty hardware is crucial for long-term implant survival. Accurate positioning ensures that loading occurs only on the portions of the implant designed to articulate with the opposing hardware components and guarantees a load distribution that is uniform and as low as possible. Implants loaded in configurations other than those intended for the specific implant design tend to develop high stresses and/or point loading conditions. This can cause implant loosening because of increased underlying bony stresses or implant damage from stresses that exceed the yield stress of the implant material. Typically, more constrained implant designs (for example, highly constrained fixed rotational axis total ankle implants versus the lightly constrained ball-and-socket hip implants) are more susceptible to damage when implanted in an improper position.

Surgical implantation of arthroplasty hardware is becoming progressively more challenging as patients opt for surgeries that minimize surgical exposure and as implant companies develop more specialized hardware designs. Advances in implant hardware have focused on restoring physiologic motion using more complex geometries and patient- or gender-specific designs. More complex implant geometry requires the axes of the implant to be aligned at specific angles relative to the native anatomy of the joint; however, the minimized surgical exposure makes it difficult (if not impossible) for the surgeon to directly visualize the anatomic landmarks required to accurately implant arthroplasty hardware. Although advances in computer-aided surgery have improved implantation accuracy, these systems are expensive and are not available in every location where joint arthroplasty is performed. It is

1: Principles of Orthopaedics

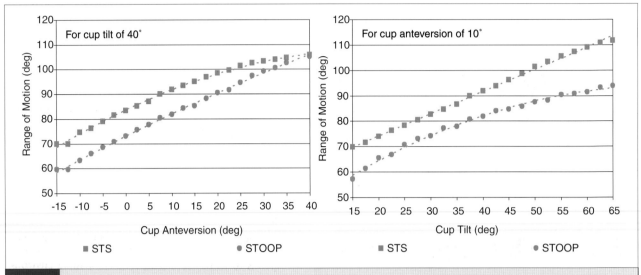

| Figure 5 | Range of motion at incipient impingement for both sit-to-stand (STS) and stooping (STOOP) dislocation challenges for (A) 40° of cup tilt as function of cup anteversion and (B) for 10° of cup anteversion as a function of cup tilt. (Reproduced with permission from Elkins JM: Biomechanics of Failure Modalities in Total Hip Arthroplasty. PhD Dissertation, The University of Iowa, 2013, p. 74.) |

recommended that a surgeon try to position the implant in a safe zone and assume that the implantation error around that location is small enough to achieve implant safety.

Safe zones can be physically tested by parametrically varying the position of implant hardware in a cadaver joint and determining the effects of the positions on implant stress. Finite element studies have made it possible to investigate a much wider parameter space, and increasing computational speed has allowed for large-scale, statistically based computer simulations (for example, Monte Carlo simulations) of the effects of implant positioning. Both cadaver and model-based studies have shown that relatively small deviations in implant version or rotation increases contact stress sufficiently to exceed the yield stress of polyethylene.[32-34] Within the same joint, the safe zone for arthroplasty hardware is a function of hardware design, joint loading activity, and patient factors such as obesity or mechanical alignment.[34-37] Therefore, what is safe for one implant design during a specific kinematic challenge (for example, walking) is not necessarily safe for other implant hardware designs or kinematic challenges (for example, standing from a sitting position).

Advanced bearing surface implants, specifically metal-on-metal implants and ceramic implants, rely on highly precise matching between the different components to preserve a microscopic lubricating fluid layer between the components. Clearance between femoral and acetabular components is ideally 100 to 200 μm in metal-on-metal implants, which is much tighter than the clearance between metal and polyethylene components. Implant malalignment that causes gapping between the components or causes the femoral neck to impinge on the edge of the cup and lever the head out of the acetabular cup will destroy the thin lubricating

layer and cause implant stresses above the yield stress of the metal. Two recent studies used finite element analysis of metal-on-metal hip bearing surfaces during a variety of kinematic challenges and with a variety of acetabular cup designs.[35,36] When the implant design or the kinematics changed, the safe zone also changed (Figure 5). This finding illustrates the challenges involved in defining an optimal implant location.

Patient-Specific Treatment and Planning

It might be reasonably argued that orthopaedic surgeons have been classifying bodies, joints, bones, and other factors into contrived groupings for many years in an attempt to cope with the complex variation in anatomy and biomechanical scenarios presented in orthopaedics. The advent of patient-specific analysis has presented innovative opportunities for analyzing and planning treatment. With advances in rapid prototyping capabilities, custom implants and patient-specific cutting guides for joint arthroplasty are now being offered by several major orthopaedic implant manufacturers.

Patient-specific analysis methods are also being used in preoperative surgical planning. The mechanical implications of nonsurgical and surgical treatment decisions can be analyzed within the context of an individual patient and a contemplated procedure. For example, in the prescription of orthotics, the widespread availability of thin, pressure-sensitive sheets has led some orthotic manufacturing companies to offer in-store evaluations of foot-floor pressure. Customized prescriptions for shoe orthotics are then made based on the sensor readings, with the objective of reducing foot-floor pressure. Techniques dating back to Ilizarov's use of external fixation frames to lengthen bone and correct malalignment are being changed by new technology. Surgeons are now aided by computerized systems that guide adjustments to a frame to achieve proper limb length and correct malalignment.[38]

Summary

As the scientific field of musculoskeletal biomechanics continues to evolve, its role in orthopaedic practice also continues to grow and change. Advances in computational power and medical imaging are making patient-specific consideration of biomechanics a reality, with implications in orthopaedic treatment, implant design, and patient rehabilitation.

Key Study Points

As assessment and modeling capabilities advance, patient-specific treatment and planning concepts are beginning to reshape the way in which orthopaedics is practiced.

- Using motion capture and computer modeling, prescribed gait modifications can be optimized to a specific patient rather than giving the patient generic instructions about a movement modification to achieve a particular mechanical goal.

- Other treatment considerations can be analyzed on a patient- and case-specific basis. Examples include assessing fracture risk based on a patient's specific bone density and architecture, planning a complex pelvic osteotomy aimed at improving femoral head coverage, and making joint replacement implant (and implantation) choices based on specific mechanical considerations.

- In the case of fixation planning, patient-specific biomechanical modeling offers opportunities to assess the relative structural merits of one fixation construct over another, including decisions about which holes in a plate need to be filled with which screws for a given fracture. This can then provide guidance in selecting the best construct to stabilize a fracture and optimize the potential for healing.

Annotated References

1. O'Keefe RJ, Jacobs JJ, Chu CR, Einhorn TA: *Orthopaedic Basic Science: Foundations of Clinical Practice*, ed 4. Rosemont, IL, American Academy of Orthopaedic Surgeons, 2007.

2. Bottlang M, Fitzpatrick DC, Augat P: *Orthopaedic Knowledge Update*, ed 10. Rosemont, IL, American Academy of Orthopaedic Surgeons, 2011, pp 59-72.

This chapter provides excellent information on musculoskeletal biomechanics along with additional background information on the topic.

3. Cole JH, van der Meulen MC: Whole bone mechanics and bone quality. *Clin Orthop Relat Res* 2011;469(8): 2139-2149.

This review article, based on a thorough search of the current literature, describes the current understanding of the relationships between bone quality and mechanical competence.

4. Chen JH, Liu C, You L, Simmons CA: Boning up on Wolff's law: Mechanical regulation of the cells that make and maintain bone. *J Biomech* 2010;43(1): 108-118.

This article describes the latest understanding of mechanobiology and the ways in which bone likely senses and responds to its day-to-day mechanical loading environment.

5. Mulvihill BM, Prendergast PJ: Mechanobiological regulation of the remodelling cycle in trabecular bone and possible biomechanical pathways for osteoporosis. *Clin Biomech (Bristol, Avon)* 2010;25(5):491-498.

The authors discuss the mechanoregulation of bone at the trabecular level, with an emphasis on the formulation of computational theories to explain phenomena.

6. Srinivasan S, Weimer DA, Agans SC, Bain SD, Gross TS: Low-magnitude mechanical loading becomes osteogenic when rest is inserted between each load cycle. *J Bone Miner Res* 2002;17(9):1613-1620.

7. Wong BL, Sah RL: Effect of a focal articular defect on cartilage deformation during patello-femoral articulation. *J Orthop Res* 2010;28(12):1554-1561.

Experiments aimed at exploring the local mechanical environment near focal articular defects of the patellofemoral joint are described.

8. Ledet EH, D'Lima D, Westerhoff P, Szivek JA, Wachs RA, Bergmann G: Implantable sensor technology: From research to clinical practice. *J Am Acad Orthop Surg* 2012;20(6):383-392.

This review article describes ways in which implantable sensor technologies have evolved and can be used to provide exquisitely accurate in vivo data unique to a given patient.

9. Kinney AL, Besier TF, Silder A, Delp SL, D'Lima DD, Fregly BJ: Changes in in vivo knee contact forces through gait modification. *J Orthop Res* 2013;31(3): 434-440.

The authors describe experiments using gait analysis to identify and modify mechanically unfavorable walking patterns in patients with knee osteoarthritis.

10. Chang A, Hayes K, Dunlop D, et al: Hip abduction moment and protection against medial tibiofemoral osteoarthritis progression. *Arthritis Rheum* 2005;52(11): 3515-3519.

11. Vincent KR, Conrad BP, Fregly BJ, Vincent HK: The pathophysiology of osteoarthritis: A mechanical perspective on the knee joint. *PM R* 2012;4(5, suppl):S3-S9.

    The authors explore the premise that unfavorable knee kinematics may contribute to the onset and/or progression of knee osteoarthritis. Changing pathologic joint mechanics with gait modification may have disease-modifying potential for medial compartment knee osteoarthritis by slowing disease progression.

12. Maulucci RA, Eckhouse RH: A real-time auditory feedback system for retraining gait. *Conf Proc IEEE Eng Med Biol Soc* 2011;2011:5199-5202.

    A new audio feedback system used with stroke patients to provide real-time feedback about gait characteristics is described. The device was tested in a small series of stroke patients and was found to be well tolerated.

13. Hunt MA, Simic M, Hinman RS, Bennell KL, Wrigley TV: Feasibility of a gait retraining strategy for reducing knee joint loading: Increased trunk lean guided by real-time biofeedback. *J Biomech* 2011;44(5):943-947.

    The authors describe a gait retraining strategy in which normal individuals were asked to walk with increasing degrees of lateral trunk lean. Increasing lateral trunk lean was shown to decrease knee adduction moment.

14. Noyes FR, Dunworth LA, Andriacchi TP, Andrews M, Hewett TE: Knee hyperextension gait abnormalities in unstable knees: Recognition and preoperative gait retraining. *Am J Sports Med* 1996;24(1):35-45.

15. Foucher KC, Hurwitz DE, Wimmer MA: Relative importance of gait vs. joint positioning on hip contact forces after total hip replacement. *J Orthop Res* 2009;27(12):1576-1582.

16. Simic M, Hunt MA, Bennell KL, Hinman RS, Wrigley TV: Trunk lean gait modification and knee joint load in people with medial knee osteoarthritis: The effect of varying trunk lean angles. *Arthritis Care Res (Hoboken)* 2012;64(10):1545-1553.

    Modifications in trunk lean were used to reduce medial compartment knee loading in 22 participants with medial knee osteoarthritis.

17. Noehren B, Scholz J, Davis I: The effect of real-time gait retraining on hip kinematics, pain and function in subjects with patellofemoral pain syndrome. *Br J Sports Med* 2011;45(9):691-696.

    The authors describe the effects of a gait retraining program designed to reduce hip adduction in runners. The particular gait modification proved effective in reducing patellofemoral pain in the runners studied.

18. Fregly BJ, Reinbolt JA, Rooney KL, Mitchell KH, Chmielewski TL: Design of patient-specific gait modifications for knee osteoarthritis rehabilitation. *IEEE Trans Biomed Eng* 2007;54(9):1687-1695.

19. Melton LJ III, Riggs BL, Keaveny TM, et al: Structural determinants of vertebral fracture risk. *J Bone Miner Res* 2007;22(12):1885-1892.

20. Anderson DD, Van Hofwegen C, Marsh JL, Brown TD: Is elevated contact stress predictive of post-traumatic osteoarthritis for imprecisely reduced tibial plafond fractures? *J Orthop Res* 2011;29(1):33-39.

    This study showed the value of a patient-specific approach to relating postoperative contact stress exposure (associated with residual fracture incongruity) with the development of posttraumatic arthritis.

21. Thomas TP, Anderson DD, Mosqueda TV, et al: Objective CT-based metrics of articular fracture severity to assess risk for posttraumatic osteoarthritis. *J Orthop Trauma* 2010;24(12):764-769.

    The authors describe a CT-based methodology for objectively quantifying fracture severity. A 100% success rate in predicting posttraumatic arthritis after tibial plafond intra-articular fractures based on severity was reported.

22. Bottlang M, Doornink J, Lujan TJ, et al: Effects of construct stiffness on healing of fractures stabilized with locking plates. *J Bone Joint Surg Am* 2010;92(suppl 2):12-22.

    This provocative study raises the question of whether a mechanical construct with locking plates may be so stiff that it impedes fracture healing. Methods are introduced to relate callus formation assessed on radiographs with the mechanical loading environment of the bone.

23. Bottlang M, Lesser M, Koerber J, et al: Far cortical locking can improve healing of fractures stabilized with locking plates. *J Bone Joint Surg Am* 2010;92(7):1652-1660.

    This article introduces a novel locking plate construct design that provides greater control over construct stiffness than is afforded by a locking plate alone. The concept of optimizing the plate construct stiffness to best promote fracture healing is addressed.

24. Mariappan YK, Glaser KJ, Ehman RL: Magnetic resonance elastography: A review. *Clin Anat* 2010;23(5):497-511.

    The authors review magnetic resonance elastography, including details about the specific mechanical, imaging, and analysis steps. Several applications for elastography and examples of the results are presented.

25. Korhonen RK, Herzog W: Depth-dependent analysis of the role of collagen fibrils, fixed charges and fluid in the pericellular matrix of articular cartilage on chondrocyte mechanics. *J Biomech* 2008;41(2):480-485.

26. Abusara Z, Seerattan R, Leumann A, Thompson R, Herzog W: A novel method for determining articular cartilage chondrocyte mechanics in vivo. *J Biomech* 2011;44(5):930-934.

    A setup is described for evaluating the deformation of individual chondrocytes in situ in a mouse knee when the knee is physiologically loaded. The system allowed the measurement of time-dependent deformation and recovery of chondrocyte shape under loading.

27. Upton ML, Gilchrist CL, Guilak F, Setton LA: Transfer of macroscale tissue strain to microscale cell regions in

the deformed meniscus. *Biophys J* 2008;95(4):2116-2124.

28. Zhang QY, Wang XH, Wei XC, Chen WY: Characterization of viscoelastic properties of normal and osteoarthritic chondrocytes in experimental rabbit model. *Osteoarthritis Cartilage* 2008;16(7):837-840.

29. Luo S, Shi Q, Zha Z, et al: Morphology and mechanics of chondroid cells from human adipose-derived stem cells detected by atomic force microscopy. *Mol Cell Biochem* 2012;365(1-2):223-231.

    The authors describe a biochemical and mechanical evaluation of chondrocytes and two chondrocyte precursors. Atomic force microscopy was used to directly measure cell stiffness, which proved to be highly dependent on cytoskeletal arrangement.

30. Moo EK, Herzog W, Han SK, Abu Osman NA, Pingguan-Murphy B, Federico S: Mechanical behaviour of in-situ chondrocytes subjected to different loading rates: A finite element study. *Biomech Model Mechanobiol* 2012;11(7):983-993.

    This article describes a multiscale finite element model that was used to investigate strain rate effects on chondrocyte viability. Based on the correlation between strain rates calculated in the model and impact-related cell death, the authors speculate that tangential strain is related to cell death.

31. Korhonen RK, Julkunen P, Wilson W, Herzog W: Importance of collagen orientation and depth-dependent fixed charge densities of cartilage on mechanical behavior of chondrocytes. *J Biomech Eng* 2008;130(2):021003.

32. Fukuda T, Haddad SL, Ren Y, Zhang LQ: Impact of talar component rotation on contact pressure after total ankle arthroplasty: A cadaveric study. *Foot Ankle Int* 2010;31(5):404-411.

    The authors describe a cadaver investigation of the effects of implant alignment on contact stresses in total ankle arthroplasty hardware. Malaligned hardware components caused point contact, increased contact stress, and increased rotational torque, all of which have the potential for increasing implant wear.

33. Espinosa N, Walti M, Favre P, Snedeker JG: Misalignment of total ankle components can induce high joint contact pressures. *J Bone Joint Surg Am* 2010;92(5):1179-1187.

    A parametric, finite element model-based investigation of the effects of implant alignment on contact stresses in total ankle arthroplasty hardware is presented. The models, which were physically validated, indicated that contact stress was particularly sensitive to implant version.

34. Li YJ, Yang GJ, Zhang LC, Cai CY, Wu LJ: Influences of head/neck ratio and femoral antetorsion on the safe-zone of operative acetabular orientations in total hip arthroplasty. *Chin J Traumatol* 2010;13(4):206-211.

    A kinematic model of total hip arthroplasty hardware was used to investigate implantation configurations that allowed for specific ranges of hip motion. The effects of head-to-neck ratio were investigated, and a greater head-to-neck ratio was found to provide larger implantation safe zones.

35. Elkins JM, Kruger KM, Pedersen DR, Callaghan JJ, Brown TD: Edge-loading severity as a function of cup lip radius in metal-on-metal total hips—a finite element analysis. *J Orthop Res* 2012;30(2):169-177.

    This article describes a large-scale, parametric, finite element model-based investigation of several hardware design parameters involving range of motion without impingement for metal-on-metal arthroplasty hardware. The results indicate the possibility that severe edge scraping may occur with various hardware geometry and implant orientations.

36. Elkins JM, O'Brien MK, Stroud NJ, Pedersen DR, Callaghan JJ, Brown TD: Hard-on-hard total hip impingement causes extreme contact stress concentrations. *Clin Orthop Relat Res* 2011;469(2):454-463.

    The authors describe a large-scale, parametric, finite element model-based investigation of the effect of implant positioning on impingement and subluxation events in metal-on-metal and ceramic-on-ceramic arthroplasty hardware. In some implantation configurations, impingement stresses exceeded material failure strengths, and scraping wear could be expected in these hard-on-hard bearings in certain implantation configurations.

37. Lombardi AV Jr, Berend KR, Ng VY: Neutral mechanical alignment: A requirement for successful TKA affirms. *Orthopedics* 2011;34(9):e504-e506.

    The authors present a review of several previous studies and discuss the ongoing debate about optimal positioning for total knee arthroplasty hardware. They conclude that there is no compelling reason to deviate from a generic safe zone because targeting that range minimized gross malalignment.

38. Rogers MJ, McFadyen I, Livingstone JA, Monsell F, Jackson M, Atkins RM: Computer hexapod assisted orthopaedic surgery (CHAOS) in the correction of long bone fracture and deformity. *J Orthop Trauma* 2007;21(5):337-342.

Chapter 6

Bearing Surface Materials for Hip and Knee Replacement

Brett R. Levine, MD, MS   Kern Singh, MD   Joshua J. Jacobs, MD

Introduction

Current joint arthroplasty implants have excellent long-term survival in hip and knee arthroplasty. As component designs have evolved, a major emphasis has been placed on improving articular bearing surface wear. Since the development of the first artificial joint arthroplasties, many materials have been used for bearing surfaces in hopes of replicating the complex environment and the biomechanics of the human body. These materials include polytetrafluoroethylene, ultra-high–molecular weight polyethylene (UHMWPE), ceramics, cobalt-chromium alloys, and highly cross-linked polyethylene (HXLPE).

To understand bearing surfaces and wear properties, it is necessary to understand the associated terminology (Table 1). A typical human joint will maintain a low coefficient of friction (ranging from 0.002 to 0.04) because of the favorable lubrication properties of articular cartilage. The goal of joint arthroplasty is to recreate the process of elastohydrodynamic lubrication (the lubricant properties determine the coefficient of friction because a constant film separates the surfaces) while minimizing the amount of time that the bearing surfaces come into direct contact with one another. Historically, replacement articulations have been limited to boundary lubrication, in which the forces involved with joint loading create a local milieu whereby the synovial fluid does not fully separate the bearing surfaces. The process of articular surface wear in total joint arthroplasty is initiated and can be accelerated by lapses of sufficient lubrication.

The process of surface wear involves five well-described mechanisms (adhesion, abrasion, third body, fatigue, and corrosion). The four classic wear modes describe the condition of the prosthesis at the time that articular wear occurs.[1] Mode 1 wear occurs when two bearing surfaces that are intended to be in contact undergo wear. Mode 2 wear describes wear generation in the setting of a primary bearing surface articulating with an unintended secondary surface (for example, polyethylene wear-through of a modular acetabular component). Mode 3 wear refers to the generation of third-body wear in which scratched surfaces may accelerate mode 1 wear rates. Mode 4 wear occurs when two secondary surfaces come in contact, such as backside wear, fretting, and taper junction mechanically assisted crevice corrosion. The material properties of the bearing surface have a substantial effect on the wear properties of a particular articulation.[2,3]

The issue of bearing surface wear has dominated joint arthroplasty research over the past two decades. The mechanisms and patterns of wear, the pathophysiology of osteolysis, and the effect of particulate debris on local tissues and surface lubrication have been extensively studied. Regardless of the specific joint, some level of bearing surface wear occurs in all articular couples. There are three broad categories of variables that affect articular wear: design (materials, geometry, and manufacture), environmental (bony structure, weight, and activity level), and combined variables (component position, surgical technique, and third-body interactions).[4] The design goals for a successful articular surface are minimizing contact stresses, balancing the amount of contact area and constraint, maintaining an acceptable range of motion, and encouraging fluid-film lubrication. Despite the most well-conceived designs, arthroplasty wear performance is often compromised by factors such as impingement, third-body damage, and the breakdown of lubricating surfaces. Similarly, the manufacturing process must be precise because mismatches in the congruency of articular couples can lead to early run-in wear; poor locking mechanisms and roughened surfaces can cause backside wear. It is important to minimize wear debris to decrease local damage from particulate-induced osteolysis and adverse local tissue reactions.

Dr. Levine or an immediate family member serves as a paid consultant to or is an employee of DePuy, Johnson & Johnson, and Zimmer; has received research or institutional support from Biomet and Zimmer; and serves as a board member, owner, officer, or committee member of the American Academy of Orthopaedic Surgeons. Dr. Singh or an immediate family member has received royalties from Pioneer and Zimmer and serves as a paid consultant to or is an employee of DePuy, Stryker, and Zimmer. Dr. Jacobs or an immediate family member has stock or stock options held in Implant Protection and has received research or institutional support from Medtronic Sofamor Danek, Nuvasive, and Zimmer.

Table 1

Tribologic Terminology

Term	Definition
Hardness	The ability to resist plastic deformation at the articular surface. A higher number indicates a harder surface. Surface treatments (ion implantation, polishing, or nitriding) can alter the hardness of a material. Common scales include Mohs, Rockwell, Vickers, and Brinell.
Scratch resistance	Related to the hardness of a material. For example, the scratch resistance of ceramic > cobalt-chromium > titanium.
Friction	The resistance to movement as two materials are in contact and relative motion. The concept of lubrication is to lower the frictional resistance to movement.
Surface roughness (R_a)	The average of the absolute value of the measured heights of deviation from the center line along the material's surface (the average of peaks and valleys along the surface). The surface roughness of articular surfaces are 0.03 μm to 0.10 μm under normal conditions but can increase 2 to 3 times (UHMWPE can increase 10-fold) with scratches and wear-related conditions.
Hydrodynamic lubrication	This occurs when articulating surfaces are fully separated by a lubricant. The viscosity of the lubricant is important to the motion of the surfaces.
Boundary lubrication	This occurs when surfaces are not fully separated because there is a very thin and surface-adherent layer between the bearings. Higher friction and wear rates are noted.
Elastohydrodynamic lubrication	The bearing surface elastically deforms, allowing the relative articulations to deform and stay congruous without plastic deformation. Low wear rates and coefficient of frictions are noted, but subsurface fatigue may be an issue.
Weeping lubrication	This occurs when one surface is porous; the elastohydrodynamic lubrication can be augmented by fluid expressed from a deforming surface. Important in articular cartilage lubrication.
Wettability	This is the ability of a surface to be wetted when in contact with a liquid (theta angle is the contact angle between the liquid drop and the solid). It is determined by adhesive and cohesive forces.
Surface tension	A property of liquids that allows the surface to support light objects/external forces. It affords the ability of a drop of water to form a spheric shape.
Viscoelasticity	The simultaneous exhibition of both viscous and elastic behaviors in a material. Such materials (plastics, not ceramics or metals) display a time-dependent behavior when a load is applied in regard to flow or creep.

Bearing Surfaces

Conventional UHMWPE

Prior to being supplanted by alternative bearing surfaces, conventional UHMWPE bearing surfaces dominated the arthroplasty market. Polyethylene is a two-phase polymer fashioned from chains of ethylene (C_2H_4) molecules organized into areas of crystalline lamella interspersed with amorphous matrix.[5] The crystalline lamella are connected to one another via tie molecules, which provide additional strength and a means for load transfer. The typical physical properties of UHMWPE used in orthopaedic applications are molecular weight, 2 to 6 million g/mole; melting temperature, 125° to 138°; tensile modulus of elasticity, 0.8 to 1.6 GPa; ultimate tensile strength, 39 to 48 MPa; and degree of crystallinity, 39% to 75%. Most UHMWPE components are fabricated from sheets or bars of GUR 1020 or GUR 1050 polyethylene resin treated with direct compression molding, hot isostatic pressing, or ram extrusion.

To summarize an important tribology concept, maximal contact stress is lowered when the modulus of elasticity of UHMWPE is decreased, thickness is increased, and the articular surface is more conforming.[6] The properties of UHMWPE have become more consistent because of the adoption of standardized sterilization techniques.

Seven classic patterns of wear damage have been described for UHMWPE surfaces: embedded debris, scratching, pitting, burnishing, surface deformation, abrasion, and delamination[7] (Figure 1). Examples of embedded debris are cement and/or metal fragments pressed into the UHMWPE, whereas scratching refers to indented lines in the direction of principal motion of the articulating components.[7] Pitting describes small, irregular areas of depression on the bearing surface, and burnishing refers to areas that visually appear to be polished. Surface deformation occurs via creep or cold flow and leads to permanent deformation of the bearing surface. Wear caused by abrasion has a more shredded appearance, as might be seen with third-body wear. Delamination is the subsurface failure of UHMWPE and is seen as polyethylene flaking.[7]

Standard UHMWPE was the gold standard for bearing surfaces in the 1970s through the 1990s. Many

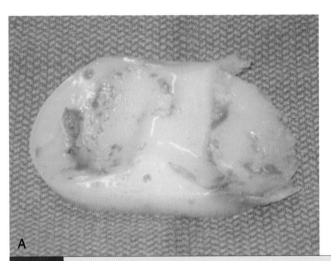 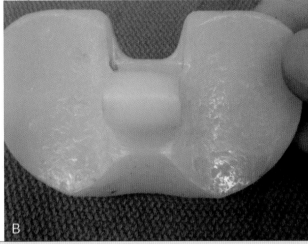

| Figure 1 | **A,** Demonstrations of clear areas of delamination and fatigue failure as significant portions of the polyethylene insert have been completely destroyed. **B,** Diffuse pitting of the surface is seen on this retrieved polyethylene liner. |

long-term follow-up studies reported good results in terms of wear and osteolysis, which were the primary concerns for limiting implant longevity[8-17] (Table 2).

Applications in Total Knee Arthroplasty

In total knee arthroplasties (TKAs) performed in the United States, the only available alternative surface for articulation is a derivative of UHMWPE. Polyethylene is used for the tibiofemoral surfaces and in resurfacing the patella. Tibial and patellar all-polyethylene components are available, but the evolution of TKA drove the development of metal-backed and modular components. The major drawback of these advances was that metal-backed components led to the use of thinner UHMWPE (which was catastrophic in some patella designs) and the potential for backside wear in modular tibial components. In addition, mobile-bearing component options exist in which the tibial articular surface is highly congruent with the femoral condyles to reduce contact stresses and maximize the contact area. The forces of increased conformity are offset by the second polyethylene articulation, with the tibial component as a rotating platform or meniscal bearing surface option. Several factors may affect the wear characteristics of polyethylene bearing surfaces in TKA, including the method of manufacture, articular surface geometry, modularity, ligamentous balancing, UHMWPE oxidation, limb alignment, and motion pattern. The multifactorial nature of polyethylene wear makes it difficult to model with computers and wear simulators.[18] Periimplant particulate-induced osteolysis has been reported to account for 25% of TKA revisions.

The manufacturing processes for UHMWPE components are important because a failure of the UHMWPE resin to fuse can introduce defects, which may result in wear damage, cracking, and delamination. Direct compression molding of liners has achieved better clinical results compared with implants machined from extruded bars. Greater levels of pitting and delamination

at the articular surface and backside wear have been reported in machined UHMWPE liners compared with those manufactured using direct compression molding.[18,19]

Articular surface geometry plays a role in wear because contact stresses vary based on the radii of curvature match of the surfaces, physiologic load, and UHMWPE thickness. In TKA liners, the maximal shear stress occurs 1 to 2 mm beneath the articular surface, where the component is weakest and susceptible to fatigue, delamination, and accelerated wear rates.[6] Additional concerns occur with component malalignment and the use of more constrained liners. Added constraint coupled with the motion pattern of directed femoral rollback can lead to tibial post wear and, possibly, fracture.

Metal-backed components were developed to reduce stress at the bone-implant interface and improve loading of the proximal tibia. Despite improved proximal load transfer, there is concern about backside wear because micromotion is often related to the design of the locking mechanism.[20] This motion may lead to burnishing, scratching, and fraying of the locking mechanism and result in wear debris of 0.32 to 0.35 μm.[18] This smaller size particle is associated with a greater volumetric load and adjacent osteolysis. Factors contributing to backside wear include the performance of the locking mechanism, the tibial baseplate surface, implant duration, and the patient's activity level. Radiation treatments to cross-link polyethylene particles, polyethylene doping with antioxidant materials, and alternative bearing surfaces are some of the modifications that have been developed to improve the wear characteristics of conventional UHMWPE.

Applications in Total Hip Arthroplasty

Conventional UHMWPE has been used extensively in total hip arthroplasty (THA) and has achieved excellent long-term results. The articular couple is often the

Table 2

Summary of Conventional UHMWPE Outcomes in THA

Study (Year)	Number of Patients	Average Age (Years)	Average Follow-up (Years)	Outcomes
Crowther and Lachiewicz (2002)[8]	56 Co-Cr	37	11	23% pelvic osteolysis, 0.15 mm/year linear wear rate, increased wear with younger age and better hip scores, and average polyethylene thickness = 7.8 mm
Eggli et al (2002)[9]	89 Co-Cr (49, 22-mm heads; 40, 32-mm heads)	66.5	5.95	Linear wear rate greater in first 2 years (run-in period); average linear wear rate = 0.11 mm/year and 0.15 mm/year for 22-mm and 32-mm heads, respectively
Kim et al (2003)[10]	80 Co-Cr (118 hips)	47	9.8	No aseptic loosening, 12% calcar and 9% acetabular osteolysis, 0.12 mm/year linear wear rate, and average polyethylene thickness = 10.7 mm
Keener et al (2003)[11]	43 Co-Cr	< 50	25	Survivorship of acetabulum at 30 years for aseptic loosening was 72%; no osteolysis data reported
Capello et al (2003)[12]	91 Co-Cr	39	11.25	47% with osteolysis around femoral stem and 12 revisions for polyethylene wear/lysis
McAuley et al (2004)[13]	488 (561 hips)	40	6.9	Average wear rate for patients younger than 50 years was 0.14 mm/year in nonrevised and 0.29 mm/year in revised components; survival for cup for any revision = 97.4%, 87.6%, and 53.8% at 5, 10, and 15 years, respectively
Singh et al (2004)[14]	36 ceramic; 2 Co-Cr	42	10	No osteolysis, cementless cups performed better, and 1 revision for extensive wear
Kearns et al (2006)[15]	221 patients; 191 Co-Cr; 90 ceramic; 18 titanium	41.1	8.4	31 patients (33 hips) revised for polyethylene wear; 24 cases of substantial osteolysis; cup survivorship with revision as end point = 98.7%, 84.6%, and 52.5% at 5, 10, and 15 years, respectively
Burston et al (2010)[16]	47 (58 hips)	39	12	26% of patients with osteolysis in one or more Gruen zones; average wear rate was ≥ 0.21 mm/year for patients younger than 50 years
McLaughlin and Leeo (2011)[17]	79 Co-Cr (94 hips)	36	16 (range, 11-18.5)	1% of cases with distal osteolysis and no aseptic femoral component loosening

Co-Cr = cobalt-chromium.

weak link, requiring revision surgery for wear, osteolysis, and subsequent aseptic loosening[15,21,22] (Figure 2). THA surfaces are inherently highly conforming, with typical clearances of approximately 0.1 mm; however, approximately 100 million microscopic UHMWPE wear particles are generated daily.[23] Finite element models have shown that with perfect conformity, the contact stresses are independent of the modulus of elasticity of UHMWPE; increasing the head size in a fixed shell size reduces the contact stresses; and the stresses are independent of the liner thickness if the head size remains fixed and the inner diameter of the cup is increased.[4] This is important because of the current emphasis on using larger diameter femoral heads to lower dislocation rates. The minimum allowable thickness of the liner is dependent on factors such as wear resistance, locking mechanism design, component orientation (vertical cups exhibit greater edge loading), head diameter, and stiffness of the acetabular component.[24]

Traditionally, wear rates of conventional UHMWPE were reported to be 0.18 mm/year for the first 5 years and then 0.1 mm/year thereafter.[6] Wear rates vary based on the patient's age and activity level, adjacent joint degenerative changes, sterilization techniques, and component positioning and design. Despite wear rates that may limit the long-term success of conventional

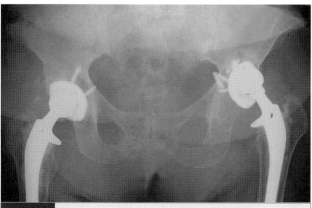

Figure 2 Supine radiograph of the hip showing eccentric polyethylene wear with osteolysis and subsequent failure of the left acetabular component at 15 years postoperatively.

UHMWPE, a recent meta-analysis showed similar outcomes in clinical and radiographic parameters compared with modern metal-on-metal implants.[25] A lower complication rate was reported in the UHMWPE group compared with patients with metal-on-metal implants who had a 3.37 times higher complication rate. A randomized clinical trial comparing conventional UHMWPE and HXLPE reported that there were no differences in cup migration, radiolucencies, or functional scores.[26] The clinical results for conventional UHMWPE in THA over the past 10 years are summarized in Table 2.

In reviewing the outcomes of conventional UHMWPE implants, it is important to consider the variability associated with changes in head size, component manufacturing, sterilization techniques, and femoral head material. Femoral head size is important in the calculation of volumetric wear ($v = \pi r^2 w$, where w = the linear wear rate and r = the radius of the femoral head). Although dislocation rates are reportedly lower with larger diameter heads, in practice it is important to consider the effect of wear, particulate debris generation, and the need for revision surgery when choosing a head size. Several studies support lower linear wear rates with direct compression molding compared with liners machined from extruded bar stock.

The sterilization and packaging of UHMWPE affects wear characteristics and survivorship. Early UHMWPE component designs were irradiated with 2.5 to 4 Mrad in a standard room air environment. The gamma irradiation sterilized the implants while creating intrasubstance free radicals from cleavage of the UHMWPE covalent bonds. These free radicals undergo oxidation in air, which leads to truncation of the large polymer chains and a reduction in fracture strength.[27] Gamma irradiation is now performed in inert environments to achieve the benefits of cross-linking without the deleterious effects of oxidation. Alternatively, diffusion of ethylene oxide gas for sterilization is possible but follows a process that is more than 40 hours in length. Gas plasma surface sterilization takes between 1.2 and 4 hours and functions by oxidizing biologic matter.[27] Increased wear rates have been reported in UHMWPE sterilized via gamma irradiation in air (0.19 mm/year) compared with a gas-plasma technique (0.097 mm/year).[28]

Highly Cross-Linked Polyethylene

Attempts to improve on the longevity of UHMWPE have led to the evolution of HXLPE options in which the components are irradiated to induce higher rates of molecular cross-linking. The amount of radiation and the method of administration have a direct effect on the properties of the polyethylene bearing surface. Radiation doses of 5, 7.5, and 10 Mrad result in improved wear properties as the dose is increased. Beyond 10 Mrad, no further improvements have been noted.[29] Similarly, mechanical properties improve from 5 to 7.5 Mrad and then decrease with elevated doses of irradiation. Advantages of HXLPE include reduced articular and backside wear rates, and greater resistance to surface pitting and delamination.

Applications in TKA

The longevity of TKA is often limited by the bearing surface. Currently, the reported rates of osteolysis after TKAs range from 5% to 20% at approximately 5- to 15-year follow-up.[29] The benefits of decreased wear associated with HXLPE have not been as widely embraced in TKA. The increased contact stresses in TKA have led to concerns related to reduced mechanical properties, including lower resistance to fatigue, fracture, and decreased ductility.[30] The strength of HXLPE can be enhanced by (1) preserving the crystalline structure by annealing the UHMWPE at temperatures below its melting point, with cycles of irradiation and annealing required to quench free radicals; (2) mechanical deformation of UHMWPE below its melting temperature, which mobilizes the crystalline phase and allows quenching of free radicals; and (3) adding scavenger agents for free radicals, with vitamin E being the most commonly used agent.[30]

Beneficial wear rates for the HXLPE liners have been reported in wear stimulation studies under optimal and adverse conditions. In a study using retrieval data from HXLPE bearing surfaces, the predominant modes of surface damage were machine mark loss and abrasion.[31] Patient weight and the conformity of the knee design were important predictors of surface damage. Concerns for mechanical failure and fracture have not been realized at short-term follow-up; however, tibial post fractures have been reported for conventional UHMWPE, and longer follow-up is needed to determine if this incidence will be greater with the diminished fatigue properties of HXLPE.

Applications in THA

The currently available options for THA liners and dual mobility femoral heads are fabricated using various proprietary methods by individual manufacturers. Typically, the process starts with ram-extruded bar

1: Principles of Orthopaedics

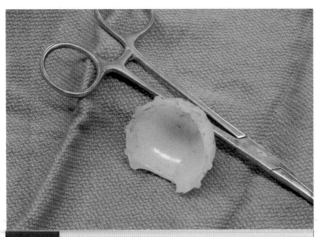

Figure 3 The lip at the rim of an HXLPE liner fractured secondary to a fall and traumatic hip dislocation. The thin cross-section of polyethylene and increased modulus of elasticity of cross-linking may make these liners susceptible to this type of injury.

stock exposed to various doses of radiation, which is then followed by thermal treatment, sterilization, and packaging. It is generally accepted that remelting decreases component strength and annealing leads to elevated oxidation levels.[32] Laboratory studies have shown reduced wear rates for HXLPE femoral heads ranging from 22 to 46 mm compared with conventional polyethylene.[33] This finding has led to the adoption of large-diameter femoral heads (> 36 mm) in THA and the acceptance of thinner polyethylene liners to reduce the rates of dislocation and limb-length discrepancy.

Further laboratory studies using adverse condition testing reported favorable results in the wear of HXLPE compared with conventional UHMWPE. This testing stressed the need for protecting the femoral head intraoperatively and minimizing the potential for third-body wear. Vertically placed acetabular components and malpositioned components leading to impingement can create increased material stress and subsequently fracture thinner HXLPE liners[34-36] (Figure 3).

Relevant clinical studies have shown equivalent functional and pain scores for conventional UHMWPE and HXLPE and substantially lower wear rates for HXLPE at midterm follow-up[20,36-41] (Table 3). Radiostereometric analysis has found wear rates of 0.005 mm/year compared with 0.037mm/year for HXLPE versus conventional UHMWPE, respectively. Overall wear reduction rates of 40% to 80% have been reported.[32] Continued follow-up is necessary to ensure that the trend toward larger diameter femoral heads does not lead to adverse outcomes.

Ceramics

Ceramics are inorganic, chemically stable material structures characterized by high wear and corrosion resistance, strength, biocompatibility, and wettability.

Compared with metal-on-polyethylene bearing surfaces, ceramic surfaces have superior lubrication, smoother surfaces, and are less susceptible to third-body wear. Early designs used in Europe had poor survivorship, with failure rates of 16% to 25% at 10-year follow-up.[42] Material and design concerns centered on high rates of aseptic loosening and ceramic fracture in 3% to 5% of patients.[42] Modern advancements, which have reduced grain size, inclusions, and grain boundaries and improved taper tolerances, provide more successful alumina materials for ceramic-on-ceramic surface bearing options[42-48] (Table 4). Such options are mainly available for THAs, with limited applications in TKA and total disk arthroplasty.

Applications in TKA

Articular surfaces that are not highly conforming may provide limited applications for ceramic bearing surfaces. The use of ceramic prostheses in the knee has been limited by concerns about component fracture. Laboratory studies have reported some success with resisting the forces generated by the knee and lower wear rates in simulator testing.[30] Although not currently in use in the United States, alumina-on-polyethylene components are available in other countries, and a 94% survivorship has been reported at 6-year follow-up.[49] No component fractures have been reported; however, these results many not apply to heavier patient populations.

Other options include alternative ceramicized bearing surfaces, such as oxygen diffusion–hardened zirconium-niobium alloy. This material may be less susceptible to catastrophic failure because it combines the potential advantages of the lower wear rate of ceramics with the strength of a metal core. Wear reduction rates of 85% have been reported in laboratory studies.[50] Early follow-up has shown good results with oxidized zirconium alloy femoral components.[51] Fatigue-related pitting and delamination are wear modes that commonly affect TKA implants, and ceramic materials may not provide an advantage in this regard.

Applications in THA
Alumina-on-Alumina Ceramics
Currently available THA options include ceramic-on-ceramic prostheses made of high-quality alumina materials with a reduced grain size. Modern components are extremely hard, are scratch resistant, maintain a low coefficient of friction, and are hydrophilic with excellent lubrication traits. These properties support the current trend of using larger diameter femoral heads because there is no clinically important increase in wear, and they provide a higher resistance to fracture and less femoral head-liner separation caused by the wettability of the alumina surface.[47] Low wear rates, 95% good or excellent results, minimal osteolysis, and 98% survivorship have been reported at 10-year follow-up using ceramic-on-ceramic bearing surfaces in THA.[52] A randomized trial reported the superiority of ceramic-on-ceramic bearing surfaces over metal-on-polyethylene

Table 3

HXLPE and Conventional UHMWPE Outcomes in THA

Study (Year)	Number of Patients	Wear Rates	Average Follow-up (Years)	Outcomes
Johanson et al[26] (2012)	60 randomized to UHMWPE or HXLPE	HXLPE = 0.005 mm/year UHMWPE = 0.056 mm/year	10	Better results found in patients treated with HXLPE and cemented stems at up to 10 years
Mutimer et al[37] (2010)	122 patients, randomized to UHMWPE or HXLPE and blinded	HXLPE = 0.05 mm/year UHMWPE = 0.26 mm/year	5.5	61 patients in each group, age 45 to 75 years; 7 dislocations and 1 revision for polyethylene wear in UHMWPE group
Calvert et al[36] (2009)	119 patients: 59 HXLPE and 60 UHMWPE	HXLPE = 0.0239 mm/year UHMWPE = 0.1276 mm/year	4	Decreased wear with HXLPE compared with UHMWPE; mean volumetric wear 13.741 mm³/year versus 60.24741 mm³/year, respectively
Bragdon et al[38] (2007)	182 patients (200 hips, HXLPE), retrospective review	0.002mm/year with 28-mm heads 0.026 mm/year with 32-mm heads	25	Survivorship of acetabulum at 30 years for aseptic loosening was 72%; no osteolysis data were reported
Campbell et al[39] (2010)	21 patients, second-generation HXLPE liners, prospective study	0.015 mm/year	2	Low level of wear noted with second-generation HXLPE compared with annealed first-generation HXLPE
Geerdink et al[40] (2009)	48 patients, 23 UHMWPE and 17 moderately cross-linked polyethylene cases analyzed	Moderately cross-linked = 0.088 mm/year UHMWPE = 0.142 mm/year	8	38% reduction in wear sustained over 8-year follow-up; less retroacetabular cyst formation in the moderately cross-lined polyethylene (12%) versus the UHMWPE (39%)
Lachiewicz et al[41] (2009)	146 hips, 90 patients with follow-up, HXLPE	Median linear wear rate = 0.028 mm/year	5.7	No difference in linear wear rate with 36-mm or 40-mm heads, but there was an increase in volumetric wear; caution suggested in using in young or active patients

surfaces, with survivorship based on liner revision of 98% and 91.3%, respectively.[42]

Early enthusiasm for ceramic-on-ceramic bearing surfaces have been tempered by the limited intraoperative options and reports of component fracture, chipping on insertion, and squeaking.[53,54] Because restoring the normal anatomy and hip biomechanics are important considerations in THA, the restricted options are a cause for concern. Fracture risk has been estimated at 1 in 2,000 to 3,000 for ceramic femoral heads and 1 in 6,000 to 8,000 for ceramic acetabular liners.[42] Revision surgery after a fracture requires a thorough synovectomy and complete debris removal. It is suggested that a ceramic ball with a metal sleeve be used with either a new ceramic or polyethylene liner at the time of revision.

Because of the brittle nature of ceramic materials, care is needed during component insertion and impaction; forceful impaction can chip the periphery of the liner and shatter the femoral head.[54] Encasing the ceramic liner within a titanium sleeve eliminates the concern for insertional chipping but may create an area for impingement.

Squeaking has been reported in 0.45% to 7% of patients with alumina-on-alumina bearing surfaces. Squeaking has been linked to the microseparation of

Table 4

Ceramic Outcomes in THA

Study (Year)	Number of Patients	Follow-up Data	Average Follow-up (Years)	Outcomes
Milošev et al[42] (2012)	487 patients MOM = 69 hips, MOP = 200 hips COC = 218 hips	Survival rates: MOP = 98.4% COC = 95.6% MOM = 87.9%	8.5	Survival for MOM was substantially worse than for the other bearing surface types.
Cai et al[43] (2012)	93 patients (113 hips), RCT COC = 51 COP = 62	Greater range of motion (6.1°) with COC larger heads	> 3	Clinical outcomes, complications, and radiographic outcomes similar between groups; only significant difference noted was in range of motion.
Kim et al[44] (2012)	127 THAs, all patients younger than 31 years	No osteolysis, squeaking, or ceramic fractures noted	14.6	Standard improvements in hip scores noted, with excellent longevity with stem and acetabular components.
Synder et al[45] (2012)	220 COC THAs (188 patients)	12-year survival was 86.4% for whole prosthesis	19.6	Very good results in 39.5% and good results in 43.6% of patients.
Chen et al[46] (2012)	413 COC THAs in Asian population	No squeaking identified in any cases	> 2	Four complications but no squeaking-related concerns.
Chevillotte et al[47] (2012)	100 COC THAs	5% incidence of squeaking reported on questionnaire	10	No component malpositioning; all squeaking hips occurred in active, heavy men; no loosening or fractures of the ceramic implants.
Yeung et al[48] (2012)	301 consecutive COC THAs, 244 with 10-year data	2.7% underwent revision surgery; survival rate of implants = 98%	10	95% of patients with excellent or good results, 4 revision for periprosthetic fracture, 1 aseptic femoral loosening, 1 femoral shortening, 2 cup revisions.

MOM = metal-on-metal, MOP = metal-on-polyethylene, COC = ceramic-on-ceramic, RCT = randomized controlled trial, COP = ceramic-on-polyethylene.

the femoral head and liner, which results in stripe wear. This scenario is typically associated with acetabular malpositioning, failure to restore hip biomechanics, and impingement.[53] Retrieval studies have shown that stripe wear and edge loading create the same milieu seen with squeaking in the laboratory (roughened articular surfaces, dry ceramic-on-ceramic articulations, and repeated forced microseparations).

Zirconia Ceramics
The addition of zirconia to alumina ceramic bearings affords a material with better resistance to crack propagation and the ability to dissipate energy. The Biolox delta (CeramTec Ag) is a newer composite ceramic bearing composed of 82% alumina, 17% zirconium oxide, 0.3% chromium oxide, and 0.6% strontium oxide.[42] This newer composite has greater fracture toughness (150%) and burst strength (160%) and maintains the same surface hardness as its alumina predecessors, with availability as a bearing against polyethylene only in the United States.[42] There have been no reported cases of femoral head fracture, and the heads are offered with greater neck length options.

Ceramic-on-Metal Articulations
Combining hard-on-hard bearing materials, the Biolox Forte (CeramTec Ag) alumina femoral heads were tested against high-carbon-wrought cobalt-chromium

alloy acetabular cups in a wear simulator study. A 100-fold decrease in wear with no bedding-in period was reported with the ceramic-on-metal versus the metal-on-metal implants.[55] No damage to the femoral heads was noted, and the surface roughness was unchanged. Because the wear rate appeared to be lower and fewer metal particles were generated, the prevalence of adverse local tissue reactions may be mitigated. A recent study reported substantially lower whole blood metal levels of chromium in ceramic-on-metal bearing materials compared with modern metal-on-metal bearing surfaces.[56] The success of this articulation has not yet been proven, and the risk of head fracture and adverse local tissue reactions has not been thoroughly evaluated.

Ceramic-on-Polyethylene

Both alumina and zirconia ceramic femoral heads with polyethylene liners have been used extensively in THA. Traditionally, the alumina heads had better wear rates and success because of fracture of the zirconia heads. Current studies of ceramic-on-polyethylene bearings have shown mixed results; however, because of the favorable biomaterial properties of ceramic heads, this type of bearing surface has remained an option for younger patients. The risk of fracture of a ceramic femoral head against a polyethylene liner appears to be lower than against a ceramic liner, and it may be more resistant to third-body wear than a cobalt-chromium head.[42]

Metal-on-Metal Implants
Cobalt-Chromium

Most metal-on-metal bearing surfaces use an alloy of cobalt-chromium combined with another element, such as molybdenum, which enhances the alloy by decreasing grain size and increasing strength. Chromium provides corrosion resistance superior to steel. Cobalt-chromium alloys are among the strongest, hardest, and most fatigue resistant metals used for replacement components. Metallic carbides from the carbon strengthen the metal and improve wear resistance.

Titanium

Titanium alloys have superior biocompatibility, strength, fracture toughness, image quality, and corrosion resistance. The ability of titanium to form a titanium dioxide film protects against wear caused by pitting and granular and crevice-type corrosion. Ti6Al4V is an alloy (grade 5 titanium alloy with 6% aluminum and 4% vanadium) that has shown increased fatigue strength and has 20% reduced elasticity to minimize the potential for stress shielding and enhance bone-to-implant load transfer. Titanium alloys have greater strength than stainless steel but have notch sensitivity that can make load-bearing materials more susceptible to cracking and scratching and thus less optimal for use as a bearing surface. Concerns about the passive release of vanadium, a cytotoxic element, have led to the introduction of alternative alloys, including niobium.

Stainless Steel

Stainless steel generally contains iron, carbon, chromium, nickel, and molybdenum. The carbon is in the form of metallic carbides, which are harder than the surrounding material. The addition of molybdenum stabilizes the carbides and provides good strength to the material. The chromium provides the adherent, protective surface oxide layer that maintains its biocompatibility. The mechanical properties of stainless steel exhibit greater ductility with elongation (threefold greater in percentage when compared with other implant metals). The disadvantages of stainless steel are lower biocompatibility and the creation of greater artifact on imaging studies.

New stainless steel alloys are engineered to increase corrosion resistance by using a nickel-free austenitic stainless alloy maintained by high nitrogen content. Nickel-free steel alloys produce higher tensile yield and fatigue strength and greater resistance to pitting and crevice corrosion than nickel-containing steel alloys. Despite these new innovations, stainless steel implants are more susceptible to galvanic and crevice corrosion, which makes them a less attractive option for modular components in total joint arthroplasty. Metal-on-metal implants were used in early THA prostheses but were later abandoned because of the success of UHMWPE and the potential tissue damage from metal debris. Casting in early designs led to large grains and poorly distributed carbides that resulted in irregular surface hardness. Design improvements have resulted in a drastic reduction in wear rates and particulate debris compared with metal-on-polyethylene articulations. Low wear rates are typically observed for metal-on-metal articulations and have been reported in the range of 1-5 μm per year.[57] Low friction and the limited size and concentration of debris in metal-on-metal bearing surfaces allow for improved implant durability[58-62] (Table 5). Under certain conditions (component malposition, hip instability, taper corrosion, lubrication breakdown, and ion hypersensitivity), however, accelerated wear and corrosion can occur with modern metal-on-metal designs.

The AAOS Technology Overview reported on a systematic review of modern metal-on-metal hip implants and made the following conclusions: (1) metal-on-metal THA and resurfacing are at a greater risk for revision than other bearing couples; (2) larger femoral heads and older age are associated with increased rates of revision with metal-on-metal THA; (3) several studies found a correlation between implant alignment and wear rates, local metal debris and adverse local tissue reactions; and (4) metal ion concentrations are elevated in metal-on-metal articulations with an undetermined clinical significance at this time.[63]

Applications in TKA

In the United States, there are no clinical applications for metal-on-metal bearing surfaces in TKA. Although there is ongoing research aimed at improving wear rates and longevity, no implantable metal-on-metal TKA prostheses are currently available.

1: Principles of Orthopaedics

Table 5				
Metal-on-Metal THA Outcomes				
Study (Year)	Number of Patients	Follow-up Data	Average Follow-up (Years)	Outcomes
Bosker et al[58] (2012)	MOM = 120 (119 patients)	39% diagnosed with pseudotumor on CT	3.6	12% revision rate; elevated serum metal ions led to a four times increase in the risk of pseudotumor
Malviya et al[59] (2011)	MOM = 50 MOP = 50	Greater satisfaction with MOM; 20% with MOM had elevated serum ion levels	2	One pseudotumor noted; elevated metal ion levels noted
Nikolaou et al[60] (2011)	MOM = 193 hips (166 patients)	13 hips were revised; metal ion levels increase for first 4 to 5 years	7	10 of 13 revisions caused by a manufacturing defect; otherwise, 98.4% survivorship
Grübl et al[61] (2007)	MOM = 105 hips (98 patients)	Survivorship 98.6%; good results reported	10	No evidence of malignancy or renal failure; no difference in long-term serum metal levels compared with prior follow-up values
Dorr et al[62] (2000)	70 MOM THAs (70 patients)	Mechanical failure rate 2%; no significant osteolysis noted	5.2	Excellent results reported with Harris hip scores; similar to MOP results, with possible wear reduction

MOM = metal-on-metal, MOP = metal-on-polyethylene

Applications in THA

Metal-on-metal bearing surfaces have a decreased rate of wear and increased toughness. This greater level of toughness allows the use of thinner liners within the same cup, affording the use of larger femoral heads and associated potential advantages (favorable clearances and wear rates and reduced dislocation rates). The larger the femoral head, the more likely a fluid-film mode of lubrication will occur and minimize articular surface wear. Additionally, the use of larger femoral heads has spurred the more widespread use of bone-conserving hip resurfacing procedures. One potential complication with the use of large metal heads relates to higher frictional torque and corrosion at the femoral head-neck junction, which may explain the problems seen more frequently with metal-on-metal THAs than with resurfacing procedures. Such complications with MOM THAs have been trunion corrosion (aka trunionosis), pseudotumor formation, component fatigue fractures, aseptic loosening, and dislocation related to local tissue destruction. Alternatively, in the AAOS Technology Overview, it was found that with hip resurfacing, the larger the femoral head the lower the risk of such complications.[63]

Despite early enthusiasm, metal-on-metal THAs have been the subject of recent controversy because of the rising rates of catastrophic failure in several metal-on-metal components. THA constructs using mono-block cobalt-chromium acetabular components have come under scrutiny because of complications associated with poor implant fixation, possible insertional deformation, and unacceptably high rates of early failure. These problems have led to the recall of many metal-on-metal THA and surface replacement devices. Although patients treated with conventional metal-on-polyethylene THAs have elevated metal levels from taper junction corrosion, these values may be increased with metal-on-metal devices because of the added wear at the articular surface.[64,65] In a well-functioning THA, serum metal levels tend to increase early, peak at 4 to 5 years after implantation, and then decrease to a steady-state level.[66] Elevated serum metal levels may accumulate at distant organs but have not been shown to be carcinogenic in patients with metal-on-metal devices. Serum metal levels are associated with transplacental transfer and are present in the milk of nursing mothers but have not been linked to teratogenic effects.[67,68]

Metallic debris is generated at a greater level in THAs when there is negative clearance because of component deformation on insertion, component malpositioning, aseptic loosening, or poor component design. Subsequent accumulation can occur and result in adverse local tissue reactions (**Figure 4**). Such reactions may cover a wide spectrum of presentations, ranging from a small fluid collection to a massive destructive le-

1: Principles of Orthopaedics

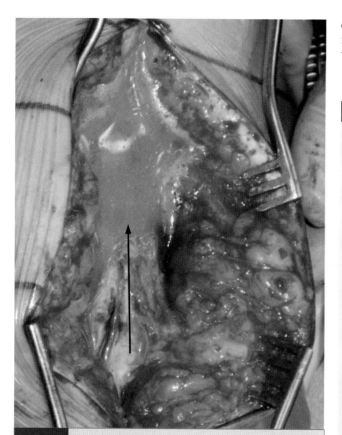

Figure 4 Photograph of an adverse local tissue reaction related to a failed metal-on-metal THA. Note the significant amount of purulent-like fluid at the top of the wound (arrow).

sion.[69] Large pseudotumors may result in local neurovascular bundle compression; abductor dysfunction; and/or a large, potential dead space after excision.[69,70] Managing these reactive masses can lead to suboptimal results, depending on the level of soft-tissue destruction. Algorithms for the evaluation of painful metal-on-metal bearing surfaces are available and include the assessment of serum metal levels and the use of hip ultrasound, metal artifact reduction sequence MRI, and hip aspiration.[69]

Although revision rates vary with metal-on-metal THAs, widespread warnings and recalls have led to a decrease in the use of these components.[71]

Summary

One of the key challenges in total joint arthroplasty is selecting the proper bearing surface that will reduce the need for complex revision surgeries. Wear and corrosion in total joint constructs is unavoidable and generates particulate debris that leads to aseptic loosening and, when present in sufficient quantities, adverse local tissue reactions. Improvements in the performance of biomaterials are needed to address the pressing issues of implant degradation and improved long-term suc-

cess. Research efforts are in place to develop new bearing surfaces to address the limitations of current devices.

Key Study Points

- The science of articular surface wear and joint lubrication remain at the forefront of total joint replacement research because the bearing surface still appears to be the weak link in the system. The perfect bearing surface does not exist; however, recent efforts continue to focus on minimizing complications and improving the wear characteristics of articular couples.

- Caution must be exercised when using alternative bearing surfaces. Articular surface wear may be reduced, but complications such as fracture, adverse local tissue reactions and aseptic loosening are now being realized with ceramic and metal-on-metal bearings.

- The idea of corrosion and potentiation of metal debris formation at a distance (articular surface from trunion) are recent concerns with modern total joint arthroplasty. The complications and adverse responses to increasing modularity and trunionosis are becoming more prevalent, leading to growing concern for new complications in total joint arthroplasty.

Annotated References

1. McKellop HA, Campbell P, Park SH, et al: The origin of submicron polyethylene wear debris in total hip arthroplasty. *Clin Orthop Relat Res* 1995;311:3-20.

2. Cooper JR, Dowson D, Fisher J, Jobbins B: Ceramic bearing surfaces in total artificial joints: Resistance to third body wear damage from bone cement particles. *J Med Eng Technol* 1991;15(2):63-67.

3. Silva M, Heisel C, Mckellop H, Schmalzried TP: *Bearing Surfaces*. Philadelphia, PA, Lippincott, Williams and Wilkins, 2007.

4. Brown TD, Bartel DL; Implant Wear Symposium 2007 Engineering Work Group: What design factors influence wear behavior at the bearing surfaces in total joint replacements? *J Am Acad Orthop Surg* 2008;16(suppl 1): S101-S106.

5. Kurtz SM: A primer on UHMWPE, in Kurtz SM, ed: *The UHMWPE Handbook*. San Diego, CA, Elsevier, 2004, pp 1-9.

6. Bartel DL, Bicknell VL, Wright TM: The effect of con-

formity, thickness, and material on stresses in ultra-high molecular weight components for total joint replacement. *J Bone Joint Surg Am* 1986;68(7):1041-1051.

7. Hood RW, Wright TM, Burstein AH: Retrieval analysis of total knee prostheses: A method and its application to 48 total condylar prostheses. *J Biomed Mater Res* 1983;17(5):829-842.

8. Crowther JD, Lachiewicz PF: Survival and polyethylene wear of porous-coated acetabular components in patients less than fifty years old: Results at nine to fourteen years. *J Bone Joint Surg Am* 2002;84(5):729-735.

9. Eggli S, z'Brun S, Gerber C, Ganz R: Comparison of polyethylene wear with femoral heads of 22 mm and 32 mm: A prospective, randomised study. *J Bone Joint Surg Br* 2002;84(3):447-451.

10. Kim YH, Oh SH, Kim JS: Primary total hip arthroplasty with a second-generation cementless total hip prosthesis in patients younger than fifty years of age. *J Bone Joint Surg Am* 2003;85(1):109-114.

11. Keener JD, Callaghan JJ, Goetz DD, Pederson DR, Sullivan PM, Johnston RC: Twenty-five-year results after Charnley total hip arthroplasty in patients less than fifty years old: A concise follow-up of a previous report. *J Bone Joint Surg Am* 2003;85(6):1066-1072.

12. Capello WN, D'Antonio JA, Feinberg JR, Manley MT: Ten-year results with hydroxyapatite-coated total hip femoral components in patients less than fifty years old: A concise follow-up of a previous report. *J Bone Joint Surg Am* 2003;85(5):885-889.

13. McAuley JP, Szuszczewicz ES, Young A, Engh CA Sr: Total hip arthroplasty in patients 50 years and younger. *Clin Orthop Relat Res* 2004;418:119-125.

14. Singh S, Trikha SP, Edge AJ: Hydroxyapatite ceramic-coated femoral stems in young patients: A prospective ten-year study. *J Bone Joint Surg Br* 2004;86(8):1118-1123.

15. Kearns SR, Jamal B, Rorabeck CH, Bourne RB: Factors affecting survival of uncemented total hip arthroplasty in patients 50 years or younger. *Clin Orthop Relat Res* 2006;453:103-109.

16. Burston BJ, Yates PJ, Hook S, Moulder E, Whitley E, Bannister GC: Cemented polished tapered stems in patients less than 50 years of age: A minimum 10-year follow-up. *J Arthroplasty* 2010;25(5):692-699.

    At a minimum 10-year follow-up, 58 consecutive polished tapered stems in patients younger than 50 years were reviewed. No stems were revised for aseptic loosening, and good or excellent results were reported in 76% of the patients. Cup wear and failure were the predominant reasons for revision in this particular cohort.

17. McLaughlin JR, Lee KR: Total hip arthroplasty with an uncemented tapered femoral component in patients younger than 50 years. *J Arthroplasty* 2011;26(1):9-15.

    Ninety-four patients younger than 50 years were treated with flat, wedge, tapered femoral stems and followed for 11 to 18.5 years after primary THA. The authors reported that 98% of the stems showed signs of osseointegration; distal femoral osteolysis was seen in one hip. Young patients achieved excellent results at a mean of 16 years after surgery.

18. Lombardi AV Jr, Ellison BS, Berend KR: Polyethylene wear is influenced by manufacturing technique in modular TKA. *Clin Orthop Relat Res* 2008;466(11):2798-2805.

19. Won CH, Rohatgi S, Kraay MJ, Goldberg VM, Rimnac CM: Effect of resin type and manufacturing method on wear of polyethylene tibial components. *Clin Orthop Relat Res* 2000;376:161-171.

20. Parks NL, Engh GA, Topoleski LD, Emperado J: The Coventry Award: Modular tibial insert micromotion. A concern with contemporary knee implants. *Clin Orthop Relat Res* 1998;356:10-15.

21. Mont MA, Maar DC, Krackow KA, Jacobs MA, Jones LC, Hungerford DS: Total hip replacement without cement for non-inflammatory osteoarthrosis in patients who are less than forty-five years old. *J Bone Joint Surg Am* 1993;75(5):740-751.

22. Jasty MJ, Floyd WE III, Schiller AL, Goldring SR, Harris WH: Localized osteolysis in stable, non-septic total hip replacement. *J Bone Joint Surg Am* 1986;68(6):912-919.

23. Muratoglu OK, Kurtz SM: *Alternative Bearing Surfaces in Hip Replacement*. New York, NY, Marcel Dekker, 2002.

24. Small SR, Berend ME, Howard LA, Tunç D, Buckley CA, Ritter MA: Acetabular cup stiffness and implant orientation change acetabular loading patterns. *J Arthroplasty* 2013;28(2):359-367.

    Four implant designs of variable stiffness were implanted into a composite pelvis at 35° or 50° of abduction. All specimens were loaded to simulate normal gait patterns, and peri-implant bone strains were measured. Stiffer components had higher localized surface strains and imbalanced load distributions. An increased abduction angle resulted in varying amounts of peri-implant bone strain.

25. Voleti PB, Baldwin KD, Lee GC: Metal-on-metal vs conventional total hip arthroplasty: A systematic review and meta-analysis of randomized controlled trials. *J Arthroplasty* 2012;27(10):1844-1849.

    A literature review found four, level I randomized controlled trials for inclusion in a meta-analysis. No substantial differences were found between patients treated with metal-on-metal and conventional THAs related to functional scores and radiographic outcomes. A 3.37 times greater rate of complications was reported in the group treated with metal-on-metal THAs. The authors recommended caution in the routine use of metal-on-metal devices in primary THAs.

26. Johanson PE, Digas G, Herberts P, Thanner J, Kärrholm J: Highly crosslinked polyethylene does not reduce aseptic loosening in cemented THA 10-year findings of a randomized study. *Clin Orthop Relat Res* 2012;470(11):3083-3093.

Sixty patients were randomized to standard UHMWPE or HXLPE THA components and followed for 10 years to assess wear rates. HXLPE was found to have a wear rate of 0.005mm/year compared with 0.056 mm/year for conventional UHMWPE. No other clinical or radiographic parameters differed between the two groups.

27. Martell JM, Berdia S: Determination of polyethylene wear in total hip replacements with use of digital radiographs. *J Bone Joint Surg Am* 1997;79(11):1635-1641.

28. Goldvasser D, Noz ME, Maguire GQ Jr, Olivecrona H, Bragdon CR, Malchau H: A new technique for measuring wear in total hip arthroplasty using computed tomography. *J Arthroplasty* 2012;27(9):1636-1640, e1.

The authors describe a new technique using CT to determine the UHMWPE wear rates in THAs. A detailed description of the three-dimensional measuring technique is reviewed.

29. Gee AO, Lee GC: Alternative bearings in total knee arthroplasty. *Am J Orthop (Belle Mead NJ)* 2012;41(6): 280-283.

The authors present a review of HXLPE, mobile bearings, and other alternative bearing surfaces in TKA.

30. Willie BM, Foot LJ, Prall MW, Bloebaum RD: Surface damage analysis of retrieved highly crosslinked polyethylene tibial components after short-term implantation. *J Biomed Mater Res B Appl Biomater* 2008;85(1): 114-124.

31. Gordon AC, D'Lima DD, Colwell CW Jr: Highly cross-linked polyethylene in total hip arthroplasty. *J Am Acad Orthop Surg* 2006;14(9):511-523.

32. Muratoglu OK, Bragdon CR, O'Connor DO, Jasty M, Harris WH: A novel method of cross-linking ultra-high-molecular-weight polyethylene to improve wear, reduce oxidation, and retain mechanical properties: Recipient of the 1999 HAP Paul Award. *J Arthroplasty* 2001; 16(2):149-160.

33. Waewsawangwong W, Goodman SB: Unexpected failure of highly cross-linked polyethylene acetabular liner. *J Arthroplasty* 2012;27(2):e1-e4.

The disadvantages of HXLPE use in THA are discussed, including a case of unexpected failure from liner fracture. Factors associated with the fractured liner included decreased mechanical properties, vertical cup placement, and a large diameter femoral head.

34. Tower SS, Currier JH, Currier BH, Lyford KA, Van Citters DW, Mayor MB: Rim cracking of the cross-linked longevity polyethylene acetabular liner after total hip arthroplasty. *J Bone Joint Surg Am* 2007;89(10):2212-2217.

35. Blumenfeld TJ, McKellop HA, Schmalzried TP, Billi F: Fracture of a cross-linked polyethylene liner: A multifactorial issue. *J Arthroplasty* 2011;26(4):e5-e8.

Fracture in a HXLPE liner is reviewed. Horizontal loading conditions were believed to have caused the failure. Liner locking mechanisms and material properties of HXLPE are reviewed in detail, particularly their relationship to component failure.

36. Calvert GT, Devane PA, Fielden J, Adams K, Horne JG: A double-blind, prospective, randomized controlled trial comparing highly cross-linked and conventional polyethylene in primary total hip arthroplasty. *J Arthroplasty* 2009;24(4):505-510.

37. Mutimer J, Devane PA, Adams K, Horne JG: Highly crosslinked polyethylene reduces wear in total hip arthroplasty at 5 years. *Clin Orthop Relat Res* 2010; 468(12):3228-3233.

A prospective, double-blinded randomized controlled trial was conducted with 122 patients to assess the wear of standard UHMWPE versus HXLPE. At mean follow-up of 5.5 years, lower wear rates were reported for the HXLPE (0.05 mm/year) compared with the standard UHMWPE (0.26 mm/year).

38. Bragdon CR, Kwon YM, Geller JA, et al: Minimum 6-year followup of highly cross-linked polyethylene in THA. *Clin Orthop Relat Res* 2007;465:122-127.

39. Campbell DG, Field JR, Callary SA: Second-generation highly cross-linked X3™ polyethylene wear: A preliminary radiostereometric analysis study. *Clin Orthop Relat Res* 2010;468(10):2704-2709.

Second-generation HXLPE liners in 19 patients were evaluated to measure wear rates and clinical outcomes and were compared with first-generation liners. Wear rates and head penetration were low at 1- to 2-year follow-ups and similar to the in vitro wear rate. Level of evidence: IV.

40. Geerdink CH, Grimm B, Vencken W, Heyligers IC, Tonino AJ: Cross-linked compared with historical polyethylene in THA: An 8-year clinical study. *Clin Orthop Relat Res* 2009;467(4):979-984.

41. Lachiewicz PF, Heckman DS, Soileau ES, Mangla J, Martell JM: Femoral head size and wear of highly cross-linked polyethylene at 5 to 8 years. *Clin Orthop Relat Res* 2009;467(12):3290-3296.

42. Milošev I, Kovač S, Trebše R, Levašič V, Pišot V: Comparison of ten-year survivorship of hip prostheses with use of conventional polyethylene, metal-on-metal, or ceramic-on-ceramic bearings. *J Bone Joint Surg Am* 2012;94(19):1756-1763.

Three different bearing surfaces, metal-on-polyethylene, ceramic-on-ceramic, and metal-on-metal, were evaluated in 487 THAs at an average follow-up of 8.5 years. Survivorship at 10 years for the metal-on-polyethylene,

1: Principles of Orthopaedics

ceramic-on-ceramic, and metal-on-metal devices were 0.984, 0.956, and 0.879, respectively. The authors concluded that a metal-on-polyethylene bearing surface is the appropriate option for older and less active patients. Level of evidence: III.

43. Cai P, Hu Y, Xie J: Large-diameter Delta ceramic-on-ceramic versus common-sized ceramic-on-polyethylene bearings in THA. *Orthopedics* 2012;35(9):e1307-e1313.

A prospective, randomized controlled trial was performed with 93 patients to evaluate a ceramic-on-ceramic device. A control group was treated with a ceramic-on-polyethylene device. The large diameter ceramic-on-ceramic device had 6.1° greater range of motion, with similar hip scores and complication rates as the ceramic-on-polyethylene device at short-term follow-up. Level of evidence: I.

44. Kim YH, Park JW, Kim JS: Cementless metaphyseal fitting anatomic total hip arthroplasty with a ceramic-on-ceramic bearing in patients thirty years of age or younger. *J Bone Joint Surg Am* 2012;94(17):1570-1575.

A review of 127 hips was performed in patients younger than 30 years at the time of surgery. All components, except one acetabular component, remained well fixed. No cases of squeaking, fracture, or osteolysis were reported. Ceramic-on-ceramic and metaphyseal filling stems appear to be successful in young patients treated with THA. Level of evidence: IV.

45. Synder M, Drobniewski M, Sibiński M: Long-term results of cementless hip arthroplasty with ceramic-on-ceramic articulation. *Int Orthop* 2012;36(11):2225-2229.

The authors reviewed 220 THAs treated with ceramic-on-ceramic prostheses (mean follow-up, 19.6 years). Overall, 12-year survival rates were 89.99% for the cup and 91.36% for the stem. Level of evidence: IV.

46. Chen WM, Wu PK, Chen CF, Huang CK, Liu CL, Chen TH: No significant squeaking in total hip arthroplasty: A series of 413 hips in the Asian people. *J Arthroplasty* 2012;27(8):1575-1579.

The squeaking rate of ceramic-on-ceramic THA implants in an Asian population was assessed from 2003 to 2009. In 413 consecutive patients, no cases of implant squeaking and four overall complications were reported. Level of evidence: IV.

47. Chevillotte C, Pibarot V, Carret JP, Bejui-Hugues J, Guyen O: Hip squeaking: A 10-year follow-up study. *J Arthroplasty* 2012;27(6):1008-1013.

The authors reviewed 100 ceramic-on-ceramic THAs at 10-year follow-up. Despite no malpositioning of the implants seen on radiographs, a 5% incidence of squeaking was reported. All the squeaking implants occurred in active, heavy men. Level of evidence: IV.

48. Yeung E, Bott PT, Chana R, et al: Mid-term results of third-generation alumina-on-alumina ceramic bearings in cementless total hip arthroplasty: A ten-year minimum follow-up. *J Bone Joint Surg Am* 2012;94(2):138-144.

The authors clinically and radiographically reviewed 301 consecutive primary THAs. Death occurred in 9.2% of patients from an unrelated cause, 2.7% underwent revision surgery, and 95% had an excellent or good result. The overall rate of implant survival was 98%, with revision for any reason as the end point. Level of evidence: IV.

49. Ezzet KA, Hermida JC, Colwell CW Jr, D'Lima DD: Oxidized zirconium femoral components reduce polyethylene wear in a knee wear simulator. *Clin Orthop Relat Res* 2004;428:120-124.

50. Laskin RS: An oxidized Zr ceramic surfaced femoral component for total knee arthroplasty. *Clin Orthop Relat Res* 2003;416:191-196.

51. Walter WL, O'Toole GC, Walter WK, Ellis A, Zicat BA: Squeaking in ceramic-on-ceramic hips: The importance of acetabular component orientation. *J Arthroplasty* 2007;22(4):496-503.

52. Akagi M, Nakamura T, Matsusue Y, Ueo T, Nishijyo K, Ohnishi E: The Bisurface total knee replacement: A unique design for flexion. Four-to-nine-year follow-up study. *J Bone Joint Surg Am* 2000;82(11):1626-1633.

53. D'Antonio JA, Capello WN, Manley MT, Naughton M, Sutton K: A titanium-encased alumina ceramic bearing for total hip arthroplasty: 3- to 5-year results. *Clin Orthop Relat Res* 2005;441:151-158.

54. Garino J, Rhaman MN, Bal BS: Reliability of modern alumina bearings in total hip replacements. *Semin Arthroplasty* 2006;17:113-119.

55. Isaac GH, Brockett C, Breckon A, et al: Ceramic-on-metal bearings in total hip replacement: Whole blood metal ion levels and analysis of retrieved components. *J Bone Joint Surg Br* 2009;91(9):1134-1141.

56. Rieker CB, Schön R, Köttig P: Development and validation of a second-generation metal-on-metal bearing: Laboratory studies and analysis of retrievals. *J Arthroplasty* 2004;19(8, suppl 3):5-11.

57. Grupp TM, Yue JJ, Garcia R Jr, et al: Biotribological evaluation of artificial disc arthroplasty devices: Influence of loading and kinematic patterns during in vitro wear simulation. *Eur Spine J* 2009;18(1):98-108.

58. Bosker BH, Ettema HB, Boomsma MF, Kollen BJ, Maas M, Verheyen CC: High incidence of pseudotumour formation after large-diameter metal-on-metal total hip replacement: A prospective cohort study. *J Bone Joint Surg Br* 2012;94(6):755-761.

A prospective review was performed on 120 metal-on-metal THAs with large diameter heads. The authors found that 39% of the patients had a pseudotumor on CT. Those with increased serum metal levels were at increased risk of pseudotumor development. Level of evidence: III.

59. Malviya A, Ramaskandhan JR, Bowman R, et al: What advantage is there to be gained using large modular metal-on-metal bearings in routine primary hip replacement? A preliminary report of a prospective randomised controlled trial. *J Bone Joint Surg Br* 2011;93(12):1602-1609.

A prospective, randomized controlled trial compared metal-on-metal THAs with a large diameter femoral head with conventional metal-on-polyethylene THAs with a 28-mm head. No clinical or radiographic differences were noted at follow-up between the groups; however, overall patient satisfaction was higher for the metal-on-metal group. Twenty percent of the metal-on-metal group had substantially elevated serum metal levels compared with one patient in the metal-on-polyethylene group. Level of evidence: I.

60. Nikolaou VS, Petit A, Debiparshad K, Huk OL, Zukor DJ, Antoniou J: Metal-on-metal total hip arthroplasty—five- to 11-year follow-up. *Bull NYU Hosp Jt Dis* 2011;69(suppl 1):S77-S83.

The authors retrospectively reviewed 166 patients (average age, 50 years) treated with metal-on-metal THAs. A 7.8% revision rate was reported. Cobalt and chromium serum levels significantly increased over the first 4 to 5 years and then stabilized before slowly decreasing. Level of evidence: IV.

61. Grübl A, Marker M, Brodner W, et al: Long-term follow-up of metal-on-metal total hip replacement. *J Orthop Res* 2007;25(7):841-848.

62. Dorr LD, Wan Z, Longjohn DB, Dubois B, Murken R: Total hip arthroplasty with use of the Metasul metal-on-metal articulation: Four to seven-year results. *J Bone Joint Surg Am* 2000;82(6):789-798.

63. Bozic KJ, Browne J, Dangles CJ, et al: Modern metal-on-metal hip implants. *J Am Acad Orthop Surg* 2012;20(6):402-406.

64. Meyer H, Mueller T, Goldau G, Chamaon K, Ruetschi M, Lohmann CH: Corrosion at the cone/taper interface leads to failure of large-diameter metal-on-metal total hip arthroplasties. *Clin Orthop Relat Res* 2012;470(11):3101-3108.

A histologic analysis of periprosthetic tissues was performed to assess adverse local tissue reactions to corrosion products. The authors concluded that metal-on-metal articulation wear may cause failure of the cone/taper fit, leading to galvanic corrosion. Level of evidence: IV.

65. Bernstein M, Desy NM, Petit A, Zukor DJ, Huk OL, Antoniou J: Long-term follow-up and metal ion trend of patients with metal-on-metal total hip arthroplasty. *Int Orthop* 2012;36(9):1807-1812.

A retrospective review of 163 prostheses was performed at a mean follow-up of 8.87 years after treatment with a second-generation metal-on-metal THA. Survivorship was found to be 91.3%, with revision for any reason as the end point. Cobalt and chromium ion levels peaked at 4 to 5 years and then gradually decreased. Level of evidence: IV.

66. Ziaee H, Daniel J, Datta AK, Blunt S, McMinn DJ: Transplacental transfer of cobalt and chromium in patients with metal-on-metal hip arthroplasty: A controlled study. *J Bone Joint Surg Br* 2007;89(3):301-305.

67. deSouza RM, Wallace D, Costa ML, Krikler SJ: Transplacental passage of metal ions in women with hip resurfacing: No teratogenic effects observed. *Hip Int* 2012;22(1):96-99.

Blood from the umbilical cord was tested in three patients with metal-on-metal resurfacing prostheses in place during pregnancy. Cobalt levels in the umbilical cord were 50% of those in the maternal blood; however, all three children were healthy and without complications. Level of evidence: IV.

68. Fabi D, Levine B, Paprosky W, et al: Metal-on-metal total hip arthroplasty: Causes and high incidence of early failure. *Orthopedics* 2012;35(7):e1009-e1016.

Early failure of metal-on-metal THAs is reported in 80 patients. Aseptic loosening was most common in 56.25% of the patients. A diagnostic algorithm is reviewed, along with two classification schemes directing treatment for metal-on-metal complications.

69. Parfitt DJ, Wood SN, Chick CM, Lewis P, Rashid MH, Evans AR: Common femoral vein thrombosis caused by a metal-on-metal hip arthroplasty-related pseudotumor. *J Arthroplasty* 2012;27(8):e9, e11.

The authors reported a single case of deep femoral vein thrombosis after metal-on-metal THA. The pressure effect from a pseudotumor led to a serious vein thrombosis and represents another potential complication of metal-on-metal THA. Level of evidence: IV.

70. Whitwell GS, Shine A, Young SK: The articular surface replacement implant recall: A United Kingdom district hospital experience. *Hip Int* 2012;22(4):362-370.

The authors review their experience with 121 ASR (DePuy) hip components after the initiation of the product recall. One year after the recall, 23 hips had been revised (an approximately 19% revision rate). Overall 5-year survivorship was 80.8%, with revision for all reasons as the end point. Level of evidence: IV.

71. Oskouian RJ, Whitehill R, Samii A, Shaffrey ME, Johnson JP, Shaffrey CI: The future of spinal arthroplasty: A biomaterial perspective. *Neurosurg Focus* 2004;17(3):E2.

1: Principles of Orthopaedics

Chapter 7

Musculoskeletal Imaging

C. Benjamin Ma, MD   Terry C.P. Lynch, MD

Introduction

Imaging has significantly enhanced the ability to diagnose musculoskeletal problems and has led to improvement in the management of musculoskeletal conditions. Plain radiography allows the diagnosis of fractures, deformity, and arthritis, which led to improved techniques in fracture fixation, deformity correction, and joint arthroplasties. MRI provides important information on soft-tissue condition and led to improvements in the management of ligament tears, rotator cuff injuries, and cartilage abnormalities. Recent advances in nuclear medicine will allow the evaluation of metabolic activity within the body, thus improving surveillance and management of cancer. In this chapter, different imaging modalities and their advantages and disadvantages for musculoskeletal imaging (Table 1) will be discussed, along with advancements and improvements of musculoskeletal imaging in different body regions.

Imaging Types

Radiography

Since its discovery in 1895, plain radiography has allowed the visualization of structures within the human body. The image produced is a projection of the amount of radiation absorbed by the structures along the course of the beam. Digital radiography is commonly used to improve diagnostic efficiency and the quality of images when compared with conventional film radiography. The process makes images portable and transferable via computers or CDs. However, there

---

are trade-offs of digital radiography versus conventional film screen radiography. Film radiography has higher spatial resolution, but the improved contrast of digital radiography allows it to have comparable diagnostic efficiency.

Plain radiography and CT are imaging modalities that rely on ionizing radiation. The scientific unit of the measurement of radiation dose, commonly referred to as the "effective dose," is the millisievert (mSv). Other radiation dose measurement units include rad, rem, Roentgen, and Sievert. Daily radiation exposure occurs from natural sources, such as the sun. The average person in the United States receives an effective dose of 3 mSv/year from naturally occurring radioactive materials and cosmic radiation. In comparison, on average, the radiation dose of a standard chest radiograph is 0.1 mSv.[1]

Computed Tomography

The principle of CT is the use of x-ray beams to produce tomographic images, or slices of an object. CT comprises multiple plain radiography images reassembled together to generate an image. These images can also be reconstructed to generate a three-dimensional image (Figure 1). In addition to generating tomographic images, CT can also be used to determine the density of the imaged structures. X-ray densities are measured in Hounsfield units (HUs) or CT numbers. Water is assigned a value of 0 HU; air, a value of –1,000 HU. Images are displayed as gray scale; denser objects are lighter. Contrary to plain radiography, good soft-tissue imaging is provided with CT scans; the gray scale can be modified ("windowed") to show data that fall within a fixed range of densities, such as bone windows or lung windows, to evaluate particular structures.

MRI and Magnetic Resonance Arthrography

MRI does not require ionizing radiation. It uses a strong magnet that generates a magnetic field and multiple coils that send and/or receive radiofrequency signals. Currently, all clinical MRI scans image the protons in hydrogen. The strength of the MRI machine is expressed in tesla (T) units. The stronger the magnet, the higher the tesla unit and the better the signal-to-noise ratio. Stronger magnets can improve imaging speed and resolution.

Conventional MRI requires a large room that is shielded to contain the magnetic field. The machine

---

Table 1

Advantages and Disadvantages of Each Imaging Modality

	Advantages	Disadvantages
Plain radiography	Most commonly used medical imaging modality Relatively inexpensive Real-time radiographic imaging, or fluoroscopy, allows instantaneous feedback on stress radiographs, angiography, and orthopaedic interventions.	Radiation exposure Not effective in soft-tissue imaging because of poor contrast resolution Magnification of the images. Measurement "standards" can be placed with the object to allow for determination of magnification. Although most medical x-ray beams do not pose a risk to a fetus, there is a small possibility that serious illness and developmental problems can occur. The actual risk depends on the type of imaging study and the trimester of pregnancy.
CT	Tomographic nature of the images with high contrast resolution Images are processed digitally; images in plane other than the one imaged can be reconstructed to give a different perspective of the object/tissue of interest. Direct measurements can be performed on the scans because there is no magnification. Can be combined with arthrography or myelography to evaluate specific joint or spinal abnormalities. Used for injections and biopsy to allow precise location of structures. Provides better delineation of bone structures than MRI.	Much higher radiation exposure than plain radiographs Subject to motion artifacts because each slice can take acquisition time up to 1 sec There is artifact with metal objects and it is difficult to image around metal prosthesis. Scans have a weight limit because patients need to lie on a scanner table. Contraindicated for pregnant patients, except in life-threatening circumstances.
MRI	Superior images of soft tissues, such as ligaments, tendons, fibrocartilage, cartilage, muscle, bone marrow, and fat MRI, similar to CT scans, has an advantage over plain radiography on obtaining tomographic images of the object of interest. More effective than CT at detecting changes in intensity within the bone marrow to diagnose osteomyelitis, malignancy, contusions, occult fractures, and stress fractures MRI contrast (gadolinium) has less allergic reaction than iodine-based media. There is no radiation exposure to the patient.	Motion blurring and metal artifacts are poorly tolerated. The examination time for MRI is much longer than for CT scans. Patients need to remain still throughout the scanning process. Sedation is often needed for pediatric patients younger than age 7 years. Metal screws, pellets, prostheses, and foreign bodies can produce significant artifact, obscuring anatomic structures. Metal suppression sequences can be used but with loss of resolution. Although MRI does not use radiation, the effect of radiofrequency and magnetic field on the fetus is unknown. It is usually recommended that a pregnant woman not have an MRI.
Ultrasound	Noninvasive at the frequencies used for diagnostic imaging Commonly used in the imaging of children and pregnant women Shows nonossified structures, such as femoral heads, to diagnose hip dysplasia and dislocation. Equipment is portable and inexpensive compared with MRI and CT equipment. Highly echogenic structures, such as a foreign body that may not be visible on radiographs, can be easily detected using ultrasound. Can be used for targeted therapy, such as injections and ablations. Useful for injections and aspirations of fluid collections Provides dynamic assessment of structures (ie, tendon and nerve subluxation).	Image quality and interpretation depend on the experience of the ultrasonographer and radiologists. Cannot image inside bone; bone cortex reflects almost all of the sound waves. Internal joint structures are not well visualized unless in a superficial location.

Table 1

Advantages and Disadvantages of Each Imaging Modality (continued)

	Advantages	Disadvantages
Nuclear medicine	Scintigraphy allows imaging of metabolic activity. Most metabolic processes involving bone have slow metabolic activity compared with soft-tissue organs, such as the kidney and the liver. Fortunately, most radioisotopes are relatively long lived. White blood cell scintigraphy can be used to diagnose osteomyelitis. Scintigraphy can be used to diagnose metastasis, stress fracture, or occult fractures.	Lack of detail and spatial resolution Limited early sensitivity to detect acute fractures in patients with slow bone metabolism; it may take several days for the bone scan to be positive to diagnose an occult femoral neck fracture. Low sensitivity can occur with lytic bone lesions, such as multiple myeloma and some metastases. Avoid in breastfeeding mothers. Nuclear agent can pass from the mother's milk to the child.

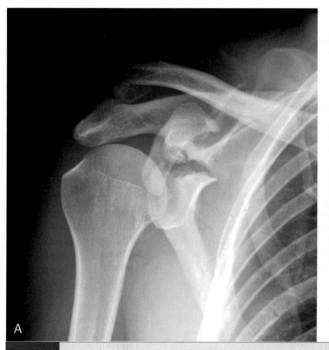 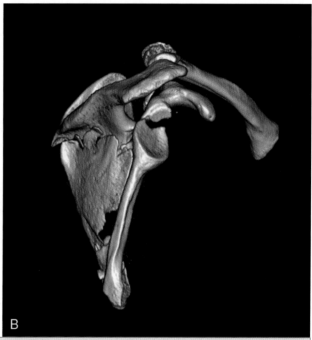

Figure 1 **A,** AP view of the scapula showing a fracture that involves the glenoid. **B,** Three-dimensional CT reconstruction of a scapular fracture.

typically has a small bore or tube whereby the patient enters to have the study performed. The machine has a weight limit, and the small bore also limits the size of the patient who can undergo the study. MRI takes longer to perform than CT and is subjected to motion artifact. Patients with claustrophobia may not tolerate conventional MRI and may require anesthesia to undergo the study.

Scanners with an open design are usually smaller machines with lower field strength; these images are of lower quality and lower resolution than those of conventional closed scanners. However, open scanners can accommodate claustrophobic patients. These machines should be used for larger joints and structures that do not require as much imaging detail.[1]

MRI is well suited for the evaluation of soft tissues. However, in certain cases, the analysis of soft tissues can be improved with the use of contrast. Contrast-enhanced MRI is performed after the intravenous injection of a gadolinium-containing compound and is commonly used in the evaluation of tumors, infections, and inflammatory conditions. Complications associated with MRI include the malfunction of electrical appliances such as pacemakers and mechanical pumps, the potential for metal objects brought into the scanner to become dangerous projectiles, the migration of metal foreign bodies in the eye or the brain, and a reaction to a patient's existing metal implants.

Magnetic resonance arthrography is performed after contrast injection for specific evaluation of joints. Di-

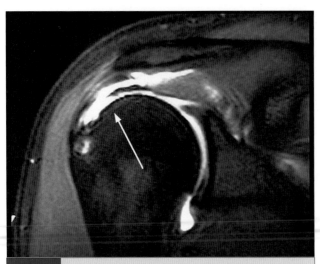

Figure 2 Direct magnetic resonance arthrography of the shoulder. The contrast clearly identifies the small rotator cuff tear of the supraspinatus tendon (arrow) with communication of the glenohumeral joint and the subacromial space.

Nuclear Medicine/Positron Emission Tomography

Nuclear imaging involves the use of radioisotope-labeled, biologically active drugs to evaluate various structures. The radioactive tracer serves as a marker of biologic activity. The images produced by scintigraphy are a collection of the radiation emissions from the isotopes.

Bone scintigraphy, commonly known as bone scans, generally is performed using diphosphonates labeled with radioactive technetium Tc 99m. The initial (transient) phase is characterized by tracer delivery to the tissue, which represents the perfusion images. The second (blood pool) phase follows the initial phase. The final (delayed) phase shows tracer accumulation in tissues with active turnover, mostly in bone undergoing growth and turnover.

Positron emission tomography (PET) is used in orthopaedic oncology. Fluorodeoxyglucose (^{18}F), or FDG, is the metabolic tracer widely used in clinical oncology. FDG accumulation reflects the rate of glucose utilization in tissue. It is transported into tissue by the same mechanisms of glucose transport and trapped in the tissue as FDG-6-phosphate. The use of FDG in the evaluation of the musculoskeletal system is based on increased glycolytic rate in pathologic tissues. High-grade malignancies tend to have higher rates of glycolysis than low-grade malignancies and have greater uptake of FDG than do low-grade or benign lesions. The FDG is typically injected intravenously, in a patient who has been fasting and who has a suitably low blood glucose level. The patient must then wait for the blood sugar to distribute and be taken up into organs that use glucose—a time during which physical activity must be kept to a minimum to minimize uptake of the radioactive sugar in muscles (this causes unwanted artifacts when the organs of interest are inside the body). The patient is then placed in the PET scanner for the actual image acquisition.

rect magnetic resonance arthrography is commonly used to diagnose labral tears in the shoulder and the hip joints, triangular fibrocartilage and ligament tears of the wrist, collateral ligament evaluation in the elbow, and postoperative evaluation of a repaired meniscus (Figure 2). With direct magnetic resonance arthrography, a dilute gadolinium-containing solution is injected into the joint. Indirect magnetic resonance arthrography is commonly used when direct injection of a joint is impractical. With indirect magnetic resonance arthrography, gadolinium is injected intravenously and allowed to travel through the vascular system to the synovium of a joint. Gadolinium contrast behaves like iodinated contrast media, but patients have less allergic reaction to gadolinium than iodine-based contrast. However, its usage is contraindicated in patients with renal insufficiency. Intravenous gadolinium can lead to irreversible renal damage, known as nephrogenic systemic fibrosis. Intravenous gadolinium should not be administered to patients on dialysis or those with a glomerular filtration rate less than 30.

Ultrasonography

Ultrasonography uses high-frequency sound waves to produce images. A transducer produces sound waves that travel through the soft tissue, and echo waves are deflected back by the tissue to the same transducer. Image resolution and beam attenuation depend on both wavelength and frequency. Doppler ultrasonography can be used to image blood vessels for flow velocity and direction. Color maps can be generated for color Doppler ultrasound.

Radiation Safety

Although imaging allows the visualization of different structures, certain risks exist. Children and fetuses are especially susceptible to ionizing radiation because of their rapidly dividing cells and growth. Radiography, CT, and bone scintigraphy produce ions that can deposit energy to organs and tissues that can damage DNA. Some tracers (such as iodine-131) have half-lives of several days and can concentrate in excreted body fluid and breast milk. Rapidly dividing tissues are the most susceptible to radiation-induced neoplasia, such as bone marrow, breast tissue, gastrointestinal mucosa, gonads, and lymphatic tissue. The risk of cancer is approximately 4% per Sievert (100 rem). The greatest risk of fetal malformation is in the first trimester and with doses > 0.1 Gy (10 rad). For risk late in pregnancy (≥ 150 days postconception), childhood malignancies such as leukemia are of concern. When obtaining radiologic studies, sensitive organs such as gonads should be shielded. It is always important to follow the ALARA principle ("as low as reasonably achievable") of dosing for pregnant women and children. The exposure to radiation decreases as an inverse square of the distance from the source. Medical personnel should wear lead aprons and be monitored using devices such as film badges. Of all imaging modalities, CT delivers the highest amount of radiation dose (5-15 mSv versus 0.1-2.0 mSv for plain radiography). CT should not be performed if other comparable imaging modalities are available. It is also important to exercise caution in performing multiple CT scans at different intervals in the same patient.

Musculoskeletal Imaging of Specific Body Parts

Shoulder

Musculoskeletal imaging is commonly used in the diagnosis of shoulder injuries, including fractures, arthritis, and soft-tissue injuries such as rotator cuff tears and instability.

Fractures

AP and axillary lateral or scapula Y views of the shoulder are commonly used to rule out shoulder fractures. More specific views, such as AP and serendipity view (45° tilted view) of the clavicle, West Point axillary lateral to diagnose bony Bankart injuries, and the Stryker notch view for Hill-Sachs lesions, are used in the diagnosis of different injuries. CT is used to evaluate the complexity of the fracture pattern, and any comminution of proximal humerus and scapula fractures. Three-dimensional reconstructions can be helpful to evaluate the joint involvement of scapular neck and body fractures.

Arthritis

For shoulder arthritis, an AP view of the glenohumeral joint or Grashey view and axillary lateral views of the shoulder can evaluate the amount of joint space narrowing. A weighted view of the AP glenohumeral joint can also evaluate signs of instability or proximal migration and inflammatory arthritis (Figure 3). Primary osteoarthritis of the shoulder usually has large inferior osteophytes seen on an AP view of the glenohumeral joint and posterior wear on the axillary lateral view. For inflammatory arthritis, there is less osteophytosis, but there will be central wear of the glenoid, osteopenia, and subchondral cyst formation. For surgical planning, CT or MRI can be obtained to evaluate the amount of glenoid wear and version. MRI allows evaluation of the condition of the rotator cuff tendon for surgical planning between conventional total shoulder replacements versus reverse shoulder replacements. Ultrasound-guided glenohumeral joint injection can increase the accuracy in intra-articular injections.

Rotator Cuff Tears and Instability

MRI is more effective than other modalities in the evaluation of soft-tissue abnormalities such as rotator cuff

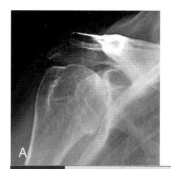
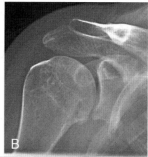

Figure 3 **A,** Plain AP radiographic view of the glenohumeral joint showing the joint space and minimal osteophytes. **B,** Weighted AP view of the glenohumeral joint of the same patient showing bone-on-bone arthritis.

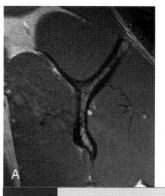
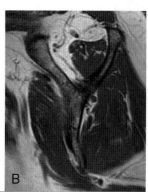

Figure 4 MRIs showing the modified Goutallier classification of fatty infiltration of the rotator cuff muscle. Grading is done on the sagittal fat-sensitive images. **A,** Grade 0: no fat in the muscle belly of all muscle groups. **B,** Grade 2: less than 50% fatty infiltration; muscle atrophy is present over the supraspinatus muscle.

tears and labral injuries and in determining size, retraction, and the tear pattern of injury. Ultrasound can allow dynamic evaluation of rotator cuff injuries and biceps mobility; however, resolution is lower and evaluation is more localized. Recent studies have highlighted the importance of muscle atrophy and fatty infiltration (Figure 4) in the muscle as negative prognostic factors in outcomes following rotator cuff repairs. The Goutallier method for evaluating the quality of the rotator cuff muscles was introduced in 1994.[2] Using CT images, the amount of fat present in the muscle was estimated. This method was later adapted for grading muscle quality on MRI scans.[3] The modified Goutallier classification system grades the muscles of the rotator cuff on the amount of fat present relative to muscle volume.

For shoulder instability, plain radiography evaluates bony deformities, such as the Hill-Sachs lesion, and anterior inferior glenoid bone loss. However, the limitation of x-ray projection makes it difficult to quantify the amount of bone loss. Three-dimensional CT scans have been recommended to evaluate the amount of

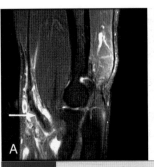 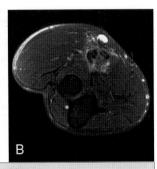

Figure 5 **A,** T2-weighted fast spin-echo sagittal image shows a complete tear of the distal biceps from the radial tuberosity. The distal tendon fragment (arrow) is thickened and undulating from retraction. Bone marrow and subcutaneous fat are reduced in signal because of fat saturation pulses, accentuating the edema in the tissues surrounding the torn biceps tendon. **B,** T2-weighted fast spin-echo axial image shows a complete tear of the distal biceps from the radial tuberosity.

glenoid bone loss when compared with other modalities, such as radiographs, MRI, and CT scans.[4] MRI and direct magnetic resonance arthrography are good to evaluate labral and ligament injuries. The ABER (abduction and external rotation) sequence is specifically performed to evaluate the anterior inferior labral structures and also the posterosuperior rotator cuff tendons when in contact with the posterior labrum. This magnetic resonance sequence is helpful to confirm the diagnosis of anterior inferior labral tears and internal impingement syndrome.[5]

Neuropathy
Ganglion cysts in the shoulder can lead to nerve compression and muscle weakness. The suprascapular nerve is the nerve most often compressed in the shoulder region. Ganglion cysts that compress the nerve at the suprascapular notch can lead to weakness in both the supraspinatus and infraspinatus muscles, whereas cysts at the spinoglenoid notch will lead to weakness in the infraspinatus muscle only. Direct magnetic resonance arthrography can evaluate the communication between the cyst and the joint, usually through a small labral tear. Indirect magnetic resonance arthrography can evaluate the presence of a dilated vein or aneurysm that can lead to nerve compression.

Elbow
Fractures
Standard radiographs of the elbow include an AP extended and lateral flexion view. For trauma imaging, an oblique lateral view for specific evaluation of the radial head is obtained. The presence of a joint effusion or hemarthrosis leads to lifting of the inferior edge of the fat contained within the coronoid fossa and produces the sail sign, whereas displacement of the fat contained within the olecranon fossa of the distal humerus allows this fat to be visualized posterior to the distal humeral condyles (posterior fat pad sign). Occult fractures are present in a significant percentage of both pediatric and adult patients with effusions, and follow-up radiographs are standard. Although MRI can detect occult fractures and bone bruises not seen on initial radiographs in patients with effusions, treatment is usually presumptive, and the utility of MRI in occult elbow fracture diagnosis is yet to be shown.[6] CT with multiplanar reformations is used for treatment planning for complex fractures of the distal humerus and the radial head.[7]

Arthritis
In the evaluation of the restricted elbow, CT can better detect intra-articular bodies and osteophytes than conventional radiographs. MRI is useful in evaluating for intra-articular bodies and has the advantage of disclosing soft-tissue abnormalities that may also produce locking, such as a thickened synovial fringe or synovial plicae.[8]

Instability and Tendinopathy
For the evaluation of elbow instability, MRI has been established as a reliable tool in assessment of the ulnar collateral ligament complex, the radial collateral ligament, the annular ligament, and the lateral ulnar collateral ligament.[9] In addition, MRI is used to evaluate biceps or triceps tendon tears (**Figure 5**) or medial or lateral epicondylitis.[10] Because of the relatively superficial position of the elbow's ligaments and tendons, sonography may be used to screen for Little Leaguer's elbow and the etiology and assessment of treatment of tennis elbow with both mixed and promising results.[11]

Neuropathy
Cubital tunnel syndrome and other neuropathies can be evaluated with MRI, both directly visualizing the nerves involved for signal and morphologic abnormalities and identifying causative factors, such as accessory anconeus epitrochlearis muscle, ganglion cysts, enthesophytes, or other masses compromising the volume of the cubital tunnel.[12]

Wrist
Fractures
Standard plain film evaluation of the wrist includes PA, oblique, and lateral views. A dedicated ulnar-deviated PA view for specific evaluation of the scaphoid is often routine because of the frequency and the consequences of occult fractures of the scaphoid. A semisupinated oblique view may reveal occult radial fractures. Secondary signs, such as obliteration or deviation of the pronator quadratus fat pad on the lateral radiograph or the scaphoid fat pad on the PA radiograph, can raise suspicion for occult fractures. Because of the frequency of missed scaphoid fractures on initial radiographs, advanced imaging with MRI, multidetector CT (MDCT), nuclear scintigraphy, or tomosynthesis are being explored in the emergency setting.[13] MDCT is often used for complex distal radius fractures. The addition of three-dimensional reconstruc-

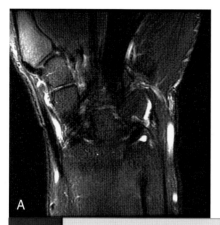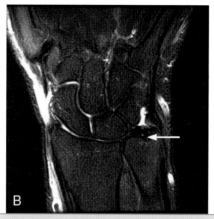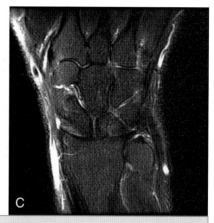

Figure 6 Triangular fibrocartilage central perforation. **A,** Extreme palmar MRI scan of the triangular fibrocartilage complex showing an intact volar radioulnar ligament. **B,** MRI scan of the triangular fibrocartilage complex halfway between the extreme volar and extreme dorsal images showing almost complete loss of the triangular fibrocartilage disk between the ulnar head and the ulnar-most aspect of the lunate. However, the distal fibers of the complex can be seen attaching to the ulnar fovea and the tip of the ulnar styloid (arrow). **C,** Dorsal MRI scan shows an intact dorsal radioulnar ligament attaching to the edge of the radius at the distal end of the sigmoid notch of the radius.

tions to the traditional two-dimensional sagittal and coronal reformations may better assess a coronal fracture line, central articular depression, and articular comminution and determine the exact number of fragments and may thus alter the surgical approach.

Instability

For evaluation of the intrinsic scapholunate and lunotriquetral ligaments of the wrist and evaluation of the triangular fibrocartilage, MDCT arthrography and magnetic resonance arthrography at 3 T have higher specificity and sensitivity when compared with conventional MRI at 1.5 T.[14] Evaluation of the triangular fibrocartilage complex by MRI at 1.5 T has been reported with sensitivities ranging from 27% to 100% and specificities from 90% to 100%. The more peripheral ulnar-sided tears and the noncommunicating partial ulnar-sided (proximal) tears, which may be more clinically significant (Figure 6), are particularly problematic in detection with MRI at 1.5 T, even with indirect arthrography.[15]

The distal radioulnar joint may be evaluated reliably with plain films, provided the lateral view is well positioned, with the volar surface of the pisiform projected between the volar surfaces of the distal pole of the scaphoid and the capitate and that the distal radius is without significant fracture deformity.[16]

Arthritis

Evaluation of the integrity of the articular cartilage within the wrist remains a challenge. Sensitivities for cartilage abnormalities of the distal radius, scaphoid, lunate, and triquetrum range from 10% to 52% using either 1.5 T or 3 T MRI machines, even with additional direct or indirect magnetic resonance arthrography. In one study, MDCT arthrography proved more sensitive than 1.5 T magnetic resonance arthrography.[17] However, for the detection of erosions from rheumatoid arthritis, even low field strength 0.2 T MRI is more sensitive than conventional radiography.[18] CT and tomosynthesis also have higher sensitivity.

Tendinopathy and Neuropathy

MRI has long been used to evaluate tendinopathy of the wrist. Increased fluid within tendon sheaths, synovial thickening, morphologic and signal abnormalities of the tendons, and scarring and thickening of the tendon sheaths all can be readily detected. Overuse syndromes such as de Quervain tenosynovitis or "baby wrist,"[19] inflammatory conditions such as rheumatoid arthritis, or even infections such as tuberculosis have been studied. Because of the relatively superficial anatomic position, sonography is gaining more attention in the evaluation of conditions such as extensor carpi ulnaris instability and impingement by volar plate fixation screws on extensor tendons.[20] MRI has also been used extensively to assess median nerve pathology in carpal tunnel syndrome and ulnar nerve pathology in the Guyon canal. Ultrasound can be useful to interrogate the wrist dynamically of superficial structures.

Tumor

Both MRI and ultrasonography can be used in the specific diagnosis of ganglion cysts, accessory muscles, foreign bodies, abscess, hemangiomas, hematomas, lipomas, tenosynovitis, tendon tears, aneurysms, and arteriovenous malformations presenting as hand masses. Solid masses such as giant cell tumor of the tendon sheath, schwannomas, and neuromas may not have a tissue-specific appearance, but differential possibilities can be narrowed significantly using these techniques.[21]

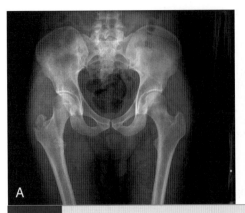
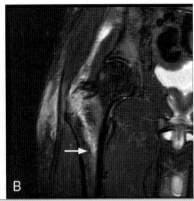
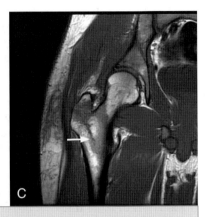

Figure 7 Intertrochanteric fracture. **A,** Plain film showing a displaced fracture of the greater trochanter apophysis. The extent of the lesion is underestimated by the plain film image. **B,** Fast spin-echo proton density-weighted coronal image shows the fracture line (arrow) extending from the base of the greater trochanter to a point midway across the intertrochanteric line; the fracture is of greater extent than the plain film suggested. **C,** Fast spin-echo T2-weighted coronal image shows the fracture line (arrow) extending from the base of the greater trochanter to a point almost completely across the intertrochanteric line, coming just short of the medial cortex, even further delineating the full extent of the fracture line. A sliding hip screw and side plate were subsequently used for fracture fixation.

Hip

Fracture

Plain film investigation for hip fractures generally includes an AP radiograph of the pelvis and a lateral view of the hip of the affected side. When the plain film study is negative, but there is inability to bear weight or other clinical findings that raise suspicion, MRI is often used in the emergency setting with abbreviated protocols to provide high sensitivity and specificity for fracture (**Figure 7**), osteonecrosis, or muscle injury.[22] When compared with bone scans, MRI is equally accurate for fracture detection but provides additional diagnoses in a substantial number of patients[22] with other pelvic fractures, such as insufficiency fractures of the sacrum or the acetabulum, muscle edema and tears, trochanteric bursitis, and hamstring tendinopathy.

Osteonecrosis

After initial plain films, MRI has become the preferred method to diagnose suspected osteonecrosis.[23] Findings such as the characteristic double line sign consisting of high signal intensity paralleling a low-intensity peripheral rim is often seen on T2-weighted images. Increased joint fluid, which is nonspecific, can be a secondary finding. Other entities need to be considered when MRI detects abnormalities of the proximal femur, including transient marrow edema of the femoral head[24] and subchondral insufficiency fractures. Distinguishing osteonecrosis from a subchondral fracture can be done by observing that in osteonecrosis, the double line forms a continuous ring.

Developmental Dysplasia of the Hip

Examination of the hip for developmental dysplasia in the pediatric population begins with dynamic and static ultrasound. The percentage of femoral head coverage, labral morphology, and superior femoral head displacement relative to the labrum and total femoral head displacement are assessed.[25] Plain film evaluation includes an assessment of the hips in AP projection with analysis of Shenton line, acetabular angles, the position of the femoral head with respect to the acetabulum using Hilgenreiner and Perkins lines, the morphology of the acetabulum, and the development and the shape of the femoral head. In the adult, acetabular depth, inclination, version, center edge angle, and femoral head sphericity are analyzed on plain films.[26]

Arthritis

Osteoarthritis is suggested on plain films by joint space narrowing, osteophytes at the femoral head neck junction or acetabular rim, subchondral cysts, subchondral sclerosis, and eventually loss of femoral head sphericity from subchondral collapse. In some patients, this process can occur prematurely or quite rapidly. In premature osteoarthritis, preexisting abnormalities such as developmental hip dysplasia, femoral acetabular impingement, or osteonecrosis are often present.[27] In rapidly occurring osteoarthritis, MRI evaluation often discloses joint effusion, diffuse bone marrow edema in the femoral head and neck, femoral head flattening, and cystlike subchondral defects. Magnetic resonance arthrography or specialized sequences may be helpful in assessing articular cartilage damage in the hip.

Femoral Acetabular Impingement and Labral Tear

The presence of a mismatch between the femoral head and neck with the acetabulum resulting in abutment of the proximal femur with the acetabulum is termed femoral acetabular impingement (FAI). This condition may lead to premature osteoarthritis. Fibrocystic changes are seen on plain films in the anterosuperior femoral neck in 33% of the patients with FAI in one study.[28] Rim ossification in the pincer type FAI and the pistol grip deformity of the femoral neck in the cam type can also be seen on plain films. MRI can assess for abnormal epiphyseal torsion angles, labral tears, and cartilage delamination in this entity. Calculation of the alpha angle as the angle subtended by the long axis femoral neck and the intersection of an idealized circle outlining the femoral head with a bony bump on the femoral neck in a specialized oblique axial plane can be supportive of the diagnosis. To evaluate hip instability or labral tears, magnetic resonance arthrography with direct injection of a gadolinium-containing compound can be done.

Total Hip Arthroplasty

In the evaluation of the painful hip after arthroplasty, the analysis of plain films for the development of radiolucency between the prosthesis and bone, between the cement and the prosthesis, or between the cement and bone should be done. Fractures of the cement, the development of sclerosis near the tip of the femoral stem, the evidence of prosthetic movement or the presence of metallic beads shed from the prosthesis can all be indicative of loosening on plain films. Plain films may also disclose stress shielding, insufficiency fractures near the femoral stem, component wear, component dislocation of the liner, or dislocation. Histiocytic response from immune reaction to prosthetic components shows a smooth endosteal scalloping on plain films. Arthrography plus aspiration and synovial biopsy to exclude infection can also disclose sinus tracts or extravasation below the intertrochanteric line. Nuclear scintigraphy, with indium-labeled white blood cells, immunoglobulin G scanning, or gallium scanning can also help in the diagnosis of periprosthetic infection.[29] Special techniques in MRI can be done to view the complications of total hip arthroplasty, such as muscle tears.[30]

Infection

In the diagnosis of a septic hip, neither ultrasound nor CT can be reliably used to exclude infection. Aspiration and synovial biopsy under either fluoroscopic guidance or ultrasonography remains essential. Work is being done using dynamic contrast-enhanced MRI to distinguish septic effusions from transient synovitis in the pediatric population.[31]

Muscles and Tendons

Abductor gluteus medius, gluteus minimus, hip adductor and rectus tendinopathies, bursitis, groin hernias, aponeurosis avulsions, athletic pubalgia, stress fractures, ischiofemoral impingement, and snapping hip can be evaluated with MRI or, in some cases, ultrasound.

Knee

Fracture

Knee fractures are commonly evaluated using orthogonal views of the tibiofemoral joint and the patella joint. AP and lateral views of the knee help rule out most of these fractures. A Merchant or skyline view of the patella can rule out dislocations or evaluate longitudinal fractures of the patella. Oblique views can be performed to evaluate fractures that are out of plane. A CT scan with coronal and sagittal reformations is recommended for comminuted and displaced tibial plateau fractures or distal femoral fractures. Three-dimensional reconstruction can help provide better visualization of the depressed articular fragments and also accurately identify the fracture plane, such as with a Hoffa fracture of the distal femur. MRI can be used to evaluate soft-tissue injuries, especially meniscus injuries with tibial plateau fractures and also associated ligament injuries.[32]

Arthritis

For arthritis of the knee, it is important to perform weight-bearing views to allow an indirect method of evaluating cartilage thickness. A bilateral flexion weight-bearing PA view, or Rosenberg view, allows better evaluation of the posterior weight-bearing surface of the tibia. The flexed PA view allows the x-ray beam to project along the posterior tibial slope to clearly evaluate the joint space. Merchant or skyline views are helpful to evaluate patellofemoral joint arthritis; however, it is important that these views are obtained at accurate knee flexion angles.

MRI has had significant improvement over the past decade in imaging cartilage lesions. Although MRI can evaluate focal cartilage injuries much better than plain radiography, we have also extended the use of MRI to evaluate the quality of cartilage. New imaging modalities such as delayed gadolinium-enhanced MRI of cartilage (dGEMRIC), T2 mapping, and T1rho mapping allow us to directly probe the biochemical composition of cartilage.[33] These techniques are developed to detect early cartilage changes, with loss of proteoglycan and organization, before loss of volume and thinning. dGEMRIC is an indirect magnetic resonance arthrography technique, where gadolinium is injected intravenously and allowed to diffuse into the joint. The amount of contrast diffusion into the cartilage matrix represents inversely the amount of proteoglycan in the articular cartilage. T2 mapping measures primarily the organization of the cartilage matrix and water content within the articular cartilage. T1rho is a novel sequence that measures the amount of proteoglycan within the cartilage (Figure 8).

Total Knee Replacement

Plain radiographs are commonly used in the evaluation of patients with total knee replacements. A change in the position of the prosthesis is a clear indication of loosening. Radiolucent lines can be present around the prosthesis; however, the diagnosis of component loosening is not as difficult as in total hip arthroplasty because the joint is more superficial, and patients will exhibit more localized pain along the loose prosthesis. The diagnosis and workup of an infected knee prosthesis is similar to the methods for total hip arthroplasty

Ligament and Meniscus Injuries

MRI has superior capabilities in the diagnosis of knee ligament and meniscus injuries. The sensitivity and the specificity for diagnosing anterior cruciate ligament in-

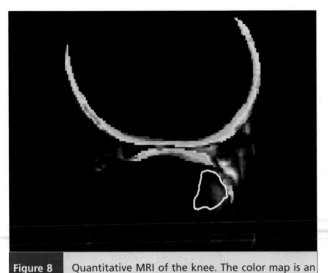

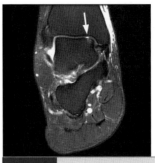

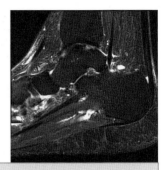

Figure 8   Quantitative MRI of the knee. The color map is an overlay to visually represent the T1rho measurement. Warmer color (red) indicates loss of proteoglycan (cartilage degeneration) whereas cold color (blue) indicates cartilage with higher content of proteoglycan. White outline indicates edema pattern.

Figure 9   Osteochondritis dissecans of the talar dome. **A,** Fast spin-echo T2-weighted coronal image of the talus shows an osteochondral defect of the talar dome. There is poorly defined subchondral edema with a full thickness articular cartilage defect (arrow) but apparently intact cortical bone. **B,** Fast spin-echo T2-weighted sagittal image of the same talus shows an osteochondral defect of the medial talar dome. The cortex appears slightly collapsed in the area of cartilage loss. In conjunction with the coronal images, the area of surface abnormality and the depth of the lesion can be ascertained.

juries are 85% and 94%, respectively, whereas for meniscus injuries the sensitivity and the specificity are 96% and 97%, respectively.[34] However, the presence of radiographic abnormalities does not mean that patients have to be symptomatic. It has been well documented that meniscus tears are present in advancing age, and arthroscopic surgery on asymptomatic meniscus tears or meniscus tears with no mechanical symptoms yields no benefits to placebo treatment. Clinicians must be careful in interpreting radiographic findings and clinical symptoms. MRI, however, is not as accurate when compared with clinical examinations in the diagnosis of chronic posterior cruciate ligament (PCL) or posterolateral corner injuries. Chronic PCL injuries can have continuity of the PCL fibers on MRI but have clinical instability. Posterolateral corner structures are quite complex, and dedicated oblique views of the posterolateral corner of the knee may be needed to diagnose these injuries.

Foot and Ankle

Standard radiographs of the tibia and the fibula include AP and lateral views. For the ankle, AP, mortise, and lateral views are obtained, and AP, oblique, and lateral images are usually obtained for the foot. Other common views are the Harris Beath axial views for the calcaneus, gravity stress views for evaluating the integrity of ankle ligaments, and weight-bearing views of the foot for evaluating acquired or congenital deformities of the foot and for interrogation of the Lisfranc joint. Specialized views are available for evaluating the calcaneal facets and the sesamoids.

Fractures

In the acute trauma setting, the decision to obtain radiographs may be determined using a standardized protocol, such as the Ottawa rules.[35] Three views are routinely obtained. The presence of a tibiotalar joint effusion detected as a teardrop sign at the anterior aspect of the joint on the lateral radiograph is associated with a significant number of radiographically occult fractures, especially if larger than 13 mm.[36] These occult fracture sites include the talar dome, the tibial overhang, the posterior rims of the distal tibia (Tillaux fracture), the medial and lateral malleoli, the tibial plafond, and the anterior process of the calcaneus.

CT with two-dimensional reconstructions can be instrumental in detecting these injuries. Three-dimensional reconstructions from MD CT data may help in surgical planning. A significant percentage, up to 45%, of occult subchondral lesions can also be detected using MRI, which are less well seen using CT. The relationship of these lesions and subsequent osteochondral defects of the talar dome is being investigated[37] (Figure 9).

Instability

In the evaluation of the ligamentous integrity of the ankle, one study demonstrated sensitivities for syndesmotic ligament injuries ranging from 45% to 62% compared with arthroscopy.[38] However, with added indirect arthrography or direct magnetic resonance arthrography, this can be improved to the 91% to 95% range.[38]

Impingement

MRI continues to have a role in the evaluation of the various impingement syndromes.[39] Soft-tissue masses can be seen in the anterolateral gutter in patients with arthroscopically confirmed anterolateral impingement in a little less than half of patients. This sensitivity improves considerably (88% to 96%) if there is fluid in the joint, either native or injected via a magnetic resonance arthrogram.[40] Sonographic arthrography and MDCT arthrography have also been studied for anterolateral impingement, with sensitivities of 85% and 97%, respectively.[41]

Tenosynovitis

Because of its superior soft-tissue contrast, MRI continues to predominate in the evaluation of tendon abnormalities. Adequate coverage is essential to include the distal insertions of the specific tendons to be interrogated (ie, flexor hallucis, posterior tibial tendon, peroneus longus) and not just limit the study to the ankle. Signal abnormalities within the tendons, fluid in the tendon sheaths, and secondary edema in subjacent bone can all be used to establish a diagnosis of tendinopathy or tenosynovitis. The amount of fluid or the extent of signal abnormality can be instrumental in distinguishing normal from pathologic findings.[42] Tendon subluxation, tears, or impingement may also be evaluated with sonography.

Infection

Plain films are obtained initially in suspected osteomyelitis and also to confirm the presence of periostitis, focal osteopenia, cortical erosion, soft-tissue edema, or soft-tissue gas or foreign bodies. Often, secondary imaging is required to definitively exclude bone infection. Nuclear scintigraphy with combined triple phase Tc-99m bone and tagged white blood cell scans can be useful in ruling out infection, especially in cases complicated by recent fracture, recent surgery, or prostheses. MRI is also used, relying on concordant signal abnormalities within the deep bone marrow on T1-weighted images (loss of normal fat signal), fluid sensitive sequences such as fat-saturated T2-weighted images or short tau inversion recovery sequences (high signal from bone marrow edema), plus enhancement after intravenous gadolinium contrast injection on fat-saturated T1-weighted images (**Figure 10**). Excluding concomitant infection in a neuropathic foot can be particularly challenging. The pattern of signal abnormality in bones may be helpful, with the signal abnormalities in the uninfected neuropathic bone confined to the immediate subcortical bone in a thin rim pattern, whereas infected bones have confluent deep marrow signal changes. Other secondary findings, such as sinus tracts, abscesses, pressure point location, and gas in the soft tissues, also can be used to distinguish the uninfected from the infected neuropathic foot.[43]

Tumors

Both MRI and sonography are used to characterize soft-tissue masses. Ganglion cysts, plantar fibromas, Morton neuromas, and lipomas can often be specifically diagnosed with MRI (**Figure 11**). However, with Morton neuroma, recurrence of tumor may be difficult to distinguish from the normal scarring process.[44]

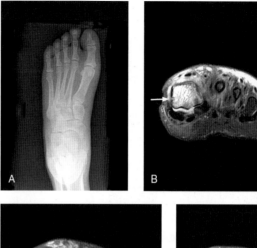
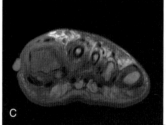
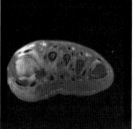

Figure 10 Osteomyelitis. **A,** Plain film of the left foot, showing edema of the great toe but no periostitis, cortical erosion, or focal osteopenia.
B, Fast spin-echo T2-weighted image showing fluid in the first metatarsophalangeal joint and deep marrow edema in the distal first metatarsal head. The cortex has a small defect at the site of penetration by a foreign body (arrow).
C, T1-weighted image showing fluid in the first metatarsophalangeal joint and deep marrow edema in the distal first metatarsal head. Deep marrow signal loss on T1-weighted images is a concordant finding with high signal on T2-weighted images in the diagnosis of osteomyelitis. However, both of these findings represent edema within the marrow, a nonspecific finding seen also in trauma and tumors. **D,** T1-weighted image after the intravenous injection of a gadolinium-based compound shows enhancement of the deep marrow of the distal first metatarsal, the synovium in the joint, and the plantar subcutaneous fat deep to the first metatarsal. These findings are all supportive of the diagnosis of osteomyelitis and possible septic arthritis.

Neuropathy

A variety of specific nerve neuropathies can be examined with MRI. Neuropathies affecting branches of the posterior tibial nerve are studied, such as the medial and lateral plantar nerves in the tarsal tunnel; Baxter neuropathy of the inferior calcaneal nerve; and jogger's foot, which is caused by entrapment of the medial plantar nerve by the abductor hallucis muscle and the master knot of Henry (chiasma plantaris), where the flexor hallucis longus and flexor digitorum longus cross. Other nerves studied with both MRI and ultrasound include the sural and superficial peroneal nerves. The physician should look for masses; scar tissue; thickened retinacu-

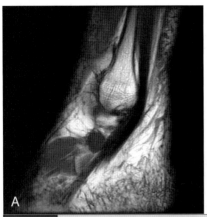
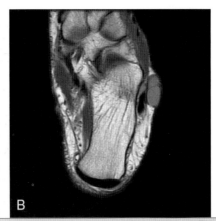
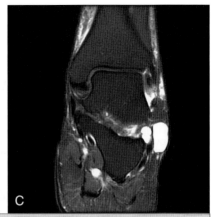

Figure 11 Ganglion cyst. **A,** T1-weighted sagittal image of the ankle shows a mass, similar but slightly darker in signal than muscle, adjacent to the peroneus brevis tendon. **B,** Proton-weighted axial image of the ankle shows the same mass, similar but slightly brighter in signal to muscle, adjacent to the peroneus brevis tendon. **C,** T2-weighted fast spin-echo coronal image of the ankle shows the same mass, with homogeneous high fluid signal, adjacent to the peroneus brevis tendon. Thin septa separate the mass into at least three compartments.

la; inflammatory conditions compressing the nerves in confined spaces such as the tarsal tunnel; neurofibromas; schwannomas of the nerves themselves; or secondary signs such as muscle atrophy, as in Baxter neuropathy involving the abductor digiti minimi muscle.

Summary

Musculoskeletal imaging has significantly enhanced the ability to diagnose, monitor, and evaluate the healing of musculoskeletal conditions. Clinicians should determine the best imaging modalities to aid in their treatment of musculoskeletal disorders.

Key Study Points

- Understand the benefits and limitations of each imaging modality: plain radiography, ultrasonography, nuclear imaging, CT, and MRI.
- Understand the importance of guidelines of radiation safety.
- Understand the importance of different imaging modalities of different conditions and body regions.

Annotated References

1. Ma CB, Steinbach LS: Musculoskeletal imaging, in Lieberman JA: *AAOS Comprehensive Orthopaedic Review*. Rosemont, IL, American Academy of Orthopaedic Surgeons, 2008, pp 137-142.

2. Goutallier D, Postel JM, Bernageau J, Lavau L, Voisin MC: Fatty muscle degeneration in cuff ruptures: Pre- and postoperative evaluation by CT scan. *Clin Orthop Relat Res* 1994;304:78-83.

3. Fuchs B, Weishaupt D, Zanetti M, Hodler J, Gerber C: Fatty degeneration of the muscles of the rotator cuff: Assessment by computed tomography versus magnetic resonance imaging. *J Shoulder Elbow Surg* 1999;8(6): 599-605.

4. Rerko MA, Pan X, Donaldson C, Jones GL, Bishop JY: Comparison of various imaging techniques to quantify glenoid bone loss in shoulder instability. *J Shoulder Elbow Surg* 2013;22(4):528-534.

   The authors compared the ability of plain radiographs, MRI, CT, and three-dimensional CT to quantify glenoid bone loss.

5. Steinbach LS: MRI of shoulder instability. *Eur J Radiol* 2008;68(1):57-71.

6. Chapman VM, Kalra M, Halpern E, Grottkau B, Albright M, Jaramillo D: 16-MDCT of the posttraumatic pediatric elbow: Optimum parameters and associated radiation dose. *AJR Am J Roentgenol* 2005;185(2): 516 -521.

7. Guitton TG, Ring D; Science of Variation Group: Interobserver reliability of radial head fracture classification: Two-dimensional compared with three-dimensional CT. *J Bone Joint Surg Am* 2011;93(21):2015-2021.

   Eighty-five orthopaedic surgeons classified 12 different radial head fractures using the Broberg and Morrey modification of the Mason classification assessing fracture line, comminution, articular surface involvement, articular stepoff or gap, central impaction, and the number of fragments. The use of three-dimensional reconstructions results in a small but substantial decrease in interobserver variation.

8. Awaya H, Schweitzer ME, Feng SA, et al: Elbow synovial fold syndrome: MR imaging findings. *AJR Am J Roentgenol* 2001;177(6):1377-1381.

9. Potter HG, Weiland AJ, Schatz JA, Paletta GA, Hotchkiss RN: Posterolateral rotatory instability of the elbow: Usefulness of MR imaging in diagnosis. *Radiology* 1997;204(1):185-189.

10. Kijowski R, De Smet AA: Magnetic resonance imaging findings in patients with medial epicondylitis. *Skeletal Radiol* 2005;34(4):196-202.

11. Struijs PA, Assendelft WJ, Kerkhoffs GM, Souer S, van Dijk CN: The predictive value of the extensor grip test for the effectiveness of bracing for tennis elbow. *Am J Sports Med* 2005;33(12):1905-1909.

12. Miller TT, Reinus WR: Nerve entrapment syndromes of the elbow, forearm, and wrist. *AJR Am J Roentgenol* 2010;195(3):585-594.

    A review of nerve entrapment syndromes of the elbow, forearm, and wrist featuring both sonographic and MRI imaging is presented.

13. Nikken JJ, Oei EH, Ginai AZ, et al: Acute wrist trauma: Value of a short dedicated extremity MR imaging examination in prediction of need for treatment. *Radiology* 2005;234(1):116-124.

14. Chhabra A, Soldatos T, Thawait GK, et al: Current perspectives on the advantages of 3-T MR imaging of the wrist. *Radiographics* 2012;32(3):879-896.

    A review of the use and findings of high field strength (3 T) MRI in evaluation of the ligaments, tendons, and articular cartilage of the wrist is presented.

15. Haims AH, Schweitzer ME, Morrison WB, et al: Internal derangement of the wrist: Indirect MR arthrography versus unenhanced MR imaging. *Radiology* 2003;227(3):701-707.

16. Mino DE, Palmer AK, Levinsohn EM: Radiography and computerized tomography in the diagnosis of incongruity of the distal radio-ulnar joint: A prospective study. *J Bone Joint Surg Am* 1985;67(2):247-252.

17. Moser T, Dosch JC, Moussaoui A, Dietemann JL: Wrist ligament tears: Evaluation of MRI and combined MDCT and MR arthrography. *AJR Am J Roentgenol* 2007;188(5):1278-1286.

18. Taouli B, Zaim S, Peterfy CG, et al: Rheumatoid arthritis of the hand and wrist: Comparison of three imaging techniques. *AJR Am J Roentgenol* 2004;182(4):937-943.

19. Anderson SE, Steinbach LS, De Monaco D, Bonel HM, Hurtienne Y, Voegelin E: "Baby wrist": MRI of an overuse syndrome in mothers. *AJR Am J Roentgenol* 2004;182(3):719-724.

20. Bianchi S, van Aaken J, Glauser T, Martinoli C, Beaulieu JY, Della Santa D: Screw impingement on the extensor tendons in distal radius fractures treated by volar plating: Sonographic appearance. *AJR Am J Roentgenol* 2008;191(5):W199-203.

21. Bianchi S, Della Santa D, Glauser T, Beaulieu JY, van Aaken J: Sonography of masses of the wrist and hand. *AJR Am J Roentgenol* 2008;191(6):1767-1775.

22. Kirby MW, Spritzer C: Radiographic detection of hip and pelvic fractures in the emergency department. *AJR Am J Roentgenol* 2010;194(4):1054-1060.

    The authors present a retrospective analysis of 92 patients referred for MRI from the emergency department. Fourteen percent of the patients with negative plain films had fractures disclosed by MRI, whereas no fracture was found in 12% of the patients with radiographs suggestive of fracture. In 43 of the 59 patients without a fracture on MRI, muscle edema or tear, trochanteric bursitis, or hamstring tendinopathy were found to account for patient symptoms.

23. Beltran J, Herman LJ, Burk JM, et al: Femoral head avascular necrosis: MR imaging with clinical-pathologic and radionuclide correlation. *Radiology* 1988;166(1 Pt 1):215-220.

24. Vande Berg BE, Malghem JJ, Labaisse MA, Noel HM, Maldague BE: MR imaging of avascular necrosis and transient marrow edema of the femoral head. *Radiographics* 1993;13(3):501-520.

25. White KK, Sucato DJ, Agrawal S, Browne R: Ultrasonographic findings in hips with a positive Ortolani sign and their relationship to Pavlik harness failure. *J Bone Joint Surg Am* 2010;92(1):113-120.

26. Clohisy JC, Carlisle JC, Beaulé PE, et al: A systematic approach to the plain radiographic evaluation of the young adult hip. *J Bone Joint Surg Am* 2008;90(suppl 4):47-66.

27. Clohisy JC, Dobson MA, Robison JF, et al: Radiographic structural abnormalities associated with premature, natural hip-joint failure. *J Bone Joint Surg Am* 2011;93(suppl 2):3-9.

    Six hundred four patients were retrospectively analyzed for causes of premature hip failure. Developmental hip dysplasia and FAI were associated with the majority of osteoarthritic hips, with significant bilaterality associated with FAI.

28. Leunig M, Beck M, Kalhor M, Kim YJ, Werlen S, Ganz R: Fibrocystic changes at anterosuperior femoral neck: Prevalence in hips with femoroacetabular impingement. *Radiology* 2005;236(1):237-246.

29. Keogh CF, Munk PL, Gee R, Chan LP, Marchinkow LO: Imaging of the painful hip arthroplasty. *AJR Am J Roentgenol* 2003;180(1):115-120.

30. Potter HG, Nestor BJ, Sofka CM, Ho ST, Peters LE,

Salvati EA: Magnetic resonance imaging after total hip arthroplasty: Evaluation of periprosthetic soft tissue. *J Bone Joint Surg Am* 2004;86(9):1947-1954.

31. Kim EY, Kwack KS, Cho JH, Lee DH, Yoon SH: Usefulness of dynamic contrast-enhanced MRI in differentiating between septic arthritis and transient synovitis in the hip joint. *AJR Am J Roentgenol* 2012;198(2): 428-433.

   Eighteen patients were evaluated using dynamic contrast-enhanced MRI with a significant difference in time enhancement curves between patients with septic arthritis and transient synovitis of the hip. The optimal time for acquisition of contrast-enhanced coronal MRI to be acquired was 3.5 minutes after injection to distinguish between the two entities.

32. Markhardt BK, Gross JM, Monu JU: Schatzker classification of tibial plateau fractures: Use of CT and MR imaging improves assessment. *Radiographics* 2009;29(2): 585-597.

33. Kurkijärvi JE, Nissi MJ, Kiviranta I, Jurvelin JS, Nieminen MT: Delayed gadolinium-enhanced MRI of cartilage (dGEMRIC) and T2 characteristics of human knee articular cartilage: Topographical variation and relationships to mechanical properties. *Magn Reson Med* 2004;52(1):41-46.

34. Magee T, Williams D: 3.0-T MRI of meniscal tears. *AJR Am J Roentgenol* 2006;187(2):371-375.

35. Verma S, Hamilton K, Hawkins HH, et al: Clinical application of the Ottawa ankle rules for the use of radiography in acute ankle injuries: An independent site assessment. *AJR Am J Roentgenol* 1997;169(3):825-827.

36. Clark TW, Janzen DL, Ho K, Grunfeld A, Connell DG: Detection of radiographically occult ankle fractures following acute trauma: Positive predictive value of an ankle effusion. *AJR Am J Roentgenol* 1995;164(5):1185-1189.

37. Griffith JF, Lau DT, Yeung DK, Wong MW: High-resolution MR imaging of talar osteochondral lesions with new classification. *Skeletal Radiol* 2012;41(4): 387-399.

   The authors present a retrospective review of 70 osteochondral defects of the talar dome and provide a new classification system based on high-quality images.

38. Kim S, Huh YM, Song HT, et al: Chronic tibiofibular syndesmosis injury of ankle: Evaluation with contrast-enhanced fat-suppressed 3D fast spoiled gradient-recalled acquisition in the steady state MR imaging. *Radiology* 2007;242(1):225-235.

39. Donovan A, Rosenberg ZS: MRI of ankle and lateral hindfoot impingement syndromes. *AJR Am J Roentgenol* 2010;195(3):595-604.

   Impingement syndromes of the ankle are reviewed, showing the differing patterns of MRI abnormalities found in anterolateral, anteromedial, posterolateral, posterior, and extra-articular impingment syndromes.

40. Rubin DA, Tishkoff NW, Britton CA, Conti SF, Towers JD: Anterolateral soft-tissue impingement in the ankle: Diagnosis using MR imaging. *AJR Am J Roentgenol* 1997;169(3):829-835.

41. Cochet H, Pelé E, Amoretti N, Brunot S, Lafenêtre O, Hauger O: Anterolateral ankle impingement: Diagnostic performance of MDCT arthrography and sonography. *AJR Am J Roentgenol* 2010;194(6):1575-1580.

   Sonography and MD CT arthrography are compared in the evaluation of anterolateral impingement. Sonography without joint injection had a sensitivity and specificity of 77% and 57% respectively, whereas CT arthrography had a sensitivity of 97% and specificity of 71% using arthroscopic findings as the reference standard.

42. Kijowski R, De Smet A, Mukharjee R: Magnetic resonance imaging findings in patients with peroneal tendinopathy and peroneal tenosynovitis. *Skeletal Radiol* 2007;36(2):105-114.

43. Ahmadi ME, Morrison WB, Carrino JA, Schweitzer ME, Raikin SM, Ledermann HP: Neuropathic arthropathy of the foot with and without superimposed osteomyelitis: MR imaging characteristics. *Radiology* 2006; 238(2):622-631.

44. Espinosa N, Schmitt JW, Saupe N, et al: Morton neuroma: MR imaging after resection—postoperative MR and histologic findings in asymptomatic and symptomatic intermetatarsal spaces. *Radiology* 2010;255(3): 850-856.

   Fibrous tissue is commonly found in postoperative intermetatarsal spaces after Morton neuroma resection and mimics the appearance of the original tumor on MRI in both asymptomatic and symptomatic patients.

Chapter 8

Patient-Centered Care: Communication Skills and Cultural Competence

Hassan R. Mir, MD   Raj D. Rao, MD

Introduction

Physicians are often attracted to the field of orthopaedics because of their interest in anatomy, biomechanics, and the scientific method. However, as most experienced practitioners will attest, mastery of these subjects alone is insufficient to achieve successful outcomes. The interpersonal and emotional aspects of patient care greatly affect every component of medical care delivery, and orthopaedic surgeons must possess effective communication skills that allow them to develop good physician-patient relationships and actively involve patients in all aspects of their care. The US Census Bureau anticipates a continued increase in population diversity: the minority population is predicted to increase from 34% in 2008 to 55% in 2050. Therefore, the ability to interact and communicate with patients must transcend various backgrounds and any expectations that patients may have.

Patient-Centered Care

Patient-centered care refers broadly to the process of involving patients and their families in decision making about individual treatment options. More specifically, the term refers to the central role of the patient in the design of changing healthcare delivery models. Studies of what patients and their families desire in a healthcare system have identified four key features of patient-centered care: "whole person" care, comprehensive communication and coordination, patient support and empowerment, and ready access.[1] Holistic care and access to care can be affected by changes in practice and through health policy. The issues of patient support and empowerment and comprehensive communication relate directly to the interactions between physicians and their patients and highlight the importance of physician education on a patient-centered approach to the physician-patient relationship.

Health literacy, which includes patients' understanding of their medical conditions and postsurgical treatment plans, has been linked to many aspects of individual health and medical care, including patient satisfaction and outcomes.[2] Orthopaedic surgeons should be aware that the terminology used and the manner in which the information is communicated to their patients can significantly affect patient understanding and emotional response to healthcare delivery.[3,4] Publications and audiovisual materials can be used to improve health literacy, but the content should ensure that the information is clearly conveyed and can be customized to the individual patient's level of comprehension.[5] Because patients respect their physicians' knowledge and counsel, physicians should educate their patients about diagnoses, treatments, and the risks and benefits of various options.

Effective communication can affect the patient's health, functional, and emotional status. Improved patient interactions can help the physician elicit important information that can improve diagnostic accuracy and enhance patient compliance by increasing the level of trust.[6,7] The physician should allow the patient to present his or her concerns by means of open-ended questions and minimal interruptions. This approach may help the physician gain insight into the patient's problems and obtain all necessary information to help narrow the list of differential diagnoses through subsequent directed questioning. Patients are also more likely to trust their physician when given the opportunity to present all of their concerns and have their questions answered. Additionally, many patients now use complementary and alternative medicines that can affect their care, and this may be unreported without a thorough interview.[8]

From a medical-legal perspective, patient-centered communication can improve the informed consent process and help reduce medical errors and malpractice litigation risk.[9,10] Many medical liability suits can be traced to breakdowns in communication, which can lead to a difference of expectations between physicians and their patients. Many lawsuits can be avoided by establishing initial patient-centered communication with good bidirectional flow of information and expectations, followed by open, honest dialogue when complications occur.

A movement toward shared decision making in medicine is occurring, with patients and their families experiencing more active involvement in the process and physician guidance.[11] This change requires effective patient-centered communication. Orthopaedic surgeons who have been educated in interview skills and information delivery can ensure a beneficial two-way interaction with all of their patients.

Communication Skills in Orthopaedics

Physicians may conduct more than 100,000 patient interviews during their careers, and the literature increasingly supports the positive influence of effective communication on various aspects of health care. Therefore, many organizations have educated medical students, residents, and practicing physicians on communication skills over the past 2 decades.[12] Although medical science continues to improve, advances in technology are unlikely to obviate the need for and the value of compassion and empathy in the physician-patient relationship. Orthopaedic surgeons and other specialists face significant daily time constraints, but education in effective verbal and nonverbal communication skills can make the time spent with their patients more effective and can improve patient relationships.

Improving Communication

A successful patient encounter requires that the patient's key concerns have been solicited and directly addressed.[11] Patient concerns can vary widely and be influenced by their values, culture, sex, and other variables.[13] To facilitate open communication, the physician should be careful to avoid a judgmental attitude and offer his or her counsel with patient feedback to ensure patient involvement and understanding.

The American Academy of Orthopaedic Surgeons (AAOS) has made substantial efforts to improve the historical patient perspective of orthopaedic surgeons as technically proficient but lacking empathy and communication skills. Patient surveys showed improvement between 1998 and 2008 (Table 1). The AAOS has partnered with the Institute for Healthcare Communication since 2003 to develop a mentoring program as well as a series of workshops that are available to enhance the communication skills of orthopaedic surgeons throughout the United States.

Communication Models

Multiple educational models have been developed to help physicians communicate and provide counsel in a more patient-centered way. The 5As model of behavioral change is an evidence-based approach that can be applied to a broad range of behaviors and health conditions.[14,15] The 5As comprise the following: (1) asking the patient about the behavior; (2) advising the patient about personal health risks; (3) assessing patient level of behavior, beliefs, and motivation; (4) assisting with the anticipation of barriers and the development of a specific action plan; and (5) arranging follow-up support. Assistance in problem solving and arranging follow-up have been shown to be the most important factors that lead to lasting change, but these are also delivered least often and may be the most challenging for orthopaedic surgeons. The 5As model has been frequently applied to health conditions such as smoking cessation and obesity, issues that often affect outcomes in orthopaedic surgery. Similarly, the model can be applied to other health conditions that require behavioral change, including musculoskeletal conditions that are managed nonsurgically, such as back pain and osteoarthritis. Postoperative results for several procedures also depend on patient adherence to rehabilitation protocols and activity restrictions.

The 4Es educational model (Figure 1) has also been used to increase patient-centered communication and improve healthcare delivery.[16] This model divides clinical care into communication tasks and biomedical tasks, which are weighted equally. The communication tasks—engagement, empathy, education, and enlistment—improve physician-patient interaction. The biomedical tasks, or the 2Fs (find it, fix it), involve making a diagnosis and then treating the problem. The 4Es model has been used more frequently than the 5As model in the education of orthopaedic surgeons about patient-centered communication because it closely parallels how surgical issues are addressed.

Engagement uses both verbal and nonverbal communication skills to establish the physician-patient relationship. Verbal interview techniques include speaking calmly, asking open-ended questions, and avoiding interruptions.[11] Nonverbal communication skills include maintaining eye contact, smiling, and sitting instead of standing to avoid appearing rushed. Empathy uses both verbal and nonverbal cues to assure the patient that his or her thoughts and feelings are understood by the surgeon in a compassionate manner and can help establish a relationship of trust that facilitates increased sharing of important information. Patient education should provide information about diagnoses and treatments in an interactive manner (using both dialogue and audiovisual aids) and ensure that the message is understood by the patient and that all alternatives have been reviewed.[2,5] Enlistment allows the patient to understand his or her active role in both the decision-making process and in the ultimate treatment outcome. Patient compliance significantly affects all treatment plans.

Table 1

Results From AAOS Survey on Patient Expectations and Perceptions on Communication

	1998 Results	2008 Results
Expectations That Remained the Same or Decreased		
Is highly trained	87%	82%
Listens to patients	85%	83%
Has successful medical results	84%	84%
Is caring and compassionate	77%	74%
Spends time answering questions	74%	74%
Delivers value/cost	70%	73%
Easy to get appointment	65%	65%
Is research oriented	39%	36%
Is prestigious	33%	31%
Accepts insurance (added in 2008)	NA	85%
Expectations That Improved		
Is highly trained	66%	75%
Spends time answering questions	35%	51%
Has successful medical results	55%	64%
Is caring and compassionate	35%	55%
Delivers value/cost	36%	50%
Easy to get appointment	28%	33%
Is research oriented	52%	64%
Is prestigious	61%	72%
Knowledge and experience	60%	71%
Overall performance	57%	67%

NA = not applicable. Arrows indicate the direction of significant differences. Percentage results are based on a scale of 1 to 5, from poor to excellent.
(Adapted from Tongue JR, Jenkins L, Wade A: Low-touch surgeons in a high-touch world. *AAOS Now* 2009;63[85]).

Incorporating Technology

Technologic advances are rapidly changing the way people interact with each other in modern society, with increasing rates of individual and mass communication occurring via e-mail, the Internet, and social media.[17] Additionally, face-to-face interactions can be interrupted frequently by using personal digital items such as mobile phones and tablets, which distract from verbal and nonverbal communication. The incorporation of new communication technology into medicine can be beneficial if done properly and without interfering with the physician-patient relationship.

Patients use the Internet to gather information about their medical conditions and healthcare providers.[18] The vast amount of medical knowledge increases exponentially and makes this task difficult; even physicians struggle to sort through all the available information.[19] In response, many physicians have established an online presence using websites and social media to educate patients about their practices and provide information about diagnoses. It is the responsibility of the physician to ensure that material posted in a publicly viewed forum is honest and accurate.

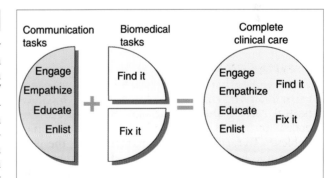

Figure 1 Illustration of the 4Es of complete clinical care, a model for physician patient communication. (Reproduced with permission from Tongue JR, Epps HR, Forese LL: Communication skills for patient-centered care: Research-based, easily learned techniques for medical interviews that benefit orthopaedic surgeons and their patients. *J Bone Joint Surg Am* 2005;87:652-658.)

Electronic communication is increasing between physicians and patients. Although electronic forms of communication such as phone calls, e-mail, texting, instant messaging, and videoconferencing, allow the rapid exchange of healthcare information, caution must be exercised. Physicians must be aware that nonverbal communication plays a large role in the exchange of medical information with audiovisual cues. This is especially important for the physical examination. Not all media allow every aspect of this exchange to occur.[20] This lack of full personal context can lead to incomplete information and incorrect conclusions and decisions. Healthcare information exchanged via newer forms of communication may also have medical-legal ramifications that are still being explored.

As electronic health records become more common, the use of computers and tablets in the patient examination room has increased.[21] Patients are using their mobile phones more frequently throughout the visit to record notes, photos, or video. Although these items may have advantages, the technology cannot be allowed to interrupt or supersede verbal and nonverbal communication, which are still central to the development of trust in the patient-physician relationship.

Adverse Events

Complications and adverse events are a reality in patient care. Shared decision making and a comprehensive and objective informed consent process prepare patients for the possibility of an unplanned adverse event. This process helps patients and their families accept the complication and prepares them for the steps necessary to address the problem. Failure to obtain appropriate informed consent is frequently cited in malpractice lawsuits. Even with suitable information and preparation, the development of a complication creates a significant amount of stress for patients, families, and physicians.

When a patient experiences an unplanned outcome, the physician often experiences myriad emotions (sadness, guilt, and/or defensiveness) irrespective of the involvement of a technical error. Similarly, the physician must remember that although patients and their families are likely to regard the complication as an error and often quickly think to assign blame, they are also experiencing mixed emotions of fear, confusion, and anger. These situations require a heightened sense of awareness and good communication skills.

Physicians should communicate with their team members to gather information, contact the patient and family, and avoid any defensive attitude.[22] It is important to discuss all aspects of the complication, including details, possible causes, and proposed treatment. An apology should be offered without accepting blame. The situation may be compounded by the physician's fear of potential litigation, but patients who receive full disclosure are more likely to maintain trust and less likely to litigate.[23,24] A sound strategy of information gathering, direct interaction, showing empathy, explaining options, and maintaining support can help with communication in these difficult situations.

Cultural Competence

The Office of Minority Health in the US Department of Health and Human Services defines cultural and linguistic competence as a set of congruent behaviors, attitudes, and policies that combine in a system, an agency, or among professionals that enables effective work in cross-cultural situations. Culture refers to integrated patterns of human behavior that include the language, thoughts, communications, actions, customs, beliefs, values, and institutions of racial, ethnic, religious, or social groups. Competence implies the capacity to function effectively as an individual and as an organization within the context of the cultural beliefs, behaviors, and needs presented by patients and their communities. The Office of Minority Health highlights social groups that influence a person's culture and self-identity, including race, ethnicity, religion, sex, sexual orientation, age, disability, and socioeconomic status.

Extensive research in cognitive psychology has identified the presence of bias in all individuals, as demonstrated by results of tests such as the Implicit Association Test (https://implicit.harvard.edu). Studies of physician attitudes reveal that very few practitioners have explicit (conscious) bias, but all physicians are prone to implicit (unconscious) bias. Bias affects how patients interpret and accept their physicians' recommendations for care. Bias also affects the recommendations that physicians make.[25] Physicians must recognize that the patient's experiences influence their attitudes. A patient's perceptions of racism and classism experienced in other healthcare settings may negatively influence the affective tone of current patient-provider communication.[26] The authors of a 2011 study showed that unconscious stereotyping and bias by healthcare providers can contribute to racial and ethnic disparities in health care.[27] An example of such bias is the common misperception that patients at a socioeconomic disadvantage tend to sue their doctors more frequently than economically advantaged patients. The authors of a recent study showed the opposite to be true: poor patients sue their physicians less often.[28]

The development of culturally competent care in a healthcare organization can enhance medical care delivery and outcomes in many ways through more effective patient-centered communication.[29] Cultural competency can help physicians deal more effectively with cultural conflicts that may occur between a patient and the clinical team and interfere with a patient-centered approach.[30] To deliver culturally competent care, clinicians must establish egalitarian goals for all of their patients, identify commonalities with their patients to counter stereotypical misinformation, and understand the perspectives of patients whose backgrounds may differ from their own. Cultural competency interventions, including the training of physicians and other healthcare professionals, have been proposed as a key strategy to help reduce healthcare disparities.[31]

Culturally Diverse Patient Populations

Cultural competence requires physicians to learn about the diverse populations they serve, which increases patient comfort and enhances communication. Medical anthropologists have criticized cultural competence efforts that divide cultures into static categories with a "list of traits."[32] The anthropologists argued that healthcare providers should be trained to be "open-minded" and willing to learn about different cultures while remembering a patient's individuality. Although this more fluid and individual approach to cultural diversity can be beneficial to the physician-patient relationship, it must be balanced with a framework that helps guide physician-patient interactions and reduces the prevalence of healthcare disparities.

Physicians should educate themselves to effectively communicate and treat patients with respect to race, ethnicity, religion, sex, sexual orientation, age, disability, and socioeconomic status. Both verbal and nonverbal communication can vary among culturally diverse groups, and constant education and practice can help physicians improve their skills. Some language barriers can be overcome through empathy and culturally appropriate nonverbal cues, but patients with limited English proficiency must be given proper access to translation services.

Improving Cultural Competence

Cultural competence can be taught using a fact-centered approach based on group characteristics that emphasizes the recognition of variation within the group, warns against ethnic stereotyping, and acknowledges that these group characteristics serve only as a first step to learning culturally competent care. This process should then evolve toward a more attitude- and skill-centered approach based on principles of cultural competence. It is important to understand the differences between stereotypes and generalizations when learning about different patient groups. Stereotypes are end points resulting from conventional and oversimplified conceptions and opinions that can be treacherous because they do not account for individual differences. Generalizations use cultural patterns as a starting point to help focus thought, with the realization that individuality must be acknowledged. A guiding principle in cultural competency education is that it may be necessary to communicate with people differently to treat them equally.[33]

Considerable variation exists in cultural competence education, with limited specific guidelines or validated evaluation methods. Currently, education programs may promote changes in providers' knowledge and attitudes, but little empirical evidence exists that such efforts reduce indicators of disparate care.[34] With increasing incorporation of cultural competence education into all levels of medical and surgical education, it is necessary to evaluate teaching methods and establish recommendations to improve outcomes.[35-38] In 2005, a successful educational model was developed that links cultural competence with patient-centered communication and medical education[39] (Table 2).

Generational differences exist regarding cultural education efforts, which may partly be the result of the increased exposure of younger populations to diversity in schools and through mass media. Some people consider generalizations such as those used in diversity education programs offensive.[40] Additionally, as diversity increases in the audience for educational programs, emphasis should be placed on principles of cultural competence rather than group generalizations because the target audience must not be assumed to be from a particular background. The AAOS has resources to help educate physicians on principles and guidelines of culturally competent care when interacting with specific patient populations.[33] Also, the amount of literature on interaction with groups from diverse backgrounds is increasing as the population of these groups in US society increases.[41]

Healthcare Disparities

Disparities in healthcare delivery and differences in diagnosis, treatment, and outcomes based on racial and ethnic backgrounds of patient populations are well established for many common clinical conditions. Given the increasing evidence for inequality, the US Congress mandated in 2003 that the Agency for Healthcare Research and Quality report on progress and opportunities to reduce healthcare disparities. The agency produces two annual reports: the *National Healthcare Quality Report* that focuses on quality, and the *National Healthcare Disparities Report* that focuses on prevailing disparities in healthcare delivery relevant to racial and socioeconomic factors in patient populations. According to the 2011 *National Healthcare Disparities Report*, racial and ethnic minorities and low-income individuals not only experience more barriers to care but also receive poorer quality of care when it is available (http://www.ahrq.gov). Although US healthcare quality and access are reported as suboptimal, especially for minority and low-income groups, the overall progress in quality enhancement is unevenly matched by improvements in access for minorities and reductions in the disparity of quality (**Figures 2** through **4**). Recognition of these problems has increased, and numerous efforts to address them have been undertaken but much work remains. Physicians can play a key role in addressing disparities by practicing culturally competent care and by advocating on behalf of their patients. A 2011 study showed that health information technology has the potential to improve quality of care and patient safety, and if carefully designed and implemented, this may also help eliminate healthcare disparities.[42]

In orthopaedic surgery, the complex reasons underlying healthcare disparities have been increasingly studied as barriers to optimal outcomes.[43-45] These studies have shown how patient-related factors contribute to the multifaceted nature of disparities in musculoskeletal care. Learning more about patient-centered care through the development of communication skills and

1: Principles of Orthopaedics

Table 2

RESPECT Model for Patient Communication and Medical Education

Skill	Definition	Behavioral Description	Examples	Relevant Evidence
Respect: show	A demonstrable attitude communicating the value and the autonomy of the patient and the validity of his or her concerns.	Nonverbal: Maintain attentive posture, appropriate eye and personal contact; follow cues regarding personal space, physical contact, and appropriate greetings. Verbal: Welcome patient to encounter, introduce self and explain role on team, ask the patient how he or she wants to be addressed, and recognize and affirm strengths and efforts.	"Hi, I'm Dr. X, and I'm looking forward to working with you." "What would you like me to call you?" "You overcame a lot to get here today!"	Disparity: African American, Hispanic, and Asian patients reported feeling less respected by their doctors than did white patients.
Explanatory model: ask	A patient's understanding of what causes his or her illness or what will help it.	Nonverbal: Give patient space to share his or her ideas by listening without judgment. Verbal: Ask patient what he or she thinks is causing or will alleviate symptoms.	"What do you or your family think is causing your symptoms?" "Why do you think this started when it did?" "What do you think will solve the problem?"	Patients and doctors often have different ideas that remain unexplored unless elicited. Without discussion, patients leave less satisfied.
Social context: ask	Effect of patient's life on illness and of illness on his or her life. Include stressors, supports, strengths, and spiritual resources that influence patient, health, or care.	Nonverbal: Show interest and pay attention. Verbal: Ask how patient's illness affects his or her life and how his or her life affects illness.	"What should I know about you to care for you best?" "What is hardest for you?" "Who helps you the most?" "What keeps you going?" "What about religion?"	Low social support predicts higher mortality post-MI. Negative health consequences follow death of spouse alleviated by presence of confiding figure.
Power: share	Access to status, control, resources, options, and ability to produce desired outcomes Power gradient favors doctors	Nonverbal: Reduce physical barriers; do not dominate the interaction; sit. Verbal: Listen; limit interruptions; build history rather than take it; use EMR to share information with patient via graphs, etc; invite open discussion of disagreement; negotiate agenda/treatment plan by eliciting preferences; empower patient, recognize strengths.	"Beside your diabetes, what else should we talk about?" "What would make your medications easier?" "Thanks for telling me that you don't agree. What do you think?"	Disparity: White physicians dominate conversation more than nonwhite patients. Self-efficacy needed to make healthy choices.
Empathy: show	Verbal and nonverbal responses that validate patients' emotions and cause them to feel understood.	Nonverbal: Listen attentively and respond accordingly. Verbal: Name and validate patients' emotions; place significance of patient's experience into words to convey specific understanding.	"That must be hard; anyone would feel that way." "This can be scary. Let's talk about it." "The injury changed everything for you."	Disparity: Doctors display less warmth with African American patients.
Concerns and/or fears: ask	Worries about symptoms, diagnosis, or treatment are often unexpressed.	Nonverbal: Head nods, etc, to encourage patient to give details. Verbal: Ask open-ended questions about fears or concerns.	"What worries you the most?" "What scares you about the medication?" "Are you worried about sex after your heart attack?"	Unvoiced concerns lead to unmet needs and patient dissatisfaction.

(continued on next page)

Table 2

RESPECT Model for Patient Communication and Medical Education (continued)

Skill	Definition	Behavioral Description	Examples	Relevant Evidence
Trust, team-building, therapeutic alliance: build, don't assume.	Relationship built on understanding, power sharing, and empathy; patient confident that doctor acts on his or her behalf.	Trust: Notice/respond to signs of distrust; elicit and respond to expectations; reassure and clarify follow-up; follow through. Therapeutic alliance: Find specific common goals; negotiate differences. Team building: Identify, enlist, and collaborate with potential members of healthcare team.	"People in my family have had the same thing." "Should we get your family involved to help us?" "We're here when you need us." "Let's make sure we answer all your questions so you feel comfortable making your decision."	Disparity: 62.8% of African Americans versus 38.4% of whites believe their doctors have experimented or would experiment on them without their consent. African American patients receive less support, partnering, and information.

EMR-electronic medical records, MI = myocardial infarction, RESPECT = respect, explanatory model, social context, power, empathy, concerns, and trust.
(Adapted with permission from Mostow C, Crosson J, Gordon S, et al: Treating and precepting with RESPECT: A relational model addressing race, ethnicity, and culture in medical training. *J Gen Intern Med* 2010;25[suppl 2]:S146-S154.)

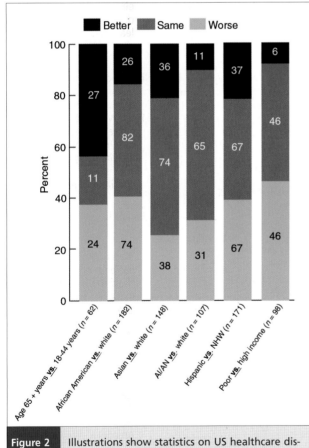

Figure 2 Illustrations show statistics on US healthcare disparities. Population's quality of care received was better than, about the same as, or worse than that of the reference group (listed after "vs."). AI = American Indian, AN = Alaska Native, NHW = non-Hispanic white. (Adapted with permission from the Agency for Healthcare Research and Quality: *2011 National Healthcare Quality and Disparities Reports.* Washington, DC, US Department of Health and Human Services (AHRQ Publication No. 12-0006), 2012.)

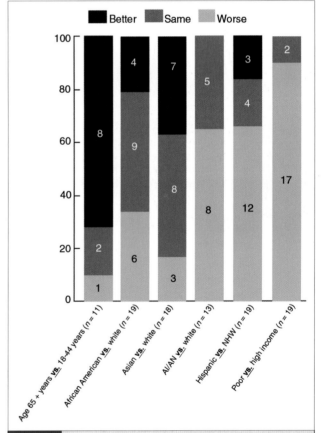

Figure 3 Illustrations show statistics on US healthcare disparities. Population's access to care received was better than, about the same as, or worse than that of the reference group (listed after "vs."). AI = American Indian, AN = Alaska Native, NHW = non-Hispanic white. (Adapted with permission from the Agency for Healthcare Research and Quality: *2011 National Healthcare Quality and Disparities Reports.* Washington, DC, US Department of Health and Human Services (AHRQ Publication No. 12-0006), 2012.)

1: Principles of Orthopaedics

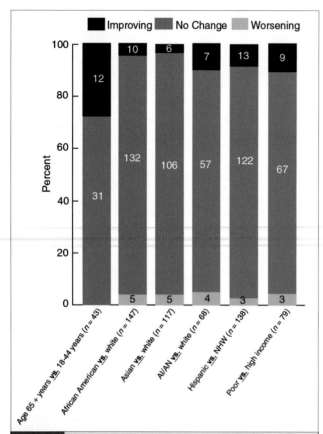

Figure 4 Illustrations show statistics on US healthcare disparities. Population's quality measures for trends over time for disparities are improving (reducing at a rate of > 1% per year), not changing (no change or change at a rate of < 1% per year) or worsening (increasing at a rate > 1% per year). Reference group is listed after "vs." AI = American Indian, AN = Alaska Native, NHW = non-Hispanic white. (Adapted with permission from the Agency for Healthcare Research and Quality: *2011 National Healthcare Quality and Disparities Reports.* Washington, DC, US Department of Health and Human Services (AHRQ Publication No. 12-0006), 2012.)

cultural competency will empower orthopaedic surgeons to build physician-patient relationships based on trust and delivery of equal-quality musculoskeletal care to all of their patients. Although the issues of communication skills and cultural competency are addressed through educational efforts by the AAOS, they are not yet universally incorporated into residency training and continuing medical education programs.

Summary

As patients become more involved in medical decision making and the healthcare system, patient-centered care must be formally taught. Communication skills are important to improve the physician-patient relationship, which remains at the center of all aspects of med-

icine irrespective of technologic advances. Excellence in effective communication should be a priority for orthopaedic surgeons because it affects all aspects of clinical care.

With an increasingly diverse patient population, physicians must become culturally competent to interact with patients who come from different backgrounds and who have various expectations. This allows physicians to treat them equally and overcome disparities in health care.

Key Study Points

- Good communication skills (verbal and nonverbal) are key in patient-physician interactions.
- Cultural competence is necessary to practice effectively in a diverse society.

Annotated References

1. Bechtel C, Ness DL: If you build it, will they come? Designing truly patient-centered health care. *Health Aff (Millwood)* 2010;29(5):914-920.

   Research conducted at the National Partnership for Women and Families suggests that a truly patient-centered healthcare system must be designed to incorporate features that matter to patients.

2. Baker DW: The meaning and the measure of health literacy. *J Gen Intern Med* 2006;21(8):878-883.

3. Bagley CH, Hunter AR, Bacarese-Hamilton IA: Patients' misunderstanding of common orthopaedic terminology: The need for clarity. *Ann R Coll Surg Engl* 2011;93(5):401-404.

   This questionnaire-based study showed that surgeons should be careful when using basic and common orthopaedic terminology to avoid misunderstanding by the patient. Educating patients in the clinic is a routine part of practice.

4. Vranceanu AM, Elbon M, Ring D: The emotive impact of orthopedic words. *J Hand Ther* 2011;24(2):112-117.

   This article discusses the emotional effect of words used by hand specialists, discusses the effect of the nomenclature chosen to describe orthopaedic diagnoses and procedures, and provides recommendations consistent with evidence-based practice.

5. Badarudeen S, Sabharwal S: Assessing readability of patient education materials: Current role in orthopaedics. *Clin Orthop Relat Res* 2010;468(10):2572-2580.

   Given the variability in the capacity of individuals seeking orthopaedic care to comprehend health-related materials, stratification of the contents of patient education materials at different levels of complexity likely will improve health literacy and enhance patient-centered communication.

6. Wilson IB, Schoen C, Neuman P, et al: Physician-patient communication about prescription medication nonadherence: A 50-state study of America's seniors. *J Gen Intern Med* 2007;22(1):6-12.

7. Schattner A, Rudin D, Jellin N: Good physicians from the perspective of their patients. *BMC Health Serv Res* 2004;4(1):26.

8. Rispler D, Sara J, Davenport L, Mills B, Iskra C: Under-reporting of complementary and alternative medicine use among arthritis patients in an orthopedic clinic. *Am J Orthop (Belle Mead NJ)* 2011;40(5):E92-E95.

   This cross-sectional study demonstrates the prevalence of complementary and alternative medicine used among orthopaedic patients and significant increases in complementary and alternative medicine reporting on the specific questionnaire than in a standard medical history.

9. Bhattacharyya T, Yeon H, Harris MB: The medical-legal aspects of informed consent in orthopaedic surgery. *J Bone Joint Surg Am* 2005;87(11):2395-2400.

10. Levinson W, Roter DL, Mulooly JP, Dull VT, Frankel RM: Physician-patient communication: The relationship with malpractice claims among primary care physicians and surgeons. *JAMA* 1997;277(7):553-559.

11. Teutsch C: Patient-doctor communication. *Med Clin North Am* 2003;87(5):1115-1145.

12. Tongue JR, Epps HR, Forese LL: Communication skills. *Instr Course Lect* 2005;54:3-9.

13. Lewis VO, McLaurin T, Spencer HT, Otsuka NY, Jimenez RL: Communication for all your patients. *Instr Course Lect* 2012;61:569-580.

   As a result of increasing malpractice litigation, physicians need to examine their communication skills. In an increasingly diverse world, social and cultural beliefs, attitudes, and behaviors have a considerable effect on the health of communities.

14. Glasgow RE, Emont S, Miller DC: Assessing delivery of the five "As" for patient-centered counseling. *Health Promot Int* 2006;21(3):245-255.

15. The Agency for Health Care Policy and Research Smoking Cessation Clinical Practice Guideline. *JAMA* 1996; 275(16):1270-1280.

16. Keller VF, Carroll JG: A new model for physician-patient communication. *Patient Educ Couns* 1994; 23(2):131-140.

17. Revankar AV, Gandedkar NH: Effective communication in the cyberage. *Am J Orthod Dentofacial Orthop* 2010;137(5):712-714.

   This article describes various modalities of Internet communication. The Internet is sculpting contemporary orthodontic visage, whether it involves interacting with a colleague through text, voice, or video; transferring patient records to distant locations; or submitting manuscripts to journals.

18. Sechrest RC: The Internet and the physician-patient relationship. *Clin Orthop Relat Res* 2010;468(10):2566-2571.

   This article reviews the development of the Internet, the core concepts that have driven the emergence and evolution of the Internet as a mass medium of information exchange, and how the healthcare industry can harness the Internet to improve the physician-patient relationship.

19. Hurwitz SR, Slawson DC: Should we be teaching information management instead of evidence-based medicine? *Clin Orthop Relat Res* 2010;468(10):2633-2639.

   Incorporation of the best evidence of busy clinical practice into the real world requires the applied science of information management. Clinicians must learn the techniques and skills to focus on finding, evaluating, and using information at the point of care.

20. Richard A: Teaching non-verbal communication skills. *Educ Prim Care* 2011;22(6):423-424.

   This study asked trainees to identify aspects of nonverbal communication, such as body language, tone, and speed. The trainees showed their control and power in directing consultation and facilitating the expression of emotion during the session.

21. Haig SV: Ethical choice in the medical applications of information theory. *Clin Orthop Relat Res* 2010; 468(10):2672-2677.

   Suggestions for maintaining high standards of practice in the face of the information technology burden include (1) increasing information technology time awareness, (2) increasing information technology goal awareness, and (3) determining how much information recorded is for financial instead of medical reasons.

22. Capozzi JD, Rhodes R: Managing medical errors. *J Bone Joint Surg Am* 2009;91(10):2520-2521.

23. Mazor KM, Simon SR, Yood RA, et al: Health plan members' views about disclosure of medical errors. *Ann Intern Med* 2004;140(6):409-418.

24. Wu AW, Cavanaugh TA, McPhee SJ, Lo B, Micco GP: To tell the truth: Ethical and practical issues in disclosing medical mistakes to patients. *J Gen Intern Med* 1997;12(12):770-775.

25. Sabin J, Nosek BA, Greenwald A, Rivara FP: Physicians' implicit and explicit attitudes about race by MD race, ethnicity, and gender. *J Health Care Poor Underserved* 2009;20(3):896-913.

26. Hausmann LR, Hannon MJ, Kresevic DM, Hanusa BH, Kwoh CK, Ibrahim SA: Impact of perceived discrimination in healthcare on patient-provider communication.

Med Care 2011;49(7):626-633.

In a cross-sectional survey at an orthopaedic Veterans Affairs clinic, African American patients more often reported perceptions of racism and classism in previous healthcare settings that may negatively influence the affective tone of subsequent patient-provider communication.

27. Stone J, Moskowitz GB: Non-conscious bias in medical decision making: What can be done to reduce it? *Med Educ* 2011;45(8):768-776.

Workshops or other learning modules about nonconscious processes can provide medical professionals with skills to reduce bias when they interact with patients from a minority group.

28. McClellan FM, White AA III, Jimenez RL, Fahmy S: Do poor people sue doctors more frequently? Confronting unconscious bias and the role of cultural competency. *Clin Orthop Relat Res* 2012;470(5):1393-1397.

This review article examines the misperception that a relationship between patient poverty and medical malpractice litigation may arise from unconscious physician bias and other social variables.

29. Shannon D: Cultural competency in health care organizations: Why and how? *Physician Exec* 2010;36(5):18-22.

Physician leaders need to understand the relevance of cultural competence. The cultural competency of their organizations needs to be strengthened to provide safer, higher quality, and more efficient health care.

30. Fiester A: What "patient-centered care" requires in serious cultural conflict. *Acad Med* 2012;87(1):20-24.

The author examined the tension that occurs when culturally sensitive issues of patient-centered care disrupt the workflow of the service; require the acknowledgement of antithetical, unsupportable values; or entail discriminatory or ad hominem practices that constitute a personal insult or affront to the provider.

31. Like RC: Educating clinicians about cultural competence and disparities in health and health care. *J Contin Educ Health Prof* 2011;31(3):196-206.

This article overviews healthcare policy as well as legislative, accreditation, and professional initiatives relating to racial and ethnic disparities in health care. Continuing medical education offerings on cultural competence and disparities are reviewed, with examples provided of available curricular resources and online courses.

32. Jenks AC: From "lists of traits" to "open-mindedness": Emerging issues in cultural competence education. *Cult Med Psychiatry* 2011;35(2):209-235.

This article explains that educators of contemporary cultural competence have rejected the list of traits approach and instead aim to produce a new kind of healthcare provider who is open-minded, willing to learn about differences, and treats each patient as an individual.

33. Jimenez RL, Lewis VO: *Culturally Competent Care Guidebook: Companion to the Cultural Competency Challenge CD-ROM.* Rosemont, IL, American Academy of Orthopaedic Surgeons, 2007.

34. Dykes DC, White AA III: Culturally competent care pedagogy: What works? *Clin Orthop Relat Res* 2011;469(7):1813-1816.

This article discusses the general approaches to culturally competent care education, the tools used in the evaluation of such endeavors, and the effect of such endeavors on caregivers and/or the outcomes of therapeutic interventions.

35. Butler PD, Swift M, Kothari S, et al: Integrating cultural competency and humility training into clinical clerkships: Surgery as a model. *J Surg Educ* 2011;68(3):222-230.

This review article uses surgery as a model to establish a set of recommendations to assist clerkship directors and curriculum committees in their efforts to ensure cultural competency and humility training in medical education over the past 2 years.

36. Smith BD, Silk K: Cultural competence clinic: An online, interactive, simulation for working effectively with Arab American Muslim patients. *Acad Psychiatry* 2011;35(5):312-316.

Preliminary data from this study support that an online, interactive patient simulation involving the care of an Arab American Muslim patient has the potential to improve the knowledge and skills of second-year medical students regarding patient care beyond the basic cultural competence curriculum.

37. Gustafson DL, Reitmanova S: How are we "doing" cultural diversity? A look across English Canadian undergraduate medical school programmes. *Med Teach* 2010;32(10):816-823.

This website and literature review shows that more research is needed to map the approaches to cultural diversity and evaluate the effectiveness of these approaches on improving physician-patient relationships, reducing health disparities, improving outcomes, and producing positive learning in physicians.

38. Harris-Haywood S, Goode T, Gao Y, et al: Psychometric evaluation of a cultural competency assessment instrument for health professionals. *Med Care* 2012.

This study evaluated the measurement properties of the Cultural Competence Health Practitioner Assessment and found that it can be used to establish associations between practitioners' cultural and linguistic competence and health outcomes as well as evaluate interventions to increase competence.

39. Mostow C, Crosson J, Gordon S, et al: Treating and precepting with RESPECT: A relational model addressing race, ethnicity, and culture in medical training. *J Gen Intern Med* 2010;25(suppl 2):S146-S154.

The specific behavioral descriptions for each component of RESPECT (respect, explanatory model, social context, power, empathy, concerns, and trust—an educational model for patient care) make it a concrete, practical, integrated model for teaching patient care. Precepting with RESPECT fosters a safe climate for residents to partner with faculty, address challenges with patients at risk, and improve outcomes.

40. Taylor P, Keeter S: *Millennials: A Portrait of Generation Next*. Washington, DC, Pew Research Center, February 2010.

    This report on the values, attitudes, behaviors, and demographic characteristics of the millennial generation was prepared by the Pew Research Center, a nonpartisan "fact tank" that provides information on the issues, attitudes, and trends shaping America and the world.

41. Hussain W, Hussain H, Hussain M, Hussain S, Attar S: Approaching the Muslim orthopaedic patient. *J Bone Joint Surg Am* 2010;92(7):e2.

    This paper reviews how cultural and religious considerations apply to orthopaedic patients who are Muslim. Understanding the fundamentals of patient beliefs and maintaining empathy to their principles will help orthopaedic surgeons provide high-quality and culturally sensitive care to their Muslim patients.

42. López L, Green AR, Tan-McGrory A, King R, Betancourt JR: Bridging the digital divide in health care: The role of health information technology in addressing racial and ethnic disparities. *Jt Comm J Qual Patient Saf* 2011;37(10):437-445.

    Several causes for disparities are amenable to interventions using health information technology, particularly innovations in electronic health records. Recommendations regarding the healthcare system and provider and patient factors can help organizations address disparities as they tailor their health information technology systems.

43. Borkhoff CM, Hawker GA, Wright JG: Patient gender affects the referral and recommendation for total joint arthroplasty. *Clin Orthop Relat Res* 2011;469(7):1829-1837.

    Patient sex plays an important role in the process of referral and recommendation for total joint arthroplasty. Female sex affects multiple steps in the process, suggesting barriers unique to women exist in the patient-physician interaction.

44. Katz JN, Lyons N, Wolff LS, et al: Medical decision-making among Hispanics and non-Hispanic whites with chronic back and knee pain: A qualitative study. *BMC Musculoskelet Disord* 2011;12:78.

    The authors assembled six focus groups of patients with chronic back or knee pain to discuss the management of their conditions and preferred roles in medical decision making. The findings suggested differences between Hispanics and non-Hispanic whites in preferred information sources and decision-making roles.

45. Hausmann LR, Hanusa BH, Kresevic DM, et al: Orthopedic communication about osteoarthritis treatment: Does patient race matter? *Arthritis Care Res (Hoboken)* 2011;63(5):635-642.

    Visits to Veterans Affairs orthopedic clinics were coded using the using the Roter Interaction Analysis System and the Informed Decision-Making model. Communication regarding the management of chronic knee and hip osteoarthritis did not vary by patient race. The findings diminish the potential role of communication in Veterans Affairs clinics as an explanation for well-documented racial disparities in arthroplasty.

1: Principles of Orthopaedics

Chapter 9
Polytrauma Care

Max Talbot, MD, FRCSC   Greg Berry, MDCM, FRCSC   Edward J. Harvey, MD, MSc

1: Principles of Orthopaedics

Introduction

In general, an understanding of the physiologic processes that affect polytraumatized patients has remained the concern of physicians other than orthopaedic surgeons. Increasingly, however, the need for early and aggressive orthopaedic care of patients with multiple traumatic injuries has made it more relevant for orthopaedic surgeons to understand the physiologic processes involved in caring for these patients. As modern battlefield techniques are adopted into civilian medicine, severely injured polytraumatized patients are surviving in greater numbers. As such, the orthopaedic care of these patients requires knowledge of intensive care and global trauma protocols. Orthopaedic surgeons must understand and integrate musculoskeletal protocols with the care and concerns of other teams of physicians. Ongoing communication and team building within the care-delivery matrix is becoming increasingly important.

Initial Assessment and Resuscitation

The principles of initial trauma management are intuitive and have remained relatively unchanged. The classic ABC mnemonic of care (airway, breathing, circulation) is still valid; ideally, however, these steps should occur concurrently. If exsanguination is occurring from a limb injury, strong consideration should be given to first controlling the catastrophic bleeding. A tourniquet is often the most efficient method to obtain temporary control of massive bleeding from open extremity wounds. Damage-control resuscitation starts at the point of injury, with the use of hypotensive resuscitation, which aims to minimize prehospital fluid adminis-

Dr. Harvey or an immediate family member has received research or institutional support from Synthes, Stryker, Smith & Nephew, and Zimmer and serves as a board member, owner, officer, or committee member of the Orthopaedic Trauma Association, the Canadian Orthopaedic Association, and the Orthopaedic Research Society. Neither of the following authors nor any immediate family member has received anything of value from or has stock or stock options held in a commercial company or institution related directly or indirectly to the subject of this chapter: Dr. Talbot and Dr. Berry.

tration. Crystalloid and colloid resuscitation should be conservative and limited by preestablished end points, such as restoration of a radial pulse. This method will minimize dilutional coagulopathy and lessen the chance of displacing established clots.

After reaching the hospital, the most severely injured trauma patients will benefit from a balanced transfusion regimen that closely approximates the composition of blood. Recent wars have provided substantial experience with massive transfusion and have resulted in the current ratio-based approach. Military and civilian retrospective studies have shown that the transfusion of high ratios of fresh frozen plasma (FFP) and platelets to packed red blood cells (PRBCs) decreases mortality in patients requiring massive transfusions.[1] A prospective trial is currently underway to validate the optimal ratio of blood products. This transfusion strategy presents challenges to logistics and resource allocation that have not been fully resolved.

It is important to note that ratio-based transfusion is required only in a small subset of patients. Efforts have been made to develop clinical scoring systems to predict massive bleeding and make early determinations about which patients will benefit from aggressive damage control resuscitation.[2] At this time, clinical judgment will serve the clinician better than any individual scoring system. Patients with more severe clinical (profound hypovolemia with large transfusion requirements) and laboratory evidence of shock and more extensive anatomic injuries will generally have a higher risk of coagulopathy and higher transfusion requirements. In such instances, the clinician should consider damage control resuscitation.

Trauma-Induced Coagulopathy

The observation that 25% of trauma patients have laboratory evidence of coagulopathy on presentation to the emergency department has led to a reappraisal of the pathophysiology of trauma-induced coagulopathy.[3] Hypothermia, acidosis, and coagulation factor dilution can be aggravating factors, but it is now clear that shock and tissue injury are the initial triggers of this condition.[4] It is postulated that hypoperfusion induces the expression of thrombomodulin by endothelial cells, which leads to protein C activation, systemic anticoagulation, and derepression of fibrinolysis.[5] Multiple studies have identified coagulopathy as an independent predictor of mortality in trauma.[5,6] More recently, coagulopathy and protein C activation have been linked to an increase in ventilator-associated pneumonia, multiple organ failure, longer mechanical ventilation, and longer stays in the intensive care unit.[6] This new understanding of the mechanisms and the consequences of trauma-induced coagulopathy has led to a reassessment of the importance of coagulopathy markers in trauma resuscitation.

Two drugs with the potential to reverse traumatic coagulopathy have been the focus of recent intense research. Recombinant factor VIIa was initially developed to treat patients with hemophilia who have antibodies to coagulation factors VIII and IX. Its potential to activate the extrinsic coagulation pathway when combined with tissue factor and to activate factor X directly at the surface of activated platelets led to its off-label use in severely traumatized patients with coagulopathy. A randomized controlled trial initially showed decreased transfusion requirements in patients with blunt (nonpenetrating) trauma; however, recombinant factor VIIa had no mortality benefit.[7] This finding led to the widespread use of recombinant factor VIIa, particularly in those with complex war injuries.[8] Early retrospective data suggested decreased mortality in civilian and military patients with traumatic injuries who were treated with recombinant factor VIIa, but larger prospective studies failed to confirm those results.[9] The use of recombinant factor VIIa has since declined considerably, and it is not currently approved by the FDA for treating patients with traumatic coagulopathy.

Tranexamic acid (TXA), an inhibitor of fibrinolysis, has been used extensively to decrease bleeding during elective surgeries and other procedures. TXA is particularly attractive because of the key role of hyperfibrinolysis in traumatic coagulopathy. Clinical Randomization of an Antifibrinolytic in Significant Hemorrhage-2 (CRASH-2) was a blinded randomized controlled trial that evaluated the role of TXA in patients with traumatic injuries.[10] More than 20,000 patients with traumatic injuries from centers in 40 countries who had active bleeding or were at risk of bleeding were included in the trial. Four-week mortality from all causes was 14.5% in the TXA group compared with 16% in the placebo group, which represents a statistically and clinically significant reduction in mortality ($P = 0.0035$). The risk of death caused specifically by bleeding was 4.9% in the TXA group compared with 5.7% in the placebo group. Subsequent analysis showed that TXA should be administered within 3 hours of injury.[11] Based on these data, TXA could potentially save more than 128,000 lives annually worldwide if it was given within 1 hour of injury.[12] It is noteworthy that no specific screening was done for hyperfibrinolysis or coagulopathy. Thromboelastography might allow clinicians to target this therapy to patients with hyperfibrinolysis, potentially producing a greater treatment effect. Interestingly, the CRASH-2 trial showed no decrease in the number of transfusions in the TXA group.

TXA has anti-inflammatory effects that may also contribute to decreasing mortality.[13] Traumatic coagulopathy is a prominent feature in traumatic combat injuries, which tend to be more severe than civilian injuries. The Military Application of Tranexamic Acid in Trauma Emergency Resuscitation (MATTERs) study retrospectively evaluated the use of TXA in 896 combat casualties requiring blood transfusions who were admitted to a medical facility at Camp Bastion, Afghanistan, over a 2-year period.[13] Despite more severe trauma, mortality in the TXA group was significantly lower (17.4% versus 23.9% [$P = 0.03$]). TXA use was independently associated with lower mortality in the subset of patients requiring massive transfusions.

It is essential to recognize the potential for trauma-induced coagulopathy in severely injured patients. Volume resuscitation should be approached with the principles of hemostatic resuscitation in mind. Institutional massive transfusion protocols are a valuable tool in ensuring a consistent approach. The administration of TXA should be considered as an adjunct to resuscitation in patients with severe bleeding.

Treatment Patterns Driven by Military Experience

The recent conflicts in Iraq and Afghanistan have given military surgeons extensive experience with injuries caused by improvised explosive devices (IEDs). The most severe injuries are sustained at close range during dismounted combat operations; multiple traumatic injuries involving mangled limbs and amputations are common and are often accompanied by pelvic fractures or intra-abdominal injuries. Advances in tactical medicine and rapid air transport often allow these patients to survive from the point of injury to a surgical facility. Tactical care on the battlefield allows medics to treat the most common causes of preventable death in a protocol-driven manner. Tourniquet application and wound packing with hemostatic dressings are the most useful interventions. Both treatments are aimed at stopping compressible hemorrhage, the most frequent cause of preventable death on the battlefield.[14]

Contrary to past medical doctrine, the prehospital application of tourniquets in current conflicts has been shown to be effective at stopping blood loss and increasing survival rates.[15] Tourniquets are an integral part of the damage control resuscitation-surgery continuum. Complications are rare and mostly consist of neurapraxias. An increased fasciotomy rate was reported when tourniquets were widely issued to US military personnel in 2005;[16] however, this is likely related to the increasing number of severe injuries cause by more sophisticated weapons and to a lower threshold for prophylactic fasciotomy before patients were evacuated from the combat theater. Extrapolation of these data to civilian medicine may be difficult. The low rate of complications from tourniquet use may not be applicable to situations in which longer periods of time elapse between tourniquet application and hospital admission.

The resuscitation of patients with multiple traumatic amputations can be extremely challenging. An aggressive application of damage control principles is essential to ensure the best outcomes. Hemodynamically unstable patients are best treated in the operating room, where resuscitation and hemorrhage control can be performed concurrently. The timing of CT has been studied. Preoperative or intraoperative CT is usually of little value because most clinically important injuries can be readily evaluated without CT.[17] Postoperative CT is useful in delineating the full extent of injuries. Determining the extent of anatomic involvement requires a consistent team approach. It is vital to swiftly control all sites of hemorrhage. Priority must be given to treating intra-abdominal injuries and unstable or open pelvic fractures. External fixation of the pelvic ring and preperitoneal packing may be indicated for stabilizing unstable pelvic fractures.[17] It is essential to achieve vascular control of all bleeding extremities while laparotomy and pelvic external fixation are ongoing. In most instances, a pneumatic tourniquet is adequate, but surgical control is necessary for the most proximal amputations. In some patients, proximal vascular control of the lower extremities is best obtained with a laparotomy. It is important to expedite the initial surgery by simultaneously performing as many of the procedures as possible.[18]

In some instances, surgical workspace is suboptimal, with two surgeons from different specialties working on each limb. Extremity procedures should be brief in a patient with overwhelming trauma. Physiology is the prime concern in a polytraumatized patient, not the complexity of the fracture. Limb injuries require control of major vessels, gross débridement, and temporary external fixation. Formal revascularization or the use of a temporary shunt can be considered for avascular extremities, depending on the patient's physiology. Débridement can be complex in patients with combat injuries. Extreme contamination and wounds in difficult anatomic areas are typical. An appreciation of the patient's physiologic status will allow the surgeon to abort the débridement before the onset of profound coagulopathy. In patients with massive trauma, it is often impossible to obtain a clean wound after the first débridement because of the need to limit physiologic insult from prolonged surgery. Staged procedures will follow at higher echelons of care.

Although war injuries are challenging to treat, high rates of survival can be expected when a mature trauma system is in place.[17,19] Severe combat injuries carry useful lessons in damage control surgery for nonmilitary surgeons who are unlikely to see mutilating injuries. In a complex case, it is easy to get drawn into the technical aspects of limb alignment and fixation, but such concerns are rarely important in a true damage control situation. All surgical procedures should be resuscitative in nature.

Extremity Trauma and Indications for Damage-Control Orthopaedics

For centuries, physicians have seen early death in polytraumatized patients; however, there was little improve-

ment in mortality rates until the modernization of intensive care and trauma resuscitation protocols. Even with better early care of these patients, unexplained morbidity and mortality existed that was sometimes attributed to the early care itself, which turned on the traumatic response cascade.[20-22] There is ongoing debate regarding whether early care contributes to complications in patients with traumatic injuries. The early hyperinflammatory response to severe trauma, which is a natural part of the healing response, is followed by a hypoinflammatory phase.[23,24] This biphasic response may result in increased morbidity during the hypoinflammatory phase. The initial trauma can cause injury to primary organs as well as an early hyperinflammatory response. Late, multiple organ dysfunctions are often associated with the second hit, particularly temporal physiologic insults that occur during the hypoinflammatory phase. Secondary endogenous and exogenous factors play a crucial role in the initiation of posttraumatic complications. Iatrogenic second hits include massive transfusions and surgical interventions that cause tissue damage, hypothermia, or blood loss. Studies have shown a higher incidence of morbidity in patients with severe pulmonary injuries or shock or in otherwise unstable patients undergoing surgery. The second hit is worsened by blood loss, sepsis, and ischemia (or conditions that cause these disorders).[25]

Applying the strategy of damage control surgery resulted in better survival rates in polytraumatized patients with abdominal injuries.[26] These principles were expanded over time with the popularization of damage-control orthopaedics (DCO). The goal of DCO is to lessen blood loss, sepsis, and ischemia. Patient selection is key, with the degree of chest trauma and brain injury among other factors that are crucial in determining a patient's viability and the applicability of DCO.[25,27]

The debate on DCO versus total early care is ongoing. Patient categories have been loosely defined to aid surgeons in choosing treatment modalities. Patients can be classified according to their overall underlying condition (Figure 1). Stable patients (grade I, cleared for surgery) usually can be taken to the operating room for early total care. Unstable patients (grade III, cardiovascular instability [systolic blood pressure < 90 mm Hg]) are taken to the operating room for management of their nonorthopaedic injuries and are treated according to the principles of DCO. Patients in extremis (grade IV, acutely life-threatening injuries) are taken to the intensive care unit where external fixation may be applied if possible. Patients in borderline condition (grade II, uncertain condition with episodes of cardiovascular instability and hypoxemia) have more problems and are more difficult to treat. These patients receive acute nonorthopaedic care in the trauma room with the resuscitation protocol. If stabilization is possible, they are taken to the operating room for DCO care. Early total care procedures usually are not appropriate for these patients regardless of the success of resuscitation.

Some authors have attempted to define borderline patients with objective laboratory or scoring benchmarks. Indications of a borderline patient include poly-

1: Principles of Orthopaedics

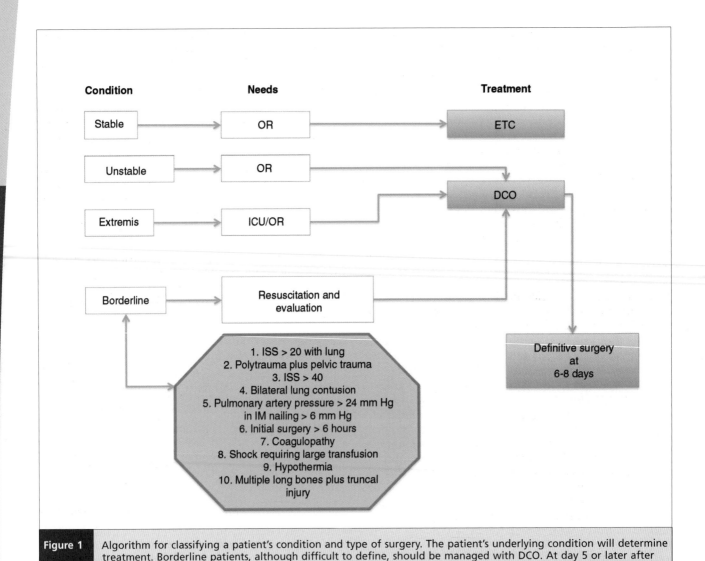

Condition   **Needs**   **Treatment**

Stable	→	OR	→	ETC
Unstable	→	OR		
Extremis	→	ICU/OR	→	DCO
Borderline	→	Resuscitation and evaluation		Definitive surgery at 6-8 days

1. ISS > 20 with lung
2. Polytrauma plus pelvic trauma
3. ISS > 40
4. Bilateral lung contusion
5. Pulmonary artery pressure > 24 mm Hg in IM nailing > 6 mm Hg
6. Initial surgery > 6 hours
7. Coagulopathy
8. Shock requiring large transfusion
9. Hypothermia
10. Multiple long bones plus truncal injury

Figure 1   Algorithm for classifying a patient's condition and type of surgery. The patient's underlying condition will determine treatment. Borderline patients, although difficult to define, should be managed with DCO. At day 5 or later after injury, DCO fixation methods can be converted to other fixation modalities. ETC = early total care, DCO = damage control orthopaedics, OR = operating room, ICU = intensive care unit, ISS = Injury Severity Score, IM = intramedullary. (Adapted with permission from Pape HC, Grimme K, Van Griensven M, et al: Impact of intramedullary instrumentation versus damage control for femoral fractures on immunoinflammatory parameters: Prospective randomized analysis by the EPOFF Study Group. *J Trauma* 2003;55[1]:7-13.)

trauma with an Injury Severity Score (ISS) greater than 20 and additional thoracic trauma, polytrauma with abdominal and/or pelvic trauma, and hemorrhagic shock (initial relative risk < 90 mm Hg) or an ISS greater than 40 without additional thoracic trauma. Bilateral lung contusions on a chest radiograph, an initial mean pulmonary arterial pressure greater than 24 mm Hg, and an increase of pulmonary arterial pressure of more than 6 mm Hg during intramedullary nailing are also indicators of a patient in borderline condition.[28] Longer procedures have been associated with multiple organ failure. Depending on the report, it appears that extremity surgery should be delayed in patients with a Glasgow Coma Scale score less than 9. Indirect measures of hypoperfusion, such as lactic acid levels or base excess, have shown some promise in diagnosing occult hypoperfusion and may play a role in better defining the borderline patient.[29] Some centers have the capability of monitoring inflammatory markers (interleukin [IL]-6, 8, 10, and 18), but the global use of these tests is not the standard of care. The role of these markers in determining patient viability and the applicability of DCO is likely to become more prominent because the markers, in particular IL-6, have been shown to be good indicators of systemic traumatic immunomodulation. High levels of inflammatory markers at the time of surgery are indicators of complicated patient care and poor outcomes.[30]

The choice and timing of procedures are also debatable. The external fixator is the primary treatment device used in DCO. External fixation decreases surgical time and blood loss, allows better visualization of the extremities, and decreases the morbidities associated with skeletal fixation. Some authors have also discussed nailing, minimally invasive plating, or various other procedures as DCO techniques.[31]

Regardless of the surgical technique, the timing of DCO versus early total care is an important factor. Much debate has centered on the fixation of femoral shaft fractures, which are a common injury in patients with polytrauma. Studies on femoral shaft fracture have shown that early femoral nailing achieves better outcomes when polytrauma is not a factor.[32] Using data reported to the National Trauma Data Bank, a 2009 retrospective study reviewed 3,069 femoral shaft fractures in polytraumatized patients who were treated with definitive fixation.[33] Definitive fixation within 12 hours of hospital admission was associated with a higher mortality rate. Femoral shaft fixation that was delayed beyond 12 hours reduced mortality by approximately 50%. This delay in treatment was particularly beneficial in patients with life-threatening abdominal injuries.

A retrospective study evaluated 766 polytraumatized patients with lung injuries and femoral fractures treated with intramedullary nailing at less than or more than 24 hours after injury.[22] In patients with severe chest trauma, there was a higher incidence of posttraumatic acute respiratory distress syndrome (33% versus 7.7%) and mortality (21% versus 4%) in the group treated with early intramedullary nailing compared with the group treated after more than 24 hours. The study authors did not stratify the findings of different (longer) time periods to treatment. In a 1999 retrospective analysis, 4,313 polytraumatized patients treated at one institution over a 24-year period were categorized into groups based on the presence or the absence of multiple organ failure.[34] In those in whom multiple organ failure developed, secondary surgery was usually performed on days 2 to 4 after injury. Using data from a level I trauma center gathered over a 12-year period, 1,362 patients with traumatic chest or head injuries and a femoral shaft fracture were stratified into several groups based on the time of treatment. Patients who were surgically treated less than 24 hours after injury did the best, and treatment 2 to 5 days after injury was associated with high complication rates. Early total care for polytraumatized patients with a femoral shaft fracture should take into account the effects of the patient's physiologic state and treatment time. Early treatment may not be the best choice for a borderline patient. Procedures done between days 2 and 5 seem to be undesirable. Patients surgically treated on or after 6 days of injury had fewer complications.[35]

Pelvic Ring Injuries

Disruption of the pelvic ring in a patient with multiple traumatic injuries is usually caused by the transfer of high-energy blunt force trauma to the bony and soft-tissue components and contents of the pelvis. This injury is associated with a high incidence of morbidity and mortality.[36,37] For a patient surviving the initial traumatic event, late mortality results from sepsis and/or multiple organ system failure, whereas survivor morbidity may include lasting urogenital, neurologic,

gastrointestinal, and musculoskeletal damage. Because of the complex nature of these injuries, a multidisciplinary approach is crucial in ensuring survival with the lowest possible morbidity.

The initial emergency department evaluation should determine possible sources of bleeding in the hemodynamically unstable patient according to Advanced Trauma Life Support principles. After thoracic, abdominal, and limb injuries have been eliminated as origins of blood loss, the pelvis must be considered a likely source in a patient with ongoing or recurrent hemodynamic instability. To save the patient's life, arrest of hemorrhage and mechanical stabilization are urgent goals. An uncommon but more lethal injury, the open pelvic fracture, must always be considered and ruled out in any patient with pelvic ring disruption. Physical examination of the perineum, rectum, and vagina is important to rule out an open pelvic fracture, which has a higher mortality rate and may alter medical management.

Imaging

Further definition of the pelvic injury can be obtained with inlet-outlet radiographic views and CT. Although plain radiographs alone can be used to classify these injuries, CT will better define all components of the injury.[38] The Young and Burgess classification of pelvic fractures is based on the instability created by the force vector applied at the moment of impact and includes four groups, which are then further subdivided. Rotationally unstable patterns include anterior-posterior compression (APC) injuries, which result in external rotational pelvic instability; lateral compression (LC) injuries, which produce internal rotation of the hemipelvis; vertical shear (VS) injuries, which are the result of an axial load through the pelvis resulting in vertical instability and displacement; and combined mechanism (CM) injuries, which have components of the other three patterns. Although this classification system cannot accurately predict a specific vascular injury, it is a useful tool in predicting likely resuscitative requirements and concomitant injuries and can help direct definitive stabilization strategies. APC injuries are more likely to be associated with solid and hollow abdominal organ injury, more profound shock, sepsis, and delayed respiratory distress syndrome, whereas LC injuries have a higher associated incidence of traumatic brain injury. Transfusion volume and mortality are highest in patients with APC injuries, followed by CM, and then LC/VS mechanisms.

Temporary Mechanical Stabilization

Historically, immediate external fixation of the pelvis was included in the management algorithm of the hemodynamically unstable patient with a pelvic ring injury.[39] This strategy was based on the supposition that the increased intrapelvic volume produced in APC and VS injuries permitted ongoing hemorrhage, which was stopped by reducing the volume available and inducing tamponade. Because cranial bleeding into the retroperitoneal space is relatively unaffected by pelvic volume

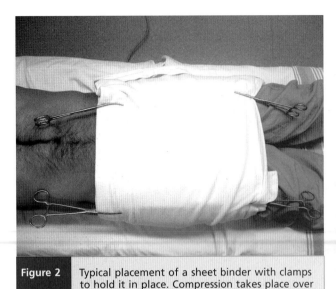

Figure 2 Typical placement of a sheet binder with clamps to hold it in place. Compression takes place over both pelvic and the greater trochanteric areas.

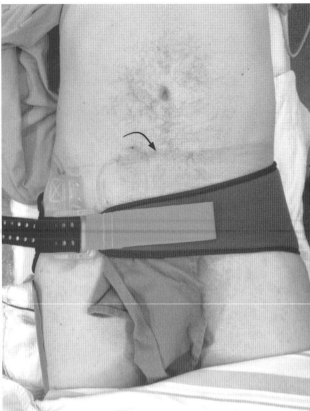

Figure 3 Photograph of a patient with a commercially available binder in place around the greater trochanters. The binder is sometimes inadvertently placed (arrow), but the greater trochanter is the best site for compression and avoiding laparotomy sites or impeding abdominal examinations.

reduction induced with external fixation and the time required for the application of an external fixation frame, formal external fixation has been largely supplanted by the use of pelvic orthotic devices or binders. Pelvic orthotic devices can take the form of a simple bed sheet or a commercial device[40] (**Figures 2 and 3**). These devices are simple, can be rapidly applied, and are effective at circumferentially constraining the pelvis to mechanically stabilize APC, VS, and some CM injuries.[41] Pelvic orthotic devices have been shown to effectively reduce volume in APC-type injuries without overreducing LC injuries.[42] In patients with APC injuries who are at higher risk of exsanguination, there is some evidence that these devices can reduce transfusion requirements, the length of the hospital stay, and mortality.[43]

The device is placed at the level of the greater trochanters, permitting access to the groin (for interventional radiology) and the abdomen (for general surgery). The device can safely remain in place for up to 190 hours without causing skin or other soft-tissue necrosis, although caution must be exercised when the involved skin has been compromised by the initial injury.[42] Additional reduction of any pelvic external rotation deformity can be achieved by binding the knees together.

Formal iliac crest or supra-acetabular external fixation is reserved for patients undergoing abdominal or thoracic surgery in the operating room or as a delayed measure to afford definitive stabilization (along with internal fixation, as needed) in some pelvic ring injury patterns. The supra-acetabular position has been shown to be mechanically advantageous.[44] The pelvic C-clamp is an external fixation device used in some centers for acute provisional stabilization of pelvic ring injuries. It differs from the other described devices in that it applies a compressive force on the posterior ring, effectively reducing fracture or dislocation seen in APC, VS, and some CM injuries.[45] In a grossly unstable pel-

vic ring, the C-clamp provides mechanical stability to allow effective preperitoneal packing. Although it can be applied using surface anatomy landmarks alone, there is a danger of intrapelvic penetration of the pins in the displaced pelvis. Most centers that regularly use this device recommend fluoroscopic imaging to avoid this complication. A safer alternative to posterior ring pin placement is gluteal pillar placement with anterior inferior iliac spine pins[46] (**Figure 4**).

Controlling Bleeding

In the absence of obvious sources of bleeding, an intervention is needed to arrest hemorrhaging in a patient with a pelvic ring injury and hemodynamic instability, either ongoing or recurrent. The three potential sources of hemorrhage are arterial, venous, and fracture surfaces. Arterial bleeding is the most difficult to control and is the primary source of lethal exsanguination. Two procedures are routinely used to treat arterial bleeding: angioembolization or preperitoneal packing. Pelvic arteriography with identification of arterial rupture and embolization has been available since the 1990s, and it has proven to be an effective method of bleeding con-

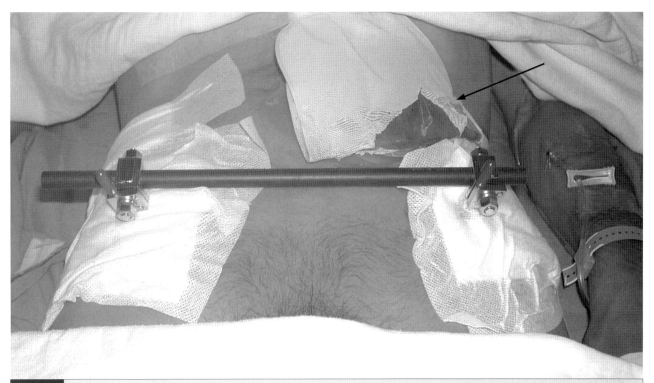

Figure 4 The use of anterior inferior iliac spine pin placement for better posterior control also avoids impingement of other abdominal procedures, such as a colostomy (arrow).

trol in the 3% to 10% of patients with pelvic fracture requiring the procedure.[47,48] The rate of successful bleeding control is approximately 90%. Repeat angiography with embolization has proven worthwhile in patients with signs of recurrent bleeding,[49,50] although the danger of systemic embolization must be taken into account. Patients with extravasation of intravenous contrast material in the pelvis seen on a CT scan (blush sign) and those older than 60 years with major pelvic trauma may require embolization.[51,52] Conversely, the absence of extravasation of intravenous contrast material on pelvic CT suggests the absence of important arterial bleeding and negates the need for angiography.[51,53]

Preperitoneal packing, rather than angiography and embolization, is used in some centers as a routine measure to control pelvic bleeding. In other centers, preperitoneal packing is reserved for patients in extremis, when treatment cannot be delayed while waiting for access to an angiography suite. Preperitoneal packing also can be used when pelvic hemorrhaging continues after angiography and embolization. The technique involves an infraumbilical midline skin and fascial incision, followed by packing of three to four abdominal sponges into the posterior pelvis at the level of the sacroiliac joints and at the pelvic cavity bilaterally to compress the major vessels contributing to exsanguination. Preperitoneal packing can be done as a stand-alone procedure (without violating the peritoneal cavity) or can be combined with a laparotomy. The abdomen is closed until the patient is returned to the operating room after

sustained hemodynamic stability and correction of all coagulopathies have been achieved. In a small number of patients, angiography and embolization will be required after packing.[54] To obtain a solid wall to pack against, stabilization of the posterior pelvic ring can be achieved with either a pelvic orthotic device or a pelvic C-clamp. When compared with an angiography-embolization protocol, a preperitoneal packing protocol in pelvic ring trauma is advantageous because there is usually more ready access to the operating room than to the angiography suite, and the need for transfusion is decreased.[55]

Pelvic trauma often results in morbidity and mortality. Routine imaging with radiographs and CT can guide resuscitation and initial stabilization strategies and predicts transfusion requirements and concomitant injuries. Pelvic orthotic devices have largely supplanted standard external fixation and C-clamp fixation in the temporary mechanical stabilization of the pelvic ring. Institutional protocols, using angiography and embolization and/or preperitoneal packing, should be established for managing hemodynamic instability caused by intrapelvic hemorrhage.

Summary

New treatment modalities and algorithms for managing polytraumatized patients have been recently proposed, mainly because of experience gained in treating injuries sustained in military combat. Newer hematologic therapies are increasingly being used in the field of trauma. There is an obvious need for transdisciplinary collaboration in treating polytraumatized patients. Although orthopaedic surgeons may not be knowledgeable about all the nuances of resuscitation, they should be aware of the most commonly used new therapies to ensure optimal care of their patients with multiple traumatic injuries.

Key Study Points

- Understand the pathophysiology of posttraumatic coagulopathy and the principles of damage-control resuscitation.

- Recognize that there is a place for tourniquet use in civilian trauma in the case of traumatic amputations or exsanguinating extremity wounds.

- Understand the principles of DCO and how this treatment fits into the overall picture of polytraumatized patients.

Annotated References

1. Brown JB, Cohen MJ, Minei JP, et al: Debunking the survival bias myth: Characterization of mortality during the initial 24 hours for patients requiring massive transfusion. *J Trauma Acute Care Surg* 2012;73(2):358-364.

   The effect on mortality of the ratio of FFP, PRBCs, and platelets was analyzed in this prospective study of 1,961 adult patients with blunt trauma and hemorrhagic shock. Six hundred four patients in the cohort received a massive transfusion (> 10 units PRBCs) in the first 24 hours after injury. The time course of mortality was specifically studied to rule out the possibility that a survival bias accounted for the decreased mortality reported in previous studies. High ratios of FFP:PRBCs and platelets:PRBCs were associated with decreased mortality at all time points, suggesting that an FFP:PRBC transfusion ratio of 1:1 is ideal.

2. Brockamp T, Nienaber U, Mutschler M, et al: Predicting on-going hemorrhage and transfusion requirement after severe trauma: A validation of six scoring systems and algorithms on the TraumaRegister DGU®. *Crit Care* 2012;16(4):R129.

   The authors present a retrospective internal and external validation of six scoring systems and algorithms (four civilian and two military systems) to predict the risk of massive transfusion at a very early stage after trauma on one single data set of severely injured patients derived from the TraumaRegister DGU database (2002-2010). Data from 56,573 patients were screened to extract one complete data set matching all variables needed to calculate all systems assessed in this study.

3. Brohi K, Singh J, Heron M, Coats T: Acute traumatic coagulopathy. *J Trauma* 2003;54(6):1127-1130.

4. Frith D, Goslings JC, Gaarder C, et al: Definition and drivers of acute traumatic coagulopathy: Clinical and experimental investigations. *J Thromb Haemost* 2010; 8(9):1919-1925.

   The authors discuss the development of a clinically relevant definition of acute traumatic coagulopathy, an impairment of hemostasis that occurs early after injury.

5. Brohi K, Cohen MJ, Ganter MT, et al: Acute coagulopathy of trauma: Hypoperfusion induces systemic anticoagulation and hyperfibrinolysis. *J Trauma* 2008;64(5): 1211-1217.

6. Cohen MJ, Call M, Nelson M, et al: Critical role of activated protein C in early coagulopathy and later organ failure, infection and death in trauma patients. *Ann Surg* 2012;255(2):379-385.

   A prospective cohort study of 203 major trauma patients was performed to assess the activity of activated protein C.

7. Boffard KD, Riou B, Warren B, et al: Recombinant factor VIIa as adjunctive therapy for bleeding control in severely injured trauma patients: Two parallel randomized, placebo-controlled, double-blind clinical trials. *J Trauma* 2005;59(1):8-18.

8. Wade CE, Eastridge BJ, Jones JA, et al: Use of recombinant factor VIIa in US military casualties for a five-year period. *J Trauma* 2010;69(2):353-359.

   A review of more than 2,000 patients entered in the Joint Theater is presented. This study was undertaken to assess how deployed physicians are using recombinant factor VIIa and its effect on casualty outcomes.

9. Hauser CJ, Boffard K, Dutton R, et al: Results of the CONTROL trial: Efficacy and safety of recombinant activated factor VII in the management of refractory traumatic hemorrhage. *J Trauma* 2010;69(3):489-500.

   This phase III randomized clinical trial evaluated the efficacy and the safety of recombinant factor VIIa as an adjunct to direct hemostasis in patients with major traumatic injuries. The authors reported on 573 patients (481 with blunt and 92 with penetrating trauma) who bled four to eight red blood cell units within 12 hours of injury and were still bleeding despite strict damage control resuscitation and surgical management. Patients were assigned to receive recombinant factor VIIa (200 μg/kg initially; 100 μg/kg at 1 hour and 3 hours) or placebo. Intensive care unit management was standardized. Primary outcome was 30-day mortality. Enrollment was terminated at 573 of 1,502 planned patients, partially because of unexpected low mortality prompted by futility analysis (10.8% versus 27.5% planned/predicted). Recombinant factor VIIa reduced blood product use but did not affect mortality compared with placebo. Modern evidence-based treatment of trauma patients lowers mortality, making outcomes studies increasingly difficult.

10. Shakur H, Roberts I, Bautista R, et al: Effects of tranexamic acid on death, vascular occlusive events, and blood transfusion in trauma patients with significant haemorrhage (CRASH-2): A randomised, placebo-controlled trial. *Lancet* 2010;376(9734):23-32.

TXA may reduce bleeding in patients undergoing elective surgery. The authors, in a randomized controlled trial, assessed the effects of the early administration of a short course of TXA acid on death, vascular occlusive events, and the receipt of blood transfusion in trauma patients.

11. Roberts I, Shakur H, Afolabi A, et al: The importance of early treatment with tranexamic acid in bleeding trauma patients: An exploratory analysis of the CRASH-2 randomised controlled trial. *Lancet* 2011; 377(9771):1096-1101, e1-e2.

The CRASH-2 trial showed that early administration of TXA safely reduces mortality from bleeding in patients with traumatic injuries. It was predicted that approximately 112,000 deaths might be averted annually if trauma patients received TXA within 3 hours of injury.

12. Ker K, Kiriya J, Perel P, Edwards P, Shakur H, Roberts I: Avoidable mortality from giving tranexamic acid to bleeding trauma patients: An estimation based on WHO mortality data, a systematic literature review and data from the CRASH-2 trial. *BMC Emerg Med* 2012;12:3.

The CRASH-2 trial showed that early administration of TXA safely reduces mortality from bleeding in trauma patients. Based on data from the CRASH-2 trial, global mortality data, and a systematic literature review, the authors estimated the number of premature deaths that might be averted worldwide every year with TXA. Based on data from the World Health Organization and their systematic literature review, the authors estimated an annual decrease of approximately 400,000 deaths in hospitalized patients with bleeding trauma. If patients received TXA within 1 hour of injury, approximately 128,000 deaths might be averted. If patients received TXA within 3 hours of injury, approximately 112,000 deaths might be averted. Country-specific estimates show that the largest numbers of averted deaths would occur in India and China.

13. Morrison JJ, Dubose JJ, Rasmussen TE, Midwinter MJ: Military Application of Tranexamic Acid in Trauma Emergency Resuscitation (MATTERs) Study. *Arch Surg* 2012;147(2):113-119.

This was a retrospective observational study comparing TXA administration with no TXA in patients receiving at least 1 unit of PRBCs. A subgroup of patients receiving massive transfusion (≥ 10 units of PRBCs) was also examined. The purpose was to characterize the contemporary use of TXA in combat injury and assess the effect of its administration on total blood product use, thromboembolic complications, and mortality.

14. Eastridge BJ, Hardin M, Cantrell J, et al: Died of wounds on the battlefield: Causation and implications for improving combat casualty care. *J Trauma* 2011; 71(1, suppl):S4-S8.

In this study, died of wounds casualties (*n* = 558) accounted for 4.56% of the military personnel not returning to duty because of battle injuries over the study period. Traumatic brain injury was the predominant injury leading to death in 83% of the patients, whereas hemorrhage from major trauma was the predominant mechan-

ism of death in 230 of 287 patients (80%). In patients with hemorrhage, the bleeding body regions that accounted for mortality were the torso (48%), an extremity (31%), and junctional areas (neck, axilla, and groin; 21%). Fifty-one percent of the casualties presented in extremis, with cardiopulmonary resuscitation at presentation. Hemorrhage is a major mechanism of death in combat injuries, underscoring the necessity for initiatives to mitigate bleeding, particularly in the prehospital environment.

15. Kragh JF Jr, Walters TJ, Baer DG, et al: Survival with emergency tourniquet use to stop bleeding in major limb trauma. *Ann Surg* 2009;249(1):1-7.

16. Kragh JF Jr, Wade CE, Baer DG, et al: Fasciotomy rates in operations enduring freedom and iraqi freedom: Association with injury severity and tourniquet use. *J Orthop Trauma* 2011;25(3):134-139.

During the period of the study (between 2003 and 2006), fasciotomy rates increased as a result of a combination of factors: increasing injury severity, increasing use of tourniquets, and increased awareness of the need to perform prophylactic fasciotomies. The authors concluded that further research is needed to determine the optimum rate of fasciotomy in a combat environment.

17. Morrison JJ, Hunt N, Midwinter M, Jansen J: Associated injuries in casualties with traumatic lower extremity amputations caused by improvised explosive devices. *Br J Surg* 2012;99(3):362-366.

IEDs pose a substantial threat to military personnel, often resulting in lower extremity amputation and pelvic injury. CT is necessary to delineate the extent of the injury, but it is unclear whether CT should be performed during or after surgery. In this study, 278 traumatic lower extremity amputations occurred in 169 combat personnel. Sixty-nine of the personnel were killed in action, 16 later died from their wounds, and 84 were wounded in action but survived. Of the 100 casualties who reached the hospital alive, 9 thoracotomies, 1 craniotomy, and 34 laparotomies were performed. All head or torso injuries that required immediate surgery were clinically apparent on admission. Higher levels of amputation were associated with greater injury burden and mortality. Intraoperative CT had little value in identifying clinically important covert injuries.

18. Benfield RJ, Mamczak CN, Vo KC, et al: Initial predictors associated with outcome in injured multiple traumatic limb amputations: A Kandahar-based combat hospital experience. *Injury* 2012;43(10):1753-1758.

An early 30-day follow-up study was performed to evaluate combat personnel with IED injuries with bilateral lower extremity amputations, with and without pelvic and perineal involvement. The results showed that the injuries were survivable. Standard measures of injury and predictors of survival bore little relationship to observed outcomes and may require reevaluation. Long-term follow-up is needed to assess the extent of functional recovery and the overall morbidity and mortality of patients with these types of IED injuries.

1: Principles of Orthopaedics

19. Beckett A, Pelletier P, Mamczak C, Benfield R, Elster E: Multidisciplinary trauma team care in Kandahar, Afghanistan: Current injury patterns and care practices. *Injury* 2012;43(12):2072-2077.

The authors report on 2,599 patients with multiple traumatic injures sustained in Afghanistan. The most common source of injury was an IED blasts (915 patients) followed by gunshot wounds (327 patients). Nineteen patients had triple amputations as a result of injuries from IEDs. One hundred twenty-seven patients received massive transfusions. The in-hospital mortality rate was 4.45%; 4,106.24 operating room hours were logged to complete 1,914 patient cases. The mean number of procedures per case in 2009 was 1.27, compared with 3.11 in 2010. Multinational and multidisciplinary care was required for the large number of severely injured patients treated at Kandahar Airfield in Afghanistan.

20. Burch JM, Ortiz VB, Richardson RJ, Martin RR, Mattox KL, Jordan GL Jr: Abbreviated laparotomy and planned reoperation for critically injured patients. *Ann Surg* 1992;215(5):476-484.

21. Henry SM, Tornetta P III, Scalea TM: Damage control for devastating pelvic and extremity injuries. *Surg Clin North Am* 1997;77(4):879-895.

22. Pape HC, Auf'm'Kolk M, Paffrath T, Regel G, Sturm JA, Tscherne H: Primary intramedullary femur fixation in multiple trauma patients with associated lung contusion—a cause of posttraumatic ARDS? *J Trauma* 1993; 34(4):540-548.

23. Pape HC, Grimme K, Van Griensven M, et al: Impact of intramedullary instrumentation versus damage control for femoral fractures on immunoinflammatory parameters: Prospective randomized analysis by the EPOFF Study Group. *J Trauma* 2003;55(1):7-13.

24. Pape HC, Marcucio R, Humphrey C, Colnot C, Knobe M, Harvey EJ: Trauma-induced inflammation and fracture healing. *J Orthop Trauma* 2010;24(9):522-525.

This article reviews the initial inflammatory response to trauma as it pertains to musculoskeletal healing.

25. Stellin G: Survival in trauma victims with pulmonary contusion. *Am Surg* 1991;57(12):780-784.

26. Rotondo MF, Schwab CW, McGonigal MD, et al: "Damage control": An approach for improved survival in exsanguinating penetrating abdominal injury. *J Trauma* 1993;35(3):375-383.

27. Townsend RN, Lheureau T, Protech J, Riemer B, Simon D: Timing fracture repair in patients with severe brain injury (Glasgow Coma Scale score < 9). *J Trauma* 1998; 44(6):977-983.

28. Pape HC, Giannoudis P, Krettek C: The timing of fracture treatment in polytrauma patients: Relevance of damage control orthopedic surgery. *Am J Surg* 2002; 183(6):622-629.

29. Crowl AC, Young JS, Kahler DM, Claridge JA, Chrzanowski DS, Pomphrey M: Occult hypoperfusion is associated with increased morbidity in patients undergoing early femur fracture fixation. *J Trauma* 2000; 48(2):260-267.

30. Sun T, Wang X, Liu Z, Chen X, Zhang J: Plasma concentrations of pro- and anti-inflammatory cytokines and outcome prediction in elderly hip fracture patients. *Injury* 2011;42(7):707-713.

In elderly patients with a hip fracture, cytokine concentrations were an independent predictor of poor outcomes. Inflammatory response played an important role in postoperative organ dysfunction.

31. Higgins TF, Horwitz DS: Damage control nailing. *J Orthop Trauma* 2007;21(7):477-484.

32. Reynolds MA, Richardson JD, Spain DA, Seligson D, Wilson MA, Miller FB: Is the timing of fracture fixation important for the patient with multiple trauma? *Ann Surg* 1995;222(4):470-481.

33. Morshed S, Miclau T III, Bembom O, Cohen M, Knudson MM, Colford JM Jr: Delayed internal fixation of femoral shaft fracture reduces mortality among patients with multisystem trauma. *J Bone Joint Surg Am* 2009; 91(1):3-13.

34. Pape H, Stalp M, Griensven M, Weinberg A, Dahlweit M, Tscherne H: Optimal timing for secondary surgery in polytrauma patients: An evaluation of 4,314 serious-injury cases. *Chirurg* 1999;70(11):1287-1293.

35. Brundage SI, McGhan R, Jurkovich GJ, Mack CD, Maier RV: Timing of femur fracture fixation: Effect on outcome in patients with thoracic and head injuries. *J Trauma* 2002;52(2):299-307.

36. Demetriades D, Karaiskakis M, Toutouzas K, Alo K, Velmahos G, Chan L: Pelvic fractures: Epidemiology and predictors of associated abdominal injuries and outcomes. *J Am Coll Surg* 2002;195(1):1-10.

37. Giannoudis PV, Grotz MR, Tzioupis C, et al: Prevalence of pelvic fractures, associated injuries, and mortality: The United Kingdom perspective. *J Trauma* 2007; 63(4):875-883.

38. Koo H, Leveridge M, Thompson C, et al: Interobserver reliability of the Young-Burgess and Tile classification systems for fractures of the pelvic ring. *J Orthop Trauma* 2008;22(6):379-384.

39. Burgess AR, Eastridge BJ, Young JW, et al: Pelvic ring disruptions: Effective classification system and treatment protocols. *J Trauma* 1990;30(7):848-856.

40. Routt ML Jr, Falicov A, Woodhouse E, Schildhauer TA: Circumferential pelvic antishock sheeting: A temporary resuscitation aid. *J Orthop Trauma* 2006;20(1, suppl): S3-S6.

41. Tan EC, van Stigt SF, van Vugt AB: Effect of a new pelvic stabilizer (T-POD®) on reduction of pelvic volume and haemodynamic stability in unstable pelvic fractures. *Injury* 2010;41(12):1239-1243.

The authors describe 15 patients with a prehospital untreated, unstable pelvic fracture with signs of hypovolemic shock treated with the T-POD device (Pyng Medical). Application of the pelvic stabilizer provided a 60% reduction in the rate of symphyseal diastasis. The patients' mean arterial pressure increased significantly from 65.3 to 81.2 mm Hg (*P* = 0.03), and the mean heart rate declined from 107 beats per minute to 94 (*P* = 0.02). In the acute setting, the T-POD device has a clear compressive effect on pelvic volume in unstable pelvic fractures.

42. Krieg JC, Mohr M, Ellis TJ, Simpson TS, Madey SM, Bottlang M: Emergent stabilization of pelvic ring injuries by controlled circumferential compression: A clinical trial. *J Trauma* 2005;59(3):659-664.

43. Croce MA, Magnotti LJ, Savage SA, Wood GW II, Fabian TC: Emergent pelvic fixation in patients with exsanguinating pelvic fractures. *J Am Coll Surg* 2007;204(5):935-942.

44. Kim WY, Hearn TC, Seleem O, Mahalingam E, Stephen D, Tile M: Effect of pin location on stability of pelvic external fixation. *Clin Orthop Relat Res* 1999;361:237-244.

45. Ganz R, Krushell RJ, Jakob RP, Küffer J: The antishock pelvic clamp. *Clin Orthop Relat Res* 1991;267:71-78.

46. Reynolds JH, Attum B, Acland RJ, Giannoudis P, Roberts CS: Anterior versus posterior pin placement of pelvic C-clamp in relationship to anatomical structures: A cadaver study. *Injury* 2008;39(8):865-868.

47. Cook RE, Keating JF, Gillespie I: The role of angiography in the management of haemorrhage from major fractures of the pelvis. *J Bone Joint Surg Br* 2002;84(2):178-182.

48. Starr AJ, Griffin DR, Reinert CM, et al: Pelvic ring disruptions: Prediction of associated injuries, transfusion requirement, pelvic arteriography, complications, and mortality. *J Orthop Trauma* 2002;16(8):553-561.

49. Fang JF, Shih LY, Wong YC, Lin BC, Hsu YP: Repeat transcatheter arterial embolization for the management of pelvic arterial hemorrhage. *J Trauma* 2009;66(2):429-435.

50. Shapiro M, McDonald AA, Knight D, Johannigman JA, Cuschieri J: The role of repeat angiography in the management of pelvic fractures. *J Trauma* 2005;58(2):227-231.

51. Ryan MF, Hamilton PA, Chu P, Hanaghan J: Active extravasation of arterial contrast agent on post-traumatic abdominal computed tomography. *Can Assoc Radiol J* 2004;55(3):160-169.

52. Kimbrell BJ, Velmahos GC, Chan LS, Demetriades D: Angiographic embolization for pelvic fractures in older patients. *Arch Surg* 2004;139(7):728-733.

53. Stephen DJ, Kreder HJ, Day AC, et al: Early detection of arterial bleeding in acute pelvic trauma. *J Trauma* 1999;47(4):638-642.

54. Burlew CC, Moore EE, Smith WR, et al: Preperitoneal pelvic packing/external fixation with secondary angio-embolization: Optimal care for life-threatening hemorrhage from unstable pelvic fractures. *J Am Coll Surg* 2011;212(4):628-637.

The authors found that preperitoneal pelvic packing and external fixation were effective in controlling hemorrhage from unstable pelvic fractures. None of the high-risk patients in this study died because of pelvic bleeding. Secondary angioembolization was needed in few patients, permitting the selective use of this resource-demanding intervention. In addition, preperitoneal pelvic packing and external fixation temporizes arterial hemorrhage, providing valuable transfer time for facilities without angiography. With other urgent surgical interventions required in more than 85% of patients, combining these procedures with preperitoneal pelvic packing and external fixation for surgical control of pelvic hemorrhage appears to optimize patient care.

55. Osborn PM, Smith WR, Moore EE, et al: Direct retroperitoneal pelvic packing versus pelvic angiography: A comparison of two management protocols for haemodynamically unstable pelvic fractures. *Injury* 2009;40(1):54-60.

1: Principles of Orthopaedics

Chapter 10
Medical Issues for the Athlete

Brian T. Feeley, MD   Sarina Behera, MD   Anthony C. Luke, MD

Introduction

The day-to-day practice of sports medicine for athletes typically involves more medical issues than orthopaedic issues. A working knowledge of these issues and of the protocols for risk concerns associated with each sport is key for physicians covering athletic events. This chapter highlights the nonorthopaedic issues that need to be considered on the field, in the training room, and at the office.

Sports Nutrition

A proper nutrition regimen is nearly as important as an athlete's training and is recognized in position statements by the American Dietetic Association, the Dietitians of Canada, and the American College of Sports Medicine.[1] With any nutrition regimen in an athlete, the goal is to achieve the appropriate caloric intake to support daily metabolic and physical demands. The timing of caloric intake should be monitored to maximize training and competition potential, especially in elite athletes.

The current recommendation for caloric intake by the US Department of Health and Human Services is approximately 2,000 calories per day (a minimum of 1,200 cal/day for women and 1,800 cal/day for men). For athletes, the caloric intake is much higher; men require up to 4,000 to 5,000 cal/day, and women require up to 2,000 to 3,000 cal/day. However, athletes typically are unable to maintain the necessary caloric intake to support their energy expenditures.[2] Low energy intake is a major nutritional concern for female athletes because a negative energy balance can lead to weight loss and disruption of the endocrine and metabolic functions. The US Department of Health and Human Services provides dietary guidelines for the energy recommendations for athletes of all levels.[3]

Physiology of Exercise

The conversion of nutrients into energy is governed by either anaerobic or aerobic mechanisms, with considerable overlap between each type. With short, high-intensity athletic events such as powerlifting or sprinting, the adenosine triphosphate/phosphocreatine system fuels high-intensity bursts that last 5 to 10 seconds. This short-term anaerobic energy system is used for activities that require up to 90 seconds of effort when adequate oxygen for aerobic activity is not available. Muscle cells primarily use glycolysis as their primary energy source, but this mechanism results in a buildup of lactate within the cells. When the lactate threshold level is reached, the ability of cells to work effectively is diminished because of increased muscle acidity and the inhibition of fatty acid breakdown, causing fatigue. The aerobic energy system is primarily used for most athletic activities. The metabolic activity takes place in the mitochondria, and carbohydrates, fats, and proteins are used as substrates for adenosine triphosphate in the presence of oxygen via the Krebs cycle and the electron transport chain.[1]

Macronutrients

Individual protein requirements vary considerably based on athletic activity, but generally should be higher than normal in athletes to help promote and maintain adequate muscle mass (Table 1). Protein is a primary contributor to tissue repair and regeneration and is the main component of the metabolic, transport, and hormonal systems. Well-planned vegetarian diets seem to effectively support athletic performance; however, this finding is not conclusive.[4] Although most vegetarian diets provide the recommended amount of daily protein, such diets often contain less protein than nonvegetarian diets, and plant-based proteins are less well digested than animal-based proteins. Therefore, the recommended protein intake for vegetarian diets should be approximately 10% higher. Protein consumption by vegans is a potential concern because their diet is limited to the amino acids lysine, threonine, tryptophan, and methionine.[5]

Ideally, carbohydrate consumption should be based on a variety of fruits, vegetables, and grains spread out among the daily training meals. The selection of healthy carbohydrates in modern society is made difficult by the convenience of prepackaged foods containing carbohydrates derived from high-fructose corn syrup. Fructose-based carbohydrates can promote de

Table 1

Recommended Intake of Macronutrients

Macronutrient	Recommended Intake	Percentage of Daily Caloric Intake
Protein	Endurance: 1.2–1.4 g/kg Strength: 1.6–1.8 g/kg	10%–35%
Carbohydrate	5–10 g/kg	40%–65%
Dietary Fat		20%–35%

(Adapted from US Department of Health and Human Services. *Dietary Guidelines of Americans.* Washington, DC, 2005. http://www.health.gov/DietaryGuidelines. Accessed April 8, 2013.)

Table 2

Important Micronutrients for Athletes

Micronutrient	Function
B vitamins (thiamin, riboflavin, niacin, B_6, folate, B_{12})	Involved in optimum energy production and the repair of muscle tissue. Folate and vitamin B_{12} are required for the production of red blood cells.
Vitamin D	Required for calcium absorption and the regulation of serum calcium and phosphate levels. Regulates the development and homeostasis of the bone. Low levels often found in indoor athletes.
Vitamins C and E	Antioxidants that inhibit oxidative stress on the muscles and other cells. May be beneficial in limiting inflammation and muscle soreness.
Calcium	Important for bone growth and the maintenance and repair of bone tissue, blood calcium levels, muscle contraction, and nerve signal generation.
Zinc	Important in the growth, building, and repair of muscle tissue, energy production, and immune status. Female athletes can have low levels.
Magnesium	Involved in the metabolism of fat and proteins, regulates membrane stability, and has important roles in multiple hormones. Athletes participating in wrestling, ballet, gymnastics, and tennis often have low levels.

novo lipogenesis, dyslipidemia, and increased visceral adiposity.[6] Sport drinks and bars should be considered supplemental to a well-balanced diet.

Dietary fat plays several important roles, including protection from injury, providing thermal insulation, and serving as a vitamin carrier. Fat is also the primary source of reserve energy in the body: plasma triglycerides can supply 30% to 80% of the energy necessary for sustained physical activity. The athlete should be encouraged to choose foods that contain essential fatty acids (such as omega-3 fatty acids) and have higher levels of unsaturated fats instead of high levels of saturated fats.

Micronutrients and Other Factors

Micronutrients play an important role in energy production, maintenance of bone and muscle health, immune function, and protection against oxidative damage. Exercise adds stress to many of these pathways, which requires maintaining an appropriate level of micronutrients at all times for physiologic health.[7] The most common vitamins and minerals considered important for athletes are listed in Table 2.

Hydration

Hydration is an often overlooked aspect of nutrition, especially during prolonged training regimens. The serious effects of dehydration, especially during hot weather, include heat stroke, heat-related illness, and death. A loss of more than 2% of body weight as a result of dehydration can result in a decrease in athletic performance; at higher levels, this loss causes mental and cognitive deficits.[8] Clinically, athletes experiencing dehydration present with muscle cramps, fatigue, and dizziness. Athletes who perspire excessively, those in hot climates, and those participating in preseason activities are more likely to experience dehydration. Hyponatremia (a serum sodium level < 135 mmol/L) can result from prolonged, heavy sweating with a concomitant failure to replenish sodium or from overhydration.

The guidelines for adequate hydration during exercise have been published by the American College of Sports Medicine, and specific guidelines for environmental activities also have been published.[8] It is recommended that fluid intake begin 4 hours before training, with a goal of drinking 5 to 7 mL per kg of body weight of either water or a sports beverage. No data

Table 3

The SCOFF Items for Screening Eating Disorders in Primary Care

(1) Do you make yourself sick because you feel uncomfortably full?

(2) Do you worry that you have lost control over how much you eat?

(3) Have you recently lost more than 15 lb in a 3-month period?

(4) Do you believe yourself to be fat when others say you are too thin?

(5) Would you say that food dominates your life?

(Reproduced with permission from Morgan JF, Reid F, Lacey JH. The SCOFF questionnaire: Assessment of a new screening tool for eating disorders. *Br Med J* 1999;319:1467-1468.)

clearly support the use of electrolyte beverages during competition to improve athletic performance, although some studies suggest that these drinks help maintain performance during endurance exercises.[8]

Caffeine and Other Supplements

The emphasis on the use of sports supplements to improve performance has increased, with an overwhelming number of products that promise muscle mass increase, fast recovery, and improved outcomes in athletic events. Despite the prevalence of these products, very few have led to improved performance. Most supplements have not shown any benefit or have dangerous side effects. Banned supplements can be identified by the World Anti-Doping Agency (http://www.wada-ama.org). Other supplements, such as sports drinks, bars, and gels, are commonly used as dietary supplements to improve recovery and have mild beneficial effects on sports performance outcomes.

Caffeine, a naturally occurring substance that stimulates the central nervous system, has had ergogenic effects in studies across multiple sports.[9] Caffeine is also theorized to decrease the perception of effort, thus allowing a higher level of effort, especially in the sedentary person.[10] Caffeine is currently on the World Anti-Doping Agency monitoring program, and the National Collegiate Athletic Association will ban any athlete with a caffeine level in urine higher than 15 µg/mL. High-energy drinks with excessive amounts of caffeine have ergolytic and potentially dangerous effects, especially when mixed with other stimulants or alcohol. Currently, creatine is the most commonly used ergogenic aid among athletes who wish to build muscle and enhance recovery. Creatine effectively improves performance in high-intensity activities, such as sprinting and weight lifting.[11] The adverse effects include fluid gain, cramps, nausea, and diarrhea. Kidney and liver dysfunction have been rarely reported, although causality is unclear. Despite these side effects, creatine is currently considered safe for healthy adults.

Eating Disorders and the Female Athlete Triad

Female athletes who participate in sports for which body image is important, such as gymnastics, dance, swimming, and figure skating, have a high prevalence of disordered eating. Eating disorders can develop in athletes across all sports and of both sexes. The clinical consequences of eating disorders include mental health problems, poor athletic performance, bradycardia and other arrhythmias, and the female athlete triad. Athletes can be evaluated for eating disorders by using the SCOFF questionnaire (Table 3), which is a brief five-question form that reliably screens for anorexia nervosa and bulimia nervosa.[11]

The female athlete triad represents the spectrum of energy availability, menstrual dysfunction, and bone mineral density. The pathologic forms of this triad result in amenorrhea, osteoporosis, and disordered eating. Research suggests osteopenia and exercise-related menstrual changes represent early diagnostic criteria for this disorder, and disordered eating is not necessarily part of the triad in all female athletes. The American College of Sports Medicine developed guidelines for the screening, diagnosis, and treatment of the female athlete triad in 1997, and updated the guidelines in 2007.[12] This model emphasizes the fact that each component can exist on its own, but the three are interrelated and can progress at different rates. Treatment for athletes with disordered eating currently focuses on a team approach that includes the physician, the family, the coach, a bone health specialist, a dietitian, and a mental health worker.[12]

Concussion

Concussion has become one of the most publicized athletic injuries, with long-term health consequences that include altered cognitive status, mental illness, and death. With the increased awareness of concussion as a significant health risk, considerable effort has been invested in improving the definition and the diagnosis of a concussion, as well as the management of postconcussion injuries. Although knowledge regarding the short-term consequences of concussions is much improved, much remains unknown about the long-term results of a single or multiple concussions.

Definition and Epidemiology

A concussion is defined as a complex pathophysiologic process induced by traumatic biomechanical forces that affect the brain.[13] The symptoms are often vague and underreported by athletes, coaches, and parents. The self-reporting of concussions has significantly increased the incidence of this condition.

Studies conducted in recent years have explored the epidemiology of concussions in athletes. In high-school sports, concussions account for almost 15% of all sports-related injuries. A review of the epidemiology of concussions in high-school athletes found that the over-

1: Principles of Orthopaedics

all injury rate was 2.5 per 10,000 athletic exposures.[14] Concussions occurred more commonly in competition than during practice, and the highest reported rates were in football (47%), girls' soccer (8%), and boys' wrestling (6%). Among football players, linemen had the highest incidence of concussions, followed by tight ends, running backs, and linebackers. However, neither the impact volume nor the intensity appeared to influence the concussion threshold level reported in high-school football players.[15]

Diagnosis and Management

The diagnosis of a concussion is made based on the mechanism of impact and the associated symptoms. The signs and symptoms of a concussion are vague and therefore are difficult to diagnose, especially in cases of a mild injury. Somatic symptoms include headache, fatigue, dizziness, nausea or vomiting, visual problems, and phonophobia. Athletes with a concussion often experience cognitive changes, including amnesia, confusion, disorientation, inability to focus, delayed verbal and motor responses, drowsiness, and reports of being "in a fog." Emotional lability and irritability are common sequelae of concussion.

The evaluation of an athlete with a concussion should begin with an initial systematic field assessment. The physician should assess and maintain adequate airway, breathing, and circulation on the field and perform a neurologic examination to evaluate for any spinal injury. After the athlete is on the sidelines, a more detailed history and physical examination are performed, with attention given to any of the previously identified symptoms discussed earlier. The player's helmet should be taken away to prevent the player from returning to the game. The Sport Concussion Assessment Tool 3rd Edition (available free online at http://bjsm.bmj.com/content/47/5/259.full.pdf) can be used on the sidelines to assess symptoms and follow the progression or the resolution of symptoms. Serial neurologic assessments also should be performed. Instructions are provided to the athlete and family for appropriate follow-up, including further neurocognitive testing when appropriate.[16]

Determining when to return to play is one of the most controversial aspects of concussion management. Expert consensus exists that any athlete suspected of having a concussion should not be allowed to return to play on the day of injury. Prior to any further athletic activity, an athlete must be entirely symptom free and cleared for play by a physician or other qualified medical professional trained in the treatment of concussions.

Postural stability and neurocognitive function tests are more sensitive than routine clinical examination for the detection of neurologic deficits. Initial treatment should emphasize physical and cognitive rest. After an athlete is completely asymptomatic for at least 24 hours, he or she may progress through a stepwise return to sports. It is strongly recommended that athletes who have sustained repeated concussions be withheld from regular sports participation for at least 7 days after symptoms have resolved, while making a gradual return to play. The effects of concussions can be cumulative, and athletes who sustain three or more concussions are much more likely to sustain a recurrent concussion, which raises questions regarding further participation in contact sports.[17,18]

Computerized concussion assessment programs have been used to provide a neurocognitive baseline for determining when athletes can return to play.[19] Although these computerized neurocognitive tests help compare athletes' results with their baseline status, the long-term efficacy of this testing method has been questioned.[20]

Long-Term Effects

The long-term effects of concussions are not well established. The long-term consequences of repeated concussions in football players have been studied.[21] Players who sustained more than three concussions reported an increased prevalence of memory problems and mild cognitive impairment compared with those who had fewer than three concussions. The results of other studies suggested an increased incidence of clinical depression in retired football players, but the association between concussion and depression is not clear in those patients.[22] Additional long-term prospective studies are needed.

Stingers

Stingers, also known as burners, are one of the most common sports injuries treated by physicians and athletic trainers. Stingers occur most commonly in football and are the result of traction or a direct impact on the nerve from the cervical root to the brachial plexus.

Mechanism of Injury

The exact mechanism of stingers is variable; they can be the result of tensile overload of the brachial plexus, stretching of the nerve root, or direct compression of the nerve root and the brachial plexus. Any of these mechanisms likely can cause similar symptoms. The C5 nerve root is most vulnerable because it is directly aligned with the upper trunk of the brachial plexus.

Presentation and Evaluation

Athletes may present with a sudden stinging or burning in the arm after a traumatic event. The athlete often leaves the field holding the arm and reporting a "dead arm" sensation. This event must be distinguished from a glenohumeral dislocation. The pain from a stinger is usually experienced in a dermatomal pattern and often lasts only seconds or minutes. The symptoms are unilateral; those with bilateral symptoms should be considered to have a spinal cord injury.

Patients with recurrent stingers or those with persistent symptoms warrant further evaluation. Although radiography is often the initial imaging study, the relative value of this examination is limited. Radiographs should be evaluated for any degenerative changes, occult facet injuries, and loss of cervical lordosis. The Torg ratio helps determine the presence of central cervical spinal stenosis, which correlates with an increased risk of complications after a stinger.[23] Advanced imaging studies are indicated in patients with persistent symptoms or recurrent stingers, and MRI has the most definitive results. In a cohort of football players with chronic stingers, 93% of players had significant disk disease or neural foraminal narrowing.[24]

Treatment

Most athletes who experience a stinger need only to rest until the symptoms resolve. Rest and NSAIDs have relieved symptoms in those with persistent pain. After the pain has resolved, rehabilitation should focus on range of motion and strength in the affected extremity. No evidence exists that equipment modification helps prevent recurrent symptoms.

Return to play is predicated on the resolution of symptoms, the restoration of full strength, and the absence of cervical spine symptoms. Athletes with brief symptoms (lasting less than 15 minutes) and complete resolution of the stinger are usually allowed to return to play unless the condition is recurrent. If the symptoms continue for more than 15 minutes, return to play is allowed the following week. If an athlete sustains more than three stingers in a season, ending that season and performing a complete evaluation should be considered.[25]

Cardiac Conditions in Athletes

Several cardiac conditions can occur in a previously healthy athlete during exercise and sports activity. The initial presentation in some of these conditions can be sudden cardiac arrest. In competitive athletes younger than 35 years, the incidence of sudden cardiac death is estimated to be less than 1 case per 100,000 per year.[26] This incidence increases with age and male sex and ranges from 1 case per 15,000 per year to 1 case per 50,000 per year in athletes older than 35 years.[27] Among the several million asymptomatic active people in the United States, it is difficult to determine who is at risk for sudden cardiac death during physical activity.

Exercise is commonly prescribed by healthcare providers to improve general wellness and cardiovascular health. Reconciling the significant health benefits of physical activity for most people with the risk of sudden cardiac death in a relatively small number of athletes is challenging. Some health conditions, including coronary artery disease and hypertrophic cardiomyopathy, are associated with sudden cardiac death in athletes of all ages.

Normal Cardiac Adaptation to Exercise

Athletes increasingly push their limits during sports participation. Intense strength and endurance training can lead to changes in heart morphology and function. Electrocardiographic changes may occur that are considered normal in athletes, including sinus bradycardia, first-degree atrioventricular block, and isolated left ventricular hypertrophy.[28] Echocardiography can reveal increased muscle mass and wall thickness in the left ventricle with or without left ventricular dilatation in highly trained athletes; this condition is referred to as athlete's heart syndrome.[29]

A left ventricular wall thickness greater than 13 mm suggests hypertrophic cardiomyopathy (HCM); however, in a small number of elite athletes, left ventricular wall thickness can range from 13 to 16 mm because of physiologic causes. Other imaging modalities, including MRI and ultrasonography, can help distinguish athlete's heart syndrome from HCM. Cessation of training also can help make the distinction between athlete's heart syndrome (the hypertrophy resolves) and HCM (the hypertrophy persists). In addition, significant anatomic variations occur between the sexes and among people of different ages and ethnicities, making it difficult to use wall thickness as the criterion to distinguish athlete's heart syndrome from HCM.

Sudden Cardiac Death

HCM is the most common cause of sudden cardiac death in competitive athletes younger than 35 years, accounting for 36% of cases (Figure 1). Other causes include congenital coronary artery anomalies (17%), arrhythmia syndromes (7%), and myocarditis (6%).[30] When a basketball player collapses on the court or a runner dies during a marathon, these cardiac conditions should be considered in the evaluation of the athlete and sometimes in his or her surviving family members. For athletes older than 35 years, the most common cause of sudden cardiac death is coronary artery disease.[27]

Hypertrophic Cardiomyopathy

HCM is an autosomal dominant condition that leads to thickening of the walls of the heart, particularly the septum. HCM generally occurs in an asymmetric manner and can lead to left ventricular outflow obstruction. Initial presentation during exercise can include chest pain, palpitations, dizziness, syncope, and/or cardiac arrest. Pediatric and adolescent patients tend to present with more severe forms of HCM than adults. More than 1,000 gene mutations have been identified in sarcomere proteins, and genetic testing can play an important role in the diagnosis of select cases. Genetic testing identifies approximately 60% of patients with HCM when there is a positive family history compared with 30% of patients without a positive family history.[31]

Congenital Coronary Artery Anomalies

Under normal conditions, the left main coronary artery arises from the left aortic sinus, and the right main coronary artery arises from the right aortic sinus. In general, if the left main coronary artery arises from the right sinus and courses between the aorta and the main pulmonary artery, the risk of ischemia and cardiac arrest is increased. The prevalence (estimated to be be-

1: Principles of Orthopaedics

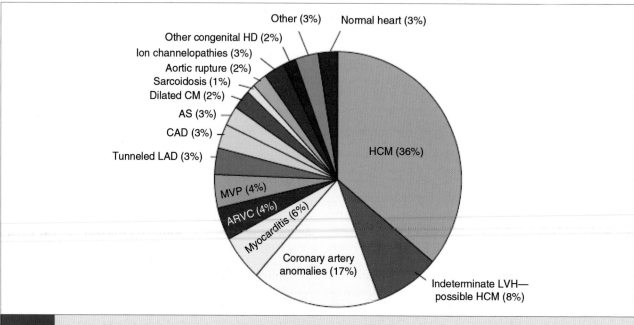

Figure 1 Chart shows the distribution of cardiovascular causes of sudden death in 1,435 young competitive athletes. From the Minneapolis Heart Institute Foundation Registry, 1980 to 2005. ARVC = arrhythmogenic right ventricular cardiomyopathy, AS = aortic stenosis, CAD = coronary artery disease, CM = cardiomyopathy, HCM = hypertrophic cardiomyopathy, HD = heart disease, LAD = left anterior descending, LVH = left ventricular hypertrophy, MVP = mitral valve prolapsed. (Data from Maron BJ, Thompson PD, Ackerman MJ, et al: Recommendations and considerations related to preparticipation screening for cardiovascular abnormalities in competitive athletes: 2007 update: A scientific statement from the American Heart Association Council on Nutrition, Physical Activity, and Metabolism. Endorsed by the American College of Cardiology Foundation. *Circulation* 2007;115[12]:1643-455.)

tween 0.1% and 0.3%) and risk of sudden death in coronary artery anomalies that are sometimes identified at autopsy have been difficult to determine.[32] Patients can be asymptomatic or present with angina, dizziness, and/or syncope with exercise. Arterial anomalies are an important and surgically preventable cause of sudden death in athletes. Without a high degree of suspicion, these anomalies can often be missed, even during echocardiography.

Arrhythmia Syndromes

Arrhythmia syndromes include heterogeneous conditions that can present as palpitations, syncope, and/or cardiac arrest in athletes. Wolff-Parkinson-White syndrome involves an accessory pathway that can participate in an atrioventricular reentry circuit, leading to tachycardia.[26] Long QT syndrome can be acquired or congenital; more than 10 gene mutations have been identified in ion channels that are involved in electrical conduction and lead to changes in the cardiac action potential.[28] Some arrhythmia syndromes are purely electrical disturbances and can sometimes be diagnosed with a baseline electrocardiogram. Other conditions are associated with structural cardiac abnormalities and include arrhythmogenic right ventricular dysplasia. In addition, ventricular arrhythmias are often the cause of sudden cardiac death in HCM. Electrocardiography and Holter monitors are commonly used to evaluate arrhythmias; however, these devices have limitations and careful evaluation by an experienced cardiologist is usually indicated.

Myocarditis

The pathology of myocarditis varies from an insidious prodrome similar to the common cold and influenza to significant inflammation of the heart, including lymphocytic infiltration of the myocardium. Acute myocarditis usually has an infectious etiology and various presentations, including chest pain, dyspnea, exercise intolerance, congestive heart failure, arrhythmias, and cardiogenic shock.[33] Athletes with myocarditis should be restricted from sports participation for at least 6 months and until the illness completely resolves. Undetected viral myocarditis that resolves without treatment can sometimes present later in life as dilated cardiomyopathy.

Coronary Artery Disease

Atherosclerotic coronary artery disease is the most common underlying cardiac condition occurring in athletes older than 35 years.[27] Although routine cardiovascular exercise is often prescribed as a method to decrease the risk factors of and improve the outcomes for coronary artery disease, intense physical exertion can transiently increase the risk of ischemia and cardiac arrest. Adults who experience sudden cardiac arrest with exercise often report angina and/or nonspecific symptoms (nausea, backache) the week before the event but may not have received adequate medical attention.[34] Older adults with established coronary artery disease should undergo a thorough cardiologic evaluation and obtain expert medical advice regarding exercise restrictions and sports participation.

Infectious Diseases in Athletes

Skin Infections

Cellulitis

Cellulitis involves a bacterial infection often resulting from a break in the skin or hematogenous transmission. Heightened vigilance is necessary to identify community-acquired methicillin-resistant *Staphylococcus aureus* (MRSA) infections, which can occur in outbreaks among athletes. The increase in rates of community-acquired MRSA is an ongoing concern. The results of a recent population study in Pennsylvania suggest that the annual incidence rate of community-acquired MRSA increased by 34% and skin and soft-tissue infections increased by 4%.[35] Concern also exists about the spread of the disease from nasal carriers. The prevalence of MRSA nasal carriers in the college student athlete population is approximately 1.8%, although it has been reported as high as 9.2% in some groups.[36] Screening all athletes for MRSA carriers is not recommended. MRSA presents most often at the elbows and the knees as a large pustule with an erythematous ring that appears aggressively and is tender to the touch. This presentation also can occur anywhere on the body, more often early in the season.[37] Abrasions sustained during sports seem to be the cause for many skin infections. Most skin infections, including small abscesses, are still usually due to *S aureus*. Carbuncles develop when infected follicles coalesce to form a deep, erythematous, painful mass.

Treatment of large, painful abscesses or carbuncles requires incision and drainage, laboratory testing of the pustule because of the high risk of MRSA, adjunct treatment with oral trimethoprim/sulfamethoxazole or clindamycin[38] for 10 days, and clinical reevaluation in 24 hours. Intravenous vancomycin is suggested if symptoms do not improve or if the infection is aggressive. If the cause is *Streptococcus*, cephalexin or azithromycin can be used for treatment. For small, benign-appearing lesions, warm compresses can be used four times per day.

Impetigo

Impctigo is caused by a skin infection resulting from group A streptococcus or *S aureus*.[40] Impetigo also can occur following a turf abrasion as a result of a secondary infection, which can present with nonbullous papules, vesicles, and pustules that burst and form a honey-colored crust. With bullous impetigo, blister-like vesicles form, with clear fluid that becomes darker, and then rupture. Ecthyma refers to ulcerated lesions with a raised yellow crust.[39]

Treatment of the nonbullous form caused by *S aureus* includes topical mupirocin three times per day for 10 days. Bullous impetigo caused by group A streptococcus is treated with cephalexin or erythromycin. If MRSA is suspected, then a course of trimethoprim/sulfamethoxazole or clindamycin for 10 days can be prescribed.

Prevention of Skin Infection Outbreaks

Athletes can return to play for wrestling or other high-contact sports when no new lesions develop for 48 hours and they have been treated with antibiotics for 72 hours. Any skin lesions should be reported to the coach or the athletic trainer. To prevent the spread of MRSA,[40] all wounds (draining, moist lesions, or healing lesions) must be covered with biooclusive prewrap and tape during competition. Athletes must practice good hygiene, including showering and washing with soap and water and using clean towels as soon as possible after play. Athletes should not share equipment, clothing, or razors. The uniforms and shared equipment should be cleaned on a routine schedule and stored in clean, dry areas. Hot tub and regular tub use should be restricted. Research on whether athletic fields may contain infectious organisms is inconclusive, and there is no indication that antimicrobial agents should be applied to playing fields.

Mononucleosis

Mononucleosis, an infectious disease caused by the Epstein-Barr virus, is spread by direct contact and through the saliva and is known to the public as "the kissing disease." The incubation period can be long, approximately 30 to 50 days. Symptoms include sore throat, fever, cervical lymphadenopathy (particularly involving the posterior cervical nodes), and splenomegaly. A complete blood count often shows more than 10% atypical lymphocytes. The heterophile antibody latex agglutination test (Monospot test) has a sensitivity of 87% (range, 79% to 95%) and a specificity of 91% (range, 82% to 99%) in patients older than 16 years.[41,42] The false-negative rate can be as high as 25% during the first week of symptoms and can range from 5% to 10% in the second week.[43]

Symptomatic treatment of mononucleosis is recommended. The patient should avoid all forms of exercise for the first 21 days after the onset of symptoms. The complication of greatest concern is atraumatic splenic rupture, which has an incidence of 0.1% to 0.2%. Most splenic ruptures occur within the first 21 days. Questions remain regarding the measurement of spleen size using ultrasonography.[42] It is recommended that athletes should not return to play unless they remain asymptomatic for at least 21 days. Up to 30% of cases can also have a coinfection of group A streptococcus pharyngitis. This infection should be treated with penicillin because 80% to 90% of individuals treated with amoxicillin develop a rash.[44]

Metabolic Diseases

Hyponatremia

Exercise-associated hyponatremia is defined as a serum sodium level less than 135 mmol/L during or up to 24 hours after prolonged physical activity[45] and is usually seen in endurance athletes. Risk factors for exercise-associated hyponatremia include slow running

1: Principles of Orthopaedics

or a performance pace of more than 4 hours for a marathon, female sex, low body mass index (< 20), excessive fluid consumption (> 3 L), and weight gain during exercise.[46] Other risk factors include event inexperience, the use of NSAIDs, and unusually hot or extremely cold environmental conditions.[45] Early signs and symptoms of exercise-associated hyponatremia can include bloating, puffiness, nausea, vomiting, and headache.[47] The athlete may appear confused and obtunded. The athlete often reports more fluid consumption (3.5 L) and can gain weight.[47] Low sodium levels can lead to seizures and death. Treatment involves fluid restriction until the onset of urination in mild cases. In severe cases, transfer to a hospital and treatment with intravenous 3% saline bolus is recommended.[45]

Rhabdomyolysis

Rhabdomyolysis occurs in athletes when muscle fibers break down, usually because of overexertion, dehydration, or heat-related illness. The breakdown of muscle cells releases myoglobin, leading to complications, including major lactic acidosis and a rapid rise in serum potassium levels, which can cause secondary lethal arrhythmias or death from acute myoglobinuric renal failure.[48] The creatine kinase level is used to detect muscle degeneration; however, creatine kinase levels may rise to approximately 5,000 U/L with exercise.[48] Creatine kinase levels can be elevated to 250,000 or higher in severe cases. Patients should be transferred to the hospital for workup because rapid decompensation can occur. Early treatment should include aggressive oral or intravenous rehydration. Dialysis is necessary if acute renal failure occurs. Usually, an athlete with a creatine kinase level of 20,000 to 50,000 U/L who is stable and has a normal serum creatinine level and good urine output recovers with oral hydration and outpatient follow-up.[49]

Sickle Cell Disease

Sickle cell disease involves mutations in the hemoglobin S gene. The prevalence of sickle cell disease is 0.2%. Approximately 8% of African Americans, 0.5% of Hispanics, and 0.2% of Caucasians have the sickle cell trait,[50] which protects against *Plasmodium falciparum* malaria. Hemoglobin S deoxygenates and polymerizes, resulting in a rigid cell shape and impaired blood flow, hemolysis, and vasoocclusive episodes. For those with the sickle cell trait, the condition is usually benign with no sickle cell crises, although an association with sudden death and rhabomyolysis has been reported.[51,52] One study reviewed 23 athlete deaths that involved a distinctive noninstantaneous collapse, with gradual deterioration over several minutes associated with vigorous or exhaustive physical exertion, usually during football conditioning drills and often in hot weather.[51] The sickle cell trait does not affect an athlete's performance or life expectancy. Screening athletes for the sickle cell trait is recommended by the National Collegiate Athletic Association, but is still controversial.[51,52]

Sickle cell crises can result in splenic infarctions, venous thromboembolism, pregnancy-related complications, increased ocular pressure and renal medullary carcinoma, microscopic and macroscopic hematuria, renal papillary necrosis, infections, or kidney stones. Sickle cell crises can occur with increased intensity of exercise, dehydration, altitude changes, asthma, and heat-related illnesses.

Environmental Issues for the Athlete

Heat-Related Injuries
Classification of Heat-Related Illness
Heat-related illnesses (Table 4) can progress along a spectrum from mild to severe. Core temperature is regulated by four main mechanisms that dissipate heat: conduction, convection, radiation, and evaporation. When the ambient temperature exceeds 35°C (94°F), the evaporation of sweat, which can be affected by high humidity, becomes the most important mechanism. Patients at risk include young athletes (because of reduced heat tolerance, longer acclimatization periods, and less sweating and voluntary fluid intake), obese athletes (because of poorer thermoregulation), athletes involved in outdoor sports with a long exercise duration (marathons, tennis, soccer, football), and individuals with medical conditions that can adversely affect heat tolerance or cause dehydration. Drug use is also a risk factor. Although not commonly enforced, cancellation of outdoor events when the ambient temperature is 28°C (82°F) is recommended by the American College of Sports Medicine.[53]

Management of Heat-Related Illness in Athletes
In serious cases of heat-related illness, core temperature must be measured rectally; oral, ear, temporal artery, and axillary temperatures are less accurate. The treatment goal is to reduce the core temperature below 40°C (104°F) as soon as possible, ideally within 30 minutes. Immersion in cold or ice water is the most effective, practical means to rapidly reduce core temperature. Early transfer to a hospital is necessary. To identify end-stage organ failure, laboratory tests for complete blood count, coagulation panel, liver function, electrolytes, renal function, urinalysis, and muscle enzymes (creatine kinase) should be ordered. Aggressive intravenous fluid rehydration can be started. Dantrolene (for malignant hyperthermia) and benzodiazepine (for seizure activity) can be used. For mild symptoms, the athlete should be moved to the shade, equipment should be removed, hydration should begin, water or ice should be applied to the groin and axilla, and the legs should be elevated to aid recovery.

In cases of environmental changes, acclimatization may take anywhere from 1 to 3 weeks. Specific preseason acclimatization guidelines for heat-related illnesses in football include modification of equipment and contact activity for the first 14 days and avoiding twice-a-day practice sessions during the first week. Younger athletes are limited to a maximum of 10 hours of exertion per week and 2 hours of exertion per practice.[54]

Table 4

Heat- and Cold-Related Injuries

Illness	Symptoms	Etiology	Management
Heat-Related			
Cramps	Presents as hyperexcitable muscles occurring during or after exercise	Unknown, although cramps seem to be associated with salt deficiency and dehydrated muscles, nonacclimatized athletes in poor condition, and supplement use (particularly stimulants and creatine)	Rehydration preferably with an electrolyte solution (can add ¼ tsp of table salt to 300–500 mL of fluids). Treat with passive stretching, rest, massage, ice, and TENS.
Syncope	Light-headedness or fainting	Dehydration and peripheral vasodilatation, causing venous pooling in lower extremities	Remove athlete from the heat and cool down with ice and water. Oral rehydration first or use IV fluids (usually normal saline).
Exhaustion	Inability to continue exercise with or without collapse	Related to dehydration and results in central fatigue and peripheral vascular dilation	Remove athlete from the heat and cool down with ice and water Oral rehydration first or use IV fluids (usually normal saline).
Heat stroke	Dizziness, lightheaded, disorientation and confusion, irritability, hyperventilation, nausea and vomiting particularly bad, fatigue and collapse	Core temperature > 40°C; can lead to end-stage organ failure	See text
Cold-Related			
Frostbite	Early pain and itching, progressing to white, cold, firm or hard tissue in the affected area	Freezing and thawing results in extracellular and intracellular ice crystal formation and cellular dehydration; vascular stasis and ischemia can occur in later stages	Avoid refreezing injury, rewarming bath at 40°–42°C (104°–108°F); provide narcotics, NSAIDs, and tetanus prophylaxis.
Trenchfoot	Pain and freezing injuries at the feet	Recurrent wet and cold exposure to the feet causes repetitive nonfreezing injury; typically temperature 0°–10°C (32°–50°F)	Rewarm when no risk of refreezing.
Hypothermia			
Mild	Confusion "umbles": stumbles, mumbles, fumbles, and grumbles	Core temperature: 32°–35°C (89°–95°F)	Passive warming with endogenous heat; general recovery expected without sequelae.
Moderate	Impaired judgment and apathy, shivering stops (31°C), muscle stiffness	Core temperature: 28°–32°C (82°–89°F)	Active rewarming often required.
Severe	Loss of consciousness (30°–32°C), decreased pulse, decreased respiratory rate, coma	Core temperature: < 28°C (82°F)	30% mortality; pulse at initial examination indicates better survival; rapid active rewarming essential

IV = intravenous, TENS = transcutaneous electrical nerve stimulation.

Cold-Related Injury

Cold-related injuries can be mild to severe and can worsen in wet conditions (Table 4). Patients who are of African descent are at risk; other risk factors include wind chill, high altitude, previous frostbite, tobacco use, altered mental status, impaired thermoregulation, and drug use (for example, anticholinergics, stimulants, marijuana, opiates). The digits, ears, nose, cheeks, and genitalia are particularly at risk. Frostbite is graded similar to burns: first-degree frostbite presents with numbness, erythema, and edema; second-degree frostbite has clear, fluid-filled blisters; third-degree frostbite shows hemorrhagic blisters; and fourth-degree frostbite presents with mottled and frozen tissue.

Immediate treatment should involve protecting the frozen tissue from further freezing or trauma. If hypothermia is a concern, immediate, rapid rewarming can be accomplished with a water bath at 40°C to 42°C (104°F to 108°F). Medications can include topical aloe vera, oral ibuprofen, and narcotics, and an oral prostaglandin to cause vasodilation should be considered. Tetanus vaccination status should be updated.

As the core temperature decreases (33°C), the individual may demonstrate impaired judgment and apathy. Sometimes the athlete may display paradoxical undressing. At 31°C, shivering stops and muscle stiffness ensues. Patients often lose consciousness at a core temperature lower than 30° to 32°C, demonstrate decreased pulse and respiratory rate, and may become comatose.

The patient with severe hypothermia must be handled gently and removed from the cold environment; wet clothing should be removed. The patient should be monitored for oxygen saturation and undergo continuous electrocardiography. If the patient has no pulse and is apneic, cardiopulmonary resuscitation can be initiated. Passive warming is performed via endogenous heat production. When hypothermia is more moderate, active warming is performed using exogenous air-warming blankets. Rapid, active internal rewarming is reserved for severe hypothermia; intravenous fluids warmed to 40°C to 43°C can be used, although lactated Ringer solution should be avoided because a cold liver cannot metabolize lactate. Extracorporeal rewarming using peritoneal dialysis or chest tube irrigation can be attempted in severe cases. If the body has been warmed to 32°C to 35°C and vital signs are absent, the patient has died.

Altitude Medicine
Acute Mountain Sickness
Acute mountain sickness is typically seen within the first 6 to 12 hours at an altitude higher than 8,000 ft. Symptoms of acute mountain sickness include headache and one of the following: gastrointestinal disturbance (nausea, vomiting, anorexia), dizziness, fatigue, or sleep disturbance. The physical examination results are usually unremarkable, and the condition is self-limited if no further ascent occurs. The initial treatment is descent (at least 1,500 to 2,000 feet). If descent is not possible, then ascent should cease and treatment with supplemental oxygen is recommended. Treatment includes oral analgesics for headache and acetazolamide and/or dexamethasone for acute symptoms.[55] Acetazolamide can be taken before ascent as a preventive measure.

High-Altitude Cerebral Edema
High-altitude cerebral edema is likely a more severe form of acute mountain sickness. Clinical symptoms include neurologic signs, ataxia, change in mental status, hallucinations, confusion, vomiting, stupor, and/or coma.

Papilledema, retinal hemorrhages, and global encephalopathy can occur. High-altitude cerebral edema can be fatal over hours to days, especially if it occurs at an altitude higher than 20,000 feet (also known as the death zone).[55] Treatment involves immediate descent to a lower altitude. If descent is not possible, the patient should be treated with supplemental oxygen and dexamethasone.

High-Altitude Pulmonary Edema
Patients with high-altitude pulmonary edema present with a dry cough, decreased exercise tolerance progressing to respiratory distress, bloody sputum, and fever. High-altitude pulmonary edema is more common in men than women, and recurrent episodes are likely. A chest radiograph shows patchy infiltrates (alveolar edema) most commonly in the right middle lobe.[56] In addition to other altitude treatments, supplemental oxygen and careful monitoring are recommended with immediate descent. Otherwise, nifedipine, glucocorticoids, acetazolamide, and inhaled salmeterol should be used for treatment.[57]

Acclimatization to altitude should ideally occur over 10 to 14 days. If ascent is necessary despite an episode of high-altitude pulmonary edema, increases in altitude should be limited to 300 m per day, with rest days every 2 to 3 days.

Summary

Medical issues are more common in sports medicine. Much of what a team physician encounters is medical rather than orthopaedic. A surgeon should be vigilant for the dietary, medical, and environmental conditions and risk factors discussed and work with the athlete's team of health providers when called for.

Key Study Points

- Recognize the symptoms of concussion and implement the restrictions and the regulations for initial concussion management.

- Be familiar with the common cardiac causes of sudden death in athletes, including HCM, congenital coronary artery anomalies, and arrhythmias.

- Heat-related injuries during sports are common and can be avoided with simple preventive measures, including proper hydration and early treatment.

Annotated References

1. Rodriguez NR, Di Marco NM, Langley S; American Dietetic Association; Dietitians of Canada; American College of Sports Medicine: American College of Sports

Medicine position stand: Nutrition and athletic performance. *Med Sci Sports Exerc* 2009;41(3):709-731.

2. Lun V, Erdman KA, Reimer RA: Evaluation of nutritional intake in Canadian high-performance athletes. *Clin J Sport Med* 2009;19(5):405-411.

3. US Department of Health and Human Services. *Dietary Guidelines of Americans.* Washington, DC, 2005. http://www.health.gov/DietaryGuidelines. Accessed April 8, 2013.

4. Tipton KD, Witard OC: Protein requirements and recommendations for athletes: Relevance of ivory tower arguments for practical recommendations. *Clin Sports Med* 2007;26(1):17-36.

5. Tipton KD, Elliott TA, Cree MG, Aarsland AA, Sanford AP, Wolfe RR: Stimulation of net muscle protein synthesis by whey protein ingestion before and after exercise. *Am J Physiol Endocrinol Metab* 2007;292(1):E71-E76.

6. Stanhope KL, Schwarz JM, Keim NL, et al: Consuming fructose-sweetened, not glucose-sweetened, beverages increases visceral adiposity and lipids and decreases insulin sensitivity in overweight/obese humans. *J Clin Invest* 2009;119(5):1322-1334.

7. Driskell J: *Vitamins and Trace Elements in Sports Nutrition.* New York, NY, CRC/Taylor & Francis, 2006.

8. Sawka MN, Burke LM, Eichner ER, et al: American College of Sports Medicine position stand: Exercise and fluid replacement. *Med Sci Sports Exerc* 2007;39(2):377-390.

9. Mohr M, Nielsen JJ, Bangsbo J: Caffeine intake improves intense intermittent exercise performance and reduces muscle interstitial potassium accumulation. *J Appl Physiol* 2011;111(5):1372-1379.

   The authors found that caffeine intake enhances fatigue resistance and reduces muscle interstitial potassium during intense intermittent exercise. Level of evidence: III.

10. Laurence G, Wallman K, Guelfi K: Effects of caffeine on time trial performance in sedentary men. *J Sports Sci* 2012;30(12):1235-1240.

    The authors found that sedentary men could exercise more after caffeine ingestion, without an accompanying increase in effort sensation, suggesting that caffeine could increase the chance that sedentary men will exercise. Level of evidence: III.

11. Baird MF, Graham SM, Baker JS, Bickerstaff GF: Creatine-kinase- and exercise-related muscle damage implications for muscle performance and recovery. *J Nutr Metab* 2012;2012:960363.

    The authors reviewed the current evidence and current opinions regarding the release of creatine kinase from skeletal muscle in response to physical activity. Level of evidence: V.

12. Nattiv A, Loucks AB, Manore MM, et al: American College of Sports Medicine position stand: The female athlete triad. *Med Sci Sports Exerc* 2007;39(10):1867-1882.

13. McCrory P, Meeuwisse W, Johnston K, et al: Consensus statement on Concussion in Sport 3rd International Conference on Concussion in Sport held in Zurich, November 2008. *Clin J Sport Med* 2009;19(3):185-200.

14. Marar M, McIlvain NM, Fields SK, Comstock RD: Epidemiology of concussions among United States high school athletes in 20 sports. *Am J Sports Med* 2012;40(4):747-755.

    The authors conducted a review of the epidemiology of concussions in high school sports. Football, hockey, girls' soccer, and wrestling had high rates of concussion. Level of evidence: IV.

15. Eckner JT, Sabin M, Kutcher JS, Broglio SP: No evidence for a cumulative impact effect on concussion injury threshold. *J Neurotrauma* 2011;28(10):2079-2090.

    The results of this accelerometer study suggested that impact volume or intensity does not influence the concussion threshold in high school football athletes. Level of evidence: II.

16. Guskiewicz KM, Broglio SP: Sport-related concussion: On-field and sideline assessment. *Phys Med Rehabil Clin N Am* 2011;22(4):603-617, vii.

    The authors of this concise review explain how to assess and evaluate athletes who have sustained a concussion during an athletic event. Level of evidence: V.

17. Guskiewicz KM, McCrea M, Marshall SW, et al: Cumulative effects associated with recurrent concussion in collegiate football players: The NCAA Concussion Study. *JAMA* 2003;290(19):2549-2555.

18. Iverson GL, Gaetz M, Lovell MR, Collins MW: Cumulative effects of concussion in amateur athletes. *Brain Inj* 2004;18(5):433-443.

19. Broglio SP, Ferrara MS, Macciocchi SN, Baumgartner TA, Elliott R: Test-retest reliability of computerized concussion assessment programs. *J Athl Train* 2007;42(4):509-514.

20. Erdal K: Neuropsychological testing for sports-related concussion: How athletes can sandbag their baseline testing without detection. *Arch Clin Neuropsychol* 2012;27(5):473-479.

    The authors reviewed the factors associated with athletes faking their baseline concussion test results to remain in the game. The authors conclude that it is difficult to fake the results of the tests and perform poorly on the examination. Level of evidence: III.

21. Guskiewicz KM, Marshall SW, Bailes J, et al: Association between recurrent concussion and late-life cognitive impairment in retired professional football players. *Neurosurgery* 2005;57(4):719-726.

22. Kerr ZY, Marshall SW, Harding HP Jr, Guskiewicz KM: Nine-year risk of depression diagnosis increases with increasing self-reported concussions in retired professional football players. *Am J Sports Med* 2012; 40(10):2206-2212.

23. Torg JS, Vegso JJ, O'Neill MJ, Sennett B: The epidemiologic, pathologic, biomechanical, and cinematographic analysis of football-induced cervical spine trauma. *Am J Sports Med* 1990;18(1):50-57.

24. Levitz CL, Reilly PJ, Torg JS: The pathomechanics of chronic, recurrent cervical nerve root neurapraxia: The chronic burner syndrome. *Am J Sports Med* 1997;25(1): 73-76.

25. Torg JS, Ramsey-Emrhein JA: Cervical spine and brachial plexus injuries: Return-to-play recommendations. *Phys Sportsmed* 1997;25(7):61-88.

26. Maron BJ, Doerer JJ, Haas TS, Tierney DM, Mueller FO: Sudden deaths in young competitive athletes: Analysis of 1866 deaths in the United States, 1980-2006. *Circulation* 2009;119(8):1085-1092.

27. Corrado D, Schmied C, Basso C, et al: Risk of sports: Do we need a pre-participation screening for competitive and leisure athletes? *Eur Heart J* 2011;32(8): 934-944.

    This report summarizes the advantages and disadvantages of preparticipation physicals for athletes of all types. Level of evidence: V.

28. Corrado D, Pelliccia A, Heidbuchel H, et al: Recommendations for interpretation of 12-lead electrocardiogram in the athlete. *Eur Heart J* 2010;31(2):243-259.

    This review focuses on the differences between normal and abnormal electrocardiograms and the resulting clinical workup required for differential diagnosis and clinical assessment. Level of evidence: V.

29. Pelliccia A, Maron BJ, Spataro A, Proschan MA, Spirito P: The upper limit of physiologic cardiac hypertrophy in highly trained elite athletes. *N Engl J Med* 1991; 324(5):295-301.

30. Maron BJ, Thompson PD, Ackerman MJ, et al: Recommendations and considerations related to preparticipation screening for cardiovascular abnormalities in competitive athletes: 2007 update. A scientific statement from the American Heart Association Council on Nutrition, Physical Activity, and Metabolism: Endorsed by the American College of Cardiology Foundation. *Circulation* 2007;115(12):1643-455.

31. Ho CY: Genetic considerations in hypertrophic cardiomyopathy. *Prog Cardiovasc Dis* 2012;54(6):456-460.

    The authors reviewed the genetic contributions to hypertrophic cardiomyopathy. The predominant gene mutations are found in the sarcomere proteins. Level of evidence: V.

32. Brothers J, Gaynor JW, Paridon S, Lorber R, Jacobs M: Anomalous aortic origin of a coronary artery with an interarterial course: Understanding current management strategies in children and young adults. *Pediatr Cardiol* 2009;30(7):911-921.

33. Elamm C, Fairweather D, Cooper LT: Pathogenesis and diagnosis of myocarditis. *Heart* 2012;98(11):835-840.

    This report reviews the underlying causes of myocarditis and the appropriate techniques to diagnose it. Level of evidence: V.

34. Parker MW, Thompson PD: Assessment and management of atherosclerosis in the athletic patient. *Prog Cardiovasc Dis* 2012;54(5):416-422.

    This report summarizes the best techniques for diagnosis and management of cardiac and peripheral arterial disease in athletes. Level of evidence: V.

35. Casey JA, Cosgrove SE, Stewart WF, Pollak J, Schwartz BS: A population-based study of the epidemiology and clinical features of methicillin-resistant *Staphylococcus aureus* infection in Pennsylvania, 2001-2010. *Epidemiol Infect* 2013;141(6):1166-1179.

    This population-based study uses electronic health record data in Pennsylvania to report that the annual incidence of community-associated MRSA increased by 34%, HA-MRSA by 7%, and skin and soft-tissue infection by 4%.

36. Rackham DM, Ray SM, Franks AS, Bielak KM, Pinn TM: Community-associated methicillin-resistant *Staphylococcus aureus* nasal carriage in a college student athlete population. *Clin J Sport Med* 2010;20(3):185-188.

    This cross-sectional study of college student athletes in East Tennessee showed that the prevalence of nasal carriage of community-acquired MRSA is estimated at 1.8%, which is similar to the general population.

37. Bowers AL, Huffman GR, Sennett BJ: Methicillin-resistant *Staphylococcus aureus* infections in collegiate football players. *Med Sci Sports Exerc* 2008;40(8): 1362-1367.

38. Forcade NA, Wiederhold NP, Ryan L, Talbert RL, Frei CR: Antibacterials as adjuncts to incision and drainage for adults with purulent methicillin-resistant *Staphylococcus aureus* (MRSA) skin infections. *Drugs* 2012; 72(3):339-351.

    This systematic review presents limited evidence that anti–MRSA antibacterial drugs provided a benefit over incision and drainage alone.

39. Pecci M, Comeau D, Chawla V: Skin conditions in the athlete. *Am J Sports Med* 2009;37(2):406-418.

40. Centers for Disease Control and Prevention (CDC): Methicillin-resistant *Staphylococcus aureus* infections among competitive sports participants—Colorado, Indiana, Pennsylvania, and Los Angeles County, 2000-2003. *MMWR Morb Mortal Wkly Rep* 2003;52(33): 793-795.

41. Ebell MH: Epstein-Barr virus infectious mononucleosis. *Am Fam Physician* 2004;70(7):1279-1287.

42. Putukian M, O'Connor FG, Stricker P, et al: Mononucleosis and athletic participation: An evidence-based subject review. *Clin J Sport Med* 2008;18(4):309-315.

43. Vidrih JA, Walensky RP, Sax PE, Freedberg KA: Positive Epstein-Barr virus heterophile antibody tests in patients with primary human immunodeficiency virus infection. *Am J Med* 2001;111(3):192-194.

44. Jaworski CA, Donohue B, Kluetz J: Infectious disease. *Clin Sports Med* 2011;30(3):575-590.

    This article reviews advances in the prevention, diagnosis, and/or management of infectious illnesses seen in athletes.

45. Hew-Butler T, Ayus JC, Kipps C, et al: Statement of the Second International Exercise-Associated Hyponatremia Consensus Development Conference, New Zealand, 2007. *Clin J Sport Med* 2008;18(2):111-121.

46. Almond CS, Shin AY, Fortescue EB, et al: Hyponatremia among runners in the Boston marathon. *N Engl J Med* 2005;352(15):1550-1556.

47. Kipps C, Sharma S, Pedoe DT: The incidence of exercise-associated hyponatraemia in the London marathon. *Br J Sports Med* 2011;45(1):14-19.

    The sodium serum results from runners in the 2006 London Marathon showed that 12.5% of healthy volunteers developed asymptomatic hyponatremia despite cool conditions, with 4 of 11 hyponatremic runners consuming more fluid and gaining more weight.

48. Eichner ER: Exertional rhabdomyolysis. *Curr Sports Med Rep* 2008;7(1):3-4.

49. Clarkson PM, Eichner ER: Exertional rhabdomyolysis: Does elevated blood creatine kinase foretell renal failure? *Curr Sports Med Rep* 2006;5(2):57-60.

50. Bonham VL, Dover GJ, Brody LC: Screening student athletes for sickle cell trait—a social and clinical experiment. *N Engl J Med* 2010;363(11):997-999.

    This reviews the National Collegiate Athletic Association's approval for mandatory testing of all Division I athletes for the sickle-cell trait.

51. Harris KM, Haas TS, Eichner ER, Maron BJ: Sickle cell trait associated with sudden death in competitive athletes. *Am J Cardiol* 2012;110(8):1185-1188.

    This review shows that 23 of 2,462 athlete deaths occurred in association with the sickle-cell trait over 31 years, with a prediliction among African American athletes.

52. Harmon KG, Drezner JA, Klossner D, Asif IM: Sickle cell trait associated with a RR of death of 37 times in National Collegiate Athletic Association football athletes: A database with 2 million athlete-years as the denominator. *Br J Sports Med* 2012;46(5):325-330.

    This review reported that the risk of death by exertion in Division I football players with the sickle-cell trait was 1 in 827. This rate was 37 times higher than in athletes without the sickle-cell trait.

53. Armstrong LE, Casa DJ, Millard-Stafford M, et al: American College of Sports Medicine position stand: Exertional heat illness during training and competition. *Med Sci Sports Exerc* 2007;39(3):556-572.

54. Bergeron MF, McKeag DB, Casa DJ, et al: Youth football: Heat stress and injury risk. *Med Sci Sports Exerc* 2005;37(8):1421-1430.

55. DeFranco MJ, Baker CL III, DaSilva JJ, Piasecki DP, Bach BR Jr: Environmental issues for team physicians. *Am J Sports Med* 2008;36(11):2226-2237.

56. Swenson ER, Maggiorini M: Salmeterol for the prevention of high-altitude pulmonary edema. *N Engl J Med* 2002;347(16):1282-1285.

57. Schoene RB: Illnesses at high altitude. *Chest* 2008;134(2):402-416.

Chapter 11

Coagulation, Blood Management, and Thromboembolism in Orthopaedic Surgery

Tessa Balach, MD   Jay R. Lieberman, MD

Introduction

Orthopaedic surgery patients comprise a heterogeneous population representing every age group and possess a variety of medical comorbidities. An understanding of bleeding and coagulation, the management of intraoperative blood loss, and the administration of blood products is necessary to enhance the care of these patients. In addition, the ability to evaluate and recognize coagulopathies preoperatively, assess patients' risk for venous thromboembolism (VTE), provide them with appropriate prophylaxis, and diagnose and treat VTE is essential.

Coagulation and Coagulopathies

The physiologic coagulation cascade is initiated when vascular endothelial injury occurs, resulting in bleeding. The initial response to endothelial injury is the formation of a platelet plug through platelet adhesion and aggregation. The simultaneous initiation of the coagulation cascade of procoagulant factors aids in hemostasis by stabilizing the platelet plug with a fibrin clot.[1] The balanced interaction between procoagulant and anticoagulant factors ensures that the hemostatic effects of the cascade are mediated and are neither insufficient nor excessive.

Dysfunction of physiologic coagulation results in disorders of clot formation and stabilization, predispos-

ing the surgical patient to excessive bleeding. Etiologies for coagulopathies include inherited qualitative platelet dysfunction (for example, von Willebrand disease), the hemophilias, and acquired coagulopathies. Acquired bleeding diatheses can result from medication use (such as aspirin or warfarin), vitamin K deficiency, or organ dysfunction (such as advanced liver disease). Thrombocytopenia, a quantitative deficiency of platelets, places a patient at increased risk of spontaneous bleeding when platelet counts are less than 10,000/μL and an increased risk of surgical bleeding when platelet counts are less than 50,000/μL to 100,000/μL.[2,3]

Evaluation of Coagulopathies

The first step in screening any surgical patient for a coagulopathy is to obtain a thorough history, which should include specific information about bleeding symptoms, systemic illnesses, medications, a personal history of bleeding, and a family history of bleeding disorders.[2-4] If a patient's history suggests a coagulopathy or abnormal bleeding, further evaluation is recommended. Initial laboratory tests include a complete blood count with smear, prothrombin time (PT), partial thromboplastin time (PTT), and international normalized ratio (INR).[3] If significant abnormalities are discovered, the patient should be referred to a hematologist for further workup of a bleeding diathesis.

Perioperative Management of Coagulopathies

After diagnosis of a coagulopathy, its management during the perioperative period is essential to appropriately control blood loss. Coagulopathies resulting from a deficiency of coagulation factors, such as the hemophilias, should be treated with the replacement of missing factors. Recombinant factor VIIa is indicated for use in patients with hemophilia (factor VII or IX inhibitors) or in those with a congenital deficiency of factor VII.[4] Medication-induced coagulopathies should be allowed to reverse, if possible (for example, preoperative discontinuation of platelet inhibitors before elective surgery). In the setting of urgent or emergent surgery,

Dr. Lieberman or an immediate family member serves as a paid consultant to or is an employee of DePuy; has received research or institutional support from Amgen and Arthrex; and serves as a board member, owner, officer, or committee member of the American Academy of Orthopaedic Surgeons and the American Association of Hip and Knee Surgeons. Neither Dr. Balach nor any immediate family member has received anything of value from or has stock or stock options held in a commercial company or institution related directly or indirectly to the subject of this chapter.

some of these coagulopathies can be treated with the administration of fresh frozen plasma. Patients who receive multiple transfusions because of massive blood loss during a surgical procedure should be evaluated intraoperatively for the development of a dilutional coagulopathy. In addition, hemostatic agents, including topical fibrin sealants, thrombin, and cellulose gels, and antifibrinolytic agents, are available to help control intraoperative bleeding.

Blood Management

Management of Perioperative Blood Loss

A preoperative estimation of surgical blood loss guides the formation of a strategy for perioperative blood management. The goals during surgery should be to emphasize hemostasis and minimize bleeding whenever possible. Intraoperative techniques and strategies such as electrocautery and hypotensive anesthesia can be used to achieve these goals. Intraoperative blood salvage systems, which return autologous blood to the patient, can be used when significant bleeding is anticipated.[5,6] These systems are contraindicated in the setting of infection or cancer.[7]

Fibrin sealants work to activate the final stages of the coagulation cascade by helping to form a more stable clot but need to be applied to a tissue bed that is dry and without active bleeding.[4] Despite this potentially challenging technical aspect, fibrin sealants can reduce blood loss and decrease the need for blood transfusions.[8] Thrombin is another topical agent that can be applied intraoperatively to wound beds. Collagen-based sponges or cellulose sheets applied topically can aid in decreasing intraoperative bleeding and are frequently combined with thrombin to further potentiate the hemostatic effects of both agents. Additional data are needed to determine if these products are a cost-effective means of decreasing blood loss.

Another strategy for managing perioperative blood loss is to ensure a patient's hemoglobin concentrations are optimized preoperatively to better tolerate acute blood loss associated with surgery. The preoperative administration of erythropoietin in the setting of total joint arthroplasty has been demonstrated to reduce the need for postoperative blood transfusion.[9,10] When combined with preoperative autologous blood donation, erythropoietin has been shown to be effective at reducing the exposure to allogeneic blood products[11] and is also useful in patients who will not accept autologous or allogeneic blood transfusions, such as Jehovah's Witnesses. In the setting of elective, noncardiac, nonvascular surgery with a high risk of bleeding, erythropoietin is indicated for patients with a hemoglobin level > 10 g/dL and ≤ 13 g/dL.[12] Recent data have demonstrated that erythropoietin and/or autologous blood donation may be cost-effective in patients who are at risk for postoperative transfusion.[13]

Tranexamic acid and aminocaproic acid are antifibrinolytic medications that aid in hemostasis by stabilizing a clot and preventing its degradation.[14] The cardiac surgery, arthroplasty, and spine literature have repeatedly shown tranexamic acid and aminocaproic acid to significantly reduce intraoperative blood loss and the subsequent need for blood transfusion.[7,14,15] The potential prothrombotic effects of these medications have not been shown to be significant. With only case reports of more serious complications, such as stroke or renal failure, the adverse effect profiles of both tranexamic acid and aminocaproic acid are significantly better than for aprotinin, an antifibrinolytic agent that is no longer available for clinical use.[14,15] Further study is needed to determine optimal dosing and administration regimens for these medications.

Transfusion of Blood Products
Red Blood Cells

The transfusion of red blood cells can be used to manage perioperative anemia. Numerous studies have sought to determine the absolute levels at which red blood cells should be transfused. A randomized, multicenter study of critical care patients found that 30-day mortality rates were similar between euvolemic patients who underwent transfusion at hemoglobin levels less than 7 g/dL compared with those who underwent transfusion at levels less than 9 g/dL; a more restrictive transfusion strategy was advocated in patients without acute myocardial infarction or unstable angina.[16] Another randomized controlled trial examined the transfusion requirements in patients after cardiac surgery and found that patients on a more restrictive transfusion strategy (to maintain a hematocrit ≥ 24%) had no significant difference in 30-day morbidity and mortality rates compared with those maintained on a more liberal transfusion strategy (to maintain a hematocrit ≥ 30%).[17] A recent Cochrane Database Review of 19 trials involving more than 6,000 patients examined transfusion thresholds and their effect on clinical outcomes. This review found that restrictive transfusion strategies did not affect the likelihood of adverse events compared with more liberal transfusion strategies and supported a transfusion threshold of 7 g/dL to 8 g/dL in most patients.[18]

The prophylactic transfusion of red blood cells in patients without risk factors for ischemia with hemoglobin levels greater than 8 g/dL is not recommended; those with risk factors for ischemia should be considered for prophylactic transfusion when hemoglobin levels are less than 10 g/dL. Risk factors for ischemia include myocardial ischemia or infarction, heart failure, chronic pulmonary disease, and chronic renal disease.[16,19-21] Euvolemic patients with symptomatic anemia, manifested by signs such as tachycardia, hypotension, or orthostatic hypotension not responsive to fluid boluses, should be considered for the transfusion of red blood cells.[20]

Platelets

Platelet dysfunction or thrombocytopenia can be managed with platelet transfusion. Patients with thrombocytopenia who are scheduled for surgery should be considered for prophylactic transfusion for platelet counts less than 50,000/μL to prevent excessive bleeding.[19,20] In addition, patients who are at increased risk of bleeding because of platelet dysfunction can be recommended for transfusion.[20]

Plasma

Plasma products such as fresh frozen plasma should be transfused in cases of massive hemorrhage and when signs of clinical coagulopathy are seen. In addition, fresh frozen plasma can be transfused to quickly reverse warfarin-induced or other acquired coagulopathies.[19,22]

Venous Thromboembolic Disease

Pathophysiology

VTE can be a serious source of morbidity and mortality. Virchow's triad of venous stasis, vascular injury, and hypercoagulability has framed the approach to the evaluation and management of patients with thromboembolic disease. In orthopaedic surgery, venous stasis and vascular injury are the most common causes of VTE.

Under normal physiologic conditions, and in the absence of a thrombophilic disorder, circulating coagulation factors are neutralized and balanced by endothelial cell surface inhibitors and circulating antiproteinases.[23] In the setting of VTE or in hypercoagulable states, the balance between thrombus formation and clot degradation is disrupted, resulting in pathologic clot formation. The most common location for pathologic thrombus formation is within the veins of the lower extremity.[23] Deep lower extremity venous thrombi that become symptomatic or embolize to the pulmonary vasculature are of most concern to the practicing orthopaedic surgeon.

Thrombophilias

Patients at increased risk for VTE events should be identified preoperatively whenever possible. The etiology of most thrombophilias falls into one of two major categories: inherited and acquired. Among the inherited causes for hypercoagulability are deficiencies of protein C, protein S, or antithrombin III; a factor V Leiden mutation; and a prothrombin gene mutation. Acquired thrombophilia can be the result of pregnancy or oral contraceptive use, nephrotic syndrome, the lupus anticoagulant, malignancy, atrial fibrillation, surgery, trauma and immobilization, or obesity.[3,21,23-25] Similar to the evaluation of patients with bleeding diatheses, a thorough history regarding prior VTE is critical. After referral to a hematologist for a more detailed evaluation of a hypercoagulable disorder, patients with a history of VTE are initially evaluated with routine blood work, including a complete blood count and chemistry evaluation that includes kidney and liver function tests. When patient history suggests a hereditary thrombo-

philia, more specific tests are ordered to evaluate for a factor V Leiden mutation, a prothrombin mutation, and the lupus anticoagulant. In addition, homocysteine, antithrombin III, protein C, and protein S levels are assessed.[21,23-26]

VTE in Orthopaedic Surgery

Orthopaedic procedures are known to be significant risk factors for the development of VTE. Rates of VTE vary considerably depending on the surgical procedure performed, the clinical scenario, and patient characteristics. The surgeon should be able to understand and estimate the risk of VTE associated with these situations and evaluate the patient for appropriate VTE prophylaxis while weighing the associated benefits and bleeding risks.

The use of VTE prophylaxis in the setting of elective total joint arthroplasty has been shown to decrease the rate of deep vein thrombosis (DVT) to 3% to 12% and that of fatal pulmonary embolus (PE) to less than 0.1%.[27-29] There is little controversy that VTE prophylaxis, in some form, should be administered to patients undergoing elective hip or knee arthroplasty. However, significant debate continues about risk stratification for patients at risk for developing VTE, the most effective mode of prophylaxis (chemical versus mechanical), the best chemoprophylactic agent (such as low molecular weight heparin, vitamin K antagonists, factor X inhibitors, thrombin inhibitors, and antiplatelet agents), as well as the duration of such treatment (10 to 14 days versus 28 days or longer).

The American College of Chest Physicians (ACCP) has published clinical practice guidelines regarding the prevention of VTE that recommended a prophylactic regimen to prevent all thromboembolic events, including asymptomatic DVT as well as fatal PE.[30] These guidelines focused more on efficacy than the bleeding risks associated with some of the chemoprophylactic regimens. In response, the American Academy of Orthopaedic Surgeons (AAOS) developed clinical practice guidelines that balanced both efficacy and safety concerns.[31]

The new evidence-based AAOS guidelines were published in September 2011 and included 10 recommendations (Table 1) related to the use of VTE prophylaxis after total joint arthroplasty. Because of a lack of evidence related to the efficacy of different prophylactic regimens in preventing symptomatic events, the guideline panel was unable to recommend a specific regimen or duration of prophylaxis. The panel did strongly recommend against screening using duplex ultrasound before discharge. New ACCP guidelines were published in February 2012 for a variety of orthopaedic procedures (Table 2), and in a shift from prior guidelines, recognized that the selection of a prophylactic regimen is a balance between efficacy and safety.[32] In this evidence-based guideline, the ACCP recommended a number of different chemoprophylactic agents and/or mechanical compression for a minimum of 14 days rather than no prophylaxis at all.[33] Both the AAOS and

1: Principles of Orthopaedics

Table 1

Summary of the American Academy of Orthopaedic Surgeon's 2011 Guideline on Preventing Venous Thromboembolic Disease in Patients Undergoing Elective Hip and Knee Arthroplasty

1. We recommend against routine postoperative duplex ultrasonography screening of patients who undergo elective hip or knee arthroplasty. **(Grade of Recommendation: Strong)**

2. Patients undergoing elective hip or knee arthroplasty are already at high risk for VTE. The practitioner might further assess the risk of VTE event by determining whether these patients had a previous VTE. **(Grade of Recommendation: Weak)** Current evidence is not clear about whether factors other than a history of previous venous thromboembolism increase the risk of VTE in patients undergoing elective hip or knee arthroplasty; therefore, we cannot recommend for or against routinely assessing these patients for these factors. **(Grade of Recommendation: Inconclusive)**

3. Patients undergoing elective hip or knee arthroplasty are at risk for bleeding and bleeding-associated complications. In the absence of reliable evidence, it is the opinion of this work group that patients be assessed for known bleeding disorders like hemophilia and for the presence of active liver disease, which further increase the risk for bleeding and bleeding-associated complications. **(Grade of Recommendation: Consensus)** Current evidence is not clear about whether factors other than the presence of a known bleeding disorder or active liver disease increase the chance of bleeding in these patients; therefore, we are unable to recommend for or against using them to assess a patient's risk of bleeding. **(Grade of Recommendation: Inconclusive)**

4. We suggest that patients discontinue antiplatelet agents (for example, aspirin, clopidogrel) before undergoing elective hip or knee arthroplasty. **(Grade of Recommendation: Moderate)**

5. We suggest the use of pharmacologic agents and/or mechanical compressive devices for the prevention of VTE in patients undergoing elective hip or knee arthroplasty and who are not at elevated risk beyond that of the surgery itself for VTE or bleeding. **(Grade of Recommendation: Moderate)** Current evidence is unclear about which prophylactic strategy (or strategies) is/are optimal or suboptimal. Therefore, we are unable to recommend for or against specific prophylactics in these patients. **(Grade of Recommendation: Inconclusive)** In the absence of reliable evidence about how long to employ these prophylactic strategies, it is the opinion of this work group that patients and physicians discuss the duration of prophylaxis. **(Grade of Recommendation: Consensus)**

6. In the absence of reliable evidence, it is the opinion of this work group that patients undergoing elective hip or knee arthroplasty, and who have also had a previous VTE, receive pharmacologic prophylaxis and mechanical compressive devices. **(Grade of Recommendation: Consensus)**

7. In the absence of reliable evidence, it is the opinion of this work group that patients undergoing elective hip or knee arthroplasty, and who also have a known bleeding disorder (for example, hemophilia) and/or active liver disease, use mechanical compressive devices for preventing VTE. **(Grade of Recommendation: Consensus)**

8. In the absence of reliable evidence, it is the opinion of this work group that patients undergo early mobilization following elective hip and knee arthroplasty. Early mobilization is of low cost, minimal risk to the patient, and consistent with current practice. **(Grade of Recommendation: Consensus)**

9. We suggest using neuraxial (such as intrathecal, epidural, and spinal) anesthesia for patients undergoing elective hip or knee arthroplasty to help limit blood loss, even though evidence suggests that neuraxial anesthesia does not affect the occurrence of venous thromboembolic disease. **(Grade of Recommendation: Moderate)**

10. Current evidence does not provide clear guidance about whether inferior vena cava (IVC) filters prevent pulmonary embolism in patients undergoing elective hip and knee arthroplasty who also have a contraindication to chemoprophylaxis and/or known residual venous thromboembolic disease. Therefore, we are unable to recommend for or against the use of such filters. **(Grade of Recommendation: Inconclusive)**

(Adapted from Mont MA, Jacobs JJ, Boggio LN, et al: Preventing venous thromboembolic disease in patients undergoing elective hip and knee arthroplasty. *J Am Acad Orthop Surg* 2011;19[12]:768-776.)

the ACCP guidelines were in agreement in recommending against VTE screening at the time of hospital discharge. The ACCP guidelines also made several suggestions, including using low-molecular-weight heparin as a chemoprophylactic agent because of its established track record with respect to efficacy, combining chemoprophylaxis with mechanical compression for prophylaxis, and continuing prophylaxis for 35 days.

This debate is not confined to the arthroplasty literature. Recent studies in the foot and ankle literature attempted to determine the rate of VTE associated with these procedures while making recommendations regarding the use of thromboprophylaxis. Several studies have found rates of DVT from less than 1% to 6% and that of PE to be less than 1% in a variety of foot and ankle surgeries ranging from trauma to arthroplasty.[34-37] All recommended against the routine use of thromboprophylaxis for these patients and emphasized the need for well-designed prospective investigations to provide more definitive guidelines for VTE prophylaxis in this subgroup of patients.[34-36]

Similarly, the incidence of VTE after arthroscopy has been examined, with rates of VTE in both knee and shoulder arthroscopy most recently reported to be less

Table 2

Summary of the American College of Chest Physicians 2012 Evidence-Based Clinical Practice Guidelines for Prevention of Venous Thromboembolism in Orthopaedic Surgery, ed 9

2.1.1   In patients undergoing total hip arthroplasty (THA) or total knee arthroplasty (TKA), we recommend use of one of the following for a minimum of 10 to 14 days rather than no antithrombotic prophylaxis: low-molecular-weight heparin (LMWH), fondaparinux, apixaban, dabigatran, rivaroxaban, low-dose unfractionated heparin (LDUH), adjusted-dose vitamin K antagonist (VKA), aspirin **(all grade 1B)**, or an intermittent pneumatic compression device (IPCD) **(Grade 1C)**.

2.1.2   In patients undergoing hip fracture surgery (HFS), we recommend use of one of the following rather than no antithrombotic prophylaxis for a minimum of 10 to 14 days: LMWH, fondaparinux, LDUH, adjusted-dose VKA, aspirin **(all grade 1B)**, or an IPCD **(Grade 1C)**.

2.2   For patients undergoing major orthopaedic surgery (THA, TKA, HFS) and receiving LMWH as thromboprophylaxis, we recommend starting either 12 h or more preoperatively or 12 h or more postoperatively rather than within 4 h or less preoperatively or 4 h or less postoperatively **(Grade 1B)**.

2.3.1   In patients undergoing THA or TKA, irrespective of the concomitant use of an IPCD or length of treatment, we suggest the use of LMWH in preference to the other agents we have recommended as alternatives: fondaparinux, apixaban, dabigatran, rivaroxaban, LDUH **(all grade 2B)**, adjusted-dose VKA, or aspirin **(all grade 2C)**.

2.4   For patients undergoing major orthopaedic surgery, we suggest extending thromboprophylaxis in the outpatient period for up to 35 days from the day of surgery rather than for only 10 to 14 days **(Grade 2B)**.

2.5   In patients undergoing major orthopaedic surgery, we suggest using dual prophylaxis with an antithrombotic agent and an IPCD during the hospital stay **(Grade 2C)**.

2.6   In patients undergoing major orthopaedic surgery and increased risk of bleeding, we suggest using an IPCD or no prophylaxis rather than pharmacologic treatment **(Grade 2C)**.

2.7   In patients undergoing major orthopaedic surgery and who decline or are uncooperative with injections or an IPCD, we recommend using apixaban or dabigatran (alternatively rivaroxaban or adjusted-dose VKA if apixaban or dabigatran are unavailable) rather than alternative forms of prophylaxis **(all grade 1B)**.

2.8   In patients undergoing major orthopaedic surgery, we suggest against using inferior vena cava (IVC) filter placement for primary prevention over no thromboprophylaxis in patients with an increased bleeding risk or contraindications to both pharmacologic and mechanical thromboprophylaxis **(Grade 2C)**.

2.9   For asymptomatic patients following major orthopaedic surgery, we recommend against Doppler (or duplex) ultrasound (DUS) screening before hospital discharge **(Grade 1B)**.

3.0   We suggest no prophylaxis rather than pharmacologic thromboprophylaxis in patients with isolated lower-leg injuries requiring leg immobilization **(Grade 2C)**.

4.0   For patients undergoing knee arthroscopy without a history of prior VTE, we suggest no thromboprophylaxis rather than prophylaxis **(Grade 2B)**.

(Reproduced with permission from Falck-Ytter Y, Francis CW, Johanson NA, et al: Prevention of VTE in orthopedic surgery patients: Antithrombotic Therapy and Prevention of Thrombosis, ed 9. American College of Chest Physicians Evidence-Based Clinical Practice Guidelines. *Chest* 2012;141[Suppl 2]:e278S-e325S.)

than 1%.[38-40] A Cochrane Database Review showed a VTE rate of less than 1% following knee arthroscopy and found no strong evidence to recommend the routine administration of thromboprophylaxis in these patients.[41]

Oncology patients represent a unique subgroup of orthopaedic patients who are considered to be at increased risk of VTE because of their cancer diagnosis. In addition, they experience increased morbidity and mortality associated with VTE.[42] In the setting of surgery for bone/soft-tissue sarcoma or metastatic bone disease, the risk of VTE must be balanced with the risk of hematoma and the resultant seeding of tumor cells. Rates of VTE in this population have been reported to range from 0% to 4% in patients managed with a variety of prophylactic regimens ranging from no prophylaxis to mechanical prophylaxis alone to chemoprophylaxis.[42-45] None of these studies provides strong recommendations for or against a specific thromboprophylactic regimen in the setting of surgery for bone and soft-tissue sarcomas or surgery for bony metastases.[42-45]

The safety and efficacy of VTE prophylaxis balanced with the risk of bleeding associated with prophylaxis is of significant concern for patients undergoing spine surgery. The risk of bleeding and the development of a postoperative epidural hematoma can result in significant and potentially irreversible neurologic injury. A recent meta-analysis of VTE after elective spine surgery found the rate of DVT to be low (1.09%) and the rate of PE to be even lower (0.06%). The rate of epidural hematoma was 0.4%, but 38% of those patients suffered a permanent neurologic deficit.[46] Data from more recent studies confirm the risk of epidural hematoma in the setting of chemoprophylaxis and suggest the need for well-designed, randomized trials to determine the role of chemoprophylaxis in spine surgery.[46-50]

1: Principles of Orthopaedics

Thromboembolic Prophylaxis

There are several options for providing patients with thromboembolic prophylaxis. A range of pharmacologic agents is available for VTE prophylaxis. Warfarin, a vitamin K antagonist, leads to decreased production of factors II, VII, IX, and X, in addition to proteins C and S. Challenges with the administration of warfarin revolve around dosing, its significant drug and dietary interactions, and the monitoring required to achieve and maintain an adequate level of anticoagulation.[49] Warfarin can be reversed with the administration of vitamin K and overcome with plasma transfusions. Low-molecular-weight heparins (for example, enoxaparin and dalteparin) and fondaparinux (an indirect factor Xa inhibitor) are administered subcutaneously once or twice daily and do not routinely require serum monitoring. Both fondaparinux and low-molecular-weight heparins have a low risk of heparin-induced thrombocytopenia.[4] New oral anticoagulants, which include factor Xa inhibitors (such as rivaroxaban) and direct thrombin inhibitors (such as dabigatran), are a class of agents that do not require monitoring and may have less risk of bleeding compared with low-molecular-weight heparins.[51,52] The safety of these drugs needs to be determined in orthopaedic clinical practice.[51] Aspirin, an antiplatelet agent, is an orally administered medication that reduces platelet adhesion and seems to reduce the rate of symptomatic VTE. Aspirin is a less powerful anticoagulant agent than the other chemoprophylactic drugs but seems to have a lower bleeding risk.

Intermittent pneumatic compression devices are a mechanical option to prevent VTE predominantly by working to decrease venous stasis. There is evidence to support that activation of the fibrinolytic system occurs with intermittent pneumatic compression devices, but it is unknown to what degree this action is clinically effective.[53] The benefits of this nonpharmacologic, noninvasive means of prophylaxis are that they are not associated with an increased risk of bleeding. Compliance with these devices is the most significant challenge associated with their use. Early mobilization and ambulation should also be considered important components of the prophylactic regimen. The availability of mobile compression devices now allows for this type of prophylaxis to be used during ambulation and after discharge from the hospital.

Inferior vena cava (IVC) filters are another nonpharmacologic but infrequently used option in the prophylaxis of PE. The indications for the use of these devices are extremely limited. Patients who cannot tolerate pharmacologic agents, who remain at high risk despite pharmacologic anticoagulation, and in whom pharmacologic anticoagulation has failed may be among the small group in whom IVC filters may be considered.[4,54] Historically, permanent IVC filters have been placed but have been associated with complications such as IVC thrombosis, erosion of the filter through the IVC walls, and the development of DVT. Retrievable filters have been developed to provide temporary prophylaxis, and early studies have shown them to be safe and effective.[54,55]

Management of Thromboembolic Events

Diagnosis

The clinical diagnosis of VTE is unreliable because the signs and symptoms of DVT or PE are often nonspecific. Possible signs and symptoms of DVT include acute calf pain, leg swelling, and a positive Homan sign. The presence of these findings during the acute postsurgical period should prompt more objective evaluation for DVT. PE can often be asymptomatic but, when of significant size, may manifest with symptoms of dyspnea, pleuritic chest pain, or syncope. Clinical signs may include transient or sustained hypoxemia, tachypnea, and persistent tachycardia.

Objective diagnostic tests should be performed for patients in whom there is sufficient clinical suspicion for VTE. Although invasive venography remains the gold standard for evaluating venous thrombosis, venous ultrasonography has been demonstrated to be sufficiently sensitive and specific for diagnosis and is the test of choice for evaluating DVT. Similarly, direct visualization of the pulmonary vasculature with angiography remains the gold standard for diagnosing PE; however, less invasive procedures with fewer associated risks have been developed and validated. Spiral CT of the chest has now become the imaging study of choice in evaluating these patients. Although this test has a high sensitivity and specificity for PE, a recent study suggests it may be too sensitive.[56] The spiral CT scan may reveal small emboli in the pulmonary vasculature that are not clinically relevant. The ventilation-perfusion (V/Q) scan compares the available ventilation capacity of the lungs with that portion of the lung being perfused using a radioactive tracer. A normal scan excludes PE, but an abnormal result is nonspecific. The V/Q scan is still indicated for patients who are unable to undergo spiral CT (for example, in those with contrast allergy or renal dysfunction).[22,57]

Treatment

The goals of treatment of VTE are to prevent PE-associated mortality and decrease the morbidity associated with DVT. Prolonged systemic chemical anticoagulation is the preferred method of treatment. The most immediate methods of achieving therapeutic anticoagulation are with intravenous unfractionated heparin, low-molecular-weight heparin, or fondaparinux. In the immediate postoperative period, rapid therapeutic anticoagulation can be associated with an increased risk of bleeding and should be avoided, if possible. Achieving more gradual therapeutic anticoagulation with the use of an unbolused heparin drip may avoid the increased risk of bleeding associated with the use of low-molecular-weight heparin, fondaparinux, or heparin boluses to achieve therapeutic anticoagulation.

Concomitant administration of an oral anticoagulant is initiated. Long-term anticoagulation is most frequently accomplished by using warfarin. New oral anticoagulants, including dabigatran and rivaroxaban may become substitutes for warfarin.[57]

The duration of treatment depends on the type and the extent of thromboembolic disease. A venous thrombosis in the deep veins proximal to the popliteal vein is treated with oral anticoagulation for 3 to 6 months, whereas the management of more distal thrombi is controversial. Perioperative PE in the absence of other risk factors for recurrent VTE is managed with 3 to 6 months of oral anticoagulation. PE in patients with hypercoagulable states or in those who have experienced recurrent PE should be managed with lifetime anticoagulation.[21,23,26] For patients who cannot tolerate anticoagulation or for those whose bleeding risk is too significant, the placement of an IVC filter may be indicated. Although the IVC filter will do little to treat existing PE, it may help to prevent future emboli.

Summary

Safe and effective treatment of orthopaedic patients demands an understanding of bleeding, coagulation, and blood management. Disorders of the normal coagulation cascade may predispose patients to increased bleeding or put them at risk for pathologic thrombosis. VTE and its sequelae can impose morbidity and mortality on patients. Future study will likely focus on further characterization of risk factors for the development of VTE associated with specific procedures, improved methods of VTE risk assessment, and the determination of the safest and most effective prophylactic regimens.

Key Study Points

- Risk factors for ischemia should be considered before the prophylactic transfusion of red blood cells in patients with asymptomatic anemia.

- AAOS guidelines for VTE prophylaxis recommend using VTE prophylaxis after total joint arthroplasty.

- The ideal perioperative VTE prophylactic regimen remains controversial.

Annotated References

1. Furie B, Furie BC: Molecular basis of blood coagulation, in Hoffman R, ed: *Hematology: Basic Principles and Practice*, ed 5. Philadelphia, PA, Churchill Livingstone/Elsevier, 2009, pp 1819-1836.

   A review of the molecular biology of coagulation factors and the coagulation cascade is presented.

2. Boller BS, Schneiderman PI: The bleeding history and differential diagnosis of purpura, in Hoffman R, ed: *Hematology: Basic Principles and Practice*, ed 5. Philadelphia, PA, Churchill Livingstone/Elsevier, 2009, pp 1851-1876.

3. Schafer AI: Approach to the patient with bleeding and thrombosis, in Cecil RL, Goldman LMD, Schafer AI, eds: *Goldman's Cecil Medicine*, ed 24. Philadelphia, PA, Elsevier/Saunders, 2012, pp 1121-1124.

   A review of the evidence-based evaluation and diagnosis of abnormalities in bleeding and coagulation is presented.

4. Reding MT, Key NS: Bleeding and thrombosis, in Hoffman R, ed: *Hematology: Basic Principles and Practice*, ed 5. Philadelphia, PA, Churchill Livingstone/Elsevier, 2009, pp 2369-2383.

5. Waters JH, Dyga RM, Waters JF, Yazer MH: The volume of returned red blood cells in a large blood salvage program: Where does it all go? *Transfusion* 2011; 51(10):2126-2132.

   This study analyzed the volume of red blood cells returned with blood salvage systems. Although that volume is high, the authors recommended selective utilization to improve efficiency and return significant volumes to a greater proportion of patients. Level of evidence: III.

6. Tse EY, Cheung WY, Ng KF, Luk KD: Reducing perioperative blood loss and allogeneic blood transfusion in patients undergoing major spine surgery. *J Bone Joint Surg Am* 2011;93(13):1268-1277.

   Multiple techniques exist in spine surgery to decrease intraoperative blood loss. Hypotension, tranexamic acid, and intrathecal morphine pumps seem to be among the best techniques.

7. Keating EM, Meding JB: Perioperative blood management practices in elective orthopaedic surgery. *J Am Acad Orthop Surg* 2002;10(6):393-400.

8. Thoms RJ, Marwin SE: The role of fibrin sealants in orthopaedic surgery. *J Am Acad Orthop Surg* 2009; 17(12):727-736.

9. Faris PM, Ritter MA, Abels RI; the American Erythropoietin Study Group: The effects of recombinant human erythropoietin on perioperative transfusion requirements in patients having a major orthopaedic operation. *J Bone Joint Surg Am* 1996;78(1):62-72.

10. Feagan BG, Wong CJ, Kirkley A, et al: Erythropoietin with iron supplementation to prevent allogeneic blood transfusion in total hip joint arthroplasty: A randomized, controlled trial. *Ann Intern Med* 2000;133(11): 845-854.

11. Bezwada HP, Nazarian DG, Henry DH, Booth RE Jr: Preoperative use of recombinant human erythropoietin before total joint arthroplasty. *J Bone Joint Surg Am* 2003;85(9):1795-1800.

12. Epogen [prescribing information]. Amgen Inc., Thousand Oaks, CA, May 2012. http://pi.amgen.com/united_states/epogen/epogen_pi_hcp_english.pdf. Accessed Sept 2, 2013.

13. Green WS, Toy P, Bozic KJ: Cost minimization analysis of preoperative erythropoietin vs autologous and alloge-

1: Principles of Orthopaedics

neic blood donation in total joint arthroplasty. *J Arthroplasty* 2010;25(1):93-96.

The authors examined the effectiveness and cost associated with perioperative blood management with erythropoietin, autologous blood donation, and allogeneic blood transfusion. Level of evidence: IV.

14. Eubanks JD: Antifibrinolytics in major orthopaedic surgery. *J Am Acad Orthop Surg* 2010;18(3):132-138.

The antifibrinolytic agents aminocaproic acid and tranexamic acid can be used in total joint arthroplasty and during pediatric and adult spine surgeries to decrease intraoperative blood loss.

15. Yang ZG, Chen WP, Wu LD: Effectiveness and safety of tranexamic acid in reducing blood loss in total knee arthroplasty: A meta-analysis. *J Bone Joint Surg Am* 2012;94(13):1153-1159.

This meta-analysis of randomized controlled trials showed tranexamic acid to be safe and effective for reducing intraoperative blood loss and the need for blood transfusions in total joint arthroplasty. Level of evidence: I.

16. Hébert PC, Wells G, Blajchman MA, et al: A multicenter, randomized, controlled clinical trial of transfusion requirements in critical care: Transfusion requirements in critical care investigators, Canadian Critical Care Trials Group. *N Engl J Med* 1999;340(6):409-417.

17. Hajjar LA, Vincent JL, Galas FR, et al: Transfusion requirements after cardiac surgery: The TRACS randomized controlled trial. *JAMA* 2010;304(14):1559-1567.

This randomized controlled trial examining transfusion strategies in cardiac surgery patients found a more restrictive strategy was not inferior to a more liberal one in regard to 30-day morbidity and mortality. Level of evidence: I.

18. Carson JL, Carless PA, Hebert PC: Transfusion thresholds and other strategies for guiding allogeneic red blood cell transfusion. *Cochrane Database Syst Rev* 2012;4:CD002042.

This Cochrane Database Review examining transfusion strategies supported the application of restricitve transfusion protocols in most patients, including those with a history of cardiovascular disease.

19. Goodnough LT: Transfusion medicine, in Cecil RL, Goldman LMD, Schafer AI, eds: *Goldman's Cecil Medicine*, ed 24. Philadelphia, PA, Elsevier/Saunders, 2012, pp 1148-1154.

A clinical update on trends and indications regarding the transfusion of blood and blood products is presented.

20. Milward PA, Brecher ME: *Conn's Current Therapy*. Philadelphia, PA, WB Saunders, 2012, pp 866-869.

The authors review the clinical application and administration of blood and blood products.

21. Whitlatch NL, Ortel TL: Thrombophilias: When should we test and how does it help? *Semin Respir Crit Care*

Med 2008;29(1):25-39.

22. Thakur NA, Czerwein JK, Butera JN, Palumbo MA: Perioperative management of chronic anticoagulation in orthopaedic surgery. *J Am Acad Orthop Surg* 2010; 18(12):729-738.

The authors discuss recommendations for the management of chronic anticoagulation in the perioperative period.

23. Lim W, Crowther MA, Ginsberg JS: Venous thromboembolism, in Hoffman R, ed: *Hematology: Basic Principles and Practice*, ed 5. Philadelphia, PA, Churchill Livingstone/Elsevier, 2009, pp 2043-2054.

24. Bauer KA: *Hematology: Basic Principles and Practice*, ed 5. Philadelphia, PA, Churchill Livingstone/Elsevier, 2009, pp 2021-2041.

25. Schafer AI: Hypercoagulable states, in Cecil RL, Goldman LMD, Schafer AI, eds: *Goldman's Cecil Medicine*, ed 24. Philadelphia, PA, Elsevier/Saunders, 2012, pp 1148-1154.

The authors provide an evidence-based approach to the diagnosis and the management of hypercoagulable states.

26. Chong LY, Fenu E, Stansby G, Hodgkinson S; Guideline Development Group: Management of venous thromboembolic diseases and the role of thrombophilia testing: Summary of NICE guidance. *BMJ* 2012;344(344): e3979.

Guidelines and recommendations about the evaluation and the treatment of thrombophilias and VTE are presented.

27. Keeney JA, Clohisy JC, Curry MC, Maloney WJ: Efficacy of combined modality prophylaxis including shortduration warfarin to prevent venous thromboembolism after total hip arthroplasty. *J Arthroplasty* 2006;21(4): 469-475.

28. Pellegrini VD Jr, Donaldson CT, Farber DC, Lehman EB, Evarts CM: The John Charnley Award: Prevention of readmission for venous thromboembolic disease after total hip arthroplasty. *Clin Orthop Relat Res* 2005;441: 56-62.

29. Won MH, Lee GW, Lee TJ, Moon KH: Prevalence and risk factors of thromboembolism after joint arthroplasty without chemical thromboprophylaxis in an Asian population. *J Arthroplasty* 2011;26(7):1106-1111.

The authors find that patients at high risk for VTE should be provided with thromboprophylaxis after total joint arthroplasty. Level of evidence: III.

30. Geerts WH, Bergqvist D, Pineo GF, et al: Prevention of venous thromboembolism: American College of Chest Physicians Evidence-Based Clinical Practice Guidelines (8th Edition). *Chest* 2008;133(6, suppl):381S-453S.

31. Johanson NA, Lachiewicz PF, Lieberman JR, et al: Prevention of symptomatic pulmonary embolism in pa-

tients undergoing total hip or knee arthroplasty. *J Am Acad Orthop Surg* 2009;17(3):183-196.

32. Falck-Ytter Y, Francis CW, Johanson NA, et al: Prevention of VTE in orthopedic surgery patients: Antithrombotic Therapy and Prevention of Thrombosis, 9th ed: American College of Chest Physicians Evidence-Based Clinical Practice Guidelines. *Chest* 2012;141(2, suppl): e278S-e325S.

    Recommendations of the ACCP for thromboembolic prophylaxis in orthopaedic surgery patients are presented.

33. Mont MA, Jacobs JJ, Boggio LN, et al: Preventing venous thromboembolic disease in patients undergoing elective hip and knee arthroplasty. *J Am Acad Orthop Surg* 2011;19(12):768-776.

    A summary of the AAOS guidelines on preventing VTE is presented.

34. Saragas NP, Ferrao PN: The incidence of venous thromboembolism in patients undergoing surgery for acute Achilles tendon ruptures. *Foot Ankle Surg* 2011;17(4): 263-265.

    This study examines the rate of venous thromboembolic disease after surgical treatment of Achilles tendon ruptures. The authors conclude that the rate of VTE is too low to recommend routine thromboprophylaxis in these patients. Level of evidence: III.

35. Pelet S, Roger ME, Belzile EL, Bouchard M: The incidence of thromboembolic events in surgically treated ankle fracture. *J Bone Joint Surg Am* 2012;94(6): 502-506.

    This study demonstrated that patients with surgically treated ankle fractures experience a rate of VTE that is low and not affected by the addition of thromboprophylaxis. The authors recommend consideration of thromboprophylaxis only in high-risk patients. Level of evidence: III.

36. Jameson SS, Augustine A, James P, et al: Venous thromboembolic events following foot and ankle surgery in the English National Health Service. *J Bone Joint Surg Br* 2011;93(4):490-497.

    The rate of thromboembolism is examined in patients undergoing a variety of foot and ankle surgeries. The authors concluded that the rate of VTE was too low to recommend the routine use of thromboprophylaxis for these patients. Level of evidence: III.

37. Barg A, Henninger HB, Hintermann B: Risk factors for symptomatic deep-vein thrombosis in patients after total ankle replacement who received routine chemical thromboprophylaxis. *J Bone Joint Surg Br* 2011;93(7): 921-927.

    The authors reviewed the rate of VTE after ankle arthroplasty and found it to be approximately 4% when low molecular weight heparin was used. Level of evidence: IV.

38. Jameson SS, James P, Howcroft DW, et al: Venous thromboembolic events are rare after shoulder surgery: Analysis of a national database. *J Shoulder Elbow Surg* 2011;20(5):764-770.

    The rate of thromboembolism is examined in patients undergoing shoulder surgery. The authors concluded that the rate of DVT and PE was too low to recommend the routine use of thromboprophylaxis for these patients. Level of evidence: II.

39. Randelli P, Castagna A, Cabitza F, Cabitza P, Arrigoni P, Denti M: Infectious and thromboembolic complications of arthroscopic shoulder surgery. *J Shoulder Elbow Surg* 2010;19(1):97-101.

    Infectious and thromboembolic complications after shoulder arthroscopy are examined. The rate of DVT was low and not further decreased with the use of thromboprophylaxis. Level of evidence: III.

40. Maletis GB, Inacio MC, Reynolds S, Funahashi TT: Incidence of symptomatic venous thromboembolism after elective knee arthroscopy. *J Bone Joint Surg Am* 2012; 94(8):714-720.

    This meta-analysis examined the rate of symptomatic VTE after knee arthroscopy. The authors found the rate to be very low and found no significant evidence to recommend the routine use of thromboprophylaxis in these patients. Level of evidence: II.

41. Ramos J, Perrotta C, Badariotti G, Berenstein G: Interventions for preventing venous thromboembolism in adults undergoing knee arthroscopy. *Cochrane Database Syst Rev* 2008;4:CD005259.

42. Ramo BA, Griffin AM, Gill CS, et al: Incidence of symptomatic venous thromboembolism in oncologic patients undergoing lower-extremity endoprosthetic arthroplasty. *J Bone Joint Surg Am* 2011;93(9):847-854.

    The rate of VTE is evaluated in orthopaedic oncology patients. The rate of thromboembolism in this patient population was low, and there was no difference in that rate among different modes of thromboprophylaxis. Level of evidence: III.

43. Mitchell SY, Lingard EA, Kesteven P, McCaskie AW, Gerrand CH: Venous thromboembolism in patients with primary bone or soft-tissue sarcomas. *J Bone Joint Surg Am* 2007;89(11):2433-2439.

44. Damron TA, Wardak Z, Glodny B, Grant W: Risk of venous thromboembolism in bone and soft-tissue sarcoma patients undergoing surgical intervention: A report from prior to the initiation of SCIP measures. *J Surg Oncol* 2011;103(7):643-647.

    This study set out to evaluate the risk of thromboembolism in patients with sarcomas. The authors identified a trend toward a decreased risk of VTE with the use of chemoprophylaxis. Level of evidence: III.

45. Ruggieri P, Montalti M, Pala E, et al: Clinically significant thromboembolic disease in orthopedic oncology: An analysis of 986 patients treated with low-molecular-weight heparin. *J Surg Oncol* 2010;102(5):375-379.

    This is a retrospective review of VTE in oncology patients treated wtih endoprosthetic reconstruction and low molecular weight heparin. The authors found the

1: Principles of Orthopaedics

rate of thromboemolism to be low with this prophylactic regimen. Level of evidence: III.

46. Sansone JM, del Rio AM, Anderson PA: The prevalence of and specific risk factors for venous thromboembolic disease following elective spine surgery. *J Bone Joint Surg Am* 2010;92(2):304-313.

    In this meta-analysis aimed at determining the rate of venous thromboembolic disease in elective spine surgery, the authors found a low rate of VTE. The use of chemoprophylaxis improved that rate, but with a higher risk of epidural hematoma. Level of evidence: II.

47. Ploumis A, Ponnappan RK, Sarbello J, et al: Thromboprophylaxis in traumatic and elective spinal surgery: Analysis of questionnaire response and current practice of spine trauma surgeons. *Spine (Phila Pa 1976)* 2010; 35(3):323-329.

    This study examined the preference of surgeons regarding prophyalxis and attempted to report a consensus protocol for thromboprophylaxis in the setting of spine trauma and elective spine surgery. Level of evidence: V.

48. Glotzbecker MP, Bono CM, Wood KB, Harris MB: Postoperative spinal epidural hematoma: A systematic review. *Spine (Phila Pa 1976)* 2010;35(10):E413-E420.

    This study defined the incidence of epidural hematoma after spine surgery to be small (< 1%) and attempted to determine the effect of thromboprophylaxis on the risk of its development. Level of evidence: IV.

49. Cheng JS, Arnold PM, Anderson PA, Fischer D, Dettori JR: Anticoagulation risk in spine surgery. *Spine (Phila Pa 1976)* 2010;35(9, suppl):S117-S124.

    This meta-analysis examined the risk of VTE in patients after spine surgery and found the rates to be low overall, with trauma patients having an increased risk. Level of evidence: III.

50. Smith JS, Fu KM, Polly DW Jr, et al: Complication rates of three common spine procedures and rates of thromboembolism following spine surgery based on 108,419 procedures: A report from the Scoliosis Research Society Morbidity and Mortality Committee. *Spine (Phila Pa 1976)* 2010;35(24):2140-2149.

    The authors present a retrospective review of data from a database and found the rates of VTE after a variety of spine surgeries to be 2% to 7%. Level of evidence: III.

51. Ageno W, Gallus AS, Wittkowsky A, et al: Oral anticoagulant therapy: Antithrombotic Therapy and Prevention of Thrombosis, 9th ed: American College of Chest Physicians Evidence-Based Clinical Practice Guidelines. *Chest* 2012;141(2, suppl):e44S-e88S.

    The authors provide an evidence-based review of the use and pharmacology of oral anticoagulants, including warfarin and the new factor Xa inhibitors.

52. Raskob GE, Gallus AS, Pineo GF, et al: Apixaban versus enoxaparin for thromboprophylaxis after hip or knee replacement: Pooled analysis of major venous thromboembolism and bleeding in 8464 patients from the ADVANCE-2 and ADVANCE-3 trials. *J Bone Joint Surg Br* 2012;94(2):257-264.

    This comparison of an oral factor Xa inhibitor, apixaban, to enoxaparin found that apixaban was more effective at preventing VTE than enoxaparin with a decreased risk of bleeding. Level of evidence: I.

53. Macaulay W, Westrich G, Sharrock N, et al: Effect of pneumatic compression on fibrinolysis after total hip arthroplasty. *Clin Orthop Relat Res* 2002;399:168-176.

54. Van Ha TG, Chien AS, Funaki BS, et al: Use of retrievable compared to permanent inferior vena cava filters: A single-institution experience. *Cardiovasc Intervent Radiol* 2008;31(2):308-315.

55. Strauss EJ, Egol KA, Alaia M, Hansen D, Bashar M, Steiger D: The use of retrievable inferior vena cava filters in orthopaedic patients. *J Bone Joint Surg Br* 2008; 90(5):662-667.

56. Parvizi J, Smith EB, Pulido L, et al: The rise in the incidence of pulmonary embolus after joint arthroplasty: Is modern imaging to blame? *Clin Orthop Relat Res* 2007;463:107-113.

57. Weitz JI: Pulmonardy embolism, in Cecil RL, Goldman LMD, Schafer AI, eds: *Goldman's Cecil Medicine*, ed 24. Philadelphia, PA, Elsevier/Saunders, 2012, pp 596-603.

    A review of the evaluation and treatment of PE is presented.

Chapter 12

Work-Related Illness, Cumulative Trauma, and Workers' Compensation

Peter J. Mandell, MD

1: Principles of Orthopaedics

Introduction

One hundred years ago, the United States had developed the world's largest economy and was still rapidly expanding its wealth. To continue that expansion, the nation needed a way to compensate employees injured at work. A no-fault workers' compensation insurance program, commonly referred to as a "grand bargain," filled that need. Workers did not have to prove employers were at fault to receive speedy and fully funded treatment, temporary cash wage replacement payments, and permanent disability awards. Employers were spared the uncertainty of civil court trials. Wisconsin was the first state to enact such a program in 1911, and Mississippi was the last in 1948.[1] In effect, these laws constituted "...the first and most enduring tort reform measure[s] in the US."[2]

The Burden of Work-Related Musculoskeletal Ailments

Approximately 116 million individuals had full-time jobs in the United States in July 2012; the unemployment rate was 8.2%.[3] Based on 2010 US Department of Labor data,[4] approximately 1,370,000 workers in the United States sustained nonfatal work injuries and illnesses severe enough to require 1 or more days away from work. The overall incidence of significant work injuries among full-time employees in the United States was 1.2%. Seven occupations were associated with a more than 3% incidence of work injuries: nursing aide, orderly, light/delivery truck driver, warehouse worker, construction laborer, big rig truck driver, and janitor. Of these seven occupations, warehouse workers had the highest number of lost workdays. The incidence of

At the time this chapter was written, Dr. Mandell or an immediate family member serves as a board member, owner, officer, or committee member of the Western Orthopaedic Association.

work injury for government workers (federal, state, county, city, public schools), including law enforcement and firefighters, was approximately two thirds higher than for private sector workers. Government landscapers with at least 1 day lost from work sustained 250% more reported injuries than comparable occupations in the private sector. Government janitorial workers sustained almost 300% more injuries, with at least 1 lost day from work, than their private sector counterparts.

For police officers, leading injury events were violent acts (such as apprehending combative suspects) and transportation incidents (such as motorcycle accidents while controlling traffic). For warehouse workers, contact with objects and equipment (for example, lacerations, punctures, being struck or crushed by an object) and overexertion were the most common accidents. Overexertion also was a leading event in injuries sustained by nursing aides, janitors, and truck drivers. In 2010, sprains, strains, and tears comprised 40% of the injuries that resulted in at least 1 day off work; more than one third of those were back injuries.[4] One eighth of sprain, strain, and tear cases involved the shoulder, and shoulder cases required more than twice as much time off work as the median of other sprain, strain, and tear cases.

Workers age 16 to 19 years, 25 to 34 years, and 45 to 54 years had work injury rates of 1.17%, 1.06%, and 1.3%, respectively.[4] The injury rate was 1.28% for men and 1.06% for women. Of workers injured in 2010, 41% were Caucasian, 11% were Hispanic, 8% were African American, and the rest were not reported.

Many studies have been published regarding the allocation of limited healthcare resources to several different diseases,[5] but few such studies focused on work-related events. The task is difficult because studies of industrial accident records indicate that 25% to 50% of nonfatal injuries and approximately 90% of deaths related to occupational disease go unreported.[6,7] The US Department of Labor data intentionally exclude farmers, farm workers, and self-employed individuals or adjustments for underreporting such groups. Correcting for those factors, it is estimated that there were approximately 8.5 million US industrial injuries in

2007, of which 2.5 million were serious enough to result in lost work days.[5] Approximately 5,600 fatalities were reported. It is estimated that the US cost of occupational injuries in 2007 was $250 billion (approximately 1.8% of the gross domestic product), including direct and indirect costs. In comparison, total costs were $432 billion for cardiovascular disease and $219 billion for cancer.[5] Total workers' compensation payouts for medical and wage replacement expenses in 2007 were $55.4 billion. The $195 billion difference between total costs and payouts to workers is one indication that workers' compensation systems do not cover the full costs of industrial accidents and illnesses.[5] State laws rarely, if ever, allow wage loss repayments to exceed 70% of preinjury base income.

Culture and Injury at Work

A 2002 analysis of a national population–based survey examined risk factors associated with work injuries.[8] Past studies had shown a greater incidence of work injuries among workers with characteristics such as low family income, rural residence, high levels of physical effort, and a history of working in awkward positions (such as frequent stooping). The study concluded that in well-run companies, which placed few constraints on their employees, workers experienced one third fewer work injuries than expected. If an employee deemed his or her work environment to be safe, injuries again decreased by one third. Conversely, work-family interference increased the risk of work injuries by more than one third. Also, the study concluded from the survey that injury risk differs as a function of race. Caucasians were injured 67% more frequently than African Americans. Those in a group titled "Other" (including Hispanics, Native Americans, and Asian Americans) were injured almost 60% more often than Caucasians. These results may have been skewed because the survey included only English-speaking adults.

A 2010 study reported on clinically based evidence of ethnic differences in recovery following distal radial fractures.[9] In general, both African Americans and Hispanics showed poorer ultimate function and greater pain scores than whites. After adjusting for sociodemographic factors and injury characteristics, the disparities for Hispanics persisted for both pain and function, whereas the outcome disparities for African Americans were no longer significant. Ethnic disparities occurred in both workers' compensation patients and those not injured at work. The authors suggested that education, body mass index, age, and sex may affect the different outcomes. The authors also found that workers' compensation patients had significantly more pain and less function than their nonwork injured counterparts. Twenty-six percent of African Americans, 14% of Hispanics, and 6% of whites reported that their fractures occurred at work—a significant difference ($P < 0.001$). Other studies have suggested that the explanation of ethnic differences in disease outcomes is multifaceted and includes factors such as poverty, lack of access to health care and information, psychologic stress, culture, lifestyle, and community environment.[9]

Treatment Outcomes in Workers' Compensation Cases

Numerous studies going back several years have reported that treatment outcomes in workers' compensation cases are worse than when that same disease or injury is treated in a nonwork injury setting. A recent study reported that lumbar fusions for diagnoses of disk degeneration, disk herniation, and/or radiculopathy in a workers' compensation setting are associated with a significant increase in disability, opiate use, prolonged work loss, and poor return-to-work status.[10] Another study indicated that workers' compensation patients achieved significantly less improvement after posterolateral lumbar fusion surgery than those not injured at work.[11] A detailed discussion about lumbar disk herniations can be found in chapter 52, Degenerative Disk Disease and Pain in the Lumbar Spine, *Orthopaedic Knowledge Update 11*.

A 2010 study determined how workers' compensation accidents affected the results of shoulder decompression or rotator cuff repair.[12] Patients in both treatment groups had significant improvement irrespective of their workers' compensation status. The results showed that although injured workers reported a significantly higher level of disability both before and after shoulder surgery, they still had statistically significant improvement 1 year after the operation.

Writing an Independent Medical Examination Report

Although the concept of a workers' compensation program ensures that injured workers do not have to prove their employers were at fault to receive workers' compensation benefits, they do need to prove that work was, at least, a partial cause of the injury. Causation requirements are easily met when a connection is made between a distinct event and bodily damage: for example, a trip and fall at work that causes an acute lumbar compression fracture. Causation is more difficult to prove when that same worker has osteoporosis and prior healed spinal compression fractures.

An orthopaedic surgeon needs to obtain a specialized history and perform a physical examination to determine whether a particular injury or illness is compensable, requires further medical treatment, and has left the employee with residual impairment. In obtaining a history, the physician must record in detail how the injury occurred. Timing can be everything in the determination of the cause for a workers' compensation case. The physician must determine if the patient reported the injury immediately or later. Researchers have noted for some time that more claims for industrial injuries are made on Mondays (25%) than on Fridays (16%), an observation known as the "Monday effect."[13] Some researchers think that a subset of workers who injure themselves on the weekend wait until they get to work on Monday to report a claim, thus receiving health coverage and wage replacement benefits. The Monday effect is more likely to occur with easily concealed injuries, such as back sprains and shoulder tendinitis, than with more obvious injuries, such as cuts and fractures. The Monday effect has long raised suspicions of worker fraud.

The patient's current complaints should be documented carefully. The physician needs to determine the source of any pain on the date of the injury and assess current pain symptoms. Close attention should be given to spreading symptoms. If the patient's records report the initial injury as a shoulder sprain but the patient now also reports neck, elbow, wrist, and hand symptoms during physical examination, the causes of pain in the later reported areas should be explored in detail. Understanding the mechanism of injury may help determine the cause of delayed symptoms in initially unreported areas. The patient's current physical limitations must be distinguished from limitations on the date of injury. How the injury has affected the worker's activities of daily living must be determined. The physician should consider the reliability of the original diagnosis. For the patient who seems to exhibit wandering pain, a list of all current complaints must be carefully compiled to avoid confusion. The worker's statements about his or her injuries should be compared with statements in the medical records.

The patient's history can provide important clues about diagnosis, causation, and prognosis—all of which the physician is expected to explore for the workers' compensation system. Did the patient sustain prior injuries to the same body part or region? Did the patient undergo prior relevant surgeries? Did he or she receive prior disability awards? Did the patient have sports-related or other non–work-related injuries that could have increased his or her vulnerability to the work injury? Does the patient have a family history of lumbar disk disease, knee instability, hand arthritis, or other issues? The patient should be assessed for other diseases and habits that can affect the musculoskeletal system, such as obesity, arthritis, diabetes, smoking, and significant alcohol consumption.

A detailed work history is also important information for the independent medical examination report. The physician needs to know the patient's work environment and activities to not only assess causation but also gauge the potential for modified work. The physician should determine the patient's length of current employment, previous work experience, job satisfaction or recent job-related changes (such as increased workload because of downsizing), and the existence of conflicts with supervisors or fellow employees or job-related stress.

For workers' compensation cases, the physical examination, including the history and physical reports, is legal evidence that is subject to great scrutiny and may have a profound effect on a patient's future. During the physical examination, the range of motion, atrophy, and motor and sensory function must be quantified, not just estimated. Tape measures, goniometers, and well-calibrated grip strength devices should be used so that objective results can be obtained. The injured and uninjured sides should be compared, when possible, to better gauge the patient's loss of particular normal function.

During the physical examination, the physician should consider a thorough differential diagnosis. Cervical disk disease can cause shoulder pain, lumbar disk disease can produce hip symptoms, and hip pathology can give rise to knee discomfort. The reliability of the patient's physical findings should be evaluated. Whether the objective findings support the patient's subjective complaints should be addressed. Nonorganic findings, such as a positive result from Waddell tests, should be noted.[14]

The patient's current and future medical treatment needs to be discussed. In many jurisdictions, final resolution of the claim includes ongoing medical interventions to cure—or at least relieve—the effects of the employee's work injury. Medical treatment recommendations should be evidence-based when possible.

Cumulative Trauma

Cumulative trauma and repetitive motion injuries are also referred to as musculoskeletal disorders or work-related musculoskeletal disorders. These terms connote an array of afflictions that seem to result from repetitive or strenuous movements: overexertion; assuming constrained, unusual, and/or prolonged postures; and other overuse events. In return for workers giving up their right to sue their employers for work-related injuries, employers agreed to accept responsibility for such conditions unless convincing evidence of other non–work-related causes exists. Some states have since limited musculoskeletal disorder claims after the grand bargain was established, but other states continue to accept them. Other causes for claimed cumulative trauma injuries may include concurrent work with a different employer, strenuous sports activities, and non–work-related accidents.

Whether repetitive stress consistently and predictably causes musculoskeletal disorders is a topic of ongoing debate in the literature. Carpal tunnel syndrome has been well studied, but the results still are not clear-cut. A scientific research paper for the German government was published in 2009 that supported categorizing carpal tunnel syndrome as an occupational disease.[15] The authors concluded that repetitive manual work tasks that involve flexion and extension at the wrist, forceful gripping, and using vibratory tools can damage the median nerve and cause carpal tunnel syndrome.[15] Also, a considerable discrepancy was noted in the results regarding computer work as a cause of carpal tunnel syndrome. Systematic and other reviews had not shown any increase in carpal tunnel risk to date.

Cumulative trauma conditions generally have similar characteristics: the neck, shoulder, carpal tunnel, back,

Table 1

Physical Examination Tests for Feigned Weakness

Test	Patient Response
The drop test	With the patient supine, the physician drops the weak or paralyzed arm over the patient's face and observes that the limb does not hit the patient.
The pain test	The physician surprises the patient with discomfort and observes that the weak or paralyzed limb moves normally.
The Hoover test	The physician places one hand under the heel of the patient's normal leg while pressing down on the weak leg and then asks the patient to lift the weak leg against resistance. If the physician feels no counterpressure under the normal heel, the patient is not trying.
The hysterical gait observation	The patient shows foot dragging rather than lifting or sudden knee buckling without falling.

knees, and feet are commonly involved. These characteristics are often nonspecific and poorly localized.[16] Usually, the onset of symptoms occurs gradually over months or years and can often require extended time for improvement. Cumulative trauma disorders may go unreported because workers do not associate their symptoms with job-related activities.[16] In many states, part of the grand bargain encompasses certain statutorily defined diagnoses that are presumed correct, including the "gun belt presumption" for police officers who have chronic low back pain and the industrially caused "cancer presumption" for firefighters who have been exposed to smoke and other toxic substances throughout their work lives.

Musculoskeletal disorders involve an average of 9 days off work compared with 7 days off for other work injuries.[17] However, the work injury rate, as measured by missed workdays between 1992 and 2007, decreased by slightly more than 50%. For musculoskeletal disorders, it decreased by 57%.[17] Some authors refer to cumulative trauma disorders as a modern-day epidemic, yet Ramazzini, the father of occupational medicine, observed in 1713 that scribes doing repetitive tasks reported "...intense fatigue in the whole arm but no remedy could relieve this and finally the whole right arm became paralyzed."[18]

More than 50% of sprain, strain, and tear injuries resulting in days away from work are classified as musculoskeletal disorders. Approximately 67% of all workers with musculoskeletal disorders are male; however, approximately 75% of carpal tunnel syndrome cases and 60% of tendinitis cases are reported by female workers. Although musculoskeletal disorders occur at higher rates in transportation, maintenance, construction, and manufacturing industries than in service occupations, 55% of carpal tunnel syndrome cases occur in the manufacturing and office work industries.

Malingering and Somatization

Malingering is at the extreme end of a spectrum of concepts that have been termed symptom magnification, exaggeration, submaximal, insincere or low effort, inappropriate pain or illness behavior, and nonorganic findings. When an orthopaedic surgeon uses such terms, the implication is that something about the patient's presentation is inconsistent.

Most studies over the past 35 years list the incidence of malingering as quite low. A survey of 48 orthopaedic surgeons and 57 neurosurgeons across the United States reported that 60% of the surgeons agreed that malingering occurred in 5% or fewer of their patients with low back pain.[19] However, 15% of the survey respondents estimated that more than 20% of their patients were feigning illness. Considerable literature exists on how to document patients who describe symptoms with little or no physical basis. An approach has been established using physical signs for low back conditions that has gained widespread acceptance.[14] The shortcomings of the physical tests were emphasized, and isolated false-positive signs may occur. For example, stocking hypesthesia may be a symptom of vascular disease, and widespread tenderness may be a symptom of osteoporosis. Isolated nonorganic signs should be ignored and significance associated with multiple positive signs.

The notion of inappropriate behavior during illness has been studied.[20] In addition to the classic signs such as stocking hypesthesia and collapsing weakness, the authors noted that bizarre pain drawings showing total body pain among other things could be used to document nonorganicity. The timing of a symptom is also important. Pain usually varies in patients with a physical disease, but patients with nonorganic symptoms have no pain-free intervals.

Pseudoneurologic findings have been discussed.[21] Patients with feigned weakness usually showed an abrupt and stepwise loss of strength. For patients with organic weakness, the loss of resistance is smooth. Physical tests for feigned weakness are presented in Table 1. With feigned sensory loss, numbness often follows the patient's own concept of his or her anatomy.[21] Almost all sensory modalities of pain, touch, and proprioception disappear at a discrete border, such as the midline or a joint. Some tests that may help document feigned sensory loss are listed in Table 2. The five-rung test (also called the five-handle position grip strength test) and rapid exchange grip strength tests are ways to document low effort.[22] The five-rung test involves a patient squeezing a hand dynamometer as hard as possible at each of the five grip settings, from smallest to largest. A normal response produces a bell-shaped strength curve.

Table 2

Physical Examination Tests for Feigned Sensory Loss

The physician applies painful stimuli to a numb area and observes the normal heart rate increase of 20 to 30 beats per minute.

The physician surprises the patient with discomfort to a numb limb and notes withdrawal.

The physician applies tuning fork vibration to the numb half of a cavity, such as the thorax or skull. Because of bone conduction, the patient should feel the vibration on the normal side.

The physician tests the great toe for proprioception and notes that the patient answers the up or down questions wrongly 100% of the time. By chance, a 50% correct answer rate is expected.

Sincere patients usually have a large variance in response among the five squeezes, peaking at the second or third rungs and dropping off significantly at the first and fifth. Low-effort patients produce a flat or flatter curve with less deviation among the five attempts.

Rapid exchange gripping also has been used to further enhance the recognition of low-effort patients.[22] The test used the rung on which the patient had the most strength during the five-rung study. A computer recorded grip strength measurements as the patient switched hands every 1.5 seconds for a total of eight times with each hand. Sincere patients had no significant differences between peak scores on the five-rung test and their results for the rapid exchange grip test. Low-effort patients had significantly greater grip strength with the rapid exchange test. Accurate identification of 91% of sincere patients and 82% of low-effort patients was reported; however, the use of any single measurement to label a patient as low effort is not advocated. Combining the results of the rapid exchange grip, the five-rung grip, and clinical impressions (that is, Waddell-like findings seen on examination) produced a more accurate characterization of low-effort patients than just a single test.

A study of the five-rung test[23] concluded that the shape of the curve was strength dependent; thus, the five-rung test may yield biased results during the assessment of sincere effort in patients with weakened hands. The five-rung test was less effective for women. However, the authors of a 2012 study offered the visual target grip test as an accurate evaluation of sincerity of effort.[24] The test tricks a patient into exerting maximal effort by providing incorrect visual feedback. The test displays a target line on a monitor and instructs the participant to reach for it with each grip repetition. The line's position is then secretly changed, which requires doubling the force necessary to reach it. Accordingly, participants are tricked into exerting more force than intended to reach the deceptive target line. Providing incorrect visual feedback caused significantly greater

increases in force during submaximal effort (69%) than during maximal effort (28%). This test effectively detected submaximal effort levels.

Other conditions can resemble malingering but are quite different and are termed somatoform pain disorders.[25] Some psychiatrists estimate that at least one half of patients seeking primary care have somatic pain as a manifestation of psychosocial distress. Most patients in the United States with somatization disorder are female. Typical somatization symptoms include headache, fibromyalgia, and back pain.

In somatization, the body is used for psychologic purposes.[26] People who cannot engage in or whose cultures do not allow open expression of psychic difficulties often communicate such issues through sometimes powerful physical symptoms.

Some patients consciously produce their disease but are motivated by unconscious reasons. These patients are similar to individuals who fear heights or crowded places but don't know why. Such patients have factitious disorders, perhaps the most famous of which is Munchausen syndrome. Those with a factitious disorder have a psychologic need to assume the role of the sick patient. As noted in a classic study: "Patients with factitious disorders can and have produced signs and symptoms of virtually any disease. The level of production can vary from a purely fictitious medical history (lying about symptoms), a simulation of signs or symptoms (such as heating a thermometer), to the actual production of disease states (administering bacterial cultures intravenously to produce septicemia). Almost all laboratory abnormalities can be produced factitiously. The only limits to factitious disorders are those of human creativity."[27] In more than three fourths of factitious disorder cases, the patient or a family member works in the healthcare field.[27] Those with a factitious disorder are often nurses, ward clerks, medical receptionists, and laboratory technicians.

Authors of a 2010 study noted that childhood events, specifically abuse and emotional trauma, have profound and enduring effects on the neuroregulatory systems that mediate illness, as well as on behavior in both childhood and adult life.[28] These authors documented relationships between traumatic stress in childhood and the leading causes of morbidity, mortality, and disability in the United States, such as cardiovascular disease, depression, obesity, smoking, alcohol and drug abuse, and chronic pain. These conclusions are based on findings from the Adverse Childhood Experiences (ACE) Study, an epidemiologic inquiry providing retrospective and prospective analyses of more than 17,000 obese patients in a medically supervised weight-loss program at Kaiser Permanente in San Diego, California. The study scrutinized the effect of traumatic experiences during the first 18 years of life on adolescent and adult medical and psychiatric disease, sexual behavior, healthcare costs, and life expectancy.[28]

In the study, 80% of the participants were Caucasian and Hispanic, 10% were African American, and 10% were Asian American; 74% had attended college; and their mean age was 57 years. Almost one half of

1: Principles of Orthopaedics

Table 3

Types of Adverse Childhood Experiences

Category	Percentage
Abuse	
Emotional—recurrent threats, humiliation	11
Physical—beating, not spanking	28
Contact sexual abuse	22
For women	28
For men	16
Household Dysfunction	
Mother treated violently	13
Household member was alcoholic or drug user	27
Household member was imprisoned	6
Household member was chronically depressed, suicidal, mentally ill, or in a psychiatric hospital	17
Not raised by both biologic parents	23
Neglect	
Physical	10
Emotional	15

the patients were men; all of the patients were middle class. The 10 categories of ACEs studied and the percentage of occurrence among the 17,000 patients are found in Table 3. The ACE score for each patient was established based on how many of the 10 different environments each individual experienced during the first 18 years of life. Approximately 33% of the patients had an ACE score of zero, but these categories were so profound that of the patients who had experienced one ACE, almost 90% had also experienced one or more additional ACE. Approximately 17% of the patients had an ACE score of 4 or higher; 11% had an ACE score of 5 or higher. Women were 50% more likely than men to have experienced five or more categories of ACE. The authors concluded that high ACE scores were the key to what, in mainstream epidemiology, appears as the natural propensity for women to have ill-defined health conditions, such as fibromyalgia, chronic fatigue syndrome, obesity, and chronic pain syndromes.[28]

A clear relationship exists between the number of unexplained symptoms a patient has and his or her ACE score.[29] A particular patient's current complaint is often only a surrogate for the real issue. The author of a classic study concluded that most behavior regarding exaggerated illness in compensation cases results from suggestion or rationalization as well as somatization,[29] and reasoned that "because any improvement in the claimant's health condition may result in denial of disability status in the future, the claimant is compelled to guard against getting well and is left with no honorable way to recover from illness."[30] In the legal system, which is often adversarial, the patient is challenged repeatedly to prove permanent illness. Consciously or subconsciously, such patients may develop a heightened awareness to the normal, minor aches and pains of daily life to justify the existence of lingering injury. A less severe interpretation of claimant behavior is offered: "Human nature being what it is, there is a tendency for the injured person to make the most (of) any complaints that he may have when examined for possible compensation.... The injured person in these circumstances has a different approach to that of a sick person coming for treatment to heal his illness. The injured person aims to 'sell his disability' and make it as large as he can to claim as much compensation as possible...this approach is understandable and to be expected. When this tendency is grossly exaggerated, it merges into malingering."[20]

Summary

The treatment and the evaluation of workers' compensation patients gives the orthopaedic surgeon the opportunity to assist the patient with his or her health and job: two of the most important aspects of life. This unique aspect of medicine requires the blending of medical and legal skills. Patients who are both ill and out of work experience added stress that can alter their responses to physical examinations, laboratory tests, and medical treatment. The doctor-patient relationship, although paramount, is shared with the employer and, many times, a lawyer. Attention to detail in the diagnosis and the examination findings is essential. The final goals are to restore the patient's health and allow him or her to return to work.

Key Study Points

- Work-related orthopaedic injuries are common and affect the health of US workers and the economy.

- Patients who sustain a work-related injury may respond differently to orthopaedic treatment but can benefit from such treatment.

- When patients do not respond as expected, the reason may be somatization.

Annotated References

1. Greenwood JG: *Disability Evaluation*. St. Louis, MO, Mosby, 1996, p. 7.

2. Hashimoto DM: The future role of managed care and capitation in worker's compensation. *Am J Law Med* 1996;22(2-3):233-261.

3. Statista: Monthly number of full-time employees in the United States from July 2012 to July 2013 (in millions, unadjusted). http://www.statista.com/statistics/192361/unadjusted-monthly-number-of-full-time-employees-in-the-us. Accessed January 18, 2013.

   This website provides up-to-date, seasonally adjusted full-time employment (> 35 hours/week) and unemployment data on a monthly basis.

4. US Department of Labor: Bureau of Labor Statistics: Nonfatal Occupational Injuries and Illnesses Requiring Days Away From Work, 2011. http://www.bls.gov/news.release/osh2.nr0.htm. Accessed January 18, 2013.

   These data provide extensive information on the incidences, case counts, diagnoses, and trends in work injuries. Figures on job types, employer categories, and the effects of age on injury rates are provided.

5. Leigh JP: Economic burden of occupational injury and illness in the United States. *Milbank Q* 2011;89(4):728-772.

   This study presents estimates of the national price of occupational injuries and illnesses in 2007. Although such costs are sizable and as high as cancer costs, workers' compensation insurance covers less than one fourth of the total cost.

6. Bonauto DK, Fan JZ, Largo TW, et al: Proportion of workers who were work-injured and payment by workers' compensation systems—10 states, 2007. *MMWR Morb Mortal Wkly Rep* 2010;59(29):897-900.

   The proportion of individuals injured at work in the 12 months of this study ranged from 4.0% to 6.9%, but insurance paid for medical treatment in only 47% to 77% of the states studied. The reasons for nonpayment need to be examined.

7. Leigh JP, Robbins JA: Occupational disease and workers' compensation: Coverage, costs, and consequences. *Milbank Q* 2004;82(4):689-721.

8. Smith TD, DeJoy DM: Occupational injury in America: An analysis of risk factors using data from the General Social Survey (GSS). *J Safety Res* 2012;43(1):67-74.

   The authors identified race, occupational category, and work-family interference as risk factors and safety climate and organizational effectiveness as protective factors for work injury.

9. Walsh M, Davidovitch RI, Egol KA: Ethnic disparities in recovery following distal radial fracture. *J Bone Joint Surg Am* 2010;92(5):1082-1087.

   Ethnic disparities have been demonstrated in the treatment of some chronic diseases. This study indicates that recovery from distal radial fracture is different between groups as well. These disparities may result from multifactorial sociodemographic factors that are present both before and after treatment. Level of evidence: II.

10. Nguyen TH, Randolph DC, Talmage J, Succop P, Travis R: Long-term outcomes of lumbar fusion among workers' compensation subjects: A historical cohort study. *Spine (Phila Pa 1976)* 2011;36(4):320-331.

    Lumbar fusion for the diagnoses of disk degeneration, disk herniation, and/or radiculopathy in a workers' compensation setting is associated with significant increase in disability, opiate use, prolonged work loss, and poor return-to-work status.

11. Carreon LY, Glassman SD, Kantamneni NR, Mugavin MO, Djurasovic M: Clinical outcomes after posterolateral lumbar fusion in workers' compensation patients: A case-control study. *Spine (Phila Pa 1976)* 2010;35(19):1812-1817.

    After controlling for covariates known to affect outcomes following lumbar fusion, patients who receive workers' compensation have significantly less improvement. Amelioration in back pain was similar between the two groups, but workers' compensation patients retained a higher level of disability after their surgeries. Level of evidence: III.

12. Holtby R, Razmjou H: Impact of work-related compensation claims on surgical outcome of patients with rotator cuff related pathologies: A matched case-control study. *J Shoulder Elbow Surg* 2010;19(3):452-460.

    One hundred ten work-related shoulder decompressions (60%) or cuff repairs (40%) were compared with 110 non–work-injured historical controls with similar diagnoses and treatments. Both groups significantly improved after surgery, although the non–work-injured group had better results. Level of evidence: III.

13. Campolieti M, Hyatt DE: Further evidence on the "Monday effect" in workers' compensation. *ILR Rev* 2006;59(3):438-450.

14. Waddell G, McCulloch JA, Kummel E, Venner RM: Nonorganic physical signs in low-back pain. *Spine (Phila Pa 1976)* 1980;5(2):117-125.

15. Giersiepen K, Spallek M: Carpal tunnel syndrome as an occupational disease. *Dtsch Arztebl Int* 2011;108(14):238-242.

    Carpal tunnel syndrome caused by work, either alone or in combination with other factors, has been well documented by epidemiologic data and is pathophysiologically plausible. However, working at a computer keyboard does not seem to raise a patient's risk for this condition.

16. Armstrong TJ: *Disability Evaluation*, ed 2. St. Louis, MO, Mosby, 2003, pp 178-190.

17. Injuries, in *The Burden of Musculoskeletal Diseases in the United States*. Rosemont, IL, American Academy of Orthopaedic Surgeons, 2011, pp 129-143.

1: Principles of Orthopaedics

A recently updated overview of the spectrum of musculoskeletal injuries in the United States, with data on prevalence, trends, location, causes, injury sites, outcomes, and the demographic characteristics of workplace injuries.

18. Ramazzini B: De morbis artificum diatriba [diseases of workers]: 1713. *Am J Public Health* 2001;91(9):1380-1382.

19. Leavitt F, Sweet JJ: Characteristics and frequency of malingering among patients with low back pain. *Pain* 1986;25(3):357-364.

20. Waddell G, Bircher M, Finlayson D, Main CJ: Symptoms and signs: Physical disease or illness behaviour? *Br Med J (Clin Res Ed)* 1984;289(6447):739-741.

21. Shaibani A, Sabbagh MN: Pseudoneurologic syndromes: Recognition and diagnosis. *Am Fam Physician* 1998;57(10):2485-2494.

22. Stokes HM, Landrieu KW, Domangue B, Kunen S: Identification of low-effort patients through dynamometry. *J Hand Surg Am* 1995;20(6):1047-1056.

23. Gutierrez Z, Shechtman O: Effectiveness of the five-handle position grip strength test in detecting sincerity of effort in men and women. *Am J Phys Med Rehabil* 2003;82(11):847-855.

24. Shechtman O, Sindhu BS, Davenport PW: Using the "visual target grip test" to identify sincerity of effort during grip strength testing. *J Hand Ther* 2012;25(3):320-329.

Participants were tricked into exerting more force than intended to reach a deceptive target line. This test effectively detected submaximal effort, although it is not safe for patients during initial therapy but may be appropriate for patients who can safely exert maximal grip force.

25. Goldberg RJ: *Current Diagnosis in Neurology*. St. Louis, MO, Mosby 1994, pp 300-304.

26. Ford CV: *The Somatizing Disorders: Illness as a Way of Life*. New York, NY, Elsevier Science Publishing Company, 1983, pp 1-2.

27. Eisendrath SJ: Factitious physical disorders. *West J Med* 1994;160(2):177-179.

28. Felitti VJ, Anda RF: The relationship of adverse childhood experiences to adult medical disease, psychiatric disorders, and sexual behavior: Implications for healthcare, in Lanius RA, Vermetten E, Pain C, eds: *The Impact of Early Life Trauma on Health and Disease—The Hidden Epidemic*. Cambridge, United Kingdom, United Kingdom University Press, 2010, pp 77-87.

T.S Eliot's haunting phrase "In my beginning is my end" capsulizes the effect of adverse childhood experiences. This chapter documents that depression, suicide, chronic pain, alcoholism, and lives cut short by two decades can all be traced back to the worst secrets of childhood.

29. Hicks A: Problems in writing medico-legal reports: I. Clinical exaggeration and malingering. *East Afr Med J* 1988;65(1):51-56.

30. Bellamy R: Compensation neurosis: Financial reward for illness as nocebo. *Clin Orthop Relat Res* 1997;336:94-106.

Chapter 13

Levels of Evidence and Grades of Recommendation

Brad Petrisor, MSc, MD, FRCSC   Mohit Bhandari, MD, PhD, FRCSC

Introduction

Evidence-based medicine requires the integration of clinical judgment and acumen, recommendations based on the best available evidence, and the incorporation of the patient's values and preferences.[1] The term *best available evidence* implies that there is a hierarchy of evidence, with studies ranging from high quality to low quality.[1] Clinical trials and research studies attempt to identify underlying truths about disease or disease processes; however, clinical research must overcome two main factors—bias and random chance—in the quest to identify these truths.[2] Bias is the systematic tendency to deviate from the truth, and, unlike random chance, bias is a modifiable factor. High-quality methodology in clinical trials reduces the introduction of bias, which can cause investigators to deviate from their attempts at identifying the truth.

This chapter will discuss the methodologic safeguards that can be incorporated into clinical research to increase the quality of the research and move the research to a higher level in the hierarchy of evidence. Research studies can become more internally valid by reducing potential sources of bias as much as possible. Historically, there have been several different systems designed to classify the hierarchy of evidence.[3] The *Journal of Bone and Joint Surgery* (American volume) and many other orthopaedic journals have incorporated a level of evidence rating for all published trials and studies.[4] However, there is more than one rating

system, and these systems do not always agree.[3] A level I (high-quality) study in one system may not correlate with a level I study in another system. Different raters may place the same study at a different level within the same system. The interrater reliability for determining the levels of evidence in the American volume of the *Journal of Bone and Joint Surgery* was determined to be high (intraclass coefficient, 0.61-0.75), but agreement was much higher for reviewers trained in epidemiology.[5] For this reason, the principles of study design and quality in generic terms will be discussed. Another potential pitfall of reporting the level of evidence of clinical trials is that it may give readers a false sense of security in incorporating the trial results into practice. It should be remembered that a high-quality level I therapeutic study does not necessarily translate into a high-quality recommendation grade for clinical practice. This requires that the study ask an important clinical question, assess the totality of the literature, and incorporate patients' values and preferences. Methods for developing grades of recommendation using the Grading of Recommendations Assessment, Development, and Evaluation (GRADE) system also are presented in this chapter.[3]

Study Designs

There are several categories of surgical literature. Some studies try to answer a question about a therapy, whereas others may seek to answer questions about a prognosis, diagnosis, harm, or economic analysis. Each area of the literature has its own hierarchy of evidence. Studies that are termed level I or the highest quality evidence in one particular category, such as therapy, may not be the highest quality evidence in the categories of prognosis or diagnosis.[6] This chapter will focus on the evidence hierarchy in the category of therapy because it encompasses most of the major study designs and is more common in orthopaedic literature.[5]

Randomized Controlled Trial

Therapy studies can be broadly categorized as those having an experimental design or those with an observational nature. The highest level of evidence in a therapy study is the randomized controlled trial, which

Dr. Petrisor or an immediate family member is a member of a speakers' bureau or has made paid presentations on behalf of Stryker; serves as a paid consultant to or is an employee of Stryker; has received research or institutional support from Stryker and Synthes; and has received nonincome support (such as equipment or services), commercially derived honoraria, or other non–research-related funding (such as paid travel) from Synthes. Dr. Bhandari or an immediate family member serves as a paid consultant to or is an employee of Amgen, Eli Lilly, Stryker, Smith & Nephew, and Zimmer and has received research or institutional support from Smith & Nephew and DePuy.

is an experimental study design. This type of design has several important methodologic safeguards to minimize bias, with the process of randomization itself being the foremost safeguard. Randomization attempts to balance the prognosis between groups within a trial. The process balances for any known prognostic variables and, more importantly, also balances for unknown prognostic variables.[7,8] Some clinical trials have used even or odd numbers or chart numbers to randomize patients; however, these methods would at best be termed pseudorandomization.[9] Randomization in and of itself is vital to reduce the bias that can be introduced into a trial with an imbalance of prognosis. In addition to randomization, concealment in the allocation of treatment groups is needed; that is, the investigators should be unable to determine the group to which a particular patient would be randomly assigned. If allocation is not concealed, the investigators could enroll patients or choose not to enroll patients based on the group to which the patients would be randomly assigned. This methodology would necessarily lead to prognostic imbalance and undermine the process of randomization.[10]

After the patients have been randomized, it is vital to maintain the prognostic balance with the process of blinding. When possible, all members of the investigative team should be blinded to treatment allocation.[10-12] Clearly, it is not possible to blind surgeons to the treatment group, and, in many instances, it is not possible to blind patients to the received treatment. However, other people involved in the study can be blinded, including the therapy staff, the clinical staff, the outcome adjudicators, the data analysts, and the writing committee.[13]

Case Series

The case series or case report is at the lowest level of the hierarchy for formal data collection. The case series is the most common study type in the orthopaedic literature.[5,14] Case series are observational and lack a control group. Most case series are often retrospective in nature and by necessity must resort to historical or literature comparisons. Reducing bias in the case series is possible by prospectively collecting the data, asking an appropriate question, using validated outcomes, and using unbiased outcome measures and adjudicators. At best, conclusions drawn from a case series are hypotheses for generating future clinical research.[15]

Case-Control Study

Above the case series in the quality hierarchy is the case-control design, an observational and retrospective study design. One of the main strengths of the case-control design is that it is useful for rare outcomes or diseases that have a low incidence rate. In many instances, the study is designed to identify the risk factors present in the development of a disease. Similarly, the study can be used to identify prognostic factors that may modify the way a disease progresses. This design is retrospective in nature because investigators identify

patients who have a particular disease or outcome and then identify control subjects (patients who do not have the disease or outcome). Study investigators assess the odds of having a risk factor associated with the identified outcome. This type of design is necessarily retrospective because the disease or the outcome has already occurred, and the investigators must look back in time to identify the risk factors. This trial design can produce findings and help identify associations between disease and risk factors, and it is a very powerful tool when the disease incidence is low or when the outcome of interest takes a long time to develop. Other potential benefits of the case-control design are that it is less expensive to conduct than a randomized controlled trial and can be done more quickly. However, the findings are only associations, meaning that investigators are not able to identify causative factors or causation per se between risk factors and the subsequent development of disease.

Cohort Design

The cohort study is the next design above the case-control study in the design hierarchy. The cohort design is observational in nature but can be very similar to the randomized trial design without the random assignment of treatments. A simple cohort trial identifies two groups of patients who differ in an exposure or a treatment. It can be used when it would be considered unethical to randomize patients to a particular treatment or exposure. For example, a prospective cohort trial could be used to assess the effect of smoking on fracture nonunion. One group of patients with a fracture who are smokers can be matched and compared with another group of patients with a fracture who are nonsmokers. The patients are matched based on known prognostic factors, such as age, fracture type, or treatment, with the groups differing only in the selected exposure. Another example is the comparison of one surgeon's treatment of tibial fractures with a second surgeon's treatment protocol. However, unknown prognostic factors are not controlled for in this type of study design, and there may be some prognostic imbalance between the groups that can affect the ultimate outcome of the trial. An imbalance in prognosis can result in an overestimation or an underestimation of the treatment effect.[2]

Study Quality

There is a hierarchy of study quality within the hierarchy of study designs. One randomized trial may be more methodologically sound than another, and it is possible that the less robust randomized trial may be downgraded to a lower quality level in the study design hierarchy. For example, trial A is a randomized trial with computer randomization and complete concealment of the treatment allocation. The trial also blinds the patient, the data collectors, the nursing teams, the physiotherapy teams, the outcomes adjudicators, and the writing committee. The outcomes observed are clearly defined and objective (for example, revision surgery or validated functional outcome measures, both generic and disease specific). The study is appropriately powered to identify a clinically important difference in outcomes. This type of study can be contrasted to trial B, a randomized trial that used a coin flip for randomization, no blinding of personnel involved in treatment allocation, and no blinding of patients. The surgeon investigator collects the outcome data using nonvalidated outcomes (the patient is doing excellent, good, fair, or poor). Trial A is more internally robust with respect to its methodology and has used appropriate techniques to minimize bias. Trial B is likely to overestimate or underestimate the truth.

Randomization and concealment of allocation are important factors in obtaining prognostic balance between groups in a randomized controlled trial. Blinding plays the important role of maintaining this prognostic balance by ensuring that the groups in the trial are treated in the same manner by different members of the care and investigative teams. Other factors, including the lack of an intention-to-treat analysis or the absence of appropriate follow-up, also can downgrade the quality and evidence level of a study.

Intention-to-Treat Analysis

An intention-to-treat analysis analyzes patients in the groups to which they were randomized, despite the treatment that they received. This type of analysis contrasts with the per protocol analysis in which investigators analyze patients to the treatment they received regardless of their randomized allocation. Intention-to-treat analysis is important for maintaining prognostic balance. For example, if a trial is devised randomizing patients with wrist fractures to treatment with Kirschner wire fixation versus locking volar plate fixation, there may be a subset of patients randomized to the Kirschner wire fixation who instead are treated with plate fixation (the surgeon may believe that a patient's bone is too osteopenic or the fracture pattern is not amenable to Kirschner wire fixation). Using the intention-to-treat analysis, this subset of patients would then be analyzed in the original treatment allocation group. The reason for this methodology is that there may be some unknown prognostic factor linking these patients that is associated with being nonamenable to wire fixation. The intention-to-treat analysis provides a more conservative estimate of the treatment effect, whereas a per-protocol analysis in this example may overestimate or underestimate the treatment effect. However, it is often useful to do both analyses so that the reader can assess the results of each.

Completion of Follow-up

The percentage of patients with completed follow-up is also a vital component in assessing the quality of a trial. For example, if only 50% of the patients return for a final assessment of functional outcomes or have unreported revision procedures, a significant number of potential outcome events will be lost or not observed. Patients may not complete follow-up assessments because of a differential in treatment effect; if a large number of patients in one group do not complete follow-up, an unknown prognostic reason could be involved. By convention, a minimum 80% follow-up rate is considered respectable for a clinical trial. However, methodologists suggest that this rate is inadequate, and all trialists should strive to approach 100% follow-up.[16]

The effect of the follow-up rate is illustrated by the following example. In a trial, 200 patients are randomized to two groups (A and B) of 100 patients each. In group A, 85 patients complete follow-up; there are five events in that group. In group B, 90 patients complete follow-up; there are eight events in that group. This would lead to an event rate of 6% in group A and 9% in group B ($P > 0.05$), which is not a statistically significant difference between the groups. However, if there are just two more patients in group B who have an event that is not assessed at follow-up, these two additional events could potentially shift the trial outcome to a statistically significant result. In small trials, which are common in orthopaedic studies (average, 80 to 100 patients), events that are undetected because of loss of follow-up can profoundly affect the result.[17] If patients are enrolled in trials to observe outcomes, it is essential that the patients complete follow-up so that the outcomes of interest can be observed.

Grading the Evidence

The GRADE Approach

The GRADE Working Group was formed in 2000 to standardize the levels of evidence and the formulation of grades of recommendation.[3] The working group is composed of healthcare workers, researchers, and opinion leaders in evidence-based medicine. The GRADE system provides a framework for the development of guidelines in a structured manner[3] (Figure 1). To develop a guideline, it is necessary to ask a well-structured question, choose an appropriate outcome, evaluate the literature, and then incorporate patients' values and preferences into a clinically relevant recommendation.[3] In some instances, the orthopaedic surgery literature has a paucity of high-quality evidence available for evaluation; however, the GRADE system will work regardless of the type of evidence used for the recommendation.

Rating the Evidence

Evidence is most commonly acquired by performing a systematic review, with a focused question and a reproducible literature search that identifies all the literature relevant to the focused question.[18] The patient population, intervention, comparator, and outcomes (known by the acronym PICO) system provides a common framework for question development.[19] The patient population for whom the guideline is being developed must be determined. Defining the population may in-

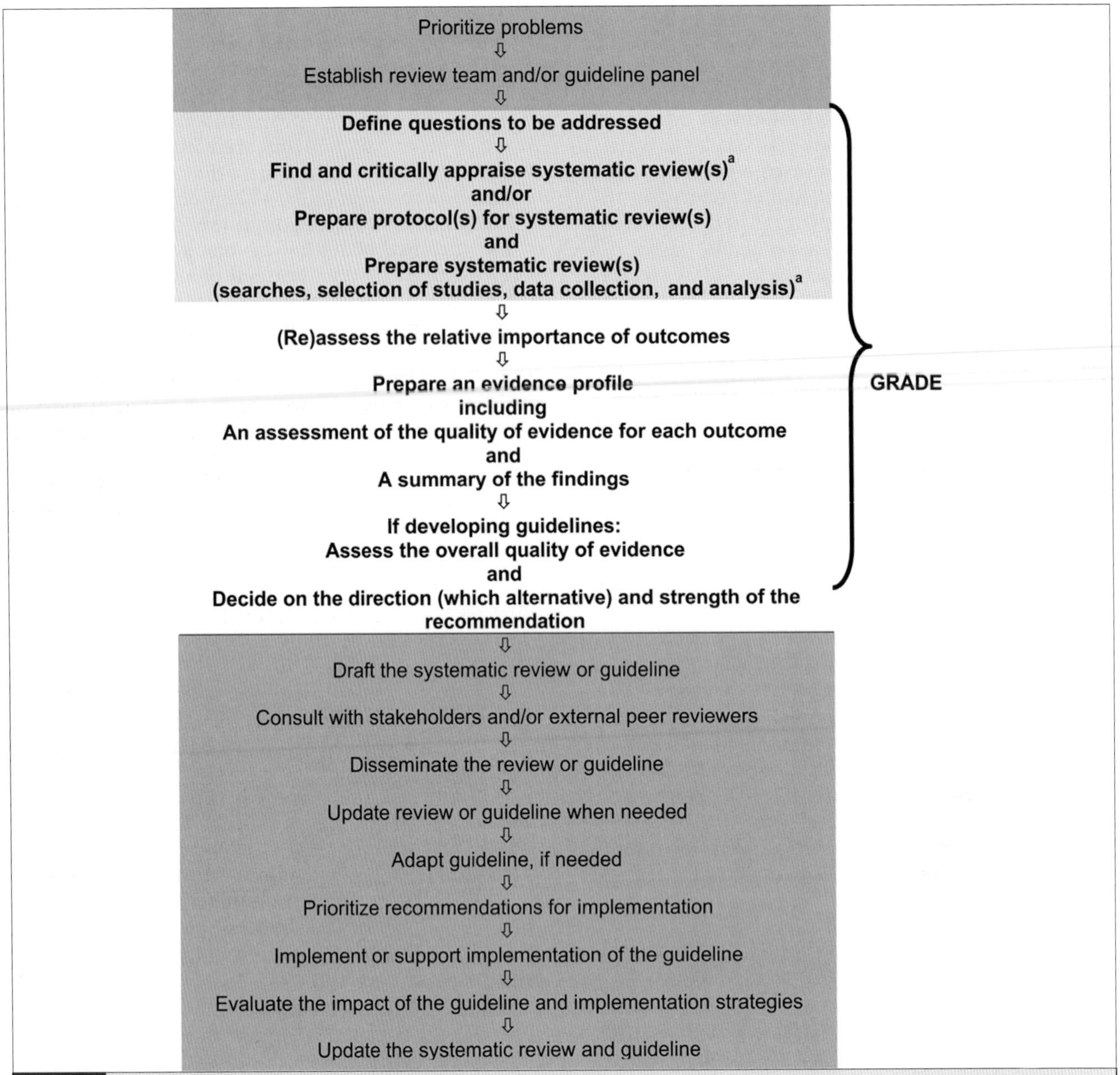

Prioritize problems
⇩
Establish review team and/or guideline panel
⇩
Define questions to be addressed
⇩
Find and critically appraise systematic review(s)[a]
and/or
Prepare protocol(s) for systematic review(s)
and
Prepare systematic review(s)
(searches, selection of studies, data collection, and analysis)[a]
⇩
(Re)assess the relative importance of outcomes
⇩
Prepare an evidence profile
including
An assessment of the quality of evidence for each outcome
and
A summary of the findings
⇩
If developing guidelines:
Assess the overall quality of evidence
and
Decide on the direction (which alternative) and strength of the
recommendation
⇩

GRADE

Draft the systematic review or guideline
⇩
Consult with stakeholders and/or external peer reviewers
⇩
Disseminate the review or guideline
⇩
Update review or guideline when needed
⇩
Adapt guideline, if needed
⇩
Prioritize recommendations for implementation
⇩
Implement or support implementation of the guideline
⇩
Evaluate the impact of the guideline and implementation strategies
⇩
Update the systematic review and guideline

Figure 1 | Illustration of the guideline development process and the role of GRADE. (Reproduced with permission from Guyatt G, Oxman AD, Akl EA, et al: GRADE guidelines: 1. Introduction—GRADE evidence profiles and summary of findings tables. *J Clin Epidemiol* 2011;64[4]:383-394.)

clude factors such as mean age, fracture type, and resource status (resource-rich or resource-poor patients). For example, asking a question about the use of biologic therapies as adjuncts to fracture repair may not have an effect in those patients who are unable to procure the use of those therapies or in healthcare systems that cannot afford their use.

The potential of several interventions for many given orthopaedic problems can confound the development of guidelines. Much of the orthopaedic literature also lacks an appropriate comparison group; therefore, it may be difficult to ascertain the appropriate comparator. In many trials in the literature, there is neither an intervention nor a comparison group. Determining the

appropriate outcome also may be difficult. For example, when assessing pelvic fracture outcomes, several different functional outcome measures have been reported in the literature, with no standard measure used by all studies.[20] This problem is also seen in other specialties, such as foot and ankle and hip and knee reconstruction.[21-24]

When developing a guideline, it is necessary to assess all patient-important outcomes as well as any potential adverse effects of various treatments.[25] It is important for content experts to formulate clinically relevant and appropriate questions and discuss all important outcomes and harms before the initiation of guideline development.[26]

Risk of Bias

After the question has been determined, it is necessary to evaluate the literature surrounding it. The GRADE Working Group suggests that the levels of evidence be ranked as follows: high quality, moderate quality, low quality, and very quality. Randomized trials are graded as high quality or moderate quality, although some trials could be further downgraded if necessary.[18] Observational studies are considered low quality or very low quality. Individual studies can be downgraded based on their risk of bias, and the total evidence can be downgraded for a lack of consistency, directness, and precision or a risk of publication bias. Evidence can by upgraded if there is a large treatment effect or a dose-response effect.[27] However, when discussing the quality of the evidence in the makeup of guidelines, the GRADE Working Group also uses the concept of quality in the form of totality of evidence. For example, several high-quality randomized trials with a low risk of bias or high internal validity may provide inconsistent or imprecise evidence for a particular outcome when the trials are compared with each other or when all the trials are evaluated together.[18]

Directness

Direct evidence as defined by the GRADE Working Group is evidence that applies directly to an investigator's question or the question put forward by the guideline committee.[28] It directly relates to the patient population of interest, compares the interventions of interest, and evaluates the patient groups with consideration of outcomes that are important to patients. Indirectness can be introduced into a trial when there are differences in the trial population and the population of interest or when the trial has no control group for comparison of outcomes. This is particularly relevant in the orthopaedic literature because many trials lack a control group.[14]

The potential for indirect evidence is illustrated by the following example. The American Academy of Orthopaedic Surgeons (AAOS) developed a clinical practice guideline on the Diagnosis and Treatment of Acute Achilles Tendon Rupture based on many studies in which the patients were not high-performance athletes.[29] If the recommendations of this AAOS guideline are applied to a population of high-performance athletes, there would be some indirectness in extrapolating the results. If the differences in the patient populations are too great, the evidence could be downgraded because of this indirectness. However, caution should be exercised in downgrading a study for indirectness in study populations, unless there is some plausible biologic rationale that one population may behave differently than another.[28] Another example of indirect evidence is applying the results of studies assessing hardware failure in osteopenic or osteoporotic patients to adolescent patients.

Consistency

Inconsistency refers to the inherent heterogeneity between studies. Systematic reviews show that several randomized controlled trials on a particular subject and having the same outcome can produce differing results. This can be caused by many factors, including differences in the patient populations, the quality of the trial, the application of an intervention, or the outcomes being assessed. An exploration of the heterogeneous factors may reveal the reason for the inconsistency; however, if the inconsistency remains unexplained, the body of literature can be downgraded for the lack of consistency.[30] The presence of inconsistency is important because it can decrease confidence in the estimate of the effect. For example, if four randomized control trials result in two trials with treatment effects in support of a given therapy and two trials with treatment effects against the same therapy, this type of inconsistency would undermine confidence in this body of literature. The literature could be downgraded for the lack of consistency.[30]

Imprecision

In general, precision is quantified by assessing the confidence interval (CI). With a 95% CI, the true treatment effect will lie within the interval 95% of the time. If a CI is significantly wide, it is an imprecise measure of the treatment effect. In individual trials, if the confidence limits cross the line of no effect, the treatment may be beneficial, may not be beneficial, or may be potentially harmful. Using the GRADE system of guideline development, if the confidence limits of a pooled estimate of effect cross a clinical threshold for recommending or not recommending a treatment, then there is a lack of precision.[31] In trials with a lack of precision, the evidence may be downgraded one or two levels. It has been suggested that with few events and confidence limits that suggest either benefit or harm, the evidence should be downgraded by two levels for imprecision.[31]

Publication Bias

Some studies with negative results or results perceived as uninteresting may not be published or may be subject to lag bias (delayed publication because of multiple rejections, with subsequent publication in more obscure journals).[32] Other authors choose to publish trials in foreign language journals. Less-than-rigorous literature search strategies may overlook these types of studies. If systematic reviews report on only positive studies, this can introduce publication bias and can lead to an overestimation of the treatment effect.[33] There may be a greater risk of publication bias with multiple, smaller randomized trials because larger trials are more likely to be published. Statistical methods for determining publication bias include the use of a funnel plot and statistical tests for asymmetry.[32]

Clinical Example

The following clinical question was formulated using the PICO format. In adult patients with a displaced

Table 1

Summary of Findings Table: Internal Fixation Versus External Fixation in Displaced Distal Radius Fractures[a]

Population: Adult Patients With Unstable Distal Radius Fractures
Intervention: Internal Fixation
Comparison: External Fixation

No. of Studies Outcomes (Design)	Limitations	Inconsistency	Indirectness	Imprecision
11 (8 RCTs) Functional outcome (DASH score)	Yes, 3 observational studies, RCTs with some limitations	Serious inconsistency, multiple patient-reported outcomes used	No serious indirectness	Some
9 (6 RCTs) Objective (grip strength)	Yes, 3 observational studies, RCTs with some limitations	Serious inconsistency, different measures obtained between trials	No serious indirectness	Some
6 (4 RCTs) Radiographic (volar tilt)	Yes, 3 observational studies, RCTs with some limitations	No serious inconsistency	No serious indirectness	Some

[a]For dichotomous outcomes, a presentation of both relative risks and absolute risks would be included. RCT = randomized controlled trial, DASH = Disabilities of the Arm, Shoulder, and Hand. Standardized mean difference is a measure of treatment effect with positive values favoring internal fixation and negative values favoring external fixation.
(Data from Wei DH, Poolman RW, Bhandari M, Wolfe VM, Rosenwasser MP: External fixation versus internal fixation for unstable distal radius fractures: A systematic review and meta-analysis of comparative clinical trials. *J Orthop Trauma* 2012;26[7]:386-394.)

distal radius fracture requiring surgical fixation, does internal fixation versus external fixation improve functional outcomes?[34] From this clinical question, a systematic literature review was identified and used to initiate the GRADE approach. From the systematic review, a table with an evidence profile and a summary of findings was created (Table 1). The table outlines the sources of the potential study limitations, inconsistencies, indirectness, and imprecision. A full summary of findings table also contains the relevant results (including relative risks and absolute risks for dichotomous outcomes) for each patient-important outcome. A quality rating for the evidence can then be obtained for each outcome.

Strength of a Recommendation

When making a recommendation, several factors, including a measure of beneficial and harmful effects, the quality of the evidence, a translation of the evidence into the clinical situation, and the baseline risk of the population in question, must be taken into account according to the GRADE Working Group. The strength of the recommendations can then be categorized as strong or weak.[26] Because the GRADE Working Group states that "a recommendation is intended to facilitate an appropriate decision in an individual patient or a population," the actual recommendation would be to do it or do not do it (strong), or probably do it or probably do not do it (weak).[3] A recommendation to "do it" would mean that most well-informed patients

would likely go ahead with the procedure; however, this would not negate the necessary conversation with the patient to offer treatment alternatives. A recommendation to "probably do it" would mean a more extensive discussion of options and a potentially greater incorporation of the patient's values and preferences into the decision.[35]

Returning to the clinical example, Table 1 suggests low-quality research supporting the use of internal locked volar plating over external fixation for treating an unstable distal radius fracture in terms of the outcome of function, grip strength, and radiographic volar tilt. The systematic review by the study investigators does not provide information on the risks associated with plate fixation (for example, a larger incision or extensor tendon rupture) versus the risks associated with external fixation (for example, pin tract infection).[34] The grade of the recommendation in favor of plate fixation would be "probably do it"; however, the treating surgeon should be aware that further high-quality research could change the recommendation, and the risks and benefits of plate fixation should be discussed with the patient, and his or her values and preferences should influence the treatment decision.

The GRADE system has been incorporated by several organizations that develop guidelines, including the World Health Organization, the Cochrane Collaboration, and the US Preventative Task Force.[36] The GRADE system uses a systematic framework for guideline development from the initiation of an appropriate clinical question to an evaluation of the literature and subsequent formulation of the guideline.[37]

Table 1

Summary of Findings Table: Internal Fixation Versus External Fixation in Displaced Distal Radius Fractures[a] (continued)

Population: Adult Patients With Unstable Distal Radius Fractures
Intervention: Internal Fixation
Comparison: External Fixation

Publication Bias	No. of Patients (Internal Fixation)	No. of patients (External Fixation)	Standardized Mean Difference (95% CI)	Quality
None detected	316	289	0.28 (0.03, 0.53)	Low
None detected	372	356	−0.28 (−0.57, 0.00)	Low
None detected	255	244	0.43 (0.11, 0.75)	Low

Summary

A number of study designs exist, each with its own strengths and weaknesses. Within studies of therapy, the randomized controlled trial is at the top level, or considered best evidence as it incorporates methodology to reduce bias, randomization being but one method. By understanding study design and study quality, it is possible to rank studies of therapy into levels of evidence. Once this is done, by incorporating the format of GRADE, it is then possible to formulate a grade of recommendation for a given treatment and the subsequent formation of clinical care guideline to aid in the evidence-based care of patients.

Key Study Points

- Gain understanding about how the GRADE working group incorporates the hierarchy of evidence.

- Gain understanding about how the GRADE working group method is used to develop a grade of recommendation.

- Gain understanding about how the incorporation of patients' preferences and values is done within the GRADE system for the development of grades of recommendation.

Annotated References

1. Sackett DL, Rosenberg WM, Gray JA, Haynes RB, Richardson WS: Evidence based medicine: What it is and what it isn't. *BMJ* 1996;312(7023):71-72.

2. Chu R, Walter SD, Guyatt G, et al: Assessment and implication of prognostic imbalance in randomized controlled trials with a binary outcome—a simulation study. *PLoS One* 2012;7(5):e36677.

   This study assessed the potential for prognostic imbalance between two arms of a randomized controlled trial. The authors concluded that the probability of prognostic balance between the two arms can be substantial in small trials.

3. Atkins D, Eccles M, Flottorp S, et al; The GRADE Working Group: Systems for grading the quality of evidence and the strength of recommendations I: Critical appraisal of existing approaches. *BMC Health Serv Res* 2004;4(1):38.

4. Wright JG, Swiontkowski MF, Heckman JD: Introducing levels of evidence to the journal. *J Bone Joint Surg Am* 2003;85(1):1-3.

5. Bhandari M, Swiontkowski MF, Einhorn TA, et al: Interobserver agreement in the application of levels of evidence to scientific papers in the American volume of the *Journal of Bone and Joint Surgery*. *J Bone Joint Surg Am* 2004;86(8):1717-1720.

6. Oxman AD, Sackett DL, Guyatt GH; The Evidence-Based Medicine Working Group: Users' guides to the medical literature: I. How to get started. *JAMA* 1993; 270(17):2093-2095.

7. Farrokhyar F, Karanicolas PJ, Thoma A, et al: Randomized controlled trials of surgical interventions. *Ann Surg* 2010;251(3):409-416.

   The authors identify potential methodologic challenges in conducting surgical randomized trials and discuss strategies to overcoming the challenges.

8. Bhandari M, Guyatt GH, Swiontkowski MF: User's guide to the orthopaedic literature: How to use an article about a surgical therapy. *J Bone Joint Surg Am* 2001;83(6):916-926.

9. Bhandari M, Guyatt GH, Lochner H, Sprague S, Tornetta P III: Application of the Consolidated Standards of Reporting Trials (CONSORT) in the fracture care literature. *J Bone Joint Surg Am* 2002;84(3):485-489.

10. Savović J, Jones H, Altman D, et al: Influence of reported study design characteristics on intervention effect estimates from randomised controlled trials: Combined analysis of meta-epidemiological studies. *Health Technol Assess* 2012;16(35):1-82.

    This study assessed the potential for bias within sequence generation, concealment of allocation, and blinding. The authors identified that bias in relationship to unclear or inadequate sequence generation, concealment of allocation, and blinding can potentially result in an overestimation or an underestimation of treatment effects.

11. Devereaux PJ, Bhandari M, Montori VM, Manns BJ, Ghall WA, Guyatt GH: Double blind, you have been voted off the island! *Evid Based Ment Health* 2002; 5(2):36-37.

12. Montori VM, Bhandari M, Devereaux PJ, Manns BJ, Ghali WA, Guyatt GH: In the dark: The reporting of blinding status in randomized controlled trials. *J Clin Epidemiol* 2002;55(8):787-790.

13. Devereaux PJ, Bhandari M, Montori VM, Manns BJ, Ghali WA, Guyatt GH: Double blind, you are the weakest link—good-bye! *ACP J Club* 2002;136(1):A11.

14. Mundi R, Chaudhry H, Sharma R, Schemitsch E, Bhandari M: What is the quality of the orthopaedic literature? *J Long Term Eff Med Implants* 2007;17(2): 103-109.

15. Guyatt GH, Sackett DL, Cook DJ; Evidence-Based Medicine Working Group: Users' guides to the medical literature: II. How to use an article about therapy or prevention: A. Are the results of the study valid? *JAMA* 1993;270(21):2598-2601.

16. Akl EA, Briel M, You JJ, et al: Potential impact on estimated treatment effects of information lost to follow-up in randomised controlled trials (LOST-IT): Systematic review. *BMJ* 2012;344:e2809.

    This study attempted to assess the reporting, extent, and actions of trialists to manage follow-up loss. The authors concluded that if different assumptions were made about patients lost to follow-up, those assumptions could change the interpretation of the trial results.

17. Thorlund K, Imberger G, Walsh M, et al: The number of patients and events required to limit the risk of overestimation of intervention effects in meta-analysis—a simulation study. *PLoS One* 2011;6(10):e25491.

    This study found that meta-analyses of small trials can introduce random error, which may result in the overestimation of the identified effects of interventions.

18. Balshem H, Helfand M, Schünemann HJ, et al: GRADE guidelines: 3. Rating the quality of evidence. *J Clin Epidemiol* 2011;64(4):401-406.

    The authors of this part of the GRADE guideline series discuss the issues involved in rating evidence for quality. The GRADE approach attempts to separate the quality of the evidence from the grade of the recommendation.

19. Guyatt GH, Oxman AD, Kunz R, et al: GRADE guidelines: 2. Framing the question and deciding on important outcomes. *J Clin Epidemiol* 2011;64(4):395-400.

    The authors of this part of the GRADE guideline series highlight the methodology behind framing a good clinical question for the development of a guideline. The method includes identifying the patient population, the interventions, the comparison groups, and all important outcomes.

20. Lefaivre KA, Slobogean GP, Valeriote J, O'Brien PJ, Macadam SA: Reporting and interpretation of the functional outcomes after the surgical treatment of disruptions of the pelvic ring: A systematic review. *J Bone Joint Surg Br* 2012;94(4):549-555.

    This study illustrates that there is substantial variability in the functional outcome scores used in reporting the surgical treatment of pelvic fractures. Some outcome scores had not been validated.

21. Goldstein CL, Schemitsch E, Bhandari M, Mathew G, Petrisor BA: Comparison of different outcome instruments following foot and ankle trauma. *Foot Ankle Int* 2010;31(12):1075-1080.

    The authors assessed different foot and ankle outcome scores and correlated foot- and ankle-specific outcome measures with validated generic functional outcome scores.

22. Farrugia P, Goldstein C, Petrisor BA: Measuring foot and ankle injury outcomes: Common scales and checklists. *Injury* 2011;42(3):276-280.

    The authors provide an update on the types of functional outcome measures used to assess ankle injury and review specific validated foot and ankle outcome measures.

23. Lau JT, Mahomed NM, Schon LC: Results of an Internet survey determining the most frequently used ankle scores by AOFAS members. *Foot Ankle Int* 2005;26(6): 479-482.

24. Bryant DM, Sanders DW, Coles CP, Petrisor BA, Jeray KJ, Laflamme GY: Selection of outcome measures for patients with hip fracture. *J Orthop Trauma* 2009; 23(6):434-441.

25. Guyatt GH, Alonso-Coello P, Vandvik PO: Experience with GRADE. *J Clin Epidemiol* 2012;65(12):1243-1244.

    This article is an introduction to the series of GRADE articles in the *Journal of Clinical Epidemiology*. It highlights the reasons for the development of a standardized grading system.

26. Guyatt GH, Oxman AD, Vist GE, et al: GRADE: An

emerging consensus on rating quality of evidence and strength of recommendations. *BMJ* 2008;336(7650): 924-926.

27. Guyatt GH, Oxman AD, Sultan S, et al: GRADE guidelines: 9. Rating up the quality of evidence. *J Clin Epidemiol* 2011;64(12):1311-1316.

   The authors discuss the GRADE system of creating guidelines and specifically look at how the system allows the quality of evidence to be uprated. The criteria used to uprate the quality of observational studies is specifically described.

28. Guyatt GH, Oxman AD, Kunz R, et al: GRADE guidelines: 8. Rating the quality of evidence—indirectness. *J Clin Epidemiol* 2011;64(12):1303-1310.

   This paper, the eighth in the series by the GRADE authors, highlights and explains the GRADE system. It specifically discusses the GRADE concept and the assessment of indirectness.

29. Chiodo CP, Glazebrook M, Bluman EM, et al: American Academy of Orthopaedic Surgeons clinical practice guideline on treatment of Achilles tendon rupture. *J Bone Joint Surg Am* 2010;92(14):2466-2468.

   The authors discuss the development of the AAOS guideline on the treatment of Achilles tendon rupture. Guidelines are provided on nonsurgical and surgical management of Achilles tendon rupture based on a focused question and a rigorous search of the literature.

30. Guyatt GH, Oxman AD, Kunz R, et al: GRADE guidelines: 7. Rating the quality of evidence—inconsistency. *J Clin Epidemiol* 2011;64(12):1294-1302.

   The authors discuss the GRADE system of guideline development and specifically address the issue of consistency. Criteria for evaluating consistency are discussed, including the assessment of the similarity of point estimates and the amount of overlap between CIs.

31. Guyatt GH, Oxman AD, Kunz R, et al: GRADE guidelines 6: Rating the quality of evidence—imprecision. *J Clin Epidemiol* 2011;64(12):1283-1293.

   The GRADE system of guideline development is discussed. The authors discuss the use and the assessment of CIs and how the quality of the evidence can be rated up or down depending on the precision of the measure of effect.

32. Guyatt GH, Oxman AD, Montori V, et al: GRADE guidelines: 5. Rating the quality of evidence—publication bias. *J Clin Epidemiol* 2011;64(12):1277-1282.

   The authors discuss the GRADE system, with a specific focus on publication bias and how it can affect the development of guidelines. Some approaches for uncovering publication bias are detailed.

33. Montori VM, Smieja M, Guyatt GH: Publication bias: A brief review for clinicians. *Mayo Clin Proc* 2000; 75(12):1284-1288.

34. Wei DH, Poolman RW, Bhandari M, Wolfe VM, Rosenwasser MP: External fixation versus internal fixation for unstable distal radius fractures: A systematic review and meta-analysis of comparative clinical trials. *J Orthop Trauma* 2012;26(7):386-394.

   The authors performed a systematic review and meta-analysis assessing external and internal fixation in treating unstable distal radius fractures. They concluded that there may be some improvement in functional outcomes with internal fixation but also suggest that both techniques may be viable. Level of evidence: II.

35. Brozek JL, Akl EA, Compalati E, et al: Grading quality of evidence and strength of recommendations in clinical practice guidelines—part 3 of 3: The GRADE approach to developing recommendations. *Allergy* 2011;66(5): 588-595.

   The authors discuss the GRADE approach for developing clinical practice guidelines. Two examples of guidelines that have used the GRADE approach in the field of allergy are discussed.

36. Guyatt G, Oxman AD, Akl EA, et al: GRADE guidelines: 1. Introduction—GRADE evidence profiles and summary of findings tables. *J Clin Epidemiol* 2011; 64(4):383-394.

   This paper provides an introduction to the GRADE approach to guideline development. The authors outline the development of the system and specifically discuss how to develop evidence profiles and tables that summarize the findings of research studies.

37. GRADE Working Group website. http://www. gradeworkinggroup.org. Accessed May 3, 2013.

   This website is available as a resource for understanding GRADE as well as providing tools for using GRADE in making recommendations.

1: Principles of Orthopaedics

Chapter 14

Orthopaedic Research: Health Research Methodology, Outcomes, and Biostatistics

Jesse Slade Shantz, MD, MBA   Saam Morshed, MD, PhD, MPH

Introduction

Orthopaedic surgeons must understand the conduct of research and the analysis of results to appropriately apply available evidence to effectively treat patients. Clinical studies become increasingly important if no evidence exists to guide treatment. As consumers and producers of clinical evidence, it is essential that orthopaedic surgeons understand that clinical research involves a compromise between the limitation of bias and the maintenance of study feasibility. This chapter uses the example of Achilles tendon rupture to highlight the basic principles of research ethics, appropriate trial design, and data analysis.[1]

Ethics and Evidence-Based Medicine

Clinical problems without literature support for a single diagnostic or treatment approach are common. Although the absence of evidence can result in marked variability and inefficiencies in the delivery of health care, the embrace of this uncertainty represents the foundation of clinical equipoise—a state in which physicians are sufficiently ambivalent in preference to prescribe one of two or more available options.[2] Equipoise is an important consideration to ethical and unbiased clinical research. In the example of an Achilles tendon rupture, equipoise would be satisfied if practitioners were willing to provide either nonsurgical or surgical care after reviewing the available literature. It follows that it is ethical to randomize patients to either treatment, with the goal of determining the more efficacious treatment.

More generally, biomedical ethics are an essential starting point for the design and performance of clinical research. Clinical trials must respect the principles of autonomy, beneficence, and nonmaleficence and place participants at minimal risk of harm.[3] These ethical principles do not limit the scope of research questions but may influence the study design that is chosen to answer a given research question. Ethical standards are upheld on an institutional level by committees dedicated to the protection of human subjects. Although such a protection committee is tasked to oversee an institution's research activities, the final responsibility lies with investigators to uphold ethical standards in their research.

A data safety and monitoring board, an independent board appointed by the study's investigators to review interim study results and incident complications, provides an additional level of patient protection in clinical trials. The data safety and monitoring board should not include investigators or those with conflicts of interest in the study outcome and should be given the power to discontinue the study based on explicit a priori cessation rules. The description of committees used to monitor and report complications has been variable in orthopaedic trials.[4]

Formulating a Research Question

A testable question based on a clinical problem without a satisfactory answer in the current literature provides the foundation for clinical research. The clear definition of several components of a clinical question is essential for the appropriate design of clinical research studies. These components include the study population, the intervention(s) being studied, the comparison or control group (if any), and the outcome to be measured.

The question, once carefully crafted, will drive the study design in several ways. In the example of an Achilles tendon rupture, there has been considerable debate in the field of orthopaedic surgery about the best treatment.[1] The central question is whether surgi-

Dr. Morshed or an immediate family member has received research or institutional support from Stryker and Synthes. Neither Dr. Shantz nor any immediate family member has received anything of value from or has stock or stock options held in a commercial company or institution related directly or indirectly to the subject of this chapter.

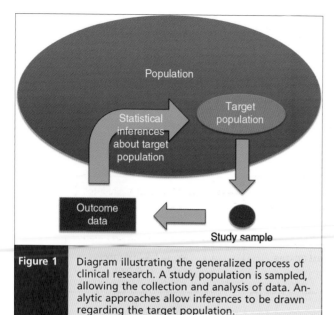

Figure 1 Diagram illustrating the generalized process of clinical research. A study population is sampled, allowing the collection and analysis of data. Analytic approaches allow inferences to be drawn regarding the target population.

cal repair or nonsurgical management of Achilles tendon ruptures leads to better outcomes. This question seems simple; however, this chapter will detail how the perspective of the investigator and the target population (for example, patients with diabetes; healthy, recreational athletes; or professional athletes) drives the study design. Each of these patient populations has unique attributes that necessitate a specific approach to treatment to ensure optimal outcomes with the fewest complications. For an athlete, rerupture of the tendon, the length of the rehabilitation period, and the amount of time before return to play would be outcomes of interest that would influence an investigator to choose a comparative trial. In diabetic patients, complications can represent a limb-threatening event, although they occur with low frequency. This factor would influence investigators to consider case-control study designs because of their statistical efficiency. Given the frequency of Achilles tendon ruptures in recreational athletes, a cost-effectiveness analysis comparing surgical and nonsurgical management might provide useful information for physicians and policymakers to best allocate finite resources efficiently. Each of these examples suggests only a few variables and illustrates that small alterations in the aims of the investigator may alter the study design.

Systematic Search of the Literature

A key component that allows the practice of evidence-based medicine is the ability to draw on previous research relevant to answering current clinical questions.[5] More specifically, an investigator must efficiently and thoroughly search for relevant literature to avoid repeating studies that have already been done. To accomplish this goal, the inclusion criteria and data to abstract must be predefined, a comprehensive search

strategy must be designed, papers should be reviewed for exclusions, relevant data from each included study should be abstracted, and results from studies should be synthesized and applied to practice.[5]

Inclusion and exclusion criteria will be mainly determined by the research question. The main goal of restricting studies included in a systematic review is to ensure that the patients represented by the study are similar to the target population desired by the investigator. Exclusion criteria limit the review of papers that investigate outmoded treatments or use lower quality study designs.

The target population is defined by characteristics of interest in that particular clinical situation and is a subset of the entire population[6] (Figure 1). For example, a surgeon prescribing a therapy plan for an elite athlete with an Achilles tendon rupture might be interested in early rehabilitation protocols. The surgeon would want to focus on trials of early rehabilitation in athletes rather than diluting the quality of data with studies including nonathletes. Failing to set focused criteria results in confusion in interpreting the outcomes of a systematic review, which can be seen in a 2010 Cochrane review of the treatment of Achilles tendon ruptures.[7] This review did not allow the separation of active and sedentary participants and led to difficulty in applying the results to each patient group.

Building a search strategy is the next component of the systematic review.[8] The goal of the investigator should be to include all relevant studies from all jurisdictions; this often requires collaboration with a medical librarian. In this way, no studies addressing the question of interest will be excluded from the analysis. It is important to register the review on an international database, such as the International Prospective Register of Systematic Reviews (PROSPERO).[9]

After assembling the potentially relevant literature, several reviewers must apply the predefined inclusion and exclusion criteria to all papers and manually search through the reference lists of reviewed papers for any missed studies. In general, reviewers should confer on the interpretation of criteria before their review and then independently evaluate each study. All disagreements should be settled by consensus. A flowchart illustrating this process as mandated by the Preferred Reporting Items for Systematic Reviews and Meta-Analyses (PRISMA)[10] statement is shown in Figure 2.

After the review, data abstraction and synthesis are generally accomplished using forms specifically designed to limit bias. The ultimate goal is to decide if the available studies are similar enough to allow statistical pooling of data or meta-analysis. Pooling similar studies combines data from multiple smaller studies with a high likelihood of false-negative results and achieves an adequately powered analysis. Often, the differences in methodology and outcome measurements make the pooling of data difficult and limit the ability to perform meta-analyses.

Despite rigorous methodology, the clinical usefulness of systematic reviews is ultimately determined by the quality of the included studies and the validity of infer-

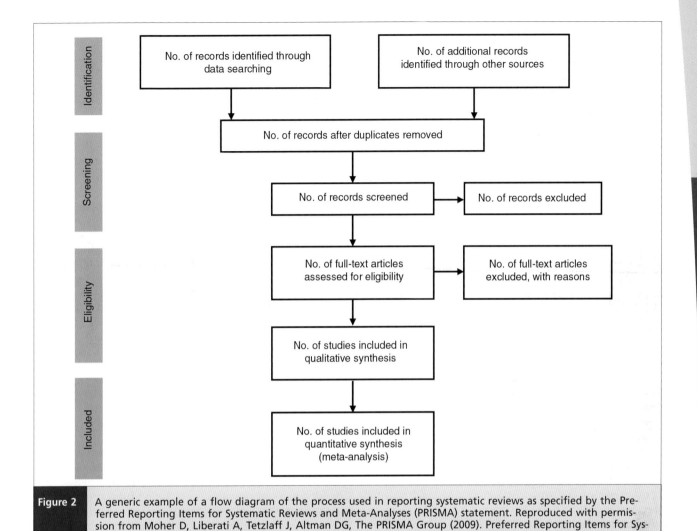

Figure 2   A generic example of a flow diagram of the process used in reporting systematic reviews as specified by the Preferred Reporting Items for Systematic Reviews and Meta-Analyses (PRISMA) statement. Reproduced with permission from Moher D, Liberati A, Tetzlaff J, Altman DG, The PRISMA Group (2009). Preferred Reporting Items for Systematic Reviews and Meta-Analyses: The PRISMA Statement. PLoS Med 6(6) e1000097. doi:10.1371/journal.pmed1000097.)

ences relevant to the target population chosen by the investigator. If the included studies are retrospective or poor in quality, the conclusions that are drawn must be cautiously interpreted. Similarly, if the patients included in the reviewed studies do not match the target population of the investigator, the study results may not accurately predict the clinical response to treatment. A well-designed search strategy may find no papers that adequately answer the clinical question. This situation provides the opportunity for a study that can help guide clinical decision making.

Bias Reduction in Clinical Research

To estimate a valid and precise answer to the study question, research studies should be designed to limit bias. Bias is defined as a systematic deviation from the true study results.[11] Unrecognized bias will result in a tendency toward erroneous study results. The most common types of bias are selection bias, information bias, and confounding bias (Table 1).

Selection Bias

Selection bias refers to systematic error in the ascertainment of study subjects, leading to a false association between an exposure and an outcome.[11] For example, in a study examining the association between Achilles tendon rerupture and basketball participation, selection bias would be introduced by using patients ascertained from a sports medicine clinic and a control group drawn from the general population. In this example, the characteristics of patients referred to a tertiary care sports clinic may be different from those of the general population, putting them at a higher risk for rerupture independent of their exposure status.

Differential loss to follow-up, a similar phenomenon in which there is a systematic deviation in the proportion of patients from study groups lost to follow-up, can potentially alter study conclusions. In the preceding example, patients involved in competitive sports may be more likely to attend future clinic appointments than patients drawn from the general population. This could artificially increase the association between basketball participation and tendon rerupture.

Table 1

Types of Bias in Clinical Trials

Type of Bias	Example(s)
Information	Patients fail to recall exposure (recall bias) or more complete records exist for patients with more severe disease (reporting bias). An assessor systematically underestimates range of motion using a goniometer.
Selection	Patients treated nonsurgically fail to attend follow-up appointments when rerupture occurs.
Confounding	Competitive sports participation increases the chances of surgical treatment and increases the chances of rerupture.

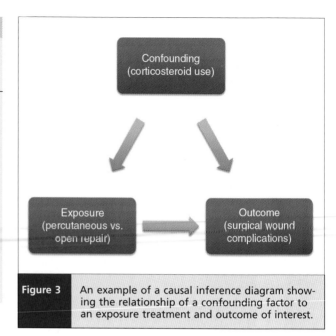

Figure 3 An example of a causal inference diagram showing the relationship of a confounding factor to an exposure treatment and outcome of interest.

Selection bias can be limited by facility-based control selection, in which the control group is drawn from the same patient population as the study group, thereby increasing the likelihood that potential confounding variables are similar in the two groups. Every effort should be made to prevent loss to follow-up.

Information Bias

Information bias results from the inaccurate classification of outcomes or flawed data collection resulting in inaccurate results.[11] Spurious conclusions resulting from measurement bias can be avoided by designing specific and reproducible information systems for data collection. Training of the study staff will increase the reproducibility of the data collected, and blinding of the assessor and the subject will improve the objectivity of measurements.[12] For example, a research coordinator may believe that surgery provides better recovery of ankle plantar flexion strength after Achilles tendon rupture. This belief may result in increased encouragement for surgically treated participants during postoperative strength testing if the participant's group assignment is known. With blinding, the predetermined beliefs of the outcome assessor cannot influence the collection of outcome data. Blinding of assessors of outcomes should be achieved wherever possible in clinical research studies to limit information bias.

Confounding Bias

Confounding bias occurs when a noncausal relationship is seen between the exposure and the outcome as a result of mixing associations with a third variable or set of variables.[13] A confounding variable is associated with both the risk factor and the outcome under study (Figure 3). For example, a study shows an association between the percutaneous treatment of Achilles tendon ruptures and wound complications. Most of the patients treated percutaneously are taking corticosteroids.

In this case, the association between corticosteroid treatment and the treatment choice and the potential for corticosteroids to impact healing and complication rates makes corticosteroid use a potential confounder of the relationship between the treatment technique and the outcome.

An important goal of clinical epidemiology is to describe an unbiased association that an exposure (such as the injury, the medical treatment, or the surgical procedure) may have with an outcome of interest. This relationship may be considered causal under certain strict conditions, with the most stringent being appropriate temporal ordering.[13] To satisfy these conditions, investigators attempt to minimize selection and information bias through rigorous study design. Randomization, restriction of enrollment, and matching are three methods that allow the control of confounding variables in clinical trials.[11]

The process of randomization, given a large sample, results in the equal allocation of known and unknown confounding factors to different treatment groups. As the incidence of a confounding factor decreases, there is a risk of unequal distribution of participants with the confounding variable to treatment groups; therefore, stratification becomes necessary. Stratification involves the separate randomization of participants with and without a given confounding factor to ensure equal distribution of that factor among treatment groups (Figure 4). Restriction involves the elimination of the effect of a confounding factor by limiting the participants to those with a single state of the confounding variable. For example, in a study of wound complications after the surgical treatment of Achilles tendon ruptures, including only those patients currently taking corticosteroids would eliminate the use of corticosteroids as a confounding factor.

Matching is another means of neutralizing confounding factors. This method involves selecting con-

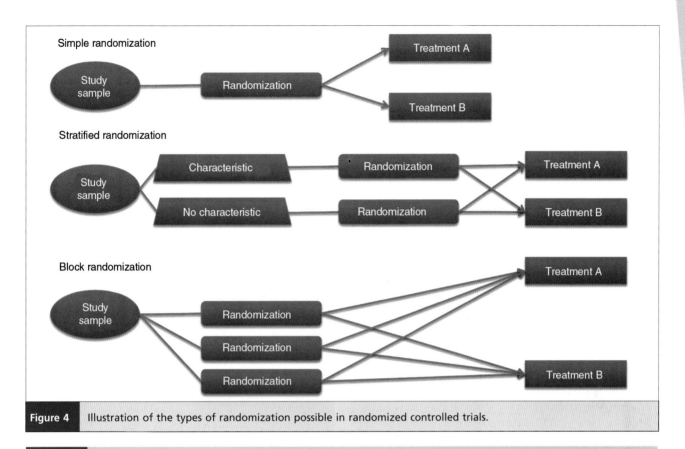

Figure 4 Illustration of the types of randomization possible in randomized controlled trials.

1: Principles of Orthopaedics

Table 2

Comparison of Analysis Methods for the Post Hoc Control of Bias in Clinical Studies

Method of Analysis	Assesses Categorical Confounding Variables	Assesses Continuous Confounding Variables	Assesses Multiple Confounding Variables Simultaneously
Stratified	Yes	No	No
Multiple regression	Yes	Yes	Yes

trol subjects based on similar characteristics. Matching can be based on one or several cofactors, such as between treated and nontreated patients in a prospective study or between participants with a positive or a negative outcome in a retrospective, case-controlled study. Age, sex, and disease severity are often used as matching criteria. Confounding also can be addressed at the analysis phase of clinical research, as will be discussed later in this chapter (Table 2).

Types of Studies

In general, two main types of clinical studies are used to investigate treatment effects: observational studies and randomized controlled trials (Figure 5). Study types are also discussed in chapter 13, Levels of Evidence and Grades of Recommendation, *Orthopaedic Knowledge Update 11*.

Observational Studies

In observational studies, participants are not randomly assigned to a treatment group. Participants are identified based on their exposure to a predetermined factor and then followed forward in time to determine the relationship between that factor and an outcome of interest (cohort study). Participants also can be identified based on an outcome, after which their exposure histories are ascertained to assess the associations of interest (case-control study). There are several types of observational study designs, each balancing the need for data and the risk of bias. In contrast, in randomized controlled trials, participants with a given set of characteristics are identified, and a treatment is randomly assigned to each participant.[14]

Randomized Controlled Trials

The randomized controlled trial is the current standard for determining causal relationships of a treatment ef-

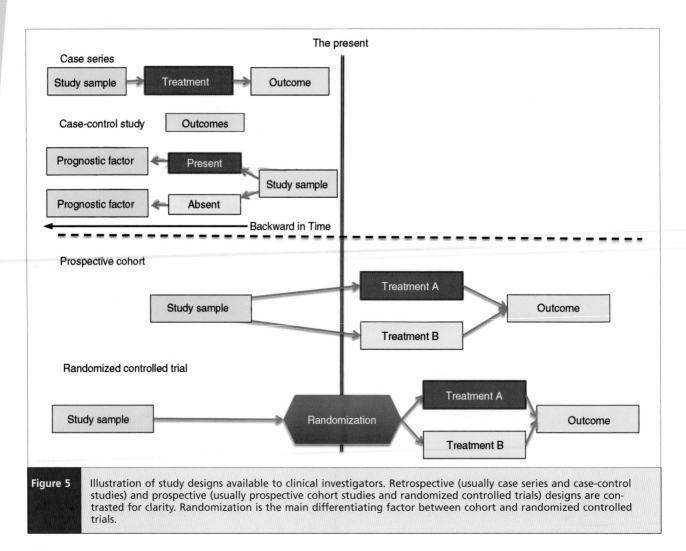

Case series

Study sample → Treatment → Outcome

Case-control study

Outcomes

Prognostic factor ← Present ← Study sample

Prognostic factor ← Absent

Backward in Time

The present

Prospective cohort

Study sample → Treatment A / Treatment B → Outcome

Randomized controlled trial

Study sample → Randomization → Treatment A / Treatment B → Outcome

Figure 5 Illustration of study designs available to clinical investigators. Retrospective (usually case series and case-control studies) and prospective (usually prospective cohort studies and randomized controlled trials) designs are contrasted for clarity. Randomization is the main differentiating factor between cohort and randomized controlled trials.

fect in clinical medicine.[15] In this study design, the investigator assigns each participant to a treatment group through a process of randomization, meaning that each participant has an equal chance of being assigned to all treatment arms.[16] Concealment of randomization is a core property of comparative trials because this process limits the bias of the investigator and the treating medical team with respect to the allocation of participants to treatment groups. This process does not eliminate the possibility of information bias if outcome assessors are not properly blinded. Randomization is intended to equally distribute (at least probabilistically) all known and unknown confounding factors among treatment groups.[13]

Randomized controlled trials, despite their methodological strengths, have several drawbacks. Performing a rigorous comparative study involves great costs and a commitment of time. It is often difficult to enroll patients in studies comparing surgical and nonsurgical treatments or in studies in which patients have preconceived treatment preferences. Randomized controlled trials often include an overly homogeneous group of patients, which makes it difficult to apply findings to diverse patient groups.

A recent randomized controlled trial of surgical versus nonsurgical management of Achilles tendon ruptures used the outcome of rerupture as a primary end point.[17] In this study, treatment variables were controlled by using identical rehabilitation protocols for the surgically and nonsurgically treated patients. Concealed randomization resulted in the equal distribution of known confounding factors; however, blinding of outcome assessors was not achieved because the treating surgeon assessed the primary outcome measure of rerupture. This may have resulted in bias in assessing rerupture; the primary outcome measure would have been better assessed by a blinded assessor. The study authors also acknowledged that the sample size may have been insufficient to detect a difference in outcomes between the two treatments.

Economic Analysis and Comparative Outcomes Research

Opportunity cost is used in the economic analysis comparing healthcare services and treatments. Essentially, economic analysis attempts to ensure that the program under study is the best way to allocate finite healthcare dollars. This can be measured by analyzing cost, cost-

Table 3

Comparison of Economic Analysis Study Designs

Type of Analysis	Allows Comparison of Two Treatments of the Same Condition	Requires Clinical Outcome Measures	Can Be Paired With Randomized Controlled Trials	Comparable Across Healthcare Domains
Cost	Yes	No	Yes	Yes/No
Cost-effectiveness	Yes	Yes	Yes	No
Cost utility	Yes	Yes	Yes	Yes

effectiveness, and cost utility (Table 3). The perspective taken is one of the fundamental decisions in economic analysis. Depending on the audience and the aims of the study, the investigator usually determines if a patient, a hospital, a health system, or a societal perspective is taken.

Cost analysis involves comparing the total cost of treatments and assumes that the efficacy of those treatments is equivalent. The units of comparison are typically currency. Only costs that are unique to one or the other treatment are considered in this analysis because common costs cancel each other. This type of analysis is useful for comparing two treatments of the same disease; however, it has limited use when attempting to influence policy regarding budget allocations between two unique clinical problems.

Cost-effectiveness studies incorporate clinical outcomes into the analysis. Units of measure tend to be expressed as cost per natural outcome unit. The more general the measure of outcome, the more easily treatments can be compared across diseases and specialties.

Cost-utility analysis takes this concept one step further and expresses the results in quality-adjusted life-years, a clinical measure that can be applied across programs and diseases. The quality-adjusted life-year represents 1 year in perfect health; any impairment in function or health status decreases the value of that year by a given fraction. For example, in one study, 1 year lived with hip arthritis would be valued at 0.49 quality-adjusted life-years based on responses by patients older than 65 years to the EuroQol Five Dimension (EQ-5D) questionnaire.[18] Cost-benefit analysis expresses the benefits of a health program in currency units. This allows the direct comparison of costs and benefits but presents the difficult task of fully valuing the monetary benefits of programs.

Prospective Cohort Studies

In a prospective cohort study, several groups are identified based on differences in an exposure of interest. The exposure can be a specific injury, a particular procedure, or a patient characteristic. The presence of a group with the exposure of interest and a control group is the main prerequisite for a prospective cohort study and differentiates this study design from the case series. Follow-up is carried out on the identified cohort of participants to look for outcomes of interest.[19]

Prospective cohort studies are similar to randomized controlled trials in all but one important characteristic: treatments are not randomly assigned. Safeguards against selection and information biases should be instituted a priori, and information should be collected on all known and measurable confounding variables for later stratification or statistical adjustment. Using these methods, research questions that do not lend themselves to randomization because of ethical or other reasons can be investigated using a cohort study design. One drawback of a prospective cohort study is the need to wait for outcomes of interest to occur. This often takes a considerable amount of time, incurs substantial expense, and presents difficulties with participant attrition.

A 2009 study comparing techniques of Achilles tendon repair prospectively enrolled patients treated with either an open or a mini-open surgical tendon repair.[20] Patients were not randomly allocated to the two treatment groups; however, they were recruited prospectively based on reported inclusion and exclusion criteria. The lack of randomization may have led to bias by the treating surgeons based on some known or unknown confounding factor, and such bias would cast doubt on the validity of the study's conclusions.

Case-Control Studies

Case-control studies are retrospective studies in which the participants are chosen based on the presence or the absence of an outcome of interest.[21] In this sense, the process of a case-control study, which identifies the presence of the outcome before the determination of factors affecting that outcome, is the reverse of a prospective study. This retrospective design allows the study of rare outcomes or those with prolonged latency periods that would not be feasible with other study designs. In this research process, cases are first identified retrospectively based on an outcome, and predetermined characteristics (for matching) of interest are included. A strict a priori definition of the methods of ascertainment of the outcome and the exposure is imperative. Control groups are composed of participants with similar characteristics who lack the outcome of interest. The composition of the control group often involves a compromise between rigor and feasibility because matching multiple characteristics will limit the number of eligible participants in the control group.

1: Principles of Orthopaedics

One limitation of case-control studies is the ability to study only one outcome of interest. There is a risk of bias in the data collected because of poor recall during patient interviews (a form of information bias) and an unequal allocation of certain factors to one of the groups (confounding bias). These limitations make it difficult to draw causal relationships between exposures and outcomes using case-control studies; however, this study design allows exploration of relationships between variables with maximal statistical efficiency, making the study of rare outcomes feasible.

A 2012 case-control study looked at the occurrence of pulmonary emboli and deep vein thromboses after Achilles tendon rupture to identify risk factors for these rare adverse events.[22] A database of 1,172 patients who had been treated for Achilles tendon rupture allowed a more precise estimation of the rate of deep vein thrombosis and pulmonary embolism after injury with minimal data collection. In this study, only nine patients had the outcome of interest, which suggests that a prospective study to assess the association between rupture and thromboembolic complications would not be feasible.

Case Series

The case series reports on the outcomes of a group of patients with similar traits who receive the same treatment.[23] Because these descriptive and often retrospective studies lack a control or comparison group, only specific inferences can be drawn from the results. Case series can be affected by selection bias because the criteria for choosing cases often are not explicitly stated. Measurement bias is an important concern because the outcome measurement is rarely blinded in case series, leading to potentially flawed outcome assessments. Despite these drawbacks, case series serve a purpose in the initial trial of a new implant or technique and may help identify safety concerns before widespread implementation. The results can be used to provide an estimate of sample size for a future randomized controlled trial. The case series can report on the natural history of a disease by reporting on disease progression in patients with a specific diagnosis.

A 2010 case series reported the results of a group of nonsurgically treated patients with Achilles tendon rupture who were managed with a functional rehabilitation protocol.[24] Functional recovery, clinical outcome, and complications were reported by the study authors; however, it is difficult to state the superiority of this method or compare the results with those of another similar study by other authors because these investigators did not evaluate a comparison treatment.[25]

Outcome Measures

Detecting treatment effects starts with selecting relevant and precise outcome measures. Treatment effects are generally quantified statistically; however, clinicians should be aware of the concept of a clinically impor-

tant difference, which is defined as the difference, from a patient's perspective, that would result in a noticeable change of outcomes for the target population. The minimally clinically important difference is a value established by clinicians based on their own experience in measuring outcomes in the condition of interest. The outcome measure must be validated for patients similar to the study's sample to ensure that the outcome construct measures the aspect of the outcome that the investigators intended to measure.[26]

The simplest outcomes to conceptualize are probably dichotomous outcomes, situations in which the outcome of interest is either present or absent. Examples are union, reoperation, infection, and survival. Many of these seemingly objective outcomes involve some judgment in the diagnosis; this introduces the risk of bias into the study. For that reason, it is desirable to assemble an adjudication committee that is blinded to treatment allocation (if possible) to democratically determine the presence or the absence of an outcome or a complication.

Patient-centered outcome measures involve determining function and the health-related quality of life.[27] Many of the current measurement instruments are self- or interview-administered questionnaires that have been rigorously validated for use in patients similar to the study population. Traditional health-related quality-of-life measures were surgeon administered, such as the Constant score for measuring shoulder function or the Harris hip score. Allowing the treating surgeon to assess outcome introduces bias. Current outcome instrument administration is standardized to decrease bias by facilitating the blinding of the assessor.

Both generic and joint disease–specific instruments are available. Generic instruments, such as the Medical Outcomes Study 36-Item Short Form and the EQ-5D, measure the overall health status of the participant and provide an estimate of the patient's functional level in society.[28,29] Each instrument has been validated in various age groups and disease states, allowing comparisons across procedures and specialties. Joint disease–specific measures include the Western Ontario McMaster Universities Osteoarthritis Index for the hip and the knee; the Disabilities of the Arm, Shoulder and Hand questionnaire for the upper extremity; and the Oswestry Low Back Pain Disability Questionnaire. All of these instruments incorporate questions that address limitations imposed by specific joint dysfunctions. Although these instruments are less generalizable to conditions outside the anatomic focus of the questionnaire, these measures are generally more sensitive to changes in function than generic outcome measures and may not be subject to the ceiling effect noted with many generic outcome instruments.

The time horizon over which measurements are taken is one consideration in outcome measurements. Clinically, surgeons can intuitively decide on the relevant time horizon for an outcome measurement based on the recovery time expected for a procedure and the expected durability of the results. For example, measuring health-related quality-of-life changes after anterior

Table 4

Types of Data and Common Statistical Tests

Dependent Variable		Independent Variable
	Two Groups	**Multiple Groups (>3)**
Categorical	Chi-square test, Fisher exact test	Chi-square
Numerical	Mann-Whitney U test, Wilcoxon signed rank test	Kruskal-Wallis test
Continuous	Student's *t* test	Analysis of variance

cruciate ligament reconstruction at only 3 month post-operatively would not be sensible because the rehabilitation period is often from 6 to 9 months. Similarly, reporting primary total hip arthroplasty survival data at 5 years does not reflect the expected 15-year survival of modern implants. Longer time horizons, however, lead to increasing challenges in patient follow-up and represent another instance of balancing the integrity of results with trial feasibility.

Analyzing Study Results

After completing follow-up on all participants or the review of the last chart, a large amount of data is available. Data can take many forms, including categorical and numerical data. Each type of data and research methodology requires appropriate statistical interrogation to draw the most accurate conclusions possible[30] (Table 4).

Categorical Data

Measurements containing two or more categories are called categorical data. This concept can be conceptualized as buckets into which observations fit, such as dead or alive; male or female; and mild, moderate, and severe disease. The simplest form of categorical data is binary data that has only two observed states, such as survival data (dead or alive).

Categorical data with more than two categories may be ordinal or nominal. Ordinal data have an obvious order and are exemplified by disease severity descriptors such as mild, moderate, and severe. Nominal data do not have an obvious order. An example of nominal data is the location of a fracture (proximal, midshaft, or distal) because these categories do not lend themselves to a natural order.

Numerical Data

Numerical data can be classified as either discrete or continuous, with the main distinction between the two forms being the restriction of values in discrete data. An example of discrete data in orthopaedic surgery trials is counting events, such as readmissions to a hospital or the number of intra-articular steroid injections. The important characteristic of this type of data is that

the separation between values is equal (for example, four injections is twice as many as two injections, whereas stage IV cartilage lesions are not necessarily twice as bad as stage II lesions).

Continuous data are obtained through measurement and can take on any measurable value based on the precision of the measuring device. Data with consistent intervals that demonstrate a normal distribution are considered normally distributed. Joint range of motion measurements determined with a goniometer are examples of continuous data. Parametric data that approximate a normal distribution with interval consistency can be illustrated by Medical Outcomes Study 36-Item Short Form scores of physical function. Nonnormally distributed numerical data such as time measurements require special consideration and statistical procedures that do not depend on the assumption of normally distributed data (Wilcoxon rank-sum test, Mann-Whitney U test).

Estimation and Hypothesis Testing

Statistical analysis of study data allows the inferences from a sample of subjects to be applied to a population of similar patients. To make such inferences, investigators and readers of scientific literature rely on estimation and hypothesis testing. With all statistical approaches, study subjects become proxies for the target population. To provide an estimate of effect, these approaches attempt to show differences or associations among variables of interest.

The process of estimation focuses on presenting the magnitude of an effect and the precision of that estimate (the sample mean and confidence interval [CI], respectively). Results are presented as a mean difference, a relative risk, or an odds ratio with a CI. A CI is a range of values that contain the target population mean with a given certainty (for example, the estimated quantity of interest will be contained within the interval 95 of 100 times for a 95% CI). The width of the CI will be determined by standard error, which is an estimate of the population standard deviation derived from variability in the sample mean estimates.

Hypothesis testing (significance testing) is based on the concept of testing the null hypothesis that the effect is zero against the alternative hypothesis that the effect is not zero. The ensuing analysis evaluates the probability (*P* value) that the data obtained could have occurred by chance. Smaller *P* values indicate a smaller probability that the observed results could have occurred by chance. Although the *P* value provides a test of the plausibility of the null and alternative hypotheses, it does not indicate the magnitude of the effect. The test statistic provides only a probability that the observed value, or one even farther from the null hypothesis, could occur by chance.

The precision of estimates and the cutpoints chosen for hypothesis testing are intended to limit the chance of error in terms of extrapolating study results to a population of interest. Two main types of error are encountered in data analysis: type I (alpha) and type II (beta) errors. Type I errors are finding an effect where, in fact, no effect exists (a false-positive result). To limit the chance of a type I error, a 95% CI or a *P* value of 0.05 are customarily selected, these values allow a 5% chance of a type I error. Type II errors, which are common in orthopaedic trials, involve finding no difference where a difference exists (a false-negative result).[31] In study design, a 10% to 20% chance of a type II error is generally accepted.

Power is defined as the probability that the study results will reject the null hypothesis if the null hypothesis is actually false. Power is related to the sample size of the study. When a lack of association or effect is reported, the reader should consider whether too few patients were enrolled to detect the effect or association of interest.

Statistical Approaches for Reducing Confounding Bias

Confounding bias can result when extraneous factors influence the observed effect of an exposure on an outcome of interest. Although rational study design can limit the effects of confounding, it is sometimes necessary to apply post hoc control for confounding variables. Subgroup analysis involves performing separate data analyses of groups within the larger study sample. For example, if an investigator believes that the risk of rerupture of the Achilles tendon after surgical or nonsurgical treatment is influenced by sex, separate analyses of rerupture rates for males and females would be appropriate. If the mean differences in rerupture rates in the male and female groups are found to be different, then statistical interaction is present, and a single, summary estimate of effect may not be appropriate. With an increasing number of confounding variables, data in each stratum become sparse and limit the use of this type of analysis.

Multiple variable regression analysis provides another method of controlling confounding factors in research studies. Regression analysis produces a linear model of data that quantifies the effect of a unit increase of each included independent variable on the dependent variable or the outcome of interest. Both continuous and categorical independent variables can be included in regression models, and, although some precision of effect estimates is lost with each included vari-

able, this method is much more statistically efficient than stratified analyses. A 2012 study investigating the association of Achilles tendon rupture with pulmonary embolism and deep vein thrombosis used logistic regression to estimate the effect of various factors on the occurrence of thromboembolic events.[22] The independent variables in the model were chosen by first performing bivariable analyses of associations with the outcome. The independent variables with sufficiently strong associations were used to build the multivariable model. One measure of a regression model's explanation of the variability in the observed data (a surrogate of robustness of the model) is expressed by the coefficient of determination (R^2) value. Other diagnostic procedures for assessing model goodness-of-fit are available and important for determining confidence in the estimates provided by a multivariable regression model. An explanation of these procedures is beyond the scope of this chapter. Consultation with a statistician is recommended when using multiple variable regression analysis.

Summary

Searching and evaluating the current literature is an essential part of evidence-based orthopaedic care. If no relevant evidence exists, it is important for investigators to develop clinical research studies to provide valid inferences regarding associations and causal relationships that will guide decision making. Increasing the methodologic quality will decrease bias at all levels of the hierarchy of evidence. Properly conducted statistical analyses clearly describe data and relationships and ultimately allow conclusions to be drawn that pertain to the target population from which the study sample originated. Clinical study design and implementation is a complex process that requires a nuanced knowledge of the clinical dilemma along with the principles of epidemiology and biostatistics. To achieve work of the highest possible quality, investigators should enlist the collaboration of experts in areas where gaps in knowledge exist.

Key Study Points

- Research methodology attempts to limit bias, a systematic deviation from the truth.

- The basis of a good comparative research question includes a well-defined study population, an intervention, a comparison group, and a validated outcome measure.

- Outcome measures should be selected carefully to ensure that they measure the effects of treatment that interest the investigator and matter to patients.

Annotated References

1. Chiodo CP, Glazebrook M, Bluman EM, et al: Diagnosis and treatment of acute Achilles tendon rupture. *J Am Acad Orthop Surg* 2010;18(8):503-510.

   A narrative review of the current treatment options for Achilles tendon rupture. Level of evidence: V.

2. Freedman B: Equipoise and the ethics of clinical research. *N Engl J Med* 1987;317(3):141-145.

3. WMA Declaration of Helsinki: Ethical Principles for Medical Research Involving Human Subjects. 2008. World Medical Association website. http://www.wma.net/en/30publications/10policies/b3. Accessed September 3, 2012.

4. Goldhahn S, Sawaguchi T, Audigé L, et al: Complication reporting in orthopaedic trials: A systematic review of randomized controlled trials. *J Bone Joint Surg Am* 2009;91(8):1847-1853.

5. Egger M, Smith GD, Altman DG: *Systematic Reviews in Health Care: Meta-Analysis in Context*, ed 2. London, England, BMJ, 2001.

6. Bhandari M, Joensson A: *Clinical Research for Surgeons*. New York, NY, Thieme, 2009.

7. Khan RJ, Carey Smith RL: Surgical interventions for treating acute Achilles tendon ruptures. *Cochrane Database Syst Rev* 2010;9:CD003674.

   In the latest update in the Cochrane library on the treatment of acute Achilles tendon rupture treatment, the authors conclude that the rerupture rate is lower in surgically repaired Achilles tendons with a corresponding increase in the rate of wound complications. Level of evidence: I.

8. Gillespie LD, Gillespie WJ: Finding current evidence: Search strategies and common databases. *Clin Orthop Relat Res* 2003;413:133-145.

9. National Institute for Health Research: PROSPERO: International Prospective Register of Systematic Reviews. York, England, PROSPERO, 2012. http://www.crd.york.ac.uk/Prospero. Accessed December 22, 2012.

   Website of the PROSPERO register of systematic reviews. This project attempts to catalogue all systematic reviews and standardize the way in which they are produced.

10. Liberati A, Altman DG, Tetzlaff J, et al: The PRISMA statement for reporting systematic reviews and meta-analyses of studies that evaluate healthcare interventions: Explanation and elaboration. *BMJ* 2009;339:b2700.

11. Szklo M, Nieto FJ: *Epidemiology: Beyond the Basics*, ed 2. Sudbury, MA, Jones and Bartlett Publishers, 2007.

12. Poolman RW, Struijs PA, Krips R, et al: Reporting of outcomes in orthopaedic randomized trials: Does blinding of outcome assessors matter? *J Bone Joint Surg Am* 2007;89(3):550-558.

13. Jewell NP: *Statistics for Epidemiology: Texts in Statistical Science Series*. Boca Raton, FL, Chapman & Hall/CRC, 2004, vol 58.

14. Katz JN, Wright JG, Losina E: Clinical trials in orthopaedics research: Part II. Prioritization for randomized controlled clinical trials. *J Bone Joint Surg Am* 2011;93(7):e30.

   The authors review the process of taking a clinical question from creation to answer and focus on the creation of randomized controlled trials in orthopaedic surgery. Subjects requiring comparative trials are explored for orthopaedic subspecialties.

15. Bederman SS, Chundamala J, Wright JG: Randomized clinical trials in orthopaedic surgery: Strategies to improve quantity and quality. *J Am Acad Orthop Surg* 2010;18(8):454-463.

   This article summarizes the challenges faced by orthopaedic surgeons attempting to plan and execute randomized controlled trials. Rather than focusing only on the specific elements of methodology, the authors catalog cultural, educational, and attitudinal reasons for the paucity of level I evidence to guide orthopaedic surgeons.

16. Boutron I, Ravaud P, Nizard R: The design and assessment of prospective randomised, controlled trials in orthopaedic surgery. *J Bone Joint Surg Br* 2007;89(7):858-863.

17. Willits K, Amendola A, Bryant D, et al: Operative versus nonoperative treatment of acute Achilles tendon ruptures: A multicenter randomized trial using accelerated functional rehabilitation. *J Bone Joint Surg Am* 2010;92(17):2767-2775.

   A recent randomized controlled trial compared surgical and nonsurgical treatment of Achilles tendon rupture. The main outcome measure was rerupture rate as determined by the treating surgeon. Randomization methodology, stratification, and blinding of assessors are all detailed in the methods section. Level of evidence: II.

18. Lawless BM, Greene M, Slover J, Kwon Y-M, Malchau H: Does age or bilateral disease influence the value of hip arthroplasty? *Clin Orthop Relat Res* 2012;470(4):1073-1078.

   This article discusses the value of a total hip arthroplasty. A decision analysis was used to allow the calculation of cost-effectiveness of the procedure. By determining a cost per quality-adjusted life-year, this procedure can be compared to other, nonmusculoskeletal medical interventions. Level of evidence: IV.

19. Bryant DM, Willits K, Hanson BP: Principles of designing a cohort study in orthopaedics. *J Bone Joint Surg Am* 2009;91(suppl 3):10-14.

1: Principles of Orthopaedics

20. Bhattacharyya M, Gerber B: Mini-invasive surgical repair of the Achilles tendon—does it reduce postoperative morbidity? *Int Orthop* 2009;33(1):151-156.

21. Busse JW, Obremskey WT: Principles of designing an orthopaedic case-control study. *J Bone Joint Surg Am* 2009;91(suppl 3):15-20.

22. Patel A, Ogawa B, Charlton T, Thordarson D: Incidence of deep vein thrombosis and pulmonary embolism after Achilles tendon rupture. *Clin Orthop Relat Res* 2012;470(1):270-274.

    An example of a large, retrospective analysis of a cohort identified by using an administrative database. The authors employ regression models to identify factors associated with thromboembolic events in Achilles tendon repairs. Level of evidence: III.

23. Kooistra B, Dijkman B, Einhorn TA, Bhandari M: How to design a good case series. *J Bone Joint Surg Am* 2009;91(suppl 3):21-26.

24. Karkhanis S, Mumtaz H, Kurdy N: Functional management of Achilles tendon rupture: A viable option for non-operative management. *Foot Ankle Surg* 2010; 16(2):81-86.

    An example from the Achilles tendon literature of a large case series. Level of evidence: IV.

25. Majewski M, Schaeren S, Kohlhaas U, Ochsner PE: Postoperative rehabilitation after percutaneous Achilles tendon repair: Early functional therapy versus cast immobilization. *Disabil Rehabil* 2008;30(20-22):1726-1732.

26. Poolman RW, Swiontkowski MF, Fairbank JC, Schemitsch EH, Sprague S, de Vet HC: Outcome instruments: Rationale for their use. *J Bone Joint Surg Am* 2009;91(suppl 3):41-49.

27. Shearer D, Morshed S: Common generic measures of health related quality of life in injured patients. *Injury* 2011;42(3):241-247.

    The authors describe and detail the appropriate application of validated clinical outcome measures for injured patients.

28. Ware JE Jr, Sherbourne CD: The MOS 36-item short-form health survey (SF-36): I. Conceptual framework and item selection. *Med Care* 1992;30(6):473-483.

29. EuroQol—a new facility for the measurement of health-related quality of life: The EuroQol Group. *Health Policy* 1990;16(3):199-208.

30. Dowrick AS, Tornetta P III, Obremskey WT, Dirschl DR, Bhandari M: Practical research methods for orthopaedic surgeons. *Instr Course Lect* 2012;61:581-586.

    This review article provides a brief review of research methods and related topics.

31. Lochner HV, Bhandari M, Tornetta P III: Type-II error rates (beta errors) of randomized trials in orthopaedic trauma. *J Bone Joint Surg Am* 2001;83(11):1650-1655.

Chapter 15

Care of the Geriatric Patient

Eric Meinberg, MD   Simon C. Mears, MD, PhD

1: Principles of Orthopaedics

Introduction

The aging of the baby boomer generation (individuals born between 1946 and 1965) means that the older segment of the population is the fastest growing. This situation presents the orthopaedic surgeon with many challenges, including caring for frail patients and those with many medical comorbidities as well as taking care of patients with osteoporotic bones, which make repair more difficult. A knowledge of basic geriatric principles is important to any orthopaedic surgeon caring for aging patients.

Demographics

Because of the aging of the baby boomers, coupled with the increased life expectancy of American adults, an ever-increasing number of geriatric patients will require management of elective and emergent orthopaedic conditions. By 2030, all baby boomers will be at least 65 years old and will fall into the geriatric age group. This segment of the population can be expected to increase by 31%, more than double the rate of younger age groups.[1] Because of better health management and decreased smoking, a woman age 65 years in 2009 can expect to live an additional 20 years. This demographic shift continues in that the number of people living beyond 100 years has increased 53% in the past 20 years and is expected to grow (Figure 1).

However, despite an increase in life expectancy, there is a significant increase in the number of comorbidities that can negatively affect an individual's health and surgical outcomes. There are 24.4% of Americans older

than 65 years who report fair or poor health, and increasing numbers of patients have heart disease, hypertension, and/or diabetes; have survived cancer; or are obese.[2] Arthritis is the most common chronic health condition, reported by 50%.[1]

Although many older patients have chronic health problems, there is also a substantial proportion of this population that remains very active. Forty percent of individuals older than 65 years report their health as very good or excellent; 35% of persons age 65 to 74 years and 24% older than 74 years report regular physical activity. Many continue to participate in high-demand activities, such as alpine skiing, cycling, swimming, and mountain climbing,[3] and there is an increasing recognition of sports injuries in the aging population.[4,5]

Preoperative Evaluation

Before orthopaedic surgery is performed, older patients should undergo a thorough medical evaluation to minimize perioperative risk. The preoperative evaluation before orthopaedic surgery is individualized and depends on the surgical team's routine practice, hospital policies, medical risk factors, and the urgency of the procedure. A more thorough evaluation is warranted in patients with multiple comorbid conditions and when the procedure is elective, whereas a targeted evaluation and intervention is needed to appropriately mitigate risk in urgent and emergent procedures.

The goal of the preoperative evaluation is simple: identify abnormalities that can be corrected to reduce the risks of surgery and shorten the subsequent recovery period. The cornerstone of this evaluation is a thorough history and physical evaluation and a review of the patient's medications. After key areas of concern are identified, targeted testing can be done to evaluate and improve modifiable conditions that the patient may have. A good preoperative evaluation should include recommendations to manage the patient's medical conditions and pain after the procedure. The routine ordering of laboratory tests and diagnostic studies, such as an electrocardiogram (ECG), without indication is of little diagnostic value and is not recommended because of its low yield.[6] Additionally, spurious positive results can lead to further testing and diagnostic dilemmas that may not benefit the patient or alter the course of care. Although abnormal test results in el-

Dr. Meinberg or an immediate family member is a member of a speakers' bureau or has made paid presentations on behalf of Synthes and Medtronic; serves as a paid consultant to or is an employee of Amgen, Medtronic, and Synthes; and serves as a board member, owner, officer, or committee member of the Northern California Chapter of the Western Orthopaedic Association. Neither Dr. Mears nor any immediate family member has received anything of value from or has stock or stock options held in a commercial company or institution related directly or indirectly to the subject of this chapter.

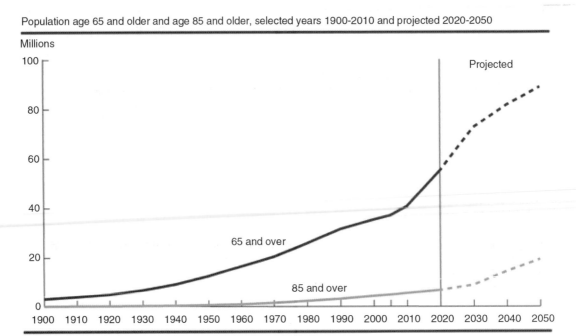

Population age 65 and older and age 85 and older, selected years 1900-2010 and projected 2020-2050

Note: These projections are based on Census 2000 results and are not consistent with the 2010 Census results. Projections based on the 2010 Census will be released in late 2012.
Reference population: These data refer to the resident population.
SOURCE: US Census Bureau, 1900 to 1940, 1970, and 1980, US Census Bureau, 1983, Table 42; 1950, US Census Bureau, 1953, Table 38, 1960, US Census Bureau, 1964, Table 155, 1990, U.S. Census Bureau, 1991, 1990 Summary Table File; 2000; US Census Bureau, 2001, *Census 2000 Summary File 1;* US Census Bureau, Table 1: Intercensal Estimates of the Resident Population by Sex and Age for the US April 1, 2000 to July 1, 2010 (US-ESTOO-INT-01); US Census Bureau, 2011. *2010 Census Summary FIle 1;* US Census Bureau, Table 2: Projections of the population by selected age groups and sex for the United States: 2010-2050 (NP2008-t2).

Figure 1 The aging population based on US census results. (http://www.agingstats.gov/Main_Site/Data/2012_Documents/Population.aspx)

derly patients are often found, they do not correlate with the risk of complications. However, simpler measures, such as the patient's American Society of Anesthesiologists physical status classification, risk of the procedure, and congestive heart failure, are predictive of postoperative complications.[7,8]

Electrocardiogram

The 2007 American College of Cardiology/American Heart Association guidelines on perioperative cardiovascular evaluation recommend a preoperative 12-lead ECG in patients scheduled to undergo surgery with any of the risk factors listed in Table 1.[9]

Chest Radiograph

An abnormal chest radiograph is more likely to be found in older patients than in the general population, especially those with a history of cardiac or pulmonary disease. In one study, only 1 of 368 patients who underwent a routine screening chest radiograph had an abnormal study.[10] A meta-analysis of routine preoperative chest radiographs involving almost 15,000 patients demonstrated only 140 unexpected abnormalities and

14 that were abnormal and for which management was changed.[11] It is unclear whether routine chest radiographs are beneficial, but they should be obtained in patients with a history of cardiopulmonary disease.

Diseases Requiring Special Consideration

Cardiac Disease

As outlined in Table 1, patients with significant or unstable cardiac disease require further evaluation and workup. This group includes those who have had a recent myocardial infarction or unstable angina. If stress testing does not demonstrate myocardial tissue at risk, surgery can proceed safely with little risk. However, those with a positive stress test will require revascularization before any elective orthopaedic procedure.

Cardiac patients without active symptoms and good functional capacity (ability to climb a flight of stairs) do not require evaluation beyond an ECG. Those with two risk factors from Table 1 also can safely undergo surgery without further workup unless it will alter management. Those with three or more risk factors,

Table 1

American College of Cardiology/American Heart Association Clinical Predictors of Increased Perioperative Cardiovascular Risk

Major Predictors That Require Intensive Management and May Lead to Delay or Cancellation of the Surgical Procedure Unless Emergent	Other Clinical Predictors That Warrant Careful Assessment of Current Status
Unstable coronary syndromes Unstable angina Severe angina Recent myocardial infarction	History of ischemic heart disease
Decompensated congestive heart failure New York Heart Association class IV Worsening heart failure New-onset heart failure	History of cerebrovascular disease
Significant arrhythmias High-grade atrioventricular block Symptomatic ventricular arrhythmias Symptomatic bradycardia New ventricular tachycardia	History of compensated heart failure or prior heart failure
Severe heart disease Severe aortic stenosis Symptomatic mitral stenosis	Diabetes mellitus
	Renal insufficiency

(Reproduced with permission from Fleisher LA, Beckman JA, Brown KA, et al: ACC/AHA 2007 guidelines on perioperative cardiovascular evaluation and care for noncardiac surgery: A report of the American College of Cardiology/American Heart Association Task Force on Practice Guidelines (Writing Committee to Revise the 2002 Guidelines on Perioperative Cardiovascular Evaluation for Noncardiac Surgery) developed in collaboration with the American Society of Echocardiography, American Society of Nuclear Cardiology, Heart Rhythm Society, Society of Cardiovascular Anesthesiologists, Society for Cardiovascular Angiography and Interventions, Society for Vascular Medicine and Biology, and Society for Vascular Surgery. *Circulation* 2007;116[17]:e418-e499.)

however, should undergo further noninvasive testing if it will alter management of the cardiac disease.[9]

Patients who had recent revascularization with a stent deserve special consideration. The risk of death or postoperative myocardial infarction is increased in those who stop antiplatelet therapy for surgery, especially if they have a drug-eluting stent because of a delay in coronary artery endothelization. Ideally, discontinuation of antiplatelet drugs should be delayed 12 months but, if necessary, can be stopped at 3 to 6 months. Those who receive a bare metal stent can stop antiplatelet therapy 4 weeks after stenting.[12] All of these patients should continue with full-strength aspirin throughout the surgical procedure and refrain from the antiplatelet drugs for as short a time as possible. Patients with drug-eluting stents are at the highest risk of thrombotic events if antiplatelet therapy is stopped. According to a guideline paper, a multidisciplinary team should measure the risk of stopping antiplatelet therapy versus the risk of bleeding if surgery must proceed.[13]

Pulmonary Disease

Patients who are being treated for asthma or chronic obstructive pulmonary disease (COPD) should be maintained on their regular medication regimens throughout the perioperative period. Those with severe COPD or asthma with physical examination findings such as wheezing, rhonchi, or rales should undergo a preoperative evaluation to identify reversible causes of postoperative pulmonary complications.[14] Alternatives to general anesthesia, such as regional blocks and epidural or spinal anesthesia, may be especially beneficial to patients with severe pulmonary disease to reduce postoperative complications. Smoking cessation more than 8 weeks before an elective surgery has resulted in a substantial reduction in pulmonary complications. Paradoxically, those who stop smoking less than 8 weeks before surgery have an increased risk of complications.[14,15]

Renal Disease

It is estimated that 5% of the US population has chronic renal disease. Geriatric patients may have acute or chronic renal failure or a combination of both conditions. It is important to note that chronic renal disease can affect both metabolic function through electrolyte imbalances and hematopoietic function, resulting in anemia and coagulopathy.

Acute renal failure must be treated before surgery and assessed by a urologist or nephrologist, and may be prerenal, intrinsic, or postrenal.

Prerenal failure causes include hypovolemia or hypotension, which result in decreased perfusion of otherwise normal functioning kidneys. Hypovolemia may be treated with an intravenous (IV) fluid bolus or a more liberal nothing-by-mouth status, allowing the patient to

1: Principles of Orthopaedics

drink clear liquids up to 3 hours before surgery. Preoperative hypotension resulting in renal dysfunction deserves a thorough evaluation before surgery, whether of an urgent or elective basis.

Intrinsic renal disease may result from infection, ischemia, or the use of nephrotoxic substances, such as aminoglycoside antibiotics or IV contrast. Treatment consists of discontinuation of the toxic substance or treating the infection that is affecting the kidney.

Postrenal failure is caused by downstream obstruction of the kidneys. Causes include renal caliculi or bladder or prostate dysfunction. Clearance of the obstruction will result in the release of a large volume of urine and allow for the recovery of renal function.

Chronic renal failure is defined as a glomerular filtration rate of less than 60 mL/min and has profound effects on perioperative morbidity and mortality. Chronic renal failure and many of its associated manifestations, including anemia, coagulopathies, and diabetes, have been identified as significant risk factors in comorbidity and mortality following total joint arthroplasty.[16] Efforts should be made to correct or normalize the metabolic and physiologic manifestations of chronic renal failure. Patients with anemia should maintain blood hemoglobin levels higher than 8 to 10 g/dL in the perioperative period. Serum potassium should remain less than 5.5 mmol/L to reduce the risk of arrhythmias; if hemodialysis is required to achieve this, the procedure should be performed 1 day before surgery to minimize fluid shifts. Medications should be reviewed with a pharmacist or an internist to ensure that there will be no medication-induced complications.

Diabetes Mellitus

Diabetes is one of the most common comorbidities and has reached pandemic status in the United States. Orthopaedic disorders such as Charcot arthropathy have been attributed to it, and a multitude of orthopaedic conditions are exacerbated by diabetes. Osteoporosis is the most common metabolic bone disease in patients with diabetes, and the cause is multifactorial. Bone mass is reduced in patients with diabetes because they tend to be more sedentary, peripheral vascular disease may contribute to lower bone vascularity and mass, and insulin's anabolic effect is absent. In addition, the effects of peripheral neuropathy and muscle deconditioning contribute to an increased fall risk.[17] Reports of increased infections and other major complications are noted throughout the literature on fracture, spine, arthroplasty, hand, and sports. Correcting associated metabolic abnormalities and normalizing blood glucose in the perioperative period can minimize complications.

Medications That Require Special Consideration

Beta Blockers

Beta-blocker medications have many potential perioperative benefits. They prevent or control arrhythmias and decrease myocardial oxygen demand. Discontinuation of beta blockers may cause rebound ischemia and complications when used for ischemic heart disease. These effects are not as significant when beta blockers are used for hypertension or migraine headaches. As a result, all patients who are on beta blockers should remain on them throughout the perioperative period and should receive them on the day of surgery, if possible. If it is determined that a patient would benefit from beta blockade during the perioperative period, it should be started early enough to be titrated to blood pressure and heart rate.[18] The use of additional beta blockade in patients undergoing high-risk surgical procedures is controversial and may lead to high rates of perioperative mortality and stroke.[19]

Other Antihypertensive Medications

Alpha-2 agonists, calcium channel blockers, angiotensin-converting enzyme (ACE) inhibitors, and diuretics may be safely continued until the day of surgery, unless there is an obvious reason, such as hypotension or hypovolemia, for them to be discontinued. Alpha-2 agonists have been shown to decrease the stress response to intubation and act as a mild anxiolytic agent during the perioperative period. Continuation of ACE inhibitors to the time of surgery increases the risk of intraoperative hypotension. Oral diuretics may affect the ability of the anesthesiologist to manage the patient's fluid balance intraoperatively, so these medications should be held the morning of surgery until the patient is able to tolerate oral intake postoperatively. Intravenous diuretics can be substituted in the perioperative period.

Corticosteroids

Surgeons who will be operating on patients who are taking glucocorticoids such as prednisone need to take special precautions before surgery. Even if taking glucocorticoids for relatively minor indications such as psoriasis or asthma, patients may have suppression of the hypothalamic-pituitary axis and are at risk for an adrenal crisis if the steroids are abruptly withdrawn or a supplemental replacement is not in place to account for the added stress of surgery. The following are general guidelines, but the patient should be evaluated by his or her internist for specific treatment recommendations: (1) Patients who have taken glucocorticoids for less than 3 weeks or have taken chronic alternate-day therapy are at low risk for adrenal suppression and should continue on their typical dose perioperatively. (2) Those who have taken the equivalent of 20 mg/day of prednisone for more than 3 weeks or have a cushingoid appearance should receive an additional perioperative stress dose of steroids. (3) Patients who have taken low doses of prednisone (5 to 20 mg/day) for more than 3 weeks should undergo further testing to evaluate the hypothalamic-pituitary axis to determine whether they require additional stress-dose steroids.

Thyroxine

Patients with hypothyroidism who receive chronic thyroxine therapy should continue to receive therapy in the perioperative period. Patients may go up to 5 to 7 days without supplementation, but if this time is exceeded, they should receive intravenous or intramuscular thyroxine at 80% of their oral dose until they are able to resume taking oral medications.

Antiplatelet Drugs

Many geriatric patients take medications that affect the normal hemostatic balance. In addition to aspirin, platelet receptor blockers such as clopidogrel and ticlopidine are administered to an increasing number of patients with a history of cardiac or thrombolic events. In patients who have received drug-eluting coronary artery stents, there is significant concern regarding catastrophic thrombosis with discontinuation before reendothelialization occurs approximately 12 months after placement. In these patients, it is recommended that platelet receptor blockers be continued except in emergencies; if discontinued, they should be restarted as quickly as possible. This group of patients should be on an aspirin regimen during this period. Because most urgent orthopaedic procedures, such as fracture fixation, do not result in critical blood loss, it is generally considered safe to continue therapy in the perioperative period.

Bisphosphonates

Many postmenopausal women are treated with bisphosphonates for chronic management of osteoporosis. The extremely long half-life of these drugs creates unique challenges in their management. Continuous use of bisphosphonates after surgery is considered safe but may be discontinued during the perioperative period if not well tolerated without any ill effects. Those who require initiation of bisphosphonate treatment following a fragility fracture may be started on this regimen immediately without any demonstrated alteration of bone healing or remodeling. Currently, it is unclear whether patients who have sustained an atypical femur fracture due to chronic bisphosphonate use would benefit from a "drug holiday" to allow for recovery of osteoclast function.

Surgical Treatment

Surgical treatment of geriatric patients presents the orthopaedic surgeon with many challenges to reduce perioperative morbidity and mortality. These patients typically have more comorbidities and frailty. Surgeries are most commonly of an urgent nature and must be performed quickly to reduce complications. Cognitive impairment can limit the types of rehabilitation with which a patient can comply. Osteoporosis is often present, and poor bone quality may affect the surgical procedure that is chosen. Because of patient frailty, there is great pressure for the surgeon to perform successful surgery and reduce the risk of reoperation.

Anesthetic Choices and Indications

Choices are available for anesthesia in the geriatric patient. Traditionally, the type of anesthetic used has not been observed to make a difference in patient outcomes.[20] It has become clear, however, that significant confounders exist in the literature. Patients with spinal anesthesia are commonly given enough supplemental medicines to also be deeply sedated at the time of their procedures.[21] In a recent randomized study, deep sedation was shown to be significantly associated with delirium when compared with light sedation.[22]

The use of regional anesthesia to augment standard techniques is also becoming popular. These techniques allow for lower doses of narcotics with fewer associated adverse effects. The use of nerve blocks in the emergency department for patients with hip fracture has been shown to reduce the need for narcotics.[23] Narcotic medicines in elderly patients lead to urinary retention, constipation, and delirium; the reduction of narcotics may reduce complications and improve outcomes as long as pain control is maintained.

Overall, the role of the anesthesiologist has expanded, and the type of anesthesia selected can affect outcomes and minimize complications after surgery; a one-size-fits-all approach is no longer applicable. Communication between the anesthesiologist, the surgeon, and the medical team is essential to allow for efficient care of the geriatric patient. Communication will lessen delays and lessen the number of cases that are cancelled.

Mitigation and Management of Blood Loss

Geriatric patients, especially those who are frail, are more likely to have chronic anemia. During major orthopaedic procedures, anemia is a major risk factor for postoperative blood transfusion.[24] The trigger for transfusion after surgery has been a subject of debate. The old standard was a goal hemaglobin of 10 g/dL. The recent Functional Outcomes in Cardiovascular Patients Undergoing Surgical Hip Fracture Repair (FOCUS) trial has provided some information that a trigger of 8.5 g/dL is safe in elderly patients after hip fracture repair.[25] The need for blood transfusion should be based on symptomatic anemia. This should be individualized in patients with severe coronary disease, renal failure, or other comorbidities that may need a higher trigger value.

Mitigation of blood loss should be considered throughout a surgical procedure. The use of tranexamic acid during major surgeries seems safe and may decrease the need for blood transfusions after surgery.[26] The surgeon should pay careful attention to detail during surgery and exercise efficiency to shorten the procedure in the geriatric patient. This should affect surgical decision making in the frail, elderly patient who may not tolerate an extensive and extended surgery.

Blood loss should first be treated with fluid management. Patients are often dehydrated when they have refrained from eating or drinking overnight. This problem is compounded in urgent or emergent procedures.

Patients with hip fractures are typically severely dehydrated at admission. IV fluid repletion is essential preoperatively and intraoperatively.[27]

Thermoregulation

All patients get cold in the operating room. The frail patient with little body mass is more prone to a lowered core temperature. Cold temperatures are associated with complications, including higher infection rates. Particular care must be taken with elderly patients in the operating room to ensure that they remain covered and warm. The use of air-warming devices is necessary and attention to detail is paramount to ensure the patient keeps his or her temperature at an optimum level throughout the procedure.

Consideration of Tissue Quality and Robust Repair

Both soft tissue and bone are weakened in the elderly patient. Periosteum and soft tissues are thinner and weaker in elderly patients than in younger patients. Frailty is associated with muscle weakness and sarcopenia, and bones often are osteoporotic. All of these factors make rehabilitation more difficult and surgical planning important in elderly patients. The surgeon needs to recognize that fixation that may be sufficient in a younger patient may not be feasible in a geriatric patient, affecting surgical decision making and possibly changing the type of repair offered. The elderly patient may do better with replacement rather than fracture fixation. These factors need to be recognized and surgical plans changed according to the individual patient.

Postoperative Treatment

Prevention of Complications

The prevention of complications is probably the most important aspect of the care of the geriatric patient. Because of their frail condition, elderly patients will more poorly tolerate errors compared with younger patients.[28,29] Each organ system is susceptible to iatrogenic injury during routine hospital care. Medicine selection must be assessed to avoid renal damage. The frail patient is unable to tolerate reoperation. Surgery should provide a reliable, long-lasting solution so that only one procedure is necessary for treatment. Some surgical complications are common in elderly patients and are described in the following sections.

Decubitus Ulcers

The skin of the elderly patient is more susceptible to pressure ulcers because of the absence of protective sensation secondary to pain, delirium, or dementia and thinner subcutaneous fat layers and hypoperfusion. A higher Braden scale rating predicts pressure ulcer formation.[30] The Braden scale is commonly used by nursing staff and evaluates sensory perception, activity, mobility, and nutrition, as well as moisture and friction at the potential ulcer site. The time to dermal injury is potentially as little as 1 to 2 hours, increasing the risk of decubitus in patients who cannot move. Ulcerations may occur on the heels or buttocks or from the edge of a splint, a cast, or a brace.

Pressure ulcers may develop in one third of elderly patients with hip fracture.[31] These ulcers often require months of healing and sometimes additional procedures. The expense related to management is tremendous to the healthcare system; ulcers are often the reason for nonpayment of the hospital by Medicare as a "never" event.[32] Prevention is the mainstay of treatment. It has been suggested that patients be turned every 2 hours.[33] In particular, splinted or numbed extremities (after the administration of a regional anesthetic) are susceptible to ulcers and must be watched. The use of prophylactic padding with a hydrocolloid dressing in high-risk patients should be considered.

Infection

Infection is a feared complication in all patients; however, elderly patients are unable to tolerate the extra antibiotics needed to fight infection or additional surgeries. Excessive or inappropriate use of antibiotics may lead to devastating *Clostridium difficile* overgrowth. As in all patients, the use of perioperative antibiotics and excellent surgical technique is needed for infection prevention. Foley catheters should be removed the day after surgery to reduce the risk of urinary tract infection. Mobilization and early incentive spirometry will help to decrease the risk of pneumonia and atelectasis.

Deep Vein Thrombosis

The geriatric patient is at risk of deep vein thrombosis after major limb surgery or trauma, especially in the lower extremity. The American College of Chest Physicians Evidence-Based Clinical Practice Guidelines and the American Academy of Orthopaedic Surgeons (AAOS) guidelines recommend prophylaxis, particularly in patients undergoing hip and knee replacement or hip fracture repair.[34,35] These recommendations also should be followed for patients who are immobilized or who have lower extremity trauma. Care must be taken in selecting agents when patients are already on blood thinners for other purposes. No information is available for those who must also continue on antiplatelet agents, although it is known that patients on oral anticoagulants for atrial fibrillation and antiplatelet drugs for a coronary stent are at high risk of bleeding.[36] In these cases, the risks of excessive bleeding must be weighed against the risk of deep vein thrombosis and individual decisions made.

Delirium

The most common complication in the perioperative period for the geriatric patient is delirium. Delirium occurs twice as often in the patient with cognitive dysfunction[27] as in those with normal cognitive function. Delirium has been shown to increase the length of hospital stay as well as morbidity and mortality.[37] The prevention of delirium in elderly patients is multifactorial.

Surgical delays in fracture patients should minimized. Careful attention to medications to prevent iatrogenically caused delirium is important. Medications have been classified by the American Geriatric Society Beers Criteria to help practitioners avoid potential unfriendly medications to the geriatric population.[38] The American Geriatrics Society has made an easy-to-use pocket list of these criteria to help avoid medications that cause delirium or other preventable side effects. In particular, anticholinergic medicines are commonly used and have a high potential for delirium in elderly patients. Attention to detail is the most important means of prevention. Other strategies to reduce delirium rates include normalization of the hospital environment, decreased sounds, and promoting sleep at night; surgery performed in a timely manner and reduced waiting times also decrease delirium rates.

The careful selection of a pain management protocol appropriate for the geriatric patient is important to minimize pain while minimizing the adverse effects of narcotic medicines. Many elderly patients also have cognitive impairment that affects both measurements of pain and influences patterns of pain medicine prescription. Fixed doses of acetaminophen are a useful adjunct to decrease pain without increasing the likelihood of delirium. Low-dose oxycodone (2.5 to 5.0 mg) can be added as needed for pain control. Care should be taken with additional medications to avoid polypharmacy and other potential drug interactions in elderly patients.

The Confusion Assessment Method is used to diagnose delirium (Table 2). The key features of delirium are a change in mental status that is acute and fluctuates. Hypoactive delirium is common and not diagnosed as often as hyperactive delirium. Although difficult to diagnose, delirium occurs often in patients with dementia. A key factor in diagnosis is examining the patient over time and referring to caregivers to help understand baseline status.

If delirium is recognized, the first action should be a determination of the cause with rectification. Electrolyte abnormalities, excessive pain, infection, or acute medical conditions should be treated. Narcotics overuse should be addressed. Delirium at night should be treated with nonpharmacologic interventions. The patient should not be left alone at night so that the use of restraints can be avoided; the environment should remain familiar. Eyeglasses and hearing aids should be used by the patient if needed.

After a careful examination and laboratory and medication reviews have been performed and if nonpharmacologic interventions have failed, the use of low-dose haloperidol can be considered. Dosage should start at 0.5 mg orally. Higher doses will lead to sedation and then a rebound effect with even worse delirium that may last for weeks. Long-acting benzodiazepams should be avoided because these will sedate the patient and lead to long-lasting delirium.

Table 2

Confusion Assessment Method

1. Acute onset and fluctuating course
2. Inattention
3. Disorganized thinking
4. Altered level of consciousness

Rehabilitation Goals

Early Mobilization, Weight Bearing, and Range of Motion

The goal of rehabilitation in the elderly patient is to restore function to the preoperative level. Because frail patients do not tolerate immobility well, every attempt should be made to allow patients to bear weight fully and have full range of motion after surgery. All patients with hip fractures should be allowed to fully bear weight after surgery.[39] Periprosthetic fractures, ankle fractures, and intra-articular fractures are problematic in this regard. If weight-bearing restrictions are required, long-term nursing care may be needed for elderly patients. Immobility leads to worse outcomes. Elderly patients have difficulty restricting weight bearing, and every attempt should be made to improve surgical fixation to allow for weight bearing as tolerated after surgical repair. Rehabilitation should not be delayed after surgery, and specialized approaches elderly patients are helpful.[40]

Osteoporosis Evaluation and Management

Osteoporosis is a common condition in frail, elderly patients. All patients older than 50 years who have had a fracture should be evaluated for osteoporosis, beginning with a dual-energy x-ray absorptiometry scan to assess bone density and an assessment of vitamin D levels. Patients with osteoporosis should be treated using a team approach. Because most patients want to avoid additional medications and are therefore reluctant to treat osteoporosis, typical compliance rates are 20%. Comprehensive programs have significantly affected the rates of compliance. A strategy for the treatment of osteoporosis in patients with fracture needs to be coordinated. This can be by the orthopaedic surgeon, by a metabolic bone clinic, or through the patient's primary care physician. Best results have been seen in managed care situations where pathways are used to encourage patients to undergo osteoporosis diagnosis and management.[41]

Comanaged Care

Rationale

The care of the elderly patient is often difficult because of multiple system failures and the many medications

1: Principles of Orthopaedics

such patients are sometimes required to take. Thus, the prevention of complications is paramount. A team approach to care through different models, with the co-management approach that allows orthopaedic surgeons to team with a hospitalist,[42] a medical doctor, or a geriatrician, has been found to have significant advantages for the patient.[43] Both teams must agree on those items for which they are responsible. For example, the orthopaedic surgeon may be in charge of the surgical wound, the surgery, weight bearing, and rehabilitation as well as deep vein thrombosis prophylaxis. The medical side of the team is responsible for making sure the patient is adequately prepared for surgery, fluid therapy, medication reconciliation, and medical management. In the comanaged care model, both teams can write orders for the patient. Communication and the use of pathways are essential to success. Communication needs to occur several times each day between teams. Weekly meetings need to occur to review care and fine-tune management.

Improved Outcomes

Comanaged care has been shown to save money and improve quality and outcomes in patients who have had a hip fracture or have undergone joint arthroplasty.[44,45] A shorter length of hospital stay and decreased complications have been shown using a hospitalist as well as with geriatric models. Comanagement has been implemented in different countries with similar results and seems to be a robust addition to the care of the elderly patient. A key element of this approach is buy-in from the hospital. An important aspect of a comanaged service is routine outcome collection and the use of this information to prove to hospital administration that better, cheaper care is being provided.

High-Energy Trauma

High-energy trauma is a particularly dangerous occurrence in the geriatric patient. Mortality rates have been found to be three times higher than in younger patients, and even minor injuries, such as clavicle fractures, can be fatal.[46] Pelvic fractures, which would be benign in the younger patient, may be lethal in the geriatric patient. Lateral compression injuries may lead to extensive blood loss and mortality.

Summary

The practicing orthopaedic surgeon needs to know basic geriatric principles. In the future, the fastest growing patient population in the area of trauma will be the geriatric patient. The avoidance of geriatric-unfriendly medications, early surgery, and medical comanagement are important to achieve optimal outcomes in this growing patient population. Reoperation must be avoided. A team approach to care is essential to improve quality, which in turn lowers costs. This includes postfracture care and the treatment of osteoporosis after fractures.

Key Study Points

- Preoperative evaluation in the geriatric patient should identify conditions that will affect surgery and then optimize the patient in a timely manner.

- Geriatric patients do not tolerate complications (either medical or surgical), and the practitioner must pay attention to detail to avoid postoperative problems.

- A comanaged approach to the geriatric patient will improve results and reduce costs of care.

Annotated References

1. Administration on Aging: *A Profile of Older Americans*. United States Department of Health and Human Services, 2011.

    This report from the Administration on Aging reviews data from the 2010 census regarding older adults in the United States.

2. National Center for Health Statistics: *Health, United States, 2011: In Brief*. Hyattsville, MD, 2012.

    This report from the Centers for Disease Control and Prevention is an annual update on health statistics across the United States.

3. Kammerlander C, Braito M, Kates S, et al: The epidemiology of sports-related injuries in older adults: A central European epidemiologic study. *Aging Clin Exp Res* 2012;24(5):448-454.

    This retrospective study analyzes the cause of sports injuries seen in 2,635 patients older than 65 years between 1994 and 2008. The authors emphasize that older adults remain active, and the prevention of injury in older adults needs to be considered.

4. Prescott JW, Yu JS: The aging athlete: Part 1, "boomeritis" of the lower extremity. *AJR Am J Roentgenol* 2012;199(3):W294-306.

    This review describes sports injury patterns in the lower extremity of older patients.

5. Quatman C, Yu JS: The aging athlete: Part 2, "boomeritis" of the upper extremity. *AJR Am J Roentgenol* 2012;199(3):W307-321.

    This review describes sports injury patterns in the upper extremity of older patients.

6. Hepner DL: The role of testing in the preoperative evaluation. *Cleve Clin J Med* 2009;76(suppl 4):S22-S27.

7. Dzankic S, Pastor D, Gonzalez C, Leung JM: The prevalence and predictive value of abnormal preoperative laboratory tests in elderly surgical patients. *Anesth Analg* 2001;93(2):301-308.

8. Liu LL, Dzankic SS, Leung JM: Preoperative electrocardiogram abnormalities do not predict postoperative car-

diac complications in geriatric surgical patients. *J Am Geriatr Soc* 2002;50(7):1186-1191.

9. Fleisher LA, Beckman JA, Brown KA, et al: ACC/AHA 2007 guidelines on perioperative cardiovascular evaluation and care for noncardiac surgery: A report of the American College of Cardiology/American Heart Association Task Force on Practice Guidelines (Writing Committee to Revise the 2002 Guidelines on Perioperative Cardiovascular Evaluation for Noncardiac Surgery) developed in collaboration with the American Society of Echocardiography, American Society of Nuclear Cardiology, Heart Rhythm Society, Society of Cardiovascular Anesthesiologists, Society for Cardiovascular Angiography and Interventions, Society for Vascular Medicine and Biology, and Society for Vascular Surgery. *J Am Coll Cardiol* 2007;50(17):e159-e241.

10. Rucker L, Frye EB, Staten MA: Usefulness of screening chest roentgenograms in preoperative patients. *JAMA* 1983;250(23):3209-3211.

11. Archer C, Levy AR, McGregor M: Value of routine preoperative chest x-rays: A meta-analysis. *Can J Anaesth* 1993;40(11):1022-1027.

12. Vandvik PO, Lincoff AM, Gore JM, et al: Primary and secondary prevention of cardiovascular disease: Antithrombotic therapy and prevention of thrombosis, 9th ed. American College of Chest Physicians Evidence-Based Clinical Practice Guidelines. *Chest* 2012;141(2, suppl):e637S-e668S.

Current guidelines for patients with coronary artery disease are reviewed. Single antiplatelet drug therapy is recommended for patients with coronary artery disease, whereas dual platelet therapy is recommended for patients within 1 year of stent procedures.

13. Korte W, Cattaneo M, Chassot PG, et al: Peri-operative management of antiplatelet therapy in patients with coronary artery disease: Joint position paper by members of the working group on Perioperative Haemostasis of the Society on Thrombosis and Haemostasis Research (GTH), the working group on Perioperative Coagulation of the Austrian Society for Anesthesiology, Resuscitation and Intensive Care (ÖGARI) and the Working Group Thrombosis of the European Society for Cardiology (ESC). *Thromb Haemost* 2011;105(5):743-749.

A consensus position is presented for antiplatelet therapy in the perioperative period. The group recommends a multidisciplinary review of each patient to optimize the risks and the benefits of continuing or stopping antiplatelet therapy for surgery.

14. Edrich T, Sadovnikoff N: Anesthesia for patients with severe chronic obstructive pulmonary disease. *Curr Opin Anaesthesiol* 2010;23(1):18-24.

An evidence-based approach for managing patients with lung disease who require surgery is presented.

15. Bushnell BD, Horton JK, McDonald MF, Robertson PG: Perioperative medical comorbidities in the orthopaedic patient. *J Am Acad Orthop Surg* 2008;16(4):216-227.

16. Bozic KJ, Lau E, Kurtz S, et al: Patient-related risk factors for periprosthetic joint infection and postoperative mortality following total hip arthroplasty in Medicare patients. *J Bone Joint Surg Am* 2012;94(9):794-800.

In 40,919 Medicare patients undergoing hip arthroplasty, rheumatologic disease (hazard ratio [HR] = 1.71), obesity (HR = 1.73), coagulopathy (HR = 1.58), and preoperative anemia (HR = 1.36) were found to be significant risk factors for periprosthetic infection.

17. Hofbauer LC, Brueck CC, Singh SK, Dobnig H: Osteoporosis in patients with diabetes mellitus. *J Bone Miner Res* 2007;22(9):1317-1328.

18. Marsland D, Colvin PL, Mears SC, Kates SL: How to optimize patients for geriatric fracture surgery. *Osteoporos Int* 2010;21(suppl 4):S535-S546.

This review paper discusses the preoperative management of geriatric patients undergoing urgent surgery.

19. Flynn BC, Vernick WJ, Ellis JE: β-Blockade in the perioperative management of the patient with cardiac disease undergoing non-cardiac surgery. *Br J Anaesth* 2011;107(suppl 1):i3-i15.

This article reviews the literature addressing the use of β-blockade for patients with coronary disease who require surgery. Although initial studies showed this method to improve outcomes, more recent studies have shown that the complications of beta blockade may outweigh the benefits.

20. Neuman MD, Silber JH, Elkassabany NM, Ludwig JM, Fleisher LA: Comparative effectiveness of regional versus general anesthesia for hip fracture surgery in adults. *Anesthesiology* 2012;117(1):72-92.

In a retrospective cohort review of 18,158 patients, the authors show an advantage to regional anesthesia over general anesthesia for elderly patients undergoing hip fracture repair.

21. Sieber FE, Gottshalk A, Zakriya KJ, Mears SC, Lee H: General anesthesia occurs frequently in elderly patients during propofol-based sedation and spinal anesthesia. *J Clin Anesth* 2010;22(3):179-183.

In a prospective observational study of 40 patients undergoing hip fracture repair with spinal anesthesia and propofol based sedation, electroencephalographic monitoring using a bispectral index showed routine sedation levels consistent with general anesthesia.

22. Sieber FE, Zakriya KJ, Gottschalk A, et al: Sedation depth during spinal anesthesia and the development of postoperative delirium in elderly patients undergoing hip fracture repair. *Mayo Clin Proc* 2010;85(1):18-26.

In this prospective randomized clinical study, light sedation with spinal anesthesia reduced postoperative delirium by 50% when compared to deep sedation in elderly patients undergoing hip fracture repair.

23. Luger TJ, Kammerlander C, Gosch M, et al: Neuroaxial versus general anaesthesia in geriatric patients for hip fracture surgery: Does it matter? *Osteoporos Int* 2010;21(suppl 4):S555-S572.

1: Principles of Orthopaedics

This review discusses the pros and cons of anesthetic choices for hip fracture repair.

24. Vochteloo AJ, Borger van der Burg BL, Mertens B, et al: Outcome in hip fracture patients related to anemia at admission and allogeneic blood transfusion: An analysis of 1262 surgically treated patients. *BMC Musculoskelet Disord* 2011;12:262.

This retrospective study shows that preoperative and postoperative anemia are independent risk factors for poor outcomes after hip fracture repair.

25. Carson JL, Terrin ML, Noveck H, et al: Liberal or restrictive transfusion in high-risk patients after hip surgery. *N Engl J Med* 2011;365(26):2453-2462.

The prospective randomized FOCUS trial shows that a restrictive transfusion threshold of 8 g/dL does not change mortality or morbidity when compared with a more liberal threshold of 10 g/dL.

26. Yang ZG, Chen WP, Wu LD: Effectiveness and safety of tranexamic acid in reducing blood loss in total knee arthroplasty: A meta-analysis. *J Bone Joint Surg Am* 2012;94(13):1153-1159.

This meta-analysis shows that tranexamic acid is safe and reduces blood loss after knee replacement.

27. Lee HB, Mears SC, Rosenberg PB, Leoutsakos JM, Gottschalk A, Sieber FE: Predisposing factors for postoperative delirium after hip fracture repair in individuals with and without dementia. *J Am Geriatr Soc* 2011; 59(12):2306-2313.

In this retrospective review of patients undergoing hip fracture repair, preexisting dementia changes the risk factors for developing delirium after surgery.

28. Makary MA, Segev DL, Pronovost PJ, et al: Frailty as a predictor of surgical outcomes in older patients. *J Am Coll Surg* 2010;210(6):901-908.

This prospective study shows that frailty predicts length of stay, complications, and discharge disposition in elderly patients undergoing surgery.

29. Higuera CA, Elsharkawy K, Klika AK, Brocone M, Barsoum WK: 2010 Mid-America Orthopaedic Association Physician in Training Award: Predictors of early adverse outcomes after knee and hip arthroplasty in geriatric patients. *Clin Orthop Relat Res* 2011;469(5):1391-1400.

This prospective study examines risk factors for complications in elderly patients undergoing hip and knee replacement.

30. Braden BJ, Maklebust J: Preventing pressure ulcers with the Braden scale: An update on this easy-to-use tool that assesses a patient's risk. *Am J Nurs* 2005;105(6):70-72.

31. Baumgarten M, Margolis DJ, Orwig DL, et al: Pressure ulcers in elderly patients with hip fracture across the continuum of care. *J Am Geriatr Soc* 2009;57(5):863-870.

32. Rosenthal MB: Nonpayment for performance? Medicare's new reimbursement rule. *N Engl J Med* 2007; 357(16):1573-1575.

33. Rich SE, Margolis D, Shardell M, et al: Frequent manual repositioning and incidence of pressure ulcers among bed-bound elderly hip fracture patients. *Wound Repair Regen* 2011;19(1):10-18.

This retrospective study questions the efficacy of frequent repositioning in preventing decubitus ulcers in nursing home patients.

34. Falck-Ytter Y, Francis CW, Johanson NA, et al: Prevention of VTE in orthopedic surgery patients: Antithrombotic Therapy and Prevention of Thrombosis, 9th ed. American College of Chest Physicians Evidence-Based Clinical Practice Guidelines. *Chest* 2012;141(2, suppl): e278S-e325S.

Guidelines are presented by the American College of Chest Physicians based on evidence-based approaches for preventing thrombotic events after orthopaedic surgery.

35. Mont MA, Jacobs JJ, Boggio LN, et al: Preventing venous thromboembolic disease in patients undergoing elective hip and knee arthroplasty. *J Am Acad Orthop Surg* 2011;19(12):768-776.

Guidelines are presented to prevent thrombotic events after hip and knee replacement surgery in an evidence-based guideline approach by the AAOS.

36. Gutierrez A, Rao SV: Atrial fibrillation and percutaneous coronary intervention: Stroke, thrombosis, and bleeding. *Curr Treat Options Cardiovasc Med* 2011; 13(3):203-214.

This review examines the use of antiplatelet medicines in patients undergoing coronary stent procedures who must be on other anticoagulants.

37. Marcantonio ER, Flacker JM, Michaels M, Resnick NM: Delirium is independently associated with poor functional recovery after hip fracture. *J Am Geriatr Soc* 2000;48(6):618-624.

38. American Geriatrics Society 2012 Beers Criteria Update Expert Panel: American Geriatrics Society updated Beers Criteria for potentially inappropriate medication use in older adults. *J Am Geriatr Soc* 2012;60(4): 616-631.

The American Geriatric Society uses an evidence-based approach to list medicines with potentially undesirable adverse effects in elderly patients.

39. Koval KJ, Sala DA, Kummer FJ, Zuckerman JD: Postoperative weight-bearing after a fracture of the femoral neck or an intertrochanteric fracture. *J Bone Joint Surg Am* 1998;80(3):352-356.

40. Bachmann S, Finger C, Huss A, Egger M, Stuck AE, Clough-Gorr KM: Inpatient rehabilitation specifically designed for geriatric patients: Systematic review and meta-analysis of randomised controlled trials. *BMJ* 2010;340:c1718.

This meta-analysis examines rehabilitation protocols for patients after hip fracture repair.

41. Dell R: Fracture prevention in Kaiser Permanente Southern California. *Osteoporos Int* 2011;22(suppl 3): 457-460.

    A 10-step program for osteoporosis treatment is presented that, when used in an effective healthcare organization, has led to a 40% reduction in fractures.

42. Phy MP, Vanness DJ, Melton LJ III, et al: Effects of a hospitalist model on elderly patients with hip fracture. *Arch Intern Med* 2005;165(7):796-801.

43. Friedman SM, Mendelson DA, Kates SL, McCann RM: Geriatric co-management of proximal femur fractures: Total quality management and protocol-driven care result in better outcomes for a frail patient population. *J Am Geriatr Soc* 2008;56(7):1349-1356.

44. Kammerlander C, Roth T, Friedman SM, et al: Orthogeriatric service—a literature review comparing different models. *Osteoporos Int* 2010;21(suppl 4):S637-S646.

    This review examines the concept of the orthogeriatric service in several patient care models.

45. Kates SL, Mendelson DA, Friedman SM: Co-managed care for fragility hip fractures (Rochester model). *Osteoporos Int* 2010;21(suppl 4):S621-S625.

    This article provides the nuts and bolts behind establishing a comanaged hip fracture program. The authors show dramatic reductions in cost and improvements in care.

46. Keller JM, Sciadini MF, Sinclair E, O'Toole RV: Geriatric trauma: Demographics, injuries, and mortality. *J Orthop Trauma* 2012;26(9):e161-e165.

    This retrospective review of elderly patients who sustain high energy trauma shows high mortality and morbidity rates in this group.

1: Principles of Orthopaedics

Section 2

Systemic Disorders

SECTION EDITOR:
Javad Parvizi, MD, FRCSC

Chapter 17
Bone and Calcium Metabolism

Parth A. Vyas, MD   Anish Potty, MD   Vinay Aggarwal, BA   Gregg Klein, MD   Joseph M. Lane, MD

Introduction

Bone is a specialized connective tissue with a high level of biologic activity. The human skeleton serves unique and vital mechanical and biologic functions, which include but are not limited to providing supporting framework; protecting vital organs; providing attachment sites to ligaments and muscles; storing minerals such as calcium, phosphorus, and sodium; and providing space for hematopoietic and lymphopoietic activities. To meet these functions effectively, bone has two distinct structural components. Cortical or compact bone is responsible for strength and resistance to tensile and sheer forces, whereas cancellous or trabecular bone has a higher surface area and is mainly responsible for metabolic and biologic functions.[1]

Composition of Bone

Bone is composed of organic matrix and inorganic minerals. The organic matrix is composed of type 1 colla-

---

---

gen and noncollagenous proteins, such as osteopontin, osteocalcin, fibronectin, thrombospondin, bone sialoprotein, growth hormones, and cytokines.[2] The inorganic portion is composed of hydroxyapatite crystals, with the composition $Ca_{10}(PO_4)_6(OH)_2$. Hydroxyapatite consists of 65% to 70% of the dry weight of bone, is responsible for its mechanical properties, and is the primary reservoir of calcium and phosphorus.[1]

Cellular Regulation of Bone and Calcium Metabolism

Osteoprogenitor cells are mesenchymal stem cells found near all bony surfaces. When stimulated by Runt-related transcription factor 2/core-binding factor subunit α-1 (RUNX2/CBFA1) transcription factor network and the Wnt/β-catenin signaling pathway, these cells are capable of differentiation to osteoblasts.

Osteoblasts synthesize, transport, and arrange the many proteins of matrix and initiate the process of mineralization. Osteoblasts have receptors that bind regulatory hormones (parathyroid hormone [PTH], vitamin D, leptin, and estrogen), cytokines, growth factors, and extracellular matrix proteins and, in turn, express several factors that regulate the differentiation and function of osteoclasts. Osteoblasts surrounded by newly deposited organic matrix transform into osteocytes; alternatively, osteoblasts remaining on the bone surface may become flattened and quiescent bone-lining cells.[1]

Osteocytes communicate with each other and the cells on the bone surface via an intricate network of cytoplasmic processes known as canaliculi, and they help control calcium and phosphate levels in the microenvironment and detect and translate mechanical forces into biologic activity (mechanotransduction).

Osteoclasts are the cells responsible for bone resorption and are derived from the same hematopoietic progenitor cells that also give rise to monocytes and macrophages. The cytokines and growth factors that regulate human osteoclast differentiation and maturation include macrophage colony-stimulating factor (M-CSF), interleukin-1 (IL-1), and tumor necrosis factor (TNF). Mature multinucleated osteoclasts (containing 6 to 12 nuclei) form from the fusion of circulating mononuclear precursors and have a limited life span (approximately 2 weeks). The osteoclast signaling pathway involves three factors: (1) the transmembrane receptor activator of nuclear factor-κB (RANK), which is expressed on osteoclast precursors; (2) RANK ligand (RANKL), which is expressed on osteoblasts and marrow stromal cells; and (3) osteoprotegerin (OPG), a secreted "decoy" receptor made by osteoblasts and several other types of cells that can bind RANKL and thus short-circuit its interaction with RANK. When stimulated by RANKL, RANK signaling activates the transcription factor NF-κB, which is essential for the generation and the survival of osteoclasts. A second important pathway involves M-CSF produced by osteoblasts and the M-CSF receptor, which is expressed by osteoclast progenitors. Activation of the M-CSF receptor stimulates a tyrosine kinase activity that is also crucial for the generation of osteoclasts. The other notable pathway is the Wnt/β-catenin pathway. Wnt proteins produced by marrow stromal cells bind to the low-density lipoprotein receptor-related protein 5 (LRP5) and LRP6 receptors on osteoblasts and thereby trigger the activation of β-catenin and the production of OPG. Osteoclasts share many characteristics of foreign body giant cells, such as their common origin from monocyte-macrophage lineage and their response to inflammatory cytokines such as TNF and IL-1. They bind to the bone surface via integrins, where they form an underlying resorption pit. The cell membrane overlying the resorption pit is thrown into numerous folds (the ruffled border). The osteoclast removes the mineral by generating an acidic environment using a proton pump system and digests the organic component by releasing proteases.[3]

Hormonal Regulation of Bone and Calcium Metabolism

All the aforementioned cellular activities are closely regulated by hormonal influences. PTH, vitamin D, and calcitonin are major hormones involved in bone mineral homeostasis, but other factors such as thyroid, insulin, insulin-like growth factor, growth hormone, and prostaglandins also play some part. The role of fibroblast growth factor-23 (FGF-23) is being discussed in relation to bone mineralization and some hypophosphatemic conditions.

Parathyroid glands identify low calcium levels in extracellular fluid and respond by secreting PTH, which then increases calcium reabsorption and decreases phosphate reabsorption in renal tubular cells. PTH also increases calcium absorption from the gut through an increased conversion of vitamin D into the active 1,25-OH metabolite. It stimulates osteoblasts directly and osteoclasts indirectly through osteoblasts. The effect of PTH on bone is dual and complex, but it ultimately increases bone resorption. The net effect of PTH is an increase in serum calcium level, when it is continuously released.[4] Intact PTH is the preferred laboratory test to evaluate PTH status in the body.

Vitamin D is either generated from the diet or is synthesized in the skin because of the effect of ultraviolet light. It is converted into 25 hydroxyvitamin D in the liver, and 25 hydroxy vitamin D is converted to 1,25 dihydroxyvitamin D (the active form) in the kidneys. Vitamin D stimulates the synthesis of calcium-binding proteins in the gut and the kidneys and promotes calcium absorption at these sites. It also promotes phosphate absorption from the gut and mineralization of the skeleton. The effects of vitamin D are not limited to bones. Recently, its influence on immunology, muscle function, and pathogenesis of some tumors has been identified. 25 hydroxyvitamin D level in serum is the preferred laboratory assay to evaluate vitamin D status.[5]

The role of FGF-23 in bone biology was first identified in human genetic and acquired rachitic diseases, such as autosomal dominant hypophosphatemic rickets, tumor-induced osteomalacia, and X-linked hypophosphatemic rickets. In these conditions, increased levels of the protein are accompanied by impaired tubular phosphate reabsorption, hypophosphatemia, low (or inappropriately normal) levels of 1,25 dihydroxyvitamin D, and impaired skeletal mineralization (rickets or osteomalacia). More recently, FGF-23 has also been shown to regulate PTH metabolism based on observations that it can suppress PTH secretion both in vitro and in vivo.[6]

Bone Quality and Density

The optimal health of the skeleton relies on both quality and quantity of bone. Bone resorption and formation are closely coordinated procedures that assist in the growth, development, and repair of microdamage to bone. Bone formation predominates during the first two to three decades of life, and peak bone mass is achieved in the third decade of life. After the fourth decade of life, bone resorption predominates, and a constant decrease in bone mass is observed. In females, a precipitous decrease in bone mass occurs around menopause because of the lack of anabolic effects of estrogen. In addition to hormonal factors, other factors such as polymorphisms in the receptors for vitamin D and LRP5/6, nutrition, physical activity, and age can also influence bone mass and bone mineral density.[1]

Bone quality is an important and independent parameter of bone health. Inadequate mineralization, most commonly a result of vitamin D deficiency, is an important bone quality issue encountered in routine clinical practice. Accumulation of microdamage as a result of the inability to repair bone wear and tear is an important bone quality issue in patients on long-term antiresorptive therapy, although bone quantity and density can be normal in such patients.

Osteopenia and Osteoporosis

Reduced bone mineral density (BMD) is prevalent in elderly individuals. Because of increased life expectancy, BMD issues can be major public health liabilities. For instance, the estimated lifetime risk of having a hip fracture and a vertebral fracture in a 50-year-old American woman is 17.5% and 15.6%, respectively. According to World Health Organization (WHO) guidelines, osteoporosis is defined as having a BMD of 2.5 standard deviations below the young normal mean, and osteopenia is defined as BMD between −1 to −2.5 standard deviations from the young normal mean.[7]

Risk Factors for Low BMD

Several factors are found to have a role in the development of osteoporosis. Calcium intake, physical activity, early menarche, and late menopause are associated with higher BMD, whereas smoking,[8] family history, white race, low body weight, and glucocorticoid intake are considered significant risk factors for the development of osteopenia or osteoporosis. Multiparity, lactation, caffeine intake, and alcoholism are also considered important risk factors, but conclusive evidence is lacking.[7]

Screening and Detection Strategies

Screening of elderly individuals for the presence of osteoporosis or osteopenia is considered an effective strategy to prevent potentially hazardous complications, such as fractures. Considerable controversies exist regarding the optimum testing interval. Dual energy x-ray absorptiometry (DEXA) scans are usually repeated at 2-year intervals in all patients and at 1 year intervals in patients who have a change in treatment.[7] Considerable data are in support of longer testing intervals in people with normal or slightly low BMD (T-score greater than −1.5).[9]

Indications for BMD Testing

BMD testing is indicated in women at least 65 years of age and men at least 70 years of age regardless of clinical risk factors; younger postmenopausal women and men age 50 to 69 years about whom there is concern based on their clinical risk factor profile; women in the menopausal transition phase if there is a specific risk factor associated with increased fracture risk, such as low body weight, prior low-trauma fracture, or medication for high risk; adults who have a fracture after age 50 years; adults with a condition (such as rheumatoid arthritis) or who are taking medication (for example, glucocorticoids in a daily dose ≥ 5 mg prednisone or equivalent for ≥ 3 months) associated with low bone mass or bone loss; anyone being considered for pharmacologic therapy for osteoporosis; anyone being treated for osteoporosis to monitor treatment effect; and anyone not receiving therapy in whom evidence of bone loss would lead to treatment.[7] DEXA is currently the most widely used method and gold standard for osteoporosis detection and follow-up. A DEXA scan is done on the hips, lumbar spine, and forearm. A peripheral DEXA scan has also been suggested because it reduces radiation exposure. The accuracy and the precision of a peripheral DEXA scan in fracture risk prediction is yet to be established.[7] In addition to DEXA, other methods such as quantitative CT and ultrasonography are described in the literature, but a lack of standards for comparison limits their use in clinical practice.

Fracture Risk Assessment

BMD is an excellent tool for detecting osteoporosis and is an effective predictor of fracture risk. Despite the high specificity of BMD, the sensitivity of DEXA is low. In addition to BMD measured by DEXA, several other factors affect an individual's probability of having a fracture. A history of low-energy fracture is a strong predictor of future fractures. In a patient with a vertebral fracture, the probability of experiencing another vertebral fracture during the first year is 19.2%, and having a vertebral fracture at baseline increases the probability of having another in 1 year by fivefold.[10] Another study has shown that persons with prior hip fractures are at three times higher risk and those hospitalized with other nonhip fractures are at 1.8 times higher risk of subsequent fractures.[11] Other significant risk factors include low body mass index, glucocorticoid exposure, a parental history of hip fracture, smoking, excessive intake of alcohol, and rheumatoid arthritis.

WHO has developed an online fracture risk assessment tool (FRAX) that incorporates all the aforementioned risk factors and calculates the probability of an individual having an osteoporotic fracture in 10 years. Treatment should be considered for patients with osteopenia in whom the 10-year risk of hip fracture is 3% or the 10-year risk of a major osteoporosis-related fracture is 20% as assessed with FRAX.[12] The National Osteoporosis Foundation (NOF) estimates that 10 million people in the United States have osteoporosis, and almost 34 million more are at increased risk because of osteopenia and other associated risk factors that may impair bone quality.[7] Thus, most patients with increased fracture risk are osteopenic, but not osteoporotic. It is the large population of osteopenic patients in which it is difficult to make treatment-related decisions; thus FRAX is an extremely helpful tool.

Treatment of Osteoporosis and Osteopenia

The primary goal of the treatment of osteoporosis is prevention of fragility fractures and the potential devastating complications resulting in increased morbidity and mortality and decreased function. Because osteoporosis is a generalized problem (throughout the skeleton), it can influence both management and outcome of almost all orthopaedic conditions, which mainly include degenerative spine and joint disorders.

There is sufficient evidence that osteoporosis treatment is most effective in terms of patient compliance when it is initiated by orthopaedic surgeons. According to a randomized controlled study, adherence to treatment occurred in 58% of patients when treatment was initiated and followed by an orthopaedic surgical team compared with 29% when primary care physicians initiated the treatment.[13] In another study of BMD testing, discussion about osteoporosis and the initiation of

Table 1

Antiosteoporotic Drugs

Antiresorptive Agents	Anabolic Agents
Bisphosphonates	Teriparatide (PTH 1-34)
Calcitonin	PTH 1-84
Estrogen	Strontium ranelate
Estrogen agonists/	(notapproved by FDA)
antagonists	
Denosumab	

PTH = parathyroid hormone.

treatment were three times higher in patients in whom BMD testing was ordered by a treating orthopaedic surgeon than in patients for whom a letter was sent to their primary care physician by the treating orthopaedic surgeon after a distal end radius fracture.[14] General guidelines for treatment are discussed in this section, but it is important to understand that an individualized approach is required for optimum management.

Nonpharmacologic Intervention

Because osteoporosis is a multifactorial disorder, its treatment requires a careful mixture of lifestyle interventions.

Diet is an important factor in maintaining bone health. In general, calcium intake between 1,000 and 1,200 mg and vitamin D intake between 600 and 800 IU is recommended to maintain positive calcium balance and reduce bone loss. A diet high in fiber and sodium can reduce calcium absorption, and the dose of calcium should be adjusted accordingly. In addition to calcium and vitamin D, magnesium, boron, vitamin C, and vitamin K are important for skeletal health, but routine supplementation for these nutrients is not recommended. It is worth noting that calcium and vitamin D requirements in elderly individuals vary considerably based on diet, ultraviolet light exposure, medicines, and underlying malabsorption; thus, it is important to monitor the serum levels of calcium, 25-hydroxyvitamin D, and PTH and periodically adjust the doses.[15]

Exercise is important in building and maintaining peak bone mass.[7] A general recommendation is that exercises should be performed two to three times per week and must include weight bearing and impact exercises. During the exercise program, care should be taken to assign loading exercises to the areas that are prone to fragility fractures, particularly the spine and the hip. Fall prevention strategies, such as balance and gait training; tai-chi; muscle conditioning; and the use of appropriate assisting devices, hip protectors, and protective flooring can make a difference in an individual's probability of having a fragility fracture. Neurologic disorders such as dementia and parkinsonism should be adequately treated.

Pharmacologic Interventions

Drugs are considered the most predictable method for treating osteoporosis (Table 1). The NOF recommends drug interventions in people with a hip or vertebral (clinical or morphometric) fracture, a T-score ≤ −2.0 at the femoral neck or spine after appropriate evaluation to exclude secondary causes, low bone mass (T-score between −1.5 and −2.0 at the femoral neck or spine), and a 10-year probability of a hip fracture ≥ 3% or a 10-year probability of a major osteoporosis-related fracture ≥ 20% based on the United States-adapted WHO algorithm.

In routine clinical practice, antiresorptive agents are usually used first to treat osteoporosis. Four bisphosphonates are approved by the FDA for osteoporosis management. Alendronate, risedronate, and ibandronate are orally administered, whereas zolendronic acid is administered intravenously. Both alendronate and risedronate treatment can reduce vertebral and hip fractures by approximately 45%. Risedronate can reduce the incidence of vertebral and hip fractures, by 70% and 41%, respectively. Ibandronate is administered as a monthly oral tablet and is comparable to alendronate and risedronate for preventing vertebral fractures, but its efficacy for hip fracture is yet to be proven. Fracture risk reduction with zolendronic acid is 35% for all fractures and 70% for vertebral fractures. Zolendronic acid is administered intravenously once per year to avoid unpleasant gastric side effects and esophagitis, and compliance is ensured. The deposition of bisphosphonates in long bones and a long physiologic half-life are responsible for a small incidence of atypical fractures.[16] Estrogen and estrogen-like agents in females can prevent bone loss, but the benefits should be carefully weighed against the potential risk for gynecologic malignancies. Of the selective estrogen receptor modulators currently approved for clinical use, only raloxifene has been approved for the prevention and treatment of osteoporosis. Raloxifene has consistently proven to increase BMD in the lumbar spine and the femoral neck by 2% to 3% and decrease levels of bone-turnover markers by 30% to 40% (levels comparable with mean levels found in premenopausal women). Raloxifene can significantly reduce the risk of vertebral fracture, but its efficacy for the prevention of hip fractures has not yet been proven.[16] Estrogen can increase bone mass and reduce fracture risk, but it is no longer used in the management of osteoporosis because it is associated with an increase in the incidence of breast and endometrial cancers.

Denosumab is a fully human monoclonal antibody against RANKL that prevents the interaction of RANKL with its receptor (RANK) on osteoclasts and osteoclast precursors and reversibly inhibits osteoclast-mediated bone resorption. Denosumab can effectively reduce the risk of vertebral fracture by 68% and hip fracture by 40%. Denosumab is promptly reversible but is also associated with atypical fractures and jaw necrosis with prolonged use.[17]

Calcitonin-salmon is FDA approved for the treatment of osteoporosis in women who are at least 5 years postmenopause. Calcitonin was found to exert its antiresorptive effects via directly reducing osteoclastic resorption and thus leads to an increase in BMD and bone strength. Furthermore, calcitonin appears to mainly target the most active osteoclasts; in contrast to most other antiresorptive agents, it does not reduce the number of osteoclasts. Its action on osteoclasts is reversible; although attenuating resorption, calcitonin treatment does not interfere markedly with bone formation, in contrast to other currently available antiresorptive agents.[18] Calcitonin reduces the risk of vertebral fracture, but evidence regarding its efficacy in the reduction of risk for hip fractures is weak.[19] It is mostly used in patients with active vertebral fracture because it does not inhibit fracture healing and has an additional benefit of pain relief.[20]

Teriparatide is indicated for use in patients in whom first-line agents fail, those with an active fracture, and for low turnover osteoporosis. Teriparatide is PTH 1-34, which is genetically engineered fractionated PTH. When administered intermittently, both PTH 1-34 and PTH 1-84 stimulate osteoblasts and produce anabolic effects on bone. After prolonged treatment, PTH also stimulates osteoclasts, but anabolic action still predominates, and the ultimate effect is bone formation.[4] The increase in BMD by PTH 1-34 daily subcutaneous dose is 13% every 2 years.[21] The risk of vertebral fracture and nonvertebral fracture is reduced by 65% and 53%, respectively. Teriparatide can also reverse potential adverse effects of long-term bisphosphonate therapy, such as osteonecrosis of the jaw and stress reaction in the cortex of the femur. It has a potential risk for osteosarcoma, proven in animal studies at doses 30 to 40 times higher than the dose in humans, but so far it has not been found to increase the risk of osteoporosis in humans using the therapeutic dose for osteoporosis. It is common practice to follow teriparatide treatment with an antiresorptive agent for 1 to 2 years to prevent loss of newly deposited bone.

Strontium ranelate is one of the anabolic agents with proven antifracture activity used in the treatment of postmenopausal osteoporosis. Its mechanism of action makes it different from other drugs because it simultaneously stimulates two reverse processes: bone formation and bone resorption. The action of the agent depends on various mechanisms, including the activation of calcium receptors, localized on osteoblasts and osteoclasts, and the influence on the OPG/RANKL system. The drug effectively prevents spinal, hip, and extravertebral fractures. The agent's antifracture efficacy within the spine does not depend on the patient's age, base BMD values, or the concentration of bone metabolism markers. As to the antifracture efficacy in the hip, it affects women with an increased bone fracture risk. Strontium ranelate increases BMD within the lumbar spine and the hip, decreases the concentrations of bone resorption markers, and increases the concentrations of bone formation markers.[22] The drug is administered in a daily 2.0-g oral dose. Although strontium ranelate use is not approved by the FDA, strontium salts are available in the United States as strontium citrate.

Over-the-counter preparations are half the weight of the recommended dose, and citrate contains half the elemental strontium than ranelate, and thus its efficacy in antiosteoporosis treatment is doubtful.

Monitoring of the patient for response to treatment is of vital importance to prevent adverse effects and ensure patient compliance. Both laboratory parameters and BMD should be periodically measured in patients on drug therapy. For treatment monitoring, the NOF recommends that a central DEXA scan be done at 2-year intervals, with reduction in the screening interval if found necessary by the clinician. All the DEXA scans should be done at the same place with the same technology and should be read by the same person to make valid comparisons. Quantitative CT can also be helpful in this regard. Peripheral DEXA or quantitative ultrasonography do not change predictably in patients undergoing treatment and thus are not recommended. Laboratory tests should be done to measure calcium and vitamin D levels. PTH level can also be a useful guide to judge serum calcium and vitamin D levels. Bone-specific alkaline phosphatase, osteocalcin, and N-terminal peptide of type 1 collagen are markers of osteoblastic function and should be elevated in patients being treated by anabolic agents. Urinary N-terminal telopeptide or serum C-terminal telopeptide are the markers of bone resorption and should decrease in patients on antiresorptive drugs. It is worth mentioning that to be valid, these tests should be done in the morning after fasting overnight and preferably at the same laboratory every time.[7]

An intelligent combination of pharmacologic and nonpharmacologic interventions, nutritional interventions, and patient education are necessary to treat an individual with osteoporosis in an optimum manner.

Osteomalacia and Rickets

Vitamin D deficiency has protean manifestations broadly termed as osteomalacia in adults and rickets in growing children. Vitamin D deficiency and insufficiency are an underestimated problem among orthopaedic surgeons, but as many as 70% of orthopaedic trauma patients have low vitamin D levels when they are evaluated. Considerable controversies exist regarding optimum vitamin D levels; a serum level of 12.5 ng/mL or below is considered deficient. However, vitamin D insufficiency exists when levels of vitamin D are not frankly depleted but are associated with increased levels of PTH (secondary hyperparathyroidism). In this state, low levels of 1,25 vitamin D lead to a decrease in serum calcium, which stimulates the parathyroid gland and leads to the production and secretion of more PTH. PTH endeavors to return serum calcium levels to normal by increasing 1-hydroxylase activity and tubular reabsorption of calcium in the kidney and by enhancing osteoclastic bone resorption, thus releasing calcium stores from the bone. Currently, vitamin D levels greater than 30 ng/mL are considered adequate in general, but some researchers even advocate levels closer to 50 ng/mL.[23]

Table 2

Classification of Rickets

Type 1	Type 2
Vitamin D deficiency or abnormal vitamin D metabolism leading to deficiency of active vitamin D (dietary deficiency or 1-hydroxylase deficiency)	Renal tubular disorders leading to defective phosphate reabsorption (Fanconi syndrome, familial hypophosphatasia, X-linked hypophosphatamic rickets)

Vitamin D deficiency in children manifests as rickets, which is characterized by the inability to mineralize bone generated by the growth plate, leading to characteristic changes and deformities in the growth plate. Malnutrition and a lack of sunlight exposure are the most common causes of rickets, but other causes exist[24] (**Table 2**).

The clinical signs of rickets depend on the age of onset and the severity of the deficiency. Rickets will be at its most severe when the deficiency coincides with a period of rapid growth. Poor mineralization of the skeleton leads to skeletal deformities that are more common in infancy, when affected children develop deformities of their weight-bearing limbs. Crawling children tend to develop forearm deformities, whereas toddlers develop genu varum (bow legs) or genu valgum (knock knees). Other clinical signs include retarded growth; swelling of the wrists, knees, and ankles; and frontal bossing of the skull. The costochondral junctions of the anterior ribs can also be affected (rickety rosary). Tooth eruption can be delayed, and if tooth enamel develops at a time of moderate hypocalcemia, it is hypoplastic. In addition, muscle weakness leads to hypotonia, and affected children are often irritable. Where vitamin D deficiency is the sole abnormality, skeletal development is not unduly delayed, but if the cause of rickets is the result of renal disease or intestinal malabsorption, then skeletal maturity is delayed.[25]

In adults, vitamin D deficiency results in impaired mineralization of bone, leading to osteomalacia. Secondary hyperparathyroidism leads to bone resorption and accelerated osteoporosis and increases the risk of fragility fractures. In adults, vitamin D deficiency is subtle and often missed because unless it is severe, it is radiologically and clinically silent. Apart from vitamin D deficiency, renal failure and oncogenic osteomalacia as a result of FGF-23 overproduction are important causes of osteomalacia in adults.

In addition to generalized osteopenia, the classic radiologic features of rickets are widening of the epiphyseal plates, with associated fraying and cupping of the metaphyses of the long bones. Because long bones develop at different stages, signs of rickets will vary in intensity in different parts of the skeleton. A radiograph of the wrist usually shows these characteristic changes. Rickets is more pronounced at the distal radius com-

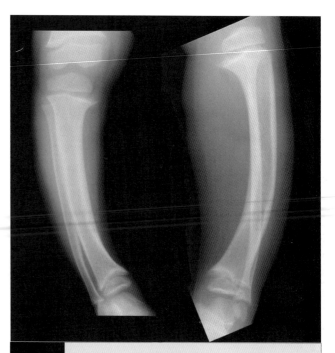

Figure 1 AP radiograph of both tibias in a child with rickets, widening of the growth plates, and lateral bowing of the tibias. (Courtesy of Robert Schneider, MD, Department of Radiology, Hospital for Special Surgery, New York, NY.)

pared with the distal ulna, as most of the growth of the radius arises from this growth plate (**Figure 1**).

Radiographs of the skeleton in patients with osteomalacia tend to be normal, although subperiosteal erosions because of secondary hyperparathyroidism can be seen on radiographs of the hand. Cortical bone may appear lamellated because of increased porosity. The classic radiographic sign of osteomalacia is a pseudofracture, or a Looser transformation zone: narrow radiolucent bands composed of unmineralized osteoid, that extend in a perpendicular fashion across the cortex. There may be an overall reduction in bone density, but equally there is often a coarsening of trabeculae. The vertebral bodies may have an amorphous ground-glass appearance. Lateral spinal radiographs may reveal a banded sclerosis seen in vertebral bodies. Condensation of trabecular bone adjacent to the vertebral end plates occurs, and this imparts an appearance of alternating bands of increased and diminished density (rugger jersey spine). This feature is secondary to hyperparathyroidism and not specific to osteomalacia[26] (**Figures 2** and **3**). If bone densitometry is performed, BMD will be reduced. In addition, in the elderly, this reduction in BMD may also be a consequence of an associated osteoporosis.

The diagnosis of rickets is based mainly on a classic radiologic and clinical picture. Vitamin D levels in serum can be confirmatory. Increased bone-specific alkaline phosphatase and secondary hyperparathyroidism are expected. Serum phosphorus level should be measured to rule out hypophosphatemia.

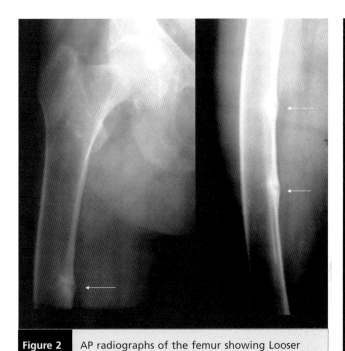

Figure 2 AP radiographs of the femur showing Looser zones (arrows). (Courtesy of Robert Schneider, MD, Department of Radiology, Hospital for Special Surgery, New York, NY.)

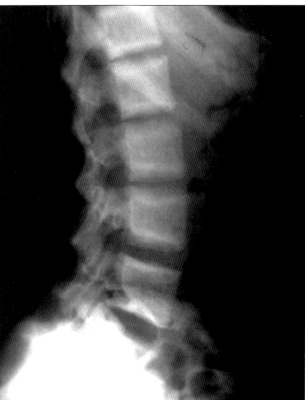

Figure 3 Lateral radiograph of the spine showing rugger jersey appearance caused by hyperparathyroidism. (Courtesy of Robert Schneider, MD, Department of Radiology, Hospital for Special Surgery, New York, NY.)

The most reliable diagnostic procedure, but one that is rarely indicated clinically, is bone biopsy and bone histomorphometry. Excessive unmineralized matrix is diagnostic of osteomalacia and rickets.

The treatment of both rickets and osteomalacia involves dosing with vitamin D, either as D_3 or D_2. Vitamin D_3 is the preferred form for supplementation because it is better absorbed. Varying doses and treatment regimens have been described, but the aim is to achieve a 25-hydroxyvitamin D level between 20 and 50 ng/mL. Supplementation with calcium is also helpful, particularly in elderly individuals, to suppress the raised PTH levels and expedite the healing process, particularly in those with a poor calcium intake. Hypophosphatemia should be corrected with phosphorus supplements to correct underlying metabolic abnormalities caused by hypophosphatemic rickets.[27]

Surgical management is rarely required in the form of corrective osteotomies except in cases of severe rickets with deformities.

Paget Disease

Paget disease of bone, also known as osteitis deformans, is characterized by an accelerated rate of abnormal bone remodeling leading to overgrowth at focal sites and mechanical bone weakness. Although capable of affecting any bone, there is a predilection for the skull, spine, pelvis, and long bones of the lower extremity. Paget disease is the second most common metabolic bone disease after osteoporosis and most commonly affects individuals older than 55 years. It is estimated to occur in 1% to 2% of the general US population, with increasing prevalence in older age groups and in men.[28] Paget disease of bone does not affect children, and the disorder juvenile Paget disease (hyperphosphatasia) is unrelated to the pathogenesis of adult Paget disease.

Current research suggests a combination of environmental and genetic influences in the development of Paget disease of bone. Environmental factors such as a viral etiology have been discussed, but further study is still required. Various gene mutations have been correlated with the development of Paget disease, with the alteration in the *SQSTM1* gene most strongly linked, although its specific role in bone metabolism is not yet fully understood.[29] It is suspected that the effect of gene mutations results in overactive osteoclast and osteoblast activity, with reports of bone formation rates six to seven times greater than normal.[30] Although bone formation is increased, the resulting lamellar structure is abnormal and mechanical strength is diminished.

Most patients with Paget disease are asymptomatic, and the diagnosis is most often made incidentally with elevated serum alkaline phosphatase or a radiograph performed for another reason. Bone biopsy is not typically needed for diagnosis. However, classic histologic findings include an increased number of osteoclasts and newly formed bone with widened lamellae and irregular cement lines, producing the characteristic mosaic pattern. The normal fatty or hematopoietic marrow spaces are also replaced by loose, highly vascularized fibrous connective tissue. Osteoclastic and osteoblastic activities eventually decrease, leaving sclerotic and deformed bones. Patients suspected of having Paget disease should undergo bone scintigraphy to evaluate the extent of disease.

The most common symptom is bone pain that is often worse at rest and relieved with movement. The pain may originate from the bone lesion itself or from bone overgrowth, leading to osteoarthritis or nerve impingement. One of the most common symptoms is low back pain because of spinal stenosis. Paget disease in the skull may also lead to hearing loss. True malignancy may develop, but the incidence is low (< 1%).[29] In patients with asymptomatic Paget disease, pharmacologic treatment is not generally necessary but patients should be monitored yearly for signs of progressive disease or impairment. Generally, therapy is indicated for asymptomatic patients when alkaline phosphatase is two to four times above the upper limit of normal.

The gold standard treatment of Paget disease of bone is with newer-generation nitrogen-containing bisphosphonates, which are capable of producing long-term remission without the toxic effects of inhibiting mineralization seen in earlier-generation bisphosphonates. Bisphosphonates reduce bone turnover by inhibiting osteoclastic bone resorption. Although bone lesions on radiographs rarely fully return to normal, the reduced bone turnover allows for new bone formation in normal lamellar structure.[31] Recent studies indicate that although intensive bisphosphonate therapy is effective in drastically normalizing serum alkaline phosphatase levels, there is no clinical advantage when compared with symptom-driven management with less aggressive bisphosphonate therapy. Calcitonin, an antiresorptive agent, is now infrequently used with the advent of newer-generation bisphosphonates and is typically reserved only when bisphosphonates are not tolerated. Analgesics are commonly used as adjunctive therapy to bisphosphonates, in addition to physical therapy, bracing, and walking aids.

The role of surgery in Paget disease includes corrective osteotomy for long bone deformity, fracture fixation, joint arthroplasty, spinal decompression, and the resection of bone tumors. Few patients require surgical treatment with the success of newer-generation bisphosphonates and effective pain management. Patients who undergo surgery are at increased risk for intraoperative complications such as increased blood loss because the bone has become abnormally hypervascular. However, patients who undergo surgery have reported improved quality of life.

Osteopetrosis

Osteopetrosis is a rare, heritable metabolic disorder caused by defective bone resorption by osteoclasts. There are multiple gene mutations linked to osteopetro-

sis, the most common being a defect in the osteoclast-specific proton-pump subunit (TCIRG1).[32] The genetic defects ultimately lead to diminished function of osteoclast carbonic anhydrase, which would normally acidify the region deep to osteoclasts and therefore allow for dissociation and resorption of the mineralized matrix. The decrease in osteoclastic activity leads to an abnormally high bone mass and density, but a decrease in mechanical bone strength leads to increased fractures. The improper resorption of bone can also cause bone growth within the medullary cavity, leaving limited space for hematopoietic cells. Thus, osteopetrosis is not solely an orthopaedic condition but may involve medical conditions such as bone marrow suppression that lead to pancytopenia and immune deficiency.

The mode of inheritance is dependent on the type of osteopetrosis. There are three primary types: rapidly progressing congenital or infantile autosomal recessive, intermediate autosomal recessive, and chronic adult autosomal dominant.[33] The congenital form is the most severe and is often lethal because of the absence of bone remodeling that results in severe bone marrow suppression. It is characterized by hepatosplenomegaly, thrombocytopenia, cranial and optic nerve palsy, osteomyelitis, and immune deficiency. Intermediate autosomal recessive osteopetrosis is characterized by recurrent fractures, short stature, neuropathies, tetanic seizures secondary to hypocalcemia, and pancytopenia.[34] The autosomal dominant form occurs more often in adults and is less severe than the congenital form. Adult forms may be asymptomatic but bone healing is delayed, fragility fractures occur, and the incidence of osteomyelitis, especially in the jaw, is increased.

The diagnosis of osteopetrosis primarily is made clinically with radiographic evaluation. There is a characteristic bone within a bone appearance and diffuse sclerosis affecting the skull, the spine, and the pelvic and appendicular bones. The diagnosis can be confirmed with genetic testing, but it is not mandatory for diagnosis. Treatment of congenital osteopetrosis involves bone marrow transplantation from an HLA-matched donor, which may potentially resolve the hematologic abnormalities and be life saving. For patients who are not candidates for bone marrow transplantation and have severe symptoms, interferon gamma-1b reportedly is an effective alternative.[35] Treatment of adult-onset osteopetrosis is largely symptomatic, and life expectancy is normal. Fractures and arthritis are prevalent in the adult-onset type, and surgical intervention with specialized drills for the unique bone type may be required to prevent delayed union or nonunion of fractures and osteomyelitis.[36]

The increased bone density seen in osteopetrosis can also result from other pathological and pharmacologically induced processes. For example, with pycnodysostosis, a lysosomal storage disease, a cysteine protease found in osteoclasts known as cathepsin K is deficient because of a mutation at chromosome 1q21.[37] Cathepsin K is responsible for the osteoclast's degradation of type I collagen and other proteins in the bone matrix.[38] In pycnodysostosis, therefore, bone is characteristically

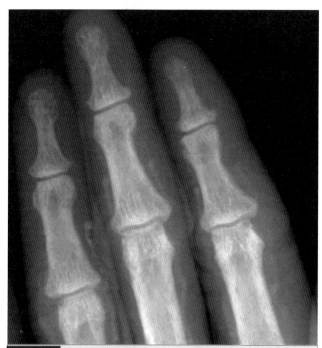

Figure 4   AP radiograph of phalanges showing subperiosteal bone resorption on the radial aspects of the middle phalanges, and arterial calcification in hyperparathyroidism from renal failure. (Courtesy of Robert Schneider, MD, Department of Radiology, Hospital for Special Surgery, New York, NY.)

osteosclerotic and prone to fractures, particularly at the extremities and the clavicle. Other signs of the disease include unusually short distal phalanges, delayed closure of skull sutures leading to a prolonged opening of the infantile fontanelle, and short stature.[37,38] Research enhancing the understanding of the role of cathepsin K in bone metabolism has led to pharmacologic developments that exploit the inhibition of the osteoclast protease to treat pathologic bone diseases. A new drug, odanacatib, is a cathepsin K inhibitor that has passed phase III clinical trials for the treatment of osteoporosis. Based on its mechanism of action, odanacatib produces a transient pycnodysostotic state and may ultimately prove useful for treating other diseases of low bone density or osteolysis. The drug shows significant promise for mainstream use in the treatment of osteoporosis by 2015.[39]

Hyperparathyroidism

The clinical picture resulting from elevated PTH levels in the serum is called hyperparathyroidism. Overactivity of the parathyroid gland that is responsible for elevated PTH level in the serum is called primary hyperparathyroidism. Examples of conditions causing primary hyperparathyroidism are parathyroid adenoma, hyperplasia, or ectopic glands. Clinical features include nephrolithiasis, proximal muscle weakness, and psychi-

atric symptoms such as anxiety, depression, and aches and pains.

When an elevated PTH level in serum is secondary to low calcium and vitamin D levels or chronic renal diseases, it is termed secondary hyperparathyroidism. In patients with chronic long-standing secondary hyperparathyroidism, regulation over secretion of PTH sometimes is lost and hypercalcemia and high PTH levels coexist. This condition is termed tertiary hyperparathyroidism and is most often seen in people with chronic renal diseases, but it is also seen in those with hypophosphatemic rickets.[40]

The skeletal changes are sometimes striking, with radiographs demonstrating osteopenia and subperiosteal resorption of the tufts and digits of the hands and feet. Brown tumor is a classic manifestation of hyperparathyroidism and can be confused with other lytic lesions, including tumors and cysts[41] (**Figure 4**).

Diagnosis and differentiation between different types of hyperparathyroidism can be made by serum levels of intact PTH, ionized calcium, phosphorus, and vitamin D. High PTH level with hypercalcemia is either primary or tertiary hyperparathyroidism. High PTH level with low or normal serum calcium levels is usually secondary hyperparathyroidism. Response to supplementation with calcium and vitamin D will help differentiate between primary and secondary hyperparathyroidism.

The treatment of primary hyperparathyroidism is mainly surgical, characterized by the removal of adenoma or adenomas or the removal of the ectopic gland. In patients who do not meet surgical criteria, bisphosphonates can be administered for suppression of osteoclasts.

Secondary hyperparathyroidism is usually reversible, provided the underlying cause is corrected. Supplementation of calcium and vitamin D is usually sufficient in most cases. Correction of underlying renal disease or malabsorption syndrome should be considered when feasible. In cases of renal failure, the active form of vitamin D (1,25 vitamin D) should be used for supplementation.[42] Tertiary hyperparathyroidism occurs when prolonged states of secondary hyperparathyroidism cannot be changed by elevating the calcium level. These situations often involve hypertrophy of all four glands. The treatment of this condition is the same as that for primary hyperparathyroidism.

Renal Osteodystrophy

The kidneys are the major regulators of mineral homeostasis, a target organ for PTH and vitamin D, and also a manufacturing site for the active form of vitamin D. Skeletal manifestation of vitamin D can result from different mechanisms. High-turnover renal osteodystrophy results from secondary hyperparathyroidism because of a lack of active 1,25 D3 dihydroxyvitamin. PTH activates osteoclast production, and excessive bone resorption occurs. The pathologic picture of patients with high-turnover renal osteodystrophy is typi-

2: Systemic Disorders

cal of hyperparathyroidism and ranges from excessive bone resorption to osteitis fibrosa cystica. Low-turnover renal osteodystrophy, which is now seen with increasing frequency, is mainly caused by aluminum toxicity, is more prevalent in patients undergoing peritoneal dialysis, and is characterized by osteomalacia. Clinical symptoms include bone pain, muscle weakness, skeletal deformities, and reduced BMD with an increased risk of fractures. In children, the typical symptoms of rickets are not unusual.

Radiologically, renal osteodystrophy may present as osteomalacia, osteosclerosis, fracture, amyloid deposition, and soft-tissue calcification and bone resorption. This clinical picture is not specific, and varieties of manifestations are common with hyperparathyroidism and rickets in children.[43]

Medical management of renal osteodystrophy consists of limitation of phosphorus intake in diet, the administration of an aluminum chelating agent (defaroxamine), and supplementation of vitamin D in its active form (calcitriol). Surgical management includes renal transplant, the fixation of pathologic fractures, reduction and fixation of slipped capital femoral epiphysis, and appropriate correction of the deformities. Multimodality management is required to treat the skeletal complications of renal osteodystrophy.[44]

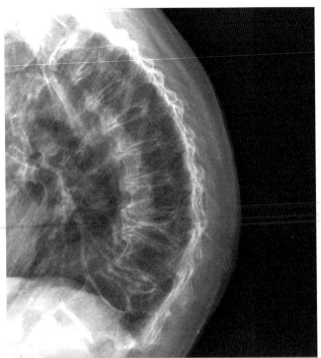

| Figure 5 | Lateral radiograph of the spine showing osteoporosis with severe compression fractures of T10 and T12, and mild compression fracture of T6. (Courtesy of Robert Schneider, MD, Department of Radiology, Hospital for Special Surgery, New York, NY.) |

Cushing Syndrome

Cushing syndrome refers to altered health secondary to prolonged exposure to elevated levels of corticosteroids. Corticosteroids have profound implications on collagen and mineral metabolism. The loss of skeletal mass may occur early in the course of glucocorticoid therapy and appears to be related to the cumulative dose of steroids, as well as to the usual risk factors for osteoporosis. The direct effects of overproduction of glucocorticoid include (1) the suppression of intestinal calcium absorption, (2) decreased renal tubular calcium resorption with increased urinary calcium excretion, and (3) suppressed osteoblast function and decreased bone formation. The indirect effects of steroids occur via secondary hyperparathyroidism. Calcium and vitamin D supplementation and antiresorptive agents have been used extensively to treat steroid-induced osteoporosis. Teriparatide, a synthetic PTH analogue, is effective in the treatment of steroid-induced osteoporosis; osteoblast dysfunction is responsible for low-turnover osteoporosis in this situation.[45]

Stress Fractures and Insufficiency Fractures

Fractures that occur in the absence of a preceding traumatic event pose unique management challenges for an orthopaedic surgeon, and underlying metabolic bone diseases may be a factor. When bone is subjected to excessive stress, it is likely to accumulate microdamage and ultimately fail. The capacity to withstand stress depends on the underlying metabolic condition and bone health. Stress causes insufficient bone to fail earlier as compared with equivalent loads in the normal population. The most common insufficiency is osteoporosis, followed by vitamin D deficiency. Osteoporotic fractures most often occur in the spine (Figure 5), the hip, and the distal end of the radius. Fatigue fracture, a variant of stress fracture, often occurs in athletes or military recruits and is most common in the metatarsals, the femoral neck, the tibia, and the pars interarticularis of the spine.

The mainstay of management of stress and insufficiency fractures is identification and treatment of underlying pathology. Complete workup for metabolic bone diseases is essential. Treatment consists of correcting the underlying insufficiency along with orthopaedic management of fractures. Fracture healing in these patients is challenging. PTH 1-84 has been shown to increase the rate of fracture healing in pelvic fractures, and the rate of union at 8 weeks was 100% in the PTH 1-84 treated group compared with 9% in the control group.[46] In another randomized controlled study, daily subcutaneous injection of teriparatide (PTH 1-34) increased the rate of healing for distal radius fractures.[47]

Osteoclasts play an important role in fracture healing, and inhibition of osteoclasts by bisphosphonates is not recommended until fracture healing is evident. Intravenous zolendronic acid at 6 weeks of fracture does not seem to inhibit fracture healing and reduces the mortality rate by 23%.

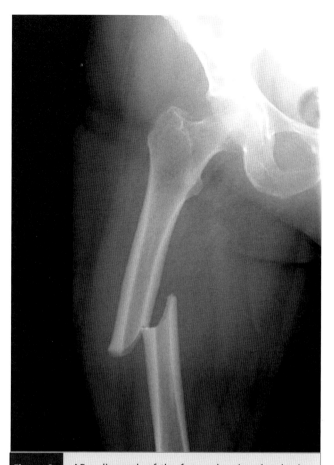

Figure 6 AP radiograph of the femur showing the classic features of an atypical fracture.

A task force appointed by the American Society for Bone and Mineral Research defined major and minor features of complete and incomplete atypical femoral fractures. According to the task force, all major features, including their location in the subtrochanteric region and the femoral shaft, transverse or short oblique orientation, minimal or no associated trauma, a medial spike when the fracture is complete, and absence of comminution, must be present to designate a femoral fracture as atypical. Minor features include fracture association with cortical thickening, a periosteal reaction of the lateral cortex, prodromal pain, bilaterality, delayed healing, comorbidities, and concomitant drug exposures including bisphosphonates, other antiresorptive agents, glucocorticoids, and proton pump inhibitors.[48] Typical radiologic features of these fractures are cortical thickening in the lateral side of the subtrochanteric region, a transverse fracture, and a medial cortical spike (Figure 6). Bilateral involvement is seen in at least 9% of people (can be a higher percentage depending on the series), and 76% of patients have prodromal pain.[49] These fractures are slow to heal and are associated with a higher rate of complications. Treatment with prophylactic surgical fixation in selected cases and teriparatide to increase bone turnover is recommended and has been successful. With the increasing awareness about this condition among clinicians, bisphosphonate therapy is closely monitored and is interspersed with drug holidays. Because bisphosphonates prevent a large number of fragility fractures and the risk of atypical fracture is very low, they will likely remain part of osteoporosis treatment at least for the near future.

Biologic agents, such as bone morphogenetic protein and dimineralized bone matrix in conjunction with bone marrow stem cells, can enhance fracture union. These agents are advantageous over conventional bone grafting because they often can be injected into the fracture site percutaneously, thus avoiding extensive surgery.

Bisphosphonate-Related Fractures

Bisphosphonates are the most common agents used to treat osteoporosis and many other metabolic bone disorders. Growing evidence favors the relationship of bisphosphonates with atypical subtrochanteric femur fractures. The estimated incidence of atypical femoral fractures increases progressively from 2 per 100,000 cases per year for 2 years of bisphosphonate use to 78 per 100,000 cases per year for 8 years of bisphosphonate use.[48] In a case-control study, bisphosphonate use was associated with fractures of the shaft and subtrochanteric region of the femur more than intertrochanteric and femoral neck fracture, with an odds ratio of 4.44.[49] The underlying mechanism is unclear, but the inability to repair wear and tear by remodeling caused by osteoclast dysfunction leads to accumulation of microdamage and ultimately a stress fracture results.

Summary

Bone is a specialized connective tissue that not only provides mechanical support but also plays a critical role in mineral homeostasis. Disorders of bone mass and/or bone quality result in compromised bone strength as manifested by low-energy fragility fractures.

Key Study Points

- A low-energy fragility fracture implies enhanced risk for additional fractures and requires treatment.

- Altered bone quality diminishes bone strength independent of bone mass.

- Both normal bone mass and bone quality depend on adequate calcium and vitamin D intake.

- Both anticatabolic (bisphosphonates, selective estrogen receptor modulators, denosumab, and calcitonin) and anabolic (teriparatide and strontium ranelate) drugs can correct osteoporosis and diminish the risk for low-energy fractures.

2: Systemic Disorders

Annotated References

1. Rosenberg AE: *Robbins and Cotran Pathologic Basis of Disease*, ed 7. Philadelphia, PA, Elsevier Saunders, 2005, pp 1274-1278.

2. Boskey AL: Noncollagenous matrix proteins and their role in mineralization. *Bone Miner* 1989;6(2):111-123.

3. Suda T, Kobayashi K, Jimi E, Udagawa N, Takahashi N: The molecular basis of osteoclast differentiation and activation. *Novartis Found Symp* 2001;232: 235-250.

4. Misiorowski W: Parathyroid hormone and its analogues—molecular mechanisms of action and efficacy in osteoporosis therapy. *Endokrynol Pol* 2011;62(1): 73-78.

   This article discusses the mechanism of action of PTH and its genetically engineered analogue PTH 1-34. The anabolic action of PTH, which is the most important desired action when its analogues are used therapeutically, is discussed in detail. Level of evidence: V.

5. Norman AW, Roth J, Orci L: The vitamin D endocrine system: Steroid metabolism, hormone receptors, and biological response (calcium binding proteins). *Endocr Rev* 1982;3(4):331-366.

6. Wesseling-Perry K: FGF-23 in bone biology. *Pediatr Nephrol* 2010;25(4):603-608.

7. National Osteoporosis Foundation: *The Clinician's Guide to Prevention and Treatment of Osteoporosis (2010)*. Washington, DC, National Osteoporosis Foundation, 2010.

   The NOF is a body of experts that sets forth guidelines from time to time for clinical practice. This guide discusses recent advances and the latest recommendations in the management of osteoporosis. Level of evidence: V.

8. Wong PK, Christie JJ, Wark JD: The effects of smoking on bone health. *Clin Sci (Lond)* 2007;113(5):233-241.

9. Gourlay ML, Fine JP, Preisser JS, et al: Bone-density testing interval and transition to osteoporosis in older women. *N Engl J Med* 2012;366(3):225-233.

   This study demonstrates that mild forms of osteopenia (T-score = −1.5) rarely progress to osteoporosis, and surveillance testing should be prolonged. Controversy exists about whether a 15-year testing interval is correct, but the idea of extending the time between retesting is well accepted.

10. Lindsay R, Silverman SL, Cooper C, et al: Risk of new vertebral fracture in the year following a fracture. *JAMA* 2001;285(3):320-323.

11. Lyles KW, Schenck AP, Colón-Emeric CS: Hip and other osteoporotic fractures increase the risk of subsequent fractures in nursing home residents. *Osteoporos Int* 2008;19(8):1225-1233.

12. Unnanuntana A, Gladnick BP, Donnelly E, Lane JM: The assessment of fracture risk. *J Bone Joint Surg Am* 2010;92(3):743-753.

    The authors discuss BMD, chemical risk factors for fracture with the use of FRAX, and bone turnover markers in the prediction of fracture risk and evaluation of patients with osteoporosis.

13. Miki RA, Oetgen ME, Kirk J, Insogna KL, Lindskog DM: Orthopaedic management improves the rate of early osteoporosis treatment after hip fracture: A randomized clinical trial. *J Bone Joint Surg Am* 2008; 90(11):2346-2353.

14. Rozental TD, Makhni EC, Day CS, Bouxsein ML: Improving evaluation and treatment for osteoporosis following distal radial fractures: A prospective randomized intervention. *J Bone Joint Surg Am* 2008;90(5): 953-961.

15. Mawer EB, Davies M: Vitamin D nutrition and bone disease in adults. *Rev Endocr Metab Disord* 2001;2(2): 153-164.

16. Gehrig L, Lane J, O'Connor MI: Osteoporosis: Management and treatment strategies for orthopaedic surgeons. *J Bone Joint Surg Am* 2008;90(6):1362-1374.

17. Cummings SR, San Martin J, McClung MR, et al: Denosumab for prevention of fractures in postmenopausal women with osteoporosis. *N Engl J Med* 2009;361(8): 756-765.

18. Karsdal MA, Henriksen K, Arnold M, Christiansen C: Calcitonin: A drug of the past or for the future? Physiologic inhibition of bone resorption while sustaining osteoclast numbers improves bone quality. *BioDrugs* 2008;22(3):137-144.

19. Kanis JA, Johnell O, Gullberg B, et al: Evidence for efficacy of drugs affecting bone metabolism in preventing hip fracture. *BMJ* 1992;305(6862):1124-1128.

20. Knopp-Sihota JA, Newburn-Cook CV, Homik J, Cummings GG, Voaklander D: Calcitonin for treating acute and chronic pain of recent and remote osteoporotic vertebral compression fractures: A systematic review and meta-analysis. *Osteoporos Int* 2012;23(1):17-38.

    This meta-analysis of 13 randomized trials demonstrated pain relief for acute compression fractures but provided no support for the use of calcitonin for the treatment of chronic pain. Level of evidence: I.

21. Han SL, Wan SL: Effect of teriparatide on bone mineral density and fracture in postmenopausal osteoporosis: Meta-analysis of randomised controlled trials. *Int J Clin Pract* 2012;66(2):199-209.

    This is a meta-analysis of eight randomized controlled trials evaluating the efficacy of once-daily subcutaneous injection of teriparatide in the treatment of postmenopausal osteoporosis. Level of evidence: I.

22. Przedlacki J: Strontium ranelate in post-menopausal osteoporosis. *Endokrynol Pol* 2011;62(1):65-72.

The antifracture efficacy of strontium ranelate was compared with that of other agents with antifracture activity. Its indications for therapy and side effects/contraindication are discussed.

23. Binkley N, Ramamurthy R, Krueger D: Low vitamin D status: Definition, prevalence, consequences, and correction. *Endocrinol Metab Clin North Am* 2010;39(2):287-301.

This review article discusses metabolism, mechanism of action, and skeletal effects of vitamin D. Topics including the normal level of vitamin D and optimum therapeutic strategies to treat vitamin D deficiency also are discussed. Level of evidence: V.

24. Rajah J, Thandrayen K, Pettifor JM: Clinical practice: Diagnostic approach to the rachitic child. *Eur J Pediatr* 2011;170(9):1089-1096.

This article discusses the clinical presentation, laboratory tests, and the radiologic picture of rickets and outlines the diagnostic approach for a child with rickets. Level of evidence: V.

25. Unuvar T, Buyukgebiz A: Nutritional rickets and vitamin D deficiency in infants, children and adolescents. *Pediatr Endocrinol Rev* 2010;7(3):283-291.

This article discusses clinical features, diagnosis, and management of vitamin D deficiency and rickets in different age groups. Level of evidence: V.

26. Reginato AJ, Coquia JA: Musculoskeletal manifestations of osteomalacia and rickets. *Best Pract Res Clin Rheumatol* 2003;17(6):1063-1080.

27. Berry JL, Davies M, Mee AP: Vitamin D metabolism, rickets, and osteomalacia. *Semin Musculoskelet Radiol* 2002;6(3):173-182.

28. Altman RD, Bloch DA, Hochberg MC, Murphy WA: Prevalence of pelvic Paget's disease of bone in the United States. *J Bone Miner Res* 2000;15(3):461-465.

29. Lodish H, Berk A, Zipursky S, Matsudaira P, Baltimore D, Darnell J: The fibrous proteins of the matrix, in *Molecular Cell Biology*, ed 4. New York, NY, WH Freeman, 2000.

30. Otto F, Thornell AP, Crompton T, et al: Cbfa1, a candidate gene for cleidocranial dysplasia syndrome, is essential for osteoblast differentiation and bone development. *Cell* 1997;89(5):765-771.

31. Komori T, Yagi H, Nomura S, et al: Targeted disruption of Cbfa1 results in a complete lack of bone formation owing to maturational arrest of osteoblasts. *Cell* 1997;89(5):755-764.

32. Tolar J, Teitelbaum SL, Orchard PJ: Osteopetrosis. *N Engl J Med* 2004;351(27):2839-2849.

33. Shapiro F: Osteopetrosis: Current clinical considerations. *Clin Orthop Relat Res* 1993;294:34-44.

34. Stark Z, Savarirayan R: Osteopetrosis. *Orphanet J Rare Dis* 2009;4:5.

35. Key LL Jr, Rodriguiz RM, Willi SM, et al: Long-term treatment of osteopetrosis with recombinant human interferon gamma. *N Engl J Med* 1995;332(24):1594-1599.

36. Landa J, Margolis N, Di Cesare P: Orthopaedic management of the patient with osteopetrosis. *J Am Acad Orthop Surg* 2007;15(11):654-662.

37. Gelb BD, Shi GP, Chapman HA, Desnick RJ: Pycnodysostosis, a lysosomal disease caused by cathepsin K deficiency. *Science* 1996;273(5279):1236-1238.

38. Motyckova G, Fisher DE: Pycnodysostosis: Role and regulation of cathepsin K in osteoclast function and human disease. *Curr Mol Med* 2002;2(5):407-421.

39. Gauthier JY, Chauret N, Cromlish W, et al: The discovery of odanacatib (MK-0822), a selective inhibitor of cathepsin K. *Bioorg Med Chem Lett* 2008;18(3):923-928.

40. Fraser WD: Hyperparathyroidism. *Lancet* 2009;374(9684):145-158.

41. Silverberg SJ, Shane E, de la Cruz L, et al: Skeletal disease in primary hyperparathyroidism. *J Bone Miner Res* 1989;4(3):283-291.

42. Unnanuntana A, Rebolledo BJ, Khair MM, DiCarlo EF, Lane JM: Diseases affecting bone quality: Beyond osteoporosis. *Clin Orthop Relat Res* 2011;469(8):2194-2206.

This review article discusses metabolic bone diseases other than osteoporosis that can impair the quality of bone and predispose an individual to fragility fractures. Level of evidence: V.

43. Tejwani NC, Schachter AK, Immerman I, Achan P: Renal osteodystrophy. *J Am Acad Orthop Surg* 2006;14(5):303-311.

44. Elder G: Pathophysiology and recent advances in the management of renal osteodystrophy. *J Bone Miner Res* 2002;17(12):2094-2105.

45. Hodgson SF: Corticosteroid-induced osteoporosis. *Endocrinol Metab Clin North Am* 1990;19(1):95-111.

46. Peichl P, Holzer LA, Maier R, Holzer G: Parathyroid hormone 1-84 accelerates fracture-healing in pubic bones of elderly osteoporotic women. *J Bone Joint Surg Am* 2011;93(17):1583-1587.

This is a prospective, randomized controlled study to evaluate the effect of PTH 1-84 on the course of pelvic fracture healing and functional outcomes in postmeno-

2: Systemic Disorders

pausal women. Twenty-one of 65 patients with pelvic fractures received PTH 1-84, and the rest served as controls. The rate and speed of healing was significantly higher in the treatment group. Level of evidence: I.

47. Aspenberg P, Genant HK, Johansson T, et al: Teriparatide for acceleration of fracture repair in humans: A prospective, randomized, double-blind study of 102 postmenopausal women with distal radial fractures. *J Bone Miner Res* 2010;25(2):404-414.

   The role of a 20-µg daily subcutaneous dose of teriparatide in acceleration of fracture healing in conservatively treated distal end radius fracture is discussed. Level of evidence: I.

48. Shane E, Burr D, Ebeling PR, et al: Atypical subtrochanteric and diaphyseal femoral fractures: Report of a task force of the American Society for Bone and Mineral Research. *J Bone Miner Res* 2010;25(11):2267-2294.

   A multidisciplinary expert group reviewed pertinent published reports concerning atypical femur fractures, as well as preclinical studies that could provide insight into their pathogenesis, and a case definition was developed to correctly identify these fractures. Level of evidence: V.

49. Lenart BA, Neviaser AS, Lyman S, et al: Association of low-energy femoral fractures with prolonged bisphosphonate use: A case control study. *Osteoporos Int* 2009; 20(8):1353-1362.

Chapter 18

Arthritis and Other Cartilage Disorders

Brian A. Klatt, MD   Antonia Chen, MD, MBA   Rocky S. Tuan, PhD

Introduction

Recent surveys performed by the Centers for Disease Control and Prevention estimate that joint disorders and arthritis affect 21% of the US population (69.9 million people).[1] Approximately 16.9 million US adults (7.9%) reported arthritis-attributable activity limitations in 2003.[2] This number was projected to increase to 17.6 million by 2005 and to 25 million (9.3% of the US adult population) by 2030[2]. Projections are based on increases in the number of patients who will suffer from arthritis as a result of an aging population and an obesity epidemic. In 2030, it is expected that a diagnosis of arthritis will be made in 67 million adults (25% of the US adult population).[2]

Cartilage plays a critical role in the normal function of articular joints. The synovial joints are lined with hyaline cartilage, which provides a low friction surface for smooth and painless movement. Articular cartilage is composed of chondrocytes and the matrix that they maintain. This matrix is composed of collagens, proteoglycans, and noncollagenous proteins. A complete and thorough discussion of the properties and function of articular cartilage can be found in chapter 3, Articular Cartilage and Intervertebral Disk, *Orthopaedic Knowledge Update 11*.

Cartilage becomes damaged and loses its function through a variety of processes. Traditional classifications have divided cartilage disorders into osteoarthritis (OA; noninflammatory) or inflammatory arthritis. The prototype inflammatory arthritis is rheumatoid arthritis

(RA), but there are numerous other types of inflammatory processes that result in arthritis. This traditional classification will serve as the structure for the chapter, but it should be noted that there is also an inflammatory component to OA. It is debated whether the inflammatory component of OA is part of the progression of the disease or the initiating event.

An understanding of the various types of arthritis will enable the orthopaedic surgeon to properly care for these patients.

Osteoarthritis

OA, also known as degenerative joint disease, is the most common cartilage disorder, and continues to be the leading cause of disability and impaired quality of life in developed countries.[3] OA is defined as the progressive loss of cartilage structure and function.

Primary OA is an idiopathic process of cartilage degeneration that occurs with normal use. This wear and tear of the joint becomes more prevalent with advancing age. Secondary OA is the development of OA because of an insult or injury that initiates and accelerates the degenerative process of OA. The age of incidence of secondary OA depends on the disease process that initiates cartilage degeneration. It can be the result of infection; traumatic joint injury; osteonecrosis; and a variety of hereditary, developmental, metabolic, and neurologic disorders.[4] An extensive list of causes of secondary OA is shown in Table 1.

Osteoarthritis Disease Progression
Changes to Cartilage
The progressive loss of cartilage is a process that involves three overlapping stages: cartilage matrix damage or alteration, chondrocyte response to tissue damage, and decline of the chondrocyte synthetic response with progressive loss of tissue.

The first phase can result from a mechanical insult, such as a traumatic high-energy impact. There is loss of proteoglycan content, and proteoglycans are found in an unaggregated form that is not bound to hyaluronate. This disrupts the matrix macromolecular framework, which makes the extracellular matrix (ECM) more permeable. The water content of the cartilage

Dr. Klatt or an immediate family member has received research or institutional support from DePuy and serves as a board member, owner, officer, or committee member of American Academy of Orthopaedic Surgeons. Dr. Chen or an immediate family member serves as a paid consultant to or is an employee of Novo Nordisk. Dr. Tuan or an immediate family member serves as a paid consultant to or is an employee of Alacer Technologies and serves as a board member, owner, officer, or committee member of the American Society for Matrix Biology Tissue Engineering and the Regenerative Medicine International Society.

Table 1

Known Causes of Joint Degeneration (Secondary Osteoarthrosis)

Cause	Presumed Mechanism
Intra-articular fracture	Damage to articular cartilage or incongruity of joint or both
High-intensity-impact joint loading	Damage to articular cartilage or subchondral bone or both
Ligament injuries	Instability of the joint
Dysplasia of joint and cartilage (developmental and hereditary)	Abnormal shape of joint or abnormal articular cartilage or both
Aseptic necrosis	Bone necrosis leads to collapse of articular surface and incongruity of joint
Acromegaly	Overgrowth of articular cartilage produces incongruity or joint or abnormal cartilage or both
Paget disease	Distortion or incongruity of joint as a result of bone remodeling
Ehlers-Danlos syndrome	Instability of joint
Gaucher disease (hereditary deficiency of enzyme glucocerebrosidase, leading to accumulation of glucocerebroside)	Bone necrosis or pathological fracture leads to incongruity of joint
Stickler syndrome (progressive, hereditary arthro-ophthalmopathy)	Abnormal development of joint or articular cartilage or both
Infection of joint (inflammation)	Destruction of articular cartilage
Hemophilia	Multiple joint hemorrhages
Hemochromatosis (excess deposition of iron in multiple tissues)	Mechanism unknown
Ochronosis (hereditary deficiency of enzyme homogentisic acid oxidase leading to accumulation of homogentisic acid)	Deposition of homogentisic acid polymers in articular cartilage
Calcium pyrophosphate deposition disease	Accumulation of calcium pyrophosphate crystals in articular cartilage
Neuropathic arthropathy (Charcot joints due to syphilis, diabetes mellitus, syringomyelia, myelomeningocele, leprosy, congenital insensitivity to pain, amylodosis)	Loss of proprioception and joint sensation results in increased impact loading and torsion, instability of joint, and intra-articular fracture

(Buckwalter JA: Articular cartilage II: Degeneration and osteoarthrosis, repair, regeneration, and transplantation. *J Bone Joint Surg Am* 1997;79[4]:612-632.)

matrix increases, which decreases matrix stiffness. This softening of the cartilage is clinically identified as chondromalacia. These changes cause the cartilage surface to fray and fibrillate, which increases the vulnerability of the joint to further mechanical insult.[5]

The second phase involves the cellular response of chondrocytes to the mechanical changes. When chondrocytes recognize tissue damage and changes to the ECM, they release or upregulate mediators that initiate a cellular response. Static and dynamic loading of cartilage results in an increase in the reactive oxygen species nitric oxide (NO), which increases chondrocyte apoptosis and premature senescence. Premature senescence is a pathologic process characterized by shortened telomeres, decreased amount of adenosine triphosphate (ATP) produced by the mitochondria, and increased β-galactosidase.[6] NO also inhibits collagen and proteoglycan synthesis by inducing the production of the cytokines interleukin-1 (IL-1) and tumor necrosis factor-α (TNF-α), which stimulate the production of

matrix metalloproteinases (MMPs) that further degrade the matrix macromolecules. As the collagen network degrades, upregulation of molecules such as aggrecan, aggrecanase-2, c-fos, c-jun, and fibronectin occur, which further weakens the mechanical properties of cartilage by destabilizing the type II collagen fiber network.[7] To combat this cartilage degradation, there is a small repair component associated with the second stage of OA that stimulates chondrocytes to synthesize macromolecules and proliferate. The repair can counteract some of the effects of the inflammatory response, although chondrocytes have minimal capability to reproduce.

The third stage of OA occurs when cartilage is unable to respond to and recover from the mechanical and chemical insult of catabolic factors, including other inflammatory mediators, such as IL-6, IL-8, and prostaglandin E$_2$. Age leads to a decline in the anabolic response of chondrocytes, and thus OA is seen more commonly in the elderly.[8]

Changes to Bone

As the cartilage degenerates, there is increased exposure of the subchondral bone. As the pressure of the cyclical joint loading impacts bone, subchondral bone increases in density and becomes sclerotic. With the exposed subchondral bone, cysts may form in the bone, which can contain myxoid, fibroid, or cartilaginous tissues. Because cartilage tissue does not easily regenerate, the joint may form osteophytes from mesenchymal stem cells that originate from periosteal tissue that are fibrous, bony, and cartilaginous outgrowths.[9] These osteophytes can help create joint space in joints such as the hip or restrict joint motion and cause contractures. They can be a source of pain at the limits of joint motion.

Changes to Periarticular Tissues

The soft tissues of the joint react to changes and the loss of cartilage. The synovium can become inflamed from the release of inflammatory factors from chondrocytes and release further chemokines and MMPs. Synovium can release collagenase and hydrolytic enzymes to further break down cartilage and stimulate vascular hyperplasia.[10] With chronic OA, the joint capsule and the ligaments become tightened and contracted. Range of motion is decreased. Muscle can also undergo atrophy with the relative inactivity of the joint because of pain.

Changes to Alignment

It has been shown that abnormal hip-knee-ankle alignment can accelerate structural changes in osteoarthritic knees; varus malalignment increases medial compartment disease fourfold, and valgus malalignment increases lateral compartment disease twofold.[11] Alignment is affected by multiple factors in the joint, including meniscal degeneration or previous meniscectomy, incompetent anterior cruciate ligament, osteophytes, and incongruous tibiofemoral contact.[12] Whether malalignment is associated with the development of OA[13] or if malalignment is a result of OA[14] is still a topic of debate. However, it has been demonstrated that malalignment can affect more than cartilage because malalignment predisposes OA patients to bone marrow lesions.[15] One study has demonstrated that greater bone marrow edema is correlated with increased pain from OA.[16]

Diagnosis of Osteoarthritis

Osteoarthritis is classically diagnosed by clinical examination and with plain radiographs. Physical examination of a joint with OA reveals joint pain, loss of motion, crepitus, joint effusion, and deformity. Findings of OA on radiographs include joint-space narrowing, osteophytes, subchondral sclerosis, and bone cysts (Table 2). The severity of symptoms does not always correlate well with radiographic findings.

Patients in the early stages of OA usually have minimal signs and symptoms, but there may be soreness and pain after excessive activity that resolves with several days of rest or a short course of anti-inflammatory medication. As the disease progresses, the symptoms can become quite life altering. Joints will be more stiff with initial motion, and there will be pain with activities of daily living, such as walking up and down stairs. With hip arthritis, stiffness in the joints can limit the ability to do simple tasks, such as putting on shoes.

Much of the current research effort to treat OA revolves around early diagnosis and treatment.[17] Research has been focused on the means to identify early OA, and some experimental techniques may gain clinical use in the evaluation of cartilage. Several new MRI techniques have been used to assess the biochemical integrity of articular cartilage, including T1rho, T2 mapping, sodium MRI, and delayed gadolinium enhanced MRI of cartilage (dGEMRIC).[18] T2 mapping and dGEMRIC have become the most commonly used imaging modalities in the clinical setting. T2 mapping is useful in evaluating cartilage after reparative procedures because it can determine if the expected normal zonal variations in healthy articular cartilage have been restored. dGEMRIC requires high doses of gadolinium contrast but has been able to show the glycosaminoglycan (GAG) concentration of cartilage. One study found that changes seen on dGEMRIC correlated well with the development of knee OA in the future.[19] In addition to MRI techniques, optical coherence tomography (OCT) may allow arthroscopic evaluation of cartilage by performing microscopic cross-sectional imaging of articular cartilage.[20,21]

Treatment of Osteoarthritis

The treatment of OA is multifaceted and can be divided into seven main categories: patient education and lifestyle modification, rehabilitation, complementary and alternative therapy, pain relievers, intra-articular injections, needle lavage, and surgical intervention. The literature for categories was evaluated in depth by a workgroup of specialists and was compiled into the clinical practice guidelines for the treatment of knee OA by the American Academy of Orthopaedic Surgeons (AAOS).[22] The levels of evidence of studies were evaluated, and recommendations were graded: A was the best, and C was the worst.

Lifestyle Modification

For early arthritis, symptoms can be treated with patient lifestyle modification. Self-management education and self-care programs are recommended to gain understanding of the disease process and suggest ways to modify activity. Specific physical therapy and exercises are also recommended, including low-impact aerobic fitness, range-of-motion exercises, and muscle strengthening. For patients who are overweight and have a body mass index of greater than 25 kg/m², weight loss is recommended using diet and exercise to unload some of the forces on the arthritic joint (Grade A recommendation with Level I evidence).

In terms of mechanical intervention, the use of an assistive walking device such as a cane or a walker can unload the joint, provide stability, and improve pain and function. Studies have shown that patellar taping may be beneficial for short-term relief of pain associated with OA.[23,24] However, it is not recommended that patients use lateral heel wedges for treating medial unicompartmental OA (Grade B recommendation with Level II evidence), and there is inconclusive advice on the use of offloading knee braces.

Pharmacologic Methods

None of the pharmacologic methods of treatment is able to restore or regenerate cartilage. Medications that are used to treat patients with OA are aimed at treating symptoms. Acetaminophen is a good pain control medication. Acetaminophen is only an analgesic; it does not possess any anti-inflammatory effects. NSAIDs can provide good pain relief for the inflammation from OA. However, the side effects associated with NSAIDs can present challenges in the treatment of elderly patients. The gastrointestinal effects are the most significant because NSAIDs are associated with the development of ulcers, and there are increased bleeding risks with long-term NSAID use. Although selective cyclooxygenase-2 inhibitors may have less gastrointestinal and bleeding side effects, they have been associated with increased cardiovascular events. The use of acetaminophen and NSAIDs is recommended by the AAOS workgroup (Grade B). Oral steroid medications

Table 2

Kellgren Scale of Osteoarthritis

Radiograph

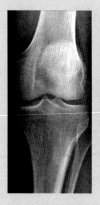 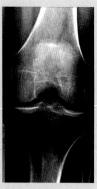 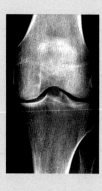 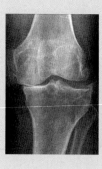 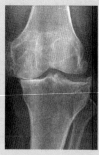

Grade	0	I	II	III	IV
Classification	Normal	Doubtful	Definite	Moderate	Severe
Description	No osteoarthritis	Minimal joint space narrowing and minute osteophytes	Possible mild joint space narrowing and definite osteophytes	Moderate joint space narrowing, moderate multiple osteophytes, some sclerosis	Severe joint space narrowing, large osteophytes, severe sclerosis, deformity of bone contour

Table 3

Viscosupplementation for the Treatment of Osteoarthritis

Trade Name	Generic Name	Source	Number of Injections	Dosage per Injection
Euflexxa	1% sodium hyaluronate	Synthetic	3	20 mg
Hyalgan	Sodium hyaluronate	Chicken combs	3-5	20 mg
Orthovisc	High molecular weight hyaluronan	Synthetic	3-4	30 mg
Supartz	Sodium hyaluronate	Chicken combs	5	25 mg
Synvisc	Hylan G-F 20	Chicken combs	3 1	16 mg 48 mg

are not routinely used to treat OA. Oral glucosamine and oral chondroitin have not demonstrated any effect in restoring cartilage, and the AAOS workgroup strongly recommends against prescribing them (Grade A).

Injections of glucocorticoids and hyaluronic acid (HA) are sometimes used to mitigate the symptoms of OA (Table 3). The AAOS workgroup recommends using corticosteroids for short-term pain relief, but the findings were inconclusive regarding the use of HA. In theory, the use of viscosupplementation, such as HA, may increase the viscosity of the existing synovial fluid and may reduce the degradation of hyaluronan in synovium and cartilage. However, studies have shown that the use of HA can cause a localized joint reaction, including erythema, effusion, swelling, and pain.[25] Some literature also warns of the hazards of using analgesic injection medications, such as bupivacaine, because they may be chondrotoxic.[26] With severe, advanced disease, the risk of damage from injections should not be of great concern. The therapeutic benefit of HA injections remains somewhat controversial.[27] In theory, exogenous HA reduces proinflammatory mediators and MMPs and stimulates chondrocytes to synthesize endogenous HA and proteoglycans.[28] However, there is a common misperception among patients that HA injections restore cartilage.

Surgical Intervention

Traditional surgical treatments of smaller cartilage defects include microfracture, cartilage transplantation, and autologous chondrocyte implantation.[29] These techniques have provided temporary relief in the restoration of small cartilage defects, but the tissue generated is fibrocartilage and is not identical to articular cartilage. The relief provided by these treatments is temporary.

There are certain scenarios for considering arthroscopy as a treatment option for OA. There are high levels of evidence (I and II) to recommend against performing arthroscopy for débriding or lavaging knee

OA. However, if there are primary symptoms of a torn meniscus or a loose body, then a partial meniscectomy or loose body removal may be warranted (Grade C).

For osteotomies, the AAOS workgroup had no conclusion on whether to perform a tibial tubercle osteotomy for symptomatic patients with isolated patellofemoral disease. However, the workgroup did support a realignment, or high tibial, osteotomy to treat active patients with malalignment and unicompartimental OA (Grade C).

Implants have been used to treat OA if there is partial joint OA or tricompartmental OA. The AAOS workgroup did not recommend using a free-floating interpositional device to treat unicompartmental OA.[22] The only reliable method of using implants to effectively treat advanced OA is by total joint arthroplasty, where the osteoarthritic articular surfaces of a joint are replaced by metal and a spacer is used to facilitate articulation. Joint arthroplasty is an option in patients with functional limitations for whom conservative measures have failed.

Cartilage Regeneration and Stem Cell Therapy

Biologic solutions through cartilage regeneration may be the future treatment of OA. Research is under way to find the appropriate cell source, the scaffold to support and organize these cells, and bioactive factors and bioreactors to support cartilage growth.

Tissue engineering seeks to form new cartilage by using chondrocytes and other renewable cell sources, such as mesenchymal and pluripotent stem cells. Pluripotent stem cells, such as embryonic stem cells (ESCs), have the potential for indefinite self-renewal and can differentiate into multiple cell types.[30] However, there are ethical concerns for using the inner cell mass of these blastocysts from embryos. Another alternative is to use a patient's own cells and use gene transduction with ESC-specific transcription factors to create ESC-like stem cells, otherwise called induced pluripotent stem cells. However, like ESCs, these cells are undifferentiated and can develop into tumors.[31] There are no

2: Systemic Disorders

Table 3				
Viscosupplementation for the Treatment of Osteoarthritis (continued)				
Duration of Pain Relief	Molecular Weight (million daltons)	Elasticity (Pa at 2.5 Hz)	Viscosity (Pa at 2.5 Hz)	Adverse Events
12 weeks	2.4-3.6	92	37	Effusion, swelling, and gastrointestinal complaints
3 to 60 days, 5 to 6 months	0.5-0.7	0.6	3	Swelling, injection site pain, and gastrointestinal complaints
22 weeks	1-2.9	60	46	Swelling, effusion, arthralgia, edema, injection site erythema, and injection site pain
6 months	0.6-1.2	9	16	Arthralgia, injection site pain
6 months	6	111	25	Effusion, injection site pain

current studies examining the use of pluripotent stem cells in the treatment of cartilage damage, but studies are currently using stem cells to treat spinal cord injury and macular degeneration.

Whatever cells are chosen must be introduced on a tissue scaffold. Tissue scaffolds are biomaterials that establish a three-dimensional structure to retain the cells and provide mechanical support to enable cartilage development over time. There are four main groups of scaffolding that may be applied for cartilage tissue engineering: (1) protein-based polymers, (2) carbohydrate-based polymers, (3) synthetic polymers, and (4) composite polymers, which combine biomaterials from the other three categories.[32]

To stimulate cells to grow within scaffolds, bioactive factors are endogenous polypeptide molecules that can be applied to constructs. Transforming growth factor-β (TGF-β) is the most common growth factor used to stimulate chondrogenesis, ECM matrix production, and mesenchymal stem cells.[33] Other members of the TGF superfamily are also responsible for stimulating cartilage repair, including TGF-β1, bone morphogenetic proteins (BMP-2 and BMP-7), TGF-β3, and cartilage-derived morphogenetic proteins (CDMP-1 and CDMP-2). TGF-β or BMP-7 can be used with insulin growth factor-1 (IGF-1) to stimulate anabolic cartilage pathways and decrease catabolic pathways. Fibroblast growth factors (FGF), specifically FGF-2 and FGF-18, bind to cell surface receptors to promote anabolic pathways and downregulate aggrecanase.[34] Platelet-derived growth factor attracts mesenchymal stem cells and can stimulate proteoglycan production and chondrocyte proliferation.[35] Platelet-rich plasma contains growth factors that may serve as an adjunct to treating OA, but too few studies have been conducted to make any meaningful conclusions in OA patients.

Finally, bioreactors are chambers that mimic physiologic conditions to facilitate chondrogenesis of a three-dimensional construct. Automated bioreactors provide mechanobiologic activation of the scaffolds seeded with cells. There are three main bioreactors that are currently used: hydrostatic, dynamic loading, and hydrodynamic bioreactors.

Gene Therapy

The use of gene therapy was first proposed to treat rheumatoid arthritis.[36] For OA, five gene therapeutic targets that enhance chondrogenesis have been extensively studied: (1) growth factors: including TGF-β, BMP, FGF, IGF-1β, and epidermal growth factor (EGF); (2) transcription factors: SOX9; (3) signal transduction molecules: SMADS; (4) proinflammatory cytokine inhibition: TNF-α and IL-1; and (5) apoptosis or senescence inhibition: Bcl-2, Bcl-XL, and inducible nitric oxide synthase (iNOS). TNF-β1 has been studied in a phase I clinical trial examining the efficacy of TissueGene-C (TG-C, TissueGene Inc.), a cell-mediated gene therapy system that contains allogenic chondrocytes that express TGF-β1. The safety of this product was established, and further studies seek to determine

the usefulness of the product in the treatment of OA.

There are multiple vectors that can be used to deliver genes, and they are divided into nonviral and viral vectors. Nonviral vectors include plasmids, liposomes, naked DNA, and complexed DNA. Unfortunately, these vectors are transient, but they are noninfectious. Viral vectors, such as adenovirus, adeno-associated virus, lentivirus, herpes simplex virus, and foamy virus, deliver the genes directly into DNA and provide stable gene expression. However, host DNA is altered, the host can react to the infectious proteins, and there can be insertional mutagenesis.

Inflammatory Arthritis

Inflammatory arthritis is a large collection of different diseases that cause joint inflammation. The diagnosis requires a complete review of the disease process profile. There are no simple clinical tests that can be used to diagnose these diseases, thus the rheumatologic history and physical examination play a critical role in diagnosis and treatment. The location of the problems and the symmetry of presentation are important disease features. For example, RA has a predilection for the wrists and the proximal joints of the hands and feet, whereas psoriatic arthritis involves the distal interphalangeal joint of the hands. The physical findings with RA tend to be symmetric, whereas other inflammatory arthritis conditions are not. Onset and chronology of the disease are important features. The onset of RA tends to present in a subacute manner, whereas septic arthritis has a rapid onset in several hours. Age, sex, and precipitating factors can also aid in diagnosis. The medical treatment of all of these diseases is beyond the expertise of the orthopaedic surgeon, and, in most cases, the involvement of a rheumatologist is essential for the proper care of the inflammatory arthritis.

Rheumatoid Arthritis

Rheumatoid factor (RF) is a set of self-reactive anti-immunoglobulin G antibodies that are detected in the blood of 80% of those with RA. RA is the most common inflammatory arthritis. The incidence of RA in the United States is 25 per 100,000 for men and 54 per 100,000 for women.[37] The definitive cause of this disease has not been determined, but the most common theory is that it is an autoimmune disease that can be stimulated in genetically susceptible individuals. An environmental antigen can trigger the initiation of the response. Rheumatoid factor is a set of self-reactive anti-immunoglobulin G antibodies that are detected in the blood of 80% of those with RA. With RA, joint destruction begins with leukocyte infiltration of the synovium, which activates type B synoviocytes that are part of the synovial pannus. This then activates transcription pathways of nuclear factor (NF)-κB, signal transducers and activators of transcription (STATs), and mitogen-activated protein kinases, which enable the upregulation of cytokines, such as TNF-α, IL-1, IL-6, and IL-17. In response to this cytokine release, multiple destructive enzymes, including MMPs (collagenase and gelatinase), cathepsins, and serine proteases (trypsin), act to destroy cartilage. Bone destruction is also activated by the same cytokines (TNF-α, IL-1, and IL-17) that upregulate receptor activator of nuclear factor-κB ligand (RANKL). With increased expression of RANKL on T cells and fibroblast-like cells, more osteoclasts are activated, which leads to bony erosions. This inflammation and invasion of the synovial pannus into articular cartilage and bone leads to the destruction of joints and causes pain and deformity.

The most common patient presentation is that of joint pain and swelling that is insidious in nature. This develops over weeks or months, where symptom duration of greater than 6 weeks is a cutoff point. Morning stiffness that lasts more than 1 hour is a hallmark symptom of RA. Joint involvement is usually symmetric in nature. RA is commonly polyarticular and often involves the wrist, the proximal interphalangeal joints of the hands, the metacarpophalangeal joints, the metatarsophalangeal joints, the elbow, the knee, the ankle, and the cervical spine. Involvement of greater than 10 joints with at least one small joint increases the likelihood of RA. As for laboratory diagnosis, patients may be positive for rheumatoid factor or anticitrullinated protein antibody, and they may have an elevated erythrocyte sedimentation rate (ESR) or C-reactive protein (CRP). The criteria for diagnosing RA is multifactorial. The American College of Rheumatology and the European League Against Rheumatism devised a classification criteria for RA. Patients who have one joint with clinical synovitis or patients with synovitis that does not have another disease explanation should be tested. Patients are scored on a numerical scale based on the following criteria, and a score of greater than 6/10 is the diagnosis of RA. The more joints involved, the higher the numerical score; one large joint = 0 points, 2 to 10 large joints = 1 point, one to three small joints = 2 points, 4 to 10 small joints = 3 points, and 10 joints with at least 1 small joint = 5 points. For serology, patients with negative rheumatoid factor or high-positive ACPA receive 3 points. If the level is elevated, patients receive 1 point. Finally, if the duration of symptoms is under 6 weeks, patients receive no points, but if the duration of symptoms are equal to or greater than 6 weeks, then patients receive 1 point.[38]

Treatment of RA has evolved over the past decade as new disease-modifying antirheumatic drugs have been introduced (**Table 4**). Historically, NSAIDs and oral corticosteroids played a large role in the treatment of RA, but there are significant side effects associated with these medications. NSAIDs have a potent role in blocking the production of prostaglandins, but gastrointestinal side effects and nephrotoxicity limit the use of NSAIDs. Additionally, NSAIDs are anticoagulants, so it is recommended that all NSAIDs be stopped 1 week before surgery. Corticosteroids inhibit the production of prostaglandins and leukotrienes. They can significantly decrease inflammation, but the side effects of corticosteroids include osteoporosis, hypertension, diabetes, and cataracts. Lower doses have fewer side effects, so low-dose oral steroids remain a part of RA medical therapy. The dosage of treatment determines whether or not a stress dose of steroids is required on the day of surgery to prevent adrenal insufficiency. Patients who take low-dose steroids (less than 7.5 mg/day) or have taken steroids for a short duration of time (less than 3 weeks) do not require a stress dose. Patients with higher dosages or longer duration of treatment should receive 50 to 100 mg of stress dose steroids on the day of surgery.

Biologic agents have revolutionized the treatment of RA. TNF-α antagonists have not only had substantial benefits on the signs and symptoms of RA but also are able to retard the radiographic progression of joint damage. These drugs work by different mechanisms, including acting as a monoclonal antibody against TNF-α or mimic the receptor for TNF-α to prevent TNF-α from working. Etanercept, infliximab, and adalimumab are TNF inhibitors approved for use in RA. Anakinra is a human recombinant anti-IL-1 receptor antagonist. Response rates to this drug were only 38%, and only modest reductions in radiographic disease progression were seen.[39,40] The use of this drug in patients with RA is limited to those with refractory disease. Abatacept and rituximab are approved for patients with active RA who have had inadequate response to other disease-modifying antirheumatic drugs or in whom treatment with an anti-TNF-α agent has failed.[41]

If medical treatment fails, those with advanced joint damage from RA may benefit from surgical treatment. Total joint arthroplasty is a reasonable and effective surgical option. Because the entire joint is affected by the inflammatory process of RA, replacement of the entire joint is recommended even if degeneration is present in only one or two compartments.

Juvenile Idiopathic Arthritis

Juvenile idiopathic arthritis (JIA) is a term that encompasses arthritis conditions in children younger than 16 years where there is no known cause. Classically, the term was used to classify all idiopathic arthritis conditions in patients younger than 16 years according to the American College of Rheumatology criteria developed in 1997.[42] This classification scheme divided childhood arthritis into three categories—pauciarticular, polyarticular, and systemic. This classification was expanded by the International League of Associations for Rheumatology in 2001 to include the following categories: systemic, polyarticular, oligoarticular, enthesitis-related, and psoriatic.[43] Undifferentiated JIA is an additional category if the presenting JIA does not fit into any of the above categories or if the presenting JIA spans multiple categories.

The epidemiology of JIA is variable, given differences in diagnostic criteria and the low frequency of the disease.[44] Studies have shown that the incidence ranges from 0.008 to 0.226 per 1,000 patients and the preva-

Table 4

Agents for Treating Rheumatoid Arthritis

Trade Name	Generic Name	Mechanism of Action	Perioperative Dosage
	Corticosteroids	Decrease production of prostaglandins and leukotrienes	≤ 7.5 mg/day = no stress dose
			Treatment < 3 weeks = no stress dose
			≥ 7.5 mg/day = 50-100 mg stress dose on the day of surgery
			Treatment > 3 weeks = 50-100 mg stress dose on the day of surgery
	NSAIDs	Prostaglandin and COX inhibitor	Stop 1 week before surgery
Actemra	Tocilizumab	Antibody against IL-6 receptor	Stop 4 weeks before surgery; resume 1-2 weeks after surgery
Arava	Leflunomide	Inhibits pyrimidine synthesis by targeting rapidly dividing cells	Minor procedures—Continue. Major procedures—Stop 2 days before surgery; resume 2 weeks after surgery
Azulfidine	Sulfasalazine	Reduces the synthesis of inflammatory mediators	Continue for all procedures
Cimzia	Certolizumab	Monoclonal antibody against TNF-α	Stop 4 weeks before surgery; resume 1-2 weeks after surgery
Cytoxan	Cyclophosphamide	Causes DNA cross-linking	Stop 4 weeks before surgery; resume 1-2 weeks after surgery
Enbrel	Etanercept	Mimics the receptor for TNF-α	Stop 2 weeks before surgery; resume 1-2 weeks after surgery
Humira	Adalimumab	Monoclonal antibodies against TNF-α	Stop 2 weeks before surgery; resume 1-2 weeks after surgery
Imuran	Azathioprine	Purine synthesis inhibitor	Stop 2 days before surgery; resume 1-3 days after surgery
Kineret	Anakinra	IL-1 receptor antagonist	Stop 1-2 days before surgery; resume 1-2 weeks after surgery
Orencia	Abatacept	Downregulates T cell lymphocytes	Stop 4 weeks before surgery; resume 1-2 weeks after surgery
Plaquenil	Hydroxychloroquine	Inhibits toll-like receptor 9 family receptors	Continue for all procedures
Remicade	Infliximab	Monoclonal antibody against TNF-α	Stop 4-6 weeks before surgery; resume 1-2 weeks after surgery
Rheumatrex	Methotrexate	Folate analog that inhibits purine metabolism or T cell activation	Continue for all procedures
Rituxan	Rituximab	Anti B cell monoclonal antibody to CD-20	Hold until B cells return to normal before surgery (may take up to 1 year), resume 4-6 weeks after surgery after wound heals
Simponi	Golimumab	Monoclonal antibody against TNF-α	Stop 4-6 weeks before surgery; resume 1-2 weeks after surgery

COX = cyclooxygenase; IL = interleukin; TNF = tumor necrosis factor.

lence ranges from 0.07 to 4.01 per 1,000 patients.[45-47] It is one of the most common chronic childhood illnesses; it affects a similar number of patients as juvenile diabetes and four times as many patients who have cystic fibrosis or sickle cell anemia.[48] Patients must be younger than 16 years at the time of diagnosis, and the duration of symptoms must last at least 6 weeks. The diagnosis of JIA is one of exclusion; there are many other causes of childhood arthritis, and there are no specific laboratory tests for JIA.

The most common JIA category is oligoarthritis JIA (oJIA),[49] which is further divided into persistent and extended subcategories. For the persistent category, four or fewer joints are affected during the disease process, but for the extended category, four or more joints are affected after 6 months. Persistent oJIA often affects one joint, which is most commonly the knee, and these patients often have a very mild disease pattern, presenting with joint swelling and some loss of motion in the knee. However, extended oJIA is more severe, and it symmetrically affects more joints (hands, wrist, and ankle), may present with chronic eye inflammation, and may also have elevated ESR and antinuclear antibody.

Polyarthritis JIA (poJIA) can be differentiated from oJIA in that five or more joints are affected in the first 6 months of the disease. There are two subcategories that are divided by the presence or the absence of rheumatoid factor: poJIA rheumatoid factor-positive patients must have two positive laboratory tests at least 3 months apart during the first 6 months of the disease. Patients positive for rheumatoid factor tend to be older females who present with symmetric small joint arthritis and are often HLA-DR4 positive. Their presentation is similar to adult patients with RA. The presentation of patients negative for poJIA rheumatoid factor is variable and can include fatigue, growth retardation, anemia, osteopenia, delay in sexual maturation, and malnutrition. The poJIA rheumatoid factor-negative diagnosis is more common, and these patients tend to do clinically better than rheumatoid factor-positive patients.

Systematic JIA is characterized by the presence of a cyclical fever that rises above 39°C and goes below 37°C for at least 2 weeks. The fever must also be accompanied by at least one of the following clinical presentations: rheumatoid rash (nonpuritic, macular, or maculopapular), generalized lymphadenopathy, serositis (peritoneal, pleural, or pericardial), and splenomegaly and/or hepatomegaly. These patients often have elevated acute-phase reactants, such as elevated ESR, CRP, and white blood cell (WBC) count, and rarely have positive rheumatoid factor or uveitis. Systematic JIA often occurs in patients younger than 6 years old and equally affects boys and girls.

The two categories that separate JIA from juvenile RA are the addition of enthesis-related arthritis and psoriatic arthritis. Patients with enthesis-related arthritis present with inflammation of soft tissue (ligaments, tendons, fascia, or joint capsule) attached to bone and arthritis, or enthesis or arthritis with at least two of the following criteria: symptomatic anterior uveitis, sacroiliac (SI) joint tenderness, or lumbosacral pain, positive human leukocyte antigen (HLA)-B27, a family history of positive HLA-B27, or the patient is a male older than 6 years at the time of onset of enthesis and/or arthritis. Most of these patients have arthritis in the peripheral joints, in comparison to the axial skeleton, and these patients may have inflammatory bowel disease. Laboratory tests for antinuclear antibody and RF are commonly negative, and imaging rarely shows changes in the SI joint or lumbosacral region until later in the disease process.

Arthritis and psoriasis are diagnosed in patients with psoriatic JIA, although the characteristic rash may not appear for many years after the presentation of arthritis. A diagnosis is made when arthritis and at least two of the following disease processes are present: nail pitting (two pits or more in one or more nails) or onycholysis (partial or full detachment of the nail from the nail bed), dactylitis (asymmetric joint swelling in a digit), or psoriasis diagnosed in a first-degree relative. The arthritis is often asymmetric and peripheral, and it often affects the small joints of the hands and feet, ankles, and knees. Approximately 20% of these patients may present with chronic anterior chamber uveitis. Table 5 summarizes the differences among the different categories of JIA.[50]

Because JIA is a diagnosis of exclusion, all other forms of arthritis must be ruled out before the diagnosis of JIA, and these patients should be followed clinically for a long period (minimum 6 weeks). After JIA is diagnosed, these patients should undergo laboratory testing and should be routinely seen in a clinic. It is also recommended that patients with JIA, except those with systemic JIA, undergo routine eye examinations every 6 months for 4 years and annually thereafter.

Treatment of JIA is similar to the anti-inflammatory and immune modulator medications used to treat RA, as described before. In children, special consideration should be taken to limit the use of oral systemic corticosteroids because their use can stunt growth and bone development. Intravenous immunoglobulin can also be used to treat patients, although specific immunoglobulins targeting cytokines currently are more commonly being used. Medications such as rilonacept and canakinumab target IL-1, and tocilizumab targets IL-6. These biologic therapies reduce inflammation and are being used to treat the different forms of JIA.[51]

Seronegative Spondyloarthropathies

Seronegative spondyloarthropathy (or seronegative spondyloarthritis) is a group of diseases that involves the axial skeleton and has negative rheumatoid factor. These diseases have a different pathophysiologic mechanism of disease than what is commonly seen in RA. The prototypical disease in this group is ankylosing spondylitis. Other diseases that are classified as seronegative spondyloarthropathies include reactive arthritis (Reiter syndrome), psoriatic arthritis, enteropathic arthritis, and juvenile-onset spondyloarthropathies.

These diseases are associated with HLA genes of the major histocompatibility complex, and this genetic component is associated with familial aggregation. These arthritis diseases generally present with oligoarthritis with asymmetric presentation, as well as sacroiliitis and spondylitis. Enthesitis, or inflammation of the insertion sites of tendons or ligaments, is also a feature of these diseases. Extra-articular features, such as involvement of the eyes, skin, and the genitourinary tract, are common.

2: Systemic Disorders

Table 5

Classification of Juvenile Idiopathic Arthritis

Classification	Number of Joints	Duration of Symptoms	Laboratory Tests	Clinical Features	Familial Trait	Other
Systematic	≥ 1	6 weeks	Elevated ESR, CRP, and WBC	Fever (≥ 39°C), rheumatoid rash (nonpuritic, pale pink, blanching, and transient), serositis, generalized lymphadenopathy, splenomegaly, or hepatomegaly		
Polyarthritis RF negative	≥ 5	6 months	Negative RF	Females, fatigue, anemia, growth retardation, osteopenia, malnutrition, and delay in sexual maturation		More common than polyarthritis RF positive
Polyarthritis RF positive	≥ 5	6 months	Positive RF HLA-DR4	Females with later onset (≥ 8 years old), symmetric small joint arthritis, and poor function outcomes		Resembles adult RA
Oligoarthritis, persistent	≤ 4	6 months		Monoarticular involvement (knee)		Most common JIA, best outcome of JIAs
Oligoarthritis, extended	≥ 4	6 months	Elevated ESR and ANA	Polyarticular involvement (hand, wrist, or ankle), younger, female, and chronic eye inflammation		Most common JIA
Enthesitis-related arthritis	≥ 1	6 weeks	HLA-B27, negative ANA and RF	Anterior uveitis, sacroiliac tenderness, lumbosacral pain, and male ≥ 6 years old,	HLA-B27"-associated disease in a first or second degree relative	
Psoriatic arthritis	≥ 1	6 weeks		Dactylitis, nail abnormalities (onycholysis or pitting); psoriatic rash may appear after 16 years old; peripheral and asymmetric arthritis of the ankles, knees, and small joints of the hands and/or feet	Psoriasis in a first-degree relative	
Undifferentiated	≥ 1	6 weeks				Does not fit any of the other categories, or the arthritis fits into more than one category

ANA = Antinuclear antibody; CRP = C-reactive protein; ESR = erythrocyte sedimentation rate; JIA = juvenile idiopathic arthritis; RA = rheumatoid arthritis; RF = rheumatoid factor; WBC = white blood cell count.

Ankylosing Spondylitis

Ankylosing spondylitis is the most common and typical form of the seronegative spondyloarthropathies; it is a chronic inflammatory disease that affects the spine and the sacroiliac joints. Normally this disease presents in the third decade of life with inflammatory back pain that is insidious in onset. Ankylosing spondylitis is diagnosed by clinical features, and the presenting features of the disease are nonspecific. The central feature of ankylosing spondylitis is inflammation at the entheses.[41] Radiographs of the SI joints show the hallmark sclerosis and erosion associated with ankylosing spondylitis. Other manifestations, such as acute anterior uveitis, a positive family history of seronegative spondyloarthritis, and a strong association with the HLA-B27 allele support the diagnosis of ankylosing spondylitis.

The cornerstone of therapy for all patients with ankylosing spondylitis is physical therapy, exercise, and education. Regular exercise is crucial to maintain proper spine function and posture. Decreased motion of the spine and kyphosis lead to significant morbidity. Pharmacologic treatment can address stiffness and muscle spasms. NSAIDs, analgesics, and muscle relaxants all play a role in treating the symptoms of ankylosing spondylitis. Because inflammation plays a role in disease progression, TNF-α antagonists, including etanercept, infliximab, and adalimumab, are approved for the treatment of ankylosing spondylitis.

Reactive Arthritis

Reactive arthritis, also known as Reiter syndrome, is an autoimmune sterile synovitis triggered by an infection of the genitourinary or the gastrointestinal tract. Data indicate that approximately 50% of reactive arthritis and undifferentiated oligoarthritis cases can be attributed to a specific pathogen by a combination of culture and serology.[41] The most common intestinal organisms include *Salmonella*, *Shigella*, or *Campylobacter*, and sexually transmitted organisms include *Chlamydia trachomatis* or *Neisseria gonorrhoeae*. Reactive arthritis characteristically involves the joints of the lower extremities in an asymmetric, oligoarticular pattern, and enthesopathy of the Achilles tendon is common. The features of anterior uveitis, urethritis (men) or cervicitis (women), and oligoarthritis are all characteristics of Reiter syndrome. Psoriatic-like cutaneous manifestations, such as circinate balanitis and keratoderma blennorrhagica, can support the diagnosis. Reactive arthritis can be self-limiting, but chronic arthritis can develop. NSAIDs are therapeutic for acute inflammation. The role of antibiotics in preventing the development of chronic synovitis is not clear.

Psoriatic Arthritis

Psoriatic arthritis is an inflammatory condition that is associated with psoriasis. The presence of skin manifestations of psoriasis is needed to reach the diagnosis. The classic findings of skin lesions, nail pitting, onycholysis, and chronic uveitis are other manifestations that can help with the diagnosis.

Up to one third of those with psoriasis develop inflammatory arthritis. This can cause pain and stiffness in the involved joints. Only 4% to 5% of those with psoriatic arthritis are positive for rheumatoid factor.[52] Psoriatic arthritis is classified among the seronegative spondyloarthropathies as a result of negative rheumatoid factor, spinal involvement, the pattern of joint involvement, the association with HLA-B27, and the extra-articular features.[41]

Psoriatic arthritis affects both the peripheral joints and the axial skeleton. There are multiple disease presentations: distal, oligoarthritis, polyarthritis, back alone, back plus distal, back plus oligoarthritis, back plus polyarthritis, remission, and arthritis mutilans. Dactylitis, or sausage digit, is a typical feature of psoriatic arthritis[41] and refers to the inflammation of an entire digit.

The treatment of psoriatic arthritis is similar to OA in some ways. Exercise and activity modification can help. For more severe symptoms, NSAIDs can be considered. Traditional disease-modifying drugs, such as methotrexate, sulfasalazine, and cyclosporine, still play a role, but TNF-α antagonists are now approved for the treatment of psoriasis and psoriatic arthritis.

Enteropathic Arthritis

This type of arthritis accompanies inflammatory bowel disease. Enteropathic arthritis occurs in 10% to 22% of patients with inflammatory bowel disease, with a higher prevalence in those with Crohn disease than with ulcerative colitis.[41] The peripheral arthritis is typically in the lower extremity, but it can manifest as an axial arthritis that is indistinguishable from ankylosing spondylitis. The axial form has an association with HLA-B27. Treatment with NSAIDs mimics that of the other seronegative spondyloarthropathies.

Crystal Deposition Diseases

The deposition of microcrystals into joints can result in damage to cartilage through acute or chronic synovitis. The two most common crystals present in crystal arthropathies are monosodium urate (MSU) and calcium pyrophosphate dihydrate (CPPD). Less frequently, calcium apatite and calcium oxalate crystal deposition can cause arthritis. Diagnosis is confirmed in the aspirate of synovial fluid. Polarized light microscopy is used to determine the difference between gout and pseudogout.

Gout

Gout is a disease caused by the deposition of MSU crystals in the joints and soft tissues of the body, and it is associated with hyperuricemia. MSU crystals are negatively birefringent needle-shaped crystals. The arthritis is more common in men and postmenopausal women, and it is both acute and chronic. Acute gouty arthritis presents with the rapid development of warmth, swelling, erythema, and pain in the involved joint. The first attack occurs in the metatarsophalangeal joint of the great toe in almost 50% of the cases. Other joints that are commonly involved include the midfoot, the ankle, the heel, and the knee. Chronic tophaceous gout usually develops after 10 years or more of acute intermittent gout. Joints become persistently uncomfortable and swollen, and there are no more pain-free periods.

The treatment of gout with colchicine and indomethacin results in quick resolution of the acute, painful symptoms. Maintenance therapy with allopurinol

2: Systemic Disorders

can reduce further attacks by decreasing the deposition of crystals in the joint.

Pseudogout

Pseudogout is a disease caused by the deposition of CPPD crystals in articular tissues. The name is derived from the symptoms of acute inflammation that can resemble a gouty attack. The deposition of crystals is usually asymptomatic, but there can be multiple presentations. In one presentation, CPPD crystals can lead to an exacerbation of OA in the involved joint. Pseudogout can also result in a severe destructive pattern that resembles neuropathic arthropathy or produce a symmetric proliferative synovitis such as RA.

Fluid analysis of the joint reveals positively birefringent rhomboid-shaped crystals. The knee is the most commonly involved joint. Chondrocalcinosis in the menisci can be seen on radiographs of the knee, which is indicative of CPPD crystals.

The treatment of acute symptoms involves the administration of NSAIDs and/or intra-articular steroid injections. There is no maintenance therapy to reduce further attacks.

Infectious Arthritis

Infectious arthritis is classified as both an inflammatory cause of arthritis and a secondary cause of OA. It is the acute process that defines it as an inflammatory arthritis. Acute infectious arthritis is also called septic arthritis. The destruction of cartilage occurs through the activation of an acute inflammatory process, such as the activation of T cells, and the production of toxins and enzymes by bacteria that in turn activates proteases such as collagenase, hyaluronidase, elastase, lipoproteinase, and lipase. If the acute process is left untreated, it can progress to complete cartilage loss in 4 weeks. Even if the acute arthritis is halted, secondary arthritis can result from damage to the cartilage.

Infection is usually a monoarticular process but can be oligoarticular or polyarticular. Diagnosis depends on an aspiration of the joint fluid and the analysis of this fluid. Greater than 50,000/mm³ nucleated cells with 90% neutrophils is usually considered diagnostic. In one study, however, greater than 50% of culture positive aspirates had synovial nucleated cell counts less than 28,000/mm³.[53]

Infection in a synovial joint occurs when bacteria gain access to the joint space. Bacteria can spread to the joint through direct access from trauma or surgery, through hematogenous spread, or through local tissues from cellulitis or osteomyelitis. Adults who develop acute septic arthritis often have an impaired immune system. RA, liver cirrhosis, chronic renal failure, malignancy, hemodialysis, HIV infection, and organ transplantation are among the immune-altering diseases that place patients at a higher risk of septic arthritis.

Nongonococcal septic arthritis is the most serious infectious arthritis. The most common organism encountered is *Staphylococcus aureus*, but group A streptococcus and *Enterobacter* are also commonly responsible for nongonococcal septic arthritis. Gonococcal arthritis differs from nongonococcal arthritis with regard to organism and presentation. The responsible organism is *Neisseria gonorrhoeae*, and gonococcal arthritis is a migratory arthritis and tenosynovitis with or without skin lesions. Patients are usually healthy, young, sexually active adults. Gonococcal cultures are often taken at extra-articular sites, and the joint fluid culture and Gram stain are typically negative.

Other less common causes of infectious arthritis should be kept in mind. Mycobacterial, fungal, and parasitic arthritis tend to present as subacute or chronic monoarticular arthritis. Viral arthritis can also result after a viral illness.

Lyme disease is an *Ixodes* tick-borne infection caused by spirochetes (*Borrelia burgdorferi*). Patients present with symptoms at one of three stages. In the early localized phase, patients often present with classic erythema migrans. In the early disseminated phase, patients commonly present with Lyme carditis or neurologic symptoms, such as sixth or seventh nerve palsy, or lymphocytic meningitis. Lyme arthritis is a late manifestation of Lyme disease, where patients often present with fever and monoarticular arthritis of the knee.[54] However, Lyme arthritis can also be found in the hip, the ankle, the wrist, or elbow. These synovial joints are affected because spirochetes invade the synovium and stimulate an immune response, which includes the accumulation of cytokines, neutrophils, immune complexes, and complement. The spirochete also induces vascularity proliferation, induces synovial hypertrophy, and stimulates chondrocytes to produce MMPs.[55]

In the classic arthritis presentation of Lyme arthritis, patients present with episodic synovitis that lasts less than 1 week and involves one to four joints; there are asymptomatic periods of 2 or more weeks between episodes. The acute pauciarticular presentation involves one to four joints continuously for less than 4 weeks. Three other clinical presentations of Lyme arthritis include migratory, polyarticular, and chronic pauciarticular presentations.[56]

The diagnosis of Lyme disease starts with a high clinical suspicion for the disease given the geographic distribution of the tick. Serological laboratory diagnosis of Lyme disease is performed using enzyme-linked immunosorbent assay and Western blot.

When a patient presents with an acutely painful native joint with a high suspicion for infectious arthritis, specific laboratory tests, including serum WBC count, ESR, and CRP, should be performed. The joint should be aspirated and sent for cell count, where special attention is paid to the synovial WBC count and differential, culture, and crystals. Patients with nongonococcal septic arthritis should be urgently treated, but the treatment method is controversial. Good results have been reported for serial aspiration, arthroscopic débridement, and arthrotomy with débridement. Antibiotics should be administered based on culture results. Culture-negative aspirates in children require aggressive treatment, even if an organism is not found. For gonococcal infections, antibiotic therapy without drainage usually suffices. Finally, for Lyme arthritis, treatment is most successful with oral antibiotics, including doxycycline, tetracycline, amoxicillin, or cefuroxime. Intravenous antibiotics, including ceftriaxone, cefotaxime, and penicillin G, can also be used.[57]

Neuropathic Arthritis

Neuropathic arthritis is a synonym for Charcot arthropathy, neurotrophic arthropathy, and neuroarthropathy. In the setting of neurologic damage, neuropathic arthritis is a destructive process that involves fractures, subluxation, and dislocation of the articular structures. Two consistent clinical features of neuropathic arthritis are the presence of significant sensory deficit and a lesser degree of pain than would be expected considering the amount of joint destruction seen on radiographs.[41]

Historically, neuropathic arthritis was seen in tertiary syphilis (tabes dorsalis). Contemporary common causes of neuropathic arthritis are diabetes, syringomyelia, spina bifida, and brain or spinal cord trauma. The typical pattern of anatomic involvement depends on the location of the neurologic impairment. In patients with diabetes, the foot is most commonly involved. Syringomyelia involves the upper extremity, and patients with spina bifida have knee, hip, ankle, and spine involvement.

The diagnosis of neuropathic arthritis is a clinical one. Plain radiographs, bone scans, and indium-111-labeled WBC scans can be useful in the diagnosis. In established disease, bone fragmentation, periarticular debris formation, and joint subluxation occur.[41] Neuropathic arthritis can be confused with infection, fracture, gout, pseudogout, osteonecrosis, or OA because affected joints often present with a fluid collection. Aspiration of a joint with neuropathic arthritis will reveal a noninflammatory fluid, and aspirates commonly produce hemorrhagic fluid.

The pathogenesis of neuropathic arthritis has not been clearly defined. The answer seems to be a combination of two separate theories. A neurovascular theory postulates that denervation alters blood flow from changes in the sympathetic regulation, and this upsets the balance in bone resorption and formation.[41] The neurotraumatic theory proposes that repeat events of minor trauma without the protection of normal pain leads to damage from further trauma and inadequate repair.[41] Recent studies have started to reveal the pathogenesis of neuropathic arthritis at a molecular level. Uncontrolled inflammation leads to an imbalance in osteoclasts and osteoblasts.[22] Several studies have shown that TNF-α and interleukins are involved in the process of bone resorption by promoting osteoclast recruitment, proliferation, and differentiation.[58] Monocytes found in neuropathic arthritis express higher levels of proinflammatory cytokines.[5] RANKL also plays a role in neuropathic arthritis, which is an important media-

tor of osteoclastogenesis and is essential in osteoclast formation and modulation.[22] There is research to support the loss of the negative-feedback mechanism in patients with diabetes. Neuropathy decreases the available amounts of calcitonin gene-related peptide and endothelial NOS that, in turn, activates RANKL.[22] Elevated glucose levels form advanced glycation end products, and the lack of a receptor for these end products leads to an increase in RANKL.[6,22]

With improved understanding of the molecular process that results in neuropathic arthritis, new treatments are being considered. Because of the role of IL-1β and TNF-α that results in aggressive and unremitting inflammation, one potential future treatment of neuropathic arthritis is anti-TNF therapy. Bisphosphonates may decrease IGF-1 and help regulate RANKL, but their clinical efficacy remains to be proven.[22] Drugs that increase receptors for advanced glycation end product levels, such as angiotensin-converting enzyme inhibitors, statins, and glitazones, may be useful in preventing or suppressing neuropathic arthritis.[22]

Summary

Arthritis affects about one fifth of the US population. OA is the most common arthritis, and the aging population and the increase in obesity are expected to lead to an epidemic of OA in the next 20 years. New understanding of the diagnosis and the pathology of OA will hopefully lead to treatments that can lessen the effect of OA.

Inflammatory arthritis is a large collection of disease processes that destroy joint cartilage and lead to disability. Biologic agents are already changing the course and severity of these diseases. Research holds great hope to treat and cure these inflammatory diseases.

Key Study Points

- An in-depth understanding of the process of cartilage degeneration in OA is leading to research that detects and treats arthritis at earlier stages, when intervention could prevent progression.

- Clinical practice guidelines with regard to the treatment of knee OA have been developed by the AAOS, and orthopaedic surgeons need to become familiar with this information. Conservative treatment must be initiated first before surgical options are considered.

- Cartilage regeneration and gene therapy are the latest frontier in joint preservation research. Knowing the challenges that are encountered in engineering solutions will help orthopaedic surgeons answer patient questions about coming innovations.

2: Systemic Disorders

Annotated References

1. Bolen J, Schieb L, Hootman JM, et al: Differences in the prevalence and severity of arthritis among racial/ethnic groups in the United States, National Health Interview Survey, 2002, 2003, and 2006. *Prev Chronic Dis* 2010; 7(3):A64.

   The authors describe the prevalence of doctor-diagnosed arthritis and its effect on activities, work, and joint pain for six racial/ethnic groups. Data are drawn from the 2002, 2003, and 2006 National Health Interview Surveys (*n* = 85,784).

2. Hootman JM, Helmick CG: Projections of US prevalence of arthritis and associated activity limitations. *Arthritis Rheum* 2006;54(1):226-229.

3. Centers for Disease Control and Prevention (CDC): Prevalence of disabilities and associated health conditions among adults—United States, 1999. *MMWR Morb Mortal Wkly Rep* 2001;50(7):120-125.

4. Buckwalter JA, Mankin HJ: Articular cartilage: Degeneration and osteoarthritis, repair, regeneration, and transplantation. *Instr Course Lect* 1998;47:487-504.

5. Uccioli L, Sinistro A, Almerighi C, et al: Proinflammatory modulation of the surface and cytokine phenotype of monocytes in patients with acute Charcot foot. *Diabetes Care* 2010;33(2):350-355.

   The authors studied the role of proinflammatory changes in the immune phenotype of monocytes in the pathogenesis of acute Charcot foot.

6. Witzke KA, Vinik AI, Grant LM, et al: Loss of RAGE defense: A cause of Charcot neuroarthropathy? *Diabetes Care* 2011;34(7):1617-1621.

   The authors compared healthy controls to patients with type 2 diabetes with and without Charcot neuropathy. Patients with Charcot neuropathy had significantly lower soluble receptor for advanced glycation end products, increased serum markers of osteocalcin, and reduced bone stiffness.

7. Lee JH, Fitzgerald JB, Dimicco MA, Grodzinsky AJ: Mechanical injury of cartilage explants causes specific time-dependent changes in chondrocyte gene expression. *Arthritis Rheum* 2005;52(8):2386-2395.

8. Mankin HJ, Grodinsky AJ, Buckwalter JA: Articular cartilage and osteoarthritis, in Einhorn TA, O'Keefe RJ, Buckwalter JA (eds): *Orthopaedic Basic Science*, ed 3. Rosemont, IL, American Academy of Orthopaedic Surgeons, 2007, pp 161-174.

9. van der Kraan PM, van den Berg WB: Osteophytes: Relevance and biology. *Osteoarthritis Cartilage* 2007; 15(3):237-244.

10. Krasnokutsky S, Attur M, Palmer G, Samuels J, Abramson SB: Current concepts in the pathogenesis of osteoarthritis. *Osteoarthritis Cartilage* 2008;16(suppl 3):S1-S3.

11. Cerejo R, Dunlop DD, Cahue S, Channin D, Song J, Sharma L: The influence of alignment on risk of knee osteoarthritis progression according to baseline stage of disease. *Arthritis Rheum* 2002;46(10):2632-2636.

12. Hunter DJ, Sharma L, Skaife T: Alignment and osteoarthritis of the knee. *J Bone Joint Surg Am* 2009; 91(suppl 1):85-89.

13. Brouwer GM, van Tol AW, Bergink AP, et al: Association between valgus and varus alignment and the development and progression of radiographic osteoarthritis of the knee. *Arthritis Rheum* 2007;56(4):1204-1211.

14. Hunter DJ, Niu J, Felson DT, et al: Knee alignment does not predict incident osteoarthritis: The Framingham osteoarthritis study. *Arthritis Rheum* 2007;56(4):1212-1218.

15. Hunter DJ, Zhang Y, Niu J, et al: Increase in bone marrow lesions associated with cartilage loss: A longitudinal magnetic resonance imaging study of knee osteoarthritis. *Arthritis Rheum* 2006;54(5):1529-1535.

16. Felson DT, McLaughlin S, Goggins J, et al: Bone marrow edema and its relation to progression of knee osteoarthritis. *Ann Intern Med* 2003;139(5, pt 1):330-336.

17. Chu CR, Williams AA, Coyle CH, Bowers ME: Early diagnosis to enable early treatment of pre-osteoarthritis. *Arthritis Res Ther* 2012;14(3):212.

   The authors review recent advances in imaging and biochemical biomarkers suitable for characterization of the preosteoarthritic joint. They discuss the implications for developing effective early treatment strategies.

18. Jazrawi LM, Alaia MJ, Chang G, Fitzgerald EF, Recht MP: Advances in magnetic resonance imaging of articular cartilage. *J Am Acad Orthop Surg* 2011;19(7): 420-429.

   The authors review biochemical-based MRI techniques; T2 mapping, T1rho, sodium MRI, and dGEMRIC. By imaging the biochemical composition of cartilage, the hope is to detect pathology earlier, intervene earlier, and thus shift management to joint preservation.

19. Owman H, Tiderius CJ, Neuman P, Nyquist F, Dahlberg LE: Association between findings on delayed gadolinium-enhanced magnetic resonance imaging of cartilage and future knee osteoarthritis. *Arthritis Rheum* 2008;58(6):1727-1730.

20. Chu CR, Lin D, Geisler JL, Chu CT, Fu FH, Pan Y: Arthroscopic microscopy of articular cartilage using optical coherence tomography. *Am J Sports Med* 2004; 32(3):699-709.

21. Chu CR, Williams A, Tolliver D, Kwoh CK, Bruno S III, Irrgang JJ: Clinical optical coherence tomography of early articular cartilage degeneration in patients with degenerative meniscal tears. *Arthritis Rheum* 2010; 62(5):1412-1420.

   The authors compare arthroscopic evaluation, OCT,

and T2-weighted MRI. They conclude that OCT can be used clinically to provide qualitative and quantitative assessments of early articular cartilage degeneration that strongly correlate with arthroscopy results.

22. Richmond J , Hunter D, Irrgang J, et al: American Academy of Orthopaedic Surgeons clinical practice guideline on the treatment of osteoarthritis (OA) of the knee. *J Bone Joint Surg Am* 2010; Apr 92(4):990-3.

23. Peter WF, Jansen MJ, Hurkmans EJ, et al: Physiotherapy in hip and knee osteoarthritis: Development of a practice guideline concerning initial assessment, treatment and evaluation. *Acta Reumatol Port* 2011;36(3): 268-281.

    A guideline steering committee consisting of 10 physiotherapists looked at 11 topics in the areas of initial assessment, evaluation, and treatment. The following recommendations were made for OA patients: education and self-management, exercise and manual therapy, supervised exercise therapy, postoperative exercise therapy, and patellar taping.

24. Hochberg MC, Altman RD, April KT, et al: American College of Rheumatology 2012 recommendations for the use of nonpharmacologic and pharmacologic therapies in osteoarthritis of the hand, hip, and knee. *Arthritis Care Res (Hoboken)* 2012;64(4):465-474.

    The authors provide up-to-date guidelines on treatments of OA of the hip, knee, and hand using systematic evidence-based literature reviews. Nonpharmacologic treatment recommendations included exercise and weight loss for hip and knee OA patients and joint protection and thermal treatment of hand OA patients. Pharmacologic treatments of all OA included acetaminophen, topical and oral NSAIDs, tramadol, and intra-articular injections. Opioids were recommended only if patients had a contraindication to total joint arthroplasty.

25. Webber TA, Webber AE, Matzkin E: Rate of adverse reactions to more than 1 series of viscosupplementation. *Orthopedics* 2012;35(4):e514-e519.

    The authors performed a retrospective study and found that patients who receive more than one series of viscosupplementation have few adverse reactions, which were defined as acute pain and swelling in the knee.

26. Chu CR, Coyle CH, Chu CT, et al: In vivo effects of single intra-articular injection of 0.5% bupivacaine on articular cartilage. *J Bone Joint Surg Am* 2010;92(3): 599-608.

    This in vivo study in rats showed reduced chondrocyte density without cartilage tissue loss six months after a single intra-articular injection of 0.5% bupivacaine. They conclude that this suggests bupivacaine toxicity.

27. Lo GH, LaValley M, McAlindon T, Felson DT: Intra-articular hyaluronic acid in treatment of knee osteoarthritis: A meta-analysis. *JAMA* 2003;290(23):3115-3121.

28. Moreland LW: Intra-articular hyaluronan (hyaluronic acid) and hylans for the treatment of osteoarthritis:

Mechanisms of action. *Arthritis Res Ther* 2003;5(2): 54-67.

29. Ventura A, Memeo A, Borgo E, Terzaghi C, Legnani C, Albisetti W: Repair of osteochondral lesions in the knee by chondrocyte implantation using the MACI® technique. *Knee Surg Sports Traumatol Arthrosc* 2012; 20(1):121-126.

    The authors conclude, through a restrospective cohort study, that matrix-induced autologous chondrocyte implantation has proven to be a safe and effective procedure to treat cartilage defects.

30. Odorico JS, Kaufman DS, Thomson JA: Multilineage differentiation from human embryonic stem cell lines. *Stem Cells* 2001;19(3):193-204.

31. Kurtz S, Ong K, Lau E, Mowat F, Halpern M: Projections of primary and revision hip and knee arthroplasty in the United States from 2005 to 2030. *J Bone Joint Surg Am* 2007;89(4):780-785.

32. Safran MR, Kim H, Zaffagnini S: The use of scaffolds in the management of articular cartilage injury. *J Am Acad Orthop Surg* 2008;16(6):306-311.

33. Fortier LA, Barker JU, Strauss EJ, McCarrel TM, Cole BJ: The role of growth factors in cartilage repair. *Clin Orthop Relat Res* 2011;469(10):2706-2715.

    The authors performed a PubMed search using chondrocyte or cartilage in combination with growth factors and their ability to synthesize extracellular growth matrix. The main growth factors that were discussed were the TGF-β superfamily, IGF-1, the FGF family, and platelet-derived growth factor.

34. Chia SL, Sawaji Y, Burleigh A, et al: Fibroblast growth factor 2 is an intrinsic chondroprotective agent that suppresses ADAMTS-5 and delays cartilage degradation in murine osteoarthritis. *Arthritis Rheum* 2009;60(7): 2019-2027.

35. Schmidt MB, Chen EH, Lynch SE: A review of the effects of insulin-like growth factor and platelet derived growth factor on in vivo cartilage healing and repair. *Osteoarthritis Cartilage* 2006;14(5):403-412.

36. Evans CH, Robbins PD, Ghivizzani SC, et al: Gene transfer to human joints: Progress toward a gene therapy of arthritis. *Proc Natl Acad Sci U S A* 2005; 102(24):8698-8703.

37. Firestein G: *Kelly's Textbook of Rheumatology*, ed 7. Philadelphia, PA, WB Saunders, 2005, pp 996-1042.

38. Aletaha D, Neogi T, Silman AJ, et al: 2010 Rheumatoid arthritis classification criteria: An American College of Rheumatology/European League Against Rheumatism collaborative initiative. *Arthritis Rheum* 2010;62(9): 2569-2581.

    The most recent classification of RA updated the 1987 American College of Rheumatology classification by focusing on the early stages of the disease. Definite RA was defined with synovitis in at least one joint without an alternate diagnosis and the following minor criteria: the site and number of joints involved, serologic findings, elevation of acute phase reactants, and the duration of symptoms.

39. Cohen SB, Moreland LW, Cush JJ, et al: A multicentre, double blind, randomised, placebo controlled trial of anakinra (Kineret), a recombinant interleukin 1 receptor antagonist, in patients with rheumatoid arthritis treated with background methotrexate. *Ann Rheum Dis* 2004; 63(9):1062-1068.

40. Bresnihan B, Newmark R, Robbins S, Genant HK: Effects of anakinra monotherapy on joint damage in patients with rheumatoid arthritis: Extension of a 24-week randomized, placebo controlled trial. *J Rheumatol* 2004;31(6):1103-1111.

41. Klippel JH, Stone JH, Crofford LJ, White PH: *Primer on the Rheumatic Diseases*, ed 13. New York, NY, Springer, 2008.

42. Giannini EH, Ruperto N, Ravelli A, Lovell DJ, Felson DT, Martini A: Preliminary definition of improvement in juvenile arthritis. *Arthritis Rheum* 1997;40(7):1202-1209.

43. Petty RE, Southwood TR, Manners P, et al: International League of Associations for Rheumatology classification of juvenile idiopathic arthritis: Second revision, Edmonton, 2001. *J Rheumatol* 2004;31(2):390-392.

44. Manners PJ, Bower C: Worldwide prevalence of juvenile arthritis why does it vary so much? *J Rheumatol* 2002; 29(7):1520-1530.

45. Manners PJ, Diepeveen DA: Prevalence of juvenile chronic arthritis in a population of 12-year-old children in urban Australia. *Pediatrics* 1996;98(1):84-90.

46. Mielants H, Veys EM, Maertens M, et al: Prevalence of inflammatory rheumatic diseases in an adolescent urban student population, age 12 to 18, in Belgium. *Clin Exp Rheumatol* 1993;11(5):563-567.

47. Tayel MY, Tayel KY: Prevalence of juvenile chronic arthritis in school children aged 10 to 15 years in Alexandria. *J Egypt Public Health Assoc* 1999;74(5-6): 529-546.

48. Gortmaker SL, Sappenfield W: Chronic childhood disorders: Prevalence and impact. *Pediatr Clin North Am* 1984;31(1):3-18.

49. Hofer M, Southwood TR: Classification of childhood arthritis. *Best Pract Res Clin Rheumatol* 2002;16(3): 379-396.

50. Gowdie PJ, Tse SM: Juvenile idiopathic arthritis. *Pediatr Clin North Am* 2012;59(2):301-327.

The authors provide a comprehensive review article on JIA, detailing the causes, the epidemiology, clinical manifestations, classifications, developments in management, complications, and long-term outcomes of JIA.

51. Ruth NM, Passo MH: Juvenile idiopathic arthritis: Management and therapeutic options. *Ther Adv Musculoskelet Dis* 2012;4(2):99-110.

There have been great developments in the management of patients with JIA; an improved classification system, patient assessment, imaging, and gene profiling have helped develop more specific treatments. Older treatments, including NSAIDs and methotrexate, are being supplemented with biologic treatments such as TNF-α inhibitors, IL-1 and IL-6 blockade, selective B cell blockade, and selective costimulation modulators.

52. Taylor W, Gladman D, Helliwell P, et al: Classification criteria for psoriatic arthritis: Development of new criteria from a large international study. *Arthritis Rheum* 2006;54(8):2665-2673.

53. McCutchan HJ, Fisher RC: Synovial leukocytosis in infectious arthritis. *Clin Orthop Relat Res* 1990;257: 226-230.

54. Smith BG, Cruz AI Jr, Milewski MD, Shapiro ED: Lyme disease and the orthopaedic implications of lyme arthritis. *J Am Acad Orthop Surg* 2011;19(2):91-100.

This review article evaluates the orthopaedic complications of Lyme disease, which should be considered in patients with mono-or pauciarticular joint pain or effusion, especially in areas with endemic Lyme disease. Treatment with antibiotics and arthroscopic synovectomy in severe cases lead to a good prognosis.

55. Puius YA, Kalish RA: Lyme arthritis: Pathogenesis, clinical presentation, and management. *Infect Dis Clin North Am* 2008;22(2):289-300, vi-vii.

56. Rose CD, Fawcett PT, Eppes SC, Klein JD, Gibney K, Doughty RA: Pediatric Lyme arthritis: Clinical spectrum and outcome. *J Pediatr Orthop* 1994;14(2):238-241.

57. Wormser GP, Dattwyler RJ, Shapiro ED, et al: The clinical assessment, treatment, and prevention of lyme disease, human granulocytic anaplasmosis, and babesiosis: Clinical practice guidelines by the Infectious Diseases Society of America. *Clin Infect Dis* 2006;43(9):1089-1134.

58. Baumhauer JF, O'Keefe RJ, Schon LC, Pinzur MS: Cytokine-induced osteoclastic bone resorption in charcot arthropathy: An immunohistochemical study. *Foot Ankle Int* 2006;27(10):797-800.

Chapter 19

Extracellular Matrix and Collagen Disorders

William V. Arnold, MD, PhD   Andrzej Fertala, PhD

Introduction

The extracellular matrix (ECM) is composed of a large number of protein molecules that are secreted by cells, with much of the three-dimensional assembly of these molecules occurring extracellularly. The ECM may be envisioned as a scaffold that holds together the cellular components of tissues and organs, but the function of the ECM goes well beyond this simple concept. Collagen proteins play a predominant role in orthopaedic-related issues because they are the main ECM constituent of bone and cartilage. A classic example of how collagen defects can cause human disease is demonstrated by mutations in type I collagen that cause osteogenesis imperfecta (discussed in chapter 66, Skeletal Dysplasias, Connective Tissue Diseases, and Other Genetic Disorders, *Orthopaedic Knowledge Update 11*). However, aberrations of other ECM components can also contribute to orthopaedic diseases. Understanding these diseases at the molecular level, and specifically how these diseases affect the ECM, may help direct future treatments of these disorders.

Chondrodysplasias: A Broad Spectrum of Diseases of Skeletal Growth

The patterning and formation of the architecture of the skeleton during fetal development is a complex and highly regulated process.[1,2] One of its initial stages involves the condensation of mesenchymal cells at sites of bone formation (**Figure 1**). In this process, mesenchymal cells differentiate into chondrocytes, which form primordial cartilage. Subsequently, the primary ossification centers are formed by degradation and mineralization of the center of the primordial cartilage. The

Dr. Arnold or an immediate family member serves as a paid consultant to or is an employee of Merck and URL Pharma; has stock or stock options held in Merck and URL Pharma; and has received research or institutional support from Stryker. Dr. Fertala or an immediate family member has received research or institutional support from Mentor Worldwide, LLC.

cortex of bone is synthesized by osteoblasts derived from the midshaft region. Subsequently, the secondary ossification centers are created in a process that involves removal of part of the embryonic cartilage. The growth plate or physis remains between structures formed within the primary and secondary ossification centers. The cartilage growth plate includes well-defined subpopulations of chondrocytes that form resting, proliferative, and hypertrophic zones characterized by a columnar arrangement of cells that form them (**Figures 1** and **2**). The biologic activity of the growth plate chondrocytes is part of the mechanism that controls bone growth and mineralization.[1,3,4]

During the physiologic process of bone development and growth, chondrocytes produce and secrete extracellular macromolecules that form the architecture of the cartilaginous ECM, signal cells via specific receptors, and serve as a reservoir for various growth factors that regulate bone development.[5] In pathologic situations caused by mutations in genes encoding these macromolecules, the processes of bone formation and growth are altered. Clinically, these pathologic situations are recognized as chondrodysplasias, a group of rare, inherited disorders of skeletal development and linear growth.[6] The clinical aspects of these chondrodysplasias are discussed in chapter 66, Skeletal Dysplasias, Connective Tissue Diseases, and Other Genetic Disorders, *Orthopaedic Knowledge Update 11*. The pathomechanisms of these diseases include the intracellular processes of biosynthesis and secretion and the extracellular processes of the formation of biologic scaffolds, receptor-mediated cell-matrix interactions, and an enzyme-dependent turnover of elements of the ECM (**Figure 3**).

Chondrodysplasias Associated With Mutations in Collagens of Cartilage

The structural integrity of cartilage and its ability to fulfill specific mechanical and biologic functions is facilitated by the presence of a unique extracellular scaffold formed by various macromolecules produced by chondrocytes (**Figure 2**). Such a scaffold not only defines the physical characteristics of cartilage but also provides a platform for the receptor-mediated attachment of cells. The biologic scaffold of cartilage is a

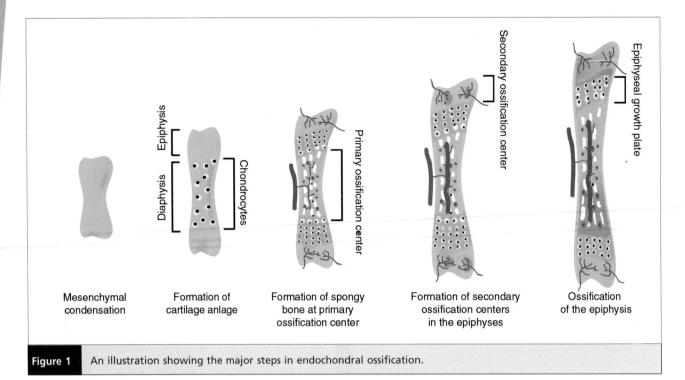

Figure 1 An illustration showing the major steps in endochondral ossification.

Mesenchymal condensation | Formation of cartilage anlage | Formation of spongy bone at primary ossification center | Formation of secondary ossification centers in the epiphyses | Ossification of the epiphysis

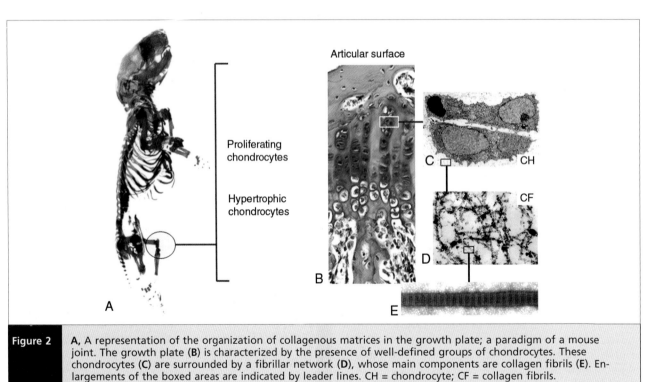

Figure 2 **A,** A representation of the organization of collagenous matrices in the growth plate; a paradigm of a mouse joint. The growth plate (**B**) is characterized by the presence of well-defined groups of chondrocytes. These chondrocytes (**C**) are surrounded by a fibrillar network (**D**), whose main components are collagen fibrils (**E**). Enlargements of the boxed areas are indicated by leader lines. CH = chondrocyte; CF = collagen fibrils.

dynamic structure whose homeostasis is maintained by the balanced processes of synthesis and degradation of its individual elements. The processes of biosynthesis and degradation are strictly regulated at different biologic levels that include gene expression; gene translation; the posttranslational modification of ECM proteins; intracellular transport and secretion of these proteins; the homotypic and heterotypic assembly of these proteins into extracellular structures; and the enzymatic degradation, turnover, and modification of these extracellular structures.[7]

Mutations associated with elements of the biologic scaffold of cartilage may affect each of these stages, thereby leading to chondrodysplasias.[6] Focusing on the

© 2014 American Academy of Orthopaedic Surgeons

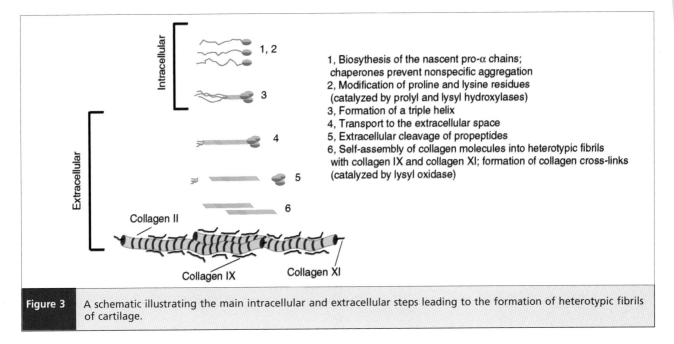

1, Biosythesis of the nascent pro-α chains;
  chaperones prevent nonspecific aggregation
2, Modification of proline and lysine residues
  (catalyzed by prolyl and lysyl hydroxylases)
3, Formation of a triple helix
4, Transport to the extracellular space
5, Extracellular cleavage of propeptides
6, Self-assembly of collagen molecules into heterotypic fibrils
  with collagen IX and collagen XI; formation of collagen cross-links
  (catalyzed by lysyl oxidase)

Figure 3 A schematic illustrating the main intracellular and extracellular steps leading to the formation of heterotypic fibrils of cartilage.

biosynthesis of collagen II, the main structural protein of cartilage, helps to illustrate the complex mechanisms involved in the pathology of diseases such as chondrodysplasias and exemplifies the challenges in developing molecular-based therapies for these diseases.[6,8,9]

Intracellular Processes of Synthesis of Procollagen II

Biosynthesis of Individual Procollagen II Chains

Collagen II belongs to a group of fibril-forming collagens with which it shares several biochemical and biophysical characteristics.[7] The collagen II protein that is assembled into the ECM is first produced as a larger, soluble procollagen II molecule that is encoded by the *COL2A1* gene. Procollagen II is produced by chondrocytes in the form of a homotrimeric protein with individual procollagen II chains that are characterized by the presence of an extended triple-helical domain flanked by the N (amino)-terminal and the C (carboxyl)-terminal globular propeptide domains (Figures 3 and 4). The telopeptides are short regions that separate the extended triple-helical collagen domain from the propeptide domains. A critical characteristic that defines the key region, namely the extended triple-helical domain, is the presence of consecutive repeats of approximately 300 amino acid triplets characterized as -G-X-Y-, in which G is the amino acid glycine, the X position is frequently occupied by the amino acid proline, and the Y position is frequently occupied by hydroxyproline, a hydroxylated form of the amino acid proline[7] (Figures 3 and 4). Before folding into a triple-helical structure, the nascent procollagen II molecules undergo posttranslational modifications that mainly include hydroxylation of proline and lysine residues pres-

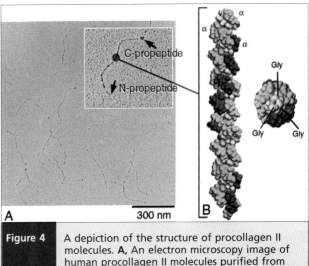

Figure 4 A depiction of the structure of procollagen II molecules. **A,** An electron microscopy image of human procollagen II molecules purified from cultures of cells that produce them. The insert depicts a procollagen II molecule in which the positions of the propeptides are indicated. Note a readily visible C-terminal propeptide. **B,** A computerized model of a fragment of the collagen triple helix. This fragment consists of three individual chains, each consisting of eight canonical -G-X-Y- triplets. A cross-section view indicates a central position of the glycine residues.

ent at the Y positions of the -G-X-Y- triplets and glycosylation of some lysine residues. Critical processes of hydroxylation are catalyzed by prolyl and lysyl hydroxylases, enzymes whose specific activities depend on the presence of ascorbic acid and iron ions.[10,11]

Assembly of the Triple-Helical Structure

Concomitant with the biosynthesis and posttranslational modifications of the nascent procollagen II

2: Systemic Disorders

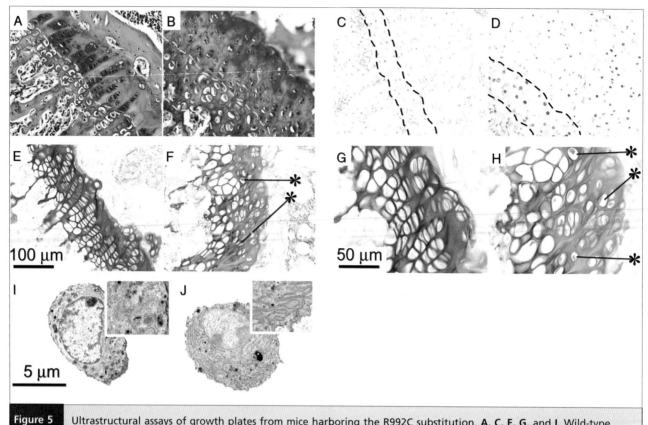

Figure 5 Ultrastructural assays of growth plates from mice harboring the R992C substitution. **A, C, E, G,** and **I,** Wild-type mouse cartilage. **B, D, F, H,** and **J,** Mutant mouse cartilage. **A** and **B,** Hematoxylin and eosin staining of the growth plates. In the mutant growth plate, the columnar arrangement of chondrocytes is altered. **C** and **D,** TdT-mediated dUTP nick-end labeling (TUNEL) of fragmented DNA. Positive labeling seen in **D** indicates the presence of fragmented DNA, an indication of apoptosis. **A, B, C,** and **D,** The dashed lines identify the hypertrophic zones of the growth plates. **E, F, G,** and **H,** Results of the immunostaining for cleaved caspase 3, yet another apoptotic marker, shown at two different magnifications. **F** and **H,** Cleaved caspase 3-positive cells are apparent in the proliferative zone. The asterisks indicate cleaved caspase 3-positive cells. **I** and **J,** Subcellular features of chondrocytes from wild type and mutant mice, respectively. Dilated ER is present in chondrocytes harboring the R992C mutant. (Reproduced with permission from Hintze V, Steplewski A, Ito H, Jensen DA, Rodeck U, Fertala A: Cells expressing partially unfolded R789C/p.R989C type II procollagen mutant associated with spondyloepiphyseal dysplasia undergo apoptosis. *Hum Mutat* 2008;29:841-851.)

chains is their assembly into a triple-helical structure, a hallmark of collagenous proteins. This process is initiated by the site-specific interactions of distinct domains localized at the C-termini of the procollagen II chains[7,11] (**Figure 3**). The assembly of individual chains is assisted by protein chaperones that prevent any premature nonspecific aggregation of the nascent procollagen II chains. The most prominent chaperones that participate in procollagen folding are heat shock protein 47 (HSP47), protein disulfide isomerase, and binding immunoglobulin protein (BiP).[9,12,13] Correctly folded procollagen molecules are characterized by the stable structure of the triple-helical domain whose thermostability depends on the presence of numerous hydrogen bonds between individual procollagen II chains. Although the formation of such hydrogen bonds depends on the presence of hydroxylated proline residues, the tight packing of the procollagen II chains into a triple helix is possible because of the presence of the glycine residues in the repeating -G-X-Y- triplet of the collagen chain (**Figure 4**). Correct folding of procollagen mole-

cules is a prerequisite for their efficient secretion from cells. Misfolded molecules are excessively accumulated intracellularly in the endoplasmic reticulum (ER). Such an excessive accumulation of proteins destined for secretion may cause ER stress, a process that frequently is associated with apoptosis of cells producing the aberrant proteins[8,9,14-17] (**Figure 5**).

Extracellular Procollagen II Processing and Self-Assembly of Collagen II Into Fibrils

Processing of Procollagen Propeptides

Upon secretion from cells, the N-terminal propeptide of procollagen II is cleaved by a group of enzymes that includes a disintegrin and metalloprotease with thrombospondin motifs (ADAMTS)-2, -3, and -14.[18,19] At the same time, the C-terminal propeptide is cleaved by enzymes belonging to the tolloid family of zinc metalloproteinases, in which procollagen C-proteinase, also described as bone morphogenetic protein-1, plays a key role.[20,21] Enzymatic cleavage of propeptides represents a critical step in the process of collagen fibril formation (**Figure 3**).

Formation of Homotypic and Heterotypic Collagen Fibrils

Enzymatic cleavage of procollagen II propeptides exposes the telopeptide region of the molecule and triggers the self-assembly of collagen II molecules into highly ordered collagen fibrils.[11] The formation of collagen fibrils is a spontaneous process driven by site-specific interactions occurring between defined regions of interacting molecules.[11,22] Electrostatic and hydrophobic interactions play a critical role in the formation of highly ordered fibrils whose distinctive morphologic feature is a well-defined periodicity (**Figures 2 and 3**). During this process, collagen II molecules coassemble with collagen IX and collagen XI to form heterotypic fibrils of cartilage. After fibrils are assembled, they are stabilized by covalent cross-links formed primarily with the involvement of lysine and hydroxylysine residues present in the triple helical regions and the telopeptides of cross-linked collagen molecules. The cross-linking process depends on the enzymatic activity of copper-dependent lysyl oxidase, an enzyme that catalyzes the formation of aldehydes from peptidyl lysine and hydroxylysine residues.[23] Properly assembled and cross-linked heterotypic collagen fibrils constitute a critical structural element of cartilage ECM (**Figure 3**).

Collagen II–Associated Diseases

Mutations in *COL2A1* are associated with chondrodysplasias, with severities ranging from profound dwarfism and lethality in utero to mild phenotypes characterized by precocious osteoarthritis. According to the revised classification of the genetic skeletal disorders proposed by the International Skeletal Dysplasia Society (ISDS), *COL2A1*-associated diseases belong to the type II collagen and similar disorders group of chondrodysplasias.[24,25] **Table 1** summarizes the main forms of the *COL2A1*-associated chondrodysplasias.

Early-Onset Osteoarthritis

Czech dysplasia, Stickler syndrome, osteonecrosis of the femoral head, spondyloepiphyseal dysplasia (SED), and Kniest dysplasia are recognized as type II collagenopathies with an arthritis phenotype. The results of a 2010 study[26] suggested that premature osteoarthritis represents a distinct phenotype associated with mutations in *COL2A1*. In addition, it is suggested that precocious osteoarthritis may develop in patients with the absence of any other characteristics indicating collagen II–related disorders. The authors of this study reported cases of early-onset osteoarthritis in individuals harboring the glycine to alanine substitution at amino acid site 204 and the glycine to serine amino acid substitution at amino acid site 393. Based on these and other exam-

ples, it can be postulated that *COL2A1* mutations may be an important element of the pathomechanism of osteoarthritis.[26]

Molecular and Cellular Mechanisms of Diseases Associated With Mutations in *COL2A1*

Anatomically, a common characteristic of chondrodysplasias associated with mutations in *COL2A1* are aberrations of skeletal growth accompanied by developmental abnormalities of the growth plates. The molecular pathomechanisms underlying these anatomic changes are complex and involve intracellular processes of synthesis and transport of procollagen molecules and extracellular processes of fibril formation and cell-matrix interaction.[9] The following sections describe the major changes observed at the molecular, cellular, and extracellular levels in cartilage of affected patients as well as in experimental conditions that include in vitro and in vivo models.

Effects of Mutations on Individual Procollagen II Molecules

Although there are more than 100 missense/nonsense mutations reported for *COL2A1*, no clear genotype-phenotype correlation has been established. Most single amino acid substitutions within the triple helical region of procollagen II are changes for glycine residues.[27] In addition, several mutations that change codons for the arginine residue present at the Y position of a -G-X-Y-triplet have also been described. Substitutions at the X positions are rarely reported, and this type of mutation is frequently associated with Stickler syndrome. Premature stop codons in the regions of *COL2A1* that encode the N-propeptide and the triple helix are also associated with Stickler syndrome, whereas those within the region that encodes the C-propeptide were found in spondyloperipheral dysplasia and the Torrance type of platyspondylic skeletal dysplasia.

Overall, it is difficult to predict the specific molecular consequences of mutations in collagen II. These consequences are broad and may cause the following conditions: (1) posttranslational overmodifications, which include overhydroxylation of proline and lysine residues and overglycosylation of the nascent procollagen II chains; (2) a decrease in the thermostability of procollagen II that prevents proper formation of the triple-helical structure at physiologic temperatures; (3) alterations of the geometry of individual procollagen II molecules by introducing a kink at the site of the mutation; (4) misalignment of individual procollagen II chains; and (5) the production of truncated chains as a result of the introduction of a premature stop codon in protein synthesis. Because of the possible intracellular degradation of misfolded or truncated mutant molecules, these changes may contribute to a decrease in the overall amount of collagen II in cartilage. Because not all mutations lead to an accelerated degradation of affected molecules, certain collagen II mutants are secreted from cells but result in the formation of aberrant

Table 1

Overview of Diseases Associated With Mutations in Collagen II

Disorder/MIM#	Gene/ Inheritance	Reported Mutation Type(s)	Observed Clinical Features	Detected Molecular and Histologic Changes
Achondrogenesis type II and hypochondro-genesis/200610	COL2A1/AD	Missense	Severe micromelic dwarfism Small chest Prominent abdomen Incomplete ossification of the vertebral bodies Disorganization of the costochondral junction	Significantly reduced amount of cartilage collagen II Overmodification of collagen II Increased amount of collagen I and collagen III
Osteonecrosis of femoral head/608805	COL2A1/AD	Missense	Progressive pain in the groin Mechanical failure of the subchondral bone Degeneration of the hip joint	Suggested changes in the fibril structure and interactions with other macromolecules of cartilage
Kniest dysplasia/156550	COL2A1/AD	Missense, splice, deletion	Short stature Round face with central depression Prominent eyes Enlargement and stiffness of joints Contractures of fingers Bell-shaped chest Myopia	Overmodification of collagen II Degeneration of chondrocytes Presence of cytoplasmic inclusions Abnormal collagen fibrils
Platyspondylic dysplasia, Torrance type/151210	COL2A1/AD	Missense, nonsense, deletions within the C propeptide	Wafer-like vertebral bodies, Severe hypoplasia of the lower ilia Short long bones with ragged metaphyses Bowing of the radius	Chondro-osseous histology is characterized by hypercellularity with slightly large chondrocytes in the resting cartilage Normal columnization with incorporation of cartilage into bone at the chondro-osseous junction
Spondyloepi-metaphyseal dysplasia Strudwick type/184250	COL2A1/AD	Missense	Disproportionate short stature Pectus carinatum Scoliosis Dappled metaphyses Retinal detachment	Dilated endoplasmic reticulum
Spondyloepiphyseal dysplasia congenita/ 183900	COL2A1/AD	Missense, splice, deletion, insertion	Short stature Shortening of proximal extremities Kyphoscoliosis and lordosis Platyspondyly Coxa vara Myopia Hearing loss	Decrease of the thermostability of collagen II mutants Atypical formation of a kink in some collagen II mutants Excessive intracellular accumulation of some thermolabile mutants Apoptosis of cells harboring some misfolded mutant collagen II Aberrations of formation of homotypic and heterotypic collagen fibrils
Spondylo-peripheral dysplasia/271700	COL2A1/AD	Nonsense in the C-terminal propeptide	Platyspondyly Severe hip changes Brachydactyly Distal shortening of ulna Myopia Hearing loss	Alteration of C propeptide-dependent association of procollagen II chains Excessive intracellular accumulation of mutant molecules
Stickler syndrome type I/108300	COL2A1/AD	Missense, deletions, splice, nonsense	High myopia Vitreoretinal degeneration Retinal detachment Cataracts Midline clefting-Pierre Robin sequence Flat midface Sensorineural or conductive hearing loss Mild SED	Truncated forms of collagen II chains

AD = autosomal dominant, SED = spondyloepiphyseal dysplasia.

extracellular fibrillar structures.[9,17,28-33]

Effects of Mutations in *COL2A1* On Cells Harboring Abnormal Procollagen Molecules

The intracellular formation of the correct triple-helical structure of procollagen II is essential for its secretion to the extracellular space.[9,17,31] Mutations associated with misfolding of the nascent chains, however, lead to the excessive accumulation of affected molecules in the endoplasmic reticulum (ER), thereby causing ER stress, a process that may trigger the unfolded protein response (UPR; **Figure 5**). The UPR involves the interaction of lumenal BiP with transmembrane stress sensors such as IRE1, ATF6, and PERK. During this process, BiP dissociates from the BiP/sensor complexes and translocates into the ER lumen, where it interacts with misfolded mutants. Dissociation of BiP activates the stress sensors and triggers downstream events that include Xbp-1 splicing and ATF6 cleavage. At the same time, accelerated biosynthesis of BiP and other molecular chaperones, such as protein disulfide isomerase, stimulates the folding of mutant molecules, whereas the overall production of proteins decreases mainly through eIF2α-dependent suppression. If the biologic events of the UPR cannot attenuate the effects of ER stress, the affected cells may undergo apoptosis.[34,35] For instance, studies have demonstrated that the presence of misfolded thermolabile R789C and R992C collagen II mutants associated with SED in humans and mice, respectively, triggers the processes of ER stress, UPR, and apoptosis[9,17,31] (**Figure 5**). Radiographic measurements of bones from mice harboring a spontaneous R992C substitution demonstrate altered growth.[36] These data exemplify the complex pathomechanism of chondrodysplasias associated with mutations in collagen II and point toward the existence of a domino effect triggered by a change at the gene level and leading to pathologies seen phenotypically at the level of bone.

In addition to causing ER stress, the presence of misfolded procollagen II chains in the ER leads to atypical interactions of these procollagens with other proteins. For example, the R789C collagen mutant binds with normal fibronectin, thereby trapping this extracellular protein inside cells and disturbing the correct formation of ECM.[37] Considering these and similar examples, it becomes quite clear that ER stress and the UPR are important consequences of mutations in genes encoding cartilage macromolecules that contribute to the pathogenesis of chondrodysplasias.[9,14,16,17,31]

The existence of the ER-related pathomechanisms offers a new possible target for developing treatment strategies for chondrodysplasias. Specifically, chemical chaperones with the potential to promote folding and the secretion of misfolded collagen II mutants were proposed as a new method to reduce ER stress.[38] Although the chaperone approach will not eliminate the mutant molecules from affected tissues, it may still offer significant therapeutic benefits. This notion is based on the possibility that the "actions" of some mutant molecules in the extracellular space may be less harmful to the tissue than their negative influence on cell functions. This concept is supported by studies that demonstrated that thermostable mutants harboring the R75C and R519C substitutions do not cause detectable ER stress.[31] Although these mutant collagens are incorporated into the ECM, their presence is associated with mild rather than severe forms of dysplasias.

Extracellular Effects of Mutations in *COL2A1*

Electron microscopy observations of cartilage from mice and affected patients harboring mutant collagen II frequently demonstrate a decrease in the number of collagen fibrils present in the extracellular space. Detailed assays show that although not all mutations alter the ability of affected collagen molecules to self-assemble into fibrils, some single amino acid substitutions completely prevent fibril formation or alter the kinetics of self-assembly. In addition, the presence of mutant molecules in a fibril negatively affects its ability to form heterotypic assemblies with wild type collagen IX.[9,17,30-33,39-41] Complex changes in the structure of the ECM formed in the presence of collagen II mutants also altered receptor-mediated cell-matrix interactions, thereby negatively affecting cartilage homeostasis.[9]

Collagen VI, Collagen IX, Collagen XI, and Collagen XXVII

In addition to collagen II, other collagen types provide additional structural elements of cartilage ECM. Collagen VI, a heterotrimer whose individual chains are encoded by the *COL6A1*, *COL6A2*, and *COL6A3* genes, is present in the pericellular region surrounding chondrocytes. The role of this protein in cartilage is not fully defined, but hypotheses have been made that it participates in the transduction of biomechanical signals.[42,43] Analyses of mice with a deletion of *COL6A1* indicate that they develop osteoarthritis, thereby suggesting the critical role of collagen VI in maintaining the integrity of cartilage.[43] In addition, mutations in *COL6A1* are also associated with ossification of the posterior longitudinal ligament of the spine.[44]

Collagen IX is a heterotrimer encoded by the *COL9A1*, *COL9A2*, and *COL9A3* genes. Together with collagen II and collagen XI, this protein participates in the formation of heterotypic fibrils, a main architectural element of the cartilage ECM. Electron microscopy shows that collagen IX decorates the surface of collagen II fibrils. Biochemical assays have determined that both collagen types are chemically cross-linked, thereby forming structurally stable collagen matrices. Chondrodysplasias associated with mutations in collagen IX are classified as the "multiple epiphyseal dysplasia and pseudoachondroplasia" group[24] (**Table 2**).

Yet another component of such complex fibrils is collagen XI. This heterotrimeric protein is encoded by the *COL11A1*, *COL11A2*, and *COL11A3/COL2A1* genes. Although the α3 (XI) chain is encoded by

2: Systemic Disorders

Table 2

Chondrodysplasias Associated With Collagen IX, Collagen X, or Collagen XI Mutations

Disorder/MIM#	Gene/Inheritance	Reported Mutation Type(s)	Observed Clinical Features	Detected Molecular and Histologic Changes
Multiple epiphyseal dysplasia type 6/ 614135	Col9A1/AD	Insertion	Early osteoarthritis Schmorl's nodes End plate irregularities Anterior osteophytes in the thoracolumbar vertebrae Normal hips	Possible alterations of formation of functional collagen IX
Stickler syndrome type IV/614134	COL9A1/AR	Nonsense, insertion	Moderate to severe sensorineural hearing loss Moderate to high myopia with vitreoretinopathy Epiphyseal dysplasia	Possible functional knockout of all collagen IX chains
Multiple epiphyseal dysplasia type 2/ 600204	COL9A2/AD	Splice	Joint pain and stiffness Mild short stature Degenerative joint disease Onset usually in childhood Mild myopathy	In-frame deletion Some variation in a muscle fiber size
Stickler syndrome type 5/614284	COL9A2/AR	Deletion	High myopia Vitreoretinal degeneration Retinal detachment Mild to moderate sensorineural hearing loss Short stature in childhood	Premature termination
Multiple epiphyseal dysplasia type 3/ 600969	COL9A3/AD	Splice	Early-onset short stature Waddling gait Stiffness and pain in the knees and other joints	In-frame deletion
Susceptibility to lumbar disk disease/603932	COL9A2; COL9A3; COL11A1/AD	Missense	Degeneration of intervertebral disks	Not reported
Metaphyseal chondrodysplasia, Schmid type/156500	COL10A1/AD	Missense, nonsense, deletion	Irregularities of the metaphyseal ends of bones of the extremities	Expansion of hypertrophic zone Expanded ER
Fibrochondro-genesis-1/ 228520	COL11A1/AR	Duplication, missense (ref.thompson)	Flat midface with a small nose Significant shortening of all limb segments but relatively normal hands and feet Bell-shaped thorax with a protuberant abdomen	Fibroblastic appearance of chondrocytes Irregular collagen fibrils
Marshall syndrome/ 154780	COL11A1/AD	Splicing	Flat or retracted midface	Possible truncated forms of affected chains Suggested incomplete formation of a triple helix
Stickler syndrome type 2/604841	COL11A1/AD	Deletion	Flat mala Abnormal vitreous architecture Congenital, nonprogressive myopia of a high degree	Predicted shortening of collagen chains
Fibrochondro-genesis-2/ 614524	COL11A2/AD, AR	Splice, deletion, insertion, missense, nonsense	Midface hypoplasia with a small nose Significant shortening of all limb segments with relatively normal hands and feet Small thorax with protuberant abdomen	Not reported

AD = autosomal dominant; AR = autosomal recessive, ER = endoplasmic reticulum.

COL2A1, the same gene that encodes procollagen II chains, it has been determined that the extent of hydroxylation and glycosylation of the α3 (XI) chain is greater than that determined for the collagen II chain. It has been shown that by forming an inner core of collagen II fibrils, collagen XI contributes to the structural integrity of the cartilage fibrillar system.[45] The International Skeletal Dysplasia Society classifies chondrodysplasias associated with collagen XI as the type XI collagen group of genetic skeletal disorders[24] (Table 2).

Collagen XXVII is a homotrimer encoded by the *COL27A1* gene. During development, this collagen type is expressed in the skin, lung, aorta, stomach, and teeth, but its expression is most notable in the proliferative zone of the growth plate. Studies in transgenic mouse models suggest that certain mutations within the triple-helical region of collagen XXVII are associated with chondrodysplasia. Electron microscopy of cartilage isolated from mice harboring mutant collagen XXVII molecules indicates that this protein plays an important role in organizing the pericellular matrix in the growth plate.[46]

Structural Aberrations of Selected Macromolecules That Interact With Cartilaginous Collagens

In addition to chondrodysplasias caused by mutations in the cartilage collagens, aberrations of proteins whose biologic activities require interactions with collagens may also alter the development of skeletal tissues. The following examples illustrate this problem.

Heat Shock Protein 47

HSP47 is a critical chaperone protein whose role has been well recognized in the intracellular folding of collagen I. Recently, it has been determined that a mutation of *SERPINH1*, a gene that encodes HSP47, is responsible for an autosomal recessive form of osteogenesis imperfecta type X, thereby indicating the importance of this chaperone in bone development.[47] The potential role of HSP47 in chondrodysplasias was investigated in a mouse model. It has been demonstrated that chondrocyte-specific inactivation of HSP47 causes a chondrodysplasia phenotype and results in pathologic endochondral bone formation. Assays of cartilage from affected mice showed a significant reduction of collagen fibrils, thereby indicating the critical role of HSP47 in cartilage development.[12]

Cartilage-Associated Protein

The hydroxylation of proline residues present at the Y position of -G-X-Y- triplets is critical for the stability of collagen triple-helical domains. However, the role of the enzyme prolyl-3-hydroxylase in the hydroxylation of proline residues present at selected X positions is less understood. One of the elements of the complex needed to hydroxylate these X-positioned proline residues is cartilage-associated protein (CRTAP).[48-50] Although this protein is found in several tissues, its presence is particularly prominent in the developing skeleton.[51] Recently, mutations in CRTAP were described in a family with osteogenesis imperfecta type VII, suggesting the important role of the hydroxylation of selected proline residues in the development of skeletal tissues.[50] An analysis of mice deficient in CRTAP revealed the development of a severe osteochondrodysplasia characterized by the shortening of long bones and osteopenia.[13]

Discoidin Domain Receptor 2

Heterotypic collagen fibrils formed by the coassembly of collagen II, collagen IX, and collagen XI are not only a critical structural element of cartilage but also an important component of a signaling mechanism that regulates the function and the behavior of chondrocytes. One of the receptors engaged in this cell-matrix interaction is discoidin domain receptor 2 (DDR2), a protein that belongs to a group of receptor tyrosine kinases. This receptor is characterized by its specificity for binding well-defined domains of the triple-helical regions of several collagen types, including collagen II and collagen X. Inactivation of DDR2 in mice alters skeletal growth with long bone shortening. In humans, mutations in DDR2 are associated with spondylometaepiphyseal dysplasia, short limb-hand type (MIM# 271665). The main clinical characteristics of this dysplasia include disproportionate short stature with short limbs, a narrow chest with pectus excavatum, brachydactyly in the hands and feet, a characteristic craniofacial appearance, and developmental delay in some but not all patients.[52]

A role for DDR2 has also been postulated in the progression of osteoarthritis. It has been suggested that collagen II fragments generated during cartilage degradation seen in osteoarthritis are able to bind to DDR2 and trigger a cascade of biologic events that leads to an increased synthesis of proinflammatory interleukin-6 and matrix-degenerating matrix metalloproteinase (MMP) 13. Such an involvement of DDR2 in the pathogenesis of osteoarthritis renders it a potential therapeutic target for limiting the progression of cartilage degeneration.[53,54]

Matrix Metalloproteinases 9 and 13

Homeostasis of skeletal tissues is maintained by the balanced physiologic processes of synthesis and degradation. Both of these processes are active during the development of skeletal tissues, and factors that disturb them can contribute to skeletal aberrations. Proteolytic enzymes play a critical role in the remodeling of skeletal tissues during their development, growth, and differentiation. Matrix metalloproteinases form a group of zinc-dependent enzymes whose common characteristic is proteolytic degradation of various ECM molecules. The critical biologic functions of this group of enzymes include the degradation of collagenous matrices and the activation of various growth factors. Mutations in MMP-9 and MMP-13 cause metaphyseal anadysplasia type 2 (MIM#613073) and type 1 (MIM#602111), respectively. These are diseases that are classified as the metaphyseal dysplasias group[24] and are characterized by severe skeletal changes that, unlike most progressive chondrodysplasias, resolve spontaneously. It was determined that the loss of function of MMP-9 or MMP-13

2: Systemic Disorders

is associated with autosomal recessive forms of metaphyseal anadysplasia, whereas dominant missense mutations in MMP-13 cause intracellular activation and autodegradation of this enzyme.[55]

Experimental Approaches to Treat Chondrodysplasias Caused by Mutations in Collagen Genes

It has been suggested that gene-based and cell-based therapies may counterbalance the pathologic changes caused by the presence of mutant collagen molecules.[13,56] Although experimental models and limited clinical trials have demonstrated the potential utility of these proposed approaches, currently there are no treatments available to eliminate the molecular effects of mutations in collagen genes. The main factors that hamper the effective implementation of proposed therapies include the inability to deliver potential blockers that would prevent the expression of these mutant proteins or vectors harboring a DNA construct that encodes the wild-type normal variants of these genes. Moreover, the delivery of therapeutic cells to the affected connective tissues in amounts relevant for successful therapies also presents a major challenge. In addition, it is unclear what therapeutic goals need to be reached as a result of cell and gene therapies to achieve a regression of pathologic changes formed in affected tissues in the presence of mutant collagen molecules. Experiments have been described that determined the minimal change in the ratio of wild-type to mutant collagen II needed to reduce the deleterious effects caused by the presence of the R789C and R992C mutants associated with SED.[9] It was demonstrated that the measurable attenuation of both intracellular and extracellular aberrations caused by the presence of these collagen II mutants is only possible by eliminating their expression entirely. Consequently, these results suggest that eliminating the pathologic intracellular and extracellular consequences of the presence of thermolabile collagen mutants with increased intracellular accumulation may not be possible by using approaches that only partially reduce the amount of mutant collagen molecules in affected tissues.

Because of these challenges, novel approaches are needed. Altering the processes that contribute to ER stress caused by the excessive intracellular accumulation of mutant collagens presents a promising therapeutic opportunity. Specifically, using chemical chaperones, compounds with the ability to prevent the misfolding of mutant collagens, may be possible to reduce ER stress and avoid apoptosis. In contrast to genetic approaches, chemical chaperones will not block the expression of misfolded mutant collagen molecules. They may, however, facilitate their folding and secretion, thereby decreasing mutant-associated intracellular stress. Such an effect has already been seen in studies performed in a cell-based model.[38] Although the chaperone approach will not eliminate mutant molecules, it may still be beneficial for affected tissues. This notion is based on the possibility that the actions of some mutant molecules in the extracellular space may be less harmful to the tissue than their negative influence on intracellular functions. This notion is further supported by studies demonstrating that thermostable mutants with R>C substitutions in positions R75C and R519C are present in the ECM but do not cause detectable ER stress, and their presence is associated with mild rather than severe dysplasias.[31]

Chondrodysplasias: A Member of the Rare Diseases Group

Chondrodysplasias represent a group of rare diseases for which no therapeutic treatments currently exist. The National Institutes of Health and the FDA recognize the growing need to intensify the basic research to identify the mechanisms behind these rare diseases and design approaches to their treatments. The urgency to move forward with research on rare diseases is not only justified by the fact that they are devastating and as a group affect a significant percentage of the US population but also because there are no treatments available for most of them. Although individually uncommon—by definition a specific rare disease affects fewer than 200,000 people in the United States—collectively these diseases are prevalent in society and contribute to major health and socioeconomic problems. Almost 7,000 rare diseases have been identified, and they affect 18 to 25 million people or 6% to 8% of the US population alone.[57] In the context of other diseases recognized as devastating in the US population, the percentage of patients with rare diseases equals that reported for patients with cancer and coronary heart disease (8.5% and 6.7% in 2010, respectively[58]). For approximately 7,000 rare diseases recognized to date, there are only about 250 treatments available, and the actual causes are known for only about 4,000 of them. The pursuit of understanding and treating these rare diseases is not purely academic. Often the insights provided by research into such rare diseases can contribute significantly to understanding other more common disorders. It is not unreasonable to postulate that information obtained from studying rare chondrodysplasias may someday contribute to a better understanding of osteoarthritis. The problems in treating these rare diseases include a poor understanding of their pathomechanisms, difficulties in identifying suitable therapeutic targets, and the fact that this group of diseases includes extremely diverse members, thereby requiring unique sets of complex scientific tools, models, skills, and experimental approaches to study each disease.

Mutations in genes encoding extracellular molecules of cartilage present a significant medical problem. For instance, mutations in the COL2A1 are not only associated with skeletal abnormalities but also with Stickler dysplasia type I, a disease associated with hearing loss, joint problems, and progressive myopia beginning in the first decade of life and causing retinal detachment and blindness.[59] In addition, mutations in collagen II have been associated with osteonecrosis of the femoral head. All patients with familial osteonecrosis according to one study[60] carried *COL2A1* mutations. Given the prevalence of osteonecrosis in total hip arthroplasty, such a finding is certainly provocative. Such opportunities to potentially apply basic science findings toward understanding more common clinical entities points to the great importance of developing gene-based etiologies for several skeletal diseases and further justifies the need to intensify relevant studies in cell-based and animal models.

Summary

Collagens are the most abundant proteins of bone and cartilage. These proteins have a typical triple-helical structure and are produced by cells in a complex step-wise fashion that requires essential intracellular and extracellular processes. Mutations in either the collagen molecules themselves or in one of the host of other molecules that are important in collagen assembly can adversely affect skeletal tissues. Numerous examples of such mutations and their subsequent effects have been presented. The treatment of the diseases that result from these mutations is challenging from both a clinical and a basic science perspective. However, the continued study of these mutations holds the promise of not only treating these diseases but also providing insight into the molecular basis of normal skeletal development and function and possibly further understanding of more common diseases such as osteoarthritis.

Key Study Points

- Collagen biosynthesis is a complex process that includes the enzymatic processing and posttranslational modification of nascent collagen chains, which are then deposited in the extracellular matrix as fibrils that provide the mechanical strength of skeletal tissues and serve as a binding platform for tissue-specific cells and proteins. Errors in any step of this process can result in disease.

- Aberrations in the structure of collagens may be caused not only by mutations in the genes encoding individual collagen chains but also mutations of the genes encoding proteins involved in collagen production or processing.

- Alterations of collagen structure are associated with several skeletal diseases, whose spectrum of severity includes mild and lethal forms. To date, no successful therapies exist to counterbalance the pathological effects of mutations affecting the structure of collagen matrices of skeletal tissues.

Annotated References

1. Lefebvre V, Bhattaram P: Vertebrate skeletogenesis. *Curr Top Dev Biol* 2010;90:291-317.

   The authors review current molecular pathways that contribute to vertebrate skeletal formation and development.

2. Baldridge D, Shchelochkov O, Kelley B, Lee B: Signaling pathways in human skeletal dysplasias. *Annu Rev Genomics Hum Genet* 2010;11:189-217.

   The authors review molecular signaling pathways that are required for skeletogenesis and how genetic mutations can affect these pathways.

3. Späth SS, Andrade AC, Chau M, Nilsson O: Local regulation of growth plate cartilage. *Endocr Dev* 2011;21:12-22.

   The authors review the current understanding of the growth plate and the molecular signals that help to regulate this process.

4. Mackie EJ, Tatarczuch L, Mirams M: The skeleton: A multi-functional complex organ. The growth plate chondrocyte and endochondral ossification. *J Endocrinol* 2011;211(2):109-121.

   The authors review the current understanding of the role of chondrocytes in the growth plate and their contribution to endochondral ossification.

5. Umlauf D, Frank S, Pap T, Bertrand J: Cartilage biology, pathology, and repair. *Cell Mol Life Sci* 2010;67(24):4197-4211.

   The authors review current findings about cartilage biology and pathology and discuss potential therapies.

6. Carter EM, Raggio CL: Genetic and orthopedic aspects of collagen disorders. *Curr Opin Pediatr* 2009;21(1):46-54.

7. Ricard-Blum S: The collagen family. *Cold Spring Harb Perspect Biol* 2011;3(1):a004978.

   The author discusses the 28 members of the collagen family of triple-helical proteins, along with the structural and functional aspects of these proteins. In addition, genetic and acquired diseases associated with collagens are presented.

8. Bateman JF, Boot-Handford RP, Lamandé SR: Genetic diseases of connective tissues: Cellular and extracellular effects of ECM mutations. *Nat Rev Genet* 2009;10(3):173-183.

9. Jensen DA, Steplewski A, Gawron K, Fertala A: Persistence of intracellular and extracellular changes after incompletely suppressing expression of the R789C (p.R989C) and R992C (p.R1192C) collagen II mutants. *Hum Mutat* 2011;32(7):794-805.

   The authors developed a molecular system in which the production of mutant collagen II could be controlled. The affected cell/matrix systems functioned normally

2: Systemic Disorders

only when the mutant collagen production was completely shut off.

10. Gorres KL, Raines RT: Prolyl 4-hydroxylase. *Crit Rev Biochem Mol Biol* 2010;45(2):106-124.

    The authors review the current understanding of the enzyme prolyl 4-hydroxylase and its role in protein modification.

11. Shoulders MD, Raines RT: Collagen structure and stability. *Annu Rev Biochem* 2009;78:929-958.

12. Masago Y, Hosoya A, Kawasaki K, et al: The molecular chaperone HSP47 is essential for cartilage and endochondral bone formation. *J Cell Sci* 2012;125(pt 5):1118-1128.

    Chondrocyte expression of the HSP47 gene was conditionally inactivated in mice, resulting in severe generalized chondrodysplasia.

13. Forlino A, Cabral WA, Barnes AM, Marini JC: New perspectives on osteogenesis imperfecta. *Nat Rev Endocrinol* 2011;7(9):540-557.

    The authors review the current understanding of autosomal dominant and autosomal recessive forms of osteogenesis imperfecta.

14. Boot-Handford RP, Briggs MD: The unfolded protein response and its relevance to connective tissue diseases. *Cell Tissue Res* 2010;339(1):197-211.

    The authors review the role of ER stress in connective tissue diseases and the role of the unfolded protein response to counter this stress.

15. Piróg-Garcia KA, Meadows RS, Knowles L, et al: Reduced cell proliferation and increased apoptosis are significant pathological mechanisms in a murine model of mild pseudoachondroplasia resulting from a mutation in the C-terminal domain of COMP. *Hum Mol Genet* 2007;16(17):2072-2088.

16. Rajpar MH, McDermott B, Kung L, et al: Targeted induction of endoplasmic reticulum stress induces cartilage pathology. *PLoS Genet* 2009;5(10):e1000691.

17. Chung HJ, Jensen DA, Gawron K, Steplewski A, Fertala A: R992C (p.R1192C) substitution in collagen II alters the structure of mutant molecules and induces the unfolded protein response. *J Mol Biol* 2009;390(2):306-318.

18. Apte SS: A disintegrin-like and metalloprotease (reprolysin-type) with thrombospondin type 1 motif (ADAMTS) superfamily: Functions and mechanisms. *J Biol Chem* 2009;284(46):31493-31497.

19. Verma P, Dalal K: ADAMTS-4 and ADAMTS-5: Key enzymes in osteoarthritis. *J Cell Biochem* 2011;112(12):3507-3514.

    The authors review the role of ADAMTS-4 and ADAMTS-5 proteinases in a human model of osteoarthritis.

20. Muir A, Greenspan DS: Metalloproteinases in Drosophila to humans that are central players in developmental processes. *J Biol Chem* 2011;286(49):41905-41911.

    The authors review the role of metalloproteinase enzymes in embryonic patterning and ECM formation.

21. Li SW, Sieron AL, Fertala A, Hojima Y, Arnold WV, Prockop DJ: The C-proteinase that processes procollagens to fibrillar collagens is identical to the protein previously identified as bone morphogenic protein-1. *Proc Natl Acad Sci USA* 1996;93(10):5127-5130.

22. Orgel JP, San Antonio JD, Antipova O: Molecular and structural mapping of collagen fibril interactions. *Connect Tissue Res* 2011;52(1):2-17.

    The authors review the binding characteristics of the fibrillar form of collagen to other ligands in the ECM.

23. Nishioka T, Eustace A, West C: Lysyl oxidase: From basic science to future cancer treatment. *Cell Struct Funct* 2012;37(1):75-80.

    The authors discuss the role of lysyl oxidase and lysyl oxidase-like proteins in tumor biology, along with the role of these proteins in the ECM and how this may affect metastases.

24. Warman ML, Cormier-Daire V, Hall C, et al: Nosology and classification of genetic skeletal disorders: 2010 revision. *Am J Med Genet A* 2011;155A(5):943-968.

    The authors present a classification of genetic disorders involving the skeletal system. The classification is based on the clinical and radiographic features of these disorders as well as their molecular pathogenesis. The classification includes 456 conditions placed into 40 groups.

25. Krakow D, Rimoin DL: The skeletal dysplasias. *Genet Med* 2010;12(6):327-341.

    The authors review the current knowledge regarding the more than 350 disorders grouped together as skeletal dysplasias.

26. Kannu P, Bateman JF, Randle S, et al: Premature arthritis is a distinct type II collagen phenotype. *Arthritis Rheum* 2010;62(5):1421-1430.

    Mutations resulting in glycine substitutions in the triple-helical domain of collagen II were found in two Australian families with an isolated arthritis phenotype. Level of evidence: V.

27. Kannu P, Bateman J, Savarirayan R: Clinical phenotypes associated with type II collagen mutations. *J Paediatr Child Health* 2012;48(2):E38-E43.

    The authors reviewed the molecular bases and phenotypic characteristics of diseases associated with mutations in collagen II. They recognized that autosomal dominant mutations in collagen II result in a spectrum of disease presentations ranging from early-onset short stature to later-onset mild phenotypes such as premature osteoarthritis. In addition, the authors pointed to the clinical importance of diagnosing collagen II mutations for accurately determining risks for affected individuals and their family members.

28. Fertala A, Ala-Kokko L, Prockop DJ: Characterization of recombinant human collagen II with Arg519-to-Cys substitution. *Ann N Y Acad Sci* 1996;785:251-253.

29. Fertala A, Ala-Kokko L, Wiaderkiewicz R, Prockop DJ: Collagen II containing a Cys substitution for arg-alpha1-519: Homotrimeric monomers containing the mutation do not assemble into fibrils but alter the self-assembly of the normal protein. *J Biol Chem* 1997; 272(10):6457-6464.

30. Fertala A, Sieron AL, Adachi E, Jimenez SA: Collagen II containing a Cys substitution for Arg-alpha1-519: Abnormal interactions of the mutated molecules with collagen IX. *Biochemistry* 2001;40(48):14422-14428.

31. Hintze V, Steplewski A, Ito H, Jensen DA, Rodeck U, Fertala A: Cells expressing partially unfolded R789C/p.R989C type II procollagen mutant associated with spondyloepiphyseal dysplasia undergo apoptosis. *Hum Mutat* 2008;29(6):841-851.

32. Steplewski A, Ito H, Rucker E, et al: Position of single amino acid substitutions in the collagen triple helix determines their effect on structure of collagen fibrils. *J Struct Biol* 2004;148(3):326-337.

33. Steplewski A, Majsterek I, McAdams E, et al: Thermostability gradient in the collagen triple helix reveals its multi-domain structure. *J Mol Biol* 2004;338(5): 989-998.

34. Schröder M, Kaufman RJ: ER stress and the unfolded protein response. *Mutat Res* 2005;569(1-2):29-63.

35. Schröder M, Kaufman RJ: The mammalian unfolded protein response. *Annu Rev Biochem* 2005;74:739-789.

36. Donahue LR, Chang B, Mohan S, et al: A missense mutation in the mouse Col2a1 gene causes spondyloepiphyseal dysplasia congenita, hearing loss, and retinoschisis. *J Bone Miner Res* 2003;18(9):1612-1621.

37. Ito H, Rucker E, Steplewski A, et al: Guilty by association: Some collagen II mutants alter the formation of ECM as a result of atypical interaction with fibronectin. *J Mol Biol* 2005;352(2):382-395.

38. Gawron K, Jensen DA, Steplewski A, Fertala A: Reducing the effects of intracellular accumulation of thermolabile collagen II mutants by increasing their thermostability in cell culture conditions. *Biochem Biophys Res Commun* 2010;396(2):213-218.

Glycerol and trimethylamine N-oxide were used to stabilize two thermolabile collagen II mutants and thereby improved cell survival by decreasing the intracellular accumulation of these mutant collagens.

39. Steplewski A, Hintze V, Fertala A: Molecular basis of organization of collagen fibrils. *J Struct Biol* 2007; 157(2):297-307.

40. Steplewski A, Brittingham R, Jimenez SA, Fertala A: Single amino acid substitutions in the C-terminus of collagen II alter its affinity for collagen IX. *Biochem Biophys Res Commun* 2005;335(3):749-755.

41. Arita M, Li SW, Kopen G, Adachi E, Jimenez SA, Fertala A: Skeletal abnormalities and ultrastructural changes of cartilage in transgenic mice expressing a collagen II gene (COL2A1) with a Cys for Arg-alpha1-519 substitution. *Osteoarthritis Cartilage* 2002;10(10): 808-815.

42. Guilak F, Alexopoulos LG, Upton ML, et al: The pericellular matrix as a transducer of biomechanical and biochemical signals in articular cartilage. *Ann N Y Acad Sci* 2006;1068:498-512.

43. Christensen SE, Coles JM, Zelenski NA, et al: Altered trabecular bone structure and delayed cartilage degeneration in the knees of collagen VI null mice. *PLoS One* 2012;7(3):e33397.

The authors compared the morphology and physical properties of bone and cartilage in mice that expressed collagen VI compared with mice without collagen VI expression. Greater effects were seen with knee joint structures with relatively minimal effects on the properties of cartilage.

44. Stetler WR, La Marca F, Park P: The genetics of ossification of the posterior longitudinal ligament. *Neurosurg Focus* 2011;30(3):E7.

The authors review the current understanding regarding the genetic factors contributing to ossification of the posterior longitudinal ligament.

45. Yingst S, Bloxham K, Warner LR, et al: Characterization of collagenous matrix assembly in a chondrocyte model system. *J Biomed Mater Res A* 2009;90(1): 247-255.

46. Plumb DA, Ferrara L, Torbica T, et al: Collagen XXVII organises the pericellular matrix in the growth plate. *PLoS One* 2011;6(12):e29422.

Mice in which the cartilage-targeted expression of a mutant collagen XXVII in which an 87-amino-acid sequence was deleted were analyzed. The resulting mice were severely dwarfed. The mutation resulted in a disruption of the pericellular matrix of the proliferative chondrocytes in the growth plate.

47. Christiansen HE, Schwarze U, Pyott SM, et al: Homozygosity for a missense mutation in SERPINH1, which encodes the collagen chaperone protein HSP47, results in severe recessive osteogenesis imperfecta. *Am J Hum Genet* 2010;86(3):389-398.

The authors report an autosomal recessive mutation in the *SEPINH1* gene that encodes the HSP47 protein. Loss of this protein results in the accumulation of procollagen I intracellularly and in the secretion of a procollagen I that is protease sensitive. Level of evidence: V.

48. Morello R, Rauch F: Role of cartilage-associated protein in skeletal development. *Curr Osteoporos Rep* 2010;8(2):77-83.

2: Systemic Disorders

The authors review recent findings regarding the role of CRTAP in collagen prolyl 3-hydroxylation and review how mutations in this protein can contribute to recessive forms of osteogenesis imperfecta.

49. Fratzl-Zelman N, Morello R, Lee B, et al: CRTAP deficiency leads to abnormally high bone matrix mineralization in a murine model and in children with osteogenesis imperfecta type VII. *Bone* 2010;46(3):820-826.

The authors report increased highly mineralized bone matrix in mice and children affected by a mutation in CRTAP, leading to findings similar to classical osteogenesis imperfecta. Level of evidence: III.

50. Morello R, Bertin TK, Chen Y, et al: CRTAP is required for prolyl 3-hydroxylation and mutations cause recessive osteogenesis imperfecta. *Cell* 2006;127(2):291-304.

51. Fernandes RJ, Farnand AW, Traeger GR, Weis MA, Eyre DR: A role for prolyl 3-hydroxylase 2 in post-translational modification of fibril-forming collagens. *J Biol Chem* 2011;286(35):30662-30669.

The authors report the results of cell culture experiments demonstrating differential preference in the 3-hydroxylation of proline at three different sites in collagen.

52. Bargal R, Cormier-Daire V, Ben-Neriah Z, et al: Mutations in DDR2 gene cause SMED with short limbs and abnormal calcifications. *Am J Hum Genet* 2009;84(1):80-84.

53. Xu L, Servais J, Polur I, et al: Attenuation of osteoarthritis progression by reduction of discoidin domain receptor 2 in mice. *Arthritis Rheum* 2010;62(9):2736-2744.

The authors present research suggesting that a decrease in the expression of DDR2 correlates with a delayed development of cartilage degeneration in a mouse model of osteoarthritis.

54. Klatt AR, Zech D, Kühn G, et al: Discoidin domain receptor 2 mediates the collagen II-dependent release of interleukin-6 in primary human chondrocytes. *J Pathol* 2009;218(2):241-247.

55. Lausch E, Keppler R, Hilbert K, et al: Mutations in MMP9 and MMP13 determine the mode of inheritance and the clinical spectrum of metaphyseal anadysplasia. *Am J Hum Genet* 2009;85(2):168-178.

56. Forlino A, Marini JC: Osteogenesis imperfecta: Prospects for molecular therapeutics. *Mol Genet Metab* 2000;71(1-2):225-232.

57. Office of Rare Diseases Research of the National Center for Advancing Translational Sciences: Rare diseases. http://rarediseases.info.nih.gov. Accessed November 4, 2013.

58. Centers for Disease Control and Prevention (CDC): http://www.cdc.gov.

59. National Center for Biotechnology Information: Online Mendelian Inheritance in Man. http://www.ncbi.nlm.nih.gov/entrez/query.fcgi?db=OMIM. Accessed November 4, 2013.

60. Liu YF, Chen WM, Lin YF, et al: Type II collagen gene variants and inherited osteonecrosis of the femoral head. *N Engl J Med* 2005;352(22):2294-2301.

Chapter 20
Muscle Disorders

George C. Babis, MD, PhD   Vasileios I. Sakellariou, MD, PhD

Introduction

The internal architecture of skeletal muscles has been found to play a substantial role in the functionality and the effectiveness of contracture. Novel methods of studying fascicle architecture and identifying functional subunits within muscle have been presented. New pathophysiologic mechanisms have been identified, and the genetic basis of most muscle disorders has been decoded.

Muscle Architecture and Function

Skeletal muscles constitute 40% to 45% of total body weight. Macroscopically, each skeletal muscle consists of parallel (biceps, triceps) or convergent (pectoralis major) fascicles that originate from bone and adjacent connective tissue and have a tendinous insertion into bone. Microscopically, skeletal muscles are composed of myocytes that are formed from the fusion of myoblasts (progenitor cells of muscle cells), which are multinucleated cells composed of myofibrils. Each myofibril is composed of the cytoplasmic proteins actin and myosin, which are arranged in a repeating unit called a sarcomere, which is the basic functional unit of the muscle fiber and is responsible for muscle contraction. Skeletal muscle fibers also contain the regulatory proteins troponin and tropomyosin, which are necessary for muscle contraction to occur.[1]

Muscle contraction occurs in response to an impulse transmitted via nerve fibers through the neuromuscular junction. Acetylcholine, a neurotransmitter, is released at the neuromuscular junction by motor neurons that cause depolarization of the skeletal muscle cells. After the cell is stimulated, ionic calcium (Ca^{2+}) is released by the sarcoplasm and interacts with troponin, which subsequently regulates the movement of tropomyosin and the exposure of myosin-binding sites on actin. Shortening of muscle then occurs as a result of adenosine triphosphate (ATP)-dependent cross-bridge cycling of myosin and actin.

The muscle fibers are categorized according to the type of myosin that is present (fast or slow) and the degree of oxidative phosphorylation of each fiber. Thus, three basic muscle types I, IIA, and IIB can be recognized. Type I fibers are slow-twitch oxidative and appear red as a result of the presence of myoglobin (oxygen binding protein). Type I fibers predominantly exist in postural muscles, and they are well suited for endurance by aerobic metabolism through the generation of ATP. They are characterized by a slow contraction rate and a relatively low strength of contraction. Type II muscle fibers are fast twitch and appear white as a result of the absence of myoglobin. They have a fast rate of contraction and a relatively high strength of contraction. Type II fibers are further subdivided into IIA and IIB, depending on their mode of energy utilization. Type IIA fibers (also called fast twitch A) are characterized by their high capacity for generating ATP by oxidation. These are resistant to fatigue but not as much as low oxidative fibers. However, type IIB fibers (also called fast twitch B) are fast glycolytic and are thus primarily anaerobic. Type IIB fibers have low myoglobin and high creatine phosphate content. They are common in muscles that require a rapid generation of power, but they fatigue easily because of lactic acid production.[2,3]

The force of the muscle contraction is proportional to the number of motor units that are activated each time. The size of the motor unit depends on the number of muscle fibers that are innervated by the nerve fiber. electromyography (EMG)-driven models can be used to assess the force of muscle contraction. Moreover, the internal architecture of a skeletal muscle plays a significant role in its functionality.[1] The authors of a 2010 study presented a novel method of studying fascicle architecture in relaxed and contracted muscles, which helps to identify functional subunits within the muscle.[4] In a 2011 study, the three-dimensional muscle architecture of the human muscle was determined in vivo by using two-dimensional ultrasound and a three-dimensional position tracker system, which enabled quantification of muscle architecture with short scan times in comparison with diffusion tensor MRI.

Dr. Babis or an immediate family member is a member of a speakers' bureau or has made paid presentations on behalf of Bristol-Myers Squibb and Pfizer Alliance; serves as a paid consultant to or is an employee of Bristol-Myers Squibb and Pfizer Alliance; and has received research or institutional support from Bayer and Amgen. Neither Dr. Sakellariou nor any immediate family member has received anything of value from or has stock or stock options held in a commercial company or institution related directly or indirectly to the subject of this chapter.

Table 1

Common Types of Inflammatory Myopathies

Muscle Disorder	Etiology	Clinical Findings
Dermatomyositis	Autoimmune reaction Infection (usually from the Epstein-Barr virus and rarely from spirochete or Lyme disease) Rhabdomyolysis as a result of statin use Paraneoplasmatic phenomena	Gottron lesions: erythematous eruptions or patches overlying the elbows, the knees, and the metacarpal and interphalangeal joints Muscle weakness symmetric proximal Severity ranges from simple deterioration to paralysis Dysphagia Pain Interstitial lung disease
Polymyositis	Lyme disease, toxoplasmosis, and other infectious pathogens Autoimmune factors Genetic factors Increased expression of MHC-I molecules on the surface of myocytes Attracted CD8 cytotoxic T cells destroy the myocytes	Muscle loss around the shoulder and the pelvis Weakness Pain Sclerodactyly Drop foot Dysphagia Increased incidence of malignancies (lung, pancreas, and ovaries)
Inclusion body myositis	Inflammation-immune reaction caused by an undetermined trigger (probably a virus or an autoimmune disorder) Abnormal accumulation of pathogenic proteins (amyloid-β, phosphorylated tau protein, and others) in aging myofibers	Progressive muscle weakness Frequent tripping and falling Drop foot Difficulties in hand tasks and dysphagia

Muscle Disorders

Inflammatory Myopathies

The term inflammatory myopathy is synonymous with dermatopolymyositis, which includes three related diseases: dermatomyositis, polymyositis, and inclusion body myositis (IBM)[6] (Table 1).

Dermatomyositis is a connective tissue disease of unknown etiology. A history of an autoimmune reaction or an infection (usually from the Epstein-Barr virus and rarely from spirochete or Lyme disease) is identified. Rhabdomyolysis as a result of statin use and paraneoplasmatic phenomena have also been indicated as possible causative factors.[7]

The clinical manifestations include skin lesions, muscle weakness, and/or pain. The skin lesions consist of erythematous eruptions or patches overlying the elbows, the knees, and the metacarpal and interphalangeal joints, which are also known as Gottron lesions. Dermal calcinosis (or calcinosis cutis) is more often seen in the juvenile form of dermatomyositis. The muscle weakness is usually symmetric and proximal, and its severity ranges from simple deterioration to paralysis. Dysphagia may occur in one third of the cases. Patients should also be evaluated for the presence of interstitial lung disease, which is frequent in both dermatomyositis and polymyositis.[8]

Polymyositis is an inflammatory myopathy with multifactorial etiology. Lyme disease, toxoplasmosis, and other infectious pathogens have been associated with polymyositis. Autoimmune and genetic factors have also been recognized. An increased expression of major histocompatibility complex-I molecules on the surface of myocytes attracts CD8 cytotoxic T cells that subsequently destroy the myocytes. Pain, weakness, and/or muscle loss around the shoulder and the pelvis are common clinical signs. Sclerodactyly, drop foot, and dysphagia are usual features. Polymyositis is also associated with increased incidence of several malignancies, especially lung, pancreas, and ovarian cancers. Interstitial lung disease is also a concern and should be periodically evaluated.[7]

IBM is another form of inflammatory myopathy. It is characterized by a different pattern of muscle weakness and wasting, which compromises both the proximal and the peripheral muscle groups.

Two types of IBMs exist: sporadic and hereditary.[9] Several theories have been presented regarding the etiology of each type. With sporadic IBM, the inflammation-immune reaction caused by an undetermined trigger (probably a virus or an autoimmune disorder) appears to cause muscle degeneration. Other authors think that an abnormal accumulation of pathogenic proteins (such as amyloid-β or phosphorylated tau protein) in aging myofibers may have a causative effect in immune system deregulation.[10] However, it is confusing that immunosuppressive medications do not improve the symptoms of sporadic IBM, as would be expected for a disease with an autoimmune etiology. The clinical manifestations of sporadic IBM consist of progressive muscle weakness, which initially presents as

Table 2

Etiologic Factors and Clinical Findings of Most Common Muscular Dystrophies

Muscle Disorder	Etiology	Clinical Findings
Duchenne muscular dystrophy (DMD)	Absence of the protein dystrophin Chromosome X (*Xp21* gene) Sporadic mutations	Progressive proximal muscle weakness Positive Gowers sign Walking aids are required by age 10 years Most patients wheelchair dependent by age 12 years Pseudohypertrophy of the calf and deltoid muscles Muscle wasting and replacement of the necrotic muscle fibers by adipose and connective tissue
Becker muscular dystrophy	Mutation in the dystrophin gene (X-linked recessive pattern) Production of a partially functional form of dystrophin	Less severe clinical manifestation Longer longevity
Congenital muscular dystrophy (CMD)	Autosomal recessive disease Mutations in genes encoding LARGE, fukutin, and fukutin-related proteins	Muscle weakness Joint deformities that progress slowly Severe brain malformations (lissencephaly and hydrocephalus)
Emery-Dreifuss muscular dystrophy	Mutations in the genes *EMD, LMNA, SYNE1, SYNE2,* and *FHL1* Absence of a transmembrane protein of the inner nuclear membrane named emerin	Joint contractures of elbows, ankles, and neck Progressive muscle wasting and weakness of the upper arms and lower legs Severe cardiac problems
Distal muscular dystrophy	Mutation in the *DYSF* gene at the 2p13.3-p13.1 locum Miyoshi myopathy: mutation of *DYSF* gene at the 2p13.3-p13.1 locum	Slow progress and a relatively late age of onset (varies from 20 to 60 years) Muscles of hands, forearms, and lower legs usually affected
Facioscapulohumeral muscular dystrophy Landouzy-Dejerine syndrome	Autosomal dominant Deletion of D4Z4 repeats at the subtelomeric region 4q35 Toxic gain of function of a putative gene called *DUX4*	Affects teenagers Weakness of the muscles of the face and the shoulder girdle
Limb-girdle muscular dystrophy	Autosomal recessive, autosomal dominant and X-linked types Defective proteins participating in the formation of a dystrophin-glycoprotein complex	Both upper arms and legs affected Muscle weakness proximal and slowly progressive Cardiopulmonary complications Death from the disease quite unusual
Oculopharyngeal muscular dystrophy	Autosomal dominant Trinucleotide repeat disorder associated with expansion of $(GCN)_{10}$ to $(GCN)_{11-17}$ at the 5' end of the coding region for PABPN1	Weakness of the extraocular muscles Blepharoptosis Dysphagia Proximal limb and facial weakness (later stages of the disease)

frequent tripping and falling, or drop foot. Difficulties with hand tasks and dysphagia usually occur during later stages of the disease.

The hereditary type comprises both autosomal dominant and recessive disorders. In the autosomal dominant form (IBM1), the quadriceps is the first muscle to be affected. In many Asian, Middle Eastern, and Jewish populations, the autosomal recessive form (IBM2), which is also known as distal myopathy with rimmed vacuoles, usually spares the quadriceps and mostly affects the leg muscles. IBM3 is associated with mutations in gene locum 17p13.1 that encodes myosin heavy chain II proteins on chromosome 17. There is

also a hereditary type related to Paget disease of bone and frontotemporal dementia caused by a mutation in a gene located at 9p13-p12 on chromosome 9.[11] Pathognomonic clinical signs and symptoms of the hereditary type include loss of balance, difficulties with heel walking and running, and weakness in the index finger.

Muscular Dystrophies

Duchenne muscular dystrophy (DMD), which is caused by the absence of the protein dystrophin, is the most common form of this group of diseases (Table 2). Dystrophin is part of a protein complex named dystrophin-glycoprotein complex that promotes the anchoring of cytoskeleton within the muscle cells, through the sarcolemma, and to the extracellular matrix that surrounds each cell. Because of defects in this assembly, contraction of the muscle leads to disruption of the outer membrane of the muscle cells and eventual weakening and wasting of the muscle.[12]

The production of dystrophin is regulated by a gene, which is located on chromosome X (*Xp21* gene),[13] which explains why predominantly male patients are affected, whereas females are carriers and have milder symptomatology. However, only two thirds of cases are inherited (in recessive pattern) and one third are new, "sporadic" mutations. Clinically, the disease becomes evident when progressive proximal muscle weakness is seen when a child begins to walk. A positive Gowers sign is characteristic of the disease and describes the way that a child helps himself or herself arise by "climbing" with the hands up to the legs to stand upright. Walking aids are required by age 10 years, whereas most patients are wheelchair dependent by age 12 years. Pseudohypertrophy of the calf and deltoid muscles is an early typical sign that progresses to muscle wasting and the replacement of the necrotic muscle fibers by adipose and connective tissue.

Becker muscular dystrophy is a variant of DMD with less severe clinical manifestations and a greater longevity. Like DMD, it is caused by a mutation in the dystrophin gene, which is inherited with an X-linked recessive pattern; but in Becker muscular dystrophy a partially functional form of dystrophin is produced, in contrast with DMD where no functional dystrophin is produced.[14]

Congenital muscular dystrophy is an autosomal recessive disease present at birth. Mutations in genes encoding laminin-a2 chain, glycosyltransferase-like protein (known as LARGE), fukutin, and fukutin-related protein have been reported as possible etiologic factors.[15,16] The disease is associated with muscle weakness and joint deformities that progress slowly. Severe brain malformations (lissencephaly and hydrocephalus) and effects in other organ systems may be present.

Emery-Dreifuss muscular dystrophy (EDMD) is characterized by joint contractures of the elbows, the ankles, and the neck; progressive muscle wasting and weakness of the upper arms and the lower legs; and severe cardiac problems caused by the absence of a transmembrane protein of the inner nuclear membrane named emerin.[17] Mutations in the genes *EMD, LMNA, SYNE1, SYNE2,* and *FHL1* are responsible for the different types of the disease (EDMD1-6).[16,18,19] Another classification is based on the pattern of inheritance, which may be X-linked, autosomal dominant, or autosomal recessive.

Distal muscular dystrophy is a non–life-threatening form of dystrophies with slow progression and a relatively late age onset, which varies from 20 to 60 years. A mutation in the *DYSF* gene at the 2p13.3-p13.1 locum is found to be responsible for this form of muscular dystrophy. Miyoshi myopathy, which is found in Japan, is related to a mutation of the DYSF gene at the 2p13.3-p13.1 locum.[20] Muscles of the hands, forearms, and lower legs are usually affected.

Facioscapulohumeral muscular dystrophy, also known as Landouzy-Dejerine syndrome, is a type of muscular dystrophy that occurs in both sexes. It has an autosomal dominant pattern of inheritance, but spontaneous mutations are also common. Two defects are required for the development of facioscapulohumeral muscular dystrophy: (1) a deletion of D4Z4 repeats at the subtelomeric region 4q35, and (2) a "toxic gain of function" of a putative gene called *DUX4*.[21] The disease affects teenagers, who have weakness of the facial muscles and the shoulder girdle.

Limb-girdle muscular dystrophy also occurs in both sexes. Autosomal recessive, autosomal dominant, and X-linked types of inheritance have been identified, with the recessive form being more common and having an earlier age of onset. The etiology is defective proteins participating in the formation of a dystrophin-glycoprotein complex. Both upper arms and legs are affected. Muscle weakness is proximal and slowly progressive. Death from the disease is quite unusual and is associated with cardiopulmonary complications.[22]

Oculopharyngeal muscular dystrophy is a trinucleotide repeat disorder associated with expansion of $(GCN)_{10}$ to $(GCN)_{11-17}$ at the 5' end of the coding region for poly(A)-binding protein nuclear 1 (PABPN1).[23] The pattern of inheritance is autosomal dominant, and the age of onset is between the fifth and sixth decades of life. Patients present with weakness of the extraocular muscles, blepharoptosis, and dysphagia. Proximal limb and facial weakness can be found during the later stages of the disease.

Myasthenias and Myasthenic Syndromes

Myasthenia gravis is an autoimmune neuromuscular disease caused by antibodies against the nicotinic acetylcholine receptors at the postsynaptic neuromuscular junction. Specific HLA types (B8 and DR3) have been found to be associated with the development of myasthenia gravis. T-helper cells are first activated by binding of the T cell receptor to the epitope, which is the acetylcholine receptor antigenic peptide fragment. T cells stimulate B cells to convert into plasma cells, which produce the antibodies against acetylcholine receptors. Patients with thymoma or other abnormalities of the thymus are predisposed to the disease.[24] Although the exact mechanism is not clarified, a possible hypothesis is that the thymus has an important role in the development of T cells and the selection of the T cell receptor, and thus it is potentially associated with myasthenia gravis.

Another form of myasthenia gravis is caused by antibodies against muscle-specific kinase protein, a necessary substance for the formation of a neuromuscular junction. Antibodies against muscle-specific kinase induce a decrease in the patency of the neuromuscular junction.[24,25] Myasthenia gravis is also associated with other autoimmune diseases, including rheumatoid arthritis, lupus, Hashimoto thyroiditis, and Graves disease.

Fatigability is the typical symptom of myasthenia gravis. Facial muscles are primarily affected, leading to blepharoptosis and diplopia. Dysphagia, dysarthria, and difficulties in breathing may also occur. The Myasthenia Gravis Foundation of America has proposed a clinical classification that includes five different classes of increasing severity, with class V being characterized by a paralysis of the respiring muscles that necessitates intubation and assisted ventilation to sustain life.[26]

Ocular myasthenia gravis is a form of myasthenia gravis limited to the muscles of the eye. Seventy-five percent of new myasthenia gravis cases present with ocular involvement (diplopia, blepharoptosis) as the initial manifestation.[27] However, in almost 80% of these cases, ocular myasthenia gravis will progress to a generalized disease.

Neuropathic Disorders

Guillain-Barré syndrome is an acute inflammatory demyelinating neuropathy that is characterized by symmetric weakness of the lower limbs that progresses in an ascending fashion with or without accompanying sensory deficits. The disease may also affect the cranial nerves and the respiratory muscles, requiring ventilator assistance.

The etiology is related to an autoimmune response against gangliosides. Myelin is therefore damaged, resulting in nerve conduction block, muscle paralysis, and sensory and autonomic dysfunction. Several infectious agents have been identified to trigger this immune reaction; the most common are *Campylobacter jejuni*, cytomegalovirus, and influenza viruses.[28,29]

Acute inflammatory demyelinating polyneuropathy is the most common form of Guillain-Barré syndrome. However, five other subtypes exist. Miller Fisher syndrome is characterized by a triad of ophthalmoplegia, ataxia, and areflexia.[30] In Chinese paralytic syndrome, the nodes of Ranvier and the axoplasm of peripheral nerves are affected. The disease is endemic to China and Mexico and has a fast recovery.[31] In acute motor sensory axonal neuropathy, the axoplasm of the peripheral nerves is affected, but recovery is very slow. Acute panautonomic neuropathy is associated with high mortality rate due to cardiovascular problems.[32] Autonomic dysfunction occurs and sweating, photophobia, nausea, dysphagia, and constipation alternating with diarrhea are the most common symptoms. Bickerstaff brainstem encephalitis is characterized by opthalmoplegia, ataxia, and hyperreflexia.[33] Although the onset of the disease is intense, prognosis is usually good.

Charcot-Marie-Tooth (CMT) disease is the most common hereditary neurologic disorder. It comprises a clinically heterogeneous group of peripheral nervous system disorders. CMT is caused by mutations that affect the myelin sheath or the nerve axon. Duplication of a region in 17p12 locum, which regulates the gene *PMP22*, is found in 80% of the cases.[34] Mutations of the gene *MFN2* induce mitochondrial dysfunction that subsequently affects neuromuscular synapses.[35]

There is a wide spectrum of clinical features related to CMT disease. The foot is usually affected first, with drop foot as the initial symptom. Muscle wasting of the lower leg, "stork leg" deformity, pes cavus (high arched foot), and claw toes are common findings. Weakness of the upper extremities, particularly the hands and the forearms, can be found at later stages of the disease. Neuropathic pain, spasmodic muscular contractions, and a loss of touch sensation may occur. Scoliosis and hip and foot deformities are common findings.

The characteristics of Guillain-Barré syndrome and CMT disease are summarized in **Table 3**.

Congenital Structural Myopathies

A summary of the congenital structural myopathies is provided in **Table 4**. Bethlem myopathy is a rare congenital myopathy with an autosomal dominant pattern of inheritance. Mutation in one of the three genes coding for type VI collagen (*COL6A1*, *COL6A2*, and *COL6A3*) is responsible for this type of muscular dystrophy.[36] Although the disease occurs during infancy, Bethlem myopathy progresses very slowly. Weakness of the proximal muscle groups of the lower extremities may cause walking difficulties and a positive Gowers sign. Contractures of the fingers and the toes are typical findings for the disease, and tiptoe walking may occur due to these contractures. The ongoing muscle cell death may cause an elevation of serum creatine kinase (CK).

Centronuclear myopathies comprise a group of myopathies characterized by abnormal location of nuclei in muscle cells. Myotubular myopathy (MTM) is the most common representative of this group of congenital myopathies. Several patterns of inheritance have been identified. X-linked recessive MTM is the most commonly diagnosed. It is caused by mutations of the *MTM1* gene at the locum Xq28 of chromosome X, which encodes for a protein named myotubularin.[37] This is a lipid phosphatase responsible for cellular transport and signaling. Non–X-linked myotubular myopathies are rare. An autosomal recessive type is caused by a mutation of the gene *BIN1*, whereas the dominant type is related to a gene named dynamin 2 (*DNM2*) that is located on chromosome 19.[38]

The clinical image is typical as for most myopathies. The neonates in the congenital type present with decreased muscle tone and significant delays in the developmental milestones. Affected individuals usually remain nonambulatory. Other clinical features include pulmonary complications as a result of weakness of the respiratory muscles, and the development of specific morphologic characteristics, such as bell-shaped thorax, scoliosis, oblong face, high arched palates, and long digits. The prognosis is poor, and affected individuals usually die in their early 50s as a result of cardiac or pulmonary conditions.

Nemaline myopathy (NEM), also known as nemaline rod myopathy, is a congenital genetically heterogeneous neuromuscular disorder. The abnormal thread-like rods in the muscle cells, which are also called

2: Systemic Disorders

Table 3		

Characteristics of the Two Most Common Neuropathic Disorders: Gullain-Barré Syndrome and Charcot-Marie-Tooth Disease

Muscle Disorder	Etiology	Clinical Findings
Guillain-Barré syndrome	Acute inflammatory demyelinating neuropathy *Campylobacter jejuni*, cytomegalovirus, and influenza viruses	Symmetric weakness of the lower limbs Progression in an ascending fashion with or without accompanying sensory deficits The disease may also affect the cranial nerves and respiratory muscles, requiring ventilator assistance.
Charcot-Marie-Tooth (CMT) disease	Mutations that affect myelin sheath or nerve axon Duplication of a region in 17p12 locum, which regulates the gene *PMP22* Mutations of the gene *MFN2* induce mitochondrial dysfunction	Foot usually affected first (drop foot) Muscle wasting of the lower leg, stork leg deformity, pes cavus, and claw toes Weakness of the upper extremities and especially of the hands and forearms at later stages of the disease Neuropathic pain Spasmodic muscular contractions Loss of touch sensation Scoliosis and hip and foot deformities common

nemaline bodies, are characteristic pathology findings for the disease. Several genetic mutations have been identified and are responsible for the various clinical forms of this entity. Six main types (NEM1-6) have been described, comprising a wide variety of clinical manifestations regarding the severity and age of onset.[39] Nemaline disease usually affects proximal muscle groups as well as bulbar and trunk muscles. Neonates are hypotonic, and developmental stages are delayed. Scoliosis occurs at an early age and progresses rapidly during puberty. Respiratory problems are present in all six types of the disease and in severe cases may be life threatening.

ZASP-related myofibril myopathy (zaspopathy) is a relatively novel type of progressive muscular dystrophy. It is caused by an A165V mutation in the *ZASP* gene, which is located at chromosome 10 and is responsible for encoding of the Z-disk-associated protein.[40] The pattern of inheritance is autosomal dominant. Zaspopathy induces a disintegration of the Z-disk of the myofibrils in the muscle cells, decreasing their contractility. Patients with this form of myofibrillar myopathy have a more distal than proximal muscle phenotype. Both anterior and posterior compartments of the lower leg are usually affected.

Myotonias/Channelopathies

Myotonia congenita is a congenital neuromuscular channelopathy with an incidence of approximately 1 case per 100,000 people. More than 80 different mutations have been reported as responsible for the development of various subtypes of the disease. Most common is a mutation in the chloride channel gene *CLCN1*, which is responsible for the formation of the chloride ion channels.[41] The pathophysiologic mecha-

nisms include instability of the channels, decreased permeability to chloride ions, and therefore prolonged muscle contractions. Another reported etiology is a defective endoplasmic retinaculum, which fails to transport the channel to the cellular surface, deteriorating also its function. The etiology and the clinical findings of common channelopathies is summarized in Table 5.

Two major forms of myotonia congenita exist: Thomsen disease, which is inherited through an autosomal dominant pattern, and Becker disease, which is inherited in an autosomal recessive pattern. These two forms differ mainly in the age of onset (early childhood for Thomsen disease and late childhood in Becker disease), and severity of muscle weakness (Becker disease may cause permanent muscle weakness, stiffness, and pain).[41]

The clinical image may vary. Early symptoms usually include frequent falls, muscle stiffness that is improved after several joint motion repetitions (warm-up effect) and difficulties in swallowing, which may be complicated with aspiration pneumonia. Permanent muscle stiffness may cause the development of chronic joint problems, gait disturbances, and injuries after a fall.

Paramyotonia congenita (von Eulenburg disease) is a rare congenital neuromuscular disorder with an incidence of 1 case per 350,000 people that is inherited with an autosomal dominant pattern. The disease is also known as paradoxical myotonia because in contrast with myotonia congenita, muscle stiffness and weakness become worse with exercise.

The etiology of paramyotonia congenita is multifactorial. Mutations in the gene *SCN4A* that interfere with the inactivation speed of the sodium channel have been reported.[42] An increase in cellular excitability is found as a result of a prolonged inward current and the pres-

Table 4

Congenital Structural Myopathies

Muscle Disorder	Etiology	Clinical Findings
Bethlem myopathy	Autosomal dominant inheritance Mutation in one of the three genes coding for type VI collagen (ie, *COL6A1*, *COL6A2*, and *COL6A3*)	Early onset Very slow progression Weakness of the proximal muscle groups of the lower extremities Walking difficulties Positive Gowers sign (climbing up the thighs with the hands) Contractures of the fingers and the toes Tiptoe walking
Myotubular myopathy (MTM)	X-linked recessive Mutations of the *MTM1* gene at the locum Xq28 of chromosome X (encoding protein myotubularin) Autosomal recessive type mutation of the gene *BIN1* Autosomal dominant type gene named dynamin 2 (*DNM2*) located on chromosome 19	Neonates with decreased muscle tone and significant delays in developmental milestones Patients nonambulatory Weakness of the respiratory muscles Development of specific morphologic characteristics: bell-shaped thorax, scoliosis, oblong face, high arched palates, long digits No good prognosis Patients die in their early 50s
Nemaline myopathy (NEM)	Nemaline bodies: abnormal thread-like rods in the muscle cells	Six main types (NEM1-6) Wide variety of clinical manifestations regarding the severity and age of onset Proximal muscle groups as well as bulbar and trunk muscles affected Neonates are hypotonic, and developmental stages are delayed Scoliosis occurs at early age and progresses rapidly.
ZASP-related myofibril myopathy	Autosomal dominant A165V mutation in the *ZASP* gene located at chromosome 10 Encoding of the Z-disk-associated protein	Both anterior and posterior compartments of the lower leg are usually affected More distal than proximal muscle phenotype

ence of a window current because of modifications of channel sensitivity to action potentials.

Clinically, muscle stiffness and weakness are much worse with exercise and sometimes induced by cold temperatures. The symptoms are typically present within the first decade of life. The face and the upper extremities are primarily affected.

Hyperkalemic periodic paralysis (HyperPP) and hypokalemic (HypoPP) periodic paralysis are rare channelopathies characterized by muscle weakness that are related to high or low serum potassium levels, respectively. Nine common mutations of the *SCN4A* gene have been described as the cause of almost 60% of HyperPP cases, but a broad genetic heterogeneity exists for at least 20% of the cases. HypoPP is related to mutations of both *SCN4A* and *CaCNA1S* genes.[43] Clinically, there is substantial overlap of these two conditions. HyperPP has an earlier age of onset (about the first decade of life), and the episodes of paralysis are comparatively of shorter duration and usually do not exceed 4 hours. HypoPP's clinical manifestations are apparent in the first or second decade of life. The epi-

sodes of muscle paralysis can be focal or generalized. There is a predilection in proximal muscle groups, but facial and respiratory muscles are not affected.

Metabolic Myopathies–Mitochondriopathies

Glycogen storage diseases (GSDs) include a large group of pathologies that are associated with defective glycogen metabolism.[44] The reported incidence of GSDs varies between 1 per 20,000 and 1 per 43,000 cases. Both genetic and acquired pathogenetic mechanisms have been found. The different types of GSDs, causative enzymatic defects, and main clinical symptomatology are summarized in Table 6.

Fibromyalgia

Fibromyalgia is a systematic disorder of the central nervous system that is associated with pain, mental impairment, and other neurologic symptoms as a result of central sensitization. The incidence of fibromyalgia is high, ranging between 2% and 4% of the population and showing a significant predilection to the female sex. The etiology is multifactorial: genetic factors, do-

Table 5

Etiology and Clinical Findings of Most Common Channelopathies

Muscle Disorder	Etiology	Clinical Findings

Myotonia congenita	Over 80 different mutations
	Most common mutation in gene *CLCN1*
	Decreased permeability to chloride ions =
	   prolonged muscle contractions
	Defective endoplasmic retinaculum
		Frequent falls
		Muscle stiffness improved after several joint motion
		   repetitions (warm-up effect)
		Difficulties in swallowing
		Chronic joint problems, gait disturbances

Paramyotonia congenita (von Eulenburg disease)	Autosomal dominant
	Mutations in the gene *SCN4A* that interfere
	   with inactivation speed of sodium channel
		Symptoms within the first decade of life
		Muscle stiffness and weakness
		Worsens with exercise and induced by cold
		   temperatures
		Face and upper extremities affected

Hyperkalemic periodic paralysis (HyperPP)	Nine common mutations of the *SCN4A* gene	Age at onset in the first decade of life Episodes of paralysis of short duration (usually do not exceed 4 hours)
Hypokalemic periodic paralysis (HypoPP)	Mutations of *SCN4A* and *CaCNA1S* genes	Age at onset in the first or second decade of life Episodes of muscle paralysis (focal or generalized) Predilection in proximal muscle groups Facial and respiratory muscles not affected

Table 6

Types of Glycogen Storage Diseases

Type	Defective Enzyme	Symptomatology
I (von Gierke disease)	Glucose-6-phosphatase	Growth failure, lactic acidosis, hyperuricemia
II (Pompe disease)	Acid maltase	Muscle weakness, heart failure, death by age 2 years (infantile variant)
III (Cori disease or Forbes)	Glycogen debrancher	Myopathy
IV (Andersen disease)	Glycogen branching enzyme	Failure to thrive, death at age 5 years
V (McArdle disease)	Muscle glycogen phosphorylase	Exercise-induced cramps, rhabdomyolysis, renal failure by myoglobinuria
VI (Hers disease)	Liver glycogen phosphorylase	Exercise-induced muscle cramps and weakness, growth retardation, hemolytic anemia
VII (Tarui disease)	Muscle phosphofructokinase	
VIII (now classified with VI; has been described as X-linked recessive)		
IX	Phosphorylase kinase	Delayed motor development, growth retardation
X (Considered a distinct condition; now classified with VI)		
XI (Fanconi-Bickel syndrome)	Glucose transporter	
XII (Red cell aldolase deficiency)	Aldolase A	Exercise intolerance, cramps

XIII	β-enolase	Exercise intolerance, cramps; increasing intensity
		   of myalgias over decades; serum creatine
		   kinase: episodic elevations; reduced with rest

0	Glycogen synthase	Occasional muscle cramping

pamine dysfunction, abnormal serotonin metabolism and/or growth hormone secretion, and psychological factors have been reported. Several stress-related disorders have been correlated with the development of fibromyalgia, such as chronic fatigue syndrome, irritable bowel syndrome, and posttraumatic stress disorder.[45,46]

The research on the pathophysiology of fibromyalgia has highlighted several potential pathways. The concept of heightened sensitivity of nociceptive systems indicates that patients demonstrate an overreaction to repetitive stimuli in the absence of an exercise-related analgesic response. Other authors have shown that patients with fibromyalgia have hyperactivity of the sympathetic nervous system and lowered adrenal response to physical or mental stimuli. Increased levels of substance P in the cerebrospinal fluid of patients with fibromyalgia is reported to be the most reproducible laboratory finding. Studies using magnetic resonance spectroscopy have shown increased glutamate/glutamine compounds in patients with fibromyalgia and increased levels of pain intensity, greater fatigue, and more symptoms of depression.[47] Reduced dopamine synthesis in the brain stem and the limbic cortex has been found in studies with positron emission tomography.[48]

Clinically, patients complain of widespread pain lasting more than 3 months that affects both proximal and distal muscle groups of the upper and lower extremities. Moreover, the American College of Rheumatology has described 18 designated points of increased tenderness and has recommended that fibromyalgia should be considered when a patient has referred pain at 11 or more of these points.

Rhabdomyolysis

Rhabdomyolysis is a clinical condition associated with severe damage to skeletal muscles. It refers to the systematic consequences caused by the release of the breakdown products of damaged muscle cells into the bloodstream.[49] The incidence of rhabdomyolysis is unclear. However, it is reported that approximately 85% of cases with major trauma will develop rhabdomyolysis, and one fifth to one half of them will eventually end up with acute kidney injury.

The etiology of rhabdomyolysis is multifactorial. Any condition that may cause severe damage to the striated muscles can possibly lead to rhabdomyolysis, including mechanical, biochemical, metabolic, and infectious diseases, and pharmaceutical factors[50,51] (Table 7). Genetic predisposition has also been reported in terms of inherited enzyme deficiencies (polymorphisms or mutations in genes encoding various cytochrome P450 isoenzymes, coenzyme Q, myophosphorlyase, CPT2, and myoadenylate deaminase) that are associated with recurrent episodes of rhabdomyolysis.[49]

The pathophysiology consists of the initial muscle cell damage, including the accumulation of sodium ions from the bloodstream that consequently cause osmotic intracellular swelling and disruption. The concentration of calcium ions is elevated and leads to continuous muscle contraction and inappropriate consumption of ATP that enter into a vicious cycle of uncontrolled ATP depletion-calcium ion influx. There is also an inflammatory response produced by neutrophil granulocytes, which contributes to the swelling of muscle tissue and release of reactive oxygen radicals. Swelling and a potential development of compartment syndrome may compromise blood supply and further damage muscle cells, leading to an abundant release of potassium and phosphate ions, myoglobulin, CK, and uric acid, which can compromise renal function and activate the coagulation system, which leads to disseminated intravascular coagulation and potentially fatal arrhythmias.[49]

Clinical manifestations of rhabdomyolysis include muscle pain, weakness, swelling, and tenderness, although "silent" cases without any muscle symptoms may exist. In more severe cases, symptomatology of hypovolemic shock may be induced from the massive transfer of intravascular fluid into muscle tissue. Abnormalities in serum electrolytes may also cause some constitutional symptoms, such as nausea or vomiting, whereas in more severe disturbances such as confusion, arrhythmias, or even coma can develop. A concentration of myoglobulin in the kidneys may cause acute kidney injury, decreased urine production, and tea-colored urine within the first 24 hours of muscle damage. The development of compartment syndrome is another potential complication caused by acute muscle swelling and is clinically manifested as pain and hypoesthesia of the affected compartment. Prognosis is dependent mainly on the underlying etiology, the severity of muscle injury, and the magnitude of complications. The mortality rate is reported to reach 20% for those who develop acute kidney injury and 60% for those with established renal impairment.[52]

Paraneoplasmic Myopathy

Lambert-Eaton myasthenic syndrome is caused by an autoimmune reaction against presynaptic voltage gated calcium channels on the presynaptic nerve terminal. These calcium channels are also found in the autonomic nervous system and the cerebellum, and this may explain the autonomic symptoms and coordination problems.

Lambert-Eaton myasthenic syndrome is often considered a type of paraneoplasmic myopathy; several types of malignant diseases and especially small cell lung cancer are found in 50% to 70% of the cases. Other autoimmune diseases, such as hypothyroidism or diabetes mellitus type I, may coexist, whereas an association with HLA DR3-B8 has also been reported.[53]

The clinical image involves a marked decrease of proximal muscle strength, especially of the lower extremities. Ocular and respiratory muscle involvement can be found in advanced stages. Bulbar muscles are rarely affected. Autonomic nervous system involvement is usually expressed with blood pressure disorders, constipation, sweating, and blurred vision.

Approach to Diagnostic/Genetic Counseling

The evaluation of a patient presenting with muscle weakness and/or pain is complex, but a systematic approach can facilitate a differential diagnosis. Determining the etiology of symptoms and localizing the anatomic site of the lesion within the neuromuscular

2: Systemic Disorders

Table 7

Etiologic Factors of Rhabdomyolysis

Pathophysiologic Mechanism	Cause of Muscle Damage		
Crush injury	Blast injury Crush syndrome Motor vehicle injuries Consistent limb pressure in a fixed position (after alcohol intoxication, prolonged surgery and/or stroke)		
Exertion	Extreme physical exercise Tetanus Seizures		
Impaired blood supply	Embolism Thrombosis Prolonged arterial clamping (resuscitation from trauma or during vascular surgery)		
Metabolic abnormalities	Hypernatremia Hypokalemia Hypocalcemia Hypophosphatemia Hyperglycemia – hyperosmolar state – ketoacidosis Hypothyroidism		
Infection	Influenza A and B Epstein-Barr virus Coxsackie virus HIV Herpes viruses Cytomegalovirus	Salmonella *Legionella pneumophila* Lyme myositis Fungal Trichinosis Toxoplasmosis	
Inflammatory diseases	Dermatomyositis Polymyositis		

Drugs and toxins	Drugs
	  Statins
	  Fibrates
	  Diuretics
	  Neuroleptics
	  Neuromuscular blocking agents
	  Selective serotonin reuptake inhibitor
	  Amphetamines, cocaine, heroin, lysergic acid diethylamide (LSD)
		Toxic agents
		  Heavy metals
		  Insect bites
		  Haff disease	

Body temperature	Hyperthermia Hypothermia		

Genetic predisposition	Glycolysis
	  Phosphofructokinase
	  Glucogen storage diseases VIII, IX, X, XI
		Lipid metabolism
		  Carnitine palmitoyltransferase I and II
		  Acyl coenzyme A dehydrogenase
		  Thiolase
			Mitochondrial
			  Succinate dehydrogenase
			  Cytochrome c oxidase
			  Coenzyme Q10

system is of paramount importance. The patient's history and physical examination have a major role in distinguishing motor impairment caused by muscle asthenia from that secondary to other etiologies. Information regarding the age of onset, sex, coexisting metabolic and rheumatic diseases, endocrinopathies, medication history, and alcohol and substance abuse are significant. A detailed neurologic examination is re-

quired to identify pathologies from the central and peripheral nervous systems. The distribution of weakness is a useful guide to differential diagnosis. An algorithm showing the steps of the diagnostic procedure based on the pattern of muscle weakness is presented in Figure 1.

Laboratory studies should include serum, urine, and cerebrospinal fluid examination and immune tests. Increased concentrations of muscle enzymes, such as CK,

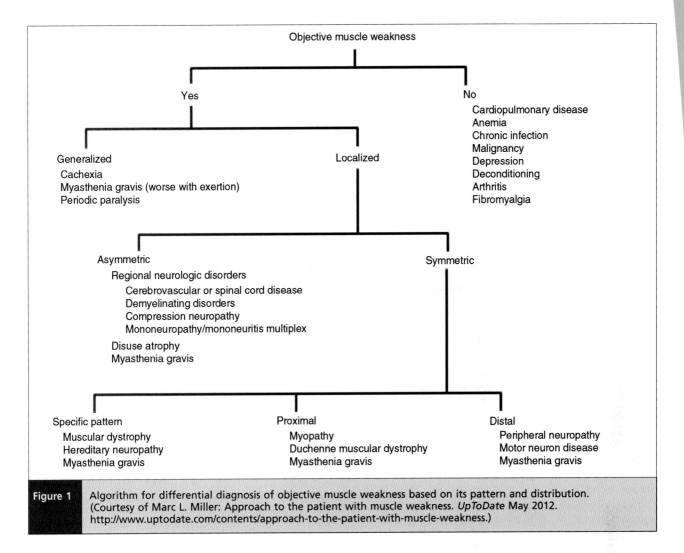

Objective muscle weakness

Yes

No
Cardiopulmonary disease
Anemia
Chronic infection
Malignancy
Depression
Deconditioning
Arthritis
Fibromyalgia

Generalized
Cachexia
Myasthenia gravis (worse with exertion)
Periodic paralysis

Localized

Asymmetric
Regional neurologic disorders
Cerebrovascular or spinal cord disease
Demyelinating disorders
Compression neuropathy
Mononeuropathy/mononeuritis multiplex
Disuse atrophy
Myasthenia gravis

Symmetric

Specific pattern
Muscular dystrophy
Hereditary neuropathy
Myasthenia gravis

Proximal
Myopathy
Duchenne muscular dystrophy
Myasthenia gravis

Distal
Peripheral neuropathy
Motor neuron disease
Myasthenia gravis

Figure 1   Algorithm for differential diagnosis of objective muscle weakness based on its pattern and distribution. (Courtesy of Marc L. Miller: Approach to the patient with muscle weakness. *UpToDate* May 2012. http://www.uptodate.com/contents/approach-to-the-patient-with-muscle-weakness.)

lactate dehydrogenase, aldolase, and transaminases (serum glutamic oxaloacetic transaminase, serum glutamic pyruvic transaminase) in serum are highly indicative of the presence of muscle disease. Specific serologic tests may reveal inflammatory myopathies or a background of connective tissue disease. Anti-histidyl-t-RNA synthetase (anti-Jo-1) antigens are specific for myositides, whereas antinuclear antibodies (anti-Sm, anti-Ro, anti-La, and anti-RNP) can be found in several rheumatic diseases.

Electrophysiologic studies, including nerve conduction velocity studies and EMG, are helpful in localizing the site of the lesion in the peripheral nerve pathway, the neuromuscular junction, or within the muscle. It is generally difficult to make distinctions between hereditary and acquired myopathies using EMG. The motor unit potentials are low and spiky. The pattern of recruitment typically becomes full with just a small firing with muscle contraction. In muscular dystrophies, large motor units on a background of small spiky units can be seen because of the presence of muscle fibers of variable diameter. In inflammatory muscle diseases (dermatomyositis, polymyositis), and nonspecific fibrillations may be seen because of muscle fiber degeneration.

In Lambert-Eaton myasthenic syndrome, EMG may demonstrate a myopathic pattern as a result of neuromuscular block. EMG should be combined with measurement of the amplitude of a compound muscle action potential evoked by nerve stimulation before and after exercise.[54]

Muscle biopsy is often necessary to confirm the diagnosis and determine the type of myopathy. Special stains have been used to reveal specific enzyme deficiencies and/or the accumulation of glycogen or lipid in glycogen or lipid storage myopathies, respectively. Electron microscopic examination is helpful to identify specific forms of myopathy (for example, IBM).

Genetic testing has been a significant tool for the diagnosis and the classification of cases with inherited myopathies and muscle dystrophies.[55,56] However, genetic heterogeneity and conventional molecular methods make the genetic assessment of most inherited myopathies a copious procedure. Algorithms aimed at reducing the number of genes qualified for possible molecular genetic testing have been proposed based on morphologic and clinical criteria (Figure 2).

Next-generation sequencing has been shown to be an efficient and effective method to facilitate diagnosis.

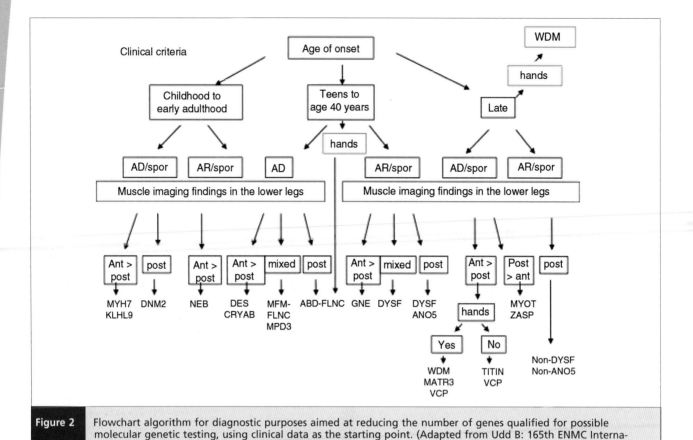

Figure 2   Flowchart algorithm for diagnostic purposes aimed at reducing the number of genes qualified for possible molecular genetic testing, using clinical data as the starting point. (Adapted from Udd B: 165th ENMC International Workshop: Distal myopathies, 6-8th February 2009, Naarden, The Netherlands. *Neuromuscul Disord* 2009;19[6]:429-438.)

DNA is first broken into a library of small fragments. These fragments are then attached to oligonucleotide adapters that facilitate the biochemistry necessary for the sequencing reaction. Genetic content among samples and germline and somatic variants of interest can be identified; single nucleotide polymorphisms, insertions and deletions (indels), copy number variants, and other structural variations may be found using this new technology. Next-generation sequencing and DNA multiplexing can be used to retrieve pathogenic mutations in cases with heterogeneous neuromuscular disorders.[55] Other researchers have used whole genome or whole exome sequencing (ES) for the genetic diagnosis of given monogenic muscle diseases.[57] However, these two methods have several disadvantages for routine molecular diagnosis, including coverage, variant analysis, validation, and price. The major drawback is that the whole exome sequencing capture library could not be customized and should be updated to incorporate novel genes.

Summary

Muscle disorders include a wide spectrum of pathologic entities, ranging from inflammatory myopathies, muscular dystrophies, and different types of myasthenic syndromes to neuropathic disorders, structural myopa-

thies, myotonias, channelopathies, mitochondriopathies, and paraneoplasmic myopathies.

Overall, the differential diagnosis of muscle disorders is a complex procedure. A systematic approach to these cases, which should follow a detailed history and clinical examination and orthological utilization of every new imaging and laboratory tool needed, will facilitate accurate diagnosis and treatment.

Key Study Points

- Abnormal accumulation of pathogenic proteins (amyloid-β, phosphorylated tau protein, and others) may have a causative effect in immune system deregulation.

- The absence of protein dystrophin is responsible for DMD. Its production is regulated by a gene located at chromosome X (*Xp21* gene). However, one third of cases comprises new sporadic mutations.

- Specific HLA types (B8 and DR3) have been found to be associated with the development of myasthenia gravis. Antibodies against muscle specific kinase induce a decrease in patency of the neuromuscular junction.

Annotated References

1. Lieber RL, Fridén J: Clinical significance of skeletal muscle architecture. *Clin Orthop Relat Res* 2001;383: 140-151.

2. Galpin AJ, Raue U, Jemiolo B, et al: Human skeletal muscle fiber type specific protein content. *Anal Biochem* 2012;425(2):175-182.

   The authors present a reliable method for human skeletal muscle fiber type specific protein analysis. They show that particular proteins exist in a hierarchal fashion throughout the continuum of skeletal muscle fiber types.

3. Pette D, Staron RS: Myosin isoforms, muscle fiber types, and transitions. *Microsc Res Tech* 2000;50(6): 500-509.

4. Stark H, Schilling N: A novel method of studying fascicle architecture in relaxed and contracted muscles. *J Biomech* 2010;43(15):2897-2903.

   The authors describe muscle architecture in more detail and compare relaxed and contracted states.

5. Rana M, Wakeling JM: In-vivo determination of 3D muscle architecture of human muscle using free hand ultrasound. *J Biomech* 2011;44(11):2129-2135.

   The authors developed and validated methods to determine in vivo muscle fascicle orientations in three dimensions using ultrasound.

6. Hak AE, de Paepe B, de Bleecker JL, Tak P-P, de Visser M: Dermatomyositis and polymyositis: New treatment targets on the horizon. *Neth J Med* 2011;69(10): 410-421.

   The authors support that there is an immune mediated inflammation involved with the development of idiopathic inflammatory myopathies. Results from the use of blockers of the lymphotoxin signaling pathway are awaited. The authors suggest that anti-B cell therapy may be a valuable therapeutic option for the treatment of refractory idiopathic inflammatory myopathies.

7. Dalakas MC, Hohlfeld R: Polymyositis and dermatomyositis. *Lancet* 2003;362(9388):971-982.

8. Mimori T, Nakashima R, Hosono Y: Interstitial lung disease in myositis: Clinical subsets, biomarkers, and treatment. *Curr Rheumatol Rep* 2012;14(3):264-274.

   Interstitial lung disease is found in nearly one half of myositis patients. Autoantibodies as well as imaging and histopathological studies are useful for the classification of interstitial lung disease in myositis and provide useful information for predicting prognosis and determining treatment.

9. Garlepp MJ, Mastaglia FL: Inclusion body myositis: New insights into pathogenesis. *Curr Opin Rheumatol* 2008;20(6):662-668.

10. Askanas V, Engel WK: Sporadic inclusion-body myosi-

tis: Conformational multifactorial ageing-related degenerative muscle disease associated with proteasomal and lysosomal inhibition, endoplasmic reticulum stress, and accumulation of amyloid-β42 oligomers and phosphorylated tau. *Presse Med* 2011;40(4, pt 2):e219-e235.

   This review article presents the newest research advances for better understanding the pathogenesis of sporadic inclusion body myositis.

11. Haubenberger D, Bittner RE, Rauch-Shorny S, et al: Inclusion body myopathy and Paget disease is linked to a novel mutation in the VCP gene. *Neurology* 2005;65(8): 1304-1305.

12. Sahenk Z, Mendell JR: The muscular dystrophies: Distinct pathogenic mechanisms invite novel therapeutic approaches. *Curr Rheumatol Rep* 2011;13(3):199-207.

   A splicing disorder related to RNA toxicity is the common mechanism for facioscapulohumeral muscular dystrophy and myotonic dystrophies.

13. Velázquez-Wong AC, Hernández-Huerta C, Márquez-Calixto A, et al: Identification of duchenne muscular dystrophy female carriers by fluorescence in situ hybridization and RT-PCR. *Genet Test* 2008;12(2):221-223.

14. Magri F, Del Bo R, D'Angelo MG, et al: Clinical and molecular characterization of a cohort of patients with novel nucleotide alterations of the dystrophin gene detected by direct sequencing. *BMC Med Genet* 2011;12:37.

   The authors analyzed a sample of patients carrying point mutations or complex rearrangements in the *DMD* gene. They report a phenotypic correlation in dystrophinopatic patients, which helps to understand the premessenger RNA maturation defects and dystrophin functional domains. The authors believe that these data could direct new therapeutic approaches relying on a more precise definition of the genetic defects.

15. Jimenez-Mallebrera C, Brown SC, Sewry CA, Muntoni F: Congenital muscular dystrophy: Molecular and cellular aspects. *Cell Mol Life Sci* 2005;62(7-8):809-823.

16. Bertini E, D'Amico A, Gualandi F, Petrini S: Congenital muscular dystrophies: A brief review. *Semin Pediatr Neurol* 2011;18(4):277-288.

   The authors provide a clinical description of the most important forms of CMD. Particular attention is paid to the main keys for a diagnostic approach, highlighting the requirement for concurrence of expertise in multiple specialties (neurology, morphology, genetics, and neuroradiology). Molecular diagnosis is significant for phenotype-genotype correlations, genetic counseling, and prognosis. Level of evidence: IV.

17. Muchir A, Worman HJ: Emery-Dreifuss muscular dystrophy. *Curr Neurol Neurosci Rep* 2007;7(1):78-83.

18. Zhang Q, Bethmann C, Worth NF, et al: Nesprin-1 and -2 are involved in the pathogenesis of Emery Dreifuss muscular dystrophy and are critical for nuclear envelope integrity. *Hum Mol Genet* 2007;16(23):2816-2833.

2: Systemic Disorders

19. Gueneau L, Bertrand AT, Jais JP, et al: Mutations of the FHL1 gene cause Emery-Dreifuss muscular dystrophy. *Am J Hum Genet* 2009;85(3):338-353.

20. Guglieri M, Magri F, Comi GP: Molecular etiopathogenesis of limb girdle muscular and congenital muscular dystrophies: Boundaries and contiguities. *Clin Chim Acta* 2005;361(1-2):54-79.

21. Tawil R, Van Der Maarel SM: Facioscapulohumeral muscular dystrophy. *Muscle Nerve* 2006;34(1):1-15.

22. Mathews KD, Moore SA: Limb-girdle muscular dystrophy. *Curr Neurol Neurosci Rep* 2003;3(1):78-85.

23. Hino H, Araki K, Uyama E, et al: Myopathy phenotype in transgenic mice expressing mutated PABPN1 as a model of oculopharyngeal muscular dystrophy. *Hum Mol Genet* 2004;13(2):181-190.

24. Spillane J, Beeson DJ, Kullmann DM: Myasthenia and related disorders of the neuromuscular junction. *J Neurol Neurosurg Psychiatry* 2010;81(8):850-857.

    This review article focuses on recent advances in the diagnosis and the treatment of disorders of the neuromuscular junction.

25. Masuda T, Motomura M, Utsugisawa K, et al: Antibodies against the main immunogenic region of the acetylcholine receptor correlate with disease severity in myasthenia gravis. *J Neurol Neurosurg Psychiatry* 2012; 83(9):935-940.

    The authors suggest that the main immunogenic region antibodies assay may be useful for predicting myasthenia gravis symptom severity, especially for discriminating between ocular and generalized types of myasthenia gravis.

26. Jaretzki A III, Barohn RJ, Ernstoff RM, et al: Myasthenia gravis: Recommendations for clinical research standards. Task Force of the Medical Scientific Advisory Board of the Myasthenia Gravis Foundation of America. *Neurology* 2000;55(1):16-23.

27. Wu X, Tuzun E, Li J, et al: Ocular and generalized myasthenia gravis induced by human acetylcholine receptor γ subunit immunization. *Muscle Nerve* 2012;45(2): 209-216.

    The authors present their findings indicating that ocular myasthenia gravis may be induced by immunity to the acetylcholine receptor γ subunit.

28. Mossberg N, Nordin M, Movitz C, et al: The recurrent Guillain-Barré syndrome: A long-term population-based study. *Acta Neurol Scand* 2012;126(3):154-161.

    The authors conclude that episodes of recurrent Guillain-Barré syndrome are shorter than in monophasic Guillain-Barré syndrome. However, no immunologic predisposing factors for recurrence beyond the previously demonstrated relationship to a weaker respiratory burst could be identified.

29. Drenthen J, Yuki N, Meulstee J, et al: Guillain-Barré syndrome subtypes related to Campylobacter infection. *J Neurol Neurosurg Psychiatry* 2011;82(3):300-305.

    The authors report that *Campylobacter jejuni* infections are strongly but not exclusively associated with axonal Guillain-Barré syndrome.

30. Roberts T, Shah A, Graham JG, McQueen IN: The Miller Fischer syndrome following campylobacter enteritis: A report of two cases. *J Neurol Neurosurg Psychiatry* 1987;50(11):1557-1558.

31. Tang XF, Zhang XJ: Guillain-Barré syndrome or "new" Chinese paralytic syndrome in northern China? *Electroencephalogr Clin Neurophysiol* 1996;101(2):105-109.

32. Akbayram S, Doğan M, Akgün C, et al: Clinical features and prognosis with Guillain-Barré syndrome. *Ann Indian Acad Neurol* 2011;14(2):98-102.

    The authors showed that Guillain-Barré syndrome is not uncommon in children younger than 2 years of age, and cerebrospinal fluid protein level might be found high in the first week of the disease in about 50% of the patients, with a higher rate of morbidity and mortality in patients with axonal involvement than in those with acute inflammatory demyelinating polyradiculoneuropathy.

33. Nagashima T, Koga M, Odaka M, Hirata K, Yuki N: Continuous spectrum of pharyngeal-cervical-brachial variant of Guillain-Barré syndrome. *Arch Neurol* 2007; 64(10):1519-1523.

34. Choi B-O, Kim NK, Park SW, et al: Inheritance of Charcot-Marie-Tooth disease 1A with rare nonrecurrent genomic rearrangement. *Neurogenetics* 2011;12(1): 51-58.

    The authors reported an Alu-Alu-mediated rearrangement with the FoSTeS by the MMBIR and a two-step rearrangement of the replication based FoSTeS/MMBIR and meiosis-based recombination that are associated with CMT disease 1A peripheral neuropathy.

35. Feely SM, Laura M, Siskind CE, et al: MFN2 mutations cause severe phenotypes in most patients with CMT2A. *Neurology* 2011;76(20):1690-1696.

    The authors report that *MFN2* mutations are found particularly likely to cause severe neuropathy that may be primarily motor or motor accompanied by prominent proprioception loss.

36. Briñas L, Richard P, Quijano-Roy S, et al: Early onset collagen VI myopathies: Genetic and clinical correlations. *Ann Neurol* 2010;68(4):511-520.

    Quantitative reverse transcription-polymerase chain reaction is a helpful tool for the identification of some mutation-bearing genes. The clinical classification proposed by the authors allows genotype-phenotype relationships to be explored.

37. Tsai T-C, Horinouchi H, Noguchi S, et al: Characterization of MTM1 mutations in 31 Japanese families with myotubular myopathy, including a patient carrying

240 kb deletion in Xq28 without male hypogenitalism. *Neuromuscul Disord* 2005;15(3):245-252.

38. Romero NB: Centronuclear myopathies: A widening concept. *Neuromuscul Disord* 2010;20(4):223-228.

The authors present particular histopathologic abnormalities associated with specific mutations that are helpful for distinguishing between nuclear centralization and nuclear internalization.

39. Olivé M, Goldfarb LG, Lee H-S, et al: Nemaline myopathy type 6: Clinical and myopathological features. *Muscle Nerve* 2010;42(6):901-907.

The authors present a unique subtype NEM6, which is phenotypically similar and probably allelic to two previously reported NEM6 pedigrees.

40. Selcen D, Engel AG: Mutations in ZASP define a novel form of muscular dystrophy in humans. *Ann Neurol* 2005;57(2):269-276.

41. Ulzi G, Lecchi M, Sansone V, et al: Myotonia congenita: Novel mutations in *CLCN1* gene and functional characterizations in Italian patients. *J Neurol Sci* 2012;318(1-2):65-71.

The authors present 12 novel mutations in *CLCN1* that may contribute to genotype-phenotype correlations of myotonia congenita.

42. Yoshinaga H, Sakoda S, Good J-M, et al: A novel mutation in *SCN4A* causes severe myotonia and school-age-onset paralytic episodes. *J Neurol Sci* 2012;315(1-2):15-19.

The authors discuss the novel mutation of the skeletal muscle sodium channel (*SCN4A*), *pI693L*, which is responsible for HypoPP and is correlated with a severe clinical form of paramyotonia congenita.

43. Matthews E, Portaro S, Ke Q, et al: Acetazolamide efficacy in hypokalemic periodic paralysis and the predictive role of genotype. *Neurology* 2011;77(22):1960-1964.

The authors showed that only half of the genotyped patients with HypoPP respond to acetazolamide, and that there is a correlation between genotype and treatment response.

44. Shin YS: Glycogen storage disease: Clinical, biochemical, and molecular heterogeneity. *Semin Pediatr Neurol* 2006;13(2):115-120.

45. Clauw DJ, Arnold LM, McCarberg BH; FibroCollaborative: The science of fibromyalgia. *Mayo Clin Proc* 2011;86(9):907-911.

The authors present new concepts regarding fibromyalgia and highlight the fact that the condition remains undiagnosed in 75% of patients. There is ongoing research to determine the role of analogous central nervous system factors in the other cardinal symptoms of fibromyalgia, such as fatigue, nonrestorative sleep, and cognitive dysfunction.

46. Schmidt-Wilcke T, Clauw DJ: Fibromyalgia: From pathophysiology to therapy. *Nat Rev Rheumatol* 2011;7(9):518-527.

The authors review the pathophysiologic mechanism related to fibromyalgia and present potential pharmacological treatments, including monoamine modulators, calcium channel modulators, and γ-aminobutyric acid modulators.

47. Valdés M, Collado A, Bargalló N, et al: Increased glutamate/glutamine compounds in the brains of patients with fibromyalgia: A magnetic resonance spectroscopy study. *Arthritis Rheum* 2010;62(6):1829-1836.

The distinctive metabolic features described in the right amygdala of patients with fibromyalgia suggest the presence of neural dysfunction in emotional processing.

48. Wood PB, Schweinhardt P, Jaeger E, et al: Fibromyalgia patients show an abnormal dopamine response to pain. *Eur J Neurosci* 2007;25(12):3576-3582.

49. Parekh R, Care DA, Tainter CR: Rhabdomyolysis: Advances in diagnosis and treatment. *Emerg Med Pract* 2012;14(3):1-15.

This review article examines the current evidence on symptoms and diagnostic methods as well as standard first-line treatments of rhabdomyolysis.

50. Dalakas MC: Toxic and drug-induced myopathies. *J Neurol Neurosurg Psychiatry* 2009;80(8):832-838.

51. Valiyil R, Christopher-Stine L: Drug-related myopathies of which the clinician should be aware. *Curr Rheumatol Rep* 2010;12(3):213-220.

Drug-related myopathies are potentially reversible in their early stages. It is important to be able to recognize toxic myopathies and discontinue therapy early before muscle damage becomes irreversible.

52. Splendiani G, Mazzarella V, Cipriani S, Pollicita S, Rodio F, Casciani CU: Dialytic treatment of rhabdomyolysis-induced acute renal failure: Our experience. *Ren Fail* 2001;23(2):183-191.

53. Takamori M: Lambert-Eaton myasthenic syndrome: Search for alternative autoimmune targets and possible compensatory mechanisms based on presynaptic calcium homeostasis. *J Neuroimmunol* 2008;201-202:145-152.

54. Meriggioli MN, Sanders DB: Advances in the diagnosis of neuromuscular junction disorders. *Am J Phys Med Rehabil* 2005;84(8):627-638.

55. Laing NG: Genetics of neuromuscular disorders. *Crit Rev Clin Lab Sci* 2012;49(2):33-48.

The authors discuss the significant role of NGS in causative genes for the different types of neuromuscular disorders. However, NGS is not good at identifying repeat expansions or copy number variations.

56. Guglieri M, Bushby K: How to go about diagnosing and managing the limb-girdle muscular dystrophies. *Neurol India* 2008;56(3):271-280.

57. Dias C, Sincan M, Cherukuri PF, et al: An analysis of exome sequencing for diagnostic testing of the genes associated with muscle disease and spastic paraplegia. *Hum Mutat* 2012;33(4):614-626.

The authors present ES as a diagnostic alternative for genetically heterogeneous disorders. They found that ES is a rapid and first-tier method to screen for mutations, although its application requires the disclosure of the extent of coverage for each targeted gene. Therefore, supplementation with second-tier Sanger sequencing for full coverage is required.

Chapter 21

Nerve Disorders

Jeffrey A. Rihn, MD   Jeremy Simon, MD   Melissa M. Guanche, MD

Introduction

The topic of nerve disorders is extensive and encompasses a wide range of pathologies and diagnoses. Disorders of the nervous system are commonly encountered in the clinical setting across all orthopaedic subspecialties. The diagnosis of such disorders can be challenging because many of the causes have similar symptoms and presentation. A thorough history and physical examination, appropriate imaging studies, electrodiagnostic studies, and laboratory work can all be helpful in reaching a diagnosis. Treatment options vary widely according to the diagnosis. Some forms of neuropathy, such as Charcot-Marie-Tooth (CMT) disease and amyotrophic lateral sclerosis (ALS), are progressive, with treatment focusing on preserving function where possible and providing symptomatic relief. Other forms of neuropathy, such as carpal tunnel syndrome, are amenable to surgical treatment. The purpose of this chapter is to provide an overview of the basic anatomy of the nervous system and the evaluation and management of common nerve disorders that are encountered in orthopaedic practice.

Anatomy of the Nervous System

At its most basic level, the nervous system is divided into the central and peripheral nervous systems. The central nervous system consists of the brain and the spinal cord and functions to initiate, send, receive, and coordinate signals that control bodily functions. The peripheral nervous system serves to transfer signals to and from the central nervous system. The basic functioning unit of the nervous system is the neuron, a cell that maintains an electrical gradient across its membrane and transmits messages using depolarizing electrical

Dr. Rihn or an immediate family member has received research or institutional support from DePuy and serves as a board member, owner, officer, or committee member of the North American Spine Society. Neither of the following authors nor any immediate family member has received anything of value from or has stock or stock options held in a commercial company or institution related directly or indirectly to the subject of this chapter: Dr. Simon and Dr. Guanche.

signals. Motor neurons transmit information from the central nervous system to the skeletal muscle and smooth muscle of the viscera. Sensory neurons transmit the information from internal and external stimuli to the central nervous system. The neuron has three main components: the cell body, the axon, and the dendrites. The dendrites receive information from other neuronal axons or external stimuli, the cell body processes the signal, and the axon transmits the signal to other neurons or end organs (skeletal muscle) through chemical or electrical synapses.

Myelin is a lipid-rich material produced by glial cells (oligodendrocytes in the central nervous system and Schwann cells in the peripheral nervous system) that surrounds axons, facilitates the rapid propagation of the electric signal, and provides structural and metabolic support of the neuron.[1] Regularly spaced interruptions in the myelin sheath, called the nodes of Ranvier, expose sodium-gated channels of the axonal membrane that allow for salutatory conduction of action potentials down the axon. The clinical effects of numerous disorders of the nervous system, including multiple sclerosis and Guillain-Barré syndrome, are the result of axonal demyelination. Not all axons in the nervous system are myelinated.

Spinal Cord

The spinal cord is organized into tracts of axons that carry information to and from the brain. It also contains interneurons that communicate signals to and from the brain and the peripheral nerves and neurons that locally control many of the body's reflexes. When looking at a cross section of the spinal cord, the peripheral white matter represents the myelinated axons of the motor and sensory tracts, and the central gray matter represents the neuronal cell bodies and unmyelinated interneurons.[2] In general, motor information is carried from the brain (motor cortex) down the spinal cord (efferent pathway), and sensory information is carried from the periphery (sensory receptors) up the spinal cord (afferent pathway). The corticospinal tracts (lateral and anterior) of the spinal cord consist of axons of the upper motor neurons that originate largely in the contralateral motor cortex of the brain.[2] Through interneurons or direct synapse, these axons carry information to the lower motor neurons, the cell bodies of which are housed in the anterior or ventral horns of the spinal cord.[3] The efferent axons of these lower motor neurons comprise the ventral root of the spinal cord that forms the spinal nerve.

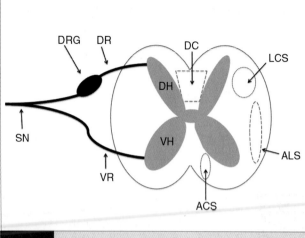

Figure 1   The cross-sectional anatomy of the spinal cord. ACS = anterior corticospinal tract, ALS = anterolateral system, DC = dorsal column tracts, DH = dorsal (posterior) horn, DR = dorsal root, DRG = dorsal root ganglion, LCS = lateral corticospinal trac, SN = spinal nerve, VH = ventral (anterior) horn, VR = ventral root.

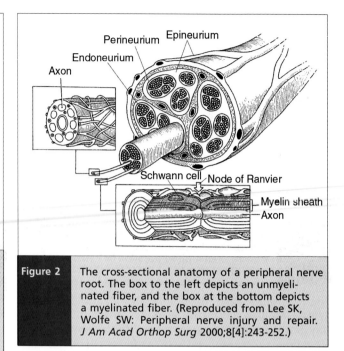

Figure 2   The cross-sectional anatomy of a peripheral nerve root. The box to the left depicts an unmyelinated fiber, and the box at the bottom depicts a myelinated fiber. (Reproduced from Lee SK, Wolfe SW: Peripheral nerve injury and repair. *J Am Acad Orthop Surg* 2000;8[4]:243-252.)

The sensory tracts of the spinal cord are divided largely into the dorsal column tracts, which carry proprioception and vibration information, and the anterolateral system, which carry pain and temperature information (spinothalamic tract).[2] The axons of the dorsal column decussate via interneurons in the brainstem, whereas the axons of the spinothalamic tract decussate via interneurons in the spinal cord, approximately two levels cranial to their entry.[3] The cell bodies of the primary sensory neurons that contribute axons to both of these sensory tracts are housed in the dorsal root ganglion (**Figure 1**).

Peripheral Nervous System

The peripheral nervous system is grossly divided into the somatic (controls skeletal muscle) and autonomic (controls visceral, smooth muscle function) nervous systems. A peripheral nerve consists of multiple neuronal axons, or nerve fibers, bundled together and surrounded by connective tissue, a vascular supply, and cellular components, including Schwann cells, fibroblasts, and macrophages.[4] The endoneurium is a layer of connective tissue that surrounds each axon and its associated Schwann cells. The neurolemma, a thin layer between the myelin sheath and the endoneurium, is the outermost layer of the Schwann cell.[4] The axons are bundled into fascicles contained within the perineurium, which contributes significantly to the tensile strength of the nerve.[5] The fascicles are bound together by the outer covering of the nerve, the epineurium. The epineurium is composed of connective tissue that functions in protecting and supporting the fascicles.[5] The inner portion of the epineurium runs between the fascicles, and the outer portion forms a sheath that surrounds the entire nerve[5] (**Figure 2**).

Nerve Injury and Healing

Peripheral nerve injury from direct compression and/or trauma is frequently encountered in orthopaedics. The varying degrees of peripheral nerve injury have been classified as neurapraxia, axonotmesis, and neurotmesis.[1-3,6] Neurapraxia represents the mildest form of nerve injury, in which there is transient loss of nerve function across the site of injury. Neurapraxia is typically caused by a compression injury that results in focal myelin damage but preservation of the axon.[5] Recovery from this type of injury is typically complete by 6 to 8 weeks after the injury.[6]

Axonotmesis is defined by damage to the nerve fibers (axons) but preservation of the supporting connective tissue structures of the nerve (endoneurium, perineurium, and epineurium).[6] This type of injury is characterized by wallerian degeneration, or degeneration of the portion of the axon distal to the injury. Recovery from this type of injury is characterized by spontaneous regeneration of the remaining axon along the preserved pathway (intact neurolemma). Although this process occurs slowly, at a rate of approximately 1 mm per day, recovery of nerve function does occur.

Neurotmesis is the most severe type of nerve injury, representing a complete transection of the nerve. This type of injury results in complete loss of motor and sensory function in the distribution of the involved nerve. In the absence of surgical repair, recovery of function does not occur.[6] Surgical repair of the nerve does increase the chance of recovery; however, recovery even with surgical repair is often incomplete. Early repair may provide better results than delayed repair.[7] For larger nerves, a microsurgical approach with grouped fascicular repair, where an attempt is made to line up and repair the fascicles rather then just lining up the

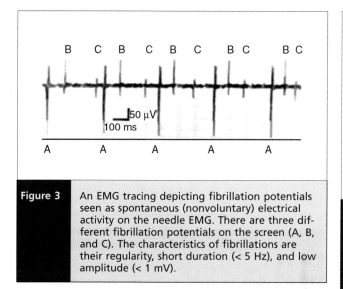

Figure 3 An EMG tracing depicting fibrillation potentials seen as spontaneous (nonvoluntary) electrical activity on the needle EMG. There are three different fibrillation potentials on the screen (A, B, and C). The characteristics of fibrillations are their regularity, short duration (< 5 Hz), and low amplitude (< 1 mV).

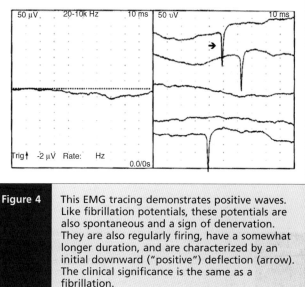

Figure 4 This EMG tracing demonstrates positive waves. Like fibrillation potentials, these potentials are also spontaneous and a sign of denervation. They are also regularly firing, have a somewhat longer duration, and are characterized by an initial downward ("positive") deflection (arrow). The clinical significance is the same as a fibrillation.

epineurium, may improve recovery, although this issue remains debatable.[7] In smaller, more distal nerves, simple repair of the epineurium has been shown to provide similar results to grouped fascicular repair.[8]

Electrodiagnostics

Electrodiagnostics can be a useful tool in the evaluation of a patient with a suspected peripheral nerve disorder. The electrodiagnostic evaluation can assess and help localize abnormalities involving the anterior horn cell, nerve root, plexus, peripheral nerve, neuromuscular junction, and muscle. The assessment is typically twofold: a nerve conduction velocity study and needle electromyography (EMG). The timing of the study always needs to be considered because nerve injuries may take up to 3 weeks to be accurately assessed by electrodiagnostics.

Nerve Conduction Velocity Study

The nerve conduction velocity study involves generating an electrical stimulus to a peripheral nerve and recording the action potential. This is done for both the sensory and the motor components of the nerve. Normal values are well described for amplitude, latency (time when depolarization begins), and conduction velocity.[9] Aberrations in any of these parameters can be indicative of a problem with that nerve. Diffuse abnormalities are indicative of peripheral neuropathy. If the abnormalities are in the distribution of a specific area of the plexus, this indicates a plexopathy. Other studies that may be used in the nerve conduction workup for peripheral neuropathy are so-called late responses. These include the F-wave, which is a response generated in a motor nerve that will travel to the anterior horn cell and fire back a response that is recorded at a distal pickup. This motor-motor response is of lower amplitude (approximately 5% of the compound motor action potential) and of longer latency. Several different

parameters are used to determine abnormalities in the F-wave response, but most commonly prolonged latency.

Electromyography

This portion of the study involves placement of a needle into the muscle. The parameters assessed are resting membrane activity, recruitment, and motor unit analysis. A muscle at rest has little spontaneous electrical activity. If an axonal lesion has occurred, characteristic findings of membrane instability called fibrillations and sharp waves will appear (**Figures 3** and **4**). The patient will be asked to voluntarily contract the muscle, and the recruitment pattern will then be assessed. If there is a block in conduction or a significant axonal lesion, the normal number of motor units will not be activated, and a pattern of decreased recruitment will be evident. By recruiting the units by asking the patient to minimally contract the muscle of interest, each unit's size, shape, and duration can be assessed. Abnormal appearances of these units may indicate a chronic process and a pattern of reinnervation. These abnormal types of motor units, with increased duration and multiple up and down deflections from the isoelectric baseline, indicate incomplete remyelination and are referred to as polyphasic motor units.

The needle portion of the study is normally performed in conjunction with the nerve conductions for a complete study. It can help to more completely characterize the problem (axonal loss, chronicity versus acuity) and assess for disorders not able to be seen on the nerve conduction velocity study, such as anterior horn cell and myopathy. Typical needle EMG screening involves five to six muscles with different nerve roots and peripheral nerve supply. Abnormalities found in specific patterns are indicative of pathology involving that region. For example, abnormalities found in the deltoid (C5-6, axillary nerve), biceps (C5-6, musculocu-

2: Systemic Disorders

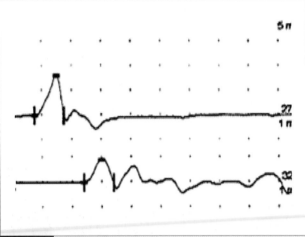

Figure 5 This tracing represents the compound motor action potentials for a nerve below and above an area of block. The first tracing (A1, top tracing) has a higher amplitude, and the duration of the response is short. The second tracing (A2, bottom tracing) shows a lower amplitude, and duration is prolonged. This represents conduction block and focal disruption of the myelin sheath.

taneous nerve), pronator teres (C5-6, median nerve) and the cervical paraspinal nerves would indicate a C6 radiculopathy.

Diagnosis

The type of injury may also be ascertained by which parameters of the nerve conduction velocity study are affected; if there is a decrease in amplitude across a specific segment and enough time has been allowed for wallerian degeneration, the pathology can be considered conduction block. Wallerian degeneration has been reported to start at approximately 3 to 5 days following the appearance of an axonal lesion.[10] A classic example seen in orthopaedics would be an ulnar neuropathy at the elbow (**Figure 5**). If a patient sustains an injury at the cubital tunnel involving the ulnar nerve, he or she may experience pain, numbness, and weakness in that distribution. If the electrodiagnostic study is the day of injury, whether the lesion is predominantly axonal or conduction block cannot be determined. It can take up to 3 weeks to find fibrillations in the most distal muscles on the needle portion and for the distal amplitudes to decrease in the nerve conduction velocity study.[11] A repeat study would be recommended at 3 weeks from the onset of injury.

In general, slowing of conduction velocity, prolonged duration of the action potential, and prolonged distal latency are indicative of a demyelinating process. After enough time has passed for wallerian degeneration, there will be a reduction in the proximal and distal compound muscle action potential amplitudes. This indicates the condition is an axonal loss process.

Table 1 shows the findings on nerve conduction velocity studies that are observed in axonal and demyelinating neuropathies.

Disorders Associated With Neuropathy

Compression Neuropathy

The most common forms of peripheral neuropathies seen in orthopaedic practice are compression neuropathies. Compression may occur intraspinally (nerve root compression) or in the periphery and may lead to demyelination, axonal loss, or both. Patients will often report sensory and/or motor deficits that will result in dermatomal/myotomal patterns distal to the site of entrapment. Physical examination will often support the symptom description, but in cases of severe pain or communication barriers, the diagnosis may not be straightforward. In these cases, referral for electrodiagnostics may be critical in confirming or refuting the diagnosis.

Common causes of intraspinal compression include herniated nucleus pulposus or stenosis. Compression secondary to epidural hematoma, abscess, lipomatosis, or tumor may also occur. Entrapment and compression neuropathies may occur in the upper and lower extremities. These conditions often require surgical decompression to prevent progression and, in many cases, to allow for neural regeneration. A classic example in the upper limb is carpal tunnel syndrome.[12] The American Academy of Orthopaedic Surgeons (AAOS) clinical practice guidelines list early surgery without conservative treatment as an option in patients with axon loss,[13] thus highlighting the importance of categorization of the median nerve injury.[14]

In the lower limbs, common peroneal neuropathy may occur with compression at the fibular head. It can mimic a lumbar radiculopathy clinically and make for a challenging diagnosis. Furthermore, common peroneal neuropathy may present atypically with involvement of the superficial motor fibers and sparing of its sensory fibers. Common peroneal neuropathy at the fibular head is the most common mononeuropathy of the lower limb. It can present atypically with selective involvement of the superficial peroneal motor fibers and sparing of the superficial peroneal sensory fibers.[15]

Compression of a peripheral nerve may lead to ischemia secondary to disruption of the vasa nervorum, flattening/squeezing of the myelin, or crush injury to the axons. Nerves may also be transected by projectiles or severed with sharp objects. In these cases, regeneration is unlikely to occur, and referral for reconstruction may be critical. Compression of the lower trunk of the brachial plexus may occur via a Pancoast tumor from growth at the apex of the lung.

Nerve conduction velocity studies in distal compressive neuropathy may reveal prolonged distal latency of the affected nerve, either sensory, motor, or both. Conduction velocity and duration may also be affected if myelin dysfunction is present. Decreased amplitude of the distal response may reflect axonal damage. If the amplitude is low above an area of compression but preserved distally, this may indicate conduction block across that segment. The needle EMG portion in the study of compression neuropathy can confirm axonal

Table 1

Common Findings on Nerve Conduction Velocity Studies

Nerve Injury	Latency	Conduction Velocity	Amplitudes	F-Wave Latency
Axonal	Normal	Normal	Reduced	Normal
Demyelinating	Prolonged	Slow	Normal or reduced	Absent or prolonged

loss by the presence of fibrillations and/or sharp waves. The presence of polyphasia suggests that the lesion is chronic and that a reinnervation process is occurring. A decreased recruitment pattern may also be noted and can be present in both conduction block as well as axonal lesions.

Neuropathies With a Genetic Basis
CMT Disease
CMT disease refers to inherited peripheral neuropathy, also referred to as hereditary motor and sensory neuropathy (HMSN). Since it was first described in late 1886, more than 50 genetic mutations have been found to cause various forms of CMT disease, with autosomal dominant, autosomal recessive, and X-linked inheritance patterns. Although numerous forms of CMT disease have been described with varying degrees of severity and clinical presentation, it has been largely divided into two groups based on nerve conduction velocity. CMT type 1 (HMSN I) is the result of demyelination and has a nerve conduction velocity that is slowed, whereas CMT type 2 (HMSN II) is the result of axonal degeneration with a near-normal nerve conduction velocity.[16] The classification of CMT disease continues to be modified as more genetic information becomes available. The two most common forms of CMT disease are CMT1A and CMT1X.[17] CMT1A has an autosomal dominant inheritance pattern and is caused by a mutation in the peripheral myelin protein gene *PMP-22* on chromosome 17 that is necessary for appropriate myelin formation by Schwann cells.[17,18] CMT1X is an X-linked form of CMT caused by a mutation in the gap junction protein β1 gene (*GJB1*), which is expressed in Schwann cells.[19] These two forms of CMT disease have a classic presentation, with the development of motor and sensory loss in adolescence or early adulthood. Typically, the distal extremities are affected most often, with early involvement of the peroneal muscles and the development of drop foot, high-arch foot (pes cavus), hammer toe deformities, and atrophy of the distal lower extremity musculature.[16] Patients walk with a high steppage gait and typically require ankle-foot orthoses. Severe forms affect the upper extremities as well, with weakness and clawing of the hands. Although motor involvement is predominant and progressive, sensory involvement is variable but typically present. Currently there is no cure for CMT disease, and treatment typically consists of maximizing function by using lower extremity orthoses.

Amyotrophic Lateral Sclerosis
Also known as Lou Gehrig disease, ALS is a rapidly progressive neurodegenerative disease of the upper and lower motor neurons that causes loss of voluntary muscle control, respiratory failure, and ultimately death, typically within 3 to 5 years from the onset of symptoms. The disease typically presents in the fifth or sixth decade of life and affects men more often than women. Although most cases of ALS occur sporadically, genetic factors are thought to play a role in all cases of ALS, and up to 10% of cases are attributed to inherited forms of the disease with familial history.[20,21] Approximately 20% of the familial cases of ALS are attributed to genetic mutations that affect the antioxidant enzyme superoxide dismutase 1 (SOD1).[20,22] Pathologic transactive response DNA binding protein, TDP-43, has recently been implicated in sporadic ALS as well as familial forms of the disease that are not associated with a SOD1 mutation.[23] Pathologically, these deficits lead to the accumulation of abnormal protein within the cytoplasm of affected neurons.[24]

The diagnosis of ALS, particularly early in the disease process, can be difficult, as other disease processes, including multiple sclerosis, stroke, and cervical spondylotic myeloradiculopathy, can mimic the early presentation of ALS. The hallmark of ALS is the involvement of both upper and lower motor neurons. Upper motor neuron findings include hyperreflexia, spasticity, ankle clonus, and positive Babinski and Hoffman signs. Lower motor neuron findings include flaccid paralysis, muscle atrophy, and fasciculations. The diagnosis of ALS is suggested by these findings in the extremities combined with dysarthria, dysphagia, and tongue atrophy and/or fasciculations attributable to cranial nerve involvement. ALS is purely a disease of motor neurons and does not affect sensation.

EMG and nerve conduction velocity studies can be helpful in the diagnosis of ALS. The sensory nerve action potentials should be normal in motor neuron disease. The motor nerve conductions should show no evidence of demyelination (normal conduction velocity and duration). A uniformly low drop in amplitude may be present in later stages of the disease. The purpose of the nerve conduction velocity studies is to exclude peripheral neuropathy, particularly multifocal mononeuropathy, which may mimic the findings of ALS.[25]

The electrodiagnostic hallmarks of ALS are signs of denervation (fibrillations and sharp waves) in at least two muscles in a limb supplied by a different peripheral nerve or root on the needle portion of the study. This

2: Systemic Disorders

should occur in multiple limbs and may also include a bulbar innervated muscle, usually the tongue. Fasciculations may be observed clinically and appear as spontaneous (not voluntarily recruited), irregularly firing motor unit potentials. There may also be polyphasic motor unit potentials diffusely in multiple limbs in a nonmyotomal pattern.

There is currently no cure for ALS. Riluzole, a sodium channel blocker that is FDA approved for the treatment of ALS, has been shown to prolong the survival of patients with ALS an average of 2 to 3 months.[26]

Infectious Neuropathies

Numerous infections have been associated with the development of neuropathy, including HIV, Lyme disease, leprosy, syphilis, and hepatitis C. The clinical manifestations of these associated neuropathies vary widely in regard to the affected neurologic pathways, the mechanism of neurologic injury, the timing of onset, and the response to treatment.

Human Immunodeficiency Virus

Antiretroviral therapy has revolutionized the treatment of HIV over the past three decades and transformed HIV from a fatal disease to a disease that is chronically managed. HIV has known neurologic effects, one of which is referred to as HIV-associated distal symmetric polyneuropathy (HIV-DSP). The incidence of HIV-DSP in patients with HIV reportedly has been as high as 60%, with onset occurring an average of 10 years after the HIV diagnosis is made.[27-29] HIV-DSP has an insidious onset, with a clinical presentation that is similar to the stocking and glove distribution observed in diabetic neuropathy, with the lower extremities affected more that the upper extremities, and with sensory function affected more than motor function.[29] Symptoms include burning, numbness, tingling, and pain in the aforementioned distribution. The mechanism of HIV-DSP is not fully understood. The neuropathy does not seem to be a direct result of the HIV virus infecting the neuron or a Schwann cell.[30] The HIV-associated glycoprotein gp120 has been shown to have Schwann cell–related neurotoxicity that affects sensory nerves.[31] The mechanism of HIV-DSP is complicated by the peripheral neuropathy that has been associated with several of the antiretroviral drugs used to treat HIV. Unlike HIV-DSP, however, drug-related peripheral neuropathy is more acute and typically resolves after discontinuing or changing the medication.[29,30] The treatment of HIV-DSP is nonspecific and is limited to medication therapy used to treat neuropathic pain.

Lyme Disease

Lyme disease is an illness caused by the spirochete *Borrelia burgdorferi* that is endemic to certain parts of the northeastern United States and transmitted to humans by Ixodes scapularis (deer tick). Three stages of Lyme disease have been described: early local, early disseminated, and late disseminated infection. Early Lyme disease is characterized by a local infection at the site of the tick bite, with approximately 80% of patients demonstrating a bullseye shaped, outwardly expanding rash referred to as erythema chronicum migrans.[32] This early stage of the disease can also cause flulike symptoms, such as fever, chills, muscle aches, and headache. If left untreated, the infection disseminates throughout the body via the bloodstream and can have devastating effects on the joints, heart, and nervous system (neuroborreliosis).

Early in the disseminated disease process, meningitis with an associated cranial neuritis and/or radiculoneuritis develops in up to 15% of patients.[33] Patients present with severe headache, neck stiffness, and varying radicular symptoms of pain, numbness, tingling, and/or weakness with loss of reflexes in one or multiple extremities. When bilateral extremities are affected, symptoms are typically worse in one than the other.[33] Cranial neuritis usually presents as unilateral or bilateral facial nerve palsy, often with associated reports of numbness or tingling on the involved side of the face.[33] Analysis of the cerebrospinal fluid shows that 90% of patients with meningitis and the aforementioned neurologic manifestations demonstrate intrathecal antibody production specific to *B burgdorferi*.[34] The neurologic deficits from cranial neuritis and radiculoneuritis typically resolve over a period of weeks to months after appropriate antibiotic treatment. Up to 30% of patients with late disseminated disease develop a chronic radiculoneuropathy with persistent burning pain, numbness, tingling, and/or weakness.[35] Unlike early radiculoneuritis, this late finding is not associated with meningitis or central nervous system involvement.[35]

The diagnosis of Lyme disease is based on clinical presentation and serologic testing of blood and/or cerebrospinal fluid. Enzyme-linked immunosorbent assay and Western blot analysis are used to test for immunoglobulin M and immunoglobulin G antibodies to *B burgdorferi*, with enzyme-linked immunosorbent assay serving more as a screening test and the Western blot analysis serving more as a definitive test. The body's antibody response can take up to 6 weeks to develop, so serologic testing may be negative in early infection. Antibodies may persist even after successful treatment or clearance of the disease, leading to false positive serologic results. Up to 10% of individuals in endemic areas are asymptomatic and seropositive.[36] Polymerase chain reaction and direct culture of the organism are also used to identify *B burgdorferi* in the cerebrospinal fluid.[34] An evidence-based review found that penicillin, ceftriaxone, cefotaxime, and doxycycline all safely and effectively treat Lyme disease that affects the nervous system in children and adults.[37] Symptomatic treatment of neuropathic symptoms is often necessary.

Leprosy

Leprosy is a chronic granulomatous disease caused by Mycobacterium leprae that directly affects the peripheral nerves, skin, and mucosa. Although relatively rare in the developed world, leprosy is still a leading cause of peripheral neuropathy in underdeveloped nations and is the most common treatable form of peripheral neuropathy worldwide.[38] Recent data indicate approximately 250,000 new cases of leprosy worldwide per year.[39] It is spread from person to person through respiratory droplets and nasal mucosa and then travels through the bloodstream. In up to 10% of patients, neurologic effects are seen in the absence of skin lesions.[38] Peripheral nerve involvement is present in up to 73% of patients at the time of diagnosis and is manifested by multifocal motor, sensory, and autonomic dysfunction.[40] Unmyelinated and small myelinated nerve fibers tend to be affected more by the granulomatous disease than large myelinated nerve fibers, and sensory function tends to be affected more than motor function.[40,41] The diagnosis of leprosy is made based on clinical presentation and the presence of acid-fast bacilli on skin lesion biopsy. Treatment involves the use of multidrug antibiotic therapy (dapsone, rifampin, and clofazimine) for 6 months to 2 years, depending on the extent of disease. A flare-up of the neurologic symptoms may occur after initiating treatment as a result of an immune response; therefore, steroids are often prescribed for a short period of time when initiating treatment to eliminate the reoccurrence of symptoms.[38]

Inflammatory Neuropathies

Acute Inflammatory Demyelinating Polyneuropathy

Acute inflammatory demyelinating polyneuropathy (AIDP; also known as Guillain-Barré syndrome) is a common and potentially life-threatening acquired peripheral polyneuropathy. This entity involves both the peripheral sensory and motor axons. The typical presentation is paresthesias in the distal extremities and/or face followed by a pattern of weakness that develops in the lower limbs and then ascends to involve the upper limbs. It may also involve cranial nerves and possibly the phrenic nerve, thus necessitating mechanical ventilation. Pain may be associated with AIDP, which can be neuritic or myotomal (burning or deep, aching). The patient will often report an antecedent illness, usually about 1 to 3 weeks before the development of weakness.[42] Several different infections have been implicated, including *Campylobacter jejuni*, Epstein-Barr virus, and cytomegalovirus,[43] but an organism is not always identified.

The history and the physical examination are extremely important in the diagnosis so that treatment can be given quickly. Reflexes in the lower extremities and/or the upper extremities are often unobtainable. Diffuse weakness of varying degrees will be present in the limbs. Sensory deficits, particularly in the distal extremities, may be present. Facial weakness and sensory deficits in the face may occur. Depending on the severity of the presentation, the patient may not be ambulatory.

The pathophysiology of AIDP is mediated by a T cell attack on the Schwann cells that may be secondary to some cross-reactivity of the antibodies against an inciting organism and similarity to the proteins on Schwann cells.[44] This process is called molecular mimicry and may be implicated in other acquired disease processes.[44] The attack on the nerve membrane and resultant inflammation leads to disruption in saltatory conduction and ultimately conduction block. The conduction block of the action potential is what leads to the motor weakness.[45]

Electrodiagnostics are also important in confirming the diagnosis. Early in the disease, the first findings may be absent or prolonged F-waves on the nerve conductions and reduced recruitment on the needle EMG. Later in the disease course, prolonged duration of the compound motor action potentials and sensory nerve action potentials will occur. Diffuse slowing of conduction velocity and prolonged distal latencies are present. This constellation of findings indicates an acquired demyelinating process.

If AIDP is suspected, the treatment is typically intravenous immunoglobulin or plasmapheresis. Supportive care is also initiated. If significant involvement occurs to the nerves supplying the muscles of respiration, the patient may be placed on a mechanical ventilator. Approximately one third of patients with AIDP will require ventilation.[46] A poorer prognosis typically occurs in older patients and patients who have rapid progression of weakness.[46]

Chronic Inflammatory Demyelinating Polyneuropathy

AIDP that shows no significant improvement may lead to the condition known as chronic inflammatory demyelinating polyneuropathy (CIDP). Instead of regaining strength and lessening paresthesias, these patients may have chronic weakness and a relapsing course.[47] These symptoms must occur in more than one limb to be considered CIDP.[47] The pathology is also autoimmune, as in AIDP. The patient must have symptoms for at least 2 months.[48] The electrodiagnostic findings are the same as in AIDP, indicating a diffuse sensory and motor demyelinating polyneuropathy. Long-term treatment involves immunosuppression, often including corticosteroids. These patients may also undergo plasmaexchange therapy and intravenous immunoglobulin, especially in patients with relapsing courses. Physical therapy, assistive devices, and pain management may be necessary over the long term.

Multifocal Motor Neuropathy

Multifocal motor neuropathy (MMN) is an autoimmune and inflammatory polyneuropathy in which the myelin sheath is attacked in multiple peripheral motor nerves. It is asymmetric, a characteristic different from many polyneuropathies. The pattern, however, will follow the distribution of peripheral nerves. Atrophy may also be present. Patients will often report deep, aching pain (myotomal) and weakness. Physical examination may demonstrate diffuse fasciculations in the muscles. Early in the disease course, the upper limbs are often involved first, a finding also different from most polyneuropathies.[49] Patients may often have drop wrist or drop foot without sensory deficits.

2: Systemic Disorders

This condition may be confused with ALS. If a careful physical examination is performed, however, the weakness will be found in the distribution of the peripheral nerves as opposed to the spinal segments in ALS. The overall prognosis is significantly better in MMN, and the patient should be referred for electrodiagnostics, which will help make the correct diagnosis. The electrodiagnostic findings in MMN are the presence of conduction block (drop in motor action potential amplitude) in multiple motor nerves. These decreases in amplitude often occur in areas not typically seen in compression neuropathy. The conduction block is also persistent, meaning repeat studies months or years later will still remain. The sensory responses should be normal, and the EMG will not demonstrate axonal loss (absence of fibrillations, sharp waves, and polyphasia).

The treatment of MMN is similar to that for CIDP and AIDP. Intravenous immunoglobulin is considered the first line of treatment.[50] Corticosteroids are also used as in CIDP, but the results are not as favorable with MMN.[51,52]

Systemic Disease

The most common neuropathy in North America is secondary to diabetes. Poor control of blood glucose carries a higher risk of developing the sequelae of diabetes. These conditions can include retinopathy, peripheral vascular disease, kidney failure, and—for purposes of this discussion—neuropathy. Diabetic polyneuropathy is categorized as displaying all the symptoms on the electrodiagnostic examination; it is a diffuse mixed sensory and motor demyelinating and axonal peripheral polyneuropathy. It is a length-dependent neuropathy in which sensory symptoms begin in the toes and progress slowly cephalad, involving the hands later in the process. Patients with diabetic peripheral polyneuropathy typically report paresthesias, dysesthesias, burning, and numbness in the distal lower extremities.[53] The electrodiagnostic findings associated with distal symmetric diabetic polyneuropathy are variable. The typical sensory nerve conduction findings show low amplitudes and prolonged distal latencies with slowing of conduction velocity. The motor amplitudes may also show prolonged latencies with a modest reduction in amplitude and slowing of conduction velocities. The needle portion may demonstrate chronic denervation in the foot intrinsic muscles, but these are not reliable by themselves to diagnose neuropathy because they may occur in patients without disease.[25] Diabetes may also affect the autonomic nervous system. Patients may develop postural hypotension from vasoconstriction inability, gastric motility problems, impotence, and other autonomic irregularities.[54]

Peripheral neuropathy frequently develops in patients with substantial kidney disease, with distal sensorimotor polyneuropathy being the type most commonly encountered. Another form, a diffuse polyneuropathy affecting both the sensory and the motor axons with features of demyelination and axonal loss, can also occur, as is seen in diabetic neuropathy.[55] The needle EMG may demonstrate abnormalities in the hand and foot intrinsics, as in diabetic neuropathy.[55] Because many patients with kidney disease may also have diabetes, it is sometimes difficult or impossible to differentiate the cause of the neuropathy using electrodiagnostics alone.

The treatment of both diabetic and uremic neuropathies includes attempts to control the underlying disease process, with a better glycemic index in diabetes and improving kidney function or performing dialysis in uremia. Symptomatic treatment may involve oral agents such as amitriptyline, gabapentin, or pregablin for neuropathic pain. These agents work by reducing "cross-talk" from nerve membrane instability.[56]

Hypothyroidism can occur from a variety of causes, but the most common is secondary to autoimmune disease and results from antibodies that block the thyroid stimulating hormone receptors and thus the production of thyroid hormone.[57] Patients may report fatigue, constipation, stiffness, weakness, and neuritic symptoms. Neuropathy may also occur in patients with hypothyroidism. The most common type of neuropathy with this disorder is carpal tunnel syndrome.[58] Carpal tunnel syndrome occurs secondary to median nerve compression from edema accumulating in the carpal tunnel from the disorder. In severe cases, diffuse fluid retention can occur and is referred to as myxedema.

Patients with hypothyroidism may also develop a peripheral polyneuropathy. The presentation will appear as paresthesias in a stocking-glove distribution in the lower and upper limbs. Electrodiagnostic testing will normally reveal a diffuse sensory and motor demyelinating and axonal peripheral polyneuropathy, as seen in diabetes and uremia.[58] Treatment is targeted toward normalizing the thyroid levels and diuresis in patients with severe edema.

Summary

Nerve disorders, which are commonly encountered in orthopaedic practice, have numerous causes and a wide range of presenting symptoms. Causes of peripheral neuropathy can be largely grouped into compression, genetic, infectious, inflammatory, and systemic illnesses. A thorough history and physical examination, laboratory studies, and electrodiagnostic testing usually allow for an accurate diagnosis. Treatment options vary widely. For many of the nerve disorders, treatment is based on symptomatic control of the neuropathic symptoms with medication. Orthoses are used to maximize function in some disorders, such as CMT disease. The diagnosis and treatment of underlying infection (Lyme disease, HIV, leprosy) or systemic illness (diabetes, kidney disease) is imperative. Surgical treatment is indicated in compression neuropathies, such as carpal tunnel syndrome, when conservative measures fail and/or evidence of axonal damage is noted on electrodiagnostic studies.

Key Study Points

- Compressive peripheral neuropathies can be treated by identifying the location of compression and surgically decompressing the affected nerve.

- The treatment of peripheral neuropathies associated with infection or systematic disease is to identify and treat the underlying pathologic process and symptomatically address the neuropathy with medical management.

- CMT disease, a peripheral neuropathy with a genetic basis, is incurable. The focus of management is maintaining function with the use of orthoses.

Annotated References

1. Rinholm JE, Bergersen LH: Neuroscience: The wrap that feeds neurons. *Nature* 2012;487(7408):435-436.

   In this article, the authors review an updated understanding of the function of myelin. Myelin not only surrounds neurons and promotes rapid conduction of the electrical signal but also supports the neuron's metabolic activity by providing the neuron with lactate, which is used to generate energy.

2. Netter FH: *Atlas of Human Anatomy.* Dover Township, NJ, CIBA-GEIGY Corp, 1989.

3. Schuenke M, Schulte E, Schumacher U: *Atlas of Anatomy: Head and Neuroanatomy.* New York, NY, Thieme, 2010, pp 9.1-9.3.

   This section of the book provides an in-depth discussion of the anatomy of the spinal cord, with descriptions and illustrations.

4. Patestas M, Gartner LP: *A Textbook of Neuroanatomy.* Malden, MA, Blackwell Publishing, Ltd, 2006, pp 3-9.

5. Lee SK, Wolfe SW: Peripheral nerve injury and repair. *J Am Acad Orthop Surg* 2000;8(4):243-252.

6. Seddon HJ: A classification of nerve injuries. *Br Med J* 1942;2(4260):237-239.

7. Murovic JA: Upper-extremity peripheral nerve injuries: A Louisiana State University Health Sciences Center literature review with comparison of the operative outcomes of 1837 Louisiana State University Health Sciences Center median, radial, and ulnar nerve lesions. *Neurosurgery* 2009;65(4, suppl):A11-A17.

8. Young L, Wray RC, Weeks PM: A randomized prospective comparison of fascicular and epineural digital nerve repairs. *Plast Reconstr Surg* 1981;68(1):89-93.

9. Bushbacher RM, Prahlow ND: *Manual of Nerve Conduction Studies*, ed 2. New York, NY, Demos Medical Publishing, 2005, pp 2-281.

10. Preston DC, Shapiro BE: *Electromyography and Neuromuscular Disorders: Clinical and Electrophysiologic Correlations*, ed 2. Amsterdam, The Netherlands, Elsevier, 2005, p 228.

11. Miller RG: Acute vs. chronic compressive neuropathy. *Muscle Nerve* 1984;7(6):427-430.

12. Pham K, Gupta R: Understanding the mechanisms of entrapment neuropathies: Review article. *Neurosurg Focus* 2009;26(2):E7.

13. Keith MW, Masear V, Chung KC, et al: American Academy of Orthopaedic Surgeons clinical practice guideline on the treatment of carpal tunnel syndrome. *J Bone Joint Surg Am* 2010;92(1):218-219.

    This article describes the evidence-based recommendations of the AAOS regarding the treatment of carpal tunnel syndrome. Early surgical treatment without conservative treatment is supported in the presence of axonal loss on electrodiagnostic testing.

14. Kodama M, Sasao Y, Tochikura M, et al: Premotor potential study in carpal tunnel syndrome. *Muscle Nerve* 2012;46(6):879-884.

    This study found that the premotor potential velocity from the second lumbrical muscle after median nerve stimulation correlated with sensory nerve conduction velocity and the severity of carpal tunnel syndrome. Level of evidence: II.

15. Annaswamy TM, Li HY: Atypical presentations of common peroneal neuropathy. *PM R* 2012;4(6):462-465.

    The authors describe two cases of common peroneal neuropathy, in which the sensory fibers of the superficial peroneal nerve are spared. The recognition of this atypical presentation can help differentiate common peroneal neuropathy from lumbar radiculopathy. Level of evidence: V.

16. Harding AE, Thomas PK: Genetic aspects of hereditary motor and sensory neuropathy (types I and II). *J Med Genet* 1980;17(5):329-336.

17. Saporta AS, Sottile SL, Miller LJ, Feely SM, Siskind CE, Shy ME: Charcot-Marie-Tooth disease subtypes and genetic testing strategies. *Ann Neurol* 2011;69(1):22-33.

    This article reviews the various genetic subtypes of CMT disease and the available testing for these subtypes. There are numerous genetic subtypes with some variation in presentation. Genetic testing and research has led to an expansion in the understanding of CMT disease and continues to expand the number of recognized subtypes. Level of evidence: III.

18. Raeymaekers P, Timmerman V, Nelis E, et al: Duplication in chromosome 17p11.2 in Charcot-Marie-Tooth neuropathy type 1a (CMT 1a). *Neuromuscul Disord* 1991;1(2):93-97.

19. Shy ME, Siskind C, Swan ER, et al: CMT1X phenotypes represent loss of GJB1 gene function. *Neurology* 2007;68(11):849-855.

20. Gros-Louis F, Gaspar C, Rouleau GA: Genetics of familial and sporadic amyotrophic lateral sclerosis. *Biochim Biophys Acta* 2006;1762(11-12):956-972.

21. Al-Chalabi A, Jones A, Troakes C, King A, Al-Sarraj S, van den Berg LH: The genetics and neuropathology of amyotrophic lateral sclerosis. *Acta Neuropathol* 2012; 124(3):339-352.

    This review article focuses on the known underlying genetic defects that are associated with amyotrophic lateral sclerosis.

22. Pasinelli P, Brown RH: Molecular biology of amyotrophic lateral sclerosis: Insights from genetics. *Nat Rev Neurosci* 2006;7(9):710-723.

23. Mackenzie IR, Bigio EH, Ince PG, et al: Pathological TDP-43 distinguishes sporadic amyotrophic lateral sclerosis from amyotrophic lateral sclerosis with SOD1 mutations. *Ann Neurol* 2007;61(5):427-434.

24. Lowe J: New pathological findings in amyotrophic lateral sclerosis. *J Neurol Sci* 1994;124(suppl):38-51.

25. Dumitru D, Amato AA, Zwarts MZ: *Electrodiagnostic Medicine*, ed 2. Philadelphia, PA, Hanley and Belfus, 2002, pp 956-957.

26. Miller RG, Mitchell JD, Moore DH: Riluzole for amyotrophic lateral sclerosis (ALS)/motor neuron disease (MND). *Cochrane Database Syst Rev* 2012;3: CD001447.

    This study is a systematic review that addresses the effectiveness of riluzole in the treatment of ALS. The authors found that riluzole is safe and prolongs the life of ALS patients by 2 to 3 months. Level of evidence: II.

27. Robinson-Papp J, Gonzalez-Duarte A, Simpson DM, Rivera-Mindt M, Morgello S; Manhattan HIV Brain Bank: The roles of ethnicity and antiretrovirals in HIV-associated polyneuropathy: A pilot study. *J Acquir Immune Defic Syndr* 2009;51(5):569-573.

28. Ellis RJ, Rosario D, Clifford DB, et al: Continued high prevalence and adverse clinical impact of human immunodeficiency virus-associated sensory neuropathy in the era of combination antiretroviral therapy: The CHARTER Study. *Arch Neurol* 2010;67(5):552-558.

    This article is a large cross-sectional, prospective analysis of HIV patients that assesses the prevalence and disability associated with HIV-associated sensory neuropathy. Level of evidence: I.

29. Evans SR, Ellis RJ, Chen H, et al: Peripheral neuropathy in HIV: Prevalence and risk factors. *AIDS* 2011;25(7): 919-928.

    The authors of this study evaluated 2,000 patients with HIV to determine prevalence and risk factors of peripheral neuropathy. There was significant peripheral neuropathy despite good control of the viral load. Advanced age and use of neurotoxic antiretroviral medications were identified as risk factors for peripheral neuropathy.

30. Pardo CA, McArthur JC, Griffin JW: HIV neuropathy: Insights in the pathology of HIV peripheral nerve disease. *J Peripher Nerv Syst* 2001;6(1):21-27.

31. Keswani SC, Polley M, Pardo CA, Griffin JW, McArthur JC, Hoke A: Schwann cell chemokine receptors mediate HIV-1 gp120 toxicity to sensory neurons. *Ann Neurol* 2003;54(3):287-296.

32. Tibbles CD, Edlow JA: Does this patient have erythema migrans? *JAMA* 2007;297(23):2617-2627.

33. Pachner AR, Steere AC: The triad of neurologic manifestations of Lyme disease: Meningitis, cranial neuritis, and radiculoneuritis. *Neurology* 1985;35(1):47-53.

34. Keller TL, Halperin JJ, Whitman M: PCR detection of *Borrelia burgdorferi* DNA in cerebrospinal fluid of Lyme neuroborreliosis patients. *Neurology* 1992;42(1): 32-42.

35. Halperin J, Luft BJ, Volkman DJ, Dattwyler RJ: Lyme neuroborreliosis: Peripheral nervous system manifestations. *Brain* 1990;113(pt 4):1207-1221.

36. Steere AC, Taylor E, Wilson ML, Levine JF, Spielman A: Longitudinal assessment of the clinical and epidemiological features of Lyme disease in a defined population. *J Infect Dis* 1986;154(2):295-300.

37. Halperin JJ, Shapiro ED, Logigian E, et al: Practice parameter: Treatment of nervous system Lyme disease (an evidence-based review). Report of the Quality Standards Subcommittee of the American Academy of Neurology. *Neurology* 2007;69(1):91-102.

38. Wilder-Smith EP, Van Brakel WH: Nerve damage in leprosy and its management. *Nat Clin Pract Neurol* 2008; 4(12):656-663.

39. Rodrigues LC, Lockwood DN: Leprosy now: Epidemiology, progress, challenges, and research gaps. *Lancet Infect Dis* 2011;11(6):464-470.

    This review article addresses the current worldwide epidemiology of leprosy and reviews current recommendations for diagnosis and treatment.

40. Vital RT, Illarramendi X, Nascimento O, Hacker MA, Sarno EN, Jardim MR: Progression of leprosy neuropathy: A case series study. *Brain Behav* 2012;2(3): 249-255.

    This is a case series of 22 patients with newly diagnosed leprosy that assesses the extent and the severity of neurologic involvment. Level of evidence: IV.

41. Jardim MR, Antunes SL, Santos AR, et al: Criteria for diagnosis of pure neural leprosy. *J Neurol* 2003;250(7): 806-809.

42. Ropper AH: The Guillain-Barré syndrome. *N Engl J Med* 1992;326(17):1130-1136.

2: Systemic Disorders

43. Jacobs BC, Rothbarth PH, van der Meché FG, et al: The spectrum of antecedent infections in Guillain-Barré syndrome: A case-control study. *Neurology* 1998;51(4):1110-1115.

44. Shahrizaila N, Yuki N: Guillain-barré syndrome animal model: The first proof of molecular mimicry in human autoimmune disorder. *J Biomed Biotechnol* 2011;2011:829129.

    This review article describes Guillain-Barré syndrome as an autoimmune disease that is triggered by molecular mimicry between GM1 gangliosides, which are cell-surface proteins expressed in neural tissue, and lipo-oligosaccharides, which are present on the cell membrane of *Campylobacter jejuni*. Antibodies to GM1 gangliosides are present in patients with Guillain-Barré syndrome. Level of evidence: V.

45. Uncini A, Kuwabara S: Electrodiagnostic criteria for Guillain-Barré syndrome: A critical revision and the need for an update. *Clin Neurophysiol* 2012;123(8):1487-1495.

    This review article discusses the electrodiagnostic criteria for acute inflammatory demyelinating polyradiculoneuropathy. Level of evidence: V.

46. Visser LH, Schmitz PI, Meulstee J, van Doorn PA, van der Meché FG; Dutch Guillain-Barré Study Group: Prognostic factors of Guillain-Barré syndrome after intravenous immunoglobulin or plasma exchange. *Neurology* 1999;53(3):598-604.

47. Koski CL, Baumgarten M, Magder LS, et al: Derivation and validation of diagnostic criteria for chronic inflammatory demyelinating polyneuropathy. *J Neurol Sci* 2009;277(1-2):1-8.

48. Barohn RJ, Kissel JT, Warmolts JR, Mendell JR: Chronic inflammatory demyelinating polyradiculoneuropathy: Clinical characteristics, course, and recommendations for diagnostic criteria. *Arch Neurol* 1989;46(8):878-884.

49. Katz JS, Wolfe GI, Bryan WW, Jackson CE, Amato AA, Barohn RJ: Electrophysiologic findings in multifocal motor neuropathy. *Neurology* 1997;48(3):700-707.

50. Patwa HS, Chaudhry V, Katzberg H, Rae-Grant AD, So YT: Evidence-based guideline: Intravenous immunoglobulin in the treatment of neuromuscular disorders: Report of the Therapeutics and Technology Assessment Subcommittee of the American Academy of Neurology. *Neurology* 2012;78(13):1009-1015.

    This is a recent evidence-based recommendation of the American Academy of Neurology regarding the treatment of neuromuscular disorders, including MMN, for which the current first-line treatment recommendation is intravenous immunoglobulin. Level of evidence: V.

51. Charles N, Benoit P, Vial C, Bierme T, Moreau T, Bady B: Intravenous immunoglobulin treatment in multifocal motor neuropathy. *Lancet* 1992;340(8812):182.

52. Nobile-Orazio E, Gallia F, Tuccillo F, Terenghi F: Chronic inflammatory demyelinating polyradiculoneuropathy and multifocal motor neuropathy: Treatment update. *Curr Opin Neurol* 2010;23(5):519-523.

    This paper reviews the current treatment recommendations for chronic inflammatory demyelinating polyradiculoneuropathy and MMN, presenting data from randomized controlled trials. The current recommendation remains intravenous immunoglobulin. Although other treatments have been studied, they are not as efficacious as intravenous immunoglobulin. Level of evidence: III.

53. Smith AG, Singleton JR: Diabetic neuropathy. *Continuum (Minneap Minn)* 2012;18(1):60-84.

    The diagnosis and treatment of diabetic neuropathy is discussed.

54. Cohen JA, Jeffers BW, Faldut D, Marcoux M, Schrier RW: Risks for sensorimotor peripheral neuropathy and autonomic neuropathy in non-insulin-dependent diabetes mellitus (NIDDM). *Muscle Nerve* 1998;21(1):72-80.

55. Krishnan AV, Kiernan MC: Uremic neuropathy: Clinical features and new pathophysiological insights. *Muscle Nerve* 2007;35(3):273-290.

56. Waszkielewicz AM, Gunia A, Słoczyńska K, Marona H: Evaluation of anticonvulsants for possible use in neuropathic pain. *Curr Med Chem* 2011;18(28):4344-4358.

    This review article describes the use of anticunvulsant medications, such as gabapentin, for treating neuropathic pain. Animal model data and clinical data are reviewed. Level of evidence: V.

57. Wartofsky L: *Harrison's Principles of Internal Medicine*, 13th ed. New York, NY, McGraw-Hill, 1994, pp 1940-1941.

58. Duyff RF, Van den Bosch J, Laman DM, van Loon BJ, Linssen WH: Neuromuscular findings in thyroid dysfunction: A prospective clinical and electrodiagnostic study. *J Neurol Neurosurg Psychiatry* 2000;68(6):750-755.

2: Systemic Disorders

Chapter 22

Musculoskeletal Oncology

John A. Abraham, MD

Clinical Presentation of Musculoskeletal Tumors

Most patients with musculoskeletal soft-tissue tumors notice a mass that is often painless. Bone tumors, however, often present as a result of pain in the affected bone, which may be accompanied by a mass, or swelling of the joint. A careful history and physical examination can raise suspicion for the presence of a tumor. Although a mass is the presenting symptom for many common traumatic and inflammatory conditions, the complaint cannot be taken lightly given how serious musculoskeletal tumors can be. For this reason, any patient reporting pain or a mass persisting longer than 6 to 8 weeks with no improvement or symptoms that worsen over time should undergo sufficient imaging studies to rule out the presence of a neoplastic condition.

Epidemiology of Musculoskeletal Tumors

According to Surveillence, Epidemiology, and End Results (SEER) data, it was estimated that the incidence of bone and soft-tissue sarcoma in the United States would be 2,810 new bone cancer cases and 10,980 new soft-tissue cancers in 2011. Previous years' data suggested that the incidence has remained relatively stable over the past 30 years. It was estimated that approximately 1,490 and 3,920 people would die from bone sarcoma and soft-tissue sarcoma, respectively, in 2011.[1] These figures suggest that sarcoma remains one of the relatively more aggressive cancers. Risk factors for sarcoma include prior radiation exposure; certain genetic conditions, including Li-Fraumeni syndrome, retinoblastoma, neurofibromatosis, Gardner syndrome, Werner syndrome, and tuberous sclerosis; and workplace exposure to vinyl chloride or dioxin. Most sarcomas, however, occur sporadically.

Initial Workup

A detailed and thorough history and multisystem physical examination must be performed. Important interview questions include smoking history, cancer screening history such as mammograms and colonoscopies, and details about the primary complaint. The deformity should be observed; size of the mass, the girth of the extremity in comparison with the contralateral side, and perfusion distal to the mass should be recorded. Manual testing of strength and neurologic function, joint range of motion, and gait should be assessed; lymph nodes should be palpated. After a careful physical examination is completed, imaging is considered as a next step in the workup. In most cases, the age of the patient provides a framework for the appropriate differential diagnosis. For example, in an adult patient older than 50 years, the threshold to consider metastatic disease is much lower than in a younger patient.

Radiology of Musculoskeletal Tumors

Plain Film

Orthogonal plain radiography represents the standard initial imaging study for any patient suspected of having a bone tumor (Figure 1). In most cases, a well-trained musculoskeletal oncologist can accurately predict diagnosis in patients with a bone lesion.[2] Modern imaging modalities can generate highly detailed images of a tumor and have other strengths, but the basis of predicting diagnosis remains the plain film. Some soft-tissue tumors may have some characteristics visible on plain film. Certain tumors, such as synovial sarcoma, can have calcifications that are visible on radiography. Some conditions that mimic tumors, such as myositis ossificans, can also be identified on plain radiography. Fatty lesions have a characteristic low density that can often be appreciated on a plain film. In any patient with a soft-tissue tumor, an initial plain film is reasonable to identify these types of findings. However, most soft-tissue lesions will require more advanced cross-sectional imaging.

Ultrasonography

Ultrasonography is advantageous in orthopaedic surgery because of its low cost and ease of use. However, its usefulness in orthopaedic oncology remains limited.

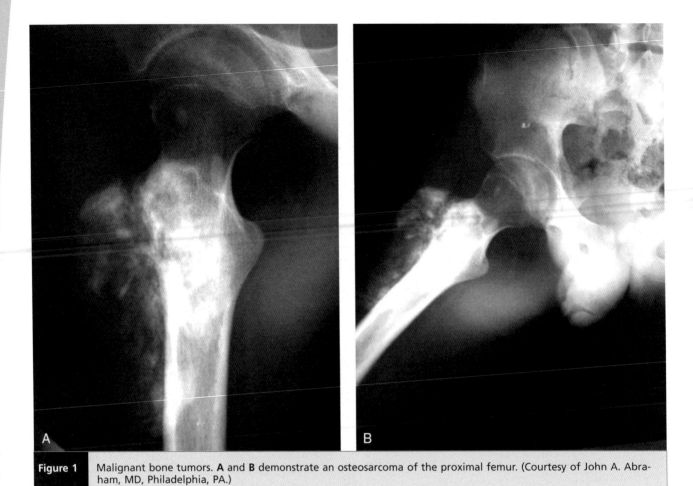

| Figure 1 | Malignant bone tumors. **A** and **B** demonstrate an osteosarcoma of the proximal femur. (Courtesy of John A. Abraham, MD, Philadelphia, PA.) |

Although ultrasonography can effectively differentiate solid and cystic lesions and may be able to conclusively identify fatty lesions, in most instances, confirmation of the diagnosis and elucidation of the anatomic details will require MRI or other cross-sectional imaging. Ultrasonography can be highly effective in determining the presence of blood flow within a lesion, which can help distinguish a vascular malformation or other vascular lesion from a tumor. Ultrasonography can be effective in conjunction with needle biopsy of soft-tissue tumors, particularly in relatively superficial and homogeneous-appearing cases.[3,4] A novel ultrasonography technique is ultrasound fusion, in which previously obtained CT or MRI data are fused with real-time ultrasonography, allowing biopsies to be performed in the ultrasound suite but retaining the diagnostic yield and accuracy of a CT-guided technique. Ultrasound fusion has the potential to improve both the speed and the ease of obtaining a musculoskeletal biopsy without compromising yield or accuracy.[5]

Magnetic Resonance Imaging

MRI is the gold standard for imaging of a primary musculoskeletal tumor. It can provide significant clues to the diagnosis and, with some tumors, such as li-

poma, can be nearly pathognomonic. MRI of extremity masses can be done with and without gadolinium contrast to evaluate the amount of blood flow. Contrast can help distinguish cystic from solid lesions and may be particularly helpful in distinguishing hematoma from neoplasm. Newer MRI techniques, which include 3T magnetic resonance dynamic contrast enhanced and magnetic resonance diffusion-weighted imaging, have been investigated with respect to their ability to help differentiate benign from malignant tumors. In one recent study, a maximum sensitivity of 87% and a sensitivity of 86% were achieved using various parameters as distinguishing thresholds.[6] Although none of these MRI techniques is accurate enough to replace tissue sampling, these data reflect the importance of this modality overall and point to potential future applications. Additionally, ultrahigh field-strength MRI is being used for musculoskeletal imaging, with clinical studies at 7T performed in neck and spine imaging. Advances in coil design may allow the application of this ultrahigh field imaging to the extremities. The advantages of this imaging modality include an increase in signal-to-noise ratio; however, the disadvantage is an exacerbation of artifact.[7] Further study will be needed to determine the precise role of ultrahigh field-strength MRI in musculoskeletal imaging.

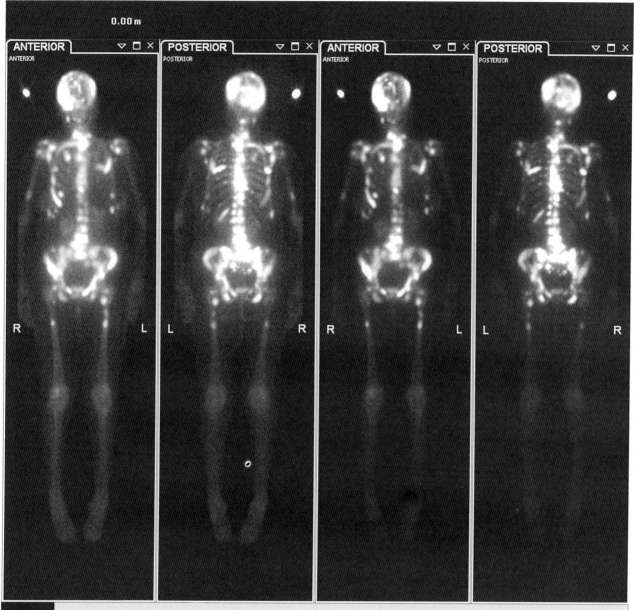

Figure 2 Detection of multiple sites of metastatic skeletal disease by a technetium Tc 99m whole body bone scan.

Bone Scan

A technetium 99 (Tc99) whole body bone scan is a useful tool for evaluating most bone lesions (**Figure 2**). With a few important exceptions, such as myeloma and purely lytic carcinoma metastases, lesions that do not demonstrate uptake are generally inert or benign. An additional advantage of a bone scan is the evaluation of additional lesions, which may suggest metastatic skeletal disease or a multifocal process. Bone scan plays an important role in the routine follow-up of patients with known skeletal metastatic disease, to identify new metastases early and potentially avert morbidity. Primary tumors of bone can present with skip metastases or bony metastatic disease that can be identified on a bone scan. Accordingly, whole body bone scan is an important staging study for any adult patient who presents with a suspected malignant bone lesion.

Fluorodeoxyglucose Positron Emission Tomography Scan

The precise role of fluorodeoxyglucose positron emission tomography (FDG-PET) scans (**Figure 3**) has not yet been determined in the management of sarcoma or other bone and soft-tissue lesions. Ideally, as a metabolic study, this type of scan would have some correlation with the histologic and behavioral characteristics of a tumor. Studies are ongoing, investigating these correlations with promising results.[8] The current major limitations are that metabolically active lesions below a

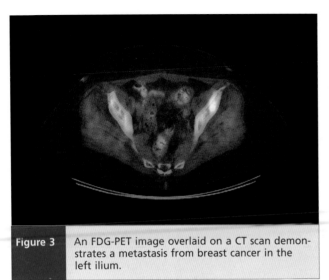

Figure 3 An FDG-PET image overlaid on a CT scan demonstrates a metastasis from breast cancer in the left ilium.

size threshold may not demonstrate FDG avidity, and the precise correlation of standardized uptake value and grade is not well established for sarcoma. However, there may be a future role for this modality in screening for metastases, estimating the effectiveness of treatment modalities by comparing pretreatment and posttreatment scans, or potentially even as an early predictor of survival.[9] One recent study demonstrated the ability of PET to measure blood flow in sarcoma, although the exact implications are unknown.[10] Further study is needed to determine the precise optimal role for PET in the management of sarcoma, and investigations are currently being performed to delineate the applications of this modality to musculoskeletal oncology.[11]

F-18 Sodium Fluoride PET Scan

F-18 sodium fluoride PET scan is gaining considerable interest for its potential application in identifying and screening for bone metastases. Radiolabeled sodium fluoride is a bone-specific radiotracer that is useful in detecting both osteolytic and osteoblastic metastases, making it more sensitive than a Tc99 bone scan, which can fail to identify purely osteolytic lesions.[12] In addition, the imaging modality of CT results in a cross-sectional image, providing significantly more anatomic detail when compared with a traditional Tc99 bone scan. Skeletal uptake of sodium fluoride occurs quickly, allowing the scan to be taken 1 hour after injection, which is another advantage over a traditional bone scan. The main drawback, however, is cost, and further study needs to be done to assess the cost-to-benefit ratio of this newer imaging modality. Nonetheless, this modality holds significant potential for future application in the imaging of bone neoplasia.

Biopsy

Biopsy of a musculoskeletal tumor is generally regarded as the last step in the diagnostic process. The major risk

of a poorly performed biopsy is contamination of the local field and subsequent alteration of the surgical procedure required to remove the entire tumor. A poorly performed biopsy can decrease or remove the possibility of successful limb salvage, in some cases necessitating amputation. Two classic studies document the risks of treatment of sarcoma in an inexperienced center compared with an experienced center.[13,14] One recent study evaluated the implementation of a set of guidelines and a control process to limit the number of incisional biopsy failures and continuously monitor a center's performance. This study demonstrated that the implementation of control measures resulted in a low proportion of inadequate, failed, or erroneous biopsies.[15] The implementation of measures such as these in high-volume referral centers further supports the notion that sarcoma management should be performed at centers specializing in sarcoma treatment.

Biopsy of musculoskeletal tumors also can be performed using an image-guided needle procedure. Although this type of procedure yields a much lower quantity of diagnostic tissue, it has the obvious benefits of avoiding a surgical procedure and the related risks, plus the added benefit of image guidance to pinpoint the locations for highest diagnostic yield. Furthermore, current data suggest that needle biopsies are not associated with seeding of the needle tract with the tumor, making this a potentially safer biopsy method than a poorly performed surgical biopsy.[16] For these reasons, many centers prefer needle biopsy as the primary modality of tissue sampling, with open surgical biopsy as a secondary procedure if a diagnosis is not obtained. To increase the safety and the likelihood of achieving an adequate diagnosis from a needle biopsy procedure, the treatment team should include skilled and specialty trained musculoskeletal radiologists and bone/soft-tissue pathologists and be directed by a musculoskeletal oncologist. The biopsy should be planned at a forum where the surgeon, the radiologist, and the pathologist can discuss each case, including patient characteristics, the ideal approach, the differential diagnosis based on radiography and advanced imaging, risks, and the protocol for tissue handling based on suspected necessary pathology studies. Several studies have evaluated the accuracy of CT-guided core needle biopsy and, in general, have demonstrated the accuracy of needle biopsy to range between 93% and 95% in skilled centers.[17,18]

In some instances, particularly for homogeneous-appearing superficial masses distant from critical or sensitive structures, an in-office needle biopsy may be performed without image guidance. This procedure should be performed only by a musculoskeletal oncologist. A core needle biopsy will generally provide a higher yield of diagnostic tissue than fine-needle aspirate.[19] However, if there is any concern that the appropriate region of a tumor may not be biopsied or there is any risk of violating nearby structures, an image-guided biopsy is preferred.

Table 1

Common Sarcoma Staging Systems

Stage	Histologic Grade	Local Extent of Disease	Systemic/Metastatic Disease Present
1. Musculoskleletal Tumor Society			
Ia	Low	Confined	No
Ib	Low	Unconfined	No
IIa	High	Confined	No
IIb	High	Unconfined	No
III	Any	Any	Yes

Stage	Histologic Grade	Size	Location (Relative to Fascia)	Systemic/Metastatic Disease Present
2. American Joint Committee on Cancer				
IA	Low	< 5 cm	Superficial or deep	No
IB	Low	≥ 5 cm	Superficial	No
IIA	Low	≥ 5 cm	Deep	No
IIB	High	< 5 cm	Superficial or deep	No
IIC	High	≥ 5 cm	Superficial	No
III	High	≥ 5 cm	Deep	No
IV	Any	Any	Any	Yes

Staging

Staging is the process of estimating a prognosis for a patient with a malignant tumor. The common staging systems for primary musculoskeletal tumors are the Musculoskeletal Tumor Society (MSTS), or Enneking staging system, and the American Joint Committee on Cancer (AJCC) staging system. The MSTS system is favored for bone tumors, whereas the AJCC system is favored for soft-tissue tumors. The important prognostic factors are considered in assigning a stage, which can be used to help choose the appropriate surgical procedure as well as estimate prognosis. Both MSTS and AJCC staging systems are described in Table 1.

Common Primary Tumors

Benign Bone Lesions

A summary listing of benign bone lesions is presented in Table 2.

Unicameral Bone Cysts

A unicameral bone cyst (UBC) is a cystic cavity at the metaphysis of bone (Figure 4). A possible etiology is increased pressure in the region of the cyst at development that leads to necrosis of local bone and then accumulation of fluid. However, the true etiology remains unknown. These lesions typically present in the first two decades of life with a 2:1 male predominance. The proximal humerus and the proximal femur are the most common sites. The lesion may be painless, but pathologic fracture can occur in up to 50% of patients and can cause significant pain. Plain radiography of a UBC is usually diagnostic. A UBC is lucent and cystic at the metaphysis of the bone with one chamber, but occasionally shows a septated appearance because of thickened cortical areas. It is central in the bone and may slightly expand the bone contour. Periosteal reaction is not seen unless in response to a fracture.

CT will show thinned cortical bone and may better define fallen fragments or pathologic fractures. MRI will show homogeneous fluid signal within the cavity. Fluid-fluid levels are usually not seen because of the absence of blood in the cavity. A bone scan will show peripheral uptake with an area of central photopenia.

Histology of the lesion shows a thin, fibrous lining with no epithelial or endothelial component. The cells are fibroblastic, and the lining may also contain scattered giant cells, mesenchymal cells, and lymphocytes, all with a bland appearance. The lining is not typically bloody unless pathologic fracture is present, and so the large lakes of red blood cells seen in aneurysmal bone cysts (ABCs) are absent. Eosinophilic fibrinous material known as cementum is sometimes seen.

Many lesions are painless and found incidentally. If imaging confirms a low level of concern for pathologic fracture, these lesions are generally observed. In the setting of a painful lesion or concern for pathologic fracture, steroid injection or curettage may be considered. Initial management, particularly in the upper extremity, is often with cyst aspiration and injection of methylprednisolone acetate. However, a recent multivariate

Table 2

Common Benign Bone Lesions

Lesion	Peak Age Group (Years)	Treatment
Cystic		
Unicameral bone cyst	5-20	Observation Methylprednisolone injection
Aneurysmal bone cyst	Younger than 20	Curettage, bone grafting
Bone forming		
Osteoid osteoma	20-30	Radiofrequency ablation
Cartilage forming		
Enchondroma	20-30	Observation
Osteochondroma	10-30	Observation Excision if symptomatic
Chondroblastoma	Younger than 20	Curettage, bone grafting
Chondromyxoid fibroma	Younger than 30	Curettage, bone grafting

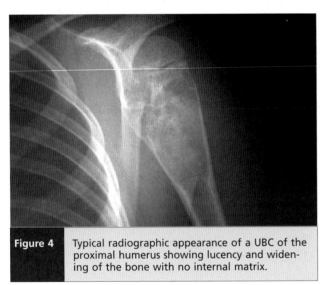

Figure 4 Typical radiographic appearance of a UBC of the proximal humerus showing lucency and widening of the bone with no internal matrix.

logistic regression analysis indicated that younger age and treatment with steroids alone are predictors of failure and suggested the injection of bone marrow aspirate as a first-line treatment of UBCs in the femur or the humerus in patients younger than 20 years.[20]

Aneurysmal Bone Cysts

An ABC is a cystic neoplasm of bone generally affecting patients younger than 20 years, with a slight female predominance. Once thought to potentially be a reactive lesion secondary to local circulatory disturbance, the etiology is now known to be a result of the translocation TRE17/USP6. It is thought that the induction of matrix metalloproteinase-9 in response to the presence of the TRE fusion protein is responsible for the pathogenesis of ABCs.[21]

Plain radiography of an ABC shows an eccentric lucent bone lesion at the metaphysis of the bone, which is bounded by a thin cortical rim. Even in the most extensive cases, a thin bony rim, or at least a portion of one, can be seen at the periphery of the cyst. The width of the cyst may be wider than that of the metaphysis, which is a distinguishing feature from UBCs, which generally do not expand wider than the metaphysis. The cyst may have multiple fluid- or blood-filled chambers separated by bony septae. Periosteal elevation and new bone formation can be seen at the junction of the cyst with normal host bone. MRI shows multiloculated fluid or blood-filled chambers, and fluid-fluid levels are a characteristic but not diagnostic feature. A soft-tissue mass can be seen on MRI. A bone scan will show uptake in the region of the lesion and may have an area of decreased uptake centrally.

An important differential diagnosis to consider in all cases of ABC is telangiectatic osteosarcoma. This variant of osteosarcoma can have a radiographic appearance similar to ABC and a similar clinical presentation. On microscopic examination, however, these malignant tumors demonstrate pleomorphic cells and atypical mitotic figures characteristic of malignancy. Malignant osteoids surrounded by osteoblasts are seen in a lacelike pattern, with malignant-appearing cells infiltrating the entire lesion. Because of the radically different treatment and prognosis of this lethal tumor, the diagnosis must be considered and ruled out in evaluating an ABC. Exposure to ionizing radiation also can lead to sarcomatous degeneration of ABCs. Additionally, rare instances of metastasis of ABC have been described and confirmed with the presence of *USP6* gene mutation in the pulmonary metastases.[22]

The treatment of ABCs has traditionally been curettage and bone grafting. This tumor is known to have a significant recurrence rate, with studies on curettage and bone grafting demonstrating up to 31% recurrence. Extended curettage, in which the entire cavity is unroofed and all surfaces of the cavity are visualized and addressed, decreases the recurrence rate compared with simple curettage performed through a small window in the bone. Factors such as young age, periarticular location, incomplete initial curettage, open physes, and high Enneking stage all have been found to be predictors of recurrence. Adjuvant therapy with agents such as alcoholic zein, phenol, liquid nitrogen, polymethyl methacrylate, high-speed burring, or argon beam have been described, but none has shown conclusive improvement in recurrence rate.

Bone-Forming and Cartilage-Forming Benign Tumors

Osteoid Osteoma

Osteoid osteoma is a painful benign bone lesion (Figure 5). In many cases the presentation is nearly diagnostic. Patients present with pain that increases over time and worsens at night and is relieved with aspirin or NSAIDs. Imaging shows an intracortical tumor, in the form of a small round lucency of less than 1.5 cm, sometimes with a central target or calcification. If not seen radiographically, the lesion can usually be seen with CT in a patient with classic presentation. The lesion is usually surrounded by a significant border of reactive bone or sclerosis. Treatment is generally with radiofrequency ablation. A newer modality of magnetic resonance-guided laser ablation has recently been shown to be less expensive.[23] In rare instances in which ablation cannot be performed, usually if the lesion is located very close to the skin or a nerve, then curettage or en bloc excision can be considered.

Osteoblastoma, a tumor that is larger than 1.5 cm and with similar although not identical histology, may not have as characteristic a symptomatology. These tumors are usually treated with curettage and bone grafting. Although osteoid osteoma and osteoblastoma were once believed to be identical tumors of different sizes, there is current evidence that these may represent distinct identities, and a recent case report challenges the notion that one can transform to the other.[24]

Enchondroma

Enchondroma is a common benign cartilage lesion of bone. The etiology in still unknown, but the idea that these tumors are displaced portions of the growth plate is a theory without any real supporting evidence and unlikely to be correct.[25] These tumors are usually incidentally found and are generally asymptomatic. In patients who present with pain and a cartilage bone lesion, it should be determined whether the pain is coming from the lesion or another source, such as rotator cuff tendinopathy or trochanteric bursitis. The cartilage matrix is identified by ring and arcs calcification on plain radiography. The effects on the bone are minimal, with limited or no endosteal scalloping and no cortical breakthrough or soft-tissue mass. In the small bones of the digits and the proximal fibula, where these lesions are common, tumors with a slightly more ag-

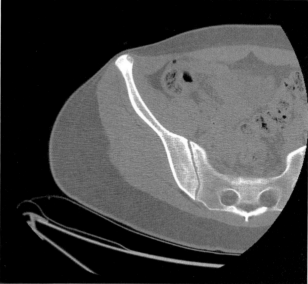

Figure 5   Osteoid osteoma. CT scan of the pelvis on the inner table of the ilium. A central lucency containing a target calcification is seen and is surrounded by dense reactive bone. This lesion was not seen on plain radiography, but a typical pattern of symptoms prompted consideration of the diagnosis, and CT scan identified the lesion.

gressive picture, such as scalloping or pathologic fracture, can still behave in a benign fashion. If radiographic and clinical features suggest a benign lesion, these tumors can be observed over time. Painful lesions or lesions with atypical radiography should raise concern for low-grade chondrosarcoma. MRI may be helpful in distinguishing these identities.[26] Clinical and radiographic factors are considered diagnostic, so biopsy is generally avoided in these tumors because of the difficulty of making an accurate diagnosis on histologic appearance alone for cartilage tumors.

Osteochondroma

Osteochondromas are benign bone lesions in which a mass of histologically normal bone projects off another bone. These lesions are capped by cartilage that has histology identical to a growth plate. These lesions may grow as a child is growing but should not change in adulthood. Imaging studies reveal a diagnostic feature of sharing the medullary canal and cancellous bone of the bone from which the lesions project. These lesions may cause symptoms of a palpable bony mass but usually are not painful unless there is an overlying secondary bursitis, impingement on a local bone, or fracture of the stalk in a pedunculated lesion. The cartilage cap is generally less than 1.5 cm thick, and any lesion with a thicker or enlarging cap should raise concern for chondrosarcomatous transformation. This is a rare occurrence in the case of solitary osteochondroma. Multiple lesions are seen in patients with hereditary multiple osteochondromatous exostoses and can cause significant bone deformity. Treatment is observation of

2: Systemic Disorders

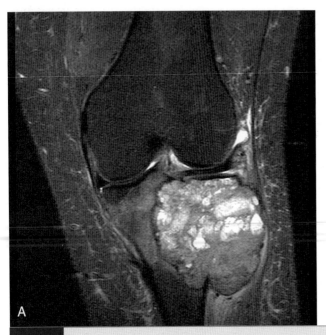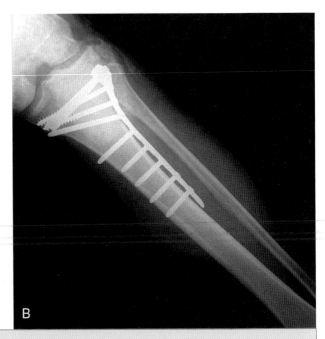

Figure 6   Giant cell tumor of bone. **A,** A large lesion remodeling the cortex of the proximal tibia and extending to the joint surface should raise concern for this diagnosis. **B,** The lesion was treated with curettage, bone grafting, and plate fixation.

asymptomatic lesions and the excision of symptomatic lesions.

Chondroblastoma

Chondroblastoma is a painful, benign lesion that has the distinguishing feature of an epiphyseal or apophyseal location. Joint pain will cause the patient to seek medical attention. On imaging, the lesion is radiolucent and may have some internal calcification. The histology shows a fibrochondroid matrix with calcification in a lacelike or chicken-wire pattern. The chondroblastic mononuclear cells have homogeneous nuclei with a longitudinal groove and a limited number of mitotic figures. Because of its location adjacent to the joint surface and incidence in a young age group, the treatment of chondroblastoma can be challenging. Curettage and bone grafting usually are curative, but in all cases consideration must be given to the effect of any procedure on the delicate adjacent cartilage surface.

Chondromyxoid Fibroma

Chondromyxoid fibroma is an eccentric, benign metaphyseal lesion. Pain, although mild, is often the presenting symptom. The lesion usually has a bubbly appearance, with sharp, well-defined margins. Histology shows myxoid and fibrous regions and, less commonly, chondroid lesions–all with a benign appearance. The tumor exhibits a lobular pattern of growth. Treatment is generally curettage and bone grafting.

Benign and Locally Aggressive Bone Lesions

Giant cell tumor of bone is a benign but locally aggressive neoplasm (**Figure 6**). A small percentage of patients

(1% to 4%) with these tumors will develop benign pulmonary metastases, which are metastatic deposits in the lung that demonstrate benign histology.[27] These tumors occur in the second to fourth decade of life and are eccentric, lytic lesions in the metaphysis of bone extending to the epiphysis. The tumor is relatively destructive and can break through the cortex or cause pathologic fracture in nearly one fifth of patients.

Giant cell tumors generally are treated with extended curettage. Initial studies with curettage and bone grafting alone have demonstrated high recurrence rates of 30% to 50%. Adjuvants in addition to curettage were introduced, all of which have some effect on lowering the recurrence rates. Cementation in lieu of bone grafting is an adjuvant therapy that provides immediate stability. Phenol's toxicity to normal tissues and difficulty in handling in the operating room environment limit its usefulness. Liquid nitrogen has been associated with a low recurrence rate on the order of 8%, but it is also associated with a high risk of fracture as a result of a relatively uncontrollable zone of injury from freezing. A high-speed burr is often used as a mechanical adjuvant to extend the curettage. To adequately perform this type of extended curettage, the cavity in the bone must be unroofed completely, and the burr used on every surface of the cavity.

Excellent results can be achieved with extended curettage, with reported recurrence rates of approximately 12%. In some tumors, particularly tumors with extensive soft-tissue extension or significant destruction of periarticular bone (Enneking grade 3), an excision and reconstruction may be preferred to extended curettage. This is particularly true in the distal radius, where excellent results can be achieved with resection of

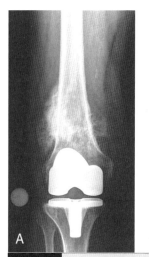
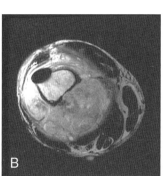
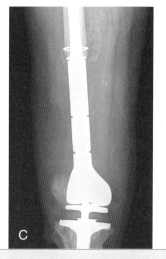
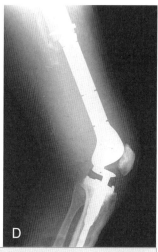

Figure 7 Distal femur osteosarcoma. **A**, Radiographic appearance before knee replacement. **B**, MRI showing large tumor mass. **C** and **D**, Postoperative images demonstrating resection and reconstruction with distal femoral endoprosthetic replacement.

aggressive giant cell tumors.[28]

Significant advances were recently made in the understanding of the pathogenesis of this disease when a critical role for the osteoclast differentiation factor, receptor activator of nuclear factor-κ B ligand (RANKL), was discovered. A fully human monoclonal antibody to RANKL, denosumab, was studied in a clinical trial in unresectable giant cell tumor, showing an 86% response rate.[29] As understanding of the basic science of this condition improves,[30] treatment of this condition is advancing and a greater role for denosumab may be identified in the future based on these results.

Malignant Bone Lesions
Osteosarcoma

Osteosarcoma is the most common sarcoma of bone. It is most frequently seen in adolescents, with an incidence in those younger than 20 years of approximately 5 per million per year in the United States, with a slight male predominance. Risk factors for osteosarcoma include Li-Fraumeni syndrome (mutation of tumor suppressor gene *p53*), Rothmund-Thomson syndrome (associated with mutation in *RECQL4*), and hereditary retinoblastoma (mutation of the retinoblastoma gene *RB1* on chromosome 13q14). This tumor can be found in association with solitary or multiple osteochondroma, solitary enchondroma or enchondromatosis (Ollier disease), multiple hereditary exostoses, fibrous dysplasia, Paget disease, chronic osteomyelitis, and bone infarcts. Tumors have been shown to develop in sites of prior exposure to ionizing radiation. Tumors that develop in sites of metallic prostheses and internal fixation have been described, but this occurrence is rare and sporadic, and the presence of these implants does not represent a causative factor (**Figure 7**). Osteosarcoma has also been associated with intravenous radium and thorium oxide use. Exposure to alkylating agents may also contribute to its development.[31]

The workup of the patient with osteosarcoma includes adequate imaging of the local site, which includes plain radiography (**Figure 8**), MRI, and in some instances CT, as well as staging studies to evaluate for metastatic disease, in the form of a chest CT scan and a Tc99 whole body bone scan. During initial evaluation of the patient, imaging of the entire bone containing the tumor is important to evaluate for the presence of skip metastases, which are distinct tumor masses occurring in the same bone. MRI is the preferred imaging modality because it is more sensitive than a bone scan for detecting skip metastases.

The understanding of the biologic basis of osteosarcoma is advancing.[32] Genetic studies have revealed complex karyotypes in osteosarcoma. Wnt signaling has been implicated as a potential therapeutic target and is currently under investigation. *WWOX* has been suggested as a potential tumor suppressor gene in osteosarcoma development, and the WWOX protein is absent or reduced in approximately 60% of the tumors studied.[33] Anti-vascular endothelial growth factor (VEGF) therapy is being investigated for metastatic disease.[34] Increasing interest in utilization of a canine model for osteosarcoma also holds promise for the future. Dogs have naturally occurring osteosarcomas that are almost identical to the human counterpart. The animal's large size and intact immune system make it an excellent model for study.[35]

Chondrosarcoma

Chondrosarcoma is the most common primary malignant bone tumor in adults, and the third most common primary bone malignancy in individuals of all ages, after osteosarcoma and Ewing sarcoma (**Figure 9**). The spectrum of cartilage tumors progressing from benign enchondroma to high-grade chondrosarcoma is a source of difficulty for both pathologists and surgeons. For these tumors, the radiographic characteristics play

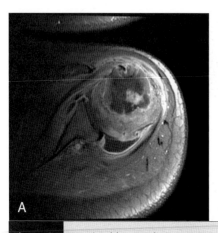
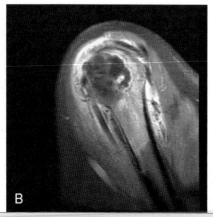
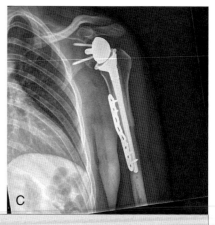

Figure 8 Proximal humeral osteosarcoma. **A** and **B**, MRI axial and sagittal views, respectively, demonstrating a destructive lesion of the proximal humerus in a 20-year-old man. **C**, Postoperative radiograph. After induction chemotherapy, a resection is performed and reconstruction is done using an allograft prosthetic composite incorporating a reverse shoulder arthroplasty.

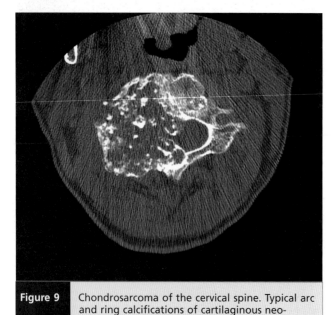

Figure 9 Chondrosarcoma of the cervical spine. Typical arc and ring calcifications of cartilaginous neoplasms are seen, along with destruction of the cortex and a soft-tissue mass. Pathology is consistent with an intermediate grade chondrosarcoma.

The treatment of chondrosarcoma is primarily wide surgical resection in the localized case. There is little or no sensitivity to conventional chemotherapy. Although chemotherapy has been used in the mesenchymal and dedifferentiated forms, based on the rationale that these forms are histologically dissimilar from the conventional type and therefore may have more sensitivity, there is poor evidence that chemotherapy has a significant clinical effect. Radiation therapy may be added for positive margins if repeat resection is not feasible, but this tumor generally has limited sensitivity to radiation therapy. The treatment of metastatic chondrosarcoma is very difficult (**Figure 10**) given that there are no highly active agents, which underscores the need for a targeted agent in the management of this tumor.

Ewing Sarcoma

Ewing sarcoma is a malignant small round cell tumor of bone; data indicate a mesenchymal stem cell derivation.[38,39] The cells are positive for CD99 and demonstrate a characteristic t(11;22) translocation. The characteristic mutation creates an EWS/Fli1 fusion protein that is critical in the pathogenesis of this tumor. However, despite the characteristic translocation and increasing understanding over the past two decades of the downstream signaling of the fusion protein,[40] a therapeutic agent targeting this pathway has not been identified. As a result, the treatment of Ewing sarcoma continues to be initiation of a multimodal chemotherapy regimen in addition to local control measures. Either wide surgical excision or radiation therapy can be used for local control, although there may be a slight local control advantage for surgical resection in extremity cases.[41] However, because this tumor usually occurs in adolescents and young adults, the risk of secondary radiation-associated sarcoma should be considered. For surgically resectable tumors that leave the patient with an acceptable level of function, surgery may represent the preferred local control measure. For unresectable tumors, or tumors for which surgery would be

almost as important a role as the histologic findings. Most experienced pathologists will finalize their evaluation of cartilage tumors only after reviewing the imaging studies to ensure that the histology and the behavior implied by imaging are consistent. For this reason, it is critical that adequate communication exists between the treating members of the team, including an expert pathologist, the radiologist, and the surgeon. Several distinct subtypes of chondrosarcoma exist: conventional, clear cell, mesenchymal, and dedifferentiated. Although attempts have been made to clarify a molecular distinction among these subtypes, the precise genetic definitions are not clear at the present time.[36,37]

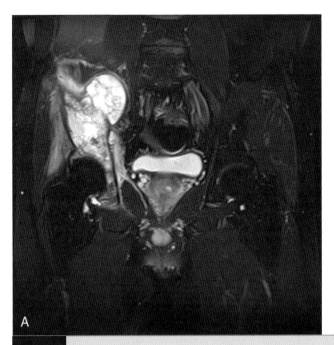
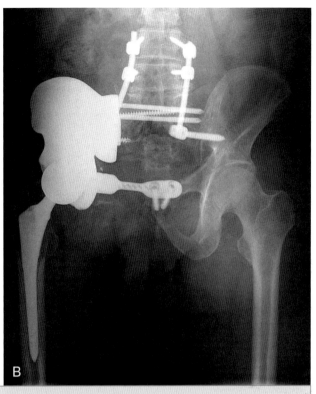

Figure 10 High-grade chondrosarcoma of the pelvis. **A,** On MRI, the mass is hyperintense on T2-weighted images. **B,** A custom endoprosthetic hemipelvis reconstruction is performed. In this case, surgical navigation is used to safely interdigitate long screws between the sacral neural foramina to achieve a stable configuration, allowing the patient to ambulate on this reconstruction.

debilitating or disfiguring, radiation therapy can be considered as the method of local control. Current treatment regimens yield 5-year survival rates of approximately 65% for localized disease.[42] Insulin-like growth factor-1 (IGF-1) targeted therapies, trabectedin (ecteinascidin 743), and epigenetically targeted therapies have all shown promise, but these therapies are not currently in use in the clinic. Work is also being done to target the EWS-FLI1 fusion product with small molecules.[43]

Myeloma

Multiple myeloma is a relatively common primary hematopoietic tumor affecting bone. The American Cancer Society estimated 20,520 new cases in the United States in 2011.[44]

Recent advancements in the pathogenesis of multiple myeloma have been made. It is now recognized that the survival and the proliferation of myeloma cells are dependent on a variety of cytokines, including interleukin-6, IGF-1, and VEGF. Myeloma cells are known to produce myeloma-derived macrophage-inflammatory factor-1α, which is responsible for upregulation of RANKL by bone marrow stromal cells, thereby activating osteoclast-mediated bone resorption. Myeloma cells also have additional bone-destroying effects of decreasing osteoprotegerin messenger RNA expression, removing the decoy inhibition effect of osteoprotegerin on osteoclast activation.[45]

The primary treatment of myeloma is chemotherapy. Induction chemotherapy is usually given with the goal of autologous or, less commonly, allogeneic progenitor stem cell transplant. Current response rates are 80% to 90% for first-line therapy and 40% to 60% in treatment of the first relapse. Novel agents introduced in the past 10 years include bortezomib, lenalidomide, and thalidomide and are associated with improved outcomes. In cases of solitary plasmacytoma, radiation therapy is generally used to treat the primary tumor.

Surgical treatment in myeloma is usually directed toward bone disease. Impending fractures, like metastatic bone disease, are treated with surgery and radiation. Bisphosphonates play an important role in reducing skeletal-related events in patients with myeloma.[46] Myeloma commonly affects the spine and can lead to painful lesions and the risk of vertebral collapse that requires surgical intervention.

Benign Soft-Tissue Lesions

Desmoid tumors, or aggressive fibromatosis, represent perhaps the most frustrating nonmalignant tumor that affects the extremities. The etiology of these tumors is unclear, and there has been debate about whether desmoid tumors represent a neoplastic or a traumatic condition. These tumors can occur in an intra-abdominal form and can also affect the abdominal wall. The tumors seem to have some response to hormonal

2: Systemic Disorders

changes, and rapid growth during pregnancy has been reported. For this reason, tamoxifen has been used, with mixed results, in the treatment of these tumors.[47] The results of local control with wide surgical excision alone are less encouraging than the results for wide surgical excision of soft-tissue sarcoma, and because of the infiltrative and locally invasive nature of the desmoid tumor, significant morbidity as a result of excision is a factor. Adjuvant modalities for local control include low-dose chemotherapy regimens and hormonal agents, as well as radiation therapy. Recent evidence suggests an improvement in local control with postoperative radiation in patients in whom a wide resection was not achieved,[48,49] but as in the case of sarcoma, required dosages are high and are associated with complications. Because of the highly variable and unpredictable course of these tumors, it has been suggested that surgical therapy should not be considered the first-line modality for these tumors. Some authors suggest a less radical initial excision and reliance on other modalities to improve local control.[50] Ongoing investigations into the biologic basis of this disease have not yielded specific targets. Tyrosine kinases have been implicated but require further study.[51] *CTNNB1*, the gene encoding β-catenin, has been found to be commonly mutated in desmoid tumors, and specific mutations may have some prognostic significance.[52]

Malignant Soft-Tissue Lesions
Soft-Tissue Sarcoma

Soft-tissue sarcomas represent a broad class of malignancies with a mesenchymal origin. The nomenclature of these tumors is based on the World Health Organization (WHO) classification.[53] In recent years, the term malignant fibrous histiocytoma has been replaced by the more accurate term undifferentiated pleomorphic sarcoma; this diagnosis refers to all sarcomas not otherwise classifiable in the WHO system. Knowledge of the specific histology is critical in understanding these tumors, because each tumor behaves in a unique fashion and has unique molecular events leading to its genesis. For localized disease, surgical excision is the mainstay of treatment, although radiation and chemotherapy are important adjuvants in specific instances (**Figure 11**). In recent years, attempts have been made to determine the molecular basis of sarcoma genesis (**Table 3**). This action is in part the result of the model paradigm for sarcoma management using targeted therapies exemplified by gastrointestinal stromal tumor (GIST). In the past two decades, activating mutations of *KIT* were found to be responsible for the development of GIST.[54] Imatinib, a tyrosine kinase inhibitor, later was used to treat GIST based on the rationale that

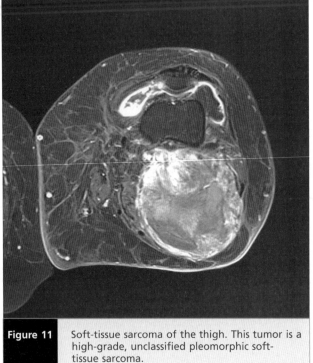

Figure 11 Soft-tissue sarcoma of the thigh. This tumor is a high-grade, unclassified pleomorphic soft-tissue sarcoma.

Table 3		
Selected Cytogenetic Events in the Development of Sarcoma		
Sarcoma	**Chromosomal Aberration**	**Resultant Fusion Protein**
Ewing sarcoma	t(11;22)(q24;q12)	EWS-FLi1 (most common)
Clear cell sarcoma	t(12;22)(q13;q12)	EWS-ATF1
Dermatofibrosarcoma protuberans	Ring chromosomes 17 and 22	COL1A1-PDGFB
Myxoid liposarcoma	t(12;16)(q13;p11)	TLS-CHOP
	t(12;22)(q13;q12)	FUS-CHOP
Synovial sarcoma	t(X;18)(p11;q11)	SYT-SSX1 or SYT-SSX2
Desmoplastic small round cell tumor	t(11;22)(p13,q12)	EWS-WT1
Alveolar soft parts sarcoma	t(X;17)(p11;q21)	ASPL-TFE3
Alveolar rhabomyosarcoma	t(2;13)(q35;q14)	PAX3-FKHR
	t(1;13)(p36;q14)	PAX7-FKHR

imatinib also inhibits KIT signaling and may therefore prove effective. Subsequent clinical trials demonstrated activity of the drug even in advanced cases of GIST, and the management of this disease, previously without any effective medical therapy, was radically changed. This success has increased the search for molecular definitions of sarcoma subtypes based on a specific genetic defect. As a result, the number of sarcomas that can be defined by a specific molecular alteration is increasing, many of which harbor balanced chromosomal translocations that generate a transcription factor-activating fusion protein. The subsequent signaling cascade provides many potential therapeutic targets, which have been the focus of the most significant sarcoma research of the past decade.

Two examples of a specific translocation leading to the identification of a targeted therapy are seen in dermatofibrosarcoma protuberans and pigmented villonodular synovitis (PVNS). Dermatofibrosarcoma protuberans is a locally aggressive skin sarcoma that carries a t(17;22) translocation, resulting in the fusion of the *COL1A1* and platelet-derived growth factor-beta (*PDGF-β*) genes. This fusion protein results in the overexpression of *PDGF-β*. Imatinib, which is an inhibitor of platelet-derived growth factor receptor-beta, has proven effective in controlling locally advanced dermatofibrosarcoma protuberans tumors. PVNS, more accurately known as giant cell tumor of synovium, is a benign but locally aggressive intra-articular lesion that is the result of a t(1;2) translocation fusing a collagen gene with colony-stimulating factor(CSF)-1, which is the gene for macrophage CSF. Imatinib and other tyrosine kinase inhibitors also inhibit the macrophage CSF receptor and have shown significant although not durable activity against PVNS. A trial is under way that is currently accruing patients to investigate the tyrosine kinase inhibitor nilotinib in patients with unresectable or recurrent PVNS.

Tyrosine kinase inhibition can also have an antiangiogenic effect, likely by inhibition of VEGF and platelet-derived growth factor receptor-beta pathways. These antiangiogenic effects are also being investigated in sarcoma. Recently studied agents include pazopanib, sunitinib, and cediranib. Pazopanib has shown enough activity in an initial European phase II study to warrant further study in a larger placebo-controlled randomized trial.[55] Both sunitinib and cediranib have shown activity in alveolar soft parts sarcoma, a disease that had previously not shown any sensitivity to conventional chemotherapy. Bevacizumab is an anti-VEGF antibody that has shown some response rate in patients with angiosarcoma, a highly vascular sarcoma derived from vessel walls.

Another pathway that has received significant attention is the mammalian target of rapamycin (mTOR), an important keystone in the PI3 and AKT signaling pathways. Rapamycin, or sirolimus, has shown benefit in patients with perivascular epithelioid cell sarcoma, a rare disease associated with upregulation of mTORC1. Other agents resulting in mTOR inhibition have generated significant interest. One such agent, ridforolimus,

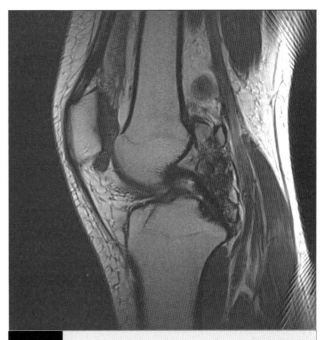

Figure 12 Pigmented villonodular synovitis of the knee. A benign intra-articular neoplasm is generally treated with synovectomy. This patient has extensive disease, seen best posteriorly adjacent to the posterior cruciate ligament.

was tested in a large phase III trial, the Sarcoma Multi-Center Clinical Evaluation of the Efficacy of Ridaforolimus trial, which enrolled patients with advanced soft-tissue or bone sarcomas. Although the final results of this trial are not yet available, the initial results of the preceding phase II trial were promising.[56]

Another important pathway in sarcoma development is the IGF-1 pathway. Multiple sarcomas, including Ewing sarcoma, alveolar soft parts sarcoma, leiomyosarcoma, synovial sarcoma, rhabdomyosarcoma, and desmoplastic small round cell tumor, have a known increase in insulin-like growth factor receptor-1 levels, which may have some role in the pathogenesis of the disease. For this reason, this is an area of high recent interest in clinical sarcoma trials. Figitumab and cixutumab, anti–insulin-like growth factor receptor-1 antibodies, have been studied in initial trials for advanced sarcoma and have shown enough promise to warrant further study. Small molecules that bind to the intracellular portion are also in development to interrupt this pathway.

Intra-articular Lesions
Pigmented Villonodular Synovitis
PVNS, or tenosynovial giant cell tumor, is an intra-articular synovial-based tumor found most commonly in the knee (**Figure 12**). It has an incidence of approximately 1.8 cases per million. The disease is monoarticular and is generally benign, although a few cases have been reported with histologically confirmed metastatic disease. The disease is seen in either localized or diffuse forms. A histologically identical variant is the giant cell

tumor of tenosynovium seen most commonly in the tendons of the hand. Although PVNS was initially thought to be an inflammatory or posttraumatic condition, recent studies have identified the overexpression of the *CSF-1* gene as the etiologic factor, supporting the concept that PVNS is a true benign neoplasm.[57] Patients with PVNS often present with recurrent hemarthroses without antecedent trauma. MRI shows a thickened synovium, with areas of low signal intensity on both T1- and T2-weighted images as a result of hemosiderin. Areas of bleeding within the hyperemic synovium will have a higher signal intensity on T1 images. The primary morbidity of PVNS is the erosion of cartilage surfaces. Additionally, bone erosions can occur, causing further joint destruction. The primary treatment before joint destruction is complete synovectomy, which can be challenging in certain joints, such as the hip or the ankle. The results of arthroscopic synovectomy are mixed, with some studies showing comparable results to open synovectomy in the knee. In cases where advanced joint destruction occurs, arthroplasty may be considered.

The addition of radiation therapy, either by standard external beam therapy or intra-articular radioisotopes, can reduce the recurrence rate with relatively low risk at moderate doses.[58] Given the recently clarified mechanism of this disease, tyrosine kinase inhibitors or other agents targeting the CSF-1 pathway are under investigation.[59] An initial proof-of-concept study using imatinib in 29 patients demonstrated some response or stable disease in 25 of 27 patients. However, in this study, 10 patients discontinued treatment because of toxicity or other reasons.[60]

Synovial Chondromatosis

Synovial chondromatosis is an intra-articular condition in which the synovium undergoes chondro-osseous metaplasia. It is unclear whether this condition represents a true neoplasm, although case reports have documented transformation to chondrosarcoma. The most common site of occurrence is the knee. As the disease progresses, ossification of the cartilage can occur, leading to osteochondromatosis. The intra-articular bodies cause pain, swelling, and mechanical symptoms. Erosion of the articular cartilage can occur. Treatment is removal of loose bodies and synovectomy. Arthroscopic or open synovectomies are both effective in relieving symptoms. In joints in which arthroscopy is not possible, or in cases with extensive chondromatosis, an open synovectomy is the preferred approach.

Advancements in Surgical Techniques

For the treatment of primary bone and soft-tissue tumors, the significance of recent medical advances has far outweighed that of surgical advancements. However, surgical techniques are continually improving. For example, there is continued progress with expandable skeletal prostheses for skeletally immature patients, but the complication rate remains high.[61] Nevertheless, these implants can provide an alternative to amputation, and research into improving these prostheses continues. One relevant recent advancement is the adaptation of computer navigation systems for use in the resection of primary bone tumors. Several centers have reported on the adaptation of commercially available surgical navigation systems to aid in particularly challenging resections, such as those in the pelvis, the spine, and the sacrum. Obvious benefits include the ability to pinpoint one's location in a complex anatomic region intraoperatively on an intraoperatively or preoperatively acquired scan. Additional potential benefits include an improved workflow in which both the surgical resection and the custom-made metallic or allograft reconstruction can be planned off a single template generated in advance of the surgery. Small-scale procedures, such as biopsies or curettages in difficult locations, can be performed using minimally invasive techniques with navigation guidance. Resection precision can potentially be increased by using such systems, allowing improved ability of the surgeon to generate a precisely defined margin. Allograft-host junctions can be more precisely mated, potentially allowing improved rates of healing (**Figure 13**). The intraoperative placement of prostheses or hardware in nonstandard locations as necessitated by the tumor resection can be potentially done with improved accuracy. Further study is needed to detail the precise roles of surgical navigation in orthopaedic oncology, but initial experience demonstrates that this technique is likely to play an important role in the future.[62]

Metastatic Disease to the Skeleton

Epidemiology

To put the extent of morbidity attributable to metastatic bone lesions in perspective, of the approximately 1.2 million new cases of cancer in the United States per year, bone metastases will develop in almost half of these cases. This staggering statistic highlights the need for understanding the processes that allow these metastases to develop. Bone metastases can result from nearly every carcinoma, although breast, lung, renal, thyroid, and prostate primary tumors represent the bulk of metastatic disease to the skeleton, together accounting for more than 80% of bone metastases.

Biology

Investigations into the biology of skeletal metastases have given significant insight into the processes required to generate a metastatic bone lesion. Multiple steps have been described, and each step represents a potential therapeutic target for interrupting this process. The current model is that the following steps need to take place for a tumor to spread from a primary site to a bone location: neovascularization, blood vessel invasion, embolism, arrest in bone compartment, tumor growth, and activation of osteoclasts.

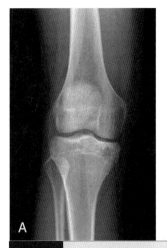
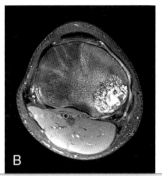
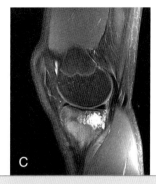
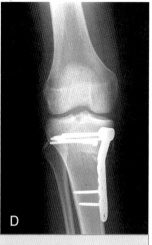

Figure 13 Clear cell chondrosarcoma of the proximal tibia. **A,** Radiographic appearance of a proximal tibia clear cell chondrosarcoma showing the epiphyseal location. **B** and **C,** MRIs show the extent of the tumor. **D,** Radiograph showing that the tumor was resected and reconstructed with an osteoarticular allograft. In this case, the allograft was sized and cut to precisely match the resection defect using computer navigation. Because of this precise matching, no visible gap is seen at the allograft-host junction site.

At initial stages of the metastatic process, micrometastases can be identified in the blood using immunohistochemical studies. It is likely that most of these cells do not survive, until the subsequent steps in the process occur. Overexpression of bone metastasis genes responsible for homing-in, invasion, angiogenesis, osteoclastogenesis, growth factor regulation, and extracellular matrix alteration complete the necessary steps to allow micrometastases in the bloodstream to implant and thrive in a bone location. The signaling pathway responsible for tumor cell proliferation and metastasis is a Raf-MEK-ERK-MAPK pathway, which is inhibited by NM-23 and Raf kinase inhibitor protein. These are therefore called metastasis suppressor genes and are a focus of investigation.[63,64]

Bone has high vascular flow in red bone marrow and contains an abundant supply of growth factors, both contributing to the high metastatic rate. Transforming growth factor (TGF)-β, IGF, fibroblast growth factor (FGF), PDGF, and bone morphogenetic protein all may play a role in promoting chemotaxis, stimulating proliferation, and preventing cell death. Cancer cells dysregulate suppression and activation of cell adhesion molecules that bind one cell tightly to another, which protects from tumor invasion. Cadherins (cell-to-like-cell), selectins (cell-to-different cell), and integrins (cell-to-matrix or cell-to-cell) are binding molecules that play an important role in this regard, either by blocking tumor invasion or promoting tumor adhesion. Matrix metalloproteinases, balanced by tissue inhibitors of metalloproteinase, are important enzymes for degrading the matrix and can help facilitate tumor cell invasion. The mobility of a tumor cell can be affected via factors such as IGF-1, IL-8, and histamine in an autocrine or paracrine fashion. Angiogenesis is also a critical stage in the development of bone metastases. Important proangiogenic factors include FGF, TGF-α, angiogenin, vascular permeability factor, and VEGF. Critical anti-angiogenic factors include angiostatin, cartilage-derived inhibitor, platelet factor-4, and tissue inhibitor of metalloproteinase.[65]

The final step in the development of bone metastases recently has been a topic of debate. After it was understood that osteoclast activation and subsequent bone resorption was the direct mechanism of bone loss secondary to activation by cancer cells, interest turned to inhibitors of this process. Bone turnover is highly regulated and normally exists in a careful balance in which osteoclast precursors are stimulated by RANK, which is produced by osteoblasts. RANK binds to RANKL, causing differentiation and osteoclastic bone resorption. Osteoprotegerin acts as an inhibitor of RANKL. Osteoclast activation by parathyroid hormone-related protein, overexpressed by cancer cells, leads to the sequence of events that dysregulates the careful balance, leading to the "hole in bone."[66,67]

Role of Bisphosphonates

The explanation of this pathway of metastatic bone disease development led to the investigation of bisphosphonate therapy in all solid tumor metastases to bone. Bisphosphonates represent a class of medications that bind to bone mineral in Howship lacunae and are taken up by osteoclasts, in which they disrupt the cytoskeleton, leading to loss of the ruffled border that is critical for the function of enzymes involved in bone resorption. Initial studies of bisphosphonate use in patients with metastatic breast carcinoma to bone showed a 23% decrease in skeletal-related events, including pathologic fracture and other morbidities related to bone metastases.[68] Since those initial findings, bisphosphonate use has been expanded to include patients with any solid tumor metastasis to bone.

The side effects and the risks associated with bisphosphonates has somewhat curtailed usage in recent years. Esophagitis, osteonecrosis of the jaw, and relatively newly described bisphosphonate-associated stress fractures have led to a discontinuation of bisphosphonate therapy in some patients. Of particular interest for orthopaedic surgeons is the risk of bisphosphonate-associated stress fractures. Although the exact incidence is unknown, the risk of developing a stress fracture of the subtrochanteric region of the femur is very low, but it has been clearly described and is associated with bisphosphonate therapy for 5 years or longer. These fractures often occur when several bisphosphonates are taken, likely representing a class effect. Several studies of these fractures have suggested surgical fixation with an intramedullary device, in addition to observation of the contralateral side.[69]

In part because of these side effects, newer medications that interrupt the same bone resorption pathway at different points have been investigated. The leading new agent is the anti-RANKL antibody denosumab, approved in 2010 for use in patients with skeletal metastases. Denosumab has become an important alternative agent for patients experiencing bisphosphonate-related side effects. Initial studies suggest a comparable decrease in skeletal-related events when compared with zoledronic acid.[70] It is currently unknown whether patients undergoing denosumab therapy have an increased risk for a femoral stress fracture. However, the risk of osteonecrosis of the jaw for both bisphosphonates and anti-RANKL antibodies is similar, despite differing mechanisms of action.

Predicting Fracture Risk

Although plain radiography is the standard for decision making, and CT scans may provide additional information in some cases, newer modalities are being promoted in more accurately determining fracture risk. The quantitative CT scan is currently the most advanced method. A graduated hydroxyapatite marker with standard densities is scanned with the patient, and the x-ray attenuation coefficient (Hounsfield unit) can be converted into an equivalent bone density for each pixel. In the area of the lesion, the bone density in a given cross-sectional area is calculated and compared with the homologous cross section on the contralateral bone (which is included in the CT field per study protocol). Structural rigidity with respect to compression, bending, and torsional rigidity is calculated at the weakest cross section and expressed as a ratio compared with the contralateral side. This information provides a calculated expected increase in fracture risk compared with unaffected or normal bone. This type of study has been validated in patients with benign bone lesions and is currently being used in patients with malignant bone lesions.[71]

Treatment of Metastatic Skeletal Disease
Nonsurgical Management

The general modalities of treatment of skeletal disease include palliative therapies with pain control medications and techniques, nonsurgical management with the patient's medical treatment alone with or without the addition of radiation therapy, bone-specific treatments such as bisphosphonates and radioactive isotopes, and surgical intervention.

Palliative measures include analgesic medications and potentially interventional procedures directed solely at reducing pain. Bone-seeking radioisotopes (strontium 89, phosphorus 32, samarium 153, rhenium 186) may help control pain related to bone lesions in certain situations. Medical therapy is specific for each primary disease.

Significant advancements have been made in the treatment of several primary tumors affecting bone. For example, renal cell carcinoma, which previously had no significant medical treatment options, now has recently approved medical therapies, such as the receptor tyrosine kinase inhibitor sunitinib, available for patients with advanced disease. Other examples include radioactive iodine treatment of thyroid cancer and octreotide in neuroendocrine tumors. In patients with a nonthreatening asymptomatic bone lesion who are receiving medical therapy that is causing stability or improvement of the overall disease and a concordant response in bone, observation alone may be adequate for the skeletal disease. For symptomatic lesions without high risk of pathologic fracture, radiation therapy is a highly effective modality of pain control. Radiation therapy also plays a critical role in conjunction with surgical intervention, by providing local control of the lesion with two main intentions: to prevent local spread of the tumor that could otherwise be facilitated by surgical manipulation of the tumor and instruments used during the surgical procedure; and to ensure the implant chosen to confer stability remains adequate over time by controlling the growth of the bone lesion locally.

Stereotactic radiosurgery is a relatively new radiation technique that has had particular implications for the management of spinal metastases. Although the precise role of this technique in the management of extremity metastases remains undefined, there is significant potential for usefulness, in particular for patients who are poor surgical candidates or patients with traditionally radiation-resistant metastases, such as those from renal cell carcinoma. Future studies will be needed to elucidate the precise role for this technique in the management of extremity metastases.

Surgical Management of Metastatic Bone Lesions

The rationale for the surgical treatment of metastatic bone lesions is to limit the amount of pain and morbidity caused by the lesion, in a manner that necessitates the shortest break from and least disruption of the overall treatment plan (**Figure 14**).

Epiphyseal and periarticular lesions generally require arthroplasty management. If the lesion is not subchondral, curettage and cementation with plate fixation for structural stability is a possibility, but the durability of the construct may not be as favorable or durable as a reconstructive procedure. In these instances, the patient's expected activity level and life span can help

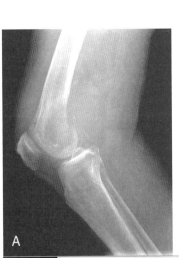
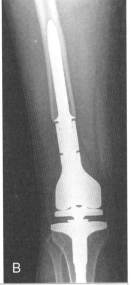

Figure 14 | Surgical treatment of metastatic disease requiring arthroplasty. **A,** Metastatic renal cell carcinoma of the distal femur extending to the joint surface. **B,** Treatment with resection and distal femoral replacement reconstruction.

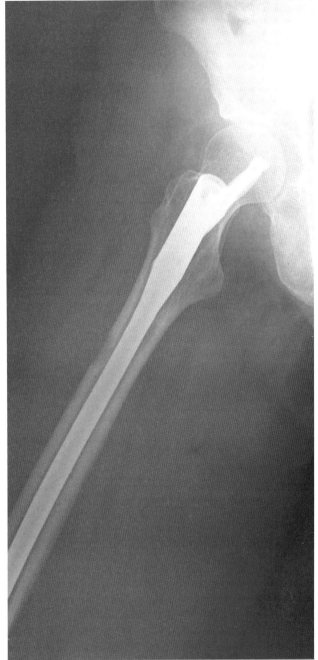

Figure 15 | Intramedullary nailing. Lateral radiograph of the femur showing intracortical metastasis from lung carcinoma imparting a high risk of pathologic fracture, treated with intramedullary nailing.

make the decision for treatment. Lesions involving the joint surface require resection and reconstruction. Modular endoprosthetic reconstructions are generally necessary to reconstruct defects generated by these resections (**Figure 15**).

Pathologic fractures can be challenging to treat. Compromised bone in addition to fracture often requires extensive stabilization or sometimes arthroplasty reconstructions. In one study comparing intramedullary nailing, curettage, and fixation versus endoprosthetic replacement in pathologic proximal femur fractures, the lowest failure rate and most durable results were found in the endoprosthetic replacement group.[72] Although this patient population is not medically well suited to tolerate large-scale surgical interventions such as resection and endoprosthetic reconstruction, the rationale is that one durable surgical intervention, even if larger scale, is far better for the overall outcome of the patient than multiple surgical attempts at solving a difficult stabilization problem. In cases where extensive bone destruction involving most of the proximal or distal portion of a long bone has occurred, resection and reconstruction with a modular endoprosthesis may be required. For this reason, careful consideration should be given to all the available options and the likelihood of success of each option before undertaking these often challenging patients.

Specific difficult anatomic locations, such as the spine and the pelvis, present additional challenges. Metastatic disease to the spine is beyond the scope of this chapter. Metastatic lesions to the pelvis and the acetabulum present unique problems not encountered in long bone disease. The primary issue is that surgical interventions in this location are often large-scale undertakings and may require extended healing times and substantial postoperative rehabilitation. Surgical procedures to address pelvic and acetabular disease are at high risk for complications and usually occur in patients who are poorly medically equipped to handle them. The patient's expected prognosis should be carefully considered to ensure that the rehabilitation and recovery period does not exceed these expectations. For

2: Systemic Disorders

these reasons, pelvic and acetabular procedures are far less commonly performed than long bone procedures. Several interventional procedures, such as radiofrequency ablation, cryotherapy, and cementation are being investigated for these difficult situations to provide some pain relief and possibly even stability, without the need for a large and highly invasive surgical procedure.

However, in some instances, it makes sense to perform a reconstructive procedure on a patient with metastatic disease to the pelvis or the acetabulum. In these instances, revision hip arthroplasty techniques are used to gain firm and stable attachment of metal implants to host bone that is not compromised by tumor infiltration. Preoperative planning is essential. Availability and proficiency in the use of acetabular augments, antiprotrusio cages, cementation, and constrained components is critical for a successful endeavor.

Summary and Future Directions

Musculoskeletal oncology is a rapidly changing field. Improvements in both diagnosis and management are increasing the ability of the orthopaedic oncologist to manage these complex problems in the extremities. New techniques may help predict fracture risk for benign and malignant tumors. The focus on a histology-specific molecular understanding of each individual sarcoma has already and should continue to open new pathways of targeted management. Newer surgical technologies are being developed that can improve oncologic resections. For patients with metastatic skeletal disease, newer agents that decrease skeletal events can significantly supplement orthopaedic oncologic procedures in maintaining the integrity of the skeleton.

Key Study Points

- Cartilage tumors are difficult to accurately grade on histologic evaluation alone; therefore, a review of the radiologic features of a tumor is critical in assigning an accurate grade.

- Determining a molecular definition for each sarcoma subtype is becoming increasingly important in soft-tissue sarcoma so as to identify specific targets and signaling pathways that can be exploited for the development of new therapeutics.

- Osteoclast activation by metastatic disease to the bone is a key step in the development of bone lesions, and inhibition of this step is an important method of controlling skeletal-related events in this patient population, either by the use of bisphosphonates or anti-RANKL antibodies.

Annotated References

1. Howlader N, Noone AM, Krapcho M, et al, eds: *SEER Cancer Statistics Review, 1975-2009 (Vintage 2009 Populations)*. Bethesda, MD, National Cancer Institute.

2. Errani C, Kreshak J, Ruggieri P, Alberghini M, Picci P, Vanel D: Imaging of bone tumors for the musculoskeletal oncologic surgeon. *Eur J Radiol* 2011.

   An up-to-date review on imaging of bone tumors considering modern modalities is presented.

3. De Marchi A, Brach del Prever EM, Linari A, et al: Accuracy of core-needle biopsy after contrast-enhanced ultrasound in soft-tissue tumours. *Eur Radiol* 2010; 20(11):2740-2748.

   The authors present a retrospective review comparing biopsy using contrast-enhanced ultrasound to final pathology results, showing a high sensitivity and specificity for this technique. Level of evidence: III.

4. Sung KS, Seo SW, Shon MS: The diagnostic value of needle biopsy for musculoskeletal lesions. *Int Orthop* 2009;33(6):1701-1706.

5. Khalil JG, Mott MP, Parsons TW III, Banka TR, van Holsbeeck M: 2011 Mid-America Orthopaedic Association Dallas B. Phemister Physician in Training Award: Can musculoskeletal tumors be diagnosed with ultrasound fusion-guided biopsy? *Clin Orthop Relat Res* 2012;470(8):2280-2287.

   A comparison of 47 patients undergoing either CT-guided or ultrasound fusion-guided biopsies demonstrated equivalent yield and accuracy, but faster scheduling and biopsy times in the ultrasound fusion group. This study highlights the promising nature of this technique. Level of evidence: II.

6. Qi ZH, Li CF, Ma XX, et al: Value of 3T magnetic resonance dynamic contrast-enhanced and diffusion-weighted imaging in differential diagnosis of musculoskeletal tumors. *Zhongguo Yi Xue Ke Xue Yuan Xue Bao* 2012;34(2):138-145.

   A Chinese study reporting results of an analysis of 63 patients with confirmed pathology using various newer MRI techniques helped identify which parameters and thresholds can best distinguish benign from malignant tumors.

7. Umutlu L, Forsting M, Ladd ME: Ultrahigh-field magnetic resonance imaging: The clinical potential for anatomy, pathogenesis, diagnosis and treatment planning in neck and spine disease. *Neuroimaging Clin N Am* 2012; 22(2):363-371, xii.

   A review of the current application of 7T MRI to neck and spine disease is presented.

8. Rakheja R, Makis W, Skamene S, et al: Correlating metabolic activity on 18F-FDG PET/CT with histopathologic characteristics of osseous and soft-tissue sarcomas: A retrospective review of 136 patients. *AJR Am J Roentgenol* 2012;198(6):1409-1416.

The authors present a retrospective study correlating the maximum standardized uptake value of specific lesions on a PET/CT scan to histologic findings at resection, showing good correlation. Level of evidence: III.

9. Herrmann K, Benz MR, Czernin J, et al: 18F-FDG-PET/CT imaging as an early survival predictor in patients with primary high-grade soft tissue sarcomas undergoing neoadjuvant therapy. *Clin Cancer Res* 2012; 18(7):2024-2031.

This small sample trial studying PET before and after one cycle of chemotherapy and correlating with overall survival shows that PET response was a significant predictor of survival, both in univariable and multivariable analysis, suggesting possible usefulness as a surrogate or intermediate clinical trial end point. Level of evidence: II.

10. Lindholm P, Sutinen E, Oikonen V, et al: PET imaging of blood flow and glucose metabolism in localized musculoskeletal tumors of the extremities. *Nucl Med Biol* 2011;38(2):295-300.

The rate of blood flow in both bone and soft-tissue sarcomas can be measured precisely using PET and labeled water, although the importance of blood flow rate is not yet well understood. Level of evidence: II.

11. Lakkaraju A, Patel CN, Bradley KM, Scarsbrook AF: PET/CT in primary musculoskeletal tumours: A step forward. *Eur Radiol* 2010;20(12):2959-2972.

The authors review current and potential future applications of PET imaging to musculoskeletal oncology.

12. Cook GJ: PET and PET/CT imaging of skeletal metastases. *Cancer Imaging* 2010;10:1-8.

The authors review the various forms of PET imaging with respect to usefulness for skeletal imaging.

13. Mankin HJ, Lange TA, Spanier SS: The hazards of biopsy in patients with malignant primary bone and soft-tissue tumors. *J Bone Joint Surg Am* 1982;64(8):1121-1127.

14. Mankin HJ, Mankin CJ, Simon MA; Members of the Musculoskeletal Tumor Society: The hazards of the biopsy, revisited. *J Bone Joint Surg Am* 1996;78(5): 656-663.

15. Biau DJ, Weiss KR, Bhumbra RS, et al: Using the CUSUM test to control the proportion of inadequate open biopsies of musculoskeletal tumors. *Clin Orthop Relat Res* 2013;471(3):905-914.

A prospective study of 116 incisional biopsies was performed according to a set of guidelines and evaluated using a control test to successfully monitor and limit the proportion of inadequate biopsies. Level of evidence: II.

16. UyBico SJ, Motamedi K, Omura MC, et al: Relevance of compartmental anatomic guidelines for biopsy of musculoskeletal tumors: Retrospective review of 363 biopsies over a 6-year period. *J Vasc Interv Radiol* 2012; 23(4):511-518, e1-e2.

A retrospective review of 363 biopsies over a 6-year period demonstrated that in cases where the needle placement breached established guidelines, no seeding of tumor along the regions of breach were seen, and no tumor recurrences could be attributed to these breaches. Level of evidence: III.

17. Dupuy DE, Rosenberg AE, Punyaratabandhu T, Tan MH, Mankin HJ: Accuracy of CT-guided needle biopsy of musculoskeletal neoplasms. *AJR Am J Roentgenol* 1998;171(3):759-762.

18. Puri A, Shingade VU, Agarwal MG, et al: CT-guided percutaneous core needle biopsy in deep seated musculoskeletal lesions: A prospective study of 128 cases. *Skeletal Radiol* 2006;35(3):138-143.

19. Rougraff BT, Aboulafia A, Biermann JS, Healey J: Biopsy of soft tissue masses: Evidence-based medicine for the musculoskeletal tumor society. *Clin Orthop Relat Res* 2009;467(11):2783-2791.

20. Sung AD, Anderson ME, Zurakowski D, Hornicek FJ, Gebhardt MC: Unicameral bone cyst: A retrospective study of three surgical treatments. *Clin Orthop Relat Res* 2008;466(10):2519-2526.

A retrospective review of 167 patients younger than 20 years treated for UBCs with either steroid injection; curettage and grafting; or injection with a combination of steroids, demineralized bone matrix, and bone marrow aspirate demonstrated the lowest failure rate in the bone marrow aspirate group. Level of evidence: III.

21. Ye Y, Pringle LM, Lau AW, et al: TRE17/USP6 oncogene translocated in aneurysmal bone cyst induces matrix metalloproteinase production via activation of NF-kappaB. *Oncogene* 2010;29(25):3619-3629.

A sophisticated molecular analysis of the role of TRE17 in the pathogenesis of ABC demonstrated that overexpression of TRE17 in preosteoblastic MC3T3 cells is sufficient to drive the formation of tumors that reproduce molecular and histologic features of ABC. This study presents a strong argument against the previously prevailing theory of a circulatory pressure disturbance as the etiology of this tumor.

22. van de Luijtgaarden AC, Veth RP, Slootweg PJ, et al: Metastatic potential of an aneurysmal bone cyst. *Virchows Arch* 2009;455(5):455-459.

23. Maurer MH, Gebauer B, Wieners G, et al: Treatment of osteoid osteoma using CT-guided radiofrequency ablation versus MR-guided laser ablation: A cost comparison. *Eur J Radiol* 2012;81(11):e1002-e1006.

A retrospective review of costs associated with CT-radiofrequency ablation versus magnetic resonance-laser ablation for treatment of osteoid osteoma in 44 patients is presented, which demonstrated a higher cost for CT-radio frequency ablation, and attributed this higher cost primarily to the higher price of the disposable radio frequency ablation probes. Level of evidence: III.

2: Systemic Disorders

24. Chotel F, Franck F, Solla F, et al: Osteoid osteoma transformation into osteoblastoma: Fact or fiction? *Orthop Traumatol Surg Res* 2012;98(6, suppl):S98-S104.

This case report details two cases that highlight a histologic distinction between osteoid osteoma and osteoblastoma aside from size. Level of evidence: V.

25. Douis H, Davies AM, James SL, Kindblom LG, Grimer RJ, Johnson KJ: Can MR imaging challenge the commonly accepted theory of the pathogenesis of solitary enchondroma of long bone? *Skeletal Radiol* 2012; 41(12):1537-1542.

A review of 240 knee MRIs in skeletally immature patients shows that none had evidence of a displaced fragment of growth plate in the metaphysis, challenging this theory regarding the etiology of enchondromas. Level of evidence: III.

26. Choi BB, Jee WH, Sunwoo HJ, et al: MR differentiation of low-grade chondrosarcoma from enchondroma. *Clin Imaging* 2013;37(3):542-547.

A retrospective series of 34 patients with confirmed enchondroma or low-grade chondrosarcoma were reviewed, and magnetic resonance parameters that can help differentiate these entities are discussed. Level of evidence: III.

27. Tubbs WS, Brown LR, Beabout JW, Rock MG, Unni KK: Benign giant-cell tumor of bone with pulmonary metastases: Clinical findings and radiologic appearance of metastases in 13 cases. *AJR Am J Roentgenol* 1992; 158(2):331-334.

28. Liu YP, Li KH, Sun BH: Which treatment is the best for giant cell tumors of the distal radius? A meta-analysis. *Clin Orthop Relat Res* 2012;470(10):2886-2894.

A meta-analysis of giant cell tumors of the distal radius showed improved results for excision of Campanacci grade 3 tumors when compared to intralesional procedures. Level of evidence: III.

29. Thomas D, Henshaw R, Skubitz K, et al: Denosumab in patients with giant-cell tumour of bone: An open-label, phase 2 study. *Lancet Oncol* 2010;11(3):275-280.

An initial single group study enrolled patients with unresectable or recurrent giant cell tumor of bone, with 30 of 35 patients demonstrating a tumor response. This study provided the rationale for a larger clinical trial of denosumab for treatment of giant cell tumor. Level of evidence: II.

30. Cowan RW, Singh G: Giant cell tumor of bone: A basic science perspective. *Bone* 2013;52(1):238-246.

A review of the biology of giant cell tumor of bone and its implications for treatment is presented.

31. Ottaviani G, Jaffe N: The etiology of osteosarcoma. *Cancer Treat Res* 2009;152:15-32.

32. Gorlick R: Current concepts on the molecular biology of osteosarcoma. *Cancer Treat Res* 2009;152:467-478.

33. Del Mare S, Kurek KC, Stein GS, Lian JB, Aqeilan RI: Role of the WWOX tumor suppressor gene in bone homeostasis and the pathogenesis of osteosarcoma. *Am J Cancer Res* 2011;1(5):585-594.

WWOX protein is absent or reduced in 60% of human osteosarcomas, as in most human tumors, making the *WWOX* gene an important tumor suppressor gene. This review detailed the current understanding of this molecule as it relates to the possible development of osteosarcoma.

34. Tanaka T, Yui Y, Naka N, et al: Dynamic analysis of lung metastasis by mouse osteosarcoma LM8: VEGF is a candidate for anti-metastasis therapy. *Clin Exp Metastasis* 2013;30(4):369-379.

A series of molecular studies on highly metastatic OS8 and parent cell lines suggests a biologically plausible rationale for anti-VEGF therapy in metastatic osteosarcoma.

35. Withrow SJ, Khanna C: Bridging the gap between experimental animals and humans in osteosarcoma. *Cancer Treat Res* 2009;152:439-446.

36. Meijer D, de Jong D, Pansuriya TC, et al: Genetic characterization of mesenchymal, clear cell, and dedifferentiated chondrosarcoma. *Genes Chromosomes Cancer* 2012;51(10):899-909.

A molecular study using array comparative genomic hybridization and tissue microarrays characterized chondrosarcoma subtype tumors. Although multiple genomic alterations were seen, none were consistent within subtype, with the exception of retinoblastoma in a large percentage of all three subtypes, suggesting a possible role for this pathway in the pathogenesis of these tumors.

37. Kim MJ, Cho KJ, Ayala AG, Ro JY: Chondrosarcoma: With updates on molecular genetics. *Sarcoma* 2011; 2011:405437.

A review of chondrosarcoma with a section regarding the current molecular understanding of these tumors and subtypes is presented.

38. Suvà ML, Riggi N, Stehle JC, et al: Identification of cancer stem cells in Ewing's sarcoma. *Cancer Res* 2009; 69(5):1776-1781.

39. Tirode F, Laud-Duval K, Prieur A, Delorme B, Charbord P, Delattre O: Mesenchymal stem cell features of Ewing tumors. *Cancer Cell* 2007;11(5):421-429.

40. Kelleher FC, Thomas DM: Molecular pathogenesis and targeted therapeutics in Ewing sarcoma/primitive neuroectodermal tumours. *Clin Sarcoma Res* 2012;2(1):6.

The molecular pathogenesis of the Ewing family of tumors is reviewed, highlighting the rationale of IGF-1R antagonists as potential therapeutic agents.

41. Bacci G, Palmerini E, Staals EL, et al: Ewing's sarcoma family tumors of the humerus: Outcome of patients treated with radiotherapy, surgery or surgery and adjuvant radiotherapy. *Radiother Oncol* 2009;93(2): 383-387.

42. Rodríguez-Galindo C, Navid F, Liu T, Billups CA, Rao BN, Krasin MJ: Prognostic factors for local and distant control in Ewing sarcoma family of tumors. *Ann Oncol* 2008;19(4):814-820.

43. Grohar PJ, Helman LJ: Prospects and challenges for the development of new therapies for Ewing sarcoma. *Pharmacol Ther* 2013;137(2):216-224.

 A review of current and future treatment options for Ewing sarcoma is presented.

44. American Cancer Society: *Cancer Facts and Figures 2012.* Atlanta, GA, American Cancer Society, 2012.

45. Raje N, Roodman GD: Advances in the biology and treatment of bone disease in multiple myeloma. *Clin Cancer Res* 2011;17(6):1278-1286.

 Multiple myeloma biology and treatment are reviewed.

46. Pozzi S, Raje N: The role of bisphosphonates in multiple myeloma: Mechanisms, side effects, and the future. *Oncologist* 2011;16(5):651-662.

 Bisphosphonate use in myeloma is reviewed.

47. Bocale D, Rotelli MT, Cavallini A, Altomare DF: Antioestrogen therapy in the treatment of desmoid tumours: A systematic review. *Colorectal Dis* 2011;13(12):e388-e395.

 A systematic review incorporated data from 168 desmoid tumors, showing some efficacy of antiestrogen treatment in about half of the patients. Level of evidence: III.

48. Rüdiger HA, Ngan SY, Ng M, Powell GJ, Choong PF: Radiation therapy in the treatment of desmoid tumours reduces surgical indications. *Eur J Surg Oncol* 2010; 36(1):84-88.

 A retrospective review of 34 consecutive patients treated with radiation alone or surgery plus radiation demonstrated a recurrence-free survival rate of 83.6% in the surgical group, and stable disease in 53% of the radiation alone group. A thallium-210 scan was used to monitor metabolic activity after radiotherapy, and it is suggested that patients with a good metabolic response to radiotherapy as determined by this method may be candidates for nonsurgical management. Level of evidence: III.

49. Baumert BG, Spahr MO, Von Hochstetter A, et al: The impact of radiotherapy in the treatment of desmoid tumours: An international survey of 110 patients. A study of the Rare Cancer Network. *Radiat Oncol* 2007;2:12.

50. Bonvalot S, Desai A, Coppola S, et al: The treatment of desmoid tumors: A stepwise clinical approach. *Ann Oncol* 2012;23(suppl 10):x158-x166.

 An algorithm is proposed for a stepwise approach to desmoid tumors, beginning with less radical treatments before treatments with associated long-term morbidity.

51. Chugh R, Wathen JK, Patel SR, et al: Efficacy of imatinib in aggressive fibromatosis: Results of a phase II multicenter Sarcoma Alliance for Research through Collaboration (SARC) trial. *Clin Cancer Res* 2010;16(19): 4884-4891.

 The results of a prospective phase II trial investigating the use of imatinib, a tyrosine kinase inhibitor, demonstrate a 1-year, progression-free survival of 66%. This result warrants further study of imatinib in the treatment of this difficult tumor. Level of evidence: II.

52. Lazar AJ, Hajibashi S, Lev D: Desmoid tumor: From surgical extirpation to molecular dissection. *Curr Opin Oncol* 2009;21(4):352-359.

53. Fletcher CD: The evolving classification of soft tissue tumours: An update based on the new WHO classification. *Histopathology* 2006;48(1):3-12.

54. Hirota S, Isozaki K, Moriyama Y, et al: Gain-of-function mutations of c-kit in human gastrointestinal stromal tumors. *Science* 1998;279(5350):577-580.

55. van der Graaf WT, Blay JY, Chawla SP, et al: Pazopanib for metastatic soft-tissue sarcoma (PALETTE): A randomised, double-blind, placebo-controlled phase 3 trial. *Lancet* 2012;379(9829):1879-1886.

 A phase III study investigated the effect of pazopanib on progression-free survival in patients with metastatic nonadipocytic soft-tissue sarcoma after failure of standard chemotherapy. Median progression free survival was significantly improved, suggesting pazopanib is a reasonable treatment option in this group of patients. Level of evidence: I.

56. Chawla SP, Staddon AP, Baker LH, et al: Phase II study of the mammalian target of rapamycin inhibitor ridaforolimus in patients with advanced bone and soft tissue sarcomas. *J Clin Oncol* 2012;30(1):78-84.

 This study is a multicenter, open-label, single-arm study phase II trial investigating the activity of ridaforolimus in patients with metastatic or unresectable bone or soft-tissue sarcomas, demonstrating favorable progression-free survival rates. Further study of this agent is warranted. Level of evidence: II.

57. West RB, Rubin BP, Miller MA, et al: A landscape effect in tenosynovial giant-cell tumor from activation of CSF1 expression by a translocation in a minority of tumor cells. *Proc Natl Acad Sci U S A* 2006;103(3):690-695.

58. Horoschak M, Tran PT, Bachireddy P, et al: External beam radiation therapy enhances local control in pigmented villonodular synovitis. *Int J Radiat Oncol Biol Phys* 2009;75(1):183-187.

59. Temple HT: Pigmented villonodular synovitis therapy with MSCF-1 inhibitors. *Curr Opin Oncol* 2012;24(4): 404-408.

 CSF-1 inhibition in the treatment of PVNS is reviewed.

60. Cassier PA, Gelderblom H, Stacchiotti S, et al: Efficacy of imatinib mesylate for the treatment of locally advanced and/or metastatic tenosynovial giant cell tumor/pigmented villonodular synovitis. *Cancer* 2012;118(6): 1649-1655.

2: Systemic Disorders

The results of the initial clinical trial using CSF-1 inhibition therapy in treatment of PVNS are reviewed. Level of evidence: III.

61. Dotan A, Dadia S, Bickels J, et al: Expandable endoprosthesis for limb-sparing surgery in children: Long-term results. *J Child Orthop* 2010;4(5):391-400.

In a retrospective study, the authors found that noninvasive expandable endoprostheses or biologic reconstruction can be used to reduce the number of surgeries in children with bone sarcomas.

62. Abraham JA: Recent advances in navigation-assisted musculoskeletal tumor resection. *Curr Orthop Pract* 2011;22(4):297-302.

Current advances in musculoskeletal tumor resection include improved precision of a planned resection or precise matching of a reconstruction to a resction defect.

63. Minn AJ, Bevilacqua E, Yun J, Rosner MR: Identification of novel metastasis suppressor signaling pathways for breast cancer. *Cell Cycle* 2012;11(13):2452-2457.

Metastasis suppressor pathways in breast cancer are reviewed.

64. Yao Y, Fang ZP, Chen H, et al: HGFK1 inhibits bone metastasis in breast cancer through the TAK1/p38 MAPK signaling pathway. *Cancer Gene Ther* 2012; 19(9):601-608.

A molecular study demonstrated that HGFK1 significantly inhibits the metastasis of breast cancer to bone by activating the TAK1/p38 MAPK signaling pathway and inhibiting RANK expression, making it a metastasis suppressor gene.

65. Zhang C, Tan C, Ding H, Xin T, Jiang Y: Selective VEGFR inhibitors for anticancer therapeutics in clinical use and clinical trials. *Curr Pharm Des* 2012;18(20): 2921-2935.

Antiangiogenic therapy in tumor growth and metastasis is reviewed.

66. Sterling JA, Edwards JR, Martin TJ, Mundy GR: Advances in the biology of bone metastasis: How the skeleton affects tumor behavior. *Bone* 2011;48(1):6-15.

The authors reviewed the current understanding of metastasis development in bone.

67. Coluzzi F, Di Bussolo E, Mandatori I, Mattia C: Bone metastatic disease: Taking aim at new therapeutic targets. *Curr Med Chem* 2011;18(20):3093-3115.

A review of new therapeutic targets for metastatic bone disease is presented.

68. Lipton A, Theriault RL, Hortobagyi GN, et al: Pamidronate prevents skeletal complications and is effective palliative treatment in women with breast carcinoma and osteolytic bone metastases: Long term follow-up of two randomized, placebo-controlled trials. *Cancer* 2000;88(5):1082-1090.

69. Banffy MB, Vrahas MS, Ready JE, Abraham JA: Nonoperative versus prophylactic treatment of bisphosphonate-associated femoral stress fractures. *Clin Orthop Relat Res* 2011;469(7):2028-2034.

A retrospective review evaluated the nonsurgical management of bisphosphonate-associated stress fractures of the subtrochanteric femur. In 83% of the nonsurgical patients, complete fractures occurred within 10 months, bolstering the argument for the prophylactic surgical management of these stress fractures. Level of evidence: IV.

70. Martin M, Bell R, Bourgeois H, et al: Bone-related complications and quality of life in advanced breast cancer: Results from a randomized phase III trial of denosumab versus zoledronic acid. *Clin Cancer Res* 2012;18(17): 4841-4849.

A secondary study of results from a randomized, double-blind, phase III trial demonstrated superiority of denosumab to zoledronic acid in decreasing skeletal-related events in metastatic breast cancer. This study demonstrated maintained health related quality of life and reduced bone complications with denosumab use. Level of evidence: I.

71. Leong NL, Anderson ME, Gebhardt MC, Snyder BD: Computed tomography-based structural analysis for predicting fracture risk in children with benign skeletal neoplasms: Comparison of specificity with that of plain radiographs. *J Bone Joint Surg Am* 2010;92(9):1827-1833.

This study details a method of quantifying the structural integrity of remaining bone in the setting of a benign skeletal lesion using CT, allowing an improved assessment of fracture risk when compared with evaluation by plain radiography, with 97% specificity. Level of evidence: I.

72. Steensma M, Boland PJ, Morris CD, Athanasian E, Healey JH: Endoprosthetic treatment is more durable for pathologic proximal femur fractures. *Clin Orthop Relat Res* 2012;470(3):920-926.

A retrospective review of 298 patients with pathologic proximal femur fractures shows a lower treatment failure rate in the endoprosthetic replacement group when compared with the intramedullary nailing group and the open reduction and internal fixation group. Level of evidence: III.

Chapter 23

Orthopaedic Infections

Jonathon K. Salava, MD   Bryan D. Springer, MD

Introduction

Infections of the musculoskeletal system can involve bone, soft tissue, and implant-related material. The development of a musculoskeletal infection can be associated with substantial morbidity and mortality and has significant financial implications to the healthcare system. Data indicate that infections of the musculoskeletal system are on the rise, and several factors are at play, including multidrug-resistant bacteria as well as poor host factors that can either predispose patients to infection and/or limit their ability to fight infection. Prevention and optimizing the environment to diminish the risk of infection are paramount to decrease the burden of an orthopaedic infection.

Surgical Site Infections: The Scope of the Problem

The Centers for Disease Control and Prevention (CDC) defines a surgical site infection (SSI) as one that occurs within 30 days of a surgical procedure or within 1 year of a surgical procedure if a material device (hardware or total joint prosthesis) has been implanted.[1] These infections are further classified as either superficial (involving the skin and subcutaneous tissue around the incision) or deep (involving fascia, muscle, bone, or the implant). Recent data by the CDC estimate that more than 300,000 SSIs are reported annually in the United States. These infections, the most common of which are hospital-acquired or nosocomial infections, result in significant morbidity, mortality, and financial strain to the healthcare system.[2]

The sequelae of an SSI often results in further surgery, longer hospitalization, increased complications, and poorer outcomes compared with patients in whom infections do not develop. The annual direct and indirect costs associated with an SSI exceed $1 billion and $10 billion, respectively, in the United States.[3] Patients in whom a SSI develops are five times more likely to be readmitted to the hospital and have double the mortality rate of patients who do not have a SSI. Because of the significant financial and detrimental patient-related outcomes for those in whom a SSI develops, much attention has been given to prevention. There are three main areas of prevention: optimization of the patient or host optimization, the type of organism, and environmental (hospital and operating room) protection (**Figure 1**). Each factor will be discussed in further detail, but the important relationship of each factor to the others should be recognized.

Surgical Care Improvement Project

In an effort to reduce the incidence of SSI, best-care practice guidelines have been implemented nationally. In response to inconsistent compliance with previous infection prevention measures, the Centers for Medicare and Medicaid Services collaborated with the CDC to develop the Surgical Care Improvement Project (SCIP). The goals of these guidelines were to reduce the incidence of SSI by 25% through the year 2012 as well as provide standard quality measures and track standards of care.[4] Six of the 10 core measures of the SCIP involve perioperative care to reduce the incidence of SSI; these six measures are listed in **Table 1**. Evidence

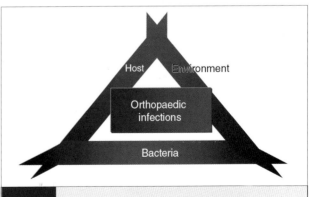

Figure 1	Interaction of the host, the environment, and bacteria all play a critical role in the development of orthopaedic infections.

Dr. Springer or an immediate family member is a member of a speakers' bureau or has made paid presentations on behalf of DePuy and serves as a paid consultant to or is an employee of Stryker and Convatec Surgical. Neither Dr. Salava nor any immediate family member has received anything of value from or has stock or stock options held in a commercial company or institution related directly or indirectly to the subject of this chapter.

Table 1

Surgical Care Improvement Project (SCIP) Guidelines That Relate to Infections

SCIP-1	Antibiotics within 1 hour of incision (2 hours for vancomycin)
SCIP-2	Receive prophylactic antibiotics consistent with recommendations
SCIP-3	Prophylactic antibiotics discontinued within 24 hours of surgery
SCIP-4	Control 6 am serum postoperative glucose
SCIP-6	Appropriate hair removal
SCIP-9	Urinary catheter removal on postoperative day 1

exists that implementation and adherence to these guidelines reduces the risk of SSIs.[5] In 2013, financial disincentives also will be applied to hospitals that do not follow and document adherence to the core measures of the SCIP guidelines.

The Microbiology of Orthopaedic Infections

The type of organism that results in a musculoskeletal infection depends on the site of the infection as well as the mechanism by which the infection was introduced. Certain types of infections are uniquely associated with certain types of organisms (for example, foot puncture wounds and *Pseudomonas*). In the overwhelming majority of orthopaedic infections, however, the underlying organism is an endogenous resident of the patient's normal skin and/or nasal flora. *Staphylococcus aureus* remains the most common organism in orthopaedic infections, accounting for up to 80% of infections. *Staphylococcus epidermidis* is the most common implant-related infection.

Recently, there has been a substantial increase in resistant bacteria, particularly methicillin-resistant *S aureus* (MRSA).[6] The cited increase in the incidence of MRSA-related infections has been attributed to the spurious use of antibiotics, poor healthcare-associated hygiene, and elective and nonelective orthopaedic surgery in immunocompromised patients. The expression of a penicillin-binding protein (PBP2a) is encoded on the *mec A* gene of *S aureus* and confers resistance to the entire antibiotic class of penicillins.

Initially only a hospital-acquired infection, MRSA has become increasingly prevalent in the community and, as a result, has been subclassified into community-acquired MRSA (CA-MRSA) and healthcare-acquired MRSA (HA-MRSA). CA-MRSA has been estimated to be present in approximately 1.3% of the general population.[6] Because it carries a gene associated with leukocidin, it has the ability to cause lysis of neutrophils, often resulting in severe soft-tissue infections. HA-MRSA generally affects chronically ill patients and those who require indwelling catheters.

MRSA has an affinity for the nares, and colonization with MRSA in the nasal passages has been shown to increase the risk of infection in patients undergoing surgery. In addition, the screening, detection, and decolonization of patients who are carriers of MRSA has been shown to reduce the associated infection risk.[7] Many institutions now routinely screen patients for nasal carriage of *S aureus* and MRSA and implement a decolonization protocol consisting of mupirocin ointment and chlorhexidine baths before surgery.

Bacterial Biofilms

Most orthopaedic infections are caused by bacteria that produce biofilm.[8] All bacteria are capable of producing a biofilm, which is a defensive and protective mechanism for bacteria to communicate and thrive on the host tissue and implants. A biofilm is further defined as a structured collection of bacteria encased in a self-produced matrix. Biofilms are resistant to antibiotics, disinfectants, phagocytosis, and other components of the host defense immune system.[9] Biofilm-associated bacterial infections are up to 100 times more resistant to antibiotics than infections that are not associated with a biofilm-producing bacteria. This resistance, however, is different from MRSA and other genetically adapted infections in that it appears to be a mechanical and metabolic resistance of the biofilm itself.

The mechanisms by which bacteria form and function in a biofilm are quite complex and only partially understood[10] (Figure 2). Biofilm formation begins with the attachment of bacterial cells to the substrate (implant or bone). The cells then aggregate and form multiple layers, secreting a protective layer or glycocalyx. The protective layer renders the cells immune to host defense mechanisms and antibiotics. After the biofilm matures, cells can detach from the biofilm and become planktonic in the surrounding milieu. This planktonic state initiates a new cycle of biofilm formation elsewhere. In addition, it appears that biofilm-associated bacteria have a unique ability to communicate with each other and provide information on nutrition and the surrounding environment that allows for safe replication and spread of the biofilm. The cell-to-cell communication also allows for the potential development of therapeutic agents aimed at preventing communication and proliferation of biofilm on materials.

The diagnosis and treatment of biofilm-associated infections can be challenging. Many biofilm-associated infections develop months or years after damage or seeding has occurred (such as after surgery). Because of the protective biofilm colony that has formed on the prosthesis or bone, traditional means of diagnosis, such as joint aspiration, often fail to yield positive cultures. There is concern, particularly regarding implant-related failures, that many causes of aseptic loosening may, in fact, be undetected septic failures caused by biofilm-related infections.

Clinically, biofilm-associated infections often remain localized, develop slowly, and rarely elicit a significant

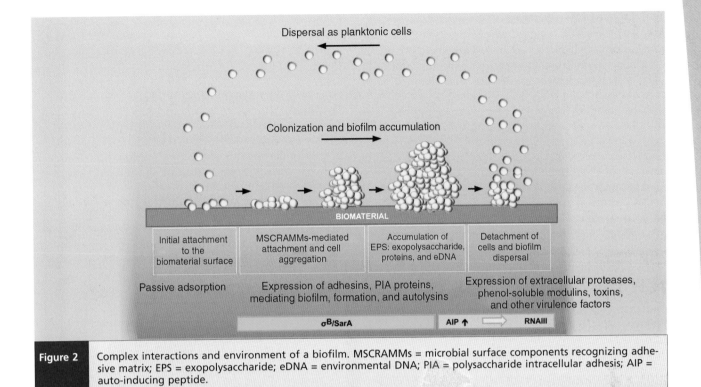

Figure 2 Complex interactions and environment of a biofilm. MSCRAMMs = microbial surface components recognizing adhesive matrix; EPS = exopolysaccharide; eDNA = environmental DNA; PIA = polysaccharide intracellular adhesis; AIP = auto-inducing peptide.

systemic response. In addition, although antibiotics can be effective against a planktonic bacterial state, they remain ineffective in curing the infection because the antibiotics cannot kill the bacteria associated with the biofilm. Thus, acute biofilm-related infections become chronic, and these chronic infections, such as periprosthetic joint infections or osteomyelitis, are the prototypical biofilm-associated infections. Eradication of these biofilm-associated infections therefore require aggressive removal of the implant material and dead bone along with sufficient high-dose antibiotics to kill planktonic bacteria and prevent the reformation of biofilm.

One of the pivotal concepts in the future treatment of biofilm-associated infections is based on the fact that bacteria are present in the surgical field from biofilm on the surfaces of bone and implants. The development of antibiofilm protective layers on prosthetic devices or antimicrobial-laden implants is the focus of much attention and research in the prevention and treatment of biofilm-related infections.

Environmental Factors Associated With Orthopaedic Infections

Most SSIs are a result of a patient's own resident skin flora, and multiple measures are in place to minimize contamination, including appropriate hand washing, antibiotic prophylaxis, surgical prep, and limiting surgical duration. Airborne bacteria in the surgical environment, however, are also associated with increased infection risk. Maximizing the physical environment and monitoring and modifying operating room behavior are two ways to limit the presence of airborne bacteria in the operating room.

Operating Room Behavior

Human behavior within the operating room has a direct link to the number of bacteria present in the environment. The microbial level in the operating room is directly related to the number of people present as well as their movement. Humans not only are reservoirs for bacteria but also shed bacteria from the skin that can attach to inanimate objects in the operating room or rapidly become airborne. These airborne bacteria then act as a source of bacterial contamination or infection.

Humans shed bacteria at different rates, and males tend to have higher shed rates than females. Thus, the number of personnel in the operating room has a direct link to the number of bacteria present in the environment, and all attempts should be made to limit the number of personnel in the operating room to only those essential to the procedure.

In addition to the number of people in the operating room, their movement within and while entering and exiting the operating room creates turbulent airflow that allows bacteria to become airborne and potentially contaminate the wound. Each time the operating room door opens during a case, the positive pressure ventilation is disrupted, limiting the effectiveness of the operating room ventilation system.[11] These factors have led the CDC to issue guidelines to limit the number of people in the operating room, minimize movement, and limit the number of door openings.[1]

2: Systemic Disorders

The Operating Room Setup

It is inevitable that bacteria will be present in the operating room environment. The three main components currently used to minimize or eliminate bacterial burden in the operating room are laminar airflow, ultraviolet light, and body exhaust suits.[12]

Most modern operating rooms are equipped with positive pressure airflow. The addition of laminar airflow allows this positive forced air to pass through a high-efficiency particle air filter to minimize the amount of airborne matter in the operating room.[13] Two laminar airflow systems, vertical and horizontal, are in current use. For laminar airflow to be effective, its path should not be obstructed. Horizontal laminar airflow forces air in a horizontal direction across the surgical site. The main limitation of horizontal airflow is the disruption of that laminar flow by personnel in the room creating turbulent flow. Vertical airflow allows filtered laminar air to be passed from the ceiling above the operating table. It is most effective when a Plexiglas shield surrounds the surgical team to minimize disruption of laminar airflow.

Numerous studies have shown the ability of ultraviolet light to diminish bacterial concentrations in the operating room and thus decrease infection rates.[14] One study demonstrated a 4.5-fold greater odds of infection in knee procedures performed without the use of ultraviolet light compared with those procedures for which ultraviolet light was used.[15]

Although ultraviolet light is simple to use and cost effective compared with other modalities, environmental concerns are associated with its use. Exposure can lead to conjunctivitis and eye damage as well as the development of skin erythema after as little as 15 minutes of exposure. It is recommended that the intensity of the ultraviolet light be kept to 25-30 $\mu W\ cm^{-2}\ S^{-1}$ to prevent overexposure. In addition, all personnel in the room should ensure that eyes and skin have appropriate protection.[16]

The use of body exhaust suits in the operating room to reduce SSIs is controversial. Exhaust suits increase the sterile coverage of the people wearing them while using paper filters to reduce the bacterial load from the operating team. The amount of reduction in bacterial load with the use of body exhaust suits has been questioned, with some studies demonstrating no reduction in bacterial counts, whereas others have shown reduction to 1 cfu/m^3. The overall reduction in infection with body exhaust suits has not been proven, and many question the cost-effectiveness of their routine use. A large study of the New Zealand registry recently found no benefit in using body exhaust suits, laminar airflow, or a combination of the two methods in reducing the rates of deep periprosthetic infection after total joint arthroplasty.[17]

The Host

The host defense system is critical in preventing and fighting infections. Many disease states alter or significantly reduce the ability of the host to fight or prevent infection, thus placing these patients at increased risk for infection. Comorbid conditions are cumulative, and each comorbid condition associated with infection increases the risk of infection by 35%. Many patients are in suboptimal health at the time leading up to surgery. Many of these disease states are modifiable, and every effort should be made to optimize the host immune system by diminishing or eliminating these modifiable conditions (**Figure 3**). Eliminating or diminishing modifiable risk factors should decrease the overall risk for the development of a deep periprosthetic infection. Three common modifiable risk factors are diabetes, obesity, and malnutrition.

Diabetes

Diabetes is associated with multiple comorbid health conditions, and affected patients have a higher complication rate and longer hospital stays after surgery. Poorly controlled diabetes (Hgb A1C > 7) and perioperative hyperglycemia thwart the ability of white blood cells to eliminate bacterial contamination. Multiple studies have shown increased rates of infection in patients with poorly controlled diabetes or perioperative hyperglycemia undergoing traumatic or elective total joint arthroplasty.

Obesity

Obesity has reached epidemic proportions in the United States. Obese patients have an increased risk of infection secondary to longer surgical times, greater surgical dissections, poorly vascularized subcutaneous tissue, a high calorie but nutritionally poor diet, inadequate antibiotic prophylaxis that is often not properly adjusted for weight, and a pathologic relationship with type II diabetes. Several studies have shown an increased risk of deep infection in obese patients after total joint arthroplasty.[18,19] Whenever possible, a patient's weight should be optimized through education, counseling, and (occasionally) surgical intervention in an attempt to decrease the risk of infection.

Malnutrition

Some groups of patients are at risk for malnutrition, including elderly patients, those with gastrointestinal disorders or cancer, and patients who abuse alcohol. It has been reported that malnourished patients had a five to seven times greater risk of infection after total joint arthroplasty than those who are not malnourished.[20] Simple blood tests before surgery can help screen patients at risk for malnutrition. Malnutrition is indicated by a total lymphocyte count less than 1,500 cells/mm³, a serum albumin level of less than 3.5 g/dL, or a transferrin level less than 200 mg/dL. Patients with preoperative malnutrition should be counseled, and strategies should be implemented to improve nutritional intake before surgery.

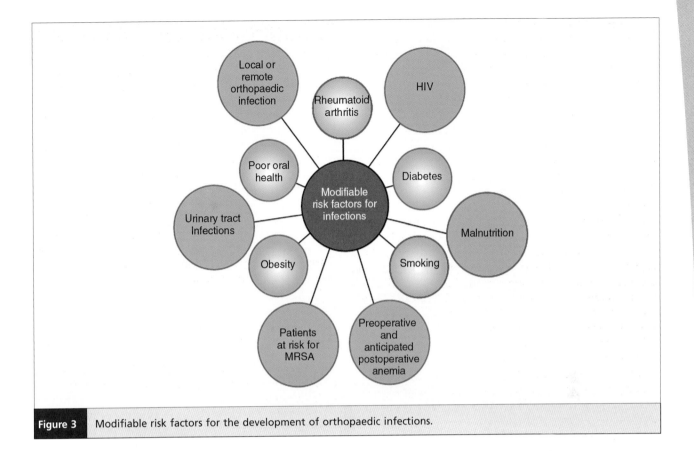

Figure 3   Modifiable risk factors for the development of orthopaedic infections.

Musculoskeletal Infection Conditions

Adult Osteomyelitis

Diagnosis

Early diagnosis of adult osteomyelitis can be crucial to patient outcomes. The diagnosis can typically be made based on the history and the physical examination alone. Therefore, it becomes important to have a high level of suspicion early on in caring for an adult patient with osteomyelitis, and several additional evaluation tools are at the surgeon's disposal to confirm, or facilitate, the diagnosis.

Laboratory evaluation is a useful tool in the workup for osteomyelitis because of its rapid results, its high sensitivity, and the ability to monitor trends. Basic serum tests typically include a white blood cell (WBC) count, erythrocyte sedimentation rate (ESR), and C-reactive protein (CRP) level. Although the WBC count is obtained routinely, it remains a poor indicator of bone infection and is not helpful in confirming or excluding osteomyelitis.[21] The CRP level and the ESR are often elevated in both acute and chronic osteomyelitis, and elevated levels of either or both should significantly raise suspicion for a diagnosis of osteomyelitis. When suspicion or the number of risk factors is low, then a normal CRP level and ESR should reassure the physician that further investigation is likely not necessary. Finally, in cases in which the suspicions of the provider conflict with the serum markers, further investigation is required.

Few additional serum markers have been evaluated as adjuncts to current laboratory testing for osteomyelitis. Leukergy and polymorphonuclear (PMN) neutrophil esterase have been mentioned in the past but have not been extensively studied nor implemented into routine practice. A more recently identified marker of possible bacterial infection is serum procalcitonin (PCT). Although the ESR and the CRP level may be more sensitive tests for osteomyelitis, PCT has potential utility in differentiating it from other noninfectious inflammatory conditions.[22,23] Although elevations of PCT are seen in such conditions, as well as trauma, its induction is lower compared with its specific induction by bacterial infections. PCT and the CRP level both have the ability to normalize rapidly following treatment and are useful in monitoring the effectiveness of treatment.

Beyond laboratory evaluation, several imaging modalities may prove to be useful in diagnosing and evaluating osteomyelitis. Conventional radiography is useful both at presentation and follow-up. Soft-tissue swelling, joint space narrowing/widening, periosteal reaction, and bone destruction may be present. It is important to remember that radiographic findings may lag 1 to 3 weeks behind the underlying pathology.[24] Ultrasound has limited use in the workup for osteomyelitis but may be useful in detecting abscess formation. CT is useful for detecting sequestrum and can sometimes demonstrate abscesses. MRI is highly sensitive and can demonstrate infectious changes to cortical bone, the medullary canal, and surrounding soft tissues

Table 2

Seven-Item Classification System

Clinical Presentation	Etiopathogenesis	Anatomy Pathology	Host Type/Age	Microorganism	Bone Defect	Soft-Tissue Defect
Acute early	Hematogenous	Rachis	$A_{a,c,i}$	Gram positive	1	0
Subacute delayed	Vasculopathy/neuropathy	Hand	$B_{a,c,i}$	Gram negative	2	cm^2
Chronic late	Trauma	Long bones	$C_{a,c,i}$	Mixed flora and/or multiresistant	3A, 3B, 3C	cm^2 B
	Temporary implant	Stage 1				
	ICS classification	Stage 2				
	Type I	Stage 3		Mycobacterium		
	Type II	Stage 4		Fungi		
	Type III	Foot		Negative		
	Permanent implant	Joint				

B = exposed bone.

as early as 2 to 3 weeks before radiographs.[25] The triphase bone scan is a sensitive test that can differentiate osteomyelitis from cellulitis, but its specificity is low. Leukocyte scintigraphy (with technetium Tc-99m or indium 111) has demonstrated increased specificity compared with a bone scan, but because of loss of sensitivity in the axial skeleton, it is recommended for use only in diagnosing chronic osteomyelitis in the appendicular skeleton. Fluorodeoxyglucose positron emission tomography (FDG-PET) has been shown to be the most sensitive technique for detecting chronic osteomyelitis, and it has greater specificity than MRI and scintigraphy, especially in the axial skeleton.[26]

The mainstay of diagnosis is the tissue sample. Although open wounds and sinus tracts are frequently sampled, they are not as reliable as bone specimens. Ideally, microbiologic diagnosis should be made with bone biopsy obtained before the initiation of antibiotic therapy. Direct bone biopsies can yield the infecting organism in 60% to 70% of needle biopsies and 90% of open biopsies. Biopsy tissue should be sent for aerobic and anaerobic cultures, and in certain scenarios, fungal and mycobacterial cultures as well. Blood cultures may also identify the organism in up to 60% of cases.

Treatment

After a diagnosis of osteomyelitis is made, treatment planning should address the goals of treatment while taking into account the extent of disease and the host's ability to handle the infection. The goal of treatment strategies includes eradication of the infection while a stable weight-bearing limb with normal mechanical axis, muscle action, and joint function is maintained. To help guide this treatment process, several classification systems have been developed, each including one or two clinical conditions. Recently, a Seven-Item Comprehensive Classification System was proposed as a more comprehensive method of describing all the relevant features of bone and joint infections[27] (Table 2). After the scope of disease and host factors are

appreciated, appropriate treatment includes thorough drainage/débridement, the elimination of dead spaces, wound protection, possible stabilization, and antimicrobial coverage. Drainage and débridement are performed down to healthy/viable bone, such that punctate bleeding is seen (paprika sign). If débridement leaves large dead spaces, then antibiotic-impregnated beads can be placed and subsequently removed after 4 to 6 weeks. Polymethyl methacrylate beads are the standard delivery agent for local antibiotics. Recent literature has demonstrated that antibiotic-impregnated bone graft substitutes, such as calcium phosphate or calcium sulfate, are just as effective in eradicating infection but require fewer surgeries after placement because of their bioabsorbable properties.[28] Dead space management also includes local or free tissue flaps and cancellous bone grafting from the iliac crest. Stabilization and soft-tissue coverage, whether it be split-thickness grafts for small defects or muscle flaps for larger defects, may also be necessary.

Beyond surgical treatment, antimicrobial therapy is also necessary for controlling and eradicating the infection. After an adequate specimen is obtained, a parenteral antibiotic regimen is initiated and targeted toward the likely pathogen. Following identification of the organism, specific antibiotics can be chosen based on the sensitivities. These are typically continued for 4 to 6 weeks beyond the final débridement, allowing for coverage of the bone with vascular soft tissue and organism eradication. Antibiotic therapy should be done in consultation with an infectious disease specialist.

Pediatric Osteomyelitis

Osteomyelitis is relatively common in children and, along with septic arthritis, accounts for up to 6 of every 1,000 pediatric hospital admissions yearly.[29] It commonly presents as an acute hematogenous process as a result of the high vascularity of growing long bones. Osteomyelitis can affect any child, regardless of health status, and is associated with dire consequences in severe cases. Therefore, the changing trends in both diagnosis and management must be recognized.

Recent studies have illustrated the changing patterns of osteomyelitis in children. *S aureus* and *Streptococcus* species are the most common pathogens, with CA-MRSA now accounting for approximately 30% to 40% of cases.[29] As seen with other types of infections, osteomyelitis caused by CA-MRSA tends to be more severe, resulting in longer hospital stays and more procedures.[30] *Haemophilus influenzae*, which has been a common etiology of osteomyelitis in the past, has become increasingly rare with the *H influenzae* type B vaccine. *Kingella kingae* has become a common fastidious pathogen in younger children, just as it has in pediatric septic arthritis.[31]

Diagnosis

In addition to symptoms and clinical findings, several laboratory markers and imaging modalities are available to assist in the diagnosis of osteoarticular infections. A WBC count is commonly obtained but may be normal in greater than 50% of cases.[32] ESR and the CRP level are also obtained, and if these are elevated (ESR > 20 mm/h, CRP > 20 mg/L), they have demonstrated superior sensitivity for osteomyelitis (94% and 95%, respectively, and 98% when combined).[33] Radiographs are not as effective as other modalities in diagnosis. MRI is the most accurate, with sensitivity and specificity much higher than radiographs or scintigraphy.[34] Some centers also use serial MRI scans in routine follow-up, but repeating these studies is useful only when patients do not respond to therapy appropriately.[35]

After the diagnosis of osteomyelitis is made, tissue is typically obtained via biopsy or aspiration for further analysis. In stable patients, cultures should ideally be performed before the administration of antibiotics. In addition to standard cultures, the tissue specimen should be inoculated into blood culture system bottles to culture *K kingae*. The development of specific polymerase chain reaction (PCR) assays has also facilitated the diagnosis of *K kingae* osteoarticular infections when routine cultures were negative.[36] In addition to identifying rare pathogens, broad-range PCR also allows for more rapid microbe identification.[37]

Treatment

The treatment of osteomyelitis in children routinely includes antibiotics and possibly surgical drainage. When deciding on empiric antibiotic therapy, the strong emergence of CA-MRSA must be taken into consideration. There has been an increase in the use of antibiotics with activity against MRSA, such as clindamycin and vancomycin.[38] Additional antibiotics with MRSA coverage used in pediatric osteomyelitis include linezolid, daptomycin, and two new cephalosporins: ceftaroline and ceftobiprole. As with septic arthritis, the duration of treatment continues to be debated. Recent data suggest that earlier transition to oral antibiotics and shorter overall antibiotic courses may not result in increased rates of treatment failure, particularly in non-MRSA cases.[39]

Adult Septic Arthritis

Diagnosis

As with all bone and joint infections, the clinical presentation of septic arthritis may be quite variable and even masked by other comorbid medical conditions. Prompt and accurate diagnosis requires a high level of suspicion. The distribution of patients affected by septic arthritis is bimodal, with a younger, sexually active group with gonococcal septic arthritis and the elderly or immunocompromised group with nongonococcal organisms. Presenting symptoms typically include rapid onset of pain, limited weight bearing and motion, and a warm joint with effusion and erythema. It is important to remember that fever and other systemic symptoms are not always present.

Laboratory and radiologic evaluation are imperative in the early workup for septic arthritis. WBC count, CRP level, and ESR are typically obtained early in the presentation. The leukocyte count may be normal in up to half of patients, whereas CRP level and ESR are almost always elevated. As mentioned previously, PCT may have a role in differentiating a pyogenic bacterial infection from other inflammatory conditions that may present as arthritis.[40] Serum should also be sent for blood cultures when septic arthritis is suspected because it may provide the only evidence of infection in up to 9% of cases.[41] Orthogonal radiographs can rule out any bony involvement, assess for joint space narrowing/widening, and identify any potential hardware in and around the joint. If there is concern about bony involvement, MRI provides an excellent assessment of the periarticular bone and soft tissues.

Joint aspiration is the most powerful tool for diagnosing septic arthritis and identifying the infectious agent. Aspiration should be performed before the administration of antibiotics. Synovial fluid gross properties are noted, and the aspirate should be sent for analyses, including cell count with differential, cultures (aerobic, anaerobic, fungal, and mycobacterial), and crystal analysis. The thresholds for septic arthritis commonly used for synovial fluid are greater than 50,000 leukocytes/µL and greater than 75% PMN leukocytes. Beyond standard culture protocols, some data suggest that direct inoculation of blood culture vials may significantly improve the detection of infection.[42] Finally, recent research has outlined the potential usefulness of PCR analysis of synovial fluid in identifying difficult pathogens in septic arthritis.[43]

Treatment

The ideal management of septic arthritis is focused on the initiation of appropriate antibiotic therapy in addition to drainage of the affected joint(s). Antibiotics should not be administered until aspiration is performed, but once administration is completed, empiric therapy should be initiated. *S aureus* and *Streptococcus* species represent the most common organisms, and ini-

2: Systemic Disorders

tial empiric antibiotics should be active against these microbes. Vancomycin is most commonly used against CA-MRSA and HA-MRSA. There is growing concern, however, regarding vancomycin resistance, such as the glycoprotein-intermediate S aureus strain.[44] Newer antibiotics such linezolid and daptomycin have already shown promise in the treatment of bone and joint infections. Others, such as ceftaroline and ceftobiprole, have also shown increased activity against MRSA and may have a role in empiric therapy. In high-risk patients, or if gram-negative bacilli are found in the synovial aspirate, a third-generation cephalosporin, such as ceftriaxone, should be added to the empiric regimen. In younger patients at risk of disseminated gonococcal infection, ceftriaxone alone may be adequate empiric treatment.

After an organism is identified, the treatment should be microbe specific. Antibiotics are typically administered parenterally for at least 1 to 2 weeks, with conversion to an active, bioavailable oral therapy if possible. Unfortunately, there is a paucity of controlled, prospective data, particularly in adult septic arthritis, regarding the best duration of antibiotics and when oral administration should begin. The only exception is for the treatment of Neisseria gonorrhoeae, for which a 1-week course of a third-generation cephalosporin is indicated.

Although no randomized controlled studies have thoroughly evaluated the modes of joint decompression, it is typically recommended. Drainage of the joint lessens the burden of infection by decreasing bacterial load, toxin levels, and PMN proteases. Options include serial arthrocentesis, arthroscopic lavage, or arthrotomy with or without synovectomy. If adequate aspiration cannot be performed, or if the joint (such as the hip) is not readily accessible, then either arthroscopic or open lavage is necessary. The optimal mode of drainage should ultimately be tailored to the patient and available resources.

Pediatric Septic Arthritis

Pediatric articular infection is a potentially devastating condition that must be ruled out in children with joint pain. The most common organisms are S aureus and Streptococcus species.[45] The incidence of H influenzae septic arthritis, however, has decreased because of the success of the H influenzae type B vaccine.[46] CA-MRSA is a common pathogen with increased virulence, and K kingae has recently been identified as a common cause of pediatric septic arthritis.[29]

Diagnosis

The tenets of diagnosis have largely remained unchanged in recent years, but newer diagnostic tools and algorithms have been introduced. The history and physical examination are mainstays in the evaluation and the workup for a septic joint. Most children present with localized pain, limited range of motion, and difficulty with weight bearing or use of an extremity (pseudoparalysis). Laboratory studies, along with the clinical evaluation, have been shown to be effective in differentiating septic arthritis from similar conditions, such as transient synovitis. Four criteria (fever ≥ 38.5° C, inability to bear weight, ESR > 40 mm/h, and leukocytosis > 12 × 10⁹ cells/L) have been developed for predicting the probability of septic arthritis (3% for one predictor, 40% for two, 93% for three, and 99.6% when all four criteria were present).[47] Despite validation in a similar follow-up population, others have not been able to demonstrate as high a level of predictability.[48] More recently, CRP level has been used to further distinguish septic arthritis from transient synovitis. A CRP level greater than 20 mg/L alone has been shown to be a strong independent risk factor for septic arthritis.[49] In combination with other criteria, it becomes an even stronger predictor of bacterial articular infection.[43,49]

Several imaging modalities are routinely used in the workup for a septic pediatric joint. Radiographs of the affected joint should always be obtained, but they are frequently negative. Ultrasound can be used with relatively high sensitivity and specificity while assessing for an effusion in suspected cases.[50,51] If seen, the fluid may then be aspirated under image guidance. MRI is also extremely sensitive and specific in differentiating septic arthritis from transient synovitis.[52] Findings in transient synovitis include contralateral effusion and the absence of bone marrow abnormalities. In septic arthritis, one would expect to find marrow changes with signal alterations and/or contrast enhancement of the soft tissues.[53] Finally, a bone scan may be useful in multifocal disease.

Treatment

As in adult septic arthritis, treatment in children includes decreasing the bacterial load and the administration of antibiotics. Initially and ideally before antibiotic administration, the joint is aspirated, with a synovial WBC count greater than 50,000 cells/mL typically indicative of septic arthritis. Decompression of the joint by aspiration plus irrigation has been described, but it is more commonly accomplished with an open arthrotomy or arthroscopy.[54,55] Empiric antibiotic therapy is typically selected to cover common local pathogens and is started as soon as the diagnostic procedures are completed. Specific guidelines regarding the length of antibiotic administration are not available, but recent trends suggest intravenous antibiotics should be given until clinical improvement is seen, typically in 5 to 7 days in most patients. The transition should then be made to oral agents for approximately 4 weeks of therapy.[56] Evidence suggests that clinical course and outcomes are improved with a 4-day supplemental course of dexamethasone after antibiotics are started.[57] With the recent emergence of K kingae as a common pathogen in pediatric septic arthritis, attention has been directed toward its specific diagnosis and management. Pediatric osteoarticular infections caused by K kingae are typically characterized by milder symptoms, and patients are younger (age 4 years or younger) when compared with those with S aureus.[58] K kingae is a fas-

Table 3

Recommendations for Tetanus Immunizations

Age (Years)	History of Tetanus Immunization	Clean, Minor Wounds	All Other Wounds (Puncture Wounds Included)
0–6	Unknown or not up to date on DTaP	DTaP	DTaP and TIG
7–10	Unknown or incomplete DTaP	Tdap and DTaP catch-up dose	Tdap and TIG
11–64	Unknown or < 3 doses, or if > 5 years since last dose	Tdap	Tdap and TIG
≥ 65	Unknown or < 3 doses	Td or Tdap (if > 10 years since last dose)[a]	Td or Tdap[a] (if 5–10 years since last dose)

[a]Adults at least 65 years of age who have or who anticipate having close contact with an infant age < 12 months and who have not previously received Tdap should receive a single dose of Tdap to protect against pertussis and reduce the likelihood of transmission; all other adults at least 65 years of age who have not previously received Tdap may be given a single dose of Tdap instead of Td.

DTaP = acellular pertussis vaccine in combination with diphtheria and tetanus toxoids; Td = tetanus-diphtheria vaccine; Tdap = tetanus toxoid, reduced diphtheria toxoid, and acellular pertussis vaccine; TI6 = tetanus immune globulin.

(Reproduced with permission from Berlin R, Carrington S: Management of pedal puncture wounds. *Clin Podiatr Med Surg* 2012;29[3]:451-458.)

tidious organism with poor growth on routine solid culture, but culture yields have significantly improved with the use of aerobic blood culture vials or kits. Although not routinely available, PCR has also been used to accurately identify *K kingae*. This is particularly true with the real-time assay specific to the potent repeat-intoxin cytotoxin.[59] MRI has also proven to be effective in differentiating *K kingae*, as epiphyseal cartilage abscesses have been identified in only *K kingae* infections.[60] In addition to joint decompression, treatment with penicillin or cephalosporins is usually successful.

Foot Puncture Wounds

Diagnosis

Foot puncture wounds can occur at a variety of stages, from a plantar laceration to cellulitis, septic arthritis, or even osteomyelitis. These wounds are commonly sustained by children and adult laborers. They are most often caused by nails, but other materials such as wood, glass, plastic, and other metals can cause this type of injury.

There are several key considerations in the workup of a puncture wound to the foot. It is important to understand the mechanism of injury because high-pressure injection-type injuries may have a deeper penetration of foreign material into the foot, requiring surgical intervention. Footwear at the time of injury should also be considered because shoes with rubber soles tend to harbor *P aeruginosa* in their warm, moist environment. A comprehensive history is essential to assess for diabetes and/or peripheral neuropathy because of increased risk of infection and delay in recognition.[61] Establishing the patient's tetanus immunization history is imperative (**Table 3**). Delays in presentation beyond 48 hours have been associated with more complications.[62] The patient should be evaluated for the presence of foreign materials, debris, devitalized tissue, neurovascular status, motion, and signs of infection (swelling, erythema, warmth to touch, fluctuation, and/or drainage).

Laboratory and radiologic evaluation may also be of benefit. For uncomplicated puncture wounds, laboratory tests may not be indicated. In cases of suspected infection, standard inflammatory/infection markers (WBC count, CRP, and ESR) should be checked, but the more valuable laboratory data will likely come from deep tissue cultures. Conventional radiographs are useful for identifying foreign bodies, fractures, and possible bony changes secondary to infection. Sonography has demonstrated an excellent ability to visualize and rule out wooden foreign bodies.[63] MRI and scintigraphy may be useful if osteomyelitis is suspected. Realizing the anatomy and the mechanism of injury will help the provider understand the more complex damage underneath a puncture wound so that the appropriate imaging is performed to prevent complications, such as foreign body migration.[64]

Treatment

The treatment of foot puncture wounds can vary along with their presentation. More benign-appearing wounds can initially be treated with soaks, elevation, rest, and irrigation. If foreign material is detected or suspected, further irrigation and débridement is warranted. In simpler wounds, antibiotic therapy is controversial, but if indicated, common organisms such as *S aureus* and *Pseudomonas* should be covered. This includes first-generation cephalosporins for clean superficial wounds and antipseudomonal agents, such as ciprofloxacin or levofloxacin, for wounds that occur through shoes.

For patients with delayed presentation or with signs of infection, both antimicrobial and surgical treatment are more aggressive. Broad-spectrum empiric therapy should be started after a tissue culture is obtained and adjusted according to identification and sensitivities. Surgical exploration, usually in the operating room setting, is recommended for the removal of foreign bodies. Abscesses should be decompressed, and necrotic tissue débrided. Additional deep cultures and biopsies should

2: Systemic Disorders

be obtained intraoperatively. The wound is typically packed to allow further drainage, and the patient refrains from bearing weight. Antibiotic duration is not well established but should follow the patient's clinical course.

Other Considerations

Wound Closure and Open Fractures

Managing the soft-tissue envelope in the presence of an open fracture can present several challenges, such as the timing of wound closure, managing open wounds, and the development of infection in the presence of an open fracture. Many of the treatment suggestions have been based on clinical judgment, with little information in the literature to make definitive recommendations on when wounds should be closed. Several considerations, including grade and location of the fracture, high-energy versus low-energy injury, fracture contamination, soft-tissue envelope, and status of the host (other injuries, smoking, diabetes, obesity) must be taken into account when making decisions regarding soft-tissue management of open fractures.

High-energy open fractures with significant soft-tissue damage and evidence of contamination should not be closed. They should be treated with aggressive irrigation and débridement of all nonviable tissue and the administration of appropriate antibiotics. A recent study has shown overall low infection rates when multiple irrigation and débridements were performed for open fractures.[65] The protocol consisted of fracture stabilization, irrigation, and débridement of the fracture and surrounding soft tissues, followed by deep cultures. Repeat irrigation and débridements were performed every 48 hours until cultures were negative, at which time wound closure or appropriate wound coverage was performed. The overall infection rate for all fracture grades was 4.3%. The overall infection rate for all type III fractures was 5.7%. Diabetes and obesity (body mass index > 30) was associated with a higher overall risk of infection.

Maintenance of Hardware in the Presence of Infection

Open fractures can pose a risk for the development of postoperative fixation. The presence of fixation hardware, acting as a foreign body, can make management of infection even more challenging. When infections occur following fracture fixation in the early postoperative period (defined as within 6 weeks from surgery), managing the infection in the presence of hardware and before fracture healing is challenging and controversial. Hardware fixation is necessary for stabilization and healing of the fracture but also is a hindrance to possible treatment and eradication of the infection, which can be a barrier to fracture healing.

Typical treatment recommendations have called for open irrigation and débridement of the fracture and local and systemic antibiotic administration, with or without hardware removal. A recent study evaluated 123 infections that developed within 6 weeks of fracture fixation.[66] These fractures were treated with open irrigation and débridement and a course of intravenous and oral antibiotics. The authors were able to achieve success (fracture union, infection eradication) in 71% of the patients. Factors associated with failure included open fractures, tobacco use, the use of intramedullary nails, *Pseudomonas* infection, and lower extremity fractures.

Periprosthetic Joint Infections

Infection following total knee and hip arthroplasty remains one of the most dreaded and difficult complications to treat. The overall incidence of infection in the literature ranges between 0.5% to 2% for primary total joint arthroplasty and 2% to 4% for revision total joint arthroplasty. According to recent studies, 16.8% of all knee revision arthroplasties and 14.8% of all hip revision arthroplasties in 2005 were performed because of infection.[67,68] The economic burden of treating a patient with an infection after total joint arthroplasty is substantial and associated with costs ranging from $60,000 to $100,000 per treatment, longer hospital stays, and a higher complication rate.[68,69] Several tools, including plain radiographs, laboratory tests, joint aspiration, advanced imaging techniques, and intraoperative testing, can assist in the diagnosis of suspected infected total knee arthroplasty (TKA). Recently, the available evidence for each diagnostic modality was evaluated, and an algorithm was proposed that can be used by clinicians in reaching the diagnosis of infection.[70] **Figures 4** and **5** demonstrate the algorithmic approach for both a high and low suspicion for infection based on the American Academy of Orthopaedic Surgeons (AAOS) clinical practice guidelines.

Despite a multitude of tests that are available, a thorough clinical history and physical examination are the mainstays of the initial evaluation. As a general rule, infection should be suspected in every patient with a painful joint arthroplasty until proven otherwise. The location and the character of pain should be noted. Sources of referred pain, such as the lumbar spine, must be ruled out. The timing of the onset of the pain should be determined.

Plain radiographs can provide useful information in the diagnosis of infection. Obtaining the patient's initial postoperative radiographs and comparing them with the most recent imaging studies is most helpful. In the setting of infection, plain radiographs may show periosteal lamination, subchondral bony resorption, progressive radiolucencies, or localized osteolysis. It is important to remember that bony destruction and lytic lesions are typically seen only after a 30% to 50% loss of bone.

Hematologic tests include the systemic WBC count, ESR, CRP level, and, more recently, an analysis of serum interleukin-6 (IL-6) level. The systemic WBC count is not a reliable indicator of TKA infections. Studies have shown that up to 70% of patients with infection may have a normal WBC count.[71]

It is important to remember that no test is 100% specific for infection. These tests generally have a high

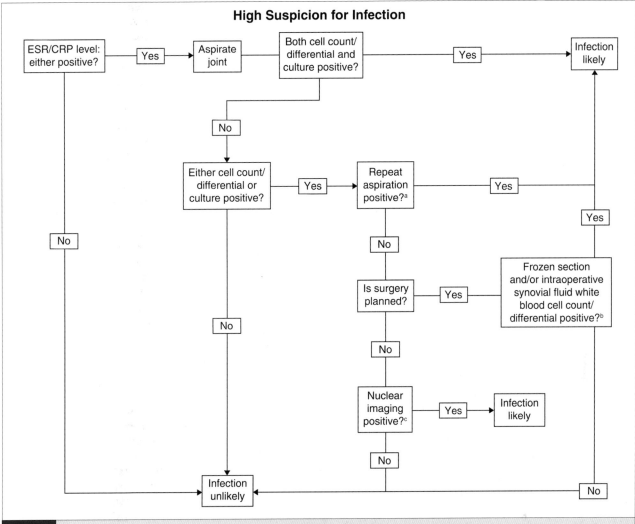

High Suspicion for Infection

Figure 4   Algorithm for treating patients with a higher probability of hip or knee periprosthetic joint infection.
[a]Perform repeat aspiration when a discrepancy exists between the probability of infection and the result of the initial aspiration culture.
[b]Perform frozen section when the diagnosis has not been established at the time of surgery; synovial fluid WBC count and differential may also be obtained intraoperatively.
[c]Nuclear imaging modalities: labeled leukocyte imaging combined with bone or marrow imaging, F-18 FDG-PET, gallium imaging, or label-leukocyte imaging.
(Reproduced from Della Valle C, Parvizi J, Bauer TW, et al: Diagnosis of periprosthetic joint infections of the hip and knee. *J Am Acad Orthop Surg* 2010;18[12]:760-770.)

sensitivity and a low specificity for infection, making them good screening tests rather than accurate predictors of infection. It is the recommendation of the AAOS workgroup that all patients with suspicion for infection have a serum ESR and CRP level performed as the initial screening test.[70]

The ESR generally peaks 5 to 7 days after surgery and will slowly return to normal in approximately 3 months. The CRP level rises within 6 hours of surgery, generally peaks 2 to 3 days after surgery, and will return to normal within 3 weeks. Neither the ESR nor the CRP level alone or in combination are sufficient to make a diagnosis of infection; the tests have a specificity of only 56%.[72] However, when used in combination, the tests are reasonably accurate for ruling out the presence of infection, with a sensitivity of 96% and a negative predictive value of 95%.[72]

The analysis of serum IL-6 level has recently gained in popularity. It generally peaks within 6 hours of surgery but can return to normal within 72 hours after surgery. The IL-6 level has been shown to have a sensitivity of 100% and a specificity of 95% for predicting the presence of infection.[73]

Joint aspiration remains one of the most effective tools for diagnosing infection; however, it can be associated with false-negative results. To minimize false-negative culture findings, the patient should not have used antibiotics within 2 to 3 weeks before the joint aspiration. A WBC count of greater than 2,500 cells/µL, with greater than 60% PMN leukocytes had a sensitiv-

2: Systemic Disorders

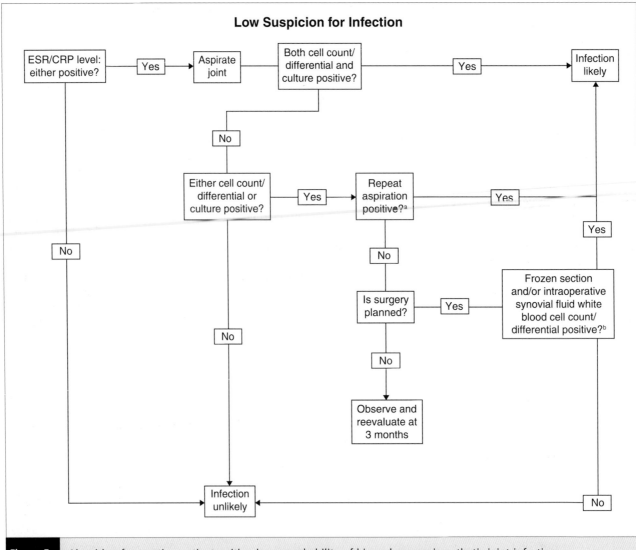

Low Suspicion for Infection

ESR/CRP level: either positive?	Yes →	Aspirate joint	Both cell count/differential and culture positive?	Yes → Infection likely

No ↓

Either cell count/differential or culture positive? → Yes → Repeat aspiration positive?[a] → Yes → (up to Infection likely) Yes

No ↓ (Repeat aspiration positive?) → No ↓

Is surgery planned? → Yes → Frozen section and/or intraoperative synovial fluid white blood cell count/differential positive?[b] → Yes (up to Infection likely)

No ↓ (Either cell count) → Infection unlikely

No ↓ (Is surgery planned?) → Observe and reevaluate at 3 months

No (ESR/CRP) → Infection unlikely

No (Frozen section) → Infection unlikely

Figure 5 Algorithm for treating patients with a lower probability of hip or knee periprosthetic joint infection.
[a]Perform repeat aspiration when a discrepancy exists between the probability of infection and the result of the initial aspiration culture.
[b]Perform frozen section when the diagnosis has not been established at the time of surgery; synovial fluid WBC count and differential may also be obtained intraoperatively.
(Reproduced from Della Valle C, Parvizi J, Bauer TW, et al: Diagnosis of periprosthetic joint infections of the hip and knee. *J Am Acad Orthop Surg* 2010;18[12]:760-770.)

ity of 98%, a specificity of 95%, and a positive predictive value of 91% in the diagnosis of infection in TKA. An aspirate of less than 2,000 cells/μL with a differential of less than 50% had a 98% negative predictive value in ruling out infection.[74] More recently, the literature has supported a variable range of synovial WBC counts and differentials in the diagnosis of periprosthetic joint infection.[75] In general, suspicion should be high when the synovial fluid WBC count is greater than 1,760 cells/μL with greater than 69% PMN leukocytes present in the differential.[76]

In the acute postoperative period, generally defined as up to 4 to 6 weeks after surgery, patients may present with pain and swelling in the joint. It can often be difficult to distinguish normal postoperative pain and

swelling from infection on physical examination in the early postoperative period. The synovial fluid cell count and differential may be elevated as a response to surgery and may not accurately reflect the presence of infection.

If traditional cell counts and differentials are used to diagnose infection in the acute postoperative period, there is concern that these values may lead to unnecessary surgery. A recent study provided information on the use of synovial fluid in the diagnosis of acute postoperative infection after TKA.[77] One hundred forty-six patients had a knee aspiration within 6 weeks of TKA. Infection was diagnosed in 19 patients. Receiver operating curves were used to determine the optimal cutoff, and it was concluded that a synovial fluid WBC count of 27,800 cells/μL had a positive predictive value of 94% and a negative predictive value of 98%. Additionally, the optimal cutoff for PMN leukocytes was 89%. CRP may be useful in the acute postoperative prosthetic joint infection workup as well, and at a threshold of 100 mg/L it has shown a negative predictive value of 91%.

Radionuclide scanning tests may be useful in diagnosing infection, particularly in equivocal situations; however, these tests are expensive, cumbersome for the patient, and lack specificity for diagnosing infection. A radioisotope labeled technetium (Tc-99m) bone scan is a measure of osteoblastic activity. Although the bone scan may be positive in the presence of infection, several other factors, including trauma, degenerative joint disease, and tumor can cause a positive result. Most importantly, radionuclide scans can stay positive for up to 12 months after surgery; they have a sensitivity and a positive predictive value in the range of 30% to 38%. Indium 111-labeled leukocyte scanning will show radionuclide accumulation in areas of WBCs. This test has been shown to have a sensitivity of 77% and a specificity of 86%.[78] Combining these two scanning tests will improve specificity, and it is generally recommended to combine the tests to improve specificity.[79]

Intraoperative testing includes the use of Gram staining and frozen-section histopathology. In general, a Gram stain is unreliable and has poor sensitivity; it should not be used alone to rule out infection.[80] It is the recommendation of the AAOS workgroup that Gram stains not be used to rule out periprosthetic joint infection.[70]

Frozen-section histopathology produces variable results.[81] It is technique dependent and relies on the experience of the pathologist to determine the presence of acute inflammation, and sampling errors often occur. Various tests show that 5 to 10 WBCs per high-power field has adequate sensitivity and specificity for diagnosing infection. The AAOS workgroup strongly recommends the use of frozen sections of peri-implant tissue in patients who are undergoing reoperation for whom the diagnosis of infection has not been established or excluded.[70] The workgroup was not able to determine a threshold (5 or 10 WBCs in a field) because the literature contains insufficient data to distinguish between the two.

New and Future Diagnostic Modalities
Leukocyte Esterase
Leukocyte esterase is an enzyme secreted by neutrophils in response to infection. Commonly used to detect infection in urinary tract infections, leukocyte esterase strips are inexpensive and widely available. A recent prospective study determined that the presence of leukocyte esterase was highly predictive of periprosthetic joint infection.[82] Synovial fluid added to the strips produced a colorimetric result in 1 to 2 minutes. When the two highest results for leukocyte esterase were included (+ or ++), the sensitivity and the specificity were 94% and 87%, respectively.

Molecular Markers for Diagnosis of Periprosthetic Joint Infection
Recently, there has been growing interest in the use of molecular genetics for diagnosing infection. Strategies can include methods to improve the sensitivity of detecting bacteria or methods that identify specific responses to infection, either by the host or the infecting organism.

PCR is used to identify the genetic material of infecting organisms. It can be used after sonication of the implants or in synovial fluid. PCR improves false-negative rates by amplification and identification of bacteria. Its major limitation, however, is the potential high false-positive rate as a result of the identification of dead or noninfectious bacteria. Improvements in PCR analysis have led to the identification of specific DNA targets for bacteria, such as the *Mec A* gene for MRSA, to lower the false-positive rates.[83] In addition, targeting RNA, genetic material that rapidly disappears after bacterial death, can lead to a lower likelihood of detecting false-positive bacterial genetic material.[84]

It appears that the host response to periprosthetic joint infection results in the secretion of specific biomarkers from neutrophils that are characteristic of periprosthetic joint infection. The identification of these specific biomarkers has shown promise in the detection of periprosthetic joint infection. A differential gene expression of neutrophils in response to periprosthetic joint infection has been identified. Several studies have now shown that microassay identification of these biomarkers (IL-6, vascular endothelial growth factor [VEGF]) were found to have very high accuracy in the diagnosis of periprosthetic joint infection.[85,86] These biomarker assays are relatively inexpensive, allow rapid identification of the infection without a false-positive rate of PCR, and can be effective even in the presence of antibiotics. The one drawback is the inability to identify the type of bacteria present.

Definition and Classification of Periprosthetic Joint Infection
Despite the multitude of tests available to evaluate patients with a suspected periprosthetic joint infection, there is no single accepted diagnostic criteria. Recently, a workgroup convened by the Musculoskeletal Infection Society analyzed all of the available evidence and proposed a new definition for periprosthetic joint infection.[87] These criteria should hopefully allow for a wide adaption of the definition of periprosthetic joint infection among clinicians.

Based on the proposed criteria, a periprosthetic joint infection exists when there is a sinus tract communicating with the joint, or a pathogen is isolated by culture from two separate tissue or fluid samples for the affected joint, or four of the following six criteria are met: (1) elevated ESR or CRP level; (2) elevated synovial leukocyte count; (3) elevated synovial leukocyte percentage; (4) presence of purulence in the affected joint; (5) isolation of a microorganism in one culture of tissue or fluid; and (6) greater than five neutrophils per

Table 4

Classification, Definition and Suggested Treatment Options for Periprosthetic Infection

Type	Description	Definition	Treatment
Type I	Positive intraoperative cultures	Two or more positive cultures obtained at surgery	Appropriate antibiotic directed therapy
Type II	Early postoperative infection	Infection within first 4 weeks after surgery	Attempted irrigation and débridement
Type III	Acute hematogenous infection	Seeding of a previously well-functioning joint	Attempted irrigation and débridement versus prosthetic removal
Type IV	Chronic (late) infection	Symptoms present for > 1 month	Prosthetic removal with two-stage exchange arthroplasty

high-power field in five high-power fields from analysis of periprosthetic tissue at ×400 magnification.

The classification system developed by Tsukayama et al[88] is widely used to classify infection following total joint arthroplasty. A type I infection involves a patient with a positive culture at the time of surgery. A type II infection is an early infection that occurs within the first month after surgery. A type III infection is a late, acute, hematogenous infection that occurs after total joint arthroplasty, with symptoms of less than 4 weeks' duration. A type IV infection is a late, chronic infection with symptoms that have persisted for more than 4 weeks. **Table 4** describes the classification system as well as the generally recommended treatment options based on the type of infection.

Several variables must be considered when choosing a treatment option. These variables include the depth and timing of the infection, the status of the soft tissues, the fixation of the prosthesis, the involved pathogenic organism, the ability of the host to fight the infection, the resources of the physician, and the patient's expectations.

Key Study Points

- Infections of the musculoskeletal system remain one of the most difficult and challenging complications in orthopaedics, and national data indicate that overall infection rates are on the rise.

- Because of the substantial morbidity and mortality associated with orthopaedic infections, much attention has been given to the prevention of infection, with guidelines such as SCIP.

- The most common infecting organisms remain *Staphylococcus* and *Streptococcus* species, with an increasing prevalence of resistant strains of *Staphylococcus* organisms (MRSA).

- New imaging modalities and diagnostic tools such as PCR are becoming widely available to aid in the diagnosis of musculoskeletal infections, but a high index of suspicion along with the history and the physical examination remain the mainstays of treatment.

Summary

Orthopaedic infections remain one of the most common and difficult conditions to treat. Recent literature would suggest that SSIs are on the rise, only adding to the continued burden of healthcare costs. Prevention is the key to minimizing the risk of orthopaedic infections. Optimizing the interaction of the host and the environment are paramount for preventing infections. Many patients in suboptimal health have modifiable health factors. It is imperative that steps be taken to maximize patient health and optimize the environment. In addition, a better understanding of bacterial defense mechanisms and biofilm environment will allow new ways to prevent and treat orthopaedic infections.

Annotated References

1. Mangram AJ, Horan TC, Pearson ML, Silver LC, Jarvis WR; Hospital Infection Control Practices Advisory Committee: Guideline for prevention of surgical site infection, 1999. *Infect Control Hosp Epidemiol* 1999; 20(4):250-278, quiz 279-280.

2. Klevens RM, Edwards JR, Richards CL Jr, et al: Estimating health care-associated infections and deaths in U.S. hospitals, 2002. *Public Health Rep* 2007;122(2): 160-166.

3. Graf K, Ott E, Vonberg RP, et al: Surgical site infections—economic consequences for the health care system. *Langenbecks Arch Surg* 2011;396(4):453-459.

   This study evaluated the economic costs associated with SSIs by reviewing 14 studies in the literature. The authors determined that an SSI almost tripled the overall healthcare costs to the patient, and often this additional cost was not covered. Level of evidence: III.

4. Thompson KM, Oldenburg WA, Deschamps C, Rupp WC, Smith CD: Chasing zero: The drive to eliminate surgical site infections. *Ann Surg* 2011;254(3):430-437.

   This study evaluated the implementation of a comprehensive program to reduce SSIs. Following institution of this protocol, the institution demonstrated a 57% decrease in the rate of SSIs and a cost savings to the hospital of more than $1 million. Level of evidence: III.

5. Rosenberger LH, Politano AD, Sawyer RG: The surgical care improvement project and prevention of postoperative infection, including surgical site infection. *Surg Infect (Larchmt)* 2011;12(3):163-168.

   This article reviews the 10 SCIP parameters developed by the CDC and the Centers for Medicare and Medicaid Services on the prevention of postoperative infection. Level of evidence: IV.

6. Patel A, Calfee RP, Plante M, Fischer SA, Arcand N, Born C: Methicillin-resistant *Staphylococcus aureus* in orthopaedic surgery. *J Bone Joint Surg Br* 2008;90(11):1401-1406.

7. Rao N, Cannella B, Crossett LS, Yates AJ Jr, McGough R III: A preoperative decolonization protocol for staphylococcus aureus prevents orthopaedic infections. *Clin Orthop Relat Res* 2008;466(6):1343-1348.

8. Arciola CR, Campoccia D, Speziale P, Montanaro L, Costerton JW: Biofilm formation in *Staphylococcus* implant infections: A review of molecular mechanisms and implications for biofilm-resistant materials. *Biomaterials* 2012;33(26):5967-5982.

   Implant infections in orthopaedics are chiefly caused by staphylococci. The ability of bacteria to grow within a biofilm enhances the ability of staphylococci to protect themselves from host defenses and antibiotic therapies. This review article discusses the complex molecular interaction of *Staphylococcus* biofilm formation and discusses potential options to fight biofilm-related infections. Level of evidence: V.

9. Patel R: Biofilms and antimicrobial resistance. *Clin Orthop Relat Res* 2005;437:41-47.

10. Costerton JW: Biofilm theory can guide the treatment of device-related orthopaedic infections. *Clin Orthop Relat Res* 2005;437:7-11.

11. Dharan S, Pittet D: Environmental controls in operating theatres. *J Hosp Infect* 2002;51(2):79-84.

12. Evans RP: Current concepts for clean air and total joint arthroplasty: Laminar airflow and ultraviolet radiation. A systematic review. *Clin Orthop Relat Res* 2011;469(4):945-953.

    This current concept review explores the available literature on the use of laminar airflow and ultraviolet light in total joint arthroplasty. There is currently a lack of high-level evidence to support the use of laminar airflow and ultraviolet light. However, the authors emphasize that higher level studies are needed to control for multiple variables before definitive decisions can be made about the use of these modalities. Level of evidence: IV.

13. Evans RP: Laminar air flow in the operating room: How effective is it in reducing infection? *AAOS Bulletin* June 2006:12-14.

14. Lidwell OM: Ultraviolet radiation and the control of airborne contamination in the operating room. *J Hosp Infect* 1994;28(4):245-248.

15. Ritter MA, Olberding EM, Malinzak RA: Ultraviolet lighting during orthopaedic surgery and the rate of infection. *J Bone Joint Surg Am* 2007;89(9):1935-1940.

16. Berg M, Bergman BR, Hoborn J: Ultraviolet radiation compared to an ultra-clean air enclosure: Comparison of air bacteria counts in operating rooms. *J Bone Joint Surg Br* 1991;73(5):811-815.

17. Hooper GJ, Rothwell AG, Frampton C, Wyatt MC: Does the use of laminar flow and spacesuits reduce early deep infection after total hip and knee replacement? The ten-year results of the New Zealand Joint Registry. *J Bone Joint Surg Br* 2011;93(1):85-90.

    For total hip replacement, there was a substantial increase in early infection in those procedures performed with the use of a spacesuit compared with those without (P < 0.0001), in those performed in a laminar-flow theater compared with a conventional theater (P < 0.003) and in those undertaken in a laminar-flow theater with a spacesuit (P < 0.001) when compared with conventional theaters without such a suit. The results were similar for total knee replacement. Level of evidence: III.

18. Malinzak RA, Ritter MA, Berend ME, Meding JB, Olberding EM, Davis KE: Morbidly obese, diabetic, younger, and unilateral joint arthroplasty patients have elevated total joint arthroplasty infection rates. *J Arthroplasty* 2009;24(6, suppl):84-88.

19. Namba RS, Paxton L, Fithian DC, Stone ML: Obesity and perioperative morbidity in total hip and total knee arthroplasty patients. *J Arthroplasty* 2005;20(7, suppl 3):46-50.

20. Greene KA, Wilde AH, Stulberg BN: Preoperative nutritional status of total joint patients: Relationship to postoperative wound complications. *J Arthroplasty* 1991;6(4):321-325.

21. Harris JC, Caesar DH, Davison C, Phibbs R, Than MP: How useful are laboratory investigations in the emergency department evaluation of possible osteomyelitis? *Emerg Med Australas* 2011;23(3):317-330.

    A literature review of 36 papers was performed to determine which laboratory tests were useful in the evaluation of osteomyelitis. WBC count was not useful in confirming or excluding osteomyelitis. A normal CRP level and ESR were helpful in ruling out osteomyelitis when there was low clinical suspicion, and confirming the need for further investigation if elevated in a patient with high suspicion. Level of evidence: III.

22. Hunziker S, Hügle T, Schuchardt K, et al: The value of serum procalcitonin level for differentiation of infectious from noninfectious causes of fever after orthopaedic surgery. *J Bone Joint Surg Am* 2010;92(1):138-148.

Serum PCT levels were evaluated in patients who had undergone orthopaedic surgery and developed a postoperative fever within 10 days of the procedure. PCT demonstrated significantly higher accuracy in diagnosing infection causes compared with the CRP level and WBC count (*P* = 0.04 at fever onset, *P* = 0.07 at day 1, and *P* = 0.003 at day 3). Level of evidence: III.

23. Schuetz P, Albrich W, Mueller B: Procalcitonin for diagnosis of infection and guide to antibiotic decisions: Past, present and future. *BMC Med* 2011;9:107.

Thirty-six studies evaluating the use of PCT in the diagnosis of bacterial infection were reviewed. Randomized controlled studies have demonstrated the effectiveness of PCT in guiding decisions to administer antibiotics to patients in intensive care units with respiratory infections or sepsis and its usefulness in monitoring trends. Level of evidence: III.

24. Lew DP, Waldvogel FA: Osteomyelitis. *Lancet* 2004; 364(9431):369-379.

25. Pineda C, Vargas A, Rodríguez AV: Imaging of osteomyelitis: Current concepts. *Infect Dis Clin North Am* 2006;20(4):789-825.

26. Termaat MF, Raijmakers PG, Scholten HJ, Bakker FC, Patka P, Haarman HJ: The accuracy of diagnostic imaging for the assessment of chronic osteomyelitis: A systematic review and meta-analysis. *J Bone Joint Surg Am* 2005;87(11):2464-2471.

27. Romanò CL, Romanò D, Logoluso N, Drago L: Bone and joint infections in adults: A comprehensive classification proposal. *Eur Orthop Traumatol* 2011;1(6): 207-217.

The authors propose a new, more comprehensive classification system for bone and joint infections in adults. The Seven-Item Comprehensive Classification System incorporates several features from previously described classification schemes in an effort to characterize all patients with any type of bone or joint infection. Level of evidence: IV.

28. McKee MD, Wild LM, Schemitsch EH, Waddell JP: The use of an antibiotic-impregnated, osteoconductive, bioabsorbable bone substitute in the treatment of infected long bone defects: Early results of a prospective trial. *J Orthop Trauma* 2002;16(9):622-627.

29. Arnold SR, Elias D, Buckingham SC, et al: Changing patterns of acute hematogenous osteomyelitis and septic arthritis: Emergence of community-associated methicillin-resistant Staphylococcus aureus. *J Pediatr Orthop* 2006;26(6):703-708.

30. Dohin B, Gillet Y, Kohler R, et al: Pediatric bone and joint infections caused by Panton-Valentine leukocidin-positive Staphylococcus aureus. *Pediatr Infect Dis J* 2007;26(11):1042-1048.

31. Yagupsky P, Porsch E, St Geme JW III: Kingella kingae: An emerging pathogen in young children. *Pediatrics* 2011;127(3):557-565.

The authors provide a thorough review of the epidemiology, pathogenesis, presentation, diagnosis, treatment, and future directions for managing *K kingae* in young children. Level of evidence: V.

32. Khachatourians AG, Patzakis MJ, Roidis N, Holtom PD: Laboratory monitoring in pediatric acute osteomyelitis and septic arthritis. *Clin Orthop Relat Res* 2003; 409:186-194.

33. Pääkkönen M, Kallio MJ, Kallio PE, Peltola H: Sensitivity of erythrocyte sedimentation rate and C-reactive protein in childhood bone and joint infections. *Clin Orthop Relat Res* 2010;468(3):861-866.

The authors prospectively monitored ESR, the CRP level, and the WBC count in pediatric patients with culture-positive osteoarticular infections. They found sensitivities of 94%, 95%, and 98% for ESR, CRP level, and combined ESR/CRP level elevation, respectively. Level of evidence: III.

34. Browne LP, Mason EO, Kaplan SL, Cassady CI, Krishnamurthy R, Guillerman RP: Optimal imaging strategy for community-acquired Staphylococcus aureus musculoskeletal infections in children. *Pediatr Radiol* 2008; 38(8):841-847.

35. Courtney PM, Flynn JM, Jaramillo D, Horn BD, Calabro K, Spiegel DA: Clinical indications for repeat MRI in children with acute hematogenous osteomyelitis. *J Pediatr Orthop* 2010;30(8):883-887.

This study demonstrated that a repeat MRI did not have a useful role in the routine follow-up of pediatric osteomyelitis, except in those cases in which a patient is not responding to standard therapy. Level of evidence: III.

36. Verdier I, Gayet-Ageron A, Ploton C, et al: Contribution of a broad range polymerase chain reaction to the diagnosis of osteoarticular infections caused by *Kingella kingae*: Description of twenty-four recent pediatric diagnoses. *Pediatr Infect Dis J* 2005;24(8):692-696.

37. Rosey AL, Abachin E, Quesnes G, et al: Development of a broad-range 16S rDNA real-time PCR for the diagnosis of septic arthritis in children. *J Microbiol Methods* 2007;68(1):88-93.

38. Herigon JC, Hersh AL, Gerber JS, Zaoutis TE, Newland JG: Antibiotic management of Staphylococcus aureus infections in US children's hospitals, 1999-2008. *Pediatrics* 2010;125(6):e1294-e1300.

This study analyzed the patterns of antibiotic use over the past decade and found that clindamycin is now the most common antibiotic prescribed for *S aureus* infections in children, including osteomyelitis. Level of evidence: IV.

39. Peltola H, Pääkkönen M, Kallio P, Kallio MJ; Osteomyelitis-Septic Arthritis Study Group: Short- versus long-term antimicrobial treatment for acute hematogenous osteomyelitis of childhood: Prospective, randomized trial on 131 culture-positive cases. *Pediatr Infect Dis J* 2010;29(12):1123-1128.

Pediatric patients with culture-positive osteomyelitis received a first-generation cephalosporin or clindamycin for 20 or 30 days with a 2- to 4-day intravenous course initially. The authors found that most children could be adequately treated for 20 days with a short initial period of intravenous antibiotics. Level of evidence: I.

40. Hügle T, Schuetz P, Mueller B, et al: Serum procalcitonin for discrimination between septic and non-septic arthritis. *Clin Exp Rheumatol* 2008;26(3):453-456.

41. Weston VC, Jones AC, Bradbury N, Fawthrop F, Doherty M: Clinical features and outcome of septic arthritis in a single UK Health District 1982-1991. *Ann Rheum Dis* 1999;58(4):214-219.

42. Hughes JG, Vetter EA, Patel R, et al: Culture with BACTEC Peds Plus/F bottle compared with conventional methods for detection of bacteria in synovial fluid. *J Clin Microbiol* 2001;39(12):4468-4471.

43. Kim H, Kim J, Ihm C: The usefulness of multiplex PCR for the identification of bacteria in joint infection. *J Clin Lab Anal* 2010;24(3):175-181.

A new multiplex PCR assay was compared to culture in detecting bacteria in synovial fluid from septic joints. Multiplex PCR offered timely (< 6 hours) detection and identification of common pathogens with better sensitivity (96% versus 74%) and similar specificity (both 100%). Level of evidence: III.

44. Hiramatsu K, Aritaka N, Hanaki H, et al: Dissemination in Japanese hospitals of strains of *Staphylococcus aureus* heterogeneously resistant to vancomycin. *Lancet* 1997;350(9092):1670-1673.

45. Young TP, Maas L, Thorp AW, Brown L: Etiology of septic arthritis in children: An update for the new millennium. *Am J Emerg Med* 2011;29(8):899-902.

The authors performed a retrospective chart review of children younger than 13 years who presented with septic arthritis to describe the etiology of septic arthritis in the postvaccination era. The most common organism was methicillin-sensitive *S aureus*, followed by CA-MRSA and *Streptococcus* pneumonia. Level of evidence: IV.

46. Luhmann JD, Luhmann SJ: Etiology of septic arthritis in children: An update for the 1990s. *Pediatr Emerg Care* 1999;15(1):40-42.

47. Kocher MS, Zurakowski D, Kasser JR: Differentiating between septic arthritis and transient synovitis of the hip in children: An evidence-based clinical prediction algorithm. *J Bone Joint Surg Am* 1999;81(12):1662-1670.

48. Sultan J, Hughes PJ: Septic arthritis or transient synovitis of the hip in children: The value of clinical prediction algorithms. *J Bone Joint Surg Br* 2010;92(9):1289-1293.

The classic criteria for differentiating septic arthritis from transient synovitis were retrospectively applied to pediatric patients in a primary care setting. The authors found that the classic criteria were not as predictive of septic arthritis in this setting, and even with the addition of the CRP level, found the probability of septic arthritis was only 59.9%. Level of evidence: III.

49. Caird MS, Flynn JM, Leung YL, Millman JE, D'Italia JG, Dormans JP: Factors distinguishing septic arthritis from transient synovitis of the hip in children: A prospective study. *J Bone Joint Surg Am* 2006;88(6):1251-1257.

50. Tsung JW, Blaivas M: Emergency department diagnosis of pediatric hip effusion and guided arthrocentesis using point-of-care ultrasound. *J Emerg Med* 2008;35(4):393-399.

51. Vieira RL, Levy JA: Bedside ultrasonography to identify hip effusions in pediatric patients. *Ann Emerg Med* 2010;55(3):284-289.

This study compared the impression of bedside hip ultrasounds, as performed by an emergency department physician, to the results of the radiology department's ultrasound. The authors found that with focused training, emergency physicians were able to identify hip effusions in pediatric patients. Level of evidence: IV.

52. Mazur JM, Ross G, Cummings J, Hahn GA Jr, McCluskey WP: Usefulness of magnetic resonance imaging for the diagnosis of acute musculoskeletal infections in children. *J Pediatr Orthop* 1995;15(2):144-147.

53. Kwack KS, Cho JH, Lee JH, Cho JH, Oh KK, Kim SY: Septic arthritis versus transient synovitis of the hip: Gadolinium-enhanced MRI finding of decreased perfusion at the femoral epiphysis. *AJR Am J Roentgenol* 2007;189(2):437-445.

54. Journeau P, Wein F, Popkov D, Philippe R, Haumont T, Lascombes P: Hip septic arthritis in children: Assessment of treatment using needle aspiration/irrigation. *Orthop Traumatol Surg Res* 2011;97(3):308-313.

Forty-three cases of septic hip arthritis were treated with needle aspiration-irrigation. Five cases required a secondary arthrotomy. CRP level less than 100, WBC count greater than 15,000, and ESR above 25 were predictive of the need for formal arthrotomy to decrease the bacterial load. Level of evidence: IV.

55. Griffet J, Oborocianu I, Rubio A, Leroux J, Lauron J, Hayek T: Percutaneous aspiration irrigation drainage technique in the management of septic arthritis in children. *J Trauma* 2011;70(2):377-383.

Fifty-two children with septic arthritis were successfully treated with percutaneous aspiration, irrigation, and drainage. Rapid clinical and biologic improvement was noted, with no long-term sequelae. Level of evidence: IV.

2: Systemic Disorders

56. Jagodzinski NA, Kanwar R, Graham K, Bache CE: Prospective evaluation of a shortened regimen of treatment for acute osteomyelitis and septic arthritis in children. *J Pediatr Orthop* 2009;29(5):518-525.

57. Harel L, Prais D, Bar-On E, et al: Dexamethasone therapy for septic arthritis in children: Results of a randomized double-blind placebo-controlled study. *J Pediatr Orthop* 2011;31(2):211-215.

    This study demonstrated that administration of a 4-day course of dexamethasone is safe and leads to a more rapid clinical improvement and a shortened hospitalization. Level of evidence: I.

58. Basmaci R, Lorrot M, Bidet P, et al: Comparison of clinical and biologic features of Kingella kingae and Staphylococcus aureus arthritis at initial evaluation. *Pediatr Infect Dis J* 2011;30(10):902-904.

    The authors compared the clinical and biologic features of children with *K kingae* and *S aureus*. Those with *K kingae* septic arthritis were younger and had shorter hospitalizations and fewer adverse events. Level of evidence: IV.

59. Ceroni D, Cherkaoui A, Ferey S, Kaelin A, Schrenzel J: *Kingella kingae* osteoarticular infections in young children: Clinical features and contribution of a new specific real-time PCR assay to the diagnosis. *J Pediatr Orthop* 2010;30(3):301-304.

    The authors performed a prospective study to define the features of osteoarticular infections in children younger than 4 years. These children presented with relatively mild to moderate clinical, radiologic, and biologic inflammatory response to *K kingae*. Specific real-time PCR demonstrated an ability to detect *K kingae* when classic isolation methods could not. Level of evidence: I.

60. Kanavaki A, Ceroni D, Tchernin D, Hanquinet S, Merlini L: Can early MRI distinguish between *Kingella kingae* and Gram-positive cocci in osteoarticular infections in young children? *Pediatr Radiol* 2012;42(1):57-62.

    Children younger than 4 years with osteoarticular infections underwent MRI, and the images from *K kingae* cases and gram-positive cocci were compared. Differences noted in the *K kingae* cases included decreased bone reaction, milder soft-tissue reaction, and the presence of epiphyseal cartilage abscesses. Level of evidence: III.

61. Lavery LA, Armstrong DG, Wunderlich RP, Mohler MJ, Wendel CS, Lipsky BA: Risk factors for foot infections in individuals with diabetes. *Diabetes Care* 2006;29(6):1288-1293.

62. Chisholm CD, Schlesser JF: Plantar puncture wounds: Controversies and treatment recommendations. *Ann Emerg Med* 1989;18(12):1352-1357.

63. Rockett MS, Gentile SC, Gudas CJ, Brage ME, Zygmunt KH: The use of ultrasonography for the detection of retained wooden foreign bodies in the foot. *J Foot Ankle Surg* 1995;34(5):478-484, discussion 510-511.

64. Firth GB, Roy A, Moroz PJ: Foreign body migration along a tendon sheath in the lower extremity: A case report and literature review. *J Bone Joint Surg Am* 2011;93(8):e38.

    The authors present the case of a 7 year old with a plantar heel puncture wound. Radiographs and limited ultrasound failed to identify the foreign body. The patient experienced proximal migration of the toothpick within the flexor hallucis longus tendon sheath with eventual skin erosion. The authors conclude that if a foreign body is suspected, then further imaging is warranted. Level of evidence: V.

65. Lenarz CJ, Watson JT, Moed BR, Israel H, Mullen JD, Macdonald JB: Timing of wound closure in open fractures based on cultures obtained after debridement. *J Bone Joint Surg Am* 2010;92(10):1921-1926.

    This retrospective study evaluated a protocol of fracture stabilization and multiple open irrigation and débridement for open fractures. With this protocol, the authors demonstrated low overall infection rates for all grades of fractures. Level of evidence: IV.

66. Berkes M, Obremskey WT, Scannell B, et al: Maintenance of hardware after early postoperative infection following fracture internal fixation. *J Bone Joint Surg Am* 2010;92(4):823-828.

    This study evaluated early postoperative infections following fracture fixation. The treatment generally consisted of open irrigation and débridement, with or without hardware removal and intravenous/oral antibiotics. Factors associated with failure included open fractures, tobacco use, the use of intramedullary nails, infection with *Pseudomonas*, and lower extremity fractures. Level of evidence: III.

67. Bozic KJ, Kurtz SM, Lau E, Ong K, Vail TP, Berry DJ: The epidemiology of revision total hip arthroplasty in the United States. *J Bone Joint Surg Am* 2009;91(1):128-133.

68. Bozic KJ, Kurtz SM, Lau E, et al: The epidemiology of revision total knee arthroplasty in the United States. *Clin Orthop Relat Res* 2010;468(1):45-51.

    This study reviewed over 60,000 revision total knee arthroplasties in the United States using the Nationwide Inpatient Sample. The most common reasons for revision were infection and aseptic loosening. Level of evidence: III.

69. Kurtz SM, Ong KL, Schmier J, et al: Future clinical and economic impact of revision total hip and knee arthroplasty. *J Bone Joint Surg Am* 2007;89(suppl 3):144-151.

70. Della Valle C, Parvizi J, Bauer TW, et al: Diagnosis of periprosthetic joint infections of the hip and knee. *J Am Acad Orthop Surg* 2010;18(12):760-770.

    This review paper provided an overview of the diagnosis of periprosthetic joint infection with an emphasis on laboratory studies and aspirations as a guideline. Level of evidence: III.

71. Della Valle CJ, Sporer SM, Jacobs JJ, Berger RA, Rosenberg AG, Paprosky WG: Preoperative testing for sepsis before revision total knee arthroplasty. *J Arthroplasty* 2007;22(6, suppl 2):90-93.

72. Austin MS, Ghanem E, Joshi A, Lindsay A, Parvizi J: A simple, cost-effective screening protocol to rule out periprosthetic infection. *J Arthroplasty* 2008;23(1):65-68.

73. Di Cesare PE, Chang E, Preston CF, Liu CJ: Serum interleukin-6 as a marker of periprosthetic infection following total hip and knee arthroplasty. *J Bone Joint Surg Am* 2005;87(9):1921-1927.

74. Leone JM, Hanssen AD: Management of infection at the site of a total knee arthroplasty. *Instr Course Lect* 2006;55:449-461.

75. Trampuz A, Hanssen AD, Osmon DR, Mandrekar J, Steckelberg JM, Patel R: Synovial fluid leukocyte count and differential for the diagnosis of prosthetic knee infection. *Am J Med* 2004;117(8):556-562.

76. Ghanem E, Parvizi J, Burnett RS, et al: Cell count and differential of aspirated fluid in the diagnosis of infection at the site of total knee arthroplasty. *J Bone Joint Surg Am* 2008;90(8):1637-1643.

77. Bedair H, Ting N, Jacovides C, et al: The Mark Coventry Award: Diagnosis of early postoperative TKA infection using synovial fluid analysis. *Clin Orthop Relat Res* 2011;469(1):34-40.

This retrospective study evaluated laboratory (ESR and CRP level) and aspiration results of patients who had early postoperative infections (< 6 weeks) and provided guidelines to diagnosis of infection in the early postoperative period. Level of evidence: III.

78. Palestro CJ, Swyer AJ, Kim CK, Goldsmith SJ: Infected knee prosthesis: Diagnosis with In-111 leukocyte, Tc-99m sulfur colloid, and Tc-99m MDP imaging. *Radiology* 1991;179(3):645-648.

79. Joseph TN, Mujtaba M, Chen AL, et al: Efficacy of combined technetium-99m sulfur colloid/indium-111 leukocyte scans to detect infected total hip and knee arthroplasties. *J Arthroplasty* 2001;16(6):753-758.

80. Morgan PM, Sharkey P, Ghanem E, et al: The value of intraoperative Gram stain in revision total knee arthroplasty. *J Bone Joint Surg Am* 2009;91(9):2124-2129.

81. Della Valle CJ, Bogner E, Desai P, et al: Analysis of frozen sections of intraoperative specimens obtained at the time of reoperation after hip or knee resection arthroplasty for the treatment of infection. *J Bone Joint Surg Am* 1999;81(5):684-689.

82. Parvizi J, Jacovides C, Antoci V, Ghanem E: Diagnosis of periprosthetic joint infection: The utility of a simple yet unappreciated enzyme. *J Bone Joint Surg Am* 2011; 93(24):2242-2248.

The authors studied the sensitivity and specificity of leukocyte esterase and found that the presence of this enzyme was strongly correlated with a diagnosis of periprosthetic joint infection.

83. Achermann Y, Vogt M, Leunig M, Wüst J, Trampuz A: Improved diagnosis of periprosthetic joint infection by multiplex PCR of sonication fluid from removed implants. *J Clin Microbiol* 2010;48(4):1208-1214.

This study evaluated the value of multiplex PCR for the detection of microbial DNA in sonication fluid from removed orthopaedic prostheses. Cases of periprosthetic joint infection in which the prosthesis (or part of it) was removed were prospectively included. The removed implant was sonicated, and the resulting sonication fluid was cultured and subjected to multiplex PCR. Of 37 periprosthetic joint infection cases, pathogens were identified in periprosthetic tissue in 24 cases (65%), in sonication fluid in 23 cases (62%), and by multiplex PCR in 29 cases (78%). Level of evidence: IV.

84. Bergin PF, Doppelt JD, Hamilton WG, et al: Detection of periprosthetic infections with use of ribosomal RNA-based polymerase chain reaction. *J Bone Joint Surg Am* 2010;92(3):654-663.

The objective of this study was to determine whether reverse transcription-quantitative polymerase chain reaction (RT-qPCR) using universal primers can be used to detect the more abundant bacterial ribosomal RNA (rRNA) as an indicator of periprosthetic infection. rRNA-based RT-qPCR demonstrated 100% specificity and positive predictive value with a sensitivity equivalent to that of intraoperative culture. Level of evidence: IV.

85. Jacovides CL, Parvizi J, Adeli B, Jung KA: Molecular markers for diagnosis of periprosthetic joint infection. *J Arthroplasty* 2011;26(6, suppl):99-103, e1.

The purpose of this study was to measure inflammatory proteins in synovial fluid from patients undergoing revision arthroplasty for septic or aseptic failure. Of 46 proteins, 5 (IL-6, IL-8, $\alpha(2)$-macroglobulin, CRP, and VEGF) had an area under the curve greater than 0.90. This prospective study has demonstrated promising results for the use of molecular markers in the diagnosis of periprosthetic joint infection. Level of evidence: IV.

86. Deirmengian C, Hallab N, Tarabishy A, et al: Synovial fluid biomarkers for periprosthetic infection. *Clin Orthop Relat Res* 2010;468(8):2017-2023.

This study evaluated the sensitivity, the specificity, and the accuracy of several potential synovial fluid biomarkers for infection and compared them with current standards of testing for periprosthetic infection. Twelve synovial fluid biomarkers had substantially higher average levels in the synovial fluid of infected versus aseptic patients. Several of these biomarkers exhibited nearly ideal sensitivity, specificity, and accuracy in this study. Level of evidence: IV.

2: Systemic Disorders

87. Parvizi J, Zmistowski B, Berbari EF, et al: New definition for periprosthetic joint infection: From the Workgroup of the Musculoskeletal Infection Society. *Clin Orthop Relat Res* 2011;469(11):2992-2994.

In order to establish consistency in the management and study of periprosthetic joint infections, the work group developed a series of major and minor criteria to better define them. The goal was to have a gold standard to improve diagnosis, treatment, surveillance, and the quality of published data.

88. Tsukayama DT, Goldberg VM, Kyle R: Diagnosis and management of infection after total knee arthroplasty. *J Bone Joint Surg Am* 2003;85(suppl 1):S75-S80.

Chapter 24

Pain Management

Jaime Baratta, MD   Kishor Gandhi, MD, MPH   Eric Schwenk, MD   Benjamin Vaghari, MD
Eugene Viscusi, MD

Introduction

Postoperative pain management following orthopaedic surgery continues to present challenges. Most recent surveys of postoperative pain continue to demonstrate that most patients experience moderate to severe pain.[1] Pain is the most common reason for readmission after ambulatory orthopaedic surgery.[2] Until recently, opioids were the primary analgesic administered after surgery; however, patients are often plagued by distressing gastrointestinal side effects.

Opioids are generally effective for nociceptive pain but not very effective for inflammatory or neuropathic pain. Therefore, opioids are particularly ineffective in relieving dynamic pain or pain related to activity or physical therapy. An understanding of the specific types of pain that a patient is experiencing is necessary to develop a rational multimodal approach. Pain following most orthopaedic procedures is more likely to be a blend of sharp, throbbing pain but often includes burning and possibly spasms. A single drug is unlikely to effectively treat this type of pain.

Recent guidelines for acute pain management support a multimodal approach.[3] These guidelines advocate around-the-clock nonopioid analgesics including acetaminophen, NSAIDs, cyclooxygenase-2 (COX-2) selective inhibitors, and local anesthetic techniques whenever possible. Opioids then become adjunctive agents. Multimodal analgesia targets specific pain pathways to enhance analgesia while minimizing opioid use (Figure 1). Early mobilization is critical to a successful outcome following surgery of the musculoskeletal system. Enhanced pain management not only improves rehabilitation but also reduces morbidity and length of hospital stay.

A small but substantial number of patients will develop chronic postsurgical pain, defined as long-term pain occurring after certain orthopaedic procedures. Total knee arthroplasty (TKA) is associated with the highest risk of chronic postsurgical pain. Although causes and preventive strategies remain elusive, chronic postsurgical pain often afflicts patients in whom pain is particularly acute, intense, and long lasting. Some experts identify nerve injury and inflammatory processes as causative factors. An intriguing current question is whether a targeted multimodal approach to pain management can reduce chronic postsurgical pain or improve pain-related outcomes weeks to months later. Studies have shown that multimodal agents such as preoperative pregabalin and preoperative and intraoperative ketamine reduce chronic pain following TKA and spine surgery, respectively.[4-6]

Patient satisfaction is intimately connected with pain management and the side effects experienced as a consequence of pain treatment. Satisfaction is an increasingly important driver for market share and payment. Patient satisfaction data are now being reported via the Hospital Consumer Assessment of Healthcare Providers and Systems (HCAHPS), also known as the CAHPS hospital survey. As part of the Affordable Care Act 2010, the Centers for Medicare and Medicaid Services (CMS) have established hospital reimbursement based on HCAHPS scores.

Analgesia for Upper Extremity Surgery

Adequate control of pain can serve to minimize hospital stays during the perioperative period, and reduced hospital stays can result in decreased nosocomial infections, fewer possible harmful medical errors, and overall improved quality of life. Regional anesthesia can be used for anesthesia and analgesia for upper extremity orthopaedic procedures. Studies have shown that patients receiving peripheral nerve block anesthesia have faster same-day recovery than those receiving general anesthesia.[7] Patients receiving selective brachial plexus

2: Systemic Disorders

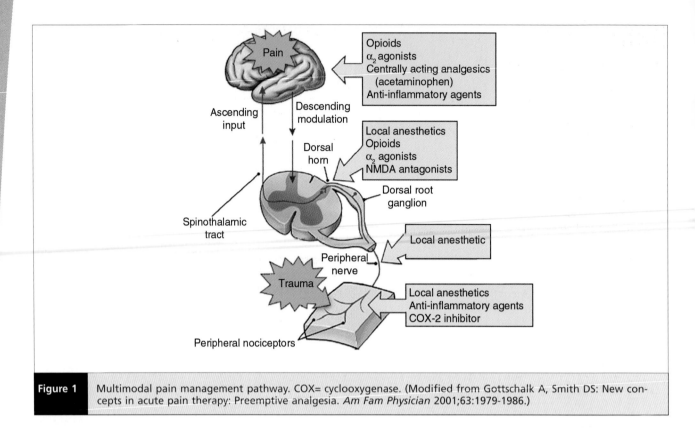

| Figure 1 | Multimodal pain management pathway. COX= cyclooxygenase. (Modified from Gottschalk A, Smith DS: New concepts in acute pain therapy: Preemptive analgesia. *Am Fam Physician* 2001;63:1979-1986.) |

blockade for shoulder surgery are significantly less likely to have pain, nausea, and vomiting, and postanesthesia care is shorter.[7] Perineural catheters (either inpatient or ambulatory) for brachial plexus blocks provide the benefit of prolonged postoperative pain control (up to 72 hours), accelerated resumption of therapy, less reliance on opioids, fewer sleep disturbances at home, and overall increased patient satisfaction at home.[8]

Selective brachial plexus blockade can be performed by using landmarks or traditional techniques (paresthesia, nerve stimulator, or ultrasound guidance). Although most traditional techniques may have unpredictable success rates, the use of ultrasound guidance leads to faster block onset and a greater success rate of upper extremity nerve blocks. Common side effects seen after brachial plexus blockade include temporary phrenic nerve blockade and diaphragmatic paralysis, hoarseness, and Horner syndrome.

The site of single-injection nerve blockade or catheter insertion for orthopaedic procedures of the upper extremity varies because of the anatomic locations of the brachial plexus (**Table 1**). The brachial plexus originates from the nerve roots of C5-T1. Interscalene nerve blocks are ideal for anesthesia/analgesia of the shoulder joint because this block will best target the suprascapular, axillary, and supraclavicular nerves (**Table 1**). Supraclavicular blocks provide a high degree of anesthesia/analgesia for elbow and hand surgery. Infraclavicular/axillary nerve blocks provide anesthesia/analgesia similar to that of supraclavicular nerve blocks but with a lower incidence of phrenic nerve paralysis,

recurrent laryngeal nerve blockade, and Horner syndrome when compared with supraclavicular blockade.

The use of perineural catheters for postoperative pain control has been studied over the past decade. Brachial plexus catheters have been shown to reduce resting and dynamic pain, sleep disturbances, opioid requirements, and opioid-related side effects.[9] Furthermore, ambulatory catheters increase home readiness and expedite hospital discharge. The perineural catheter can then be attached to an inpatient or ambulatory pump. The concentration and rate of local anesthetic infusions are best adjusted to minimize motor blockade and adverse local anesthetic toxicity. Patient selection and education are critical before ambulatory catheters are used for surgery. It is recommended that patients be given verbal and written instructions for the management and the removal of ambulatory catheters.[9] It is not uncommon for leakage or dislodgement of catheters to occur at the insertion site, resulting in secondary block failure. Oral opioids can be administered to minimize analgesic gaps.

As an alternative to peripheral nerve blocks and perineural catheters, local wound infiltration analgesia and infusions have also been investigated for analgesia after orthopaedic surgeries.[10] Wound infiltration analgesia involves infiltration of the tissue at the end of surgery and, when applicable, catheters with continuous infusions can be inserted under direct vision by the surgeon. Initial investigations performed for subacromial and glenohumeral joint catheters showed that these modalities led to modest improvements in pain control when compared with placebo.[11,12] However, a case se-

Table 1

Indications for Peripheral Nerve Blocks

Peripheral Nerve Block	Indications
Interscalene block (Roots/trunks of brachial plexus)	Shoulder arthroscopy Rotator cuff repair Shoulder arthroplasty Fracture of humeral neck
Supraclavicular block (Divisions of brachial plexus)	Total elbow replacement Ulnar nerve repair Hand surgery
Infraclavicular/axillary block (Cords/terminal nerves of brachial plexus)	Total elbow replacement Carpel tunnel repair Hand/digit surgery
Lumbar plexus block	Total hip replacement Open reduction and internal fixation of acetabular fracture Total knee replacement Quadriceps repair
Femoral nerve block	Total knee replacement Anterior cruciate ligament repair Quadriceps repair Adjuvant to sciatic block for foot/ankle surgery
Sciatic nerve block	Total ankle replacement Foot/ankle surgery Metatarsal amputation Adjuvant to femoral block for total knee replacement

ries published in 2007 showed a direct correlation between periarticular joint infusions and postarthroscopic glenohumeral chondrolysis in the upper extremity.[13] Postarthroscopic glenohumeral chondrolysis involves the deterioration of articular cartilage with a high-volume local anesthetic, leading to loss of hyaline cartilage in the shoulder joints. Patients with an intra-articular catheter after shoulder surgeries showed signs of shoulder stiffness, shoulder crepitus independent of range of motion, pain, and radiographic glenohumeral joint space narrowing. These cases have resulted in litigation and a warning against using intra-articular catheters in the shoulder joint.

Analgesia for Lower Extremity Surgery

Neuraxial Anesthesia

Surgical procedures involving the lower extremity are amenable to regional anesthetic techniques, including spinal, epidural, and peripheral nerve blocks. Although a spinal anesthetic is the most common neuraxial technique used, a combined spinal-epidural anesthetic may be used for longer procedures, and postoperative analgesia may be provided.

It is well known that neuraxial anesthesia, when compared with general anesthesia, has been shown to decrease postoperative morbidity and mortality after major surgery by reducing cardiac and pulmonary complications, the length of surgery, the need for transfusion, postoperative nausea and vomiting, and the inci-

dence of thromboembolic disease in patients undergoing total joint arthroplasty. However, neuraxial anesthesia/analgesia is not without risks, which include postoperative backache, postdural puncture headache, local anesthetic systemic toxicity, total spinal anesthesia, neurologic injury, and spinal/epidural hematoma. The most significant complication is that of neurologic dysfunction secondary to spinal/epidural hematoma. Although the precise incidence is unknown, the literature cites an incidence of less than 1 in 150,000 epidurals and less than 1 in 220,000 spinal procedures.[14] Given the risk of spinal/epidural hematoma, familiarity with each patient's preoperative medications as well as the plan for postoperative anticoagulation and communication with the anesthesiologist is imperative. In addition, patients with preexisting neurologic conditions may not be ideal candidates for regional techniques. Although localized infection is not a contraindication, it is recommended that the risks and benefits of neuraxial anesthesia be assessed in the patient with bacteremia. Also, patients with scoliosis, morbid obesity, prior back surgery with the placement of hardware, and severe osteoarthritis may not be ideal candidates for neuraxial anesthesia.

Spinal and Epidural Analgesia

Spinal analgesia may be used as part of a multimodal technique for postoperative analgesia following lower extremity surgery with the addition of opioids or clonidine (an α-2 agonist) to the intrathecal mixture, although the analgesic efficacy of spinal analgesia is limited by the lack of titratability as well as the side effect profile of each drug. The advantages of epidural analgesia are demonstrated most clearly with TKA; studies have shown improved early rehabilitation, better pain control, and decreased morphine consumption without any impairment of motor function compared with intravenous patient-controlled anesthesia with morphine.[15] Although conflicting data exist, preemptive epidural analgesia may decrease the incidence of postoperative phantom limb pain following lower extremity amputation.[16] Side effects of epidural analgesia include nausea, vomiting, respiratory depression, urinary retention, hypotension, and pruritus. However, the use of epidural analgesia may decrease the incidence of postoperative pulmonary, cardiovascular, and infectious complications, as well as decrease the length of hospital stays. Nonetheless, there are limitations to the efficacy of epidural analgesia, including hypotension, the risk of epidural hematoma and abscess formation, and incompatibility with anticoagulation, as well as impaired motor function and interference with rehabilitation.

Peripheral Nerve Blocks

Postoperative analgesia for lower extremity surgery can be achieved by a variety of peripheral nerve blocks (Table 1), which are advantageous over epidural analgesia because of their ability to decrease urinary retention and hypotension. When continuous peripheral nerve blocks were compared, regardless of catheter location, the analgesia provided was superior to that of opioid analgesia with the added benefit of fewer opioid-related side effects.[17] The most significant risk associated with peripheral nerve block is nerve injury; however, nerve injury is often temporary, and the incidence is estimated at approximately 1:5000.[18] In addition, peripheral nerve blocks may cause persistent muscular weakness or interfere with rehabilitation.

A lumbar plexus block involves unilateral blockade of the first four lumbar spinal nerves, which give rise to the lateral femoral cutaneous, femoral, and obturator nerves and results in analgesia suitable for surgery involving the hip, the knee, or the quadriceps. Continuous lumbar plexus block has been shown to improve pain control, enhance patient satisfaction, and reduce opioid requirements as well as opioid side effects when compared with patient-controlled anesthesia following total hip arthroplasty and open reduction and internal fixation of acetabular fractures.[19,20] Compatibility with anticoagulation and the risk of neurologic injury secondary to hematoma are similar to that of neuraxial blockade.

The femoral nerve supplies motor innervation to the quadriceps muscle and cutaneous innervation to the anteromedial thigh and knee and the medial aspect of the lower leg and foot and is ideal for postoperative pain control following knee surgery. A femoral nerve block may result in quadriceps weakness, which increases the risk of falls and may interfere with rehabilitation; however, because of easy compressibility, the risk of hematoma formation is much less than that with lumbar plexus block. Single-injection femoral nerve block has been shown to provide improved analgesia, decreased opioid requirements, early rehabilitation, and decreased length of hospital stay following TKA when compared to systemic opioids.[21] Femoral nerve block has also resulted in improved pain scores and reduced opioid requirements compared with a sham block following anterior cruciate ligament repair.[22] Compared with epidural analgesia, continuous femoral nerve block results in a better side effect profile as well as a lower risk of irreversible nerve damage secondary to hematoma formation.

The sciatic nerve provides sensory innervation to the posterior thigh and knee as well as the entire leg and foot below the knee, with the exception of the medial lower leg and ankle and motor innervation to the hamstring and all lower extremity muscles below the knee. The side effect profile and the risk of hematoma formation is similar to that of femoral nerve blocks, and the risk of falls secondary to an insensate lower extremity is increased with the use of combined femoral and sciatic nerve blocks. The utility of adding a sciatic nerve block to a femoral nerve block for postoperative pain relief following TKA is controversial. Sciatic nerve blocks, with or without the addition of femoral or saphenous nerve block, show the most benefit for surgery of the lower leg below the knee. Continuous sciatic nerve blocks have been shown to decrease postoperative pain, reduce opioid requirements, and increase patient satisfaction, as well as facilitate earlier discharge following foot and ankle surgery.[23] In addition, continuous sciatic blocks are compatible with portable local anesthetic infusion pumps, thus allowing continued pain control upon discharge and subsequent decreased pain, opioid use and related side effects, sleep disturbances, and improved satisfaction.[24]

Intra-articular Local Anesthetic Infusion

Intra-articular local anesthetic injection involves infiltration of local anesthetic directly into the tissues of the surgical field. Infusions of local anesthetic have been used alone as well as with NSAIDs and epinephrine. The simplicity and the speed of placement as well as the avoidance of motor blockade has driven increasing interest in this technique as a mode of postoperative analgesia following total joint arthroplasty.

Currently, conflicting data exist regarding the efficacy of intra-articular local anesthetic infusions compared with neuraxial and peripheral nerve block techniques. One study showed that a multimodal intra-articular infusion of ropivacaine, ketorolac, and epinephrine provided improved analgesia and decreased opioid consumption following TKA compared with low-dose epidural ropivacaine combined with parenteral ketorolac.[25] In studies examining efficacy in patients undergoing bilateral TKA (where one knee receives intra-articular local anesthetic infusion and the other knee received either no injection or normal saline placebo), the results have been conflicting, with one study showing lower visual analog scale scores and im-

Table 2

Nonopioid Analgesics and Commonly Used Dosing for Orthopaedic Procedures

Drug	Preoperative Dose	Route of Administration	Time Before Surgery	Postoperative Dose
NSAIDs				
Ketorolac	15-30 mg	PO/IV	30 min – 2 hours	15-30 mg every 6 hours
Ibuprofen	600-800 mg	PO		800 mg every 6 hours
COX-2 Inhibitors				
Celecoxib	200 mg or 400 mg	PO	30 min – 2 hours	200 mg × 1
Antineuropathic				
Gabapentin	600–1,200 mg	PO	30 min – 2 hours	600 mg BID (up to 48 hours)
Pregabalin	75-300 mg	PO	30 min – 2 hours	75 mg-150 mg BID
Acetaminophen (PO or IV)	1 g	PO/IV	30 min – 2 hours	1 g every 6 hours (weight > 50 kg)

PO = by mouth, IV = intravenous, BID = twice daily, TID = three times daily.

proved range of motion in the injection group and the other study showing no improvement in pain scores, patient satisfaction, or range of motion in either group.[26,27] Still, studies have shown that continuous intra-articular local anesthetic infusions can result in improved pain control and reduced opioid requirements following total joint arthroplasty.[28] At this time, there are insufficient data to compare the efficacy of intra-articular local anesthetic infusions with the current gold standards of postoperative pain control as continuous peripheral nerve blocks following total joint arthroplasty; thus, further studies are needed.

Pain Management in the Opioid-Tolerant Patient

Persistent postsurgical pain with reduced health-related quality of life up to 1 year after total hip arthroplasty and TKA is common.[29] These patients typically take chronic opioids and present with extremes of tolerance (reduced analgesic effects of opioids) before surgery. The development of tolerance with chronic opioid use results from desensitization of opioid antinociceptive pathways and can be attributed to the desensitization of the μ-opioid receptor and second-messenger systems (protein kinase and G-protein) at the cellular level. Opioid tolerance in patients with chronic pain can usually be addressed by increasing the dose of opioids. Chronic opioid users often require a twofold to threefold increase in perioperative opioids when compared with opioid-naïve patients.

Appropriate management strategy of patients with opioid tolerance involves identifying these patients before surgery and carefully assessing preoperative opioid requirements. Perioperative management involves careful planning that uses multimodal drug regimens. During the preoperative period, patients may receive acetaminophen, celecoxib, gabapentin, or pregabalin

(Table 2). Both gabapentin and pregabalin act to inhibit the $\alpha_2\delta$ subunit on the presynaptic voltage-gated calcium channel and attenuate the neuronal sensitization response. Perioperative use of pregabalin in total knee replacement has been shown to decrease opioid consumption and the incidence of neuropathic pain at 3 and 6 months after surgery.[4]

Intraoperative ketamine, an N-methyl-D-aspartate antagonist, when given during spine surgery, was shown to reduce total morphine consumption and pain intensity up to 6 weeks after surgery with no differences in side effects compared with placebo.[6] Alternatively, an intraoperative single bolus of methadone (0.2 mg/kg) has also shown a 50% reduction in postoperative opioid consumption and pain scores at 48 hours after surgery for complex spine procedures.[30]

Opioid-tolerant patients may see maximal benefits with regional anesthesia techniques using continuous neuraxial and peripheral nerve catheters for orthopaedic procedures. Postoperative management will require supplemental opioids to control breakthrough pain as well as prevent acute withdrawal from opioids. This may be met with systemic opioids, such as with patient-controlled analgesia. However, it is helpful to maintain preoperative doses of extended-release opioids during the perioperative course. Postoperative ketamine infusions (up to 4 days) have also proven successful in decreasing opioid requirements and improving analgesia in patients with chronic pain and opioid tolerance.

Intravenous Nonopioid Analgesics

Nonopioid analgesics are an important adjunct to opioid-based medications in perioperative analgesia because they help reduce overall opioid use and subsequent deleterious side effects (Table 2). Intravenous nonopioid analgesics include acetaminophen, ke-

2: Systemic Disorders

Table 3

Suggested Dosing for Oral Opioids in the Postoperative Period

Drug	Dose (mg)	Frequency (hours)	Duration (hours)
Hydrocodone/acetaminophen	10/325	Every 4-6	4-8
Hydromorphone	2-4	Every 3-4	3-4
Oxycodone immediate release	5-10	Every 4-6	3-4
Oxycodone/acetaminophen	10/325	Every 4-6	3-4
Morphine sulfate	10-30	Every 3-4	2-4
Oxymorphone immediate release	10-20	Every 4-6	7-11

torolac, and ibuprofen. Acetaminophen functions via the inhibition of cyclooxygenase, which is similar to NSAIDs, but with little to no peripheral activity. Acetaminophen is both an effective analgesic and a potent antipyretic agent. Intravenous administration is advantageous in patients unable to take pills by mouth and when a more rapid analgesic effect is desired. Although intravenous administration of analgesics has been demonstrated to produce higher plasma levels of acetaminophen and a trend toward reduced postanesthesia care unit stay than oral doses, a recent study in patients undergoing knee arthroscopy ultimately showed no change in overall pain scores.[31]

Intravenous acetaminophen is usually dosed at 1,000 mg every 6 hours for a maximum daily dose of 4,000 mg in those age 13 years and older who weigh more than 50 kg. For children aged 2 to 12 years or adults who weigh less than 50 kg, dosing is weight based at 15 mg/kg every 6 hours with a total daily dose of 75 mg/kg. Studies have shown that intravenous acetaminophen is both safe and efficacious compared with placebo and has shown significant reductions in pain scores and opioid consumption when administered for 24 hours postoperatively in patients undergoing major orthopaedic surgery.[32,33] Overall, acetaminophen has a proven record of safe use with minimal side effects; however, hepatotoxicity is always a concern, although more often in the elderly.

Two commonly used intravenous NSAIDs in the perioperative period are ketorolac and ibuprofen. Both medications are nonspecific cyclooxygenase inhibitors that, unlike acetaminophen, have potent peripheral anti-inflammatory properties. Common dosing strategies for ketorolac include one-time injections of 30 mg intravenously or 30-60 mg intramuscularly or 30 mg intravenously every 6 hours for up to 5 days in patients without significant renal disease. Previous studies have shown conflicting results on both the most effective timing and the dose of ketorolac in orthopaedic patients; however, when given as a standing intravenous medication, ketorolac demonstrates clear improvement in pain scores and reductions in opioid consumption during the postoperative period in patients undergoing lumbar decompression surgery.[34]

Intravenous ibuprofen is commonly dosed in a range of 400 mg to 800 mg every 6 hours. A multicenter, randomized, double-blinded, placebo-controlled trial revealed that 800 mg intravenous dose of ibuprofen every 6 hours when given throughout the perioperative period is effective at reducing pain scores and opioid consumption in adult orthopaedic patients.[35] Another study involving both orthopaedic and abdominal surgeries showed that 800 mg every 6 hours was more effective at reducing pain scores than the 400 mg dosing regimen, although both were noteworthy for gastrointestinal side effects.[36]

Oral Analgesics

As patients progress to the postoperative period, their analgesics are often switched from the intravenous formulation to the oral formulation. Oral opioids are an important component of many patients' analgesic regimens, and those most commonly used include hydrocodone, hydromorphone, oxycodone, morphine, and oxymorphone (**Table 3**). Typically, this transition occurs on the first or second postoperative day after pain has been reasonably controlled with intravenous medications and patients are tolerating a liquid diet.

Hydrocodone is one of the most frequently prescribed opioid analgesics, although the potential for abuse is high, and it is commonly paired with acetaminophen or aspirin. It is reliably absorbed, with onset at 35 minutes and peak plasma concentration occurring after 80 minutes. Hydromorphone is five times more potent than morphine with a slightly shorter duration of action and is effective for moderate to severe pain. Oxycodone, available in both sustained-release and immediate-release forms, is also reliably absorbed with onset at 35 minutes. It is also commonly paired with acetaminophen for greater analgesic benefit. However, caution must be used when drugs are combined with acetaminophen (not to exceed 4 g per day). Acetaminophen can be dosed around-the-clock, rather than as needed, and given separately from oxycodone so that the potential for exceeding 4 g of acetaminophen is greatly reduced. Both hydrocodone and oxycodone

2: Systemic Disorders

have a duration of 3.5 to 4 hours. Morphine is also an option, but it is limited by poor absorption and extensive hepatic first-pass metabolism. It is also available in sustained-release formulations. Oxymorphone, with peak effect in 30 minutes, is a metabolite of oxycodone that is 10 times more potent than morphine and can cause significant nausea and vomiting. It is available as a sustained-release formulation and an immediate-release formulation.

Several oral nonopioid medications can provide effective analgesia and potentially decrease consumption of opioids and their side effects. NSAIDs, such as ketorolac and ibuprofen, and COX-2 inhibitors, such as celecoxib, may decrease opioid requirements after surgery. They do not cause opioid-type side effects, such as nausea, vomiting, and pruritus. These benefits should be weighed against potential side effects, including poor wound healing, gastrointestinal irritation, decreased platelet function, and renal impairment.

Gabapentin and pregabalin, anticonvulsants with analgesic properties that act via inhibition of $\alpha_2\delta$ subunit on the presynaptic voltage-gated calcium channel and attenuation of the neuronal sensitization response, can be an effective addition to a multimodal regimen. Gabapentin reduces postoperative pain scores and opioid usage, and pregabalin has been shown to reduce chronic neuropathic pain and opioid consumption and promote better range of motion during the first 30 days after TKA.[4] Side effects include sedation and confusion.

A Potential Novel Agent in Regional Analgesia

Given the limited duration, efforts have been made to increase the duration of analgesia provided by local anesthetics. Recently the FDA approved liposomal bupivacaine for single-dose wound infiltration in postoperative pain relief among patients undergoing hemorrhoidectomy and bunionectomy. Liposomal bupivacaine increases the duration of action of local anesthetic via slow release from a multivesicular liposome over 96 hours and delays the peak plasma concentration compared with plain bupivacaine administration. In multicenter, double-blinded studies, liposomal bupivacaine significantly reduced pain scores and opioid consumption for the first 72 hours following hemorrhoidectomy, whereas similar results were seen in the first 24 hours following first metatarsal bunionectomy.[37] Although more research will be needed regarding the utility of liposomal bupivacaine with regard to peripheral nerve blockade and neuraxial analgesia, there is certainly the potential to decrease the need for continuous catheters and external pumps.

Summary

Aggressive pain management using a multimodal approach is now considered standard treatment. With careful planning, multimodal techniques instituted preoperatively will reduce postoperative pain. Accurate assessment of the characteristics of pain will direct rational drug choices while minimizing side effects. Better pain management in the postoperative setting will likely improve patient satisfaction and facilitate faster discharge from the hospital.

Key Study Points

- A multimodal approach to perioperative pain management following orthopaedic surgery is key. An around-the-clock regimen of acetaminophen, NSAIDs or COX-2 inhibitors, neuropathic agents, and local anesthetics with opioids as an adjunct is the current recommendation in acute pain management.

- It is imperative to identify opioid-tolerant patients and those with chronic pain prior to surgery because they can be challenging to treat. A multimodal analgesic plan should be developed to address perioperative pain management because chronic postsurgical pain is common.

Annotated References

1. Apfelbaum JL, Chen C, Mehta SS, Gan TJ: Postoperative pain experience: Results from a national survey suggest postoperative pain continues to be undermanaged. *Anesth Analg* 2003;97(2):534-540.

2. Coley KC, Williams BA, DaPos SV, Chen C, Smith RB: Retrospective evaluation of unanticipated admissions and readmissions after same day surgery and associated costs. *J Clin Anesth* 2002;14(5):349-353.

3. American Society of Anesthesiologists Task Force on Acute Pain Management: Practice guidelines for acute pain management in the perioperative setting: An updated report by the American Society of Anesthesiologists Task Force on Acute Pain Management. *Anesthesiology* 2012;116(2):248-273.

   A summary of the most recent American Society of Anesthesiologists guidelines for perioperative acute pain management, emphasizing a multimodal approach is presented.

4. Buvanendran A, Kroin JS, Della Valle CJ, Kari M, Moric M, Tuman KJ: Perioperative oral pregabalin reduces chronic pain after total knee arthroplasty: A prospective, randomized, controlled trial. *Anesth Analg* 2010;110(1):199-207.

   Patients who received pregabalin 300 mg preoperatively had a lower incidence of chronic neuropathic pain at 3 and 6 months after TKA and less opioid consumption at 30 days.

5. Burke SM, Shorten GD: Perioperative pregabalin improves pain and functional outcomes 3 months after

lumbar discectomy. *Anesth Analg* 2010;110(4):1180-1185.

The authors randomized patients to pregabalin or placebo and found that pregabalin decreased pain during the immediate postoperative period and at 3 months.

6. Loftus RW, Yeager MP, Clark JA, et al: Intraoperative ketamine reduces perioperative opiate consumption in opiate-dependent patients with chronic back pain undergoing back surgery. *Anesthesiology* 2010;113(3):639-646.

This prospective, double-blind, randomized trial demonstrated less opioid consumption in the intraoperative ketamine group compared to placebo following back surgery.

7. Hadzic A, Williams BA, Karaca PE, et al: For outpatient rotator cuff surgery, nerve block anesthesia provides superior same-day recovery over general anesthesia. *Anesthesiology* 2005;102(5):1001-1007.

8. Ilfeld BM: Continuous peripheral nerve blocks: A review of the published evidence. *Anesth Analg* 2011;113(4):904-925.

The authors reviewed the published literature on continuous peripheral nerve blocks and looked at benefits, complications, and risks.

9. Ilfeld BM, Enneking FK: Continuous peripheral nerve blocks at home: A review. *Anesth Analg* 2005;100(6):1822-1833.

10. Ganapathy S, Brookes J, Bourne R: Local infiltration analgesia. *Anesthesiol Clin* 2011;29(2):329-342.

The authors provide an evidence-based review of wound infiltration analgesia for various surgical procedures.

11. Savoie FH, Field LD, Jenkins RN, Mallon WJ, Phelps RA II: The pain control infusion pump for postoperative pain control in shoulder surgery. *Arthroscopy* 2000;16(4):339-342.

12. Barber FA, Herbert MA: The effectiveness of an anesthetic continuous-infusion device on postoperative pain control. *Arthroscopy* 2002;18(1):76-81.

13. Hansen BP, Beck CL, Beck EP, Townsley RW: Postarthroscopic glenohumeral chondrolysis. *Am J Sports Med* 2007;35(10):1628-1634.

14. Horlocker TT, Wedel DJ, Rowlingson JC, et al: Regional anesthesia in the patient receiving antithrombotic or thrombolytic therapy: American Society of Regional Anesthesia and Pain Medicine Evidence-Based Guidelines (Third Edition). *Reg Anesth Pain Med* 2010;35(1):64-101.

The authors discuss the most recent evidence-based practice guidelines delineated by the American Society of Regional Anesthesia and Pain Medicine regarding the safe and appropriate use of regional anesthesia for patients receiving anticoagulation therapy.

15. Capdevila X, Barthelet Y, Biboulet P, Ryckwaert Y, Rubenovitch J, d'Athis F: Effects of perioperative analgesic technique on the surgical outcome and duration of rehabilitation after major knee surgery. *Anesthesiology* 1999;91(1):8-15.

16. Gottschalk A, Smith DS: New concepts in acute pain therapy: Preemptive analgesia. *Am Fam Physician* 2001;63(10):1979-1984.

17. Richman JM, Liu SS, Courpas G, et al: Does continuous peripheral nerve block provide superior pain control to opioids? A meta-analysis. *Anesth Analg* 2006;102(1):248-257.

18. Fowler SJ, Symons J, Sabato S, Myles PS: Epidural analgesia compared with peripheral nerve blockade after major knee surgery: A systematic review and meta-analysis of randomized trials. *Br J Anaesth* 2008;100(2):154-164.

19. Siddiqui ZI, Cepeda MS, Denman W, Schumann R, Carr DB: Continuous lumbar plexus block provides improved analgesia with fewer side effects compared with systemic opioids after hip arthroplasty: A randomized controlled trial. *Reg Anesth Pain Med* 2007;32(5):393-398.

20. Chelly JE, Casati A, Al-Samsam T, Coupe K, Criswell A, Tucker J: Continuous lumbar plexus block for acute postoperative pain management after open reduction and internal fixation of acetabular fractures. *J Orthop Trauma* 2003;17(5):362-367.

21. Wang H, Boctor B, Verner J: The effect of single-injection femoral nerve block on rehabilitation and length of hospital stay after total knee replacement. *Reg Anesth Pain Med* 2002;27(2):139-144.

22. Mulroy MF, Larkin KL, Batra MS, Hodgson PS, Owens BD: Femoral nerve block with 0.25% or 0.5% bupivacaine improves postoperative analgesia following outpatient arthroscopic anterior cruciate ligament repair. *Reg Anesth Pain Med* 2001;26(1):24-29.

23. White PF, Issioui T, Skrivanek GD, Early JS, Wakefield C: The use of a continuous popliteal sciatic nerve block after surgery involving the foot and ankle: Does it improve the quality of recovery? *Anesth Analg* 2003;97(5):1303-1309.

24. Ilfeld BM, Morey TE, Wang RD, Enneking FK: Continuous popliteal sciatic nerve block for postoperative pain control at home: A randomized, double-blinded, placebo-controlled study. *Anesthesiology* 2002;97(4):959-965.

25. Andersen KV, Bak M, Christensen BV, Harazuk J, Pedersen NA, Søballe K: A randomized, controlled trial comparing local infiltration analgesia with epidural infusion for total knee arthroplasty. *Acta Orthop* 2010;81(5):606-610.

A randomized trial comparing the efficacy of multimodal intra-articular infusion of a ketorolac, epinephrine, ropivacaine mixture and epidural ropivacaine with intravenous ketorolac in TKA is discussed. Both infusions ran at 4 mL/h, and the intra-articular group demonstrated superior pain relief and decreased opioid consumption.

26. Mullaji A, Kanna R, Shetty GM, Chavda V, Singh DP: Efficacy of periarticular injection of bupivacaine, fentanyl, and methylprednisolone in total knee arthroplasty: A prospective, randomized trial. *J Arthroplasty* 2010; 25(6):851-857.

    The authors discuss a randomized trial examining the efficacy of periarticular injection of bupivacaine, fentanyl, methylprednisolone mixture during bilateral TKA resulting in better pain scores, improved range of motion, and superior quadriceps recovery in the injected knee.

27. Joo JH, Park JW, Kim JS, Kim YH: Is intra-articular multimodal drug injection effective in pain management after total knee arthroplasty? A randomized, double-blinded, prospective study. *J Arthroplasty* 2011;26(7): 1095-1099.

    A prospective, randomized, double-blinded trial comparing intra-articular multimodal injection in one knee and saline placebo in the contralateral knee during bilateral TKA showed no improvement in patient pain and satisfaction, range of motion, or blood loss.

28. Bianconi M, Ferraro L, Traina GC, et al: Pharmacokinetics and efficacy of ropivacaine continuous wound instillation after joint replacement surgery. *Br J Anaesth* 2003;91(6):830-835.

29. Liu SS, Buvanendran A, Rathmell JP, et al: A cross-sectional survey on prevalence and risk factors for persistent postsurgical pain 1 year after total hip and knee replacement. *Reg Anesth Pain Med* 2012;37(4): 415-422.

    This multi-institutional study investigated the effect of chronic pain after hip and knee replacement surgery on quality of life.

30. Gottschalk A, Durieux ME, Nemergut EC: Intraoperative methadone improves postoperative pain control in patients undergoing complex spine surgery. *Anesth Analg* 2011;112(1):218-223.

    This randomized study in spine surgery showed that a single bolus of methadone before skin incision improved pain control.

31. Brett CN, Barnett SG, Pearson J: Postoperative plasma paracetamol levels following oral or intravenous paracetamol administration: A double-blind randomised controlled trial. *Anaesth Intensive Care* 2012;40(1): 166-171.

This study demonstrates that although intravenous acetaminophen leads to higher plasma levels relative to oral dosing, there was no change in postanesthesia care unit pain scores in patients after knee arthroscopy.

32. Sinatra RS, Jahr JS, Reynolds L, et al: Intravenous acetaminophen for pain after major orthopedic surgery: An expanded analysis. *Pain Pract* 2012;12(5):357-365.

    Expanded analysis of intravenous acetaminophen continues to demonstrate reductions in pain scores and opioid consumption in patients undergoing major orthopaedic surgery.

33. Jahr JS, Breitmeyer JB, Pan C, Royal MA, Ang RY: Safety and efficacy of intravenous acetaminophen in the elderly after major orthopedic surgery: Subset data analysis from 3, randomized, placebo-controlled trials. *Am J Ther* 2012;19(2):66-75.

    A study examining the effects of intravenous acetaminophen in elderly patients is presented. The results indicate that intravenous acetaminophen is both safe and effective in this population.

34. Cassinelli EH, Dean CL, Garcia RM, Furey CG, Bohlman HH: Ketorolac use for postoperative pain management following lumbar decompression surgery: A prospective, randomized, double-blinded, placebo-controlled trial. *Spine (Phila Pa 1976)* 2008;33(12): 1313-1317.

35. Singla N, Rock A, Pavliv LA: A multi-center, randomized, double-blind placebo-controlled trial of intravenous-ibuprofen (IV-ibuprofen) for treatment of pain in post-operative orthopedic adult patients. *Pain Med* 2010;11(8):1284-1293.

    The authors found that administration of intravenous ibuprofen before and after surgery led to a reduction of pain and morphine use in patients undergoing orthopaedic surgery.

36. Southworth S, Peters J, Rock A, Pavliv L: A multicenter, randomized, double-blind, placebo-controlled trial of intravenous ibuprofen 400 and 800 mg every 6 hours in the management of postoperative pain. *Clin Ther* 2009; 31(9):1922-1935.

37. Candiotti K: Liposomal bupivacaine: An innovative nonopioid local analgesic for the management of postsurgical pain. *Pharmacotherapy* 2012;32(9, suppl): 19S-26S.

    This article discusses the utility of liposomal bupivacaine, including current approaches to pain management and how liposomal bupivacaine is currently used.

2: Systemic Disorders

Section 3

Upper Extremity

SECTION EDITOR:

William N. Levine, MD

Chapter 25

Shoulder Trauma: Bone

John-Erik Bell, MD, MS   Edwin R. Cadet, MD

Proximal Humeral Fractures

Proximal humeral fractures account for approximately 4% to 5% of all fractures.[1,2] Fracture patterns vary based on the mechanism of injury and bone density at the time of injury. In patients older than 60 years, proximal humeral fractures are caused by low-energy trauma;[3] these fractures are often considered fragility fractures and serve as a clinical indication of existing osteopenia or osteoporosis. When warranted, the patient should be evaluated and treated for osteoporosis as part of fracture management. In younger patients without osteopenia, proximal humeral fractures can be the result of high-energy trauma, and greater consideration is given to humeral head preservation with fracture osteosynthesis in this patient population. Although most proximal humeral fractures are minimally displaced and are treated nonsurgically, the management of displaced proximal humeral fractures is controversial.

Presentation

The affected extremity and chest may exhibit visual evidence of trauma (ecchymosis or swelling). Careful evaluation for additional injuries and the cause for trauma is important, especially with high-energy trauma and in elderly patients with cognitive deficits or in the setting of unwitnessed trauma. A thorough neurovascular examination must be performed to identify injury to the neighboring neurovascular structures, particularly in the setting of fracture-dislocations. The most commonly encountered neurologic injuries following a proximal humeral fracture are axillary and/or suprascapular neurapraxias.[4]

Anatomy and Vascularity

The four anatomic parts of the proximal humerus are the humeral head, the greater tuberosity, the lesser tuberosity, and the surgical neck.[5,6] The average humeral neck-shaft angle measures approximately 140°.[7] Humeral head version is quite variable depending on

which anatomic landmarks are used.[8,9] Thirty degrees has traditionally been considered normal humeral head retroversion.

Historically, the anterior humeral circumflex artery was considered to be the dominant vascular supply to the humeral head; however, recent studies have demonstrated that the posterior humeral circumflex artery plays a greater role in supplying blood to the proximal humerus.[10,11] The authors of one study argued that the posterior and anterior humeral circumflex arteries are equally important in humeral head perfusion.[10] They noted that the posterior humeral circumflex artery was consistently larger in diameter than the anterior humeral circumflex artery. The vascularity of the proximal humerus was quantitatively assessed in a cadaver study; the posterior humeral circumflex artery was found to contribute 64% of the blood supplied to the proximal humerus, whereas the anterior humeral circumflex artery contributes just 36%.[11] Regardless, the vascular supply to the articular head segment plays a critical role in determining proper management and the outcome of proximal humeral fractures.

Classification

Proximal humeral fractures have been classified based on the anatomic location of the fracture. With the Codman classification, the proximal humerus was divided into the four anatomic parts based on epiphyseal lines as discussed previously.[5,6] This classification scheme was expanded to include the presence of fracture displacement and angulation to define the severity of the fracture pattern.[5] With the Neer classification, a fracture part was defined as a fragment displaced more than 1 cm or angulated more than 45°. The probability of humeral head necrosis increases with the severity of the fracture. The AO classification is used less frequently than the Neer and Codman classification systems and emphasizes determination of whether vascularity to the articular fragment is significantly compromised. Type A is an extra-articular, unifocal fracture that involves one of the tuberosities with or without a concomitant metaphyseal fracture. Type B is an extra-articular, bifocal fracture or fracture-dislocation with tuberosity and metaphyseal involvement. Type C is a fracture or a fracture-dislocation of the articular surface; this type is considered the most severe because the vascular supply is thought to be at the greatest risk of injury, making the humeral head susceptible to the development of osteonecrosis (Figure 1).

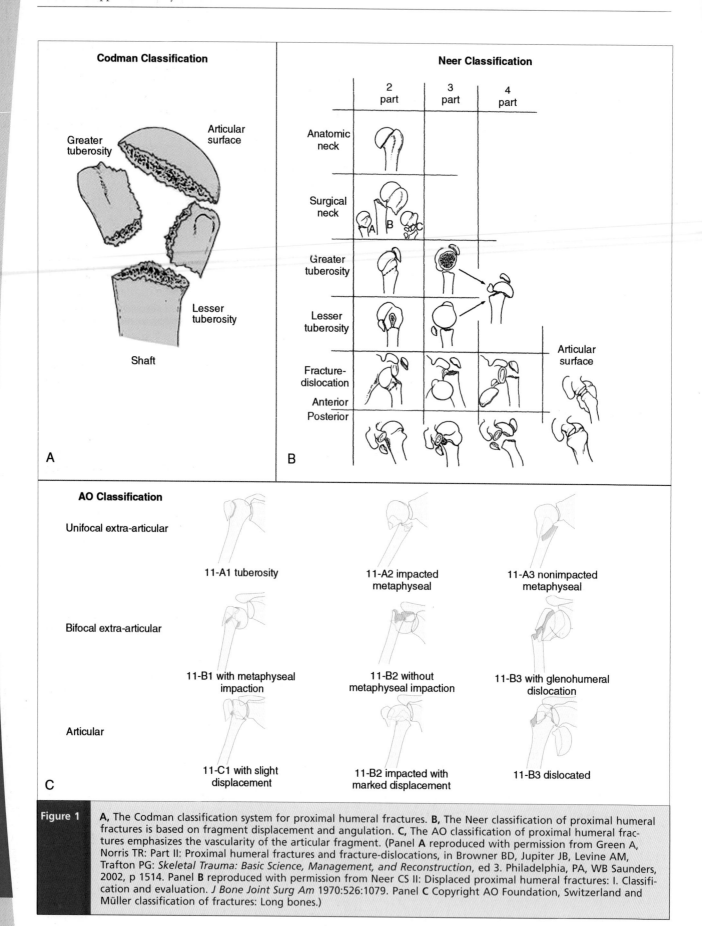

Codman Classification

Greater tuberosity

Articular surface

Lesser tuberosity

Shaft

A

Neer Classification

	2 part	3 part	4 part
Anatomic neck			
Surgical neck	A B C		
Greater tuberosity			
Lesser tuberosity			Articular surface
Fracture-dislocation Anterior Posterior			

B

AO Classification

Unifocal extra-articular

11-A1 tuberosity

11-A2 impacted metaphyseal

11-A3 nonimpacted metaphyseal

Bifocal extra-articular

11-B1 with metaphyseal impaction

11-B2 without metaphyseal impaction

11-B3 with glenohumeral dislocation

Articular

11-C1 with slight displacement

11-B2 impacted with marked displacement

11-B3 dislocated

C

Figure 1   **A,** The Codman classification system for proximal humeral fractures. **B,** The Neer classification of proximal humeral fractures is based on fragment displacement and angulation. **C,** The AO classification of proximal humeral fractures emphasizes the vascularity of the articular fragment. (Panel **A** reproduced with permission from Green A, Norris TR: Part II: Proximal humeral fractures and fracture-dislocations, in Browner BD, Jupiter JB, Levine AM, Trafton PG: *Skeletal Trauma: Basic Science, Management, and Reconstruction*, ed 3. Philadelphia, PA, WB Saunders, 2002, p 1514. Panel **B** reproduced with permission from Neer CS II: Displaced proximal humeral fractures: I. Classification and evaluation. *J Bone Joint Surg Am* 1970:526:1079. Panel **C** Copyright AO Foundation, Switzerland and Müller classification of fractures: Long bones.)

Imaging and Fracture Classification

Fracture classification can be performed using plain radiographs, advanced imaging, or a combination of both. A trauma radiographic series for proximal humeral fractures should include a true AP view of the affected shoulder obtained in the plane of the scapula, a scapular Y or outlet view, and axillary views. Several studies have assessed the interobserver and intraobserver reliability of plain radiographs and CT scans in defining proximal humeral fractures using the Neer or the AO classification systems.[12-15] Although additional imaging is routinely used to further characterize these fractures, it has been shown that the addition of CT and three-dimensional imaging did not improve interobserver reproducibility of either the Neer or the AO classification systems.[15,16] In addition, the interobserver reproducibility of the Neer classification had a mean kappa coefficient of 0.52 with plain radiographs alone and 0.50 with radiographs and CT scans.[12] There was a slight increase in intraobserver reliability when CT was added to plain radiographic interpretation (0.64 versus 0.72); however, no increase in interobserver reproducibility was observed with the addition of CT.

Nonsurgical Management

Nonsurgical management is chosen for most proximal humeral fractures depending on factors such as fracture displacement, patient age and comorbidities, and bone quality. The goals of nonsurgical management are to provide a period of brief immobilization to allow for fracture consolidation, followed by a period of progressive passive and active-assisted range of motion. Serial radiographs are taken during the early postinjury period to monitor fracture displacement. Active range of motion and strengthening exercises are instituted when signs of osseous union occur, usually between 6 and 8 weeks. Potential negative sequelae of nonsurgical management for significantly displaced proximal humeral fractures include symptomatic nonunion, malunion, and osteonecrosis of the humeral head.

Surgical Management

When surgery is chosen, the choice of approach and fixation technique depends on the viability of the articular segment, the surgeon's ability to achieve and sustain an acceptable reduction, the ability to achieve adequate medial calcar support, bone quality, patient age and comorbidities, and the patient's ability to comply with postoperative restrictions and rehabilitation. Young, active patients with a valgus-impacted, three- and/or four-part proximal humeral fracture with adequate bone quality or two-part greater and lesser tuberosity and surgical neck fracture patterns are candidates for osteosynthesis with transosseous suture fixation, locked plating, intramedullary nailing, or percutaneous pinning techniques (Figure 2). Hemiarthroplasty is recommended for patients with four-part proximal humeral fractures in whom anatomic reduction cannot be achieved intraoperatively; patients with moderate or severe osteopenia that can compromise osteosynthesis

fixation techniques; patients with Neer four-part fracture-dislocations; and patients with malunion, nonunion, hardware failure, or osteonecrosis of the humeral head following osteosynthesis. Reverse total shoulder arthroplasty (RTSA) may be appropriate in patients with lower physical demands and those older than 70 years with poor bone quality.[17]

Greater and Lesser Tuberosity Fractures

Two-part greater tuberosity fractures account for approximately 15% of displaced proximal humeral fractures with or without anterior glenohumeral joint dislocation.[18] Two-part greater tuberosity fractures are defined as displaced when the fragment is displaced more than 1.0 cm; however, less tolerance of displacement for the greater tuberosity also has been indicated. Surgical management has been recommended for fracture fragments displaced 5 mm or greater. Osteosynthesis of greater tuberosity fractures with displacement greater than 5 mm in athletes and heavy laborers has been advocated.[19]

Traditionally, open reduction and internal fixation (ORIF) of fractures of the greater tuberosity via an anterosuperior, deltoid-splitting approach has yielded good results. A deltopectoral approach may be used with greater tuberosity fractures with substantial distal cortical extension. Arthroscopic techniques have been used to treat these fractures.[20] Open and arthroscopic fixation techniques include transosseous suture repair, suture anchor configurations similar to rotator cuff repair techniques, the use of cannulated screws via arthroscopic-assisted or open approaches, and tension band constructs. The degree of osteopenia and comminution present will often guide the surgical approach when managing these fractures.

Two-part lesser tuberosity fractures occur less often than two-part greater tuberosity fractures and often occur in conjunction with posterior glenohumeral dislocations (for example, seizure) or may represent a physeal fracture-avulsion of the subscapularis in the adolescent patient population. Arthroscopic fixation techniques with smaller avulsion lesser tuberosity fractures have been reported. Larger fragments are generally reduced via open techniques, and fixation is achieved with interfragmentary screws (Figure 3). Comminuted fragments may be surgically managed with transosseous sutures or modern suture anchor techniques similar to rotator cuff repair, as described previously for greater tuberosity fractures.

Surgical Neck Fractures

Surgical management of surgical neck fractures is indicated for a fracture pattern exhibiting significant displacement, polytrauma, comorbid ipsilateral upper extremity injuries (such as floating shoulder), vascular compromise, open fractures, metastatic fractures, or fractures for which nonsurgical management was unsuccessful. The advent of proximal humeral locking plates provides a good option to ensure rigid fracture stabilization, particularly in the setting of osteopenic

3: Upper Extremity

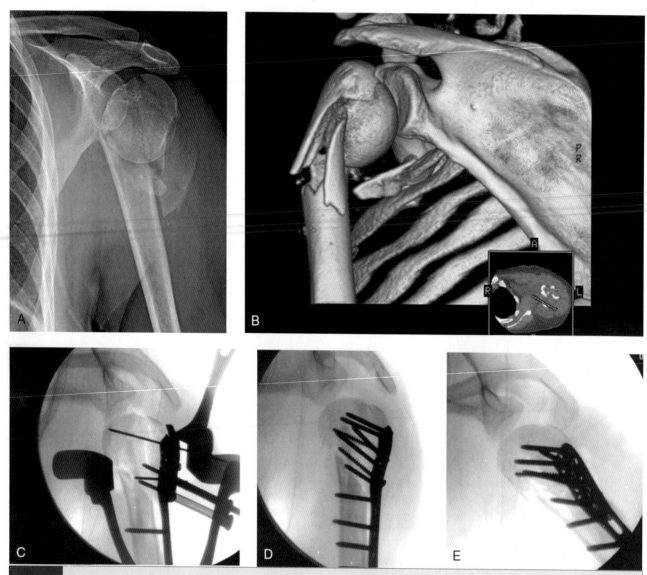

Figure 2 AP radiograph (**A**) and three-dimensional CT scan (**B**) of a displaced, comminuted three-part proximal humeral fracture in a 55-year-old woman. Open reduction and internal fixation with proximal locking plate and fibular strut allograft with medial calcar augmentation is shown in **C** through **E**. Provisional wire fixation is first achieved (**C**), followed by locking plate application as seen on the AP (**D**) and axillary (**E**) fluoroscopic images.

bone and early mobilization (Figure 4). Fixed-angled locking plates neutralize forces exerted on fracture fragments from the pull of the rotator cuff and the surrounding musculature to provide rigid fixation so that mobilization can begin in the early postoperative period. Other surgical options include intramedullary nailing, blade plate fixation, suture fixation (in the setting of osteopenic bone), and percutaneous pinning.

Open Reduction and Internal Fixation With Precontoured Locking Plates

The development of locking plate technology has provided a successful technique in the management of proximal humeral fractures. Successful ORIF of displaced proximal humeral fractures requires medial sup-

port via an anatomic reduction of the metaphysis, inferomedial screw placement along the calcar of the proximal humerus, or augmented support of the medial column with a structural endosteal implant.[21,22] The mean Constant scores were compared in a study of patients age 55 years or older with three- or four-part proximal humeral fractures treated with locked plating or hemiarthroplasty.[23] At a mean 36-month follow-up, significantly higher mean Constant shoulder scores were found in the locking plate group ($P < 0.001$). Despite the higher complication rate in the locked plate group, better outcomes were achieved with locked plating than with hemiarthroplasty, especially in patients with three-part fractures. Of 38 patients in the locking plate group, 6 developed osteonecrosis following sur-

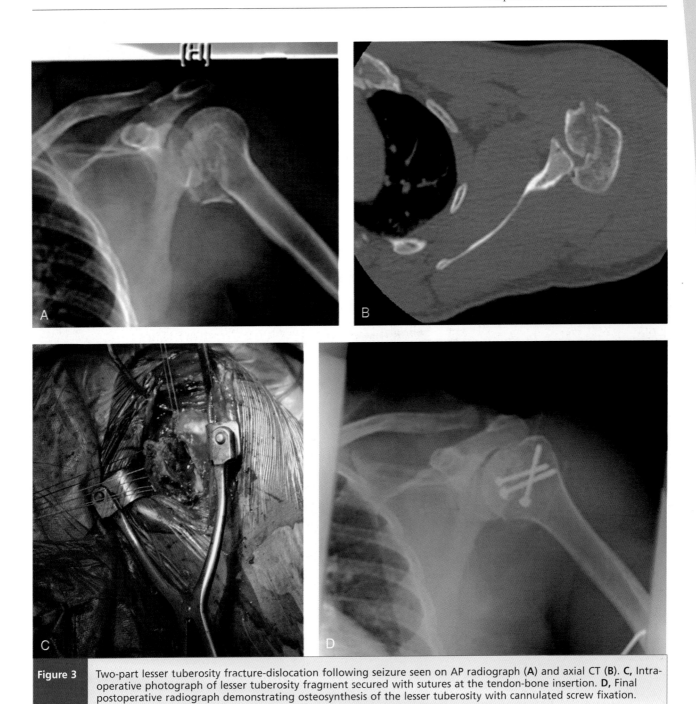

Figure 3 Two-part lesser tuberosity fracture-dislocation following seizure seen on AP radiograph (**A**) and axial CT (**B**). **C**, Intraoperative photograph of lesser tuberosity fragment secured with sutures at the tendon-bone insertion. **D**, Final postoperative radiograph demonstrating osteosynthesis of the lesser tuberosity with cannulated screw fixation.

gery, 6 had evidence of screw perforation of the humeral head, 4 had loss of fixation, and 3 developed wound infection. In contrast, 7 of 48 patients in the hemiarthroplasty group had nonunion of the tuberosity fragments, and 3 patients developed wound infection. The authors of this study noted that loss of fixation in the locking plate group was seen only in patients with initial varus malalignment of more than 20°. Proper surgical technique is essential, as complication rates as high as 40% have been cited using the locking plate technique for treating proximal humeral fractures.[24]

In a randomized controlled trial, clinical improvements in quality-of-life measures and range of motion were noted in patients treated with precontoured locking plates for displaced, three-part proximal humeral fractures compared with patients treated nonsurgically; however, the authors did not find a statistically significant difference in those measures.[25] Both groups experienced a statistically significant decline in quality-of-life measures when compared with the preinjury state. Despite acceptable fracture reduction achieved in 86% of the patients, the locking plate group had a 30% complication rate requiring either minor or major surgery compared with 3% in the nonsurgical group. Complications included infection, postoperative stiffness, screw perforation, nonunion, and osteonecrosis.

3: Upper Extremity

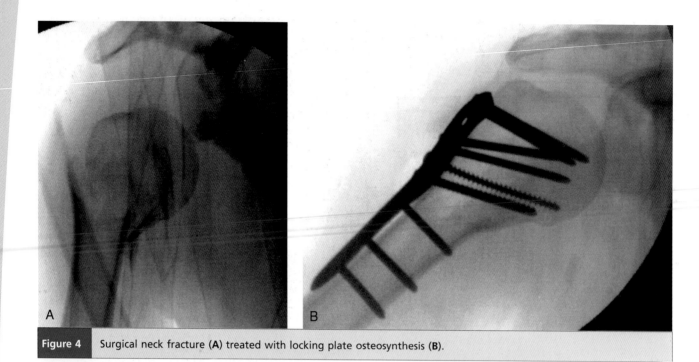

Figure 4 Surgical neck fracture (**A**) treated with locking plate osteosynthesis (**B**).

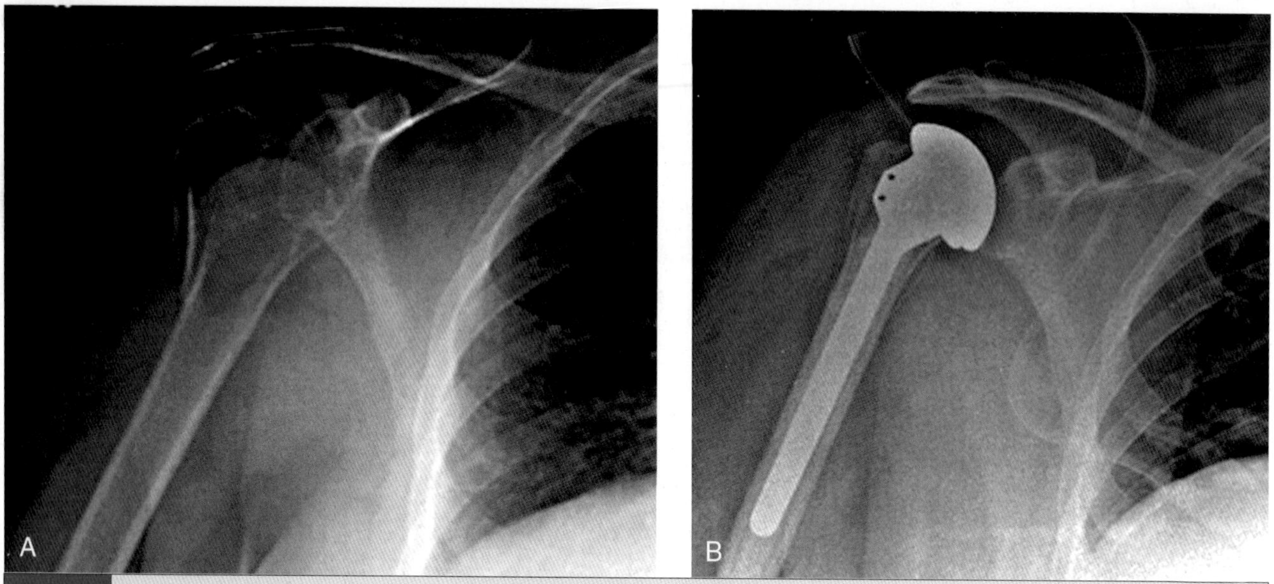

Figure 5 Head-split, four-part proximal humeral fracture (**A**) in a 62-year-old, right-handed woman treated with hemiarthroplasty (**B**). Note anatomic tuberosity position.

Only one patient in the nonsurgical group progressed to a nonunion, and an additional patient required surgery for subacromial impingement secondary to symptomatic tuberosity malunion.

Hemiarthroplasty

Hemiarthroplasty generally is recommended for patients with four-part proximal humeral fractures with poor bone quality that compromises osteosynthesis fixation techniques; head-splitting fractures; inability to obtain acceptable reduction; and/or malunion, non-

union, hardware failure, or osteonecrosis of the humeral head following osteosynthesis[17] (Figure 5). Hemiarthroplasty serves as a viable option for pain relief following displaced four-part proximal humeral fractures; however, the affected shoulder rarely returns to its baseline level of function, specifically regarding range of motion. The authors of a 2011 study found that hemiarthroplasty improved outcome measures related to quality of life in patients 2 years following hemiarthroplasty for four-part proximal humeral fractures compared with patients treated nonsurgically.[26] There was no significant difference with regard

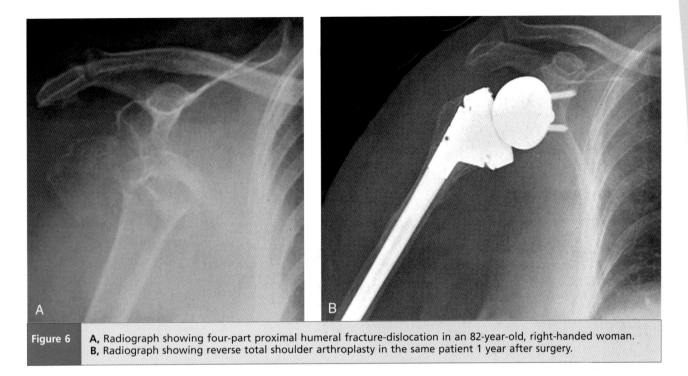

Figure 6 A, Radiograph showing four-part proximal humeral fracture-dislocation in an 82-year-old, right-handed woman. B, Radiograph showing reverse total shoulder arthroplasty in the same patient 1 year after surgery.

to Constant scores, range of motion (forward elevation ranged between 90° and 95°), or additional surgery between the groups. The outcomes of early management of proximal humeral fractures with hemiarthroplasty in 808 patients (810 hemiarthroplasties) were reported in another study.[27] At a mean follow-up of 3.7 years, mean active forward elevation was 105.7°, mean abduction was 92.4°, and external rotation was 30.4°; these results were similar to those of other reports.[27-29] The Constant score was identified for 560 patients in eight papers, and the mean Constant score in patients who underwent humeral hemiarthroplasty was 56.6 out of 100 (range, 11 to 98).

Some studies have reported no significant improvements in range of motion, pain relief, and subjective patient scores when comparing patients treated with hemiarthroplasty versus nonsurgical management. In a randomized controlled trial of 50 patients assigned to either nonsurgical management or hemiarthroplasty for four-part proximal humeral fractures, no significant differences in Constant and Simple Shoulder Test scores between the groups were found.[30] The nonsurgical group had greater abduction strength at 3 and 12 months; however, by 12 months, no difference was found with regard to pain relief between the two groups.

Reverse Total Shoulder Arthroplasty

The potential risk of tuberosity nonunion has given rise to the increasing use of RTSA for the treatment of displaced comminuted four-part fractures. RTSA was initially introduced to treat rotator cuff arthropathy.[31] In contrast to the benefits of anatomic humeral head replacement, the main benefits associated with RTSA are the ability to achieve active forward elevation even

with tuberosity union failure and the addition of glenoid resurfacing. Resurfacing the glenoid with the glenosphere component can potentially prevent the painful sequelae of glenoid erosion and medialization that can occur with resurfacing the humeral head in isolation (Figure 6).

A cohort of 43 patients with three- or four-part proximal humeral fractures was treated with RTSA in a prospective study.[32] At an average 22-month follow-up, mean active forward elevation and external rotation with the arm in abduction were 97° and 30°, respectively. The mean Constant score was 44. Complications included neurapraxias (5 patients), most of which resolved; reflex sympathetic dystrophy (3 patients); anterior dislocation of the implant (1 patient); displacement of the tuberosities (19 patients); and scapular notching (10 patients). The authors concluded that adequate clinical results could be achieved with RTSA in patients with three- or four part fractures, despite loss of reduction of the tuberosities. The authors of a 2010 study reported the clinical and radiographic findings of 36 patients at a mean follow-up of 6.6 years who underwent RTSA for displaced Neer, three- and four-part proximal humeral fractures.[33] They reported slight reductions in Constant scores when compared to one-year postoperative values (a decrease from 55 to 53). Furthermore, the authors found an alarming rate of radiographic evidence of glenoid loosening (63%) in this patient population; however, only one patient had loosening of the baseplate at 12-year follow-up.

A series of 40 patients with complex three- or four-part proximal humeral fractures who underwent either hemiarthroplasty or RTSA was studied retrospectively.[34] Twenty-one patients underwent hemiarthroplasty with a standard cemented stem and 19 under-

3: Upper Extremity

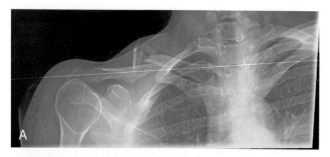

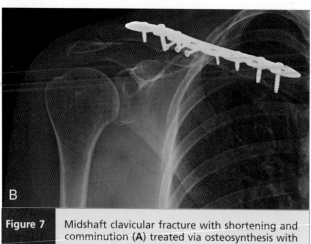

| **Figure 7** | Midshaft clavicular fracture with shortening and comminution (**A**) treated via osteosynthesis with a precontoured plate (**B**). |

went RTSA using a reverse prosthesis with a cemented stem. The mean follow-up period for the hemiarthroplasty and RTSA groups was 16.5 and 12.4 months, respectively. Constant scores, active abduction, and forward elevation were higher in the RTSA group compared with the hemiarthroplasty group (53, 91°, 97.5° versus 39, 60°, 53.5°, respectively). However, external rotation was greater in the hemiarthroplasty group (13.5° versus 9°, respectively). Thirty-three patients were available for follow-up. In the hemiarthroplasty group, radiographs showed failed tuberosity healing in 3 of 17 patients (18%). In the RTSA group, 15 of 16 patients (94%) demonstrated radiographic evidence of scapular notching; however, no cases of glenosphere loosening were reported.

Clavicle Fractures

Midshaft Clavicular Fractures

The most common location for a clavicle fracture is at the midshaft region. Historically, nonunion rates as low 0.8% were cited for midshaft clavicular fractures. With such low reported rates of nonunion, nonsurgical management for midshaft clavicle fractures was historically recommended. However, recent literature has suggested higher incidences of nonunion that are associated with certain patient and fracture-pattern risk factors, including age, female sex, fracture displacement (shortening of more than 20 mm) and fracture comminution.[35] The

Canadian Orthopaedic Trauma Society reported the results of a multicenter trial that compared nonsurgical with surgical management for displaced, midshaft clavicular fractures. Higher union rates, greater patient satisfaction, and shorter time to union in the surgical group despite higher complication (34%) and reoperation (18%) rates were reported.[36] Furthermore, it was demonstrated that greater than 2.0 cm of shortening following displaced midshaft clavicle fractures treated without surgery led to higher patient dissatisfaction with regard to perceived shoulder function.[37]

Osteosynthesis of midshaft clavicular fractures is most commonly achieved with plate fixation techniques. Precontoured or contoured locked or dynamic compression plates provide rigid stability that affords early mobilization in the early postoperative period (Figure 7). Precontoured plates may lead to less plate irritation and the need for hardware removal than contoured plates.[38] Issues of hardware irritability and the risk of iatrogenic neurovascular injury has led to continuing debate on the location of ideal clavicle plate placement. The two most common sites for plate placement for midshaft clavicular fractures are either superior or anteroinferior. Despite the advantages conferred by anteroinferior clavicle plate placement with regard to hardware prominence and the risk of injury to the underlying neurovascular structure, biomechanical studies have suggested that superior plating may be advantageous for biomechanical stability when assessing for bending stiffness and load to failure of the fixation construct.[39]

Intramedullary nailing also provides another surgical option when managing midshaft clavicular fractures.[40] Intramedullary nailing may provide the advantages of less surgical dissection when compared with plate fixation; however, complications such as medial or lateral cortical perforation, malunion, nonunion, hardware irritation, and the need for hardware removal also may be encountered with intramedullary nailing techniques.[41]

Distal Third Clavicular Fractures

Fractures involving the distal third of the clavicle account for 10% to 15% of all clavicle fractures and are difficult to treat.[42] Distal clavicular fractures are characterized based on the location relative to the coracoclavicular ligaments. Type I distal clavicular fractures occur lateral to the coracoclavicular ligaments and medial to the acromioclavicular ligaments. These fractures are usually minimally displaced and, in general, are treated nonsurgically. Type III fractures have acromioclavicular, intra-articular extension without significant ligamentous injury and are considered stable fracture patterns that render nonsurgical management appropriate.

Type II fractures are either located medial (type IIA) or in between (type IIB) the coracoclavicular ligaments and compromise the suspensory ligamentous support of the shoulder girdle. The distal fragment displaces inferiorly and medially secondary to the weight of the

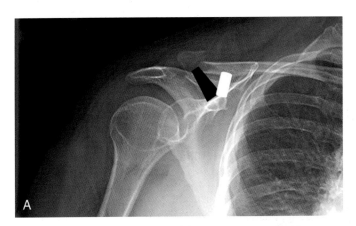

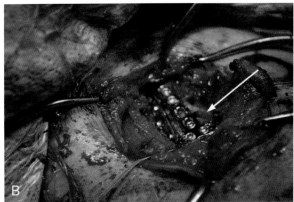

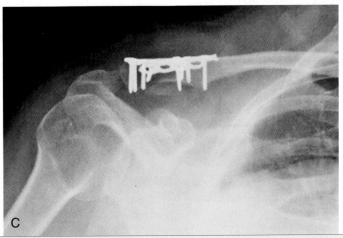

Figure 8   **A,** Preoperative radiograph showing a fracture of the distal clavicle. Note the trapezoid (black trapezoid) and co-noid (white cylinder) ligaments. **B,** Intraoperative photograph of dual plate construct demonstrating superior T-shaped and longitudinal locking plates. **C,** Postoperative radiograph.

shoulder girdle and deforming muscular forces. When compared with type I and III distal clavicular fractures, type II fractures are most at risk for the development of a nonunion. The authors of one study reported 45% delayed union and 30% nonunion in type II fractures treated nonsurgically.[43] Given the reported high rate of nonunion, surgical management is often recommended.

The optimal treatment of distal clavicular fractures remains controversial. Several options are available for patients undergoing surgical treatment of type II distal clavicular fractures (Figure 8). These options include internal fixation with coracoacromial ligament transfer,[18] hook plate,[44] double plate fixation[45] (Figure 8), and distal clavicular excision with coracoclavicular ligament reconstruction. However, some of these procedures are associated with significant failure rates and hardware complications necessitating surgical removal.[44,46]

Medial Third Clavicular Fractures

Medial third clavicular fractures are the least common of clavicle fractures. Most of these fractures represent physeal fracture-dislocations that occur lateral to the sternoclavicular joint complex. The direction of fracture displacement will often guide management. Frac-

tures of the medial third of the clavicle that are displaced anteriorly are often tolerated well and are treated nonsurgically. Fractures that are displaced posteriorly may cause life-threatening compromise to the adjacent mediastinal structures. In these scenarios, emergent closed reduction is attempted, with open reduction and stabilization reserved when reduction via closed measures fail. Thoracic surgery consultation is recommended when performing closed reduction and open reduction and stabilization techniques for medial clavicular fractures. A myriad of techniques have been described for the surgical management of these fractures, including osteosynthesis with modern plating techniques or sternoclavicular joint reconstruction with the use of either suture and/or graft augmentation, with or without medial clavicle excision.[47]

Scapula and Glenoid Fractures

Evaluation and Classification

Fractures of the scapula are typically the result of high-energy trauma and account for approximately 1% of all fractures and 5% of all shoulder fractures.[48,49] Asso-

3: Upper Extremity

ciated injuries are found in up to 90% of patients with scapula fractures, including ipsilateral upper extremity (50%), thoracic injury (80%), head injury (48%), and spinal injury (26%). A complete physical examination is critical to identify these potentially serious injuries. This should include an examination of the shoulder and a neurovascular examination of the ipsilateral upper extremity. Radiographic evaluation should consist of both standard shoulder trauma radiographs as well as a chest x-ray to evaluate for thoracic trauma such as pneumothorax, pulmonary contusion, or rib fractures. A three-dimensional CT scan is the best study to characterize the scapula fracture itself and determine optimal treatment.[50,51] Specific fracture locations include the glenoid fossa, the glenoid neck, the scapular body, the acromion, the coracoid, and combined injuries to the superior shoulder suspensory complex. The modified Ideberg classification is used to classify patterns of injury when the injury involves the glenoid articular surface (Figure 9).

Scapular Body Fractures

Most scapular body fractures should be treated nonsurgically, but the treatment of significantly displaced fractures is controversial, and good results have been reported with surgical treatment as well.[52] Both nonsurgical and surgical treatment have been effective, but no level I evidence exists to determine which is superior. A 2011 level III study found that surgical treatment resulted in rates of healing, return to work, pain, and complications similar to those of nonsurgical treatment.[53] Another study reported that isolated scapular body fractures healed without surgical treatment and resulted in function similar to the contralateral side and the uninjured general population, but the results in polytrauma patients were worse than in patients with isolated fractures.[54] Nonsurgical treatment typically consists of sling use for 7 to 10 days until a patient is comfortable without the support. Passive range of motion, pendulums, and pulleys can be initiated at that point for the first 4 to 6 weeks. A strengthening program begins at 6 to 8 weeks.

Glenoid Neck Fractures

Glenoid neck fractures are extra-articular but can result in significant displacement of the entire glenohumeral joint in some cases. Most glenoid neck fractures can be treated nonsurgically, and in the absence of additional fracture or ligamentous injury, these fractures are stable. Fractures that are displaced more than 1 cm and more than 40° may be unstable as a result of associated additional injury to the superior shoulder suspensory complex and have historically been considered for surgery in young, active patients. Recent literature has suggested that the threshold for surgery should be at least 2 cm of displacement, however.[53] Multiple case series of glenoid neck fractures treated both nonsurgically and surgically have shown mixed results, making definite conclusions impossible to draw. The results of nonsurgical treatment are mixed, with a 100% incidence of residual pain and

33% incidence of weakness.[55] Nevertheless, surgical treatment is also accompanied by significant morbidity, and the large dissection and scarring can also cause residual symptoms. It has not been definitively shown that surgical treatment results in significant improvement over these mixed nonsurgical results.

Surgical approaches for the fixation of glenoid neck and body fractures are generally performed from the posterior aspect of the shoulder. The modified Judet approach (Figure 10, A and B) can be used to expose the scapular body and the scapular spine in addition to the glenoid neck and the posterior glenohumeral joint. It is a utilitarian approach that runs transversely along the scapular spine and vertically along the medial scapular border. The deltoid is reflected superiorly and laterally from the scapular spine, and the infraspinatus is reflected laterally on its neurovascular pedicle, exposing the body of the scapula. The scapula is repaired using a combination of plates and screws (Figure 10, C through E). An alternative approach involves a vertical incision in the posterior axillary fold and exploits the interval between the infraspinatus and the teres minor, but the quadrilateral space must be protected. This approach gives excellent access to the glenoid neck, but more medial exposure of the scapular body is limited.

Glenoid Fossa Fractures

The treatment of intra-articular fractures is controversial and is still most commonly nonsurgical, but there are more well-defined surgical indications for these fracture types compared with glenoid neck or scapular body fractures. Any type I fracture that results in glenohumeral instability and most fractures with intra-articular stepoff of 5 mm or more should be considered for surgical repair.[56,57] Type Ia fractures can be repaired arthroscopically or through an anterior deltopectoral approach with either suture anchors or screws (Figure 11). Depending on the fracture pattern and location, more comminuted fractures can be treated with a posterior approach or a combined anterior-posterior approach in complex cases. A recent study reported on 33 patients with intra-articular glenoid fractures displaced more than 4 mm.[57] At mean follow-up of 27 months after surgical treatment, 87% of the patients were pain free and reported good functional outcomes and a low complication rate.[57] Improvement in articular congruity has been shown to result in good outcomes, with up to 80% to 90% good and excellent results when reduced to within 2 mm of anatomic alignment.[56,58]

Floating Shoulder Injuries

The superior shoulder suspensory complex consists of the glenoid, the coracoid, the distal clavicle, the acromion, the coracoclavicular ligaments, and the acromioclavicular ligaments and provides stability to the entire shoulder and upper extremity. Instability results if two elements of this complex are disrupted.[59] The combination of a clavicle fracture and a glenoid neck fracture decreases overall stability by 31%.[60] Despite this defini-

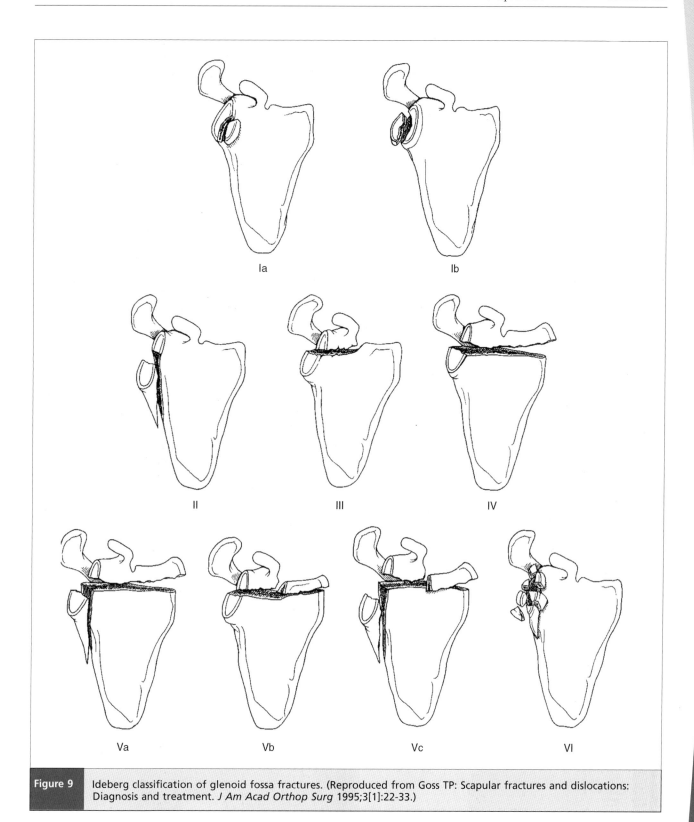

Ia   Ib

II   III   IV

Va   Vb   Vc   VI

Figure 9   Ideberg classification of glenoid fossa fractures. (Reproduced from Goss TP: Scapular fractures and dislocations: Diagnosis and treatment. *J Am Acad Orthop Surg* 1995;3[1]:22-33.)

tion of instability, surgical indications are controversial because outcomes are mostly similar in both surgically and nonsurgically treated floating shoulder injuries. A series of patients with floating shoulder injuries were retrospectively reviewed and at 35 months postinjury, those treated surgically had a mean Constant score of 76 and those treated nonsurgically had a Constant score of 71.[61] Nonsurgical treatment of floating shoulder injuries achieved satisfactory results, even with clavicle displacement of more than 10 mm and scapular displacement of more than 5 mm, with results comparable to those of nondisplaced fractures.[62,63]

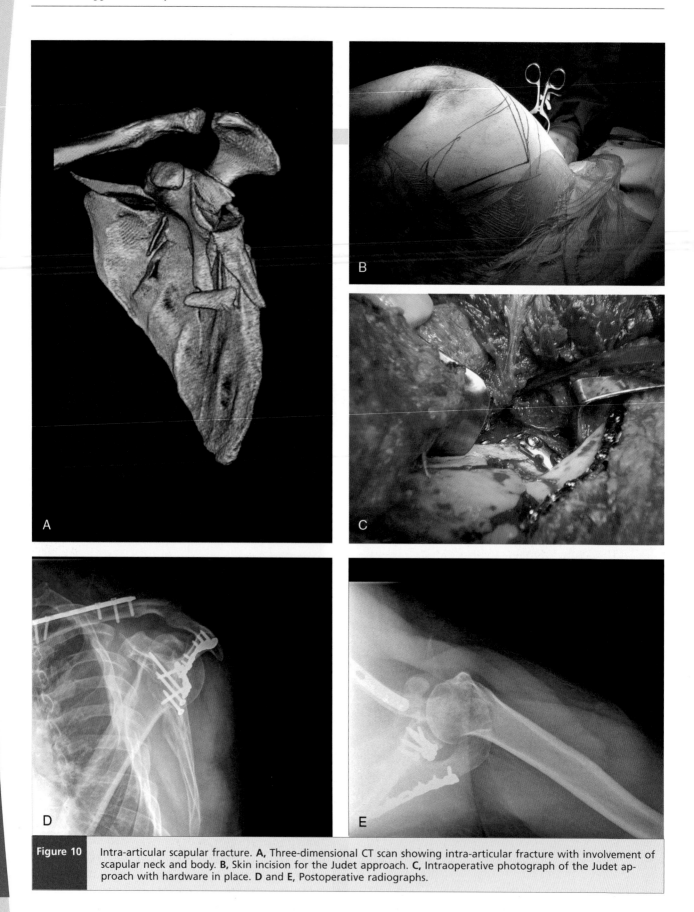

Figure 10 Intra-articular scapular fracture. **A,** Three-dimensional CT scan showing intra-articular fracture with involvement of scapular neck and body. **B,** Skin incision for the Judet approach. **C,** Intraoperative photograph of the Judet approach with hardware in place. **D** and **E,** Postoperative radiographs.

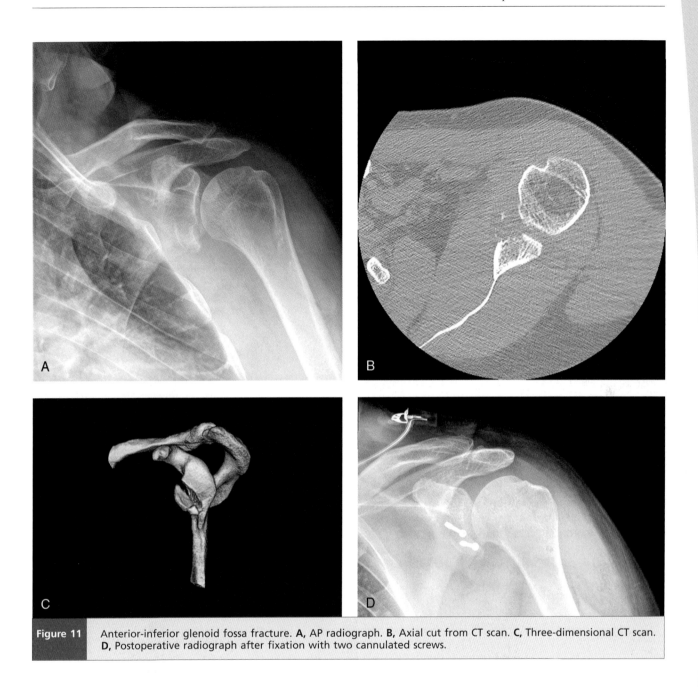

Figure 11 Anterior-inferior glenoid fossa fracture. **A,** AP radiograph. **B,** Axial cut from CT scan. **C,** Three-dimensional CT scan. **D,** Postoperative radiograph after fixation with two cannulated screws.

Humeral Shaft Fractures

Evaluation and Classification

Humeral shaft fractures account for about 3% of all fractures and occur in a bimodal distribution. These fractures occur most often in elderly patients as a result of low-energy trauma such as falls, but a substantial number also occur via a high-energy mechanism in young trauma patients.[64] The upper extremity should be specifically evaluated for additional injuries, and a thorough neurovascular examination should be performed.

Orthogonal radiographs of the ipsilateral shoulder and elbow, including the forearm, should always be part of the humeral shaft fracture evaluation. Advanced imaging is usually not necessary. Humeral shaft fractures are described as proximal third, middle third, or distal third and patterns include transverse, spiral, oblique, and comminuted. A 2012 retrospective study comparing surgical and nonsurgical treatment found similar healing rates and complication rates between the two groups, with an additional 5.3% radial nerve injuries resulting from surgery.[65] Authors of a 2010 study found that nonunion and malunion rates were higher in the surgically treated group.[66] A 2012 Cochrane review comparing surgical versus nonsurgical treatment of humeral shaft fractures was unable to find evidence from prospective randomized studies to determine which intervention is preferred or to compare complications or outcomes.[67]

3: Upper Extremity

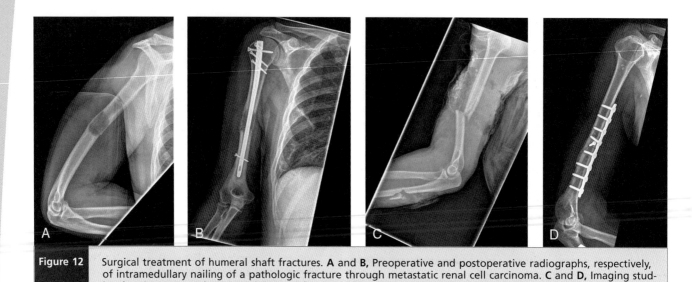

Figure 12 Surgical treatment of humeral shaft fractures. **A** and **B**, Preoperative and postoperative radiographs, respectively, of intramedullary nailing of a pathologic fracture through metastatic renal cell carcinoma. **C** and **D**, Imaging studies showing open reduction and internal fixation with a 4.5 mm limited contact dynamic compression plate open humeral shaft fracture associated with open forearm fracture.

Nonsurgical Treatment

Most of these fractures should be treated nonsurgically with a functional brace.[68] The functional brace aligns the fracture via gravity and hydrostatic pressure. Significant deformity is well tolerated because the shoulder has such a large arc of motion that it can compensate functionally. Generally, 20° of anterior angulation, 30° of varus, and shortening of 2 to 3 cm is acceptable and results in restoration of function. A study of 620 humeral shaft fractures found nonunion rates of less than 2% for closed fractures, with low rates of malunion and good functional outcomes.[68] Another study reported 95% good to excellent results with functional bracing.[69]

Surgical Treatment

Despite the excellent results of nonsurgical treatment, there are several strong indications for the surgical treatment of humeral shaft fractures, including pathologic fractures, open fractures, ipsilateral upper extremity fractures (such as a forearm fracture), fractures with neurovascular injuries, fractures in polytrauma patients, and the failure of nonsurgical treatment (Figure 12). Treatment options include plate fixation, intramedullary nailing, and external fixation. Plate fixation typically consists of a 4.5-mm dynamic compression plate and can be performed through either a posterior, a lateral, or an anterolateral approach depending on the fracture location and surgeon preference. Intramedullary nailing can be performed either antegrade or retrograde but has been associated with increased rates of shoulder pain, secondary to damage to the rotator cuff during antegrade insertion.

Several recent studies have compared nailing versus plating. The authors of a 2012 study evaluated nailing versus plating of humeral shaft fractures in Medicare patients using administrative claims and found that nail fixation was more prevalent than plating and had no

difference in complication rates.[70] Another study compared nailing and plating; no significant difference in outcomes or complications were found between the groups.[71] In another comparison study of nailing and plating, a higher rate of good and excellent results and a tendency for earlier union were found in the plating group.[72] A 2011 Cochrane review comparing dynamic compression plating with locked intramedullary nailing for humeral shaft fractures found no difference in nonunion rate, surgical time, blood loss, iatrogenic radial nerve injury, return to preinjury occupation by 6 months, or American Shoulder and Elbow Surgeons scores between plating and nailing. The review did show a statistically significant increase in shoulder impingement after nailing (relative risk = 0.12) and found that nails were removed more frequently than plates (relative risk = 0.17).[73]

Management of Radial Nerve Palsy

Radial nerve palsy is a common associated injury of humeral shaft fractures. The incidence of radial nerve palsy after humeral shaft fracture is 11% based on a large systematic review of more than 4,000 fractures.[74] The rate is significantly higher in distal third fractures (23.6%) compared with proximal third fractures (1.8%). The nerve recovers at an average of 7 weeks in 70% of cases.[74,75] Therefore, the current recommendation is nonsurgical management in the setting of a closed humeral fracture with radial nerve palsy at presentation. Similarly, radial nerve palsy following fracture manipulation or splinting will generally recover spontaneously. The primary indication for immediate exploration is an open humeral shaft fracture. Electrodiagnostic testing at a minimum of 4 weeks after injury can provide a baseline for assessing later nerve recovery. A repeat test at 3 to 4 months after injury can be obtained if no return of brachioradialis or wrist extensor function is evident on examination, because these should recover first in a high radial nerve palsy. Typically, brachioradialis function should recover by 3 months, extensor digitorum communis function by 6 months, and extensor pollicis longus function may take 9 to 12 months to return. Surgical exploration may be warranted if there is no evidence of brachioradialis function at 4 months after fracture occurrence. A meta-analysis compared initial surgical versus nonsurgical management of radial nerve palsies with acute humeral shaft fractures. The authors found no improvement in nerve recovery in patients treated with early surgery and less morbidity in the nonsurgical group.[76] They concluded that recovery from radial nerve palsy is not improved by early surgery. A decision analysis of radial nerve injury in humeral shaft fracture was performed, and it was concluded that radial nerve palsies should be observed initially except in cases of open fracture or concomitant forearm injury.[77]

Summary

Although there are many new technologies available for the management of fractures around the shoulder, additional research is needed in many areas to determine not only which implants should be used for which fractures but also for which fractures surgical treatment offers significant advantages over nonsurgical treatment. As discussed in this chapter, the role of nonsurgical treatment remains controversial for displaced proximal humeral fractures, midshaft clavicular fractures, scapula fractures, and humeral shaft fractures. When surgery is chosen, new implants such as proximal humeral locking plates and RTSA have widened the choices and offered potentially improved outcomes for select patients and fracture patterns but at the high cost of increased complication rates. What is most clear from a thorough literature review in these areas is that more research is needed to help define surgical indications and implant choices for these common yet difficult fractures.

Key Study Points

- New technology, including locking plate fixation and RTSA, offers surgeons more options than ever for difficult proximal humeral fractures, but indications and technique are important because complication rates associated with these new techniques are high.

- Recent literature supports the consideration of surgical stabilization for midshaft clavicular fractures displaced by more than 2 cm, but there is still a role for nonsurgical treatment.

- Most scapular fractures should be treated nonsurgically, provided the glenohumeral joint remains concentrically reduced.

Annotated References

1. Green A, Norris T: Proximal humeral fractures and fracture dislocations, in Browner BD, Jupiter J, Levine A, Trafton P, eds: *Skeletal Trauma*, ed 3. Philadelphia, PA, Saunders, 2003.

2. Stimson BB: *A Manual of Fractures and Dislocations*, ed 2. Philadelphia, PA, Lea & Febiger, 1947.

3. Solberg BD, Moon CN, Franco DP, Paiement GD: Locked plating of 3- and 4-part proximal humerus fractures in older patients: The effect of initial fracture pattern on outcome. *J Orthop Trauma* 2009;23(2): 113-119.

4. Visser CP, Coene LN, Brand R, Tavy DL: Nerve lesions in proximal humeral fractures. *J Shoulder Elbow Surg* 2001;10(5):421-427.

5. Neer CS II: Displaced proximal humeral fractures: I. Classification and evaluation. *J Bone Joint Surg Am* 1970;52(6):1077-1089.

6. Codman E: *The Shoulder: Rupture of the Supraspinatus Tendon and Other Lesions in or About the Subacromial Bursa*. Boston, MA, Privately Printed, 1934.

7. Takase K, Yamamoto K, Imakiire A, Burkhead WZ Jr: The radiographic study in the relationship of the glenohumeral joint. *J Orthop Res* 2004;22(2):298-305.

8. Boileau P, Bicknell RT, Mazzoleni N, Walch G, Urien JP: CT scan method accurately assesses humeral head retroversion. *Clin Orthop Relat Res* 2008;466(3): 661-669.

9. Hernigou P, Duparc F, Hernigou A: Determining humeral retroversion with computed tomography. *J Bone Joint Surg Am* 2002;84(10):1753-1762.

10. Duparc F, Muller JM, Fréger P: Arterial blood supply of the proximal humeral epiphysis. *Surg Radiol Anat* 2001;23(3):185-190.

11. Hettrich CM, Boraiah S, Dyke JP, Neviaser A, Helfet DL, Lorich DG: Quantitative assessment of the vascularity of the proximal part of the humerus. *J Bone Joint Surg Am* 2010;92(4):943-948.

   The authors present a controlled laboratory study of 24 cadaver human shoulder specimens in a quantitative assessment of blood supply to the humeral head. The authors note that the posterior humeral circumflex artery provided 64% of the blood supply to the humeral head compared with 36% via the anterior circumflex artery.

12. Bernstein J, Adler LM, Blank JE, Dalsey RM, Williams GR, Iannotti JP: Evaluation of the Neer system of classification of proximal humeral fractures with computerized tomographic scans and plain radiographs. *J Bone Joint Surg Am* 1996;78(9):1371-1375.

3: Upper Extremity

53. Jones CB, Sietsema DL: Analysis of operative versus nonoperative treatment of displaced scapular fractures. *Clin Orthop Relat Res* 2011;469(12):3379-3389.

One hundred eighty-two scapular fractures were retrospectively reviewed, of which 31 were treated with ORIF and compared with a series of 31 matched controls treated nonsurgically. There was no difference in return to work, pain, or complications between the surgical and nonsurgical groups. Level of evidence: III.

54. Gosens T, Speigner B, Minekus J: Fracture of the scapular body: Functional outcome after conservative treatment. *J Shoulder Elbow Surg* 2009;18(3):443-448.

55. Pace AM, Stuart R, Brownlow H: Outcome of glenoid neck fractures. *J Shoulder Elbow Surg* 2005;14(6):585-590.

56. Kavanagh BF, Bradway JK, Cofield RH: Open reduction and internal fixation of displaced intra-articular fractures of the glenoid fossa. *J Bone Joint Surg Am* 1993;75(4):479-484.

57. Anavian J, Gauger EM, Schroder LK, Wijdicks CA, Cole PA: Surgical and functional outcomes after operative management of complex and displaced intra-articular glenoid fractures. *J Bone Joint Surg Am* 2012;94(7):645-653.

Thirty-three patients with displaced intra-articular glenoid fractures were retrospectively reviewed. At mean 27-month follow-up, all patients had fracture union, 87% were pain free, and 90% had returned to preinjury level of work and activity.

58. Mayo KA, Benirschke SK, Mast JW: Displaced fractures of the glenoid fossa: Results of open reduction and internal fixation. *Clin Orthop Relat Res* 1998;347:122-130.

59. Goss TP: Double disruptions of the superior shoulder suspensory complex. *J Orthop Trauma* 1993;7(2):99-106.

60. Williams GR Jr, Naranja J, Klimkiewicz J, Karduna A, Iannotti JP, Ramsey M: The floating shoulder: A biomechanical basis for classification and management. *J Bone Joint Surg Am* 2001;83-A(8):1182-1187.

61. van Noort A, te Slaa RL, Marti RK, van der Werken C: The floating shoulder: A multicentre study. *J Bone Joint Surg Br* 2001;83(6):795-798.

62. DeFranco MJ, Patterson BM: The floating shoulder. *J Am Acad Orthop Surg* 2006;14(8):499-509.

63. Edwards SG, Whittle AP, Wood GW II: Nonoperative treatment of ipsilateral fractures of the scapula and clavicle. *J Bone Joint Surg Am* 2000;82(6):774-780.

64. Ekholm R, Adami J, Tidermark J, Hansson K, Törnkvist H, Ponzer S: Fractures of the shaft of the humerus: An epidemiological study of 401 fractures. *J Bone Joint Surg Br* 2006;88(11):1469-1473.

65. Mahabier KC, Vogels LM, Punt BJ, Roukema GR, Patka P, Van Lieshout EM: Humeral shaft fractures: Retrospective results of non-operative and operative treatment of 186 patients. *Injury* 2013;44(4):427-430.

A retrospective analysis of surgical versus nonsurgical treatment of humeral shaft fractures is presented. Time to union and complication rates were similar between the groups. A radial nerve palsy was present in 5.3% of the surgically treated fractures after the surgery.

66. Denard A Jr, Richards JE, Obremskey WT, Tucker MC, Floyd M, Herzog GA: Outcome of nonoperative vs operative treatment of humeral shaft fractures: A retrospective study of 213 patients. *Orthopedics* 2010;33(8).

This was a retrospective study of 213 patients comparing surgical and nonsurgical treatment of humeral shaft fractures. Although a significant increase in malunion and nonunion was found in the nonsurgical group, there was no difference in time to union, infection, or radial nerve palsy.

67. Gosler MW, Testroote M, Morrenhof JW, Janzing HM: Surgical versus non-surgical interventions for treating humeral shaft fractures in adults. *Cochrane Database Syst Rev* 2012;1:CD008832.

This systematic review of surgical versus nonsurgical treatment of humeral shaft fractures in adults shows that there are insufficient data to make a recommendation regarding surgical treatment for humeral shaft fractures.

68. Sarmiento A, Zagorski JB, Zych GA, Latta LL, Capps CA: Functional bracing for the treatment of fractures of the humeral diaphysis. *J Bone Joint Surg Am* 2000;82(4):478-486.

69. Koch PP, Gross DF, Gerber C: The results of functional (Sarmiento) bracing of humeral shaft fractures. *J Shoulder Elbow Surg* 2002;11(2):143-150.

70. Chen F, Wang Z, Bhattacharyya T: Outcomes of nails versus plates for humeral shaft fractures: A Medicare cohort study. *J Orthop Trauma* 2013;27(2):68-72.

This administrative claims study, using Medicare claims data, compared nailing and plating of humeral shaft fractures. In this elderly population, nails were more commonly used than plates, had a shorter anesthesia time, and there was no difference in reoperation rates or mortality. Level of evidence: II.

71. Heineman DJ, Poolman RW, Nork SE, Ponsen KJ, Bhandari M: Plate fixation or intramedullary fixation of humeral shaft fractures. *Acta Orthop* 2010;81(2):216-223.

This meta-analysis compared nailing and plating of humeral shaft fractures. No significant differences were found in complication rate, union rate, infection, nerve palsy, or the need for additional surgery.

72. Singisetti K, Ambedkar M: Nailing versus plating in humerus shaft fractures: A prospective comparative study. *Int Orthop* 2010;34(4):571-576.

The authors present a prospective study of nailing versus plating of humeral shaft fractures in 20 patients. Improved outcomes were seen in the plating group compared with the nailing group.

73. Kurup H, Hossain M, Andrew JG: Dynamic compression plating versus locked intramedullary nailing for humeral shaft fractures in adults. *Cochrane Database Syst Rev* 2011;6:CD005959.

   This Cochrane review compared nailing and plating of humeral shaft fractures. There was a significant increase in shoulder pain and the need for hardware removal in the nailing group but no significant difference in operative time, nerve injury, return to preinjury occupation, or radial nerve palsy.

74. Shao YC, Harwood P, Grotz MR, Limb D, Giannoudis PV: Radial nerve palsy associated with fractures of the shaft of the humerus: A systematic review. *J Bone Joint Surg Br* 2005;87(12):1647-1652.

75. Ring D, Chin K, Jupiter JB: Radial nerve palsy associated with high-energy humeral shaft fractures. *J Hand Surg Am* 2004;29(1):144-147.

76. Liu GY, Zhang CY, Wu HW: Comparison of initial nonoperative and operative management of radial nerve palsy associated with acute humeral shaft fractures. *Orthopedics* 2012;35(8):702-708.

   This systematic review of the literature compared initial surgical versus nonsurgical treatment of radial nerve palsy associated with humeral shaft fracture. Surgical treatment resulted in no improvement in radial nerve function compared with nonsurgical treatment, and nonsurgically treated patients had fewer complaints about treatment.

77. Bishop J, Ring D: Management of radial nerve palsy associated with humeral shaft fracture: A decision analysis model. *J Hand Surg Am* 2009;34(6):991-996, e1.

3: Upper Extremity

Chapter 26

Shoulder Reconstruction

Charles M. Jobin, MD   Louis U. Bigliani, MD

Introduction

Shoulder reconstruction has advanced significantly over the last decade, with improved anatomic shoulder arthroplasty designs, the expanding use of reverse shoulder arthroplasty, a better understanding of arthroplasty failure modes, and corresponding developments in implant design and fixation strategies. Nevertheless, the time-proven concepts of re-creating anatomic relationships and soft-tissue balancing continue to be the foundation for shoulder reconstruction. Understanding the many etiologies of glenohumeral arthrosis helps the surgeon guide treatment and plan proper surgical approaches for successful patient outcomes.

Glenohumeral Joint Disorders

Numerous disease processes, pathologic biomechanics, and injury patterns cause glenohumeral joint disorders. The most common disorders include osteoarthritis, inflammatory arthritis, osteonecrosis, posttraumatic arthritis, rotator cuff tear arthropathy (RCTA), septic arthritis, postcapsulorrhaphy arthropathy, and iatrogenic arthropathy. Each disorder has characteristic presentations, examination findings, radiographic characteristics, and treatment strategies.

Osteoarthritis is the most frequent cause of disability in the United States, with a prevalence that increases with age, with occurrence typically after the sixth decade of life, and affects women more often than men. Shoulder osteoarthritis is less prevalent than osteoarthritis of the knee and the hip but can be equally debilitating. Osteoarthritis is the most common degenerative process in the shoulder. The classic presentation includes progressive atraumatic symptoms of pain, loss of motion, morning stiffness, and concomitant loss of strength. Radiographic signs of shoulder osteoarthritis include osteophyte formation, loss of joint space, subchondral sclerosis, and osseous cyst formation. Poste-

rior glenoid wear and posterior humeral subluxation are common findings in later stages of the disease. Surgical treatment includes débridement, capsular release, surface replacement or hemiarthroplasty, and total shoulder replacement.

Rheumatoid arthritis is an inflammatory process characterized by a synovial disease that erodes the glenohumeral articulation. Painful motion, polyarticular disease, and loss of motion are common. The radiographic findings include periarticular erosions, subchondral cysts, osteopenia, and central glenoid wear, with medialization of the humeral head in advanced disease. Nearly 50% of patients with rheumatoid arthritis have a thinned or torn rotator cuff, compared with only 5% of patients with primary osteoarthritis. When surgical reconstruction is considered, the degree of glenoid erosion and the status of the rotator cuff must be taken into account. Patients with rheumatoid arthritis and preserved joint space may benefit from arthroscopic synovectomy, whereas patients with rheumatoid arthritis in later stages benefit from arthroplasty.

Osteonecrosis is a less frequent disease of the shoulder and in younger patients often occurs with deep, unexplained shoulder pain. It may be idiopathic or posttraumatic, or it may result from steroid usage, alcoholism, sickle cell disease, lupus, Gaucher disease, caisson disease from deep-water diving decompression, vascular compromise, and chemotherapy or irradiation. Osteonecrosis is likely caused by disruption of the vascular supply to the humeral head, which is shared between the anterior and posterior humeral circumflex arteries.[1] This subchondral osteonecrosis leads to cartilage collapse and loss. If the humeral head collapses and loses its sphericity, secondary arthritis of the glenoid may develop. Treatment is guided by a careful assessment of the etiology of the osteonecrosis and reversal of the offending cause, if possible, followed by radiographic assessment of subchondral collapse and glenoid involvement. Classification is based on a modified Ficat scheme, and core decompression is performed as an early intervention before significant subchondral collapse,[2] whereas hemiarthroplasty or surface replacement may benefit patients with unipolar disease, and total shoulder replacement is reserved for shoulders in which the glenoid has become secondarily involved.

RCTA is the secondary development of arthrosis in the setting of a massive rotator cuff tear and is characterized by proximal humeral migration, arthrosis, and rotator cuff insufficiency. The pathogenesis is multifactorial and includes a loss of normal mechanics and disruption of biologic nutritional factors. With massive cuff tears, the rotator cuff force couple is lost, resulting in proximal head migration from unrestrained pull of the deltoid. Nutritional pathways are likely disturbed with loss of watertight joint space, disuse osteopenia, altered cartilage forces, and changes in cartilage water content and glycosaminoglycan arrangement. Calcium phosphate crystals have been identified in RCTA, but it is unknown if they represent a primary derangement leading to RCTA or if these crystals are secondary to the process of RCTA.[1] With the development of RCTA, the humeral head may remain contained within the coracoacromial arch or escape anterosuperiorly. Radiographic findings include acetabularization of the acromion, femoralization of the humeral head, superior eccentric glenoid wear, and coracoid base erosion. Treatment depends on the degree of pain, motion preserved, humeral head containment, function of the subscapularis, and involvement of the glenoid. Contained RCTA with preserved forward elevation of more than 90° may be treated with hemiarthroplasty alone, whereas patients with a loss of containment or pseudoparalytic motion may benefit from reverse shoulder arthroplasty.

Posttraumatic arthritis is a mixed group of disorders resulting from osseous, cartilaginous, and soft-tissue trauma. Tuberosity malunion with altered rotator cuff forces may lead to glenohumeral arthrosis. Intra-articular fractures with step-off or gapping may lead to arthrosis. Iatrogenic arthritis secondary to anterior stabilization procedures is known as postcapsulorrhaphy arthropathy. It is characterized by significant stiffness with loss of external rotation and typical posterior glenoid wear from eccentric forces on the glenoid. Anterior tightening procedures and subscapularis advancements, such as the Putti-Platt and Magnuson-Stack procedures, commonly lead to this type of arthritis. Shoulder reconstruction for postcapsulorrhaphy arthropathy is complicated by a contracted and scarred subscapularis and a propensity for humeral posterior subluxation. Full subscapularis release, possible tendon Z-lengthening, undersizing the humeral head, and posterior capsule imbrication are strategies to improve soft-tissue balance and motion.

Chondrolysis is a devastating disease that infrequently occurs after routine arthroscopy, local analgesic catheter insertion, infection, or thermal capsular procedures.[3] The chondral loss is rapid and devastating, and the workup should rule out infection as a potential cause. The treatment of these patients, who are typically younger, is controversial, with some surgeons recommending total shoulder replacement to offer the most predictable successful outcome in the midterm while acknowledging the risks of glenoid component loosening, polyethylene wear, and glenoid bone loss. Others advocate biologic glenoid resurfacing with or without humeral head replacement to improve function, reduce pain, and preserve glenoid bone stock for future replacement surgery when the patient is older.

Nonsurgical Treatment

Nonsurgical treatment of glenohumeral arthritis is recommended initially, although data on its effectiveness are inconclusive. Activity modification, anti-inflammatory medications, and physical therapy are first-line treatments. Secondary treatments include steroid injections, local analgesics, and viscosupplementation. Other options, such as acupuncture, electrical stimulation, ultrasound therapy, magnetic therapy, and glucosamine and chondroitin sulfate supplements, are offered but not well studied. A multimodal approach combining these nonsurgical treatments should be used in all patients before surgical care.

Physical therapy is commonly used for the treatment of glenohumeral arthritis to preserve motion and optimize function. No well-designed studies demonstrate a benefit of specific therapy for shoulder arthritis, although empiric evidence suggests its usefulness. A meta-analysis of therapy for all shoulder conditions found improvements in pain and function with therapy, but less improvement in motion.[4]

Pharmacotherapy with analgesics; NSAIDs; opioids; opioid-like drugs, and neuromodulators such as antidepressants, anticonvulsants, and muscle relaxants is frequently used for arthritis-related shoulder pain. The use of disease-modifying antirheumatic drugs (DMARDs) has significantly decreased the incidence of shoulder arthroplasty in patients with rheumatoid arthritis. Meta-analyses have demonstrated better pain relief with NSAIDs than with acetaminophen. Cyclooxygenase-2 selective NSAIDs have the benefit of reduced gastrointestinal side effects but are costly. A Cochrane systematic review of these agents for the treatment of inflammatory arthritis failed to demonstrate an advantage of combination therapy over monotherapy.[5]

Intra-articular glenohumeral steroid injections have not been effectively compared with placebo or local analgesics. Steroids likely reduce inflammatory processes and synovial symptoms. Guidelines for steroid injection are based on level IV evidence often confounded by the coadministration of local analgesics such as bupivacaine, which has an independent effect on chondrocyte viability. Steroid injections also risk subcutaneous fat atrophy, bacterial arthritis, hemarthrosis, and ligament and tendon attrition. Nevertheless, steroid injections likely benefit patients with conditions such as adhesive capsulitis and subacromial bursitis and therefore may have a role in the treatment of an acute exacerbation of an osteoarthritic shoulder condition.

Viscosupplementation for shoulder pain has been proven mildly effective in a double-blinded, randomized saline-controlled trial of 3 or 5 weekly sodium hyaluronate injections. Pain improved modestly over a 26-week period. Subgroup analysis demonstrated that patients with osteoarthritis benefited from viscosupplementation, whereas other groups did not.[6] These results mirror the results of viscosupplementation studies in other joints such as the knee.

Joint-Preserving Treatment

Joint-preserving surgical treatment of shoulder arthritis is a viable option before arthroplasty for mild disease, especially in younger adults in whom implant longevity is a concern or in situations in which the arthritis is localized to a focal area of chondral loss. Cartilage-preserving options include capsular release, glenohumeral débridement, and synovectomy. Cartilage restoration procedures include microfracture of focal chondral lesions, osteochondral autograft, autologous chondrocyte implantation, osteochondral allograft, and glenoid biologic resurfacing. The effectiveness of these treatments remains inconclusive, and there are no high-quality studies to support their widespread use at this time.

Arthroscopic débridement of glenohumeral arthritis is successful in short-term to midterm follow-up. The removal of loose debris, the resection of unstable cartilage flaps or degenerative labral tears, and microfracture chondroplasty of unipolar full-thickness cartilage lesions on the glenoid or the humeral head are reasonable treatments for younger adults with failed nonsurgical treatment. Good to excellent short-term results have been reported in 80% of patients with a concentric articulation and without loss of radiographic joint space.[7] Microfracture creates a fibrocartilage scar that does not rejuvenate hyaline cartilage. Negative prognostic factors for microfracture include full-thickness cartilage lesions greater than 2 cm², bipolar chondral lesions, workers' compensation, and follow-up greater than 2.5 years.[8]

Arthroscopic débridement and circumferential capsular release are beneficial procedures to regain motion and reduce pain in mild to moderate osteoarthritis with stiffness. Capsular release causes a reduction in joint contact pressures that likely results in reduced pain. A study of nine patients demonstrated temporary improvements in motion and pain for up to 1 year, delaying the need for arthroplasty.[9] Capsular release loses effectiveness at midterm follow-up, and many patients require conversion to arthroplasty.

The results of osteochondral autograft for full-thickness humeral head and glenoid chondral lesions demonstrate improved Constant scores at 2.5 years but also progression of osteoarthritic radiographic changes.[10] Autologous chondrocyte implantation in the shoulder has been reported only in a single case study with 3-month follow-up, and the long-term results are unknown.[11] Fresh osteochondral allografts have been used to fill large engaging Hill-Sachs lesions, resurface humeral head osteochondral lesions, and rebuild the anterior glenoid in patients with severe bone loss from anterior instability.[12] These structural and biologically active allografts have the advantages of no donor site morbidity and no limitation in size; however, the disadvantages are limited chondrocyte viability, potential immunogenicity and disease transmission, and concern regarding long-term osseous incorporation.

Biologic interposition without metallic humeral resurfacing has been studied with an acellular human dermal scaffold to resurface the glenoid. The follow-up results at more than 2 years were mixed, with similar rates of success and failure. Nearly 25% of the patients required conversion to arthroplasty, and only 25% demonstrated retention of interposed tissue on MRI.[13] A study of patients younger than 60 years with severe osteoarthritis demonstrated significant improvement in 75% of the patients with glenoid resurfacing with a porcine small intestine submucosa scaffold.[14] Histologic examination demonstrated viable cartilage cells, suggesting cartilage ingrowth into the scaffold tissue. Failures were seen in patients who had preoperative flattening of the humeral head.

Hemiarthroplasty

Hemiarthroplasty was developed more than 50 years ago for the treatment of nonreconstructible proximal humeral fractures. The indications for hemiarthroplasty include treatment of primary glenohumeral osteoarthritis in younger adults in whom the longevity of a glenoid component is of concern, arthritic conditions in which the glenoid bone stock is inadequate for implantation of a component, RCTA, inflammatory arthropathy with a contained humeral head, and osteonecrosis of the humeral head without secondary involvement of the glenoid. Stemless or short-stem humeral resurfacing arthroplasty is an option that theoretically better recreates proximal humeral geometry and preserves metaphyseal bone. The indications and long-term outcomes of these resurfacing designs remain poorly defined.

Hemiarthroplasty is a viable option in younger patients in whom a glenoid component could be at risk for early loosening or wear. Hemiarthroplasty with concentric reaming of the glenoid, known as "ream and run," is an option, but follow-up studies demonstrated that men older than 60 years had better results than younger adults, and pain relief was delayed up to 1.5 years postoperatively.[15] A study of patients younger than 55 years with 10-year follow-up demonstrated 92% implant survival with total shoulder arthroplasty (TSA) compared with 72% for hemiarthroplasty. Glenoid components were deemed at risk for loosening or had loosened in nearly 30% of the TSA patients, whereas nearly 50% of the hemiarthroplasty patients had moderate to severe glenoid arthritis.[16] Not only is survivorship improved with TSA, but most comparative studies demonstrated superior pain relief and improved function with TSA and a low 1.7% revision rate for all-polyethylene glenoid components at 43-month follow-up.[17]

Clinical success and survivorship of hemiarthroplasty are likely affected by preoperative and patient-specific factors. Understanding glenoid morphology is critical to the success of hemiarthroplasty. Centralized glenoid wear without posterior wear or static posterior humeral subluxation leads to improved midterm outcomes.[18] However, a recent long-term study (17.9-year follow-up) demonstrated poor patient satisfaction (25%) following hemiarthroplasty for glenohumeral

3: Upper Extremity

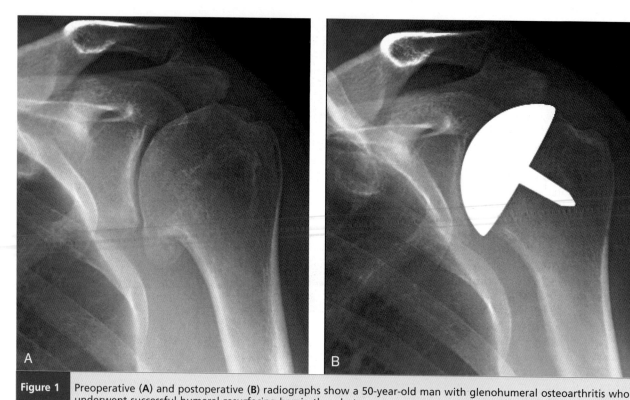

Figure 1 Preoperative (**A**) and postoperative (**B**) radiographs show a 50-year-old man with glenohumeral osteoarthritis who underwent successful humeral resurfacing hemiarthroplasty.

osteoarthritis irrespective of glenoid morphology.[19] Ten-year survivorship of hemiarthroplasty is affected by diagnosis, with almost 100% survival in rheumatoid arthritis, 94% in osteonecrosis and primary osteoarthritis, 81% in RCTA, and 77% in fracture sequelae.[20] Younger age and obesity are risk factors for hemiarthroplasty revision.

Resurfacing hemiarthroplasty is an attractive option because metaphyseal bone is preserved, and anatomic re-creation of proximal humeral geometry is theoretically easier[21] (Figure 1). Prerequisites for resurfacing arthroplasty include adequate bone stock to support the implant, minimal and concentric glenoid wear, and lack of posterior humeral subluxation. Surface replacement is technically demanding because malpositioning of the implant is possible without a medullary guide. Overstuffing the glenohumeral joint by increasing head size and lateralizing the humerus often leads to rapid progression of glenoid pain, stiffness, and rotator cuff dysfunction. Certain patient populations may benefit from humeral resurfacing designs. Patients with rheumatoid arthritis with total elbow stemmed prostheses may be at risk for humeral shaft fracture if a proximal humeral stem is implanted adjacent to the total elbow stem. Stemless designs also match proximal humeral geometry in situations of malunion where geometric constraints of the humeral shaft axis can be bypassed and the head replacement can be placed anatomically. Original reports of the Copeland implant had encouraging functional and radiographic results with only 3% loosening.[22] Other studies failed to reproduce these successful results and found moderate glenoid erosion in 12%

of the patients and age-adjusted Constant scores lower than expected.[23]

Hemiarthroplasty with biologic resurfacing is an option in younger adults with significant osteoarthritis. Interposition material, such as lateral meniscal allograft, Achilles tendon allograft, fascia lata autograft, and anterior capsule, all have been used. Follow-up at 2 to 15 years after hemiarthroplasty with glenoid biologic resurfacing demonstrated good functional outcome scores but continued glenoid erosion with medialization of approximately 7 mm. Poor results were demonstrated with interposition of the anterior capsule, whereas Achilles tendon allograft had the best outcome.[24] One recent report of 19 patients treated with hemiarthroplasty with glenoid meniscal allograft resurfacing found an alarming revision rate of 32%, with most requiring conversion to TSA.[25]

Hemiarthroplasty is an option for nonreconstructible proximal humeral fractures. The results depend largely on tuberosity healing in an anatomic position to restore rotator cuff function. The outcomes are heterogeneous, and systematic reviews reveal nearly a 40% dissatisfaction rate.[26] Motion after hemiarthroplasty is bimodal, with some patients regaining nearly full forward elevation with tuberosity healing and other patients with tuberosity failure having pseudoparalytic shoulders. Patients older than 70 years may be candidates for reverse shoulder replacement with a more predictable return of moderate forward elevation and reliable pain relief. Proximal humeral nonunion and malunion may be treated with hemiarthroplasty, but tuberosity healing remains a major concern, and outcomes were less than satisfactory in more than one half of the patients in a 2012 study.[27]

Total Shoulder Arthroplasty

TSA continues to be the most effective treatment of glenohumeral arthritis, with more than 95% of patients obtaining symptomatic relief. TSA rates continue to increase in the United States, doubling in frequency every 7 years. TSA survivorship is greater than 85% at 15-year follow-up.[28] Indications for TSA include glenohumeral arthritis with failed nonsurgical treatment, glenohumeral arthritis with a reparable supraspinatus tendon tear, inflammatory arthropathy with an intact rotator cuff, posttraumatic arthritis, postcapsulorrhaphy arthritis, and failed hemiarthroplasty with glenoid wear. Contraindications include an irreparable rotator cuff tear, RCTA, inability to implant a stable glenoid prosthesis, septic arthritis, and possibly a dysfunctional rotator cuff or deltoid. The most common TSA failure mode is glenoid component aseptic loosening, followed by rotator cuff dysfunction in the long term. Factors that contribute to component loosening include edge loading on the glenoid prosthesis, component malposition, polyethylene wear osteolysis, and insufficient bony support for the glenoid prosthesis. The management of posterior glenoid wear and posterior humeral subluxation during TSA are surgical dilemmas. Optimizing the longevity of glenoid fixation will be an area of research focus in the future.

Patient age is an important factor that guides clinical decision-making regarding the treatment of glenohumeral osteoarthritis. Concern over glenoid component loosening, bone loss, and the need for revision surgery in younger adults make surgeons hesitant to implant a glenoid component. Studies on complication rates, implant survival, hemiarthroplasty conversion rates to TSA, and glenoid loosening rates in younger patients are helping define algorithms for the surgical care of younger adults. One study on patients younger than 50 years demonstrated a high conversion rate (15%) from hemiarthroplasty to TSA for painful glenoid arthritis, with unsatisfactory results in 60% of hemiarthroplasty patients. Revision-free survival rates for hemiarthroplasty and TSA were 85% and 97% at 10 years and 75% and 84% at 20 years, respectively.[29]

Secondary rotator cuff dysfunction following TSA is another risk that should factor into surgical decision making. A multicenter study found rotator cuff dysfunction rates of 0% at 5 years, 16% at 10 years, and 55% at 15 years.[30] Clinical and radiographic outcomes were negatively affected by rotator cuff dysfunction. These high rates of rotator cuff dysfunction should elicit concern when TSA implantation is considered in younger patients. Another multicenter retrospective study with a minimum follow-up of 8 years found 28% polyethylene glenoid component migration, with an overall complication rate of 11% and a revision rate of 8% among TSA patients.[31]

Component positioning and soft-tissue balancing are important for the outcome of TSA (Figure 2). Contrac-

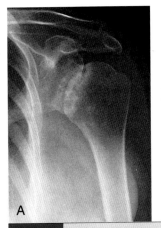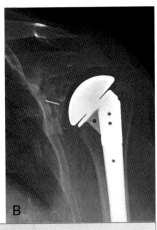

Figure 2 Total shoulder arthroplasty radiographs show glenohumeral arthritis (**A**) and successful total shoulder arthroplasty with re-creation of proximal humeral geometry and a well-cemented, pegged, all-polyethylene glenoid component (**B**).

ture of anterior soft tissues likely contributes to increased posterior glenoid contact stresses and posterior glenoid bony erosion, leading to increasing glenoid retroversion and posterior translation of the humeral head. Reconstruction of the osteoarthritic shoulder attempts to re-create bony anatomy to restore biomechanics and the soft-tissue balance. Prosthetic designs have evolved to better match the proximal humeral anatomy and relationship of the head, tuberosities, and shaft in attempts to appropriately tension the rotator cuff, provide stability, and allow full motion (Figure 3). Head inclination, retroversion, and medial-posterior offset from the canal axis are more easily re-created with third-generation prostheses that have eccentric head options. A CT osteology study of normal shoulders found head inclination of 41°, head thickness of 19 mm, head diameter of 46 mm, medial offset of 7 mm, and posterior offset of 2 mm.[32]

The glenohumeral kinematics after anatomic TSA do not match native glenohumeral motion. The native scapulohumeral rhythm comprises a 2:1 ratio of glenohumeral to scapulothoracic motion, with slight superior head translation during the first 30° of glenohumeral abduction. Kinematics after TSA with a radially mismatched glenoid has been evaluated in vivo and does not perfectly re-create ball-and-socket motion.[33] The contact point on the glenoid component is highly variable and not at the center of the glenoid. During shoulder abduction of 45° and 90°, the contact point tends to migrate posterosuperiorly in 77% of patients. This finding mimics glenoid component retrieval studies that have found increased polyethylene wear in the posterior quadrant of radially mismatched glenoids.[34] Posterior humeral subluxation and posterior glenoid wear are common problems in shoulder osteoarthritis, and the management of these asymmetric forces on the glenoid is challenging. Risk factors for glenoid component lucency include younger age at index procedure, dominant arm, early radiographic lucency, a metal-

3: Upper Extremity

tial studies of these constructs had unfavorable outcomes, with high rates of component loosening.[50,51] Relative indications for bone grafting include uneven wear that cannot be accommodated by reaming, insufficient bone volume to support the glenoid component, medialization of more than 1 cm of the joint line, more than 20° of retroversion, and potential component penetration of the glenoid vault with anticipated version correction.[51] Augmented glenoid components are prosthetic solutions to glenoid bone loss, but their durability is relatively unknown. One study demonstrated fair to poor patient satisfaction with continued joint instability, and the authors recommended the discontinuation of augmented glenoid components.[50]

Glenoid dysplasia is characterized by more than 25° of retroversion and is commonly associated with dysplastic development. Glenoid dysplasia is different from the biconcave glenoid associated with osteoarthritis because the dysplastic articulation often maintains stability. In glenoid dysplasia, there is hypertrophy of the posterior soft tissues; even though the center of the humeral head lies posterior to the scapular plane, it is often contained within the glenoid surface arc. TSA is a viable option for treating painful dysplasia with mild version correction, and hemiarthroplasty is an option if the glenoid bone stock will not support a glenoid component.[52]

Humeral stem designs are evolving to preserve proximal metaphyseal bone and increase implant longevity through osseous ingrowth. Press-fit stems have loosening rates of 5% to 10%, and the use of proximal ingrowth stems has improved these rates in the midterm.[53] Ingrowth stems have the disadvantages of stress shielding, proximal bone resorption, and difficult revision because of secure ingrowth. Fully cemented stems have similar disadvantages complicating revision and increasing proximal stress shielding. A recent randomized controlled trial demonstrated improved pain, function, and strength with fully cemented stems compared with uncemented stems, suggesting less symptomatic micromotion and improved rotational stability.[54]

Lesser tuberosity osteotomy (LTO) may be advantageous for subscapularis function after TSA compared with subscapularis tenotomy or subscapularis peel off the tuberosity. A retrospective comparative study found that LTO had higher clinical outcome scores and lower rates of subscapularis tendon tear or ultrasound attenuation compared with tenotomy repairs.[55] However, a recent randomized controlled trial of LTO versus subscapularis peel demonstrated no difference in the healing rates, subscapularis fatty infiltration, or clinical outcomes.[56] Osseous union of LTO is nearly 100% in most studies, but subscapularis function remains equivocal. Biomechanically, LTO repair is stronger than soft-tissue or transosseous tenotomy repair under cyclic loading.[57] Osteotomy likely provides improved glenoid surgical exposure and faster initial biomechanical strength, but whether LTO has significant clinical benefits over tenotomy remains controversial.

Venous thromboembolic events after shoulder arthroplasty may occur at a higher rate than previously reported (0.5%). A prospective cohort study of 100 patients following shoulder arthroplasty with Doppler ultrasound found a 13% deep vein thrombosis (DVT) rate, with one half occurring in the operated upper extremity and the other half in the lower extremities.[58] This DVT rate is comparable to rates after total hip arthroplasty. Symptomatic pulmonary embolism and fatal pulmonary embolism were very rare at 2% and 1%, respectively. DVT prophylaxis is recommended in high-risk patients, but it is unknown if routine pharmacologic DVT prophylaxis should be given.

Computer-assisted or computer-navigated TSA may play a role in the optimization of component positioning. Computer simulation of glenoid implantation can predict the amount of glenoid retroversion that can be corrected without peg penetration.[49] Computer-assisted TSA is safe and provides real-time surgeon feedback on glenoid reamer version with improved implantation accuracy.[59] Trials comparing glenoid component positioning using patient-specific instruments versus standard surgical instruments are ongoing.

Rotator Cuff Tear Arthropathy

RCTA is a constellation of pathology, including rotator cuff insufficiency, degenerative arthropathy, and varying degrees of superior head migration with containment or escape. Surgical treatment may include arthroscopic débridement with possible tuberoplasty and biceps tenotomy in contained RCTA with a concentric head or arthroplasty. The outcome of arthroscopic treatment is unpredictable.

Unconstrained anatomic TSA is contraindicated in RCTA because of evidence of early glenoid loosening from the "rocking horse" effect. Hemiarthroplasty is recommended for younger patients with relatively active lifestyles or in patients with rheumatoid arthritis who maintain forward elevation of more than 90°. The results of hemiarthroplasty are improved if the subscapularis is intact, preoperative elevation is maintained, and the humeral head is centered and contained.[60] Laterally extended RCTA heads are designed to articulate with the acromion and may reduce friction. A decision tree has been established to help define the treatment of irreparable rotator cuff tears with arthroplasty or joint preservation (Figure 6).

Outcomes from hemiarthroplasty for RCTA are mixed depending on patient expectations and the duration of follow-up. In the midterm, hemiarthroplasty has a satisfaction rate of nearly 85%. However, the risk of continued erosion of the glenoid and acromion, along with the limited improvement in shoulder motion and the development of humeral instability, continues to be a long-term concern. At 5 years postoperatively, only 67% of RCTA hemiarthroplasties were considered successful.[61] A cost analysis of hemiarthroplasty versus reverse total shoulder arthroplasty (RTSA) for RCTA found that RTSA could be cost-effective with lower implant cost because of the significant health utility gained adjusted for the utility lost as a result of complications.[62]

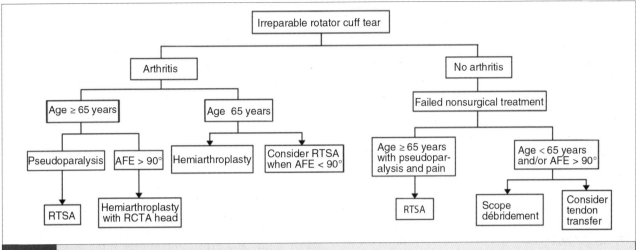

Figure 6 Treatment algorithm for irreparable rotator cuff tear. Patients at least 65 years of age with rotator cuff tear arthropathy (RCTA) and pseudoparalysis are excellent candidates for reverse total shoulder arthroplasty (RTSA); those that maintain active forward elevation (AFE) may be candidates for hemiarthroplasty. If there is no arthritis, then RTSA should be reserved for patients who have pseudoparalysis because satisfaction is decreased if preoperative motion is greater than 90°. (Adapted from Izquierdo R, Voloshin I, Edwards S, et al: Treatment of glenohumeral osteoarthritis. *J Am Acad Orthop Surg* 2010;18[6]:375-382.)

RTSA is ideally reserved for the older patient with RCTA and pseudoparalysis. RTSA is indicated when there is loss of head containment within the coracoacromial arch. The results from RTSA for RCTA are excellent, with complication rates of less than 5%, compared with other etiologies such as fracture sequelae and revision arthroplasty, which have complication rates approaching 50%.[63] Patients with a pseudoparalytic shoulder can expect to achieve 120° or more of forward elevation. External rotation, as well as internal rotation behind the back, may continue to be limited. Pain relief and American Shoulder and Elbow Surgeons (ASES) and Constant scores consistently are improved compared with preoperative levels.

Reverse Total Shoulder Arthroplasty

RTSA was designed to treat rotator cuff–deficient shoulders. Improved understanding of the biomechanics of the rotator cuff–deficient shoulder and reverse arthroplasty have facilitated the development of modern reverse implant designs. The indications for RTSA include a pseudoparalytic RCTA shoulder, uncontained RCTA, fracture sequelae with a dysfunctional or a deficient rotator cuff, and revision arthroplasty with a deficient rotator cuff. Relative indications for RTSA are expanding to include irreparable rotator cuff tears and arthritis with an intact but grossly dysfunctional rotator cuff. The contraindications for RTSA include a dysfunctional deltoid, neurologic impairment of the axillary nerve, and young patient age, although no true age limit is known at this time.

Original RTSA implant designs in the 1970s were constrained and had high failure rates secondary to component loosening, which led to the development of a semiconstrained design. The newer designs transferred the center of rotation medially and lengthened the humerus to re-tension the deltoid and soft tissues. These mechanical changes afford increased compression of the reverse articulation, lengthening of the deltoid lever arm, and recruitment of more deltoid fibers for shoulder abduction (**Figure 7**). A more medial center of rotation reduces shear forces across the baseplate-bone interface and leads to improved implant fixation longevity.[63]

Modern RTSA is effective at reducing pain and improving function in a variety of shoulder disorders. The authors of a 2006 study stratified reverse arthroplasty outcomes and revision rates by diagnosis in 45 patients with RCTA, fracture sequelae, or revision arthroplasty. Overall forward elevation increased from 55° preoperatively to 121° postoperatively, Constant scores increased from 17 to 58 points, and 78% of the patients were satisfied, with 67% having no pain or slight pain.[63]

There is a diagnosis-dependent only effect on RTSA outcomes. A recent study of 191 patients found that posttraumatic arthritis and revision arthroplasty etiologies had less improvement and higher complication rates compared with RCTA, arthritis with cuff tear, or irreparable massive cuff tear without arthritis.[64] Lower satisfaction is found after RTSA for irreparable cuff tears if preoperative forward elevation is greater than 90°.[65] RTSA for inflammatory arthritis has similarly good functional and pain relief outcomes, but higher rates of acromial fractures near 15% and cemented stem loosening approaching 10% were found at 3-year follow-up.[66] RTSA in patients with Parkinson disease results in poor functional outcomes, although pain relief is good.

The optimal biomechanical reverse shoulder arthroplasty implant design is still unknown. Many factors contribute to a successful arthroplasty, and numerous

3: Upper Extremity

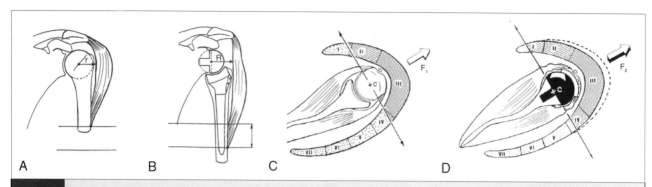

Figure 7 Biomechanics of reverse total shoulder arthroplasty. The reverse total shoulder arthroplasty (**B** and **D**) improves the mechanical advantage of the native deltoid muscle (**A** and **C**) to abduct the arm by increasing the deltoid level arm length from *r* to *R* by medializing the center of rotation. Medializing the center of rotation also recruits more anterior and posterior deltoid muscle zones (I and IV) for abduction. Lengthening the arm (*L*) tensions the deltoid to optimize the muscle force-length relationship. (Adapted with permission from Boileau P, Watkinson D, Hatzidakis AM, Hovorka I: The Grammont reverse shoulder prosthesis: Results in cuff tear arthritis, fracture sequelae, and revision arthroplasty. *J Shoulder Elbow Surg* 2006;15[5]:527-540.)

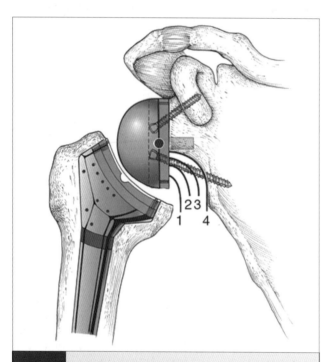

Figure 8 Scapular notching at the inferior glenoid neck after reverse shoulder replacement is a common complication. The Sirveaux grading of notching was described to help define the risk of baseplate loosening. Grade 1: notching involves only the lateral pillar; grade 2: notching contacts the inferior screw; grade 3: notching extends beyond the inferior screw; grade 4: notching extends to the baseplate central peg. (Adapted from Cheung E, Willis M, Walker M, Clark R, Frankle MA: Complications in reverse total shoulder arthroplasty. *J Am Acad Orthop Surg* 2011;19[7]:439-449.)

sion, optimized bone-implant forces to increase fixation longevity, and low wear rates to minimize osteolysis and aseptic loosening.

The factors that affect soft-tissue tension, most importantly in the deltoid, include the height of humeral stem implantation, the thickness of the polyethylene insert, and the inferior position of the glenosphere. The factors that affect impingement-free motion include glenosphere position and tilt, lateralization of the center of rotation, increased glenosphere size to provide clearance, and the depth and the diameter of the humeral socket. The factors that reduce baseplate-bone shear and torque forces include a center of rotation near the bone-implant interface, inferior baseplate tilt, the lack of an eccentric baseplate peg, and reduced impingement levering forces. Articulation compression is a stability factor and is affected by soft-tissue tension, rotator cuff integrity, humeral lateral offset, humeral component inclination, arm abduction angle, and humeral component version. Many of these factors are determined by the implant design, but many can be modified by the surgeon and will affect the outcome.

Component positioning is critical to reduce scapular notching (**Figure 8**). An inferiorly placed glenosphere at the inferior margin of the glenoid reduces the rates of glenoid notching and corresponds with improved subjective outcomes.[67] Notching may be a combination of mechanical impingement and a biologic response to repetitive trauma and polyethylene debris. More valgus humeral socket designs demonstrate higher rates of scapular notching compared with less valgus designs. Implant retrieval studies demonstrate polyethylene rim damage from direct contact with inferior baseplate screws as a source of polyethylene debris and osteolysis.

Soft-tissue tension and deltoid tension significantly affect forward elevation postoperatively.[68,69] If the arm is shortened or the deltoid tension is not properly restored, forward elevation is impaired. Excessive arm lengthening may cause acromial insufficiency fractures,

outcome measures exist. Biomechanically, a successful RTSA has a low dislocation risk, improved motion before impingement, mechanically advantageous muscle vectors for increased strength, balanced soft-tissue ten-

especially in patients with osteoporosis or inflammatory arthritis; can cause deltoid fatigue or dysfunction; and can contribute to tension neuropathies.[70] Instability remains a significant risk in RTSA, with rates between 2% and 30%. Efforts to reduce instability include increased soft-tissue tension in both the vertical and horizontal directions, retentive polyethylene liners, and more valgus humeral component positioning. Subscapularis repair during RTSA does not appear to lessen the risk of dislocation,[71] although initial reports suggested improved stability.

Lateralization of the center of rotation through bony structural grafting or implant design is an option to improve impingement-free motion, improve the articulation compression and stability, and augment deficient glenoid bone. Metallic lateralization has increased torque and shear forces at the bone-metal interface. Metallic lateral offset glenosphere designs have slightly higher revision rates (10%) compared with medialized designs.[72] Glenoid structural bone grafting to lateralize the baseplate using autologous humeral head or allograft during RTSA has shown encouraging results in terms of graft incorporation and baseplate fixation. Autologous structural grafting with extended peg baseplates have shown 98% incorporation by CT scan and improved internal rotation and reduced scapular notching (20%) compared with nonlateralized historic controls.[73]

The long-term outcomes of RTSA are relatively unknown. One study demonstrated 91% survival of the prosthesis at 10 years, with most revisions occurring within the first 3 years. The authors of the study also found an ominous decrement in function at 6 years postoperatively, with only 60% of the patients maintaining a Constant score greater than 30 or a pain score less than 10 at 10 years postoperatively.[74] The deltoid muscle may fatigue or stretch over time and become less effective at arm elevation. The revision rates for RTSA remain high (5% to 15%), even among experienced surgeons. The most common reason for revision is instability, but wound complications and glenoid component complications are also major contributors to revision.

Revision Shoulder Arthroplasty

The incidence of revision arthroplasty will likely increase over the next decade as the rate of primary shoulder arthroplasty continues to increase. The reasons for failure can be divided into three groups: soft-tissue problems, such as rotator cuff tear or cuff dysfunction; osseous concerns of bone loss or glenoid arthritis; and implant complications, including malposition, polyethylene wear, loosening, and oversizing or undersizing of components. Arthroplasty failures are often multifactorial with significant soft-tissue scarring. An analysis of outcomes by failure etiology found that soft-tissue reconstruction had worse outcomes than implant revision.[75] Overall, nearly 50% of the revisions had poor to fair results.

A review of hemiarthroplasty and TSA revision rates

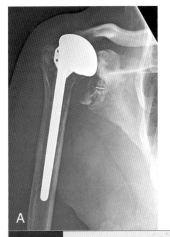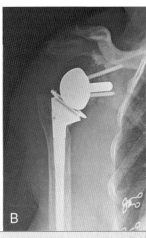

Figure 9 A failed total shoulder arthroplasty with anterosuperior escape and a loose glenoid component (**A**) can be revised to a reverse total shoulder arthroplasty (**B**). Structural bone grafting was required because of medialization and loss of glenoid bone stock. (Ccourtesy of Leesa Galatz, MD, St. Louis, MO.)

demonstrated a higher rate of conversion of hemiarthroplasty to TSA (8%) for symptomatic glenoid arthritis compared with revision for a loose polyethylene TSA component (2%).[17] Outcomes from hemiarthroplasty conversion to TSA have been modest and less successful than primary TSA. Conversions to TSA are stiffer and require more frequent revision surgery, and more than 30% are unsatisfactory. Conversion of a failed hemiarthroplasty to TSA as a result of instability or stem loosening has worse outcomes compared with hemiarthroplasty conversion to TSA for glenoid arthritis.[76]

The failure of TSA most commonly occurs because of aseptic glenoid component loosening. When adequate glenoid bone stock remains and there is a functional rotator cuff, reimplantation of a new polyethylene component is often possible. In patients with deficient glenoid bone and a functional rotator cuff, the glenoid component may be removed and the glenoid cavity bone grafted. TSA conversion to a hemiarthroplasty has a 90% satisfaction rate despite graft resorption and medial head migration.[77]

Revision to RTSA has become a valuable option in patients with a failed shoulder arthroplasty and an irreparable rotator cuff tear or deficient tuberosities. Shoulders that were once deemed unreconstructable may now be salvaged with RTSA (**Figure 9**). A functional deltoid and sufficient glenoid bone stock for implantation of a baseplate are required. A review of failed hemiarthroplasty for fracture sequelae revised to RTSA demonstrated improvements in ASES scores and forward elevation with 70% good or excellent results.[78]

The treatment of periprosthetic shoulder infection is controversial. It is unknown if débridement and retention of components, single-stage revision, an antibiotic spacer, two-stage revision with an antibiotic spacer, or resection arthroplasty is most successful in eradicating an infection. A multicenter retrospective review of 44 periprosthetic shoulder infections found 95% eradication with similar rates for resection, two-staged reimplantation, and placement of a permanent antibiotic spacer, although worse clinical outcomes were found with resection arthroplasty.[79] A single-stage revision study of infected RTSAs found 90% eradication.[80] A study of two-stage revision with antibiotic spacer placement found that infection was eradicated in more than 82% of the patients, and 43% of the patients preferred to permanently retain the antibiotic spacer.[81] Débridement and the retention of components gives the best functional outcome but risks recurrent infection, whereas resection arthroplasty remains a salvage effort to relieve pain or eradicate a deep infection.

Evidence-Based Guidelines

The American Academy of Orthopaedic Surgeons has published a clinical practice guideline on the treatment of glenohumeral osteoarthritis.[82] Because of the lack of high-quality evidence, few recommendations were made. Injectable viscosupplementation has weak support in the literature. TSA and hemiarthroplasty are both good options, but TSA is preferable to hemiarthroplasty. Keeled or pegged glenoid components are both viable options, and surgeons should perform more than two TSAs per year to avoid complications. The consensus recommendations included that venous thromboembolism prophylaxis should be used for shoulder arthroplasty, and an irreparable rotator cuff tear is a contraindication for TSA. Notably, the committee was unable to recommend physical therapy, pharmacotherapy, injectable corticosteroids, arthroscopic treatments, biologic interposition with allograft or autograft, or concomitant biceps tenotomy or tenodesis, nor did the committee establish a preference for subscapularis tenotomy versus lesser tuberosity osteotomy. Many areas of glenohumeral arthritis treatment remain in need of high-quality research.

A Cochrane systematic review of shoulder osteoarthritis compared nonsurgical to surgical treatments, and because of the lack of nonsurgical control patients, there was a poor level of evidence to support surgical treatment.[83] TSA did have improved patient outcome scores and shoulder function compared with hemiarthroplasty. TSA also has better cost-effectiveness than hemiarthroplasty for the treatment of osteoarthritis.[84] TSA provides a greater increase in quality-adjusted life-years (QALYs), with less cost per QALY gained. TSA is therefore preferred over hemiarthroplasty for both patient benefit and payer cost reasons.

Summary/Future Directions

The future directions of shoulder reconstruction will likely involve an emphasis on joint preservation treatments using disease-modifying agents, gene therapy, growth factors, and cartilage regeneration techniques. Improved glenoid component longevity will be a focus of research attention to solve the problem of loosening and osteolysis. Finally, computer-navigated arthroplasty will likely become part of shoulder reconstruction. There remains a dearth of high-quality evidence to support the most basic principles in shoulder reconstruction. Future studies that focus on evidence-based medicine will likely affect shoulder reconstruction for decades to come.

Key Study Points

- Despite significant advances in arthroplasty design, soft-tissue balancing and subscapularis healing remain critical components.
- RTSA has revolutionized shoulder surgery for the management of the pseudoparalytic shoulder.
- Because of the increased incidence of RTSA, there will likely be an epidemic of failed RTSAs that will pose significant soft-tissue, bony, and functional challenges for surgeons in the future.

Annotated References

1. Hettrich CM, Boraiah S, Dyke JP, Neviaser A, Helfet DL, Lorich DG: Quantitative assessment of the vascularity of the proximal part of the humerus. *J Bone Joint Surg Am* 2010;92(4):943-948.

   A cadaver study found that the posterior humeral circumflex artery provides 64% of the blood supply to the humeral head. Level of evidence: V.

2. Mont MA, Maar DC, Urquhart MW, Lennox D, Hungerford DS: Avascular necrosis of the humeral head treated by core decompression: A retrospective review. *J Bone Joint Surg Br* 1993;75(5):785-788.

3. Yeh PC, Kharrazi FD: Postarthroscopic glenohumeral chondrolysis. *J Am Acad Orthop Surg* 2012;20(2):102-112.

   This review found that postarthroscopic glenohumeral chondrolysis is a rare complication associated with proud suture anchors, thermal devices, and intra-articular pain pumps. Level of evidence: V.

4. Marinko LN, Chacko JM, Dalton D, Chacko CC: The effectiveness of therapeutic exercise for painful shoulder conditions: A meta-analysis. *J Shoulder Elbow Surg* 2011;20(8):1351-1359.

   This meta-analysis found that therapeutic exercise is an effective treatment of painful shoulder conditions. Level of evidence: II.

5. Ramiro S, Radner H, van der Heijde DM, Buchbinder R, Aletaha D, Landewé RB: Combination therapy for pain management in inflammatory arthritis: A

Cochrane systematic review. *J Rheumatol Suppl* 2012; 90:47-55.

A systematic Cochrane review found insufficient evidence to establish the value of combination therapy over monotherapy for pain management in inflammatory arthritis. Level of evidence: IV.

6. Blaine T, Moskowitz R, Udell J, et al: Treatment of persistent shoulder pain with sodium hyaluronate: A randomized, controlled trial. A multicenter study. *J Bone Joint Surg Am* 2008;90(5):970-979.

7. Weinstein DM, Bucchieri JS, Pollock RG, Flatow EL, Bigliani LU: Arthroscopic debridement of the shoulder for osteoarthritis. *Arthroscopy* 2000;16(5):471-476.

8. Cameron BD, Galatz LM, Ramsey ML, Williams GR, Iannotti JP: Non-prosthetic management of grade IV osteochondral lesions of the glenohumeral joint. *J Shoulder Elbow Surg* 2002;11(1):25-32.

9. Richards DP, Burkhart SS: Arthroscopic debridement and capsular release for glenohumeral osteoarthritis. *Arthroscopy* 2007;23(9):1019-1022.

10. Scheibel M, Bartl C, Magosch P, Lichtenberg S, Habermeyer P: Osteochondral autologous transplantation for the treatment of full-thickness articular cartilage defects of the shoulder. *J Bone Joint Surg Br* 2004;86(7): 991-997.

11. Romeo AA, Cole BJ, Mazzocca AD, Fox JA, Freeman KB, Joy E: Autologous chondrocyte repair of an articular defect in the humeral head. *Arthroscopy* 2002;18(8): 925-929.

12. Provencher MT, Ghodadra N, LeClere L, Solomon DJ, Romeo AA: Anatomic osteochondral glenoid reconstruction for recurrent glenohumeral instability with glenoid deficiency using a distal tibia allograft. *Arthroscopy* 2009;25(4):446-452.

13. de Beer JF, Bhatia DN, van Rooyen KS, Du Toit DF: Arthroscopic debridement and biological resurfacing of the glenoid in glenohumeral arthritis. *Knee Surg Sports Traumatol Arthrosc* 2010;18(12):1767-1773.

This case series of arthroscopic débridement and biologic resurfacing of the glenoid had 28% unsatisfactory results in pain relief and functional improvement in glenohumeral osteoarthritis in the intermediate term. Level of evidence: IV.

14. Savoie FH III, Brislin KJ, Argo D: Arthroscopic glenoid resurfacing as a surgical treatment for glenohumeral arthritis in the young patient: Midterm results. *Arthroscopy* 2009;25(8):864-871.

15. Gilmer BB, Comstock BA, Jette JL, Warme WJ, Jackins SE, Matsen FA: The prognosis for improvement in comfort and function after the ream-and-run arthroplasty for glenohumeral arthritis: An analysis of 176 consecutive cases. *J Bone Joint Surg Am* 2012;94(14):e102.

A prospective study of ream and run hemiarthroplasty in 176 shoulders found subjective improvements after 1.5 years postoperatively and the best results in older male patients with good prior function. Level of evidence: II.

16. Bartelt R, Sperling JW, Schleck CD, Cofield RH: Shoulder arthroplasty in patients aged fifty-five years or younger with osteoarthritis. *J Shoulder Elbow Surg* 2011;20(1):123-130.

This study compared TSA to hemiarthroplasty in adults younger than 55 years and found improved implant survivorship, long-term pain relief, and motion after TSA compared with hemiarthroplasty. Level of evidence: IV.

17. Radnay CS, Setter KJ, Chambers L, Levine WN, Bigliani LU, Ahmad CS: Total shoulder replacement compared with humeral head replacement for the treatment of primary glenohumeral osteoarthritis: A systematic review. *J Shoulder Elbow Surg* 2007;16(4):396-402.

18. Levine WN, Djurasovic M, Glasson JM, Pollock RG, Flatow EL, Bigliani LU: Hemiarthroplasty for glenohumeral osteoarthritis: Results correlated to degree of glenoid wear. *J Shoulder Elbow Surg* 1997;6(5):449-454.

19. Levine WN, Fischer CR, Nguyen D, Flatow EL, Ahmad CS, Bigliani LU: Long-term follow-up of shoulder hemiarthroplasty for glenohumeral osteoarthritis. *J Bone Joint Surg Am* 2012;94(22):e1641-e1647.

This long-term follow-up of a cohort of 28 patients who underwent hemiarthroplasties for arthritis found only 25% satisfaction at an average of 17 years' follow-up. Level of evidence: IV.

20. Gadea F, Alami G, Pape G, Boileau P, Favard L: Shoulder hemiarthroplasty: Outcomes and long-term survival analysis according to etiology. *Orthop Traumatol Surg Res* 2012;98(6):659-665.

A retrospective study of 272 patients who underwent hemiarthroplasty found the best results with osteonecrosis, good results with rheumatoid arthritis and primary osteoarthritis in patients younger than 50 years, and the worst results with rotator cuff tear and fracture sequelae. Level of evidence: IV.

21. Thomas SR, Sforza G, Levy O, Copeland SA: Geometrical analysis of Copeland surface replacement shoulder arthroplasty in relation to normal anatomy. *J Shoulder Elbow Surg* 2005;14(2):186-192.

22. Levy O, Copeland SA: Cementless surface replacement arthroplasty (Copeland CSRA) for osteoarthritis of the shoulder. *J Shoulder Elbow Surg* 2004;13(3):266-271.

23. Al-Hadithy N, Domos P, Sewell MD, Naleem A, Papanna MC, Pandit R: Cementless surface replacement arthroplasty of the shoulder for osteoarthritis: Results of fifty Mark III Copeland prosthesis from an independent center with four-year mean follow-up. *J Shoulder Elbow Surg* 2012;21(12):1776-1781.

This retrospective review of 53 humeral resurfacing replacements found similar functional results to stemmed hemiarthroplasty and a low revision rate at 4-year

3: Upper Extremity

follow-up but a high rate of glenoid erosion. Level of evidence: IV.

24. Krishnan SG, Nowinski RJ, Harrison D, Burkhead WZ: Humeral hemiarthroplasty with biologic resurfacing of the glenoid for glenohumeral arthritis: Two to fifteen-year outcomes. *J Bone Joint Surg Am* 2007;89(4):727-734.

25. Lee BK, Vaishnav S, Rick Hatch GF III, Itamura JM: Biologic resurfacing of the glenoid with meniscal allograft: Long-term results with minimum 2-year follow-up. *J Shoulder Elbow Surg* 2013;22(2):253-260.

    This series of hemiarthroplasty with meniscal allograft glenoid resurfacing for osteoarthritis found inconsistent 4-year results, with a mean visual analog scale pain score of 3.5 and a 32% complication rate. Level of evidence: IV.

26. Kontakis G, Koutras C, Tosounidis T, Giannoudis P: Early management of proximal humeral fractures with hemiarthroplasty: A systematic review. *J Bone Joint Surg Br* 2008;90(11):1407-1413.

27. Duquin TR, Jacobson JA, Sanchez-Sotelo J, Sperling JW, Cofield RH: Unconstrained shoulder arthroplasty for treatment of proximal humeral nonunions. *J Bone Joint Surg Am* 2012;94(17):1610-1617.

    This series of shoulder arthroplasty for humeral nonunion demonstrated decreased pain and improved function but less than 50% satisfaction, with inconsistent tuberosity healing resulting in poor functional outcome. Level of evidence: IV.

28. Cil A, Veillette CJ, Sanchez-Sotelo J, Sperling JW, Schleck CD, Cofield RH: Survivorship of the humeral component in shoulder arthroplasty. *J Shoulder Elbow Surg* 2010;19(1):143-150.

    This series of 1,584 shoulder arthroplasties found humeral stem survivorship of 95%, 92%, and 88% at 2, 5, and 20 years, respectively. Younger age, male gender, posttraumatic arthritis, uncemented stem, and metal-backed glenoid increased humeral component failure. Level of evidence: IV.

29. Sperling JW, Cofield RH, Rowland CM: Minimum fifteen-year follow-up of Neer hemiarthroplasty and total shoulder arthroplasty in patients aged fifty years or younger. *J Shoulder Elbow Surg* 2004;13(6):604-613.

30. Young AA, Walch G, Pape G, Gohlke F, Favard L: Secondary rotator cuff dysfunction following total shoulder arthroplasty for primary glenohumeral osteoarthritis: Results of a multicenter study with more than five years of follow-up. *J Bone Joint Surg Am* 2012;94(8):685-693.

    This retrospective review of 518 TSA long-term outcomes found increased rotator cuff dysfunction and reduced clinical and radiographic outcomes over time. Preoperative infraspinatus fatty infiltration and superior tilt of the glenoid component were negative prognostic factors. Level of evidence: IV.

31. Favard L, Katz D, Colmar M, Benkalfate T, Thomazeau H, Emily S: Total shoulder arthroplasty—arthroplasty for glenohumeral arthropathies: Results and complications after a minimum follow-up of 8 years according to the type of arthroplasty and etiology. *Orthop Traumatol Surg Res* 2012;98(4, suppl):S41-S47.

    A retrospective study found anatomic TSA had a high risk of glenoid loosening (28%), making the authors hesitant to use cemented polyethylene glenoid components, especially in young patients. Level of evidence: IV.

32. Robertson DD, Yuan J, Bigliani LU, Flatow EL, Yamaguchi K: Three-dimensional analysis of the proximal part of the humerus: Relevance to arthroplasty. *J Bone Joint Surg Am* 2000;82(11):1594-1602.

33. Massimini DF, Li G, Warner JP: Glenohumeral contact kinematics in patients after total shoulder arthroplasty. *J Bone Joint Surg Am* 2010;92(4):916-926.

    This in vivo study of TSA joint contact mapping found that joint kinematics are not simple ball-and-socket mechanics. The superior-posterior glenoid quadrant has the most articular contact. Level of evidence: IV.

34. Nho SJ, Ala OL, Dodson CC, et al: Comparison of conforming and nonconforming retrieved glenoid components. *J Shoulder Elbow Surg* 2008;17(6):914-920.

35. Edwards TB, Labriola JE, Stanley RJ, O'Connor DP, Elkousy HA, Gartsman GM: Radiographic comparison of pegged and keeled glenoid components using modern cementing techniques: A prospective randomized study. *J Shoulder Elbow Surg* 2010;19(2):251-257.

    This randomized clinical study of pegged versus keeled glenoid components during TSA for osteoarthritis found increased rates of glenoid lucency with keeled components (46%) compared with pegged components (15%) at 2-year follow-up. Level of evidence: I.

36. Walch G, Young AA, Boileau P, Loew M, Gazielly D, Molé D: Patterns of loosening of polyethylene keeled glenoid components after shoulder arthroplasty for primary osteoarthritis: Results of a multicenter study with more than five years of follow-up. *J Bone Joint Surg Am* 2012;94(2):145-150.

    This multicenter study of TSA with all-polyethylene keeled components found 30% loosening rates with minimum 5-year follow-up. Loosening was associated with reaming of subchondral bone, component malposition, and glenoid deformity. Level of evidence: III.

37. Fox TJ, Cil A, Sperling JW, Sanchez-Sotelo J, Schleck CD, Cofield RH: Survival of the glenoid component in shoulder arthroplasty. *J Shoulder Elbow Surg* 2009;18(6):859-863.

38. Collin P, Tay AK, Melis B, Boileau P, Walch G: A ten-year radiologic comparison of two-all polyethylene glenoid component designs: A prospective trial. *J Shoulder Elbow Surg* 2011;20(8):1217-1223.

    This prospective cohort study found no difference in glenoid component lucency between flat-back and convex-back glenoid all-polyethylene designs. Young age, hand dominance, and poor implantation influenced glenoid lucency. Level of evidence: II.

39. Tammachote N, Sperling JW, Vathana T, Cofield RH, Harmsen WS, Schleck CD: Long-term results of cemented metal-backed glenoid components for osteoarthritis of the shoulder. *J Bone Joint Surg Am* 2009; 91(1):160-166.

40. Boileau P, Avidor C, Krishnan SG, Walch G, Kempf JF, Molé D: Cemented polyethylene versus uncemented metal-backed glenoid components in total shoulder arthroplasty: A prospective, double-blind, randomized study. *J Shoulder Elbow Surg* 2002;11(4):351-359.

41. Lawrence TM, Ahmadi S, Sperling JW, Cofield RH: Fixation and durability of a bone-ingrowth component for glenoid bone loss. *J Shoulder Elbow Surg* 2012; 21(12):1764-1769.

    This case series of TSA examines the use of an ingrowth glenoid component for deficient glenoid bone stock. With 11-year follow-up, there was a high rate of revision for glenoid loosening, and a high rate of glenoid lucency if unrevised. Level of evidence: IV.

42. Throckmorton TW, Zarkadas PC, Sperling JW, Cofield RH: Pegged versus keeled glenoid components in total shoulder arthroplasty. *J Shoulder Elbow Surg* 2010; 19(5):726-733.

    This retrospective review of pegged versus keeled glenoid components found that radiolucencies develop over time, but there was no difference in clinical or radiographic outcomes between pegged and keeled components at midterm follow-up. Level of evidence: IV.

43. Rahme H, Mattsson P, Wikblad L, Nowak J, Larsson S: Stability of cemented in-line pegged glenoid compared with keeled glenoid components in total shoulder arthroplasty. *J Bone Joint Surg Am* 2009;91(8):1965-1972.

44. Wirth MA, Loredo R, Garcia G, Rockwood CA Jr, Southworth C, Iannotti JP: Total shoulder arthroplasty with an all-polyethylene pegged bone-ingrowth glenoid component: A clinical and radiographic outcome study. *J Bone Joint Surg Am* 2012;94(3):260-267.

    This series of TSA with an anchor peg glenoid component found evidence of bone between the flanges of the polyethylene central peg in 68% of the components at 3-year follow-up. Level of evidence: IV.

45. Wirth MA, Klotz C, Deffenbaugh DL, McNulty D, Richards L, Tipper JL: Cross-linked glenoid prosthesis: A wear comparison to conventional glenoid prosthesis with wear particulate analysis. *J Shoulder Elbow Surg* 2009;18(1):130-137.

46. Shapiro TA, McGarry MH, Gupta R, Lee YS, Lee TQ: Biomechanical effects of glenoid retroversion in total shoulder arthroplasty. *J Shoulder Elbow Surg* 2007; 16(3, suppl):S90-S95.

47. Iannotti JP, Greeson C, Downing D, Sabesan V, Bryan JA: Effect of glenoid deformity on glenoid component placement in primary shoulder arthroplasty. *J Shoulder Elbow Surg* 2012;21(1):48-55.

    A clinical series of glenoid retroversion of more than 10° found near 40% failure with placement of a pegged glenoid component to within 10° of the ideal position by asymmetric reaming without center peg perforation. Level of evidence: IV.

48. Iannotti JP, Norris TR: Influence of preoperative factors on outcome of shoulder arthroplasty for glenohumeral osteoarthritis. *J Bone Joint Surg Am* 2003;85(2): 251-258.

49. Nowak DD, Bahu MJ, Gardner TR, et al: Simulation of surgical glenoid resurfacing using three-dimensional computed tomography of the arthritic glenohumeral joint: The amount of glenoid retroversion that can be corrected. *J Shoulder Elbow Surg* 2009;18(5):680-688.

50. Rice RS, Sperling JW, Miletti J, Schleck C, Cofield RH: Augmented glenoid component for bone deficiency in shoulder arthroplasty. *Clin Orthop Relat Res* 2008; 466(3):579-583.

51. Hill JM, Norris TR: Long-term results of total shoulder arthroplasty following bone-grafting of the glenoid. *J Bone Joint Surg Am* 2001;83(6):877-883.

52. Bonnevialle N, Mansat P, Mansat M, Bonnevialle P: Hemiarthroplasty for osteoarthritis in shoulder with dysplastic morphology. *J Shoulder Elbow Surg* 2011; 20(3):378-384.

    Hemiarthroplasty for shoulder osteoarthritis with glenoid dysplasia gives satisfactory results at medium-range follow-up. Level of evidence: IV.

53. Throckmorton TW, Zarkadas PC, Sperling JW, Cofield RH: Radiographic stability of ingrowth humeral stems in total shoulder arthroplasty. *Clin Orthop Relat Res* 2010;468(8):2122-2128.

    This series of proximally coated humeral ingrowth stems for TSA showed few radiolucencies (7%) and no loosening at midterm follow-up. Level of evidence: IV.

54. Litchfield RB, McKee MD, Balyk R, et al: Cemented versus uncemented fixation of humeral components in total shoulder arthroplasty for osteoarthritis of the shoulder: A prospective, randomized, double-blind clinical trial. A JOINTs Canada Project. *J Shoulder Elbow Surg* 2011;20(4):529-536.

    This randomized controlled trial of cemented versus uncemented humeral stems during TSA found that cemented stems had better quality of life, strength, and range of motion up to 2 years postoperatively. Level of evidence: I.

55. Scalise JJ, Ciccone J, Iannotti JP: Clinical, radiographic, and ultrasonographic comparison of subscapularis tenotomy and lesser tuberosity osteotomy for total shoulder arthroplasty. *J Bone Joint Surg Am* 2010;92(7): 1627-1634.

    This retrospective comparative study of tenotomy and osteotomy found that lesser tuberosity osteotomy had

3: Upper Extremity

better clinical outcomes, a lower rate of subscapularis tendon tear or attrition, and universal healing. Level of evidence: III.

56. Lapner PL, Sabri E, Rakhra K, Bell K, Athwal GS: Healing rates and subscapularis fatty infiltration after lesser tuberosity osteotomy versus subscapularis peel for exposure during shoulder arthroplasty. *J Shoulder Elbow Surg* 2013;22(3):396-402.

     This randomized controlled trial of lesser tuberosity osteotomy versus subscapularis peel tenotomy found no significant difference in radiologic healing, muscle fatty changes, and clinical outcomes. Level of evidence: I.

57. Ponce BA, Ahluwalia RS, Mazzocca AD, Gobezie RG, Warner JJ, Millett PJ: Biomechanical and clinical evaluation of a novel lesser tuberosity repair technique in total shoulder arthroplasty. *J Bone Joint Surg Am* 2005; 87(suppl 2):1-8.

58. Willis AA, Warren RF, Craig EV, et al: Deep vein thrombosis after reconstructive shoulder arthroplasty: A prospective observational study. *J Shoulder Elbow Surg* 2009;18(1):100-106.

59. Nguyen D, Ferreira LM, Brownhill JR, et al: Improved accuracy of computer assisted glenoid implantation in total shoulder arthroplasty: An in-vitro randomized controlled trial. *J Shoulder Elbow Surg* 2009;18(6): 907-914.

60. Goldberg SS, Bell JE, Kim HJ, Bak SF, Levine WN, Bigliani LU: Hemiarthroplasty for the rotator cuff-deficient shoulder. *J Bone Joint Surg Am* 2008;90(3):554-559.

61. Sanchez-Sotelo J, Cofield RH, Rowland CM: Shoulder hemiarthroplasty for glenohumeral arthritis associated with severe rotator cuff deficiency. *J Bone Joint Surg Am* 2001;83(12):1814-1822.

62. Coe MP, Greiwe RM, Joshi R, et al: The cost-effectiveness of reverse total shoulder arthroplasty compared with hemiarthroplasty for rotator cuff tear arthropathy. *J Shoulder Elbow Surg* 2012;21(10):1278-1288.

     This cost-effectiveness study demonstrated that RTSA had potential utility over hemiarthroplasty for the treatment of CTA, especially when the cost of the reverse implant was decreased to less than $7,000, providing cost of less than $50,000 per QALY. Level of evidence: IV.

63. Boileau P, Watkinson D, Hatzidakis AM, Hovorka I: Neer Award 2005: The Grammont reverse shoulder prosthesis. Results in cuff tear arthritis, fracture sequelae, and revision arthroplasty. *J Shoulder Elbow Surg* 2006;15(5):527-540.

64. Wall B, Nové-Josserand L, O'Connor DP, Edwards TB, Walch G: Reverse total shoulder arthroplasty: A review of results according to etiology. *J Bone Joint Surg Am* 2007;89(7):1476-1485.

65. Boileau P, Gonzalez JF, Chuinard C, Bicknell R, Walch G: Reverse total shoulder arthroplasty after failed rotator cuff surgery. *J Shoulder Elbow Surg* 2009; 18(4):600-606.

66. Hattrup SJ, Sanchez-Sotelo J, Sperling JW, Cofield RH: Reverse shoulder replacement for patients with inflammatory arthritis. *J Hand Surg Am* 2012;37(9):1888-1894.

     A retrospective review of 19 reverse shoulder arthroplasties for inflammatory arthritis and deficient rotator cuff demonstrated very good results, with near 90% satisfaction and a mean visual analog scale pain score of 1, flexion of 138°, an ASES score of 76, and a Simple Shoulder Test score of 8. Level of evidence: IV.

67. Lévigne C, Boileau P, Favard L, et al: Scapular notching in reverse shoulder arthroplasty. *J Shoulder Elbow Surg* 2008;17(6):925-935.

68. Jobin CM, Brown GD, Bahu MJ, et al: Reverse total shoulder arthroplasty for cuff tear arthropathy: The clinical effect of deltoid lengthening and center of rotation medialization. *J Shoulder Elbow Surg* 2012;21(10): 1269-1277.

     This prospective cohort of RTSA for RCTA found improved forward elevation with increased deltoid lengthening. Level of evidence: II.

69. Lädermann A, Walch G, Lubbeke A, et al: Influence of arm lengthening in reverse shoulder arthroplasty. *J Shoulder Elbow Surg* 2012;21(3):336-341.

     This retrospective review of RTSA found that increased arm lengthening correlated with improved forward elevation and that arm shortening had loss of active elevation. Level of evidence: IV.

70. Cheung E, Willis M, Walker M, Clark R, Frankle MA: Complications in reverse total shoulder arthroplasty. *J Am Acad Orthop Surg* 2011;19(7):439-449.

     This review of RTSA demonstrated that the most common complications include neurologic injury, periprosthetic fracture, hematoma, infection, scapular notching, dislocation, mechanical baseplate failure, and acromial fracture. Level of evidence: IV.

71. Clark JC, Ritchie J, Song FS, et al: Complication rates, dislocation, pain, and postoperative range of motion after reverse shoulder arthroplasty in patients with and without repair of the subscapularis. *J Shoulder Elbow Surg* 2012;21(1):36-41.

     This case-control study of subscapularis repair after RTSA demonstrated no effect on complications, dislocations, range of motion, or pain relief with subscapularis repair. Level of evidence: IV.

72. Frankle M, Levy JC, Pupello D, et al: The reverse shoulder prosthesis for glenohumeral arthritis associated with severe rotator cuff deficiency: A minimum two-year follow-up study of sixty patients surgical technique. *J Bone Joint Surg Am* 2006;88(suppl 1, pt 2):178-190.

73. Boileau P, Moineau G, Roussanne Y, O'Shea K: Bony increased-offset reversed shoulder arthroplasty: Minimizing scapular impingement while maximizing glenoid

fixation. *Clin Orthop Relat Res* 2011;469(9):2558-2567.

Structural bone grafting of the glenoid during reverse shoulder arthroplasty lateralizes the baseplate and has low rates of inferior scapular notching, improved shoulder rotation, and no evidence of prosthetic instability. Level of evidence: IV.

74. Guery J, Favard L, Sirveaux F, Oudet D, Mole D, Walch G: Reverse total shoulder arthroplasty: Survivorship analysis of eighty replacements followed for five to ten years. *J Bone Joint Surg Am* 2006;88(8):1742-1747.

75. Dines JS, Fealy S, Strauss EJ, et al: Outcomes analysis of revision total shoulder replacement. *J Bone Joint Surg Am* 2006;88(7):1494-1500.

76. Sassoon AA, Rhee PC, Schleck CD, Harmsen WS, Sperling JW, Cofield RH: Revision total shoulder arthroplasty for painful glenoid arthrosis after humeral head replacement: The nontraumatic shoulder. *J Shoulder Elbow Surg* 2012;21(11):1484-1491.

This series of revision TSA after failed hemiarthroplasty found decreased pain and increased motion with worse outcome if the stem was revised or if there was instability associated with the subscapularis dysfunction. Level of evidence: IV.

77. Scalise JJ, Iannotti JP: Bone grafting severe glenoid defects in revision shoulder arthroplasty. *Clin Orthop Relat Res* 2008;466(1):139-145.

78. Levy J, Frankle M, Mighell M, Pupello D: The use of the reverse shoulder prosthesis for the treatment of failed hemiarthroplasty for proximal humeral fracture. *J Bone Joint Surg Am* 2007;89(2):292-300.

79. Romanò CL, Borens O, Monti L, Meani E, Stuyck J: What treatment for periprosthetic shoulder infection? Results from a multicentre retrospective series. *Int Orthop* 2012;36(5):1011-1017.

This retrospective analysis shows comparable infection eradication rates after two-stage revision, resection arthroplasty, or permanent spacer implant for the treatment of septic shoulder prosthesis. Level of evidence: IV.

80. Beekman PD, Katusic D, Berghs BM, Karelse A, De Wilde L: One-stage revision for patients with a chronically infected reverse total shoulder replacement. *J Bone Joint Surg Br* 2010;92(6):817-822.

This review found that one-stage revision arthroplasty for infected reverse arthroplasty reduces the cost and duration of treatment and had a 90% rate of eradication of infection and good functional outcomes. Level of evidence: IV.

81. Jawa A, Shi L, O'Brien T, et al: Prosthesis of antibiotic-loaded acrylic cement (PROSTALAC) use for the treatment of infection after shoulder arthroplasty. *J Bone Joint Surg Am* 2011;93(21):2001-2009.

This series of shoulder arthroplasty infections managed by antibiotic spacer found 82% infection eradication. Forty-three percent of the patients declined a second-stage procedure because of acceptable function and pain relief. Level of evidence: IV.

82. Izquierdo R, Voloshin I, Edwards S, et al: Treatment of glenohumeral osteoarthritis. *J Am Acad Orthop Surg* 2010;18(6):375-382.

This clinical practice guideline based on a systematic review found that management of glenohumeral osteoarthritis remains controversial, and the scientific evidence on this topic can be significantly improved. Level of evidence: V.

83. Singh JA, Sperling J, Buchbinder R, McMaken K: Surgery for shoulder osteoarthritis: A Cochrane systematic review. *J Rheumatol* 2011;38(4):598-605.

This Cochrane systematic review of shoulder arthroplasty versus nonsurgical treatment found poorly controlled studies of nonsurgical treatment, but TSA was associated with better shoulder function compared with hemiarthroplasty. Level of evidence: V.

84. Mather RC III, Watters TS, Orlando LA, Bolognesi MP, Moorman CT III: Cost effectiveness analysis of hemiarthroplasty and total shoulder arthroplasty. *J Shoulder Elbow Surg* 2010;19(3):325-334.

A cost-utility analysis of TSA versus hemiarthroplasty found that TSA is a cost-effective procedure, with greater utility and a lower overall cost. Level of evidence: II.

Shoulder Instability and Rotator Cuff Disease

Sara Edwards, MD   Leesa M. Galatz, MD

Shoulder Instability

The shoulder is the most frequently dislocated joint. Diagnosis and treatment of patients with shoulder instability are common problems facing orthopaedic surgeons and continue to evolve. Physical examination of the shoulder is an important facet.

Video 27.1: Physical Examination of the Shoulder. Jordan M. Case, MD; Sandeep Mannava, MD; Stephanie G. Cheetham, BA; Benjamin Long, MS; Allston J. Stubbs, MD (14.43 min)

Anatomy

Stability of the shoulder joint is the result of the interaction of static and dynamic stabilizers. Static constraints include the osteochondral anatomy of the glenoid and the humerus, including the glenoid labrum and capsule, the glenohumeral ligaments, and the coracohumeral ligaments. Dynamic stabilizers include the rotator cuff and the long head of the biceps tendon.

Static stability is primarily maintained by the congruency of the glenohumeral joint, the labrum, and the ligaments about the shoulder. The glenohumeral joint has a ball-and-socket configuration with a mismatch between the two radii of curvature. The relatively unconstrained relationship is unique to the shoulder and allows the shoulder to obtain a large excursion and

range of motion. The fibrocartilaginous glenoid labrum serves to deepen the socket of the glenoid, providing additional stability. The labrum also serves as an attachment site for the glenohumeral capsule and ligaments and the long head of the biceps tendon. It also decreases the glenoid radius of curvature to more closely match the humeral curvature. The glenohumeral ligaments are discrete thickenings of the capsule (Figure 1) that tighten and relax in various degrees of motion.

The dynamic stabilizers of the shoulder include the rotator cuff, the scapular stabilizers, and the long head of the biceps tendon. Proprioceptive feedback in the form of neurologic connectivity between the dynamic and static stabilizers provides further stability to the shoulder. Disruption or subtle dysfunction of any of the stabilizers may lead to shoulder instability and pain.

Biomechanics

Traumatic anterior instability typically occurs when excessive force is placed on the arm in an abducted and externally rotated position. This position stretches or

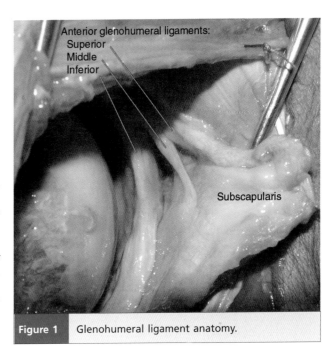

Anterior glenohumeral ligaments:
Superior
Middle
Inferior

Subscapularis

Figure 1 Glenohumeral ligament anatomy.

Dr. Galatz or an immediate family member serves as an unpaid consultant to Tornier and serves as a board member, owner, officer, or committee member of the American Shoulder and Elbow Surgeons, the American Orthopaedic Association, and the American Academy of Orthopaedic Surgeons. Neither Dr. Edwards nor any immediate family member has received anything of value from or has stock or stock options held in a commercial company or institution related directly or indirectly to the subject of this chapter.

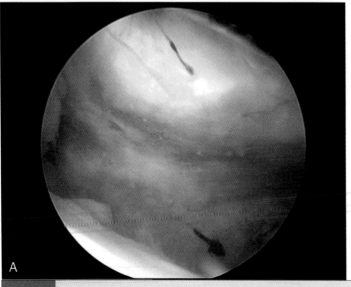
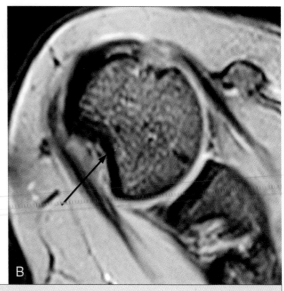

Figure 2 **A,** An arthroscopic image of an engaging Hill-Sachs lesion. **B,** Axial MRI of the same lesion (arrow) engaging the anterior rim of the glenoid, with external rotation and anterior translation.

tears the anteroinferior glenohumeral ligament. With dislocation, the anterior labrum, the capsule (ligaments), and occasionally the anterior glenoid rim fail. The capsule also may be avulsed from the humeral insertion; this occurrence is known as humeral avulsion of the glenohumeral ligament (HAGL).

Posterior dislocations occur with the arm in a forward flexed, adducted position. The structures at risk for failure are the posterior capsulolabral complex and the posterior glenoid rim.

Repetitive submaximal stress to the ligaments can produce a pathologic increase in joint range of motion. This atraumatic instability pattern often is associated with underlying generalized laxity or instability in multiple joints. Occasionally, underlying scapulothoracic mechanics will be dysfunctional. Proprioception is often abnormal in these patients as well.

Humeral and glenoid bone loss in patients with anterior instability can increase the failure rates of standard arthroscopic instability repair techniques. Reports have noted unacceptable recurrent instability following arthroscopic repair in patients with substantial bone loss.[1] A biomechanical study demonstrated a significant decrease in anterior shoulder stability with bone loss of 21% of the glenoid.[2] Chronic recurrent instability can lead to attritional bony changes of the anterior glenoid that may require bony augmentation to reconstruct. Acute defects typically have identifiable bone that is amenable to repair at the time of surgery.

Humeral bone loss from a Hill-Sachs lesion or a reverse Hill-Sachs lesion can contribute to instability as a result of the loss of the radius of curvature of the humeral head, which precipitates engagement of the humeral lesion with the glenoid with a smaller arc of motion (an engaging Hill-Sachs lesion; Figure 2). A recent biomechanical study demonstrated that with a 25% Hill-Sachs defect, significant differences were noted in joint translation, capsular force, and bony contact force. However, the findings also suggested that an isolated humeral defect, after anatomic labral and capsular repair, is not a risk factor for recurrent instability.[3]

The rotator cuff provides dynamic stability by providing a force couple in both the transverse and coronal planes. Loss of the coronal force couple results in superior head migration but not necessarily loss of function. The transverse force couple, composed of the subscapularis, infraspinatus, and teres minor muscles, provides anterior-posterior stability. Loss of the transverse force couple results in a pathologic increase in translation or subluxation of the humeral head toward the rotator cuff deficiency and can result in a functional loss of abduction.

The long head of the biceps tendon is thought to provide a dynamic stabilizing force for abduction, flexion, and rotation. Recent attention to the biceps as a source of pain has led to an increased incidence of biceps tenotomy and tenodesis. The success of these procedures, even in younger patients, has led to controversy regarding the importance of the role of the long head of the biceps tendon in stabilization.

Classification

Instability is often classified on the basis of timing, the direction of instability, and etiology. Instability can occur in one plane or in multiple directions. It can result from an acute traumatic event or recurrent microtrauma that causes pathology over time.

Anterior Instability

The most common direction of shoulder dislocation is anterior. Subluxation events that are not true dislocations may occur and may result in recurrent instability and intra-articular pathology. Anterior dislocations and subluxations can cause injury of the glenoid labrum

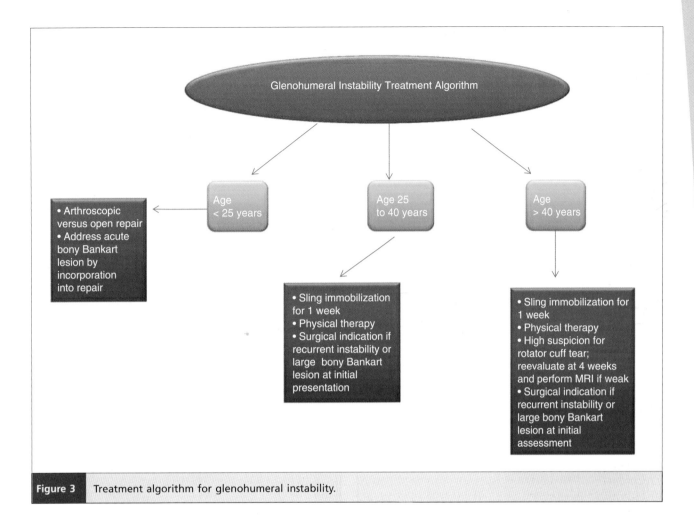

Glenohumeral Instability Treatment Algorithm

Age < 25 years
- Arthroscopic versus open repair
- Address acute bony Bankart lesion by incorporation into repair

Age 25 to 40 years
- Sling immobilization for 1 week
- Physical therapy
- Surgical indication if recurrent instability or large bony Bankart lesion at initial presentation

Age > 40 years
- Sling immobilization for 1 week
- Physical therapy
- High suspicion for rotator cuff tear; reevaluate at 4 weeks and perform MRI if weak
- Surgical indication if recurrent instability or large bony Bankart lesion at initial assessment

Figure 3 Treatment algorithm for glenohumeral instability.

(Bankart lesion), injury of the anterior glenoid rim (bony Bankart lesion), injury of the glenohumeral ligaments by tearing or stretching, or HAGL. Additional damage to soft tissue, cartilage, the humeral head, the rotator cuff, and the glenoid cavity can occur at the time of the initial dislocation or with repeated instability. A magnetic resonance arthrogram is the most sensitive radiographic study for detecting labral tears and cartilage lesions. An increasing number of subluxations and dislocations correlates with the prevalence of labral and cartilage lesions.[4]

Treatment

Following diagnosis of a shoulder dislocation, closed reduction of the joint is attempted (Figure 3). Typically, pain medication and sedatives are given in a monitored setting in the emergency department. An intra-articular lidocaine block is also an effective analgesic for reduction. The Milch method of gentle traction and manipulation has recently been found to be more successful than the Stimson method for reducing a shoulder dislocation, providing a success rate of 82% compared with 28% on the first attempt.[5] A neurovascular examination should be completed both before and after reduction, with care taken to document any nerve injury. If a closed reduction attempt is unsuccessful, either a closed or an open

reduction should be performed in the operating room with the patient under general anesthesia. Following the reduction, the patient's shoulder should be immobilized in a sling. Recent evidence suggests that immobilization in a neutral position or internal rotation is as effective as immobilization in external rotation.[6]

Natural History

The treatment of acute, traumatic anterior shoulder instability in the young, active patient is controversial. Traditional nonsurgical treatments, such as physical therapy and prolonged sling immobilization in either internal or external rotation, do not alter the recurrent dislocation rate. Recurrence rates as high as 92% have been reported with nonsurgical treatment.[7] Patients with large bony defects at the time of injury have a higher risk of recurrence. Multiple recurrent dislocations also increase the intra-articular pathology and the amount of bone loss identified on MRI.[4]

Although the rate of recurrent dislocation is high, this risk decreases with age.[8] Patients older than 40 years have an increased risk of rotator cuff tears and neurologic injury, particularly to the axillary nerve. In patients older than 60 years, dislocation is positively correlated with greater tuberosity fracture, a rotator cuff tear, and neurologic injury.[9]

3: Upper Extremity

Recent evidence supports offering surgical intervention (either arthroscopic or open) to patients younger than 22 years with a first-time dislocation because of the high recurrent instability rates. Randomized prospective data suggest that patients treated with an arthroscopic Bankart repair after initial dislocation had an 82% reduction in the risk of recurrent instability.[10] Surgical practices have been evolving over the past 10 years, with more than 68% of surgeons offering surgery to patients age 16 to 25 years with a first-time dislocation.

Osteoarthritis is noted to develop in patients with shoulder instability. A 5- to 20-year follow-up study of patients treated with open Bankart repair noted early signs of osteoarthritis preoperatively in 26% of the patients. After treatment, the osteoarthritis progressed in 32% of the treated patients. The progression of osteoarthritis was correlated with the number of preoperative subluxations and the total number of preoperative dislocations. Male patients as well as patients with glenoid bone deficit were at increased risk for the progression of osteoarthritis.[11]

Arthroscopic Versus Open Repair

Anterior shoulder instability can be treated with either open or arthroscopic stabilization. Multiple studies have reported excellent results for open repair with recurrent instability of approximately 5%. First-generation arthroscopic repair techniques (staples or tacks) resulted in inferior rates of success, with recurrent instability of 15% to 33%.[10] The advent of suture anchors and the improvement of arthroscopic repair techniques have resulted in a 90% to 96% success rate.[10,12-15] A recent study noted that 90% of surgeons now prefer arthroscopic repair as the initial procedure of choice.[16] A randomized prospective trial comparing open and arthroscopic repair for recurrent anterior shoulder instability showed that the two groups had similar outcome scores and rates of recurrence.[17]

A recent study of long-term outcomes of patients treated with acute arthroscopic repair following dislocation with a mean follow-up of 11 years (range, 9 to 13 years) noted a recurrent dislocation rate of 14.3%, with all patients requiring revision surgery. Nine patients in this series (21%) noted intermittent subluxation.[15] Another prospective series examined patients treated with arthroscopic Bankart repair at 8-year follow-up and found that 35% sustained a recurrent dislocation. Patients treated with two or fewer suture anchors had a higher dislocation rate than patients treated with three or four suture anchors.[18]

Recurrent Instability Following Surgery

Instability following surgery occurs secondary to repeat trauma, large bony defects on the glenoid or the humerus, capsular laxity and redundancy, failure of healing of the labrum, malunion of the labrum, or an unrecognized HAGL lesion.

Recent evidence suggests that arthroscopic anteroinferior capsular repair techniques using a low anteroinferior 5:30 clock position have similar outcomes to open procedures.[19] Another study, comparing patient outcomes following revision arthroscopic Bankart repair to patient outcomes following primary arthroscopic Bankart repair, found subjective outcomes to be significantly lower for the revision procedure than for the index procedure, although the recurrent dislocation rates were comparable.[20]

Patients with glenoid bone lesions incorporated into the arthroscopic repair did significantly better, with a 93% success rate.[21] The quality of the bone fragment and the chronicity of repair are also important because repair of the attritional fragments in patients with multiple dislocations is associated with a higher rate of failure.[22] For contact athletes, a recurrence rate of 89% was noted in patients with a lesion to the anterior glenoid rim of 20% to 30% when treated with arthroscopic labral repair and capsular shift alone.

For defects of the anterior glenoid involving more than 25% to 30% of the joint surface, a bony procedure is often necessary. The Latarjet procedure, which transfers the coracoid process to the glenoid bony defect, has been shown to have a low recurrence rate.[23] The coracoid process serves to extend the glenoid rim and enhance the arc available for translation before dislocation. The conjoined tendon functions as a sling to resist anterior humeral translation when the arm is abducted and externally rotated. The transferred coracoid process and the conjoined tendon tension the lower subscapularis and reinforce the deficient anteroinferior capsule. Other techniques, such as the Bristow procedure, bone grafting with iliac crest graft, and allograft use with the femoral head or distal tibia, have been used as well. Postoperative arthrosis and limitations in shoulder motion are concerns following nonanatomic coracoid reconstruction, and care should be taken to counsel patients accordingly. Recently, coracoid bone resorption has been reported following the Latarjet procedure, although the clinical significance is unknown.[24]

Osteochondral allograft, remplissage, or infraspinatus transfer into the defect may be considered for Hill-Sachs lesions larger than 25% of the total surface area of the glenoid cavity. Humeral arthroplasty or bone graft at the time of the index procedure should be strongly considered for lesions larger than 40% of the total surface area of the glenoid cavity.

Posterior Instability

Posterior shoulder dislocations are less common than anterior dislocations and are commonly missed. Mechanisms of injury include trauma to the anterior aspect of the shoulder, seizure, electrocution, or an indirect force applied through an adducted and flexed arm.

Acute and Recurrent Posterior Dislocation

Posterior dislocations, once reduced, are usually self-limited. After a short period of immobilization in external rotation, physical therapy is recommended. Approximately 17% of patients will develop a recurrent dislocation in the first year following a dislocation. Recurrent dislocation is highest in patients younger than 40 years, patients with a seizure disorder, and patients with large humeral head defects.[25] The diagnosis is often missed. Vigilance in obtaining axillary shoulder radiographs is essential to avoid missing this diagnosis. Occasionally, a CT scan is needed if plain radiographs are inconclusive.

Surgical Treatment

Surgery is reserved for patients with recurrent posterior instability or recurrent pain with posterior loading of the arm (such as occurs in the action of a football lineman or a weight lifter). The repair should address the torn posterior labrum and/or bony defect, capsular redundancy, and ligament tears. Both open and arthroscopic approaches have documented success.

Chronic Posterior Dislocation

After several weeks of posterior dislocation (unreduced), the bone of the humeral head and the posterior glenoid will erode. If the dislocation is left untreated, a closed reduction is unlikely to be successful, and open repair will be required. Preoperative planning with a CT scan can help anticipate bony defects that need to be addressed in surgery. To improve stability, subscapularis or lesser tuberosity transfer into the reverse Hill-Sachs lesion, osteochondral bone grafting, segmental humeral head replacement, or humeral head replacement can be performed. Iliac crest bone graft can be used to reconstruct glenoid deficits.

Humeral head replacement is indicated for chronic dislocations in which the patient has developed clinically significant osteoarthritis, osteonecrosis with head collapse, or damage of more than 50% of the humeral head.

Multidirectional Instability

Multidirectional instability (MDI) is a term used to describe symptomatic instability in more than one plane. Patients with MDI often demonstrate symptoms in other joints as well as generalized ligamentous laxity. There is usually no acute trauma before the onset of symptoms, and the patient does not experience a true dislocation. MDI can be secondary to poor scapulohumeral mechanics, genetic hyperlaxity (Ehlers-Danlos syndrome), and/or rotator cuff dysfunction.

Comparison with the unaffected side will help identify instability and increased motion in multiple planes. Anterior or posterior apprehension tests are often positive in the direction of laxity. Load and shift testing is often positive. Inferior instability is often present and is characterized by a positive sulcus sign in both neutral positioning of the arm and external rotation. MRI arthrography often shows a patulous capsule and a normal labrum.

Nonsurgical Treatment

The mainstay of treatment of MDI is nonsurgical and includes activity modification, along with abstaining from the aggravating sport. Nonsurgical results have been variable, with success rates as high as 80%.

Surgical Treatment

Open capsular shift has been successful in the management of MDI, with reported success rates as high as 88%. Arthroscopic capsular shift techniques also demonstrate promising results, with success rates of 85% to 88%. A recent retrospective review of symptomatic athletes with MDI who underwent an arthroscopic shift demonstrated good results, with 91% of patients having full range of motion, 98% having normal strength, and 86% being able to return to their sport.[26]

Rotator Cuff Disease

Rotator cuff disease encompasses many common causes of shoulder pain. Ranging from tendinitis to a full-thickness tear, often with accompanying degenerative changes of the glenohumeral joint, rotator cuff pathology generates a multitude of clinical issues, including nonsurgical versus surgical care, how to repair, when to repair, and how to manage irreversible changes that preclude repair. In addition, biologic strategies to enhance tendon healing have become a prominent topic of research. In spite of the increased commercial availability of these products, their role in tendon healing and their effect on outcomes remain unclear.

Natural History

Understanding the natural history of rotator cuff disease and the likelihood of tear progression influences clinical decision making. Efforts to address these issues provide a basis for formulating indications for nonsurgical and surgical treatment, as well as determining the optimal timing for treatment.

Muscle tissue is designed to bear load. The biologic health of a muscle depends on its mechanical environment. Muscles that are unloaded atrophy, accumulate fat, and undergo fibrotic changes (Figure 4). This fact is particularly relevant in the setting of rotator cuff tears because many tears are either asymptomatic or treated nonsurgically, leaving some portion of the muscle unloaded for a period of time. In a retrospective review of 1,688 patients, fatty changes of the supraspinatus correlated with patient age, the size of the tear, and a longer delay between the onset of symptoms and the diagnosis of a tear.[27] Moderate fatty changes were identified 3 years after the onset of symptoms, and severe changes occurred 5 years after the onset of symptoms. Fatty accumulation in the infraspinatus correlated with the same patient factors and was moderate at 2.5 years and severe at 4 years after the onset of symptoms.[28] Taken together, these studies highlight the development of irreversible changes, specifically atrophy, fat accumulation, and fibrosis. Therefore, consideration should be given to early repair in patients younger than 60 years or patients of working age with symptomatic tears before the aforementioned irreversible changes render the tear irreparable.

Not all rotator cuff tears initiate directly adjacent to the biceps tendon. In a study of 360 shoulders, tears oc-

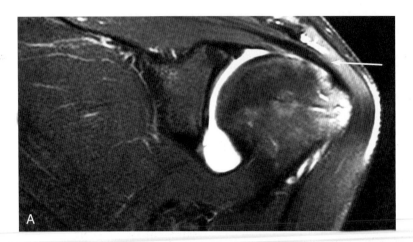

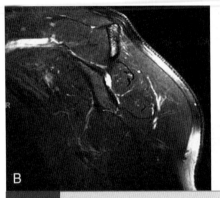

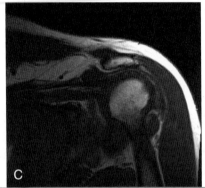

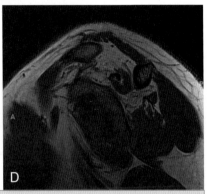

Figure 4 Representative MRI of the rotator cuff. **A,** Coronal MRI showing normal supraspinatus muscle and tendon (arrow). **B,** Sagittal MRI showing normal supraspinatus, infraspinatus, teres minor, and subscapularis muscles. **C,** Coronal MRI of a chronic tear with retraction associated with atrophy, fatty accumulation, and fibrosis. **D,** Sagittal MRI of a chronic tear with retraction demonstrating severe atrophy and fatty accumulation.

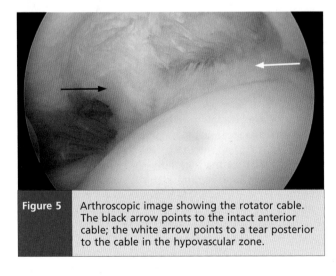

Figure 5 Arthroscopic image showing the rotator cable. The black arrow points to the intact anterior cable; the white arrow points to a tear posterior to the cable in the hypovascular zone.

ceps in the relatively hypovascular zone within the rotator cable (Figure 5). In a similar study, fatty degeneration correlated with the proximity to the biceps tendon.[30] Tears that extended anteriorly to the biceps groove were more likely to have fatty degeneration of the supraspinatus, and fatty degeneration of the infraspinatus was dependent on the overall tear size. These studies suggest that in many tears, some tendon containing the anterior aspect of the rotator cable is preserved and protects against fatty change by maintaining some load-bearing ability. When this area is torn, the muscles are more vulnerable to rapid degenerative and atrophic changes.

Rotator cuff tears progress in size over time. In addition, in the setting of an asymptomatic cuff tear, the onset of pain is associated with an increase in tear size. In a group of patients followed prospectively, pain development in a previously painless tear had a corresponding increase in tear size, a decrease in the American Shoulder and Elbow Surgeons (ASES) score, and loss of motion.[31] In another prospective population study, workers without shoulder pain were followed to determine the risk factors for the development of shoulder pain.[32] Age was the number one factor, but a work position with the shoulder overhead and abducted was also a factor.

curred most commonly 15 to 16 mm posterior to the biceps tendon, and the anterior extent of the tear was an average of 8 mm posterior to the biceps tendon.[29] Evaluation of all sizes of tears had similar findings, indicating that tears generally begin posterior to the bi-

Biomechanics

The purpose of the rotator cuff is to keep the humeral head centered on the glenoid cavity during shoulder motion. Arising from the scapula, the rotator cuff muscles converge to insert on the tuberosities, providing a centering vector as the deltoid fires with its superiorly directed vector. In the setting of a malfunctioning or an insufficient rotator cuff, the humeral head is pulled superiorly. In the early stages, this occurrence is primarily a dynamic finding associated with muscle activation; however, fixed proximal migration can occur in later stages.

Theoretically, the purpose of a rotator cuff repair is to restore muscle function. A repair has a high likelihood of relieving the pain associated with a tear. Strength restoration is not as reliable. One study attempted to evaluate the mechanical results after rotator cuff repair.[33] Twenty-one patients were evaluated for up to 2 years after a repair and were compared with a matched control group. Although pain relief and satisfaction scores were high, the repaired shoulders remained weaker than the control shoulders; on biplane radiographs the humeral heads were found to be positioned more superiorly. Further work is necessary to determine how to maximize strength and mechanics.

Nonsurgical Treatment

Nonsurgical treatment of rotator cuff tears includes pain medication, physical therapy and rehabilitation, activity modification, and steroid injections. Although it is certainly possible to control pain and improve function in the short term, risk assessment for tear progression and the development of chronic irreversible changes should influence the decision. A few studies have recently evaluated the structural and functional outcomes of rotator cuff tears treated nonsurgically and uniformly found progression in tear size in a varying percentage of patients.

In a retrospective review of 24 patients followed for 27 to 61 months (median, 42 months), 25% had an increase in tear size.[34] MRI evaluation showed that the other tears were the same or smaller. No pretreatment scores were available for comparison. Another group of 61 patients prospectively followed for 25 to 39 months revealed that 49% of the tears increased in size on ultrasound evaluation; 43% were the same, and 8% were smaller.[35] Ten new tears were discovered, which accounted for 24% of the intact rotator cuffs (patients had bilateral ultrasound examinations). The only factor that correlated with an increase in tear size was the presence of significant pain. A long-term, 13-year follow-up study of 65 patients with a tear treated nonsurgically showed that 88% had slight or no pain, and 72% had no difficulties with activities of daily living.[36] Younger patients had worse final assessment scores. These studies emphasize the importance of surveillance in the setting of a rotator cuff tear treated nonsurgically, especially in younger patients.

Table 1

Factors Associated With Failure of Rotator Cuff Healing

Older age

Increased tear size

Fatty infiltration of muscle

Muscle atrophy

Tendon length and retraction

Surgical Treatment

Rotator cuff repair has historically led to predictably good and excellent results, even in the long term.[37,38] Studies of open, mini-open, and arthroscopic repairs report excellent pain relief, improvement in functional outcome scores, and overall patient satisfaction. A 16-year follow-up of 75 patients demonstrated some decline in measures.[39] The average age at the time of surgery was 52 years, and the average age at the time of follow-up was 72 years. Only 37% of the patients were pain free at final follow-up, and 43% had some impairment in function.

In the past several years, much of the research related to the rotator cuff has centered on tendon healing and the relationship of healing to functional outcomes. Factors associated with healing (Table 1), both patient related and surgeon related, are beginning to surface, yet controversy still remains. Specifically, there has been a shift toward arthroscopic repair, such that it is now the most common approach. In addition, some surgeons have shifted toward double-row repair, using additional anchors and fixation to improve the biomechanical strength of the repair. In spite of this, patient biology has an important effect on healing and is likely the most important factor with regard to healing.

The controversy over single-row versus double-row repair is at the forefront of recent research[40-47] (Table 2). A level I prospective randomized study[40] comparing the two methods evaluated patients on the basis of anatomic outcome and the Western Ontario Rotator Cuff and ASES scores. Smaller tears and double-row repairs had a greater healing rate. Single-row repairs led to 67% healing versus 78% in the double-row repair group. However, there were no differences in the functional or quality-of-life outcome scores between the groups.

A systematic review of single-row versus double-row repairs[48] evaluated seven level I or level II studies, comparing the efficacy of these two repair techniques. There were no differences in ASES, University of California–Los Angeles, or Constant scores. Failure to heal occurred in 43% of the single-row group and 27% of the double-row group ($P = 0.057$). Although not statistically significant, this finding suggests a trend toward better healing in the double-row group. Another systematic review had similar conclusions.[49] Double-row

3: Upper Extremity

Table 2

Summary of Level I and Level II Studies Comparing Single-Row and Double-Row Repairs

Study	Level of Evidence	Tear Recurrence, %		Postoperative ASES Score		Postoperative Constant Score	
		SR	DR	SR	DR	SR	DR
Aydin et al[41]	II					82.2	78.8
Burks et al[42]	I	10%	20%	85.9	85.5	77.8	74.4
Charousset et al[43]	II	60%	39%			80.7	82.7
Franceschi et al[44]	I	46%	31%				
Grasso et al[45]	I					100.5	104.9
Koh et al[46]	I	63%	30%	85.9	83.4	85.4	82.5
Lapner et al[40]	I	33%	22%	87.9	89.3	85.6	86.3
Park et al[47]	II			91.6	93.0	76.7	79.7

ASES = American Shoulder and Elbow Surgeons, SR = single-row repair, DR = double-row repair.

fixation may have some structural benefit in larger tears, but there was no difference in clinical outcomes. Not surprisingly, a cost-effectiveness analysis of single-row versus double-row repair found that double-row repair was not cost effective.[50] This conclusion was dependent largely on the cost of the anchors.

The relationship between healing and outcomes is controversial; multiple studies have not found a correlation between healing and outcomes.[51-53] On the other hand, many other studies have shown a difference. In one study of 66 patients with massive tears repaired with an arthroscopic suture bridge technique,[54] the failure rate was 42.2%. Retraction and fatty infiltration were associated with failure of healing. Structural failure in this study was associated with lower functional outcome scores. Another study of 206 patients that compared single-row repair to two methods of double-row repair found not only a higher failure rate in single-row repairs but also better functional outcomes in all patients in the study whose tears healed.[55] Some of these differences between studies could be a function of the method of evaluation. Some outcome scores are more patient based, whereas others are more physician directed. This difference may explain the findings to a certain extent, yet the relationship remains controversial.

The time course of healing or failure to heal is also a focus of recent investigation. One study found that healing actually increased over a 5-year period.[56] With repeated imaging using ultrasound at regular intervals over the time period, the percentage of intact rotator cuffs increased. However, this finding is an exception. Most studies document an increase in rotator cuff defects with time. In addition, most have found a high percentage of failure very early after repair. In one such study,[57] 95 patients were followed over 11 years. The overall failure rate was 33%. Seventy-four percent of these failures occurred within the first 3 months. Eleven percent of the failures occurred between 3 and 6

months. Fourteen percent of the failures occurred between 2 and 5 years and were related to sports or traumatic events. Overall, the clinical results remained stable over time. A smaller study of 22 patients[58] found an overall failure rate of 41%, with 7 of 9 failures occurring within the first 3 months. Together, these studies highlight the potential importance of structural or biologic augmentation soon after repair.

Biologic Augmentation of Rotator Cuff Repair

Despite improvements in repair techniques, the failure rate after rotator cuff repair, especially in older patients and in the setting of larger, retracted tears, remains unacceptably high.[37,59,60] Tendon healing is characterized by a reparative process rather than a regenerative process.[61] Tendon healing generates scar tissue, which gains about one half to one third of the structural properties of normal tendon. Material viscoelastic properties become only one tenth of normal, substantiating the fact that the healing tissue has poorly organized, inferior properties compared with normal tendon. This finding has generated a surge of interest in biologic augmentation. Several graft augmentation devices are currently available, but little evidence substantiates their efficacy. Platelet-rich plasma has also been evaluated, but most randomized studies have not shown a benefit. This section will review the most recent studies regarding the use of currently available products.

The purpose of an extracellular matrix patch is twofold. It can be used to augment a tendon-to-bone repair, and it can be used to bridge an irreparable defect. Biologic and synthetic grafts are available (Table 3), but there is little evidence to support their use at this time. One randomized prospective study using a porcine intestinal submucosal graft showed worse results in the patients with graft augmentation.[62] The product generated a noninfectious inflammatory reaction in several patients. One of the problems identified involved

Table 3			

Scaffold Devices With FDA Clearance for Rotator Cuff Repair

(A) ECM

Product Name	ECM Type	ECM Source	Marketed by
Restore	SIS	Porcine	Depuy Orthopaedics
CuffPatch	SIS (cross-linked)	Porcine	Organogenesis
GraftJacket	Dermis	Human	Wright Medical
ArthroFlex	Dermis	Human	Arthrex
Conexa	Dermis (α-Gal–reduced)	Porcine	Tornier
TissueMend	Dermis (fetal)	Bovine	Stryker Orthopaedics
Zimmer Collagen Repair	Dermis (cross-linked)	Porcine	Zimmer
Bio-Blanket	Dermis (cross-linked)	Bovine	Kensey Nash
OrthADAPT Bioimplant	Pericardium (cross-linked)	Equine	Pegasus Biologics

(B) Synthetic

Product Name	Material	Marketed by
SportMesh Soft Tissue Reinforcement	Poly(urethaneurea)	Biomet Sports Medicine
X-Repair	Poly-L-lactide	Synthasome
Biomerix RCR Patch	Polycarbonate poly(urethaneurea)	Biomerix

(C) Hybrid

Product Name	Material	Marketed by
OrthADAPT PR Bioimplant	Equine pericardium (cross-linked) with woven polymer	Pegasus Biologics

ECM = extracellular matrix; SIS = small intestinal submucosa
(Reproduced with permission from Richetti ET, Aurora A, Iannotti JP, Derwin KA: Scaffold devices for rotator cuff repair. *J Shoulder Elbow Surg* 2012;21(2):251-265.)

the preparation of the material because some DNA isotope remained in the graft tissue, which caused the inflammatory reaction. The authors advised against using this product. A second randomized, prospective study involved using a porcine dermal graft to reinforce repairs of chronic supraspinatus and infraspinatus tears.[63] The investigators showed better outcome scores and healing in the augmented repair group.

A recent study of 24 patients who had interposition of a human dermal graft in the setting of a massive, irreparable tear showed some promising results.[64] Follow-up was a minimum of 2 years, with an average of 3 years. Repair integrity was evaluated by ultrasound, and outcome and pain scores all improved. One tear recurred because of noncompliance with postoperative rehabilitation. The repair was intact in 76% of the patients. Another study used a polycarbonate polyurethane patch to augment an open rotator cuff repair in 10 patients. One patient had a persistent tear 1 year after surgery. All patients improved clinically.[65] Neither of these studies had a control group, but, nevertheless, these studies suggest a potential benefit of initial repair augmentation. Further high-level studies are needed to define indications for graft use because these results

may not be better than repair or débridement without augmentation.

Platelet-rich plasma has been suggested as a potential biologic augmentation product primarily on the basis of its growth factor contents. Platelets are best known for their role in hemostasis but also contain a multitude of growth factors, which could potentiate tendon healing. Some preparations contain white blood cells, whereas others do not. An alternative product is platelet-rich fibrin matrix (PRFM). In this preparation, calcium chloride is added to the centrifugation, which causes the formation of a fibrin matrix with the platelets inside. Ideally, this matrix creates a scaffold with a slower growth factor release after reabsorption.

A randomized, prospective study using PRFM in 88 patients showed no difference in Constant scores or MRI findings between patients with the matrix augmentation and the control patients.[66] Another randomized controlled trial using PRFM showed no differences in strength, healing, vascularity, or clinical outcome scores.[67] In fact, a regression analysis suggested that PRFM actually decreased healing in this study. A level II cohort study showed no improvement in clinical or structural outcomes with the use of PRFM.[68]

3: Upper Extremity

Some promising results do exist. In a nonrandomized study of 40 patients, 20 treated with PRFM and 20 without, the patients treated with PRFM showed no difference in clinical outcomes but a higher healing rate in tears larger than 3 cm.[69] A randomized controlled trial using platelet-rich plasma in 53 patients showed some modest improvements in pain during the very early postoperative period.[70] Follow-up MRI showed no differences in the healing rates of the tears, however. Overall, there is little evidence at this time to support the routine use of platelet-rich plasma or PRFM in rotator cuff repair. Its ability to enhance tendon healing and its cost effectiveness are unsubstantiated.

Summary

The field of tendon research is rapidly expanding. Rotator cuff repair is a common surgical procedure, and questions regarding the method of repair, the timing of repair, and biologic augmentation fuel interesting research studies. Although both good and bad prognostic factors for nonsurgical and surgical treatment have been discovered, more studies are needed to outline and refine the available treatment strategies.

Key Study Points

- Significant bone defects of the glenoid (> 25%) lead to unacceptably high rates of failure of arthroscopic labral repair.

- Growing evidence suggests that earlier intervention should be considered for full-thickness rotator cuff tears in younger patients who have not yet developed significant tendon retraction, fatty infiltration, and atrophy.

- Despite the tremendous commercial availability of biologic augmentation for rotator cuff repair, little evidence supports its widespread use at this time.

Annotated References

1. Burkhart SS, De Beer JF: Traumatic glenohumeral bone defects and their relationship to failure of arthroscopic Bankart repairs: Significance of the inverted-pear glenoid and the humeral engaging Hill-Sachs lesion. *Arthroscopy* 2000;16(7):677-694.

2. Itoi E, Lee SB, Berglund LJ, Berge LL, An KN: The effect of a glenoid defect on anteroinferior stability of the shoulder after Bankart repair: A cadaveric study. *J Bone Joint Surg Am* 2000;82(1):35-46.

3. Sekiya JK, Jolly J, Debski RE: The effect of a Hill-Sachs defect on glenohumeral translations, in situ capsular

forces, and bony contact forces. *Am J Sports Med* 2012; 40(2):388-394.

In this controlled laboratory study, it was demonstrated that, with capsular restoration, a Hill-Sachs defect of 25% or less did not significantly alter recurrent instability. The Hill-Sachs lesion did increase the in situ forces in the capsule as well as the glenohumeral contact force.

4. Kim DS, Yoon YS, Yi CH: Prevalence comparison of accompanying lesions between primary and recurrent anterior dislocation in the shoulder. *Am J Sports Med* 2010;38(10):2071-2076.

There are significantly more Bankart lesions and bony defects in patients with recurrent instability compared with patients with first-time dislocation. Level of evidence: III.

5. Amar E, Maman E, Khashan M, Kauffman E, Rath E, Chechik O: Milch versus Stimson technique for nonsedated reduction of anterior shoulder dislocation: A prospective randomized trial and analysis of factors affecting success. *J Shoulder Elbow Surg* 2012;21(11):1443-1449.

The success of reduction without sedation was superior for the Milch method compared with the Stimson method. Level of evidence: I.

6. Liavaag S, Brox JI, Pripp AH, Enger M, Soldal LA, Svenningsen S: Immobilization in external rotation after primary shoulder dislocation did not reduce the risk of recurrence: A randomized controlled trial. *J Bone Joint Surg Am* 2011;93(10):897-904.

Immobilization in external rotation does not reduce the rate of recurrent dislocation for patients with a first-time traumatic dislocation. Level of evidence: I.

7. Wheeler JH, Ryan JB, Arciero RA, Molinari RN: Arthroscopic versus nonoperative treatment of acute shoulder dislocations in young athletes. *Arthroscopy* 1989;5(3):213-217.

8. Hovelius L, Olofsson A, Sandström B, et al: Nonoperative treatment of primary anterior shoulder dislocation in patients forty years of age and younger: A prospective twenty-five-year follow-up. *J Bone Joint Surg Am* 2008;90(5):945-952.

9. Robinson CM, Shur N, Sharpe T, Ray A, Murray IR: Injuries associated with traumatic anterior glenohumeral dislocations. *J Bone Joint Surg Am* 2012;94(1): 18-26.

This prospective trauma database study examining 3,633 patients demonstrated greater prevalence of rotator cuff tear, neurologic injury, and/or greater tuberosity fracture following shoulder dislocation. Level of evidence: II.

10. Robinson CM, Jenkins PJ, White TO, Ker A, Will E: Primary arthroscopic stabilization for a first-time anterior dislocation of the shoulder: A randomized, double-blind trial. *J Bone Joint Surg Am* 2008;90(4):708-721.

11. Ogawa K, Yoshida A, Matsumoto H, Takeda T: Outcome of the open Bankart procedure for shoulder instability and development of osteoarthritis: A 5- to 20-year

follow-up study. *Am J Sports Med* 2010;38(8):1549-1557.

This cohort study of 163 patients (167 joints) undergoing the open Bankart procedure found that most postoperatively detected osteoarthritis developed before surgery. The development and the progression of osteoarthritis cannot be prevented by surgery. However, over 20 years the development of osteoarthritis was very slow. Level of evidence: III.

12. Kim SH, Ha KI, Cho YB, Ryu BD, Oh I: Arthroscopic anterior stabilization of the shoulder: Two to six-year follow-up. *J Bone Joint Surg Am* 2003;85(8):1511-1518.

13. Carreira DS, Mazzocca AD, Oryhon J, Brown FM, Hayden JK, Romeo AA: A prospective outcome evaluation of arthroscopic Bankart repairs: Minimum 2-year follow-up. *Am J Sports Med* 2006;34(5):771-777.

14. Marquardt B, Witt KA, Liem D, Steinbeck J, Pötzl W: Arthroscopic Bankart repair in traumatic anterior shoulder instability using a suture anchor technique. *Arthroscopy* 2006;22(9):931-936.

15. Owens BD, DeBerardino TM, Nelson BJ, et al: Long-term follow-up of acute arthroscopic Bankart repair for initial anterior shoulder dislocations in young athletes. *Am J Sports Med* 2009;37(4):669-673.

16. Malhotra A, Freudmann MS, Hay SM: Management of traumatic anterior shoulder dislocation in the 17- to 25-year age group: A dramatic evolution of practice. *J Shoulder Elbow Surg* 2012;21(4):545-553.

There is a trend among orthopaedic surgeons to offer surgery to young patients with a first-time dislocation.

17. Bottoni CR, Smith EL, Berkowitz MJ, Towle RB, Moore JH: Arthroscopic versus open shoulder stabilization for recurrent anterior instability: A prospective randomized clinical trial. *Am J Sports Med* 2006;34(11):1730-1737.

18. van der Linde JA, van Kampen DA, Terwee CB, Dijksman LM, Kleinjan G, Willems WJ: Long-term results after arthroscopic shoulder stabilization using suture anchors: An 8- to 10-year follow-up. *Am J Sports Med* 2011;39(11):2396-2403.

Long-term results (8- to 10-year follow-up) of arthroscopic Bankart repair showed that approximately one third of the patients experienced recurrent dislocation. The presence of a Hill-Sachs defect or fewer than three suture anchors might increase the chance of redislocation. Level of evidence: IV.

19. Bartl C, Schumann K, Paul J, Vogt S, Imhoff AB: Arthroscopic capsulolabral revision repair for recurrent anterior shoulder instability. *Am J Sports Med* 2011;39(3):511-518.

Arthroscopic capsulolabral revision repair via the anteroinferior 5:30 clock position achieves comparable results with open revision repairs with a low recurrent instability rate. Level of evidence: IV.

20. Krueger D, Kraus N, Pauly S, Chen J, Scheibel M: Subjective and objective outcome after revision arthroscopic stabilization for recurrent anterior instability versus initial shoulder stabilization. *Am J Sports Med* 2011;39(1):71-77.

Revision arthroscopic shoulder stabilization has lower clinical outcomes compared with primary arthroscopic shoulder stabilization. Level of evidence: III.

21. Sugaya H, Moriishi J, Kanisawa I, Tsuchiya A: Arthroscopic osseous Bankart repair for chronic recurrent traumatic anterior glenohumeral instability. *J Bone Joint Surg Am* 2005;87(8):1752-1760.

22. Boileau P, Villalba M, Héry JY, Balg F, Ahrens P, Neyton L: Risk factors for recurrence of shoulder instability after arthroscopic Bankart repair. *J Bone Joint Surg Am* 2006;88(8):1755-1763.

23. Schmid SL, Farshad M, Catanzaro S, Gerber C: The Latarjet procedure for the treatment of recurrence of anterior instability of the shoulder after operative repair: A retrospective case series of forty-nine consecutive patients. *J Bone Joint Surg Am* 2012;94(11):e75.

Coracoid transfer as described by Latarjet can effectively restore anterior glenohumeral shoulder stability if previous surgical procedures have been unsuccessful. Patients with instability and pain preoperatively have lower measures on outcome scores postoperatively. Level of evidence: IV.

24. Griesser MJ, Harris JD, McCoy BW, et al: Complications and re-operations after Bristow-Latarjet shoulder stabilization: A systematic review. *J Shoulder Elbow Surg* 2013;22(2):286-292.

The authors found that shoulder surgery for osseous stabilization using the Bristow-Latarjet technique has a complication rate of 30%. Recurrent anterior dislocation and subluxation rates were 2.9% and 5.8%, respectively.

25. Robinson CM, Seah M, Akhtar MA: The epidemiology, risk of recurrence, and functional outcome after an acute traumatic posterior dislocation of the shoulder. *J Bone Joint Surg Am* 2011;93(17):1605-1613.

This retrospective review of 112 patients with posterior dislocations demonstrates a low risk of repeat dislocation (17%). Patients have persistent deficits in shoulder function within the first two years after injury. Level of evidence: II.

26. Baker CL III, Mascarenhas R, Kline AJ, Chhabra A, Pombo MW, Bradley JP: Arthroscopic treatment of multidirectional shoulder instability in athletes: A retrospective analysis of 2- to 5-year clinical outcomes. *Am J Sports Med* 2009;37(9):1712-1720.

27. Melis B, DeFranco MJ, Chuinard C, Walch G: Natural history of fatty infiltration and atrophy of the supraspinatus muscle in rotator cuff tears. *Clin Orthop Relat Res* 2010;468(6):1498-1505.

Moderate fatty infiltration of the supraspinatus occurs 3 years after the onset of symptoms of rotator cuff dis-

3: Upper Extremity

ease. Severe fatty infiltration appears 5 years after the onset of symptoms. Level of evidence: IV.

28. Melis B, Wall B, Walch G: Natural history of infraspinatus fatty infiltration in rotator cuff tears. *J Shoulder Elbow Surg* 2010;19(5):757-763.

   Moderate fatty infiltration appears 2.5 years after the onset of symptoms. Severe fatty infiltration was seen 4 years after the onset of symptoms. Level of evidence: IV.

29. Kim HM, Dahiya N, Teefey SA, et al: Location and initiation of degenerative rotator cuff tears: An analysis of three hundred and sixty shoulders. *J Bone Joint Surg Am* 2010;92(5):1088-1096.

   In this study, 360 shoulder ultrasounds were evaluated for tear location and initiation. Degenerative rotator cuff tears likely originate in the region 15 to 16 mm posterior to the biceps tendon.

30. Kim HM, Dahiya N, Teefey SA, Keener JD, Galatz LM, Yamaguchi K: Relationship of tear size and location to fatty degeneration of the rotator cuff. *J Bone Joint Surg Am* 2010;92(4):829-839.

   Fatty degeneration of the rotator cuff muscle is closely associated with tear size and location. If the tear extends to the anterior cable just posterior to the biceps tendon, fatty infiltration of the supraspinatus is more likely to be present.

31. Mall NA, Kim HM, Keener JD, et al: Symptomatic progression of asymptomatic rotator cuff tears: A prospective study of clinical and sonographic variables. *J Bone Joint Surg Am* 2010;92(16):2623-2633.

   The development of pain in the presence of a previously asymptomatic rotator cuff tear is associated with an increase in tear size. Larger tears are more likely to increase in size. Level of evidence: III.

32. Bodin J, Ha C, Petit Le Manac'h A, et al: Risk factors for incidence of rotator cuff syndrome in a large working population. *Scand J Work Environ Health* 2012;38(5):436-446.

   This large Scandinavian study evaluated 3,710 workers for the incidence of rotator cuff–related pain in a working population. Age was the strongest predictor for the development of rotator cuff–related symptoms. Working with the arm in an abducted position was the major work-related risk factor for both men and women.

33. Bey MJ, Peltz CD, Ciarelli K, et al: In vivo shoulder function after surgical repair of a torn rotator cuff: Glenohumeral joint mechanics, shoulder strength, clinical outcomes, and their interaction. *Am J Sports Med* 2011;39(10):2117-2129.

   Rotator cuff repair of a supraspinatus tear does not fully restore normal glenohumeral joint mechanics and shoulder strength, even in the setting of a healed repair. Level of evidence: IV.

34. Fucentese SF, von Roll AL, Pfirrmann CW, Gerber C, Jost B: Evolution of nonoperatively treated symptomatic isolated full-thickness supraspinatus tears. *J Bone Joint Surg Am* 2012;94(9):801-808.

   The authors confirmed that the size of small rotator cuff tears usually does not change over a short period. No surgical treatment led to no increase in size of rotator cuff tears over a 3.5-year period.

35. Safran O, Schroeder J, Bloom R, Weil Y, Milgrom C: Natural history of nonoperatively treated symptomatic rotator cuff tears in patients 60 years old or younger. *Am J Sports Med* 2011;39(4):710-714.

   In this study, 51 patients with 61 rotator cuff tears were followed for tear progression by ultrasound. One half of the patients age 60 years or younger had an increase in tear size 2 to 3 years after the index ultrasound. Level of evidence: IV.

36. Kijima H, Minagawa H, Nishi T, Kikuchi K, Shimada Y: Long-term follow-up of cases of rotator cuff tear treated conservatively. *J Shoulder Elbow Surg* 2012;21(4):491-494.

   In this study, 103 rotator cuff tears were treated nonsurgically. At 13 years after the diagnosis, 90% of the patients had no pain or only slight pain, and about 70% had no disturbance in activities of daily living. Younger patients had more significant pain and disorder. Level of evidence: II.

37. Galatz LM, Ball CM, Teefey SA, Middleton WD, Yamaguchi K: The outcome and repair integrity of completely arthroscopically repaired large and massive rotator cuff tears. *J Bone Joint Surg Am* 2004;86(2):219-224.

38. Galatz LM, Griggs S, Cameron BD, Iannotti JP: Prospective longitudinal analysis of postoperative shoulder function: A ten-year follow-up study of full-thickness rotator cuff tears. *J Bone Joint Surg Am* 2001;83(7):1052-1056.

39. Borgmästars N, Paavola M, Remes V, Lohman M, Vastamäki M: Pain relief, motion, and function after rotator cuff repair or reconstruction may not persist after 16 years. *Clin Orthop Relat Res* 2010;468(10):2678-2689.

   In this study, 75 patients were followed an average of 16 years after rotator cuff repair. The early high functional scores did not persist. Range of motion and strength both decreased to less than the preoperative values. However, long-term pain relief occurred in most patients. Level of evidence: IV.

40. Lapner PL, Sabri E, Rakhra K, et al: A multicenter randomized controlled trial comparing single-row with double-row fixation in arthroscopic rotator cuff repair. *J Bone Joint Surg Am* 2012;94(14):1249-1257.

   There were no significant differences in functional or quality-of-life outcomes in comparing single-row and double-row fixation techniques. Smaller initial tear size and double-row fixation were associated with higher healing rates. Level of evidence: I.

41. Aydin N, Kocaoglu B, Guven O: Single-row versus double-row arthroscopic rotator cuff repair in small- to medium-sized tears. *J Shoulder Elbow Surg* 2010;19(5):722-725.

The authors concluded that arthroscopic repair of the rotator cuff using the double-row technique showed no significant differences in clinical outcomes compared with single-row repair. Level of evidence: II.

42. Burks RT, Crim J, Brown N, Fink B, Greis PE: A prospective randomized clinical trial comparing arthroscopic single- and double-row rotator cuff repair: Magnetic resonance imaging and early clinical evaluation. *Am J Sports Med* 2009;37(4):674-682.

43. Charousset C, Grimberg J, Duranthon LD, Bellaiche L, Petrover D: Can a double-row anchorage technique improve tendon healing in arthroscopic rotator cuff repair? A prospective, nonrandomized, comparative study of double-row and single-row anchorage techniques with computed tomographic arthrography tendon healing assessment. *Am J Sports Med* 2007;35(8):1247-1253.

44. Franceschi F, Ruzzini L, Longo UG, et al: Equivalent clinical results of arthroscopic single-row and double-row suture anchor repair for rotator cuff tears: A randomized controlled trial. *Am J Sports Med* 2007;35(8):1254-1260.

45. Grasso A, Milano G, Salvatore M, Falcone G, Deriu L, Fabbriciani C: Single-row versus double-row arthroscopic rotator cuff repair: A prospective randomized clinical study. *Arthroscopy* 2009;25(1):4-12.

46. Koh KH, Kang KC, Lim TK, Shon MS, Yoo JC: Prospective randomized clinical trial of single- versus double-row suture anchor repair in 2- to 4-cm rotator cuff tears: Clinical and magnetic resonance imaging results. *Arthroscopy* 2011;27(4):453-462.

The authors concluded that the clinical results and the retear rates associated with double-row suture anchor repair with an additional medial suture anchor did not differ statistically from those associated with single-row repairs with two lateral suture anchors in patients with medium or large tears of the rotator cuff. Level of evidence: I.

47. Park JY, Lhee SH, Choi JH, Park HK, Yu JW, Seo JB: Comparison of the clinical outcomes of single- and double-row repairs in rotator cuff tears. *Am J Sports Med* 2008;36(7):1310-1316.

48. DeHaan AM, Axelrad TW, Kaye E, Silvestri L, Puskas B, Foster TE: Does double-row rotator cuff repair improve functional outcome of patients compared with single-row technique? A systematic review. *Am J Sports Med* 2012;40(5):1176-1185.

This is a systematic review of level I or II clinical evidence studies that compared single-row and double-row fixation rotator cuff repair. Functional outcome scores did not differ between single-row and double-row repairs. The double-row repairs had a trend toward a lower recurrence rate, although the data did not reach statistical significance.

49. Saridakis P, Jones G: Outcomes of single-row and double-row arthroscopic rotator cuff repair: A systematic review. *J Bone Joint Surg Am* 2010;92(3):732-742.

Single-row and double-row rotator cuff repair groups were compared in this systematic review. Double-row repair appears to offer a benefit in terms of structural healing. However, there is little evidence to support any functional differences between the two techniques in terms of outcome scores; one exception may be patients with tears larger than or equal to 3 cm. There may be some benefits secondary to the structural healing.

50. Genuario JW, Donegan RP, Hamman D, et al: The cost-effectiveness of single-row compared with double-row arthroscopic rotator cuff repair. *J Bone Joint Surg Am* 2012;94(15):1369-1377.

A cost-effectiveness analysis of single-row and double-row rotator cuff repair was performed. A double-row repair was not found to be cost effective.

51. Boughebri O, Roussignol X, Delattre O, Kany J, Valenti P: Small supraspinatus tears repaired by arthroscopy: Are clinical results influenced by the integrity of the cuff after two years? Functional and anatomic results of forty-six consecutive cases. *J Shoulder Elbow Surg* 2012;21(5):699-706.

This case series demonstrated that arthroscopic repair of small supraspinatus tears leads to excellent clinical and anatomic results at a mean 35 months after surgery. Healing occurred in 71.8% of the patients. Failure of healing had no significant effect on the clinical results. Level of evidence: IV.

52. Toussaint B, Schnaser E, Bosley J, Lefebvre Y, Gobezie R: Early structural and functional outcomes for arthroscopic double-row transosseous-equivalent rotator cuff repair. *Am J Sports Med* 2011;39(6):1217-1225.

This study compared rotator cuff repair techniques. A transosseous-equivalent double-row rotator cuff repair yields results that compare favorably with those reported for other double-row techniques. Level of evidence: IV.

53. Tashjian RZ, Hollins AM, Kim HM, et al: Factors affecting healing rates after arthroscopic double-row rotator cuff repair. *Am J Sports Med* 2010;38(12):2435-2442.

In this study, 48 patients (49 shoulders) were followed after arthroscopic double-row repair. The healing rates were 67% in single-tendon tears and 36% in multitendon tears. Age and longer duration of follow-up were correlated with poorer tendon healing. Level of evidence: IV.

54. Kim JR, Cho YS, Ryu KJ, Kim JH: Clinical and radiographic outcomes after arthroscopic repair of massive rotator cuff tears using a suture bridge technique: Assessment of repair integrity on magnetic resonance imaging. *Am J Sports Med* 2012;40(4):786-793.

In this study, 66 patients with massive rotator cuff tears were followed after a repair using a suture bridge technique; 42.4% of the patients had recurrence of the tear. The structural failures had a significant effect on clinical outcomes compared with the healed group. Recurrence of the tear was correlated with fatty infiltration of the infraspinatus and a greater degree of retraction. Level of evidence: III.

3: Upper Extremity

55. Mihata T, Watanabe C, Fukunishi K, et al: Functional and structural outcomes of single-row versus double-row versus combined double-row and suture-bridge repair for rotator cuff tears. *Am J Sports Med* 2011; 39(10):2091-2098.

This study compared single-row repair to two different double-row techniques. The double-row techniques led to a lower incidence of recurrence of the tear. Patients with recurrent tears had inferior functional scores compared with those without recurrence of the tear. Level of evidence: III.

56. Gulotta LV, Nho SJ, Dodson CC, et al: Prospective evaluation of arthroscopic rotator cuff repairs at 5 years: Part I. Functional outcomes and radiographic healing rates. *J Shoulder Elbow Surg* 2011;20(6):934-940.

In this prospective cohort study, 193 patients were followed prospectively in a rotator cuff registry. Fifty-five percent of the patients originally enrolled returned for evaluations at midrange follow-up (2 to 5 years). The results were good, and ultrasound healing rates appeared to increase with time. Level of evidence: II.

57. Kluger R, Bock P, Mittlböck M, Krampla W, Engel A: Long-term survivorship of rotator cuff repairs using ultrasound and magnetic resonance imaging analysis. *Am J Sports Med* 2011;39(10):2071-2081.

Long-term survivorship of rotator cuff repair was evaluated by MRI and ultrasound. The majority of recurrent tears occurred in the first 3 months after repair. Level of evidence: III.

58. Miller BS, Downie BK, Kohen RB, et al: When do rotator cuff repairs fail? Serial ultrasound examination after arthroscopic repair of large and massive rotator cuff tears. *Am J Sports Med* 2011;39(10):2064-2070.

In this study, 22 patients with tears larger than 3 cm underwent arthroscopic repair and were followed sequentially after surgery; 41% had recurrent tears. The majority of the recurrent tears occurred within 3 months after surgery. No recurrent tears occurred after 6 months. Level of evidence: III.

59. Lafosse L, Brozska R, Toussaint B, Gobezie R: The outcome and structural integrity of arthroscopic rotator cuff repair with use of the double-row suture anchor technique. *J Bone Joint Surg Am* 2007;89(7):1533-1541.

60. Boileau P, Brassart N, Watkinson DJ, Carles M, Hatzidakis AM, Krishnan SG: Arthroscopic repair of full-thickness tears of the supraspinatus: Does the tendon really heal? *J Bone Joint Surg Am* 2005;87(6):1229-1240.

61. Galatz LM, Sandell LJ, Rothermich SY, et al: Characteristics of the rat supraspinatus tendon during tendon-to-bone healing after acute injury. *J Orthop Res* 2006; 24(3):541-550.

62. Iannotti JP, Codsi MJ, Kwon YW, Derwin K, Ciccone J, Brems JJ: Porcine small intestine submucosa augmentation of surgical repair of chronic two-tendon rotator cuff tears: A randomized, controlled trial. *J Bone Joint Surg Am* 2006;88(6):1238-1244.

63. Barber FA, Burns JP, Deutsch A, Labbé MR, Litchfield RB: A prospective, randomized evaluation of acellular human dermal matrix augmentation for arthroscopic rotator cuff repair. *Arthroscopy* 2012;28(1):8-15.

Forty-two patients were followed in a prospective randomized study evaluating the efficacy of a cellular human dermal matrix augmentation of large rotator cuff tears. The augmented repairs showed better ASES and Constant scores and had a greater healing rate as evaluated by MRI. Level of evidence: II.

64. Gupta AK, Hug K, Berkoff DJ, et al: Dermal tissue allograft for the repair of massive irreparable rotator cuff tears. *Am J Sports Med* 2012;40(1):141-147.

A prospective observational study of 24 patients was performed. The patients had an interposition repair of a massive rotator cuff tear using human dermal allograft. The patients demonstrated a significant improvement in pain, range of motion, and strength. Subjective outcome scores also improved. There was no comparison group in this study. Level of evidence: IV.

65. Encalada-Diaz I, Cole BJ, Macgillivray JD, et al: Rotator cuff repair augmentation using a novel polycarbonate polyurethane patch: Preliminary results at 12 months' follow-up. *J Shoulder Elbow Surg* 2011;20(5): 788-794.

In this study, 10 patients with supraspinatus tears underwent an open rotator cuff repair augmented with a polycarbonate polyurethane patch. The patch was well tolerated, and no major complications were noted. There was a 10% tear recurrence rate at the 12-month point. Level of evidence: IV.

66. Castricini R, Longo UG, De Benedetto M, et al: Platelet-rich plasma augmentation for arthroscopic rotator cuff repair: A randomized controlled trial. *Am J Sports Med* 2011;39(2):258-265.

This is a prospective randomized study evaluating augmentation of rotator cuff repair with autologous PRFM. There were no statistically significant differences in the Constant score or in MRI tendon scores. This study does not support the use of autologous PRFM for augmentation of a double-row repair. Level of evidence: I.

67. Rodeo SA, Delos D, Williams RJ, Adler RS, Pearle A, Warren RF: The effect of platelet-rich fibrin matrix on rotator cuff tendon healing: A prospective, randomized clinical study. *Am J Sports Med* 2012;40(6):1234-1241.

This is a prospective randomized clinical study evaluating 69 patients who underwent rotator cuff repair. The experimental group received PRFM at the repair site. The repairs augmented with PRFM had no demonstrable improvement in healing, vascularity, strength, or clinical rating scales. In fact, regression analysis suggested that PRFM may have a negative effect on healing. Level of evidence: II.

68. Weber SC, Kauffman JI, Parise C, Weber SJ, Katz SD: Platelet-rich fibrin matrix in the management of arthroscopic repair of the rotator cuff: A prospective, randomized, double-blind study. *Am J Sports Med* 2013;4(2): 263-270.

Sixty consecutive rotator cuff repairs were randomized to receive or not receive platelet-rich fibrin matrix during surgery. There was no difference in outcome scores or healing between the groups.

69. Barber FA, Hrnack SA, Snyder SJ, Hapa O: Rotator cuff repair healing influenced by platelet-rich plasma construct augmentation. *Arthroscopy* 2011;27(8):1029-1035.

This study evaluated the use of PRFM in rotator cuff repair in a case-control study. PRFM appeared to lower tear recurrence rates in this study. There were no clinical differences between the two groups. Level of evidence: III.

70. Randelli P, Arrigoni P, Ragone V, Aliprandi A, Cabitza P: Platelet rich plasma in arthroscopic rotator cuff repair: A prospective RCT study, 2-year follow-up. *J Shoulder Elbow Surg* 2011;20(4):518-528.

This prospective, randomized controlled trial evaluated the use of platelet-rich plasma in patients undergoing arthroscopic rotator cuff repair. The only major difference was reduced pain in the first postoperative month. There were no significant differences in healing. There were no statistically significant differences in functional outcome scores. Level of evidence: I.

Video Reference

27.1: Case JM, Mannava S, Cheetham SG, Long B, Stubbs AJ: Video. *Physical Examination of the Shoulder.* Available at http://orthoportal.aaos.org/emedia/singleVideoPlayer.aspx?resource=EMEDIA_OSVL_12_27. Accessed January 15, 2014.

3: Upper Extremity

Chapter 28

Shoulder and Elbow Disorders in the Athlete

Christopher S. Ahmad, MD   William N. Levine, MD

The Shoulder

The shoulder (specifically the labrum and the rotator cuff) is at great risk for injury given the tremendous forces placed on it during the throwing motion. Although an isolated event can cause injury, it is more common for overhead athletes to sustain injury following repetitive microtrauma during years of throwing.

The throwing motion has been classified into five stages: wind-up, early cocking, late cocking, acceleration, and deceleration with follow-through (Figure 1). An understanding of the arm position and progression through this cycle can help predict where injury may occur in the throwing shoulder. For example, in early to late cocking, the shoulder is placed in maximal abduction and external rotation, which places the capsule and posterosuperior rotator cuff at risk for injury. This hyperexternal rotation position is necessary, however, to develop the forces necessary for the internal rotators to generate velocity in the acceleration phase. The arm develops speeds of nearly 7,000° per second during the throwing motion. These forces are dissipated through the bony and soft-tissue structures of the shoulder, putting them at risk for injury throughout the throwing motion.

The shoulder range of motion necessary to generate these forces while also keeping the humeral head centered on the glenoid is afforded by the synchrony of the static and dynamic stabilizers of the shoulder. The static stabilizers include the glenohumeral ligaments and the capsule. The dynamic stabilizers include the rotator cuff, the biceps tendon, and the scapular stabilizers. The generalized ligamentous laxity afforded by the capsule and the ligaments allows the necessary range of motion for the humeral head to move in the glenohu-

meral joint to develop the velocity and forces necessary for effective throwing. Repetitive overuse/microtrauma can lead to breakdown of any of the static stabilizers, the dynamic stabilizers, or the scapular stabilizers (latissimus dorsi, rhomboids, or serratus anterior muscles).

Adaptive Changes in the Throwing Shoulder

In a study of asymptomatic college baseball players, the authors determined that bony adaptive changes are present in humeral anatomy to account for the increased external rotation and decreased internal rotation commonly found in overhead athletes;[1] in a study of 298 Amateur Athletic Union baseball players, the authors thought that soft-tissue adaptive changes in the capsule accounted for similar findings.[2] Regardless of the etiology, adaptive changes in the developing shoulder allow increased external rotation and therefore increased efficiency of the throwing motion over time. These adaptive changes also are at play in the development of pathology.

Shoulder Instability

Shoulder instability occurs when the humerus subluxates or dislocates in relation to the glenoid. This type of instability is less common in the throwing athlete, who instead will report pain, weakness, or neurologic symptoms ("dead arm" syndrome).[3]

The etiology of shoulder instability in the throwing athlete remains controversial. Repetitive microtrauma has been suggested as a cause leading to stretching of the anterior capsule, allowing increased translation of the humeral head on the glenoid. Another proposed etiology is contraction of the posterior capsule (as demonstrated on physical examination with decreased internal rotation) that leads to increased anterior translation and potential pathologic changes (anterior labral tears, superior labrum anterior to posterior [SLAP] tears). Although the exact etiology remains undetermined, the physical examination can help to delineate the treatable conditions in the symptomatic throwing shoulder. Posterior capsular contracture should be identified and addressed with a proper rehabilitation program (sleeper's stretch, for example). Increased anterior translation (symptomatic) can be treated with a rehabilitation pro-

Dr. Ahmad or an immediate family member serves as a paid consultant to or is an employee of Acumed and Arthrex and has received research or institutional support from Arthrex, Major League Baseball, and Stryker. Dr. Levine or an immediate family member has received research or institutional support from Stryker and serves as a board member, owner, officer, or committee member of the American Orthopaedic Association.

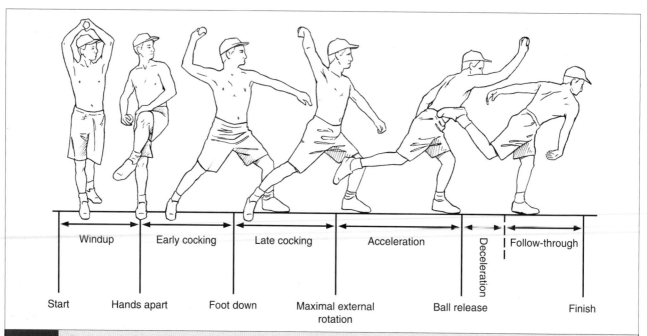

Figure 1 Schematic of the stages of the throwing motion. (Reproduced from Bernstein J, Pepe M, Kaplan L: Shoulder and elbow disorders in the athlete, in Flynn JM, ed: *Orthopaedic Knowledge Update 10*. Rosemont, IL, American Academy of Orthopaedic Surgeons, 2011, pp 315-324.)

gram designed to stabilize the rotator cuff and the periscapular muscles. Because of the complex and intricate anatomic relationships of the soft tissues of the glenohumeral joint, surgery is reserved for the recalcitrant, painful shoulder that does not respond to a well-supervised and patient-compliant rehabilitation program. Surgery is directed toward the pathology. If an anterior labral tear or other soft-tissue injury has occurred, then primary repair will be performed; however, the results are not always predictably good, so athletes need to be counseled. Posterior capsular contractures are almost always treated nonsurgically and only on rare occasions will surgical release be required.

Superior Labrum/Biceps Tendon

Because of its direct connection to the superior labrum, the long head of the biceps tendon also may play a role in stabilizing the glenohumeral joint. During the late cocking phase, the long head of the biceps tendon contributes to the torsional stability of the humerus. After sectioning of the long head of the biceps tendon, the anteroinferior structures demonstrate more strain.[4] Loading of the biceps tendon also demonstrates decreased anteroposterior translation of the humerus.[5] Therefore, it is clear that the long head of the biceps tendon also plays a role in anterior stability.

SLAP tears have been classified into many types,[6-8] but the critical aspect for clinicians is to determine whether the superior labral-biceps anchor is unstable or if the tear extends into the biceps tendon (Figure 2). Furthermore, defining a SLAP tear can be challenging,

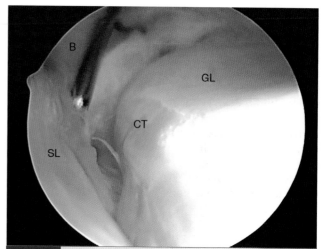

Figure 2 Arthroscopic view of a right shoulder type II SLAP tear in a 22-year-old right-handed male pitcher. The probe is pulling the superior labral tear away from the glenoid. GL = glenoid; B = biceps; SL = superior labrum; CT = cartilage thinning (from repetitive trauma). (Courtesy of the Columbia University Center for Shoulder, Elbow, and Sports Medicine, New York, NY.)

even for experienced shoulder and sports medicine surgeons reviewing arthroscopic videos at different time points.[9]

Despite technologic advances, return to play following SLAP repair is not predictable, with a high percentage of professionals unable to return to their prior level.[10] Nonsurgical management involving rotator cuff

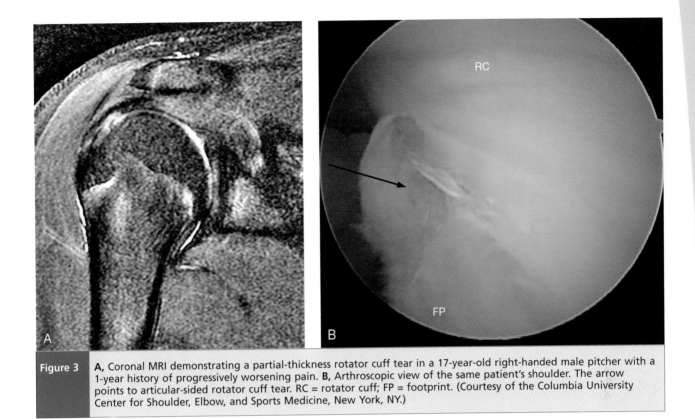

Figure 3 **A,** Coronal MRI demonstrating a partial-thickness rotator cuff tear in a 17-year-old right-handed male pitcher with a 1-year history of progressively worsening pain. **B,** Arthroscopic view of the same patient's shoulder. The arrow points to articular-sided rotator cuff tear. RC = rotator cuff; FP = footprint. (Courtesy of the Columbia University Center for Shoulder, Elbow, and Sports Medicine, New York, NY.)

and periscapular rehabilitation can lead to successful outcomes in a similar percentage of athletes (approximately 66%).[11] Biceps tenodesis has been suggested as an alternative to SLAP repair in a recent study, although the patients included were an older cohort so this finding remains controversial at this time.[12]

Rotator Cuff/Internal Impingement

Unlike internal impingement of the rotator cuff, impingement syndrome (external impingement) typically occurs from subacromial spurring and is associated with bursitis. Internal impingement occurs during the extreme throwing motion (abduction, external rotation, and extension) between the rotator cuff (posterior supraspinatus, anterior infraspinatus) and the postero-superior glenoid/labrum. The net result of this contact if it becomes pathologic is the development of articular-sided rotator cuff tears and SLAP tears (Figure 3). Some think that these tears are adaptive in nature and necessary for elite throwers to have the rotation necessary to generate the force and velocity for effective throwing.

The diagnosis of internal impingement can be made with a physical examination. The apprehension test (shoulder abduction, external rotation, and especially extension) will cause pain as opposed to the true sense of instability found in patients with instability. This pain will diminish when the test is repeated with only abduction and external rotation (elimination of extension by bringing the arm in front of the plane of the body). These patients also typically have loss of internal rotation compared with their dominant side. Gleno-

humeral internal rotation deficit (GIRD) is defined as a loss of 20° or more of internal rotation of the throwing shoulder compared with the nonthrowing shoulder.[13-15] Studies have shown that although bony adaptive changes (as mentioned previously) play a substantial role in the change in the external rotation/internal rotation arc, there are soft-tissue changes that account for GIRD. Stretching programs have been found to be successful in the nonsurgical management of GIRD.[16,17]

Management of the shoulders of athletes with GIRD is challenging. All reasonable nonsurgical options should be used, including activity modification, anti-inflammatory medications, corticosteroid injections, evaluation of the pitching motion for poor form and mechanics, a period of cessation from throwing, and a supervised stretching program dedicated to stretch the posterior capsule. Surgical intervention should be reserved only for the recalcitrant athlete, who should receive counseling about the unpredictable outcomes of surgery in this patient cohort (mini-open rotator cuff repair, arthroscopic repair, or arthroscopic débridement).[18-20]

Acromioclavicular Joint

The acromioclavicular (AC) joint is a diarthrodial joint composed of the lateral clavicle, the medial acromion, and the stabilizing ligaments (AC joint capsule and the more medial coracoclavicular ligaments: conoid and trapezoid). AC joint separations occur from trauma and are not typically found in overhead athletes. Instead, the AC joint is prone to injury from repetitive stress and highly prone to the development of degener-

3: Upper Extremity

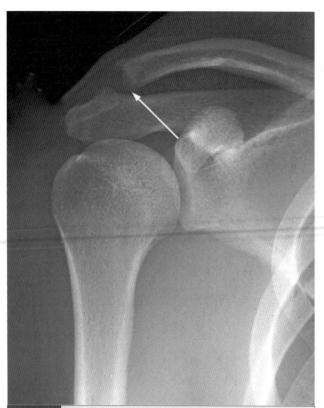

Figure 4 AP radiograph showing distal clavicle osteolysis in a 25-year-old man who plays minor league baseball. Note the relative joint space widening and the erosion of the superior clavicle. (Courtesy of the Columbia University Center for Shoulder, Elbow and Sports Medicine, New York, NY.)

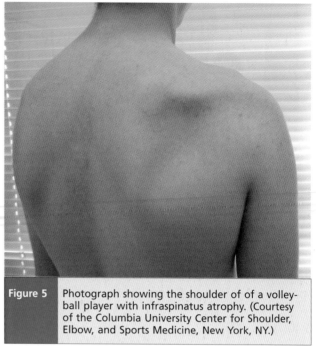

Figure 5 Photograph showing the shoulder of of a volleyball player with infraspinatus atrophy. (Courtesy of the Columbia University Center for Shoulder, Elbow, and Sports Medicine, New York, NY.)

ative changes.[21] In addition, osteolysis of the distal clavicle (weightlifter's shoulder) occurs, which likewise can lead to pain in the anterosuperior shoulder.

Physical examination will demonstrate pain directly over the AC joint, pain with cross-body adduction (pain must still occur over the AC joint, however), pain with extension and internal rotation (reaching for bra or back pocket), and a positive active-compression test (superficial pain registered by the patient with resisted forward elevation while the arm is in 90° of forward flexion, 10° to 15° of adduction, and maximal internal rotation (thumbs down).

Radiographs will typically show widening of the AC joint with erosions of the distal clavicle and are pathognomonic for osteolysis (also referred to as weightlifter's shoulder; Figure 4).

Treatment of the symptomatic AC joint typically involves NSAIDs, rest, rotator cuff strengthening, and occasionally a corticosteroid injection directly into the AC joint. Ultrasound-assisted injections may increase the efficacy of the injection, but no long-term studies currently exist to support routine use. If nonsurgical management of the symptomatic AC joint fails, either arthroscopic or open AC joint débridement is recommended.

Suprascapular Nerve

Suprascapular neuropathy should be suspected in young throwing athletes or those involved in sports such as volleyball, baseball, tennis, and swimming. The suprascapular nerve can be compressed in the thrower's shoulder in two clinical scenarios in these athletes. The first is in conjunction with a SLAP tear and an associated paralabral cyst that can compress the suprascapular nerve. The second, rarer situation is compression of the suprascapular nerve secondary to infraspinatus hypertrophy that develops in volleyball players.

The history is important in these athletes because they will typically describe a characteristic dull pain, 3 to 4 cm medial to the posterolateral corner of the acromion, that can be exacerbated by throwing. In addition, they may report weakness, decreased control, and decreased performance. A physical examination can detect subtle atrophy in the supraspinous and/or infraspinous fossae (Figure 5). Determining the location of the atrophy will help guide the clinician regarding the source of the compression. If the supraspinatus and infraspinatus are involved, then the compression is more proximal at the suprascapular notch. If only the infraspinatus is involved, however, then the compression is more distal at the spinoglenoid notch.

MRI should be performed to evaluate for labral tears and associated paralabral cysts. Most athletes with suprascapular neuropathy can be managed nonsurgically. A large, compressing paralabral cyst can be aspirated with or without ultrasound guidance, which may eliminate the symptoms. When symptoms persist despite appropriate nonsurgical management, arthroscopic SLAP repair and cyst decompression are recommended. Because of the advances made in shoulder arthroscopy, open cyst excision is rarely necessary.

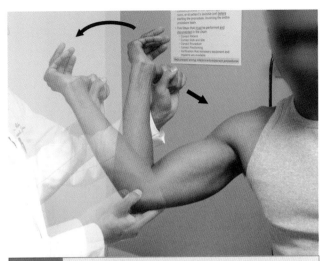

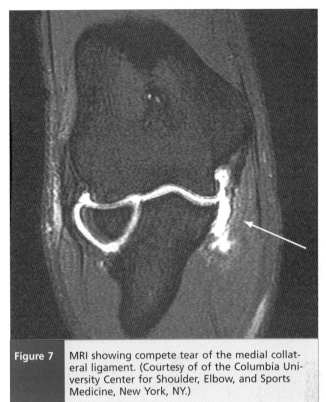

Figure 6 The moving valgus stress test. The arrows indicate the valgus stress applied to the elbow while moving the elbow from flexion to extension. (Reproduced from Ahmad CS: Elbow throwing injuries and the throwing athlete, in Galatz LM, ed: *Orthopaedic Knowledge Update: Shoulder and Elbow*, ed 3, Rosemont, IL, American Academy of Orthopaedic Surgeons, 2008, pp 451-460.)

Figure 7 MRI showing compete tear of the medial collateral ligament. (Courtesy of of the Columbia University Center for Shoulder, Elbow, and Sports Medicine, New York, NY.)

The Elbow

Medial Collateral Ligament Injuries

Overhead athletes (most commonly baseball pitchers) subject the elbow to tremendous repetitive valgus forces that can cause a medial collateral ligament (MCL) injury. The valgus torque in the elbow is highest during the acceleration phase of throwing. The MCL complex consists of three ligaments. The anterior oblique is the strongest and the primary stabilizer to valgus stress.[22,23] It is functionally composed of anterior and posterior bands that provide a reciprocal function in resisting valgus stress through the range of elbow flexion-extension motion.[23,24] The anterior band is taut in extension, and the posterior band is tight in flexion. The flexor carpi ulnaris is a primary dynamic contributor to valgus stability, and the flexor digitorum superficialis is a secondary stabilizer.[25] The olecranon also acts as an elbow valgus stress stabilizer, and aggressive olecranon resection puts the MCL at risk for injury. The throwing motion is considered a process involving a kinetic chain of elements that functions to optimize the efficiency of proximal segments and decrease force loads seen at smaller, distal segments such as the elbow. Weakness, imbalance, or stiffness within the kinetic chain can cause a risk of elbow injury. For example, significant GIRD of the shoulder has been observed in players sustaining MCL injuries.

Patients with MCL injuries experience medial elbow pain that occurs during the acceleration phase of throwing. Symptoms often are insidious in onset and felt with throwing greater than 50% to 75% of maximal effort and result in decreased velocity and throwing accuracy. Acute injuries may present suddenly with

a pop, sharp pain, and an inability to continue throwing. Physical examination demonstrates tenderness with direct palpation of the ligament. The moving valgus stress test is the most useful physical examination maneuver specific for MCL injury and is performed with valgus stress applied to the elbow while the arm is moved through an arc of flexion and extension (Figure 6). The subjective feeling of apprehension, instability, or pain localized to the MCL at a flexion arc of 70° to 120° indicates an MCL injury. Valgus stress radiographs may be used to measure the medial joint line opening, and an opening greater than 3 mm has been considered diagnostic of valgus instability.[26,27] Baseline mild increased valgus elbow laxity has been observed in uninjured, asymptomatic dominant elbows of professional baseball pitchers.[28] Conventional MRI is capable of identifying thickening within the ligament from chronic injury or more obvious full-thickness tears (Figure 7). Magnetic resonance arthrography improves the diagnosis of partial undersurface tears.[29] Dynamic ultrasonography is capable of detecting increased laxity with valgus stress.[30] Although no accepted classification has been established, tears are often considered full thickness or partial thickness. It should be noted that many asymptomatic pitchers will have abnormal features on MRI and radiographs; therefore, imaging serves to assist in the diagnosis of symptomatic valgus insufficiency.

Nonsurgical treatment includes a period of rest from throwing, flexor-pronator strengthening, optimizing throwing mechanics, emphasis on correcting muscle imbalances or weakness in the entire kinetic chain,

3: Upper Extremity

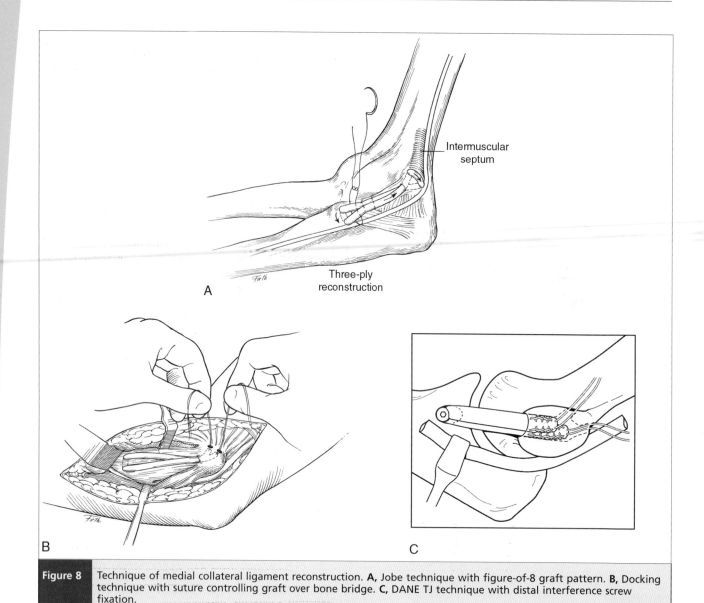

Intermuscular
septum

Three-ply
reconstruction

A

B

C

Figure 8 Technique of medial collateral ligament reconstruction. **A,** Jobe technique with figure-of-8 graft pattern. **B,** Docking technique with suture controlling graft over bone bridge. **C,** DANE TJ technique with distal interference screw fixation.

shoulder glenohumeral internal rotation restoration followed by a progressive throwing program, or even changing position to decrease throwing demands. Platelet-rich plasma is currently being investigated as a method to enhance the healing of the MCL without surgery, but there is no evidence to indicate that it is ready for widespread use.

Indications for surgery include a failure of nonsurgical treatment and patient willingness to comply with the necessary rehabilitation. Direct surgical repair is an option in some cases and most favorable with ligament-type avulsion injuries in young athletes in whom chronic changes in the entire ligament have not developed and who may have a less predictable future in baseball. Most commonly, however, surgery consists of MCL reconstruction. Several surgical techniques currently used for MCL reconstruction include the modified Jobe technique, the docking technique, and the hybrid interference screw technique (Figure 8). Most

current techniques use a muscle-splitting approach through the flexor-pronator mass to expose the injured MCL. Converging tunnels are made both on the ulna (at the sublime tubercle) and on the humeral epicondyle.[27] A palmaris longus graft is weaved through the tunnels in a figure-of-8 fashion, tensioned, and sutured to the adjacent periosteum or native ligament for fixation. Ipsilateral gracilis can also be used in the case of a small or absent palmaris.

The docking technique is a modification of the Jobe technique that simplifies graft passage, tensioning, and fixation.[31] The ulnar tunnels are created similar to the Jobe technique at the sublime tubercle. The inferior humeral tunnel is connected to two small exit tunnels. The graft is then passed through the ulnar tunnel and then the graft length is adjusted so both graft limbs, each with a whipstitched suture at the end, may be tensioned into the humeral tunnel. The sutures are then tied over the bony bridge on the humeral epicondyle

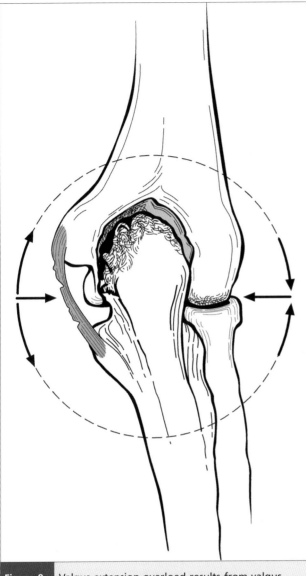

Figure 9   Valgus extension overload results from valgus torque resisted by the medial ulnar collateral ligament and shear forces developed in the posteromedial ulnohumeral joint.

for fixation. A hybrid technique achieves ulnar-sided fixation in a single bone tunnel with an interference screw and humeral fixation using the docking technique.[26] This technique is less technically demanding because the required number of drill holes is reduced. Less dissection through a muscle-splitting approach is afforded because only a single central tunnel is required rather than two tunnels with an intervening bony bridge on the ulna. With a single tunnel, the posterior ulnar tunnel closest to the ulnar nerve is avoided. Finally, graft passage is less difficult with an interference screw in a single tunnel. At this time, however, there are no long-term studies demonstrating the efficacy of this modification.

Complications include ulnar nerve injury, medial antebrachial cutaneous nerve injury, ulnar or epicondylar

fracture, stiffness, and failure to achieve the preinjury level of throwing. A recent systematic review of published reports of ulnar collateral ligament reconstruction in overhead athletes revealed that 83% of patients had an excellent result.[32] There was an overall complication rate of 10%; postoperative ulnar neuropathy was the most common complication.

Valgus Extension Overload

Valgus torque, combined with deceleration, produces high compression and shear forces acting on the posterior medial olecranon and the posterior medial trochlea (Figure 9). The pathologic consequences to shear and compression are chondral erosion and osteophyte formation localized to the posteromedial tip of the olecranon and the trochlea. The pathology of posteromedial elbow impingement is one of the most common diagnoses (occurring in 78% of injured athletes requiring surgery [baseball players and other overhead athletes, for example]).[33,34]

The pathomechanics of posteromedial impingement have been studied in cadaver models. MCL laxity causes altered contact forces medially between the trochlea and the olecranon with simulated valgus forces.[35] These data suggest that patients with symptomatic valgus extension overload and posterior medial impingement may have underlying valgus instability, even though MCL pain may not be the presenting symptom.

Symptoms related to posteromedial impingement include a decrease in throwing velocity and accuracy and difficulty warming up. Sensations of locking or catching suggest loose bodies or a chondral injury. For isolated posteromedial impingement, elbow pain is localized to the posteromedial aspect of the olecranon and usually occurs just after ball release during the deceleration phase of throwing as the elbow approaches full extension. Posterior osteophytes may limit full elbow extension. Patients often will have had a history of MCL injury. Pain during the acceleration phase of throwing may indicate a combined MCL injury.

Local tenderness over the posteromedial olecranon is elicited. The extension impingement test is performed by the examiner forcing the relaxed patient's flexed elbow into terminal extension. Reproduction of posterior or posteromedial pain similar to the pain felt while throwing is considered positive. Simultaneous valgus load during the maneuver often increases the pain, whereas varus stress diminishes the pain. The MCL must be evaluated in all throwers presenting with medial elbow pain using direct palpation and the moving valgus stress test.[36]

AP, lateral, oblique, and axillary views of the elbow may reveal posteromedial olecranon osteophytes and/or loose bodies (Figure 10). Several views have been described to better visualize the posterior compartment, but CT scans with three-dimensional reconstructions currently are the gold standard. Three-dimensional surface renderings can demonstrate the overall morphologic changes, loose bodies, and osteophyte fragmenta-

3: Upper Extremity

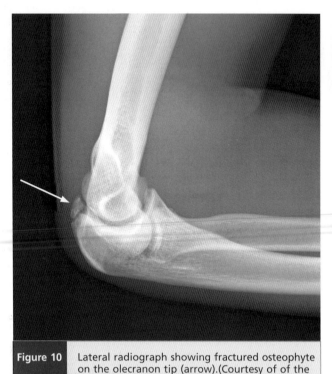

Figure 10 Lateral radiograph showing fractured osteophyte on the olecranon tip (arrow).(Courtesy of of the Columbia University Center for Shoulder, Elbow, and Sports Medicine, New York, NY.)

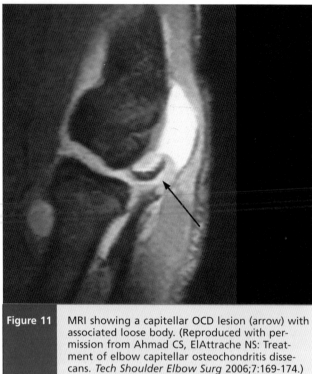

Figure 11 MRI showing a capitellar OCD lesion (arrow) with associated loose body. (Reproduced with permission from Ahmad CS, ElAttrache NS: Treatment of elbow capitellar osteochondritis dissecans. *Tech Shoulder Elbow Surg* 2006;7:169-174.)

tion. Sometimes a fractured osteophyte is observed, particularly in a symptomatic patient. MRI is also informative, especially if MCL pathology is suspected.

An initial course of nonsurgical treatment consists of activity modification with a period of rest from throwing, intra-articular cortisone injections, and NSAIDs. Pitching mechanics should be evaluated and instruction instituted to correct flaws in technique that may be contributing to the injury. After a period of rest, a progressive throwing program is instituted under the supervision of experienced therapists and trainers. Surgical treatment is indicated for those patients who have persistent symptoms despite nonsurgical management and wish to return to the same level of competition. In a report of professional baseball players who underwent olecranon débridement, 25% developed valgus instability and eventually required MCL reconstruction.[33] Subsequent basic science studies have demonstrated that excessive olecranon resection increases the demands on the MCL during valgus stress and increases valgus instability.[35,37] Basic science and clinical experience therefore indicate that MCL insufficiency can develop following posteromedial decompression. Current recommendations, therefore, are to limit olecranon resection to osteophytes only and avoid removal of the normal olecranon. It has also been demonstrated that existing MCL insufficiency created in cadavers causes contact alterations in the posteromedial compartment that may be the cause of symptomatic chondrosis and osteophyte formation, which eventually manifests as valgus extension overload.[25] In addition, osteophyte formation may contribute to elbow stability in the setting of MCL injury; therefore, removal of the bony im-

pingement may convert an asymptomatic MCL into a painful valgus instability.

Capitellar Osteochondritis Dissecans

The combination of abnormal radiocapitellar compressive forces and limited vascularity of the capitellum supplied by end arteries are responsible for the development of osteochondritis dissecans (OCD).[38] Repetitive compressive forces are generated by either large valgus stresses on the elbow during throwing or racket swinging or from constant axial compressive loads on the elbow, such as those endured by gymnasts. The capitellum is supplied by two end arteries coursing from posterior to anterior that are branches of the radial recurrent and interosseous recurrent arteries.[39]

Patients with symptomatic OCD experience lateral elbow pain, stiffness, and mechanical symptoms of locking or catching by unstable cartilage or intra-articular loose bodies. Physical examination demonstrates tenderness over the radiocapitellar joint, and loss of range of motion with a 15° to 20° flexion contracture is common. Radiographs may be negative early in the disease process, but as the condition progresses, flattening, sclerosis, and lucencies of the capitellum will become apparent. In suspected cases of OCD, an MRI should be obtained to determine the location, size, and stability of a possible OCD lesion (Figure 11).

The management of OCD lesions is based primarily on the demands of the patient; the size, location, and stability of the overlying cartilage; and the status of the capitellar growth plate.[40,41] Several classification systems based on radiographic[42] and arthroscopic[40] findings have been proposed, but none has been universally adopted. A useful classification includes three stages. In stage 1, the osteochondral fragment is intact, stable, and nondisplaced. Treatment is nonsurgical and includes elbow rest. In stage 2, the osteochondral fragment is partially separated and documented both radiographically and arthroscopically. Treatment is surgical; for smaller lesions, arthroscopic débridement is performed. Fragment fixation has been advocated by some for this stage, although the healing potential of fixed fragments and the clinical results of the procedure are often unpredictable.[42,43] Extension of the lesion into the lateral margin of the capitellum is associated with a potentially poorer prognosis. The lateral column of the capitellum supports large compressive forces when the elbow is stressed in valgus or with axial loading. Lesions that do not involve a substantial portion of the lateral buttress of the capitellum and do not engage the radial head are treated with microfracture or drilling. With lateral column involvement of more than approximately 6 to 7 mm, the absence of a lateral buttress allows engagement of the radial head in the defect that inhibits healing and may lead to accelerated radiocapitellar arthrosis. Osteochondral restoration by means of osteochondral autograft is beneficial in this setting.

In stage 3, the fragment is fully displaced and has become a loose body; débridement, drilling, or osteochondral replacement is indicated. If the loose osteochondral piece is shown to be acutely displaced in a patient with previously documented OCD, reduction and fixation is an option. The results of fixation, however, are inconsistent. The treatment guidelines are similar to those of stage 2 lesions.

Longitudinal studies have documented that 50% of patients with radiocapitellar OCD will eventually develop osteoarthritis.[44] Newer techniques, including osteochondral grafting (mosaicplasty), may change the long-term degenerative process. Return to sports following treatment of capitellar OCD has varied.

Radiocapitellar Plica

Posterolateral elbow impingement can be caused by a thickened radiocapitellar plica.[45,46] The plica can cause chondral erosion on the radial head and capitellum.[45] Symptoms include painful clicking or catching, and effusions.[45] Pain can be reproduced with the plica impingement test performed with a valgus load on the elbow and passive flexion with the forearm in pronation. A painful snap is indicative of a positive test. A posterior plica can be examined by the extension-supination maneuver, bringing the elbow to full extension while applying a valgus stress with the forearm in supination.[45] Arthroscopic excision of the plica has high success rates.[46]

Lateral Epicondylitis

Lateral epicondylitis is the most common elbow disorder in patients seeking medical attention, affects 50% of all recreational tennis players, and is the most common elbow injury in golfers. Risk factors for tennis players include heavy racquets, inappropriate grip size, high string tension, and poor technique. The disorder most often occurs in the fourth decade of life. The extensor carpi radialis brevis (ECRB) is the most commonly involved tendon, but the extensor digitorum communis, the extensor radialis longus, and the extensor carpi ulnaris also may be involved. Microtrauma from repetitive activity results in characteristic pathology of histopathologic angiofibroblastic hyperplasia.[47,48]

Patients report pain just below the lateral epicondyle and demonstrate tenderness over the ECRB insertion. Pain is reproduced with maximum passive wrist flexion, gripping, resisted long finger extension, and resisted wrist extension while the elbow is fully extended. Grip strength is often decreased compared with the unaffected side. Radial nerve entrapment can present concomitantly in up to 5% of patients with lateral epicondylitis. Radiographs are typically normal, but calcium deposits in the tendon are occasionally seen, especially if prior treatment included cortisone injections. MRI may show increased signal and degeneration at the tendon origin but is not necessary for the diagnosis.

Nonsurgical treatment is always attempted and includes rest, NSAIDs, counterforce bracing, physical therapy, swing or activity modifications, and cortisone injections. Physical therapy focuses on extensor stretching and strengthening. Counterforce bracing is believed to limit muscle fatigue and redistribute force into the muscle belly rather than the tendon origin. Platelet-rich plasma injections, although controversial, show promise as a possible therapeutic modality for lateral epicondylitis.[49]

Indications for surgery include pain that interferes with daily activities and occupation and the failure of nonsurgical treatment of up to 6 months. Contraindications include inadequate nonsurgical treatment, inability to comply with rehabilitation, active infection, or severe ankylosis of the elbow. Open ECRB release, débridement, and repair remain reliable options. More recently, arthroscopic débridement of the ECRB has been advocated. Success rates with surgery are as high as 85%. The complications of surgery include iatrogenic lateral ulnar collateral ligament injury, which leads to pain and posterolateral rotatory instability. Iatrogenic posterior interosseous nerve and median nerve injuries have been reported with arthroscopic release.[50]

Medial Epicondylitis

Medial epicondylitis occurs much less frequently than lateral epicondylitis. The dominant extremity is involved 75% of the time and the condition is caused by repetitive wrist flexion or forearm pronation activities. It is common in golfers, baseball pitchers, racquet sports, football, weightlifting, and occupations such as carpentry and plumbing.[51] The pronator teres and the flexor carpi radialis are most affected. Patients report pain localized to the medial epicondyle that is increased by resisted forearm pronation or wrist flexion activities. Physical examination demonstrates tenderness at the tendon origin on the medial epicondyle. Pain is reproduced with resisted forearm pronation and wrist

3: Upper Extremity

flexion. A flexion contracture may be present. Radiographs are normal but occasionally show calcium deposits in the tendon. MRI may show increased signal and degeneration at the tendon origin. Nonsurgical treatment includes rest, ice, NSAIDs, ultrasound, counterforce bracing, and corticosteroid injections followed by guided rehabilitation and return to sport. Throwing and swing modification and racquet/equipment modifications also should be considered. Indications for surgery include pain that limits function and interferes with daily activities and occupation in the setting of failure of nonsurgical treatment of 6 months. The open surgical technique involves excision of the pathologic portion of the tendon, enhancement of the vascular environment, and reattachment of the origin of the flexor-pronator muscle group. The success rates with surgery are 80% to 95%, although objective strength deficits may persist.

Distal Biceps Tendon Ruptures

Biceps tendon ruptures are most common in the dominant elbow of physically active middle-aged men,[52] and the risk is greater in those who smoke or are on anabolic steroids.[53] The mechanism of injury involves a flexed elbow subjected to a rapid, unexpected eccentric load during attempted biceps contraction. Degenerative tendinopathy from decreased vascularity or tendon impingement may predispose to rupture.[54]

Patients often feel a pop and pain localized to the anterior elbow, with subsequent swelling and ecchymosis. Physical examination findings include proximal retraction of the muscle belly with a change in contour. Weakness and pain, primarily in supination, are characteristic. The hook test is sensitive for biceps ruptures.[55] The test is performed by asking the patient to actively flex the elbow to 90° while sitting or standing and fully supinate the forearm to its end point of supination. The examiner then uses the index finger to feel beneath the lateral edge of the biceps tendon in an attempt to hook the tendon. The test is negative if the finger can be inserted 1 cm beneath the tendon and positive when there is no cord-like structure that can be hooked. Sensitivity, specificity, positive predictive value, and negative predictive value were all 100%, including examinations for partial tendon ruptures.[55] MRI is used if the diagnosis is unclear, if the tear is thought to be at the myotendinous junction, to evaluate retraction in a chronic tear, or for a suspected partial biceps tendon rupture. MRI technique with the elbow flexed, abducted, and supinated improves the diagnosis of partial- and full-thickness distal biceps tears.

Nonsurgical management should be considered in patients with significant medical comorbidities and perioperative surgical risk, both of which are uncommon in individuals with distal biceps tendon tears. Nonsurgical treatment, however, results in decreased elbow flexion strength, supination strength, and upper extremity endurance.[56]

Several surgical options exist for repairing the biceps tendon, including the approach and fixation strategy.

The single-incision, anterior approach uses the interval between the brachioradialis and the pronator teres at the proximal aspect of the forearm. The posterior interosseous nerve must be protected by limiting forceful lateral retraction and keeping the arm supinated. The two-incision technique was developed in an attempt to minimize the risk of neurologic injury associated with the single-incision technique. Through an anterior incision, the biceps tendon is identified and the most distal end of the tendon is débrided. With the forearm in supination, a blunt hemostat is advanced along the medial border of the radial tuberosity to the dorsolateral aspect of the proximal forearm. Contact with the ulnar periosteum is avoided to reduce the potential for heterotopic ossification and radioulnar synostosis. A second incision is made over the hemostat, and the common extensor muscle mass and supinator muscles are split down to the radial tuberosity with the forearm in maximal pronation.

Fixation of the tendon can be achieved with bone tunnels, suture anchors, interference screws, or cortical buttons. Various modes of failure have been reported with the bone tunnel technique, including suture breakage and cutting through the bony bridge at the suture-bone interface.[57] The cortical button technique has been demonstrated to have the highest peak load to failure in multiple studies[57-59] and better strength to cyclic loading.[58,59] Postoperatively, patients are traditionally immobilized in a posterior splint for the first 1 to 2 weeks. Light strengthening is resumed at approximately 8 weeks, with an expected return to heavy activities at 3 to 5 months after surgery (depending on the patient). Currently, there is a trend to early range of motion following distal biceps tendon repairs. One study concluded that immediate postoperative range of motion after repair of the distal biceps tendon leads to early gain of extension and has no deleterious effect on healing or strength.[60]

Complications associated with the single-incision technique include radial nerve injury that often resolves. The two-incision repair decreases the incidence of radial nerve injury but has a higher risk of proximal radioulnar synostosis. A muscle-splitting approach instead of the original technique of subperiosteal ulnar dissection reduces the incidence of radioulnar synostosis. Chronic proximal retraction of the ruptured tendon may preclude anatomic reattachment because of a loss of tendon length.

Triceps Tendon Rupture

Injury to the triceps tendon is rare and is seen in body builders, middle-aged men, or debilitated patients. Risks include steroid injections for olecranon bursitis, anabolic steroids, inflammatory or systemic conditions, and previous triceps surgery. Ruptures occur most commonly at the origin of the lateral head of the triceps and less so through the triceps muscle belly or musculotendinous junction. Usually the anconeus expansion is intact.[61,62] The mechanism of injury is an eccentric load to a contracting triceps. Patients present with acute swelling, ecchymosis, and pain. After the swelling subsides, a palpable gap and extensor weakness are observed. Neurologic examination must be performed to assess possible compartment syndrome and cubital tunnel syndrome. Radiographs are used to assess possible olecranon fracture. MRI is used to identify partial tears and muscle or musculotendinous junction tears.

Nonsurgical management is considered only for elderly, sedentary patients who do not require extension strength and are too ill to undergo surgery. Acute repair is performed via a straight posterior incision. Locking sutures in the tendon are passed through drill holes in the olecranon. Complications include failure of the repair, elbow stiffness, and ulnar nerve injury.

Summary

Shoulder and elbow disorders in athletes typically fall into injury patterns related to repetitive overuse or acute traumatic injuries. In addition, specific sporting activites such as baseball pitching have predictable injury patterns. Therefore, understanding the various pathomechanics of sport-specific injuries has become a great advantage to the clinician. Successful and appropriate treatment relies critically on detailed history and physical examination features with supporting imaging studies.

Key Study Points

- Overuse injuries of the shoulder and the elbow are common and increasing in incidence in overhead athletes.

- Controversy exists with respect to SLAP tears and fixation. There is a growing trend to either treat nonsurgically or consider biceps tenodesis in some athletes.

- MCL reconstruction of the elbow leads to a successful outcome in a high percentage of athletes.

Annotated References

1. Reagan KM, Meister K, Horodyski MB, Werner DW, Carruthers C, Wilk K: Humeral retroversion and its relationship to glenohumeral rotation in the shoulder of college baseball players. *Am J Sports Med* 2002;30(3):354-360.

2. Levine WN, Brandon ML, Stein BS, Gardner TR, Bigliani LU, Ahmad CS: Shoulder adaptive changes in youth baseball players. *J Shoulder Elbow Surg* 2006;15(5):562-566.

3. Burkhart SS, Morgan CD, Kibler WB: Shoulder injuries in overhead athletes: The "dead arm" revisited. *Clin Sports Med* 2000;19(1):125-158.

4. Rodosky MW, Harner CD, Fu FH: The role of the long head of the biceps muscle and superior glenoid labrum in anterior stability of the shoulder. *Am J Sports Med* 1994;22(1):121-130.

5. Itoi E, Newman SR, Kuechle DK, Morrey BF, An KN: Dynamic anterior stabilisers of the shoulder with the arm in abduction. *J Bone Joint Surg Br* 1994;76(5):834-836.

6. Andrews JR, Carson WG Jr, McLeod WD: Glenoid labrum tears related to the long head of the biceps. *Am J Sports Med* 1985;13(5):337-341.

7. Maffet MW, Gartsman GM, Moseley B: Superior labrum-biceps tendon complex lesions of the shoulder. *Am J Sports Med* 1995;23(1):93-98.

8. Snyder SJ, Karzel RP, Del Pizzo W, Ferkel RD, Friedman MJ: SLAP lesions of the shoulder. *Arthroscopy* 1990;6(4):274-279.

9. Gobezie R, Zurakowski D, Lavery K, Millett PJ, Cole BJ, Warner JJ: Analysis of interobserver and intraobserver variability in the diagnosis and treatment of SLAP tears using the Snyder classification. *Am J Sports Med* 2008;36(7):1373-1379.

10. Neri BR, ElAttrache NS, Owsley KC, Mohr K, Yocum LA: Outcome of type II superior labral anterior posterior repairs in elite overhead athletes: Effect of concomitant partial-thickness rotator cuff tears. *Am J Sports Med* 2011;39(1):114-120.

    The authors reported on 23 elite overhead athletes who underwent arthroscopic SLAP repair and found only 57% were able to return to their preinjury level of performance. Level of evidence: III.

11. Edwards SL, Lee JA, Bell JE, et al: Nonoperative treatment of superior labrum anterior posterior tears: Improvements in pain, function, and quality of life. *Am J Sports Med* 2010;38(7):1456-1461.

    Nonsurgical management of documented SLAP tears in this series led to return to preinjury level of performance in 66% of athletes. However, 20 patients (51%) in this series failed nonsurgical management. Level of evidence: IV.

12. Boileau P, Parratte S, Chuinard C, Roussanne Y, Shia D, Bicknell R: Arthroscopic treatment of isolated type II SLAP lesions: Biceps tenodesis as an alternative to reinsertion. *Am J Sports Med* 2009;37(5):929-936.

13. Kibler WB, Sciascia A, Thomas SJ: Glenohumeral internal rotation deficit: Pathogenesis and response to acute throwing. *Sports Med Arthrosc* 2012;20(1):34-38.

    The authors defined GIRD as a loss of 20 or more degrees of internal rotation and the total arc of motion deficit as a loss of 8° total arc difference.

14. Wilk KE, Macrina LC, Fleisig GS, et al: Correlation of glenohumeral internal rotation deficit and total rotational motion to shoulder injuries in professional baseball pitchers. *Am J Sports Med* 2011;39(2):329-335.

    One hundred twenty-two professional baseball pitchers were examined over three seasons, and pitchers with GIRD were nearly twice as likely to be injured and require subsequent surgery than those without GIRD. Major league pitchers were also more likely miss more games than minor league players. Level of evidence: IV.

15. Myers JB, Laudner KG, Pasquale MR, Bradley JP, Lephart SM: Glenohumeral range of motion deficits and posterior shoulder tightness in throwers with pathologic internal impingement. *Am J Sports Med* 2006;34(3): 385-391.

16. Aldridge R, Stephen Guffey J, Whitehead MT, Head P: The effects of a daily stretching protocol on passive glenohumeral internal rotation in overhead throwing collegiate athletes. *Int J Sports Phys Ther* 2012;7(4): 365-371.

    The authors showed that passive stretching of the posterior capsule in collegiate baseball players (5 days/week × 12 weeks) led to statistically significant increases in internal rotation and total arc of motion. Level of evidence: I.

17. Shanley E, Thigpen CA, Clark JC, et al: Changes in passive range of motion and development of glenohumeral internal rotation deficit (GIRD) in the professional pitching shoulder between spring training in two consecutive years. *J Shoulder Elbow Surg* 2012;21(11): 1605-1612.

    Range of motion was altered between seasons of pitching in this study of 33 asymptomatic baseball pitchers over two seasons. Because humeral retrotorsion was controlled, these changes were due to soft-tissue adaptations.

18. Mazoué CG, Andrews JR: Repair of full-thickness rotator cuff tears in professional baseball players. *Am J Sports Med* 2006;34(2):182-189.

19. Namdari S, Baldwin K, Ahn A, Huffman GR, Sennett BJ: Performance after rotator cuff tear and operative treatment: A case-control study of major league baseball pitchers. *J Athl Train* 2011;46(3):296-302.

    Thirty-three Major League Baseball pitchers were identified who had undergone rotator cuff repair surgery and were found to have a steady decline in performance. They did not return to their preinjury level of performance. Unfortunately, in this database review study, several variables, including the type of procedure and postoperative rehabilitation, were not determined. Level of evidence: III.

20. Reynolds SB, Dugas JR, Cain EL, McMichael CS, Andrews JR: Débridement of small partial-thickness rotator cuff tears in elite overhead throwers. *Clin Orthop Relat Res* 2008;466(3):614-621.

21. Wright RW, Steger-May K, Klein SE: Radiographic findings in the shoulder and elbow of Major League Baseball pitchers. *Am J Sports Med* 2007;35(11):1839-1843.

22. Callaway GH, Field LD, Deng XH, et al: Biomechanical evaluation of the medial collateral ligament of the elbow. *J Bone Joint Surg Am* 1997;79(8):1223-1231.

23. Regan WD, Korinek SL, Morrey BF, An KN: Biomechanical study of ligaments around the elbow joint. *Clin Orthop Relat Res* 1991;271:170-179.

24. Morrey BF, An KN: Articular and ligamentous contributions to the stability of the elbow joint. *Am J Sports Med* 1983;11(5):315-319.

25. Park MC, Ahmad CS: Dynamic contributions of the flexor-pronator mass to elbow valgus stability. *J Bone Joint Surg Am* 2004;86(10):2268-2274.

26. Conway JE: The DANE TJ procedure for elbow medial ulnar collateral ligament insufficiency. *Tech Shoulder Elbow Surg* 2006;7:36-43.

27. Thompson WH, Jobe FW, Yocum LA, Pink MM: Ulnar collateral ligament reconstruction in athletes: Muscle-splitting approach without transposition of the ulnar nerve. *J Shoulder Elbow Surg* 2001;10(2):152-157.

28. Ellenbecker TS, Mattalino AJ, Elam EA, Caplinger RA: Medial elbow joint laxity in professional baseball pitchers: A bilateral comparison using stress radiography. *Am J Sports Med* 1998;26(3):420-424.

29. Hill NB Jr, Bucchieri JS, Shon F, Miller TT, Rosenwasser MP: Magnetic resonance imaging of injury to the medial collateral ligament of the elbow: A cadaver model. *J Shoulder Elbow Surg* 2000;9(5):418-422.

30. Sasaki J, Takahara M, Ogino T, Kashiwa H, Ishigaki D, Kanauchi Y: Ultrasonographic assessment of the ulnar collateral ligament and medial elbow laxity in college baseball players. *J Bone Joint Surg Am* 2002;84(4):525-531.

31. Rohrbough JT, Altchek DW, Hyman J, Williams RJ III, Botts JD: Medial collateral ligament reconstruction of the elbow using the docking technique. *Am J Sports Med* 2002;30(4):541-548.

32. Vitale MA, Ahmad CS: The outcome of elbow ulnar collateral ligament reconstruction in overhead athletes: A systematic review. *Am J Sports Med* 2008;36(6): 1193-1205.

33. Andrews JR, Timmerman LA: Outcome of elbow surgery in professional baseball players. *Am J Sports Med* 1995;23(4):407-413.

34. Reddy AS, Kvitne RS, Yocum LA, Elattrache NS, Glousman RE, Jobe FW: Arthroscopy of the elbow: A long-term clinical review. *Arthroscopy* 2000;16(6):588-594.

35. Kamineni S, ElAttrache NS, O'Driscoll SW, et al: Medial collateral ligament strain with partial posteromedial olecranon resection: A biomechanical study. *J Bone Joint Surg Am* 2004;86(11):2424-2430.

36. O'Driscoll SW, Lawton RL, Smith AM: The "moving valgus stress test" for medial collateral ligament tears of the elbow. *Am J Sports Med* 2005;33(2):231-239.

37. Kamineni S, Hirahara H, Pomianowski S, et al: Partial posteromedial olecranon resection: A kinematic study. *J Bone Joint Surg Am* 2003;85(6):1005-1011.

38. Singer KM, Roy SP: Osteochondrosis of the humeral capitellum. *Am J Sports Med* 1984;12(5):351-360.

39. Haraldsson S: On osteochondrosis deformas juvenilis capituli humeri including investigation of intra-osseous vasculature in distal humerus. *Acta Orthop Scand Suppl* 1959;38:1-232.

40. Baumgarten TE, Andrews JR, Satterwhite YE: The arthroscopic classification and treatment of osteochondritis dissecans of the capitellum. *Am J Sports Med* 1998;26(4):520-523.

41. Mihara K, Tsutsui H, Nishinaka N, Yamaguchi K: Nonoperative treatment for osteochondritis dissecans of the capitellum. *Am J Sports Med* 2009;37(2):298-304.

42. Takahara M, Mura N, Sasaki J, Harada M, Ogino T: Classification, treatment, and outcome of osteochondritis dissecans of the humeral capitellum. *J Bone Joint Surg Am* 2007;89(6):1205-1214.

43. Larsen MW, Pietrzak WS, DeLee JC: Fixation of osteochondritis dissecans lesions using poly(l-lactic acid)/poly(glycolic acid) copolymer bioabsorbable screws. *Am J Sports Med* 2005;33(1):68-76.

44. Bauer M, Jonsson K, Josefsson PO, Lindén B: Osteochondritis dissecans of the elbow: A long-term follow-up study. *Clin Orthop Relat Res* 1992;284:156-160.

45. Antuna SA, O'Driscoll SW: Snapping plicae associated with radiocapitellar chondromalacia. *Arthroscopy* 2001;17(5):491-495.

46. Kim DH, Gambardella RA, Elattrache NS, Yocum LA, Jobe FW: Arthroscopic treatment of posterolateral elbow impingement from lateral synovial plicae in throwing athletes and golfers. *Am J Sports Med* 2006;34(3):438-444.

47. Kraushaar BS, Nirschl RP: Tendinosis of the elbow (tennis elbow): Clinical features and findings of histological, immunohistochemical, and electron microscopy studies. *J Bone Joint Surg Am* 1999;81(2):259-278.

48. Nirschl RP, Pettrone FA: Tennis elbow: The surgical treatment of lateral epicondylitis. *J Bone Joint Surg Am* 1979;61(6):832-839.

49. Gosens T, Peerbooms JC, van Laar W, den Oudsten BL: Ongoing positive effect of platelet-rich plasma versus corticosteroid injection in lateral epicondylitis: A double-blind randomized controlled trial with 2-year follow-up. *Am J Sports Med* 2011;39(6):1200-1208.

This prospective randomized study (100 patients) showed significant improvement using platelet-rich plasma compared with steroids for the treatment of lateral epicondylitis even 2 years after the injections. Level of evidence: I.

50. Carofino BC, Bishop AT, Spinner RJ, Shin AY: Nerve injuries resulting from arthroscopic treatment of lateral epicondylitis: Report of 2 cases. *J Hand Surg Am* 2012;37(6):1208-1210.

The authors reported two major complications of arthroscopic lateral epicondylitis surgery with a complete transection of the posterior interosseous nerve and a partial laceration of the median nerve. Level of evidence: V.

51. Gabel GT, Morrey BF: Operative treatment of medical epicondylitis: Influence of concomitant ulnar neuropathy at the elbow. *J Bone Joint Surg Am* 1995;77(7):1065-1069.

52. Morrey BF, Askew LJ, An KN, Dobyns JH: Rupture of the distal tendon of the biceps brachii: A biomechanical study. *J Bone Joint Surg Am* 1985;67(3):418-421.

53. Safran MR, Graham SM: Distal biceps tendon ruptures: Incidence, demographics, and the effect of smoking. *Clin Orthop Relat Res* 2002;404:275-283.

54. Seiler JG III, Parker LM, Chamberland PD, Sherbourne GM, Carpenter WA: The distal biceps tendon. Two potential mechanisms involved in its rupture: Arterial supply and mechanical impingement. *J Shoulder Elbow Surg* 1995;4(3):149-156.

55. O'Driscoll SW, Goncalves LB, Dietz P: The hook test for distal biceps tendon avulsion. *Am J Sports Med* 2007;35(11):1865-1869.

56. Baker BE, Bierwagen D: Rupture of the distal tendon of the biceps brachii: Operative versus non-operative treatment. *J Bone Joint Surg Am* 1985;67(3):414-417.

57. Kettler M, Tingart MJ, Lunger J, Kuhn V: Reattachment of the distal tendon of biceps: Factors affecting the failure strength of the repair. *J Bone Joint Surg Br* 2008;90(1):103-106.

58. Mazzocca AD, Burton KJ, Romeo AA, Santangelo S, Adams DA, Arciero RA: Biomechanical evaluation of 4 techniques of distal biceps brachii tendon repair. *Am J Sports Med* 2007;35(2):252-258.

59. Bisson LJ, de Perio JG, Weber AE, Ehrensberger MT, Buyea C: Is it safe to perform aggressive rehabilitation after distal biceps tendon repair using the modified 2-incision approach? A biomechanical study. *Am J Sports Med* 2007;35(12):2045-2050.

3: Upper Extremity

Treatment

Nonsurgical Treatment

Patients without a mechanical block to forearm rotation have a good outcome when early ROM is initiated. Prolonged immobilization results in a higher degree of residual stiffness. Early aspiration and local anesthetic injection into the elbow offer no long-term benefit in the management of radial head fractures without a block to rotation.[4] Although most patients with moderately displaced radial head fractures have good long-term results,[5,6] one series reported that 12% of the patients had a poor early outcome from nonsurgical treatment and required early intervention in the form of a radial head excision.[7]

Surgical Treatment

An examination under anesthesia is helpful to test the integrity of the collateral ligaments. The radial head can be approached using a posterior or a lateral skin incision (followed by an extensor digitorum communis–splitting approach or a Kocher approach) depending on surgeon preference and the presence of concomitant injuries requiring treatment. If the lateral collateral ligament (LCL) is injured, a Kocher approach between the anconeus and extensor carpi ulnaris muscles should be considered because it facilitates ligament repair. If the LCL is intact, an approach that splits the common extensor origin is preferred because it allows better exposure of the anterolateral quadrant of the radial head, which is most commonly fractured, and preservesthe lateral ulnar collateral ligament, avoiding iatrogenic posterolateral and varus instability.

Radial Head Fragment Excision

Fragment excision can be considered for small, unreconstructable partial articular fractures of the radial head. A progressive loss of concavity-compression stability occurs with larger fragment size, limiting this option to fragments smaller than 25% of the articulation. Limited outcome studies are available for radial head fragment excisions performed either open or arthroscopically.[8]

Radial Head Excision

Long-term outcome studies of radial head excision show that most patients have substantial evidence of radiographic arthritis and an increased valgus carrying angle of the elbow.[9] In spite of these findings, the functional outcomes of most patients following radial head excision have been good.[10,11] Proximal migration of the radius is common with radial head excision[12] and may result in symptomatic ulnar impaction syndrome at the wrist if there is concomitant disruption of the interosseous membrane, also known as the Essex-Lopresti injury. Excision of the radial head has been associated with impingement of the radial neck on the ulna, which is termed proximal radioulnar impingement syndrome. Because of the frequency of associated ligamentous and osseous injuries in patients with comminuted radial head fractures, the importance of the radial head for load transfer, and the stabilizing role of the radial head for both the elbow and the forearm, primary radial head excision should be performed with caution. Because the outcome of delayed radial head excision has been reported to have good results, radial head excision is most commonly performed as a late treatment option when other nonsurgical or surgical treatments have failed.

Open Reduction and Internal Fixation

Open reduction and internal fixation (ORIF) is indicated for displaced radial head fractures when stable fixation is possible and surgery is indicated because of the presence of a mechanical block to motion, associated elbow fractures, or ligamentous injuries requiring treatment. ORIF of displaced noncomminuted fractures of the radial head has provided good or excellent outcomes in most series (Figure 1). Nonrandomized studies have shown patients treated with ORIF to have better outcomes and a lower rate of osteoarthritis compared with patients treated with primary radial head excision.[13,14] One study showed that ORIF of simple partial articular fractures had better results than complete articular fractures or fractures with more than three displaced fragments.[15] Plates should be placed on the nonarticulating portion of the radial head to avoid impingement with the proximal radioulnar joint during forearm rotation. Plate fixation has a higher incidence of rotational stiffness than low-profile countersunk screws placed obliquely from the radial head into the radial neck.

Radial Head Arthroplasty

Radial head arthroplasty is indicated in patients with comminuted displaced radial head fractures where stable internal fixation is not possible. Factors to consider are the presence of associated ligamentous and osseous injuries and osteoporosis, which increase the risk of failure of internal fixation (Figure 2). Although the early and medium-term results of most currently available radial head designs have been good, the long-term results are unknown.[16-18] In patients with elbow instability, monopolar radial head replacements have been shown to provide improved concavity-compression stability of the radiocapitellar joint compared with a bipolar design.[19,20] Stress shielding has been reported with well-fixed noncemented stems. Loose nonsmooth noncemented stem designs have been associated with pain and are a common reason for revision surgery.[21,22] Radiolucencies around smooth noncemented stems were not correlated with clinical outcome.[23]

Correct radial head implant diameter and thickness are key to providing a good outcome. Radial head implants whose diameter is too large have been associated with the development of trochlear erosions, whereas implants that are too thick have been associated with capitellar wear and postoperative stiffness.[24] The excised radial head should be used to judge implant size. The space between the capitellum and the radial head prosthesis should not be used to evaluate radial head

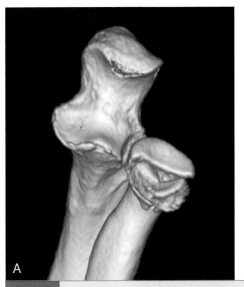
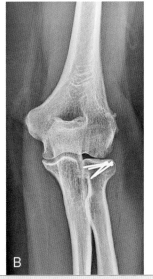
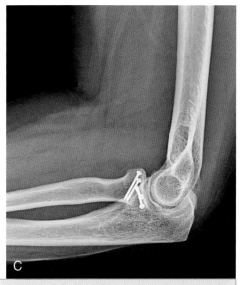

Figure 1   A three-dimensional CT reconstruction (**A**) of a Mason type II radial head fracture is shown. Follow-up radiographs (**B** and **C**) at 2 years after surgery demonstrate healing of the fracture after ORIF with countersunk screws.

length because many patients have a concomitant LCL injury. The radial head should articulate approximately 2 mm distal to the tip of the coronoid at the level of the proximal radioulnar joint.[25] The medial ulnohumeral joint space should be parallel on intraoperative fluoroscopy;[26] however, overlengthening by 6 mm can easily be missed on imaging.[27] Contralateral radiographs have been shown to be useful to quantify radial head overlengthening postoperatively because of the side-to-side consistency of radial head morphology.[28]

Complications

Radiographic malunion and nonunion are common with nonsurgical treatment but are often asymptomatic. Intra-articular osteotomy has recently been reported to be effective for symptomatic malunion of partial articular fractures of the radial head.[29] Persistent pain or mechanical symptoms can be effectively managed with radial head excision or arthroplasty.

Radiographic osteoarthritis is common with both nonsurgical and surgical management of radial head fractures but does not correlate with functional outcome.[10,11,23,24] Clinically significant osteoarthritis can be managed with radial head excision; however, radial head excision should be performed with caution in patients with concomitant ulnohumeral arthritis. Radiocapitellar replacement arthroplasty has been shown to restore elbow kinematics when the medial collateral ligament (MCL) is intact.[30] Good short-term outcomes have been reported; however, the long-term efficacy of this procedure remains unknown.

Forearm and elbow stiffness is common in patients with radial head fractures because of capsular contracture or the development of heterotopic ossification. Although therapy and splinting are typically effective, surgical management may be required for persistent contractures that are functionally disabling. Prominent

hardware after ORIF and improper sizing of a radial head arthroplasty are frequent causes of stiffness that require surgical management.

Complex Elbow Instability

The elbow is one of the most commonly dislocated joints in the body, with elbow dislocation having an annual incidence of approximately 5.2 per 100,000 per year.[31] Elbow dislocations can be classified as simple or complex. A simple dislocation is defined as an elbow dislocation with soft-tissue injury only. Conversely, a complex dislocation involves associated fractures, such as fractures of the radial head, the capitellum, or the ulna.

Complex elbow dislocations, or fracture-dislocations, are some of the most technically difficult injuries to manage. These injuries can broadly be classified into three patterns: (1) terrible triad injuries characterized by radial head and coronoid fractures with elbow dislocation caused by a posterolateral rotatory instability pattern; (2) varus posteromedial instability; and (3) Monteggia-type injuries and associated variants, such as transolecranon fracture-dislocations. Stabilizing the elbow joint to allow early ROM is of paramount importance in managing these injuries.

A detailed history, a physical examination, and applicable imaging are essential in establishing the diagnosis and developing a treatment plan. Generally, standard elbow radiographs are sufficient to establish the diagnosis; however, CT is usually required to develop a treatment plan. Initial management should consist of closed reduction to decrease pain, minimize soft-tissue swelling, and allow for more accurate interpretation of radiographs. The definitive surgical management of complex elbow instabilities varies with the classification and mag-

3: Upper Extremity

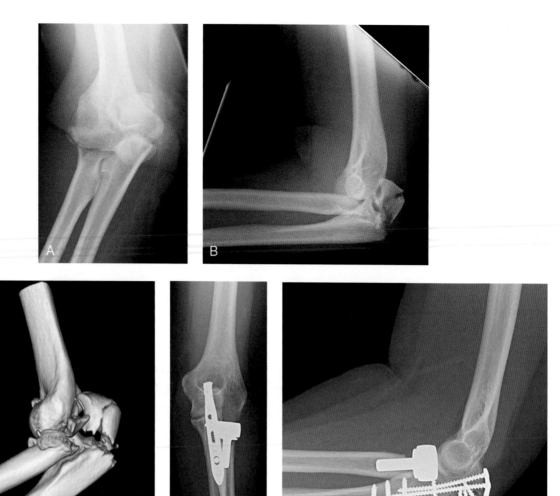

Figure 2 Preoperative AP (**A**) and lateral (**B**) radiographs and a three-dimensional CT reconstruction (**C**) show a left-sided transolecranon fracture-dislocation with a comminuted nonreconstructible radial head fracture. **D** and **E**, ORIF of the proximal ulna and radial head arthroplasty were performed using a modular, noncemented radial head replacement.

nitude of the injury. Most patients with elbow fracture-dislocations will require surgical treatment.

Terrible Triad Injuries

The term terrible triad injury of the elbow was coined because of the historically poor outcomes of this injury. However, a systematic surgical approach and better understanding of elbow anatomy and instability have led to improved outcomes.

The mechanism of injury in terrible triad injuries is thought to be related to posterolateral rotatory instability. Recently, however, the authors of a biomechanical study offered an alternative mechanism of injury in which forearm pronation is associated with a terrible triad injury and forearm supination is associated with simple dislocation.[32]

Patient history and physical examination are important to determine the mechanism of injury, associated injuries, neurovascular status, and skin integrity. Prereduction and postreduction radiographs should be carefully examined to characterize the fracture and assess the congruency of the elbow. Advanced imaging (CT) is typically obtained to assist with fracture classification and characterization.

The individual components of the terrible triad injury can be classified to aid in the surgical management of this injury. For radial head fractures, several classification systems exist, which were described earlier. The McKee classification of LCL injuries includes six patterns.[33] The most common injury pattern involves proximal avulsion of the LCL from the isometric point on the lateral epicondyles.

Two classification schemes describe coronoid fracture patterns. The Regan and Morrey classification is

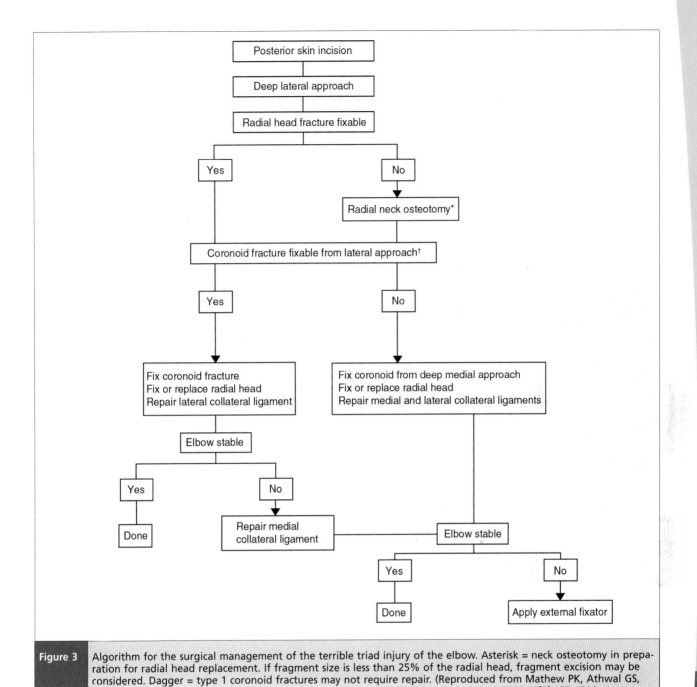

Figure 3 Algorithm for the surgical management of the terrible triad injury of the elbow. Asterisk = neck osteotomy in preparation for radial head replacement. If fragment size is less than 25% of the radial head, fragment excision may be considered. Dagger = type 1 coronoid fractures may not require repair. (Reproduced from Mathew PK, Athwal GS, King GJ: Terrible triad injury of the elbow: Current concepts. *J Am Acad Orthop Surg* 2009;17[3]:137-151.)

based on the percentage of the coronoid fragment height on a lateral elbow radiograph.[34] The O'Driscoll classification system is based on the size and the location of the fracture fragments: type 1 involves transverse fractures of the tip of the coronoid, type 2 involves a fracture of the anteromedial facet of the coronoid process, and type 3 involves a fracture of the coronoid at its base. Type 2 fractures can be further subdivided into anteromedial rim fractures; rim and tip fractures; and fractures involving the sublime tubercle, which is the attachment of anterior bundle of the MCL.[35] This classification recognizes that not all coronoid fractures are in the coronal plane and helps differentiate the complex patterns of injury.

A small subset of terrible triad injuries may be managed nonsurgically if strict criteria are met: the elbow must be concentrically reduced, the radial head fracture must not meet surgical indications, the coronoid fracture must be small, and the elbow must be sufficiently stable to allow early ROM.[36,37]

Most terrible triad injuries require surgical management. A systematic approach helps to address the critical components of this injury[37] (Figure 3). This approach includes fixation or replacement of the radial head, fixation of the coronoid fragment, and repair of the LCL. After these procedures have been performed,

3: Upper Extremity

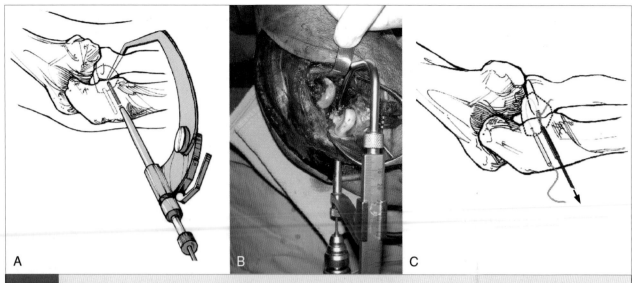

Figure 4 Illustration (**A**) and photograph (**B**) show a targeting device used to assist in drill hole placement for retrograde screws or suture fixation of a coronoid fracture. **C,** Suturing of the coronoid fragment is most frequently done through the lateral arthrotomy, after which the sutures are drawn through drill holes (arrow) exiting the subcutaneous border of the ulna. (Reproduced from Mathew PK, Athwal GS, King GJ: Terrible triad injury of the elbow: Current concepts. *J Am Acad Orthop Surg* 2009;17[30]:137-151.)

the elbow is intraoperatively assessed for stability, preferably with fluoroscopy, to determine if MCL repair or rarely an external fixator is required.

The goals of treatment of the radial head fracture are to have a stable construct to allow the radial head to function as an elbow stabilizer and to permit early mobilization. The treatment options include ORIF and radial head arthroplasty. On occasion, an associated radial neck fracture will require stabilization. Radial head excision is contraindicated in patients with complex elbow instability.

Coronoid fractures associated with terrible triad injuries are typically Regan and Morrey type I or II. Type I coronoid fractures usually do not require repair. Elbow joint stability is not significantly improved following repair of a small tip fracture.[38] With larger coronoid fragments, fixation is usually achieved with sutures, suture anchors, screws, or rarely, a plate. The authors of a recent biomechanical study[39] demonstrated superior strength and coronoid fragment stability with screws placed retrograde, posterior to anterior, compared with anterior-to-posterior screws. The authors concluded that retrograde coronoid fixation was biomechanically superior and technically easier. In patients with coronoid fracture comminution, an alternative is to reattach the fragments and the anterior capsule to the coronoid process using transosseous sutures. Suture fixation was found to be clinically superior to suture anchors and ORIF in a 2011 study[40] (Figure 4). The authors of the study reported improved stability and lower nonunion rates with suture fixation in 40 consecutive patients treated surgically for terrible triad injuries.

Terrible triad injury outcome studies reveal an average flexion of 132° and an average extension deficit of 16°. Forearm supination could be restored to 62° and

forearm pronation to 76°. In a recent literature review, most of the patients (71%) were rated as having good or excellent outcomes at final follow-up (106 of 150 patients) according to the Mayo Elbow Performance Score or the Broberg-Morrey score.[41] Risks associated with terrible triad injuries include residual instability, arthritis, heterotopic ossification, stiffness, neuropathy, infection, malunion, and nonunion.[41]

Postoperatively, the arm is placed into a splint at 90° of flexion. Supervised early motion should begin 3 to 5 days after surgery.[42] Active flexion and extension ROM is initiated within a stable arc. Active forearm rotation is conducted in 90° or more of flexion. In patients with tenuous stability, an overhead rehabilitation protocol may be used.[42]

The position of forearm rotation depends on the status of the medial and lateral ligaments. For example, in patients with an intact MCL, the elbow is splinted in pronation to protect the lateral repair. In patients with an unrepaired MCL tear, the elbow may be splinted in supination.

Varus Posteromedial Rotatory Instability

Varus posteromedial rotatory instability is hypothesized to occur when an axial load is applied to the extended pronated arm, resulting in varus and posteromedial rotation of the forearm. This instability pattern results in an anteromedial coronoid process fracture and rupture of the LCL and the posterior bundle of the MCL. Fractures of the radial head with this injury pattern are uncommon but do occur.

If an anteromedial facet fracture of the coronoid is not discovered and is left untreated, the ulnohumeral

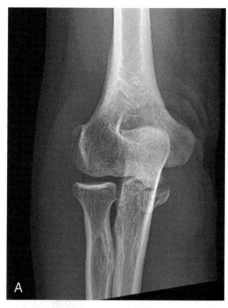
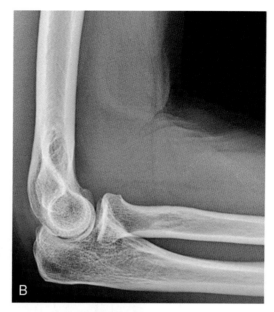
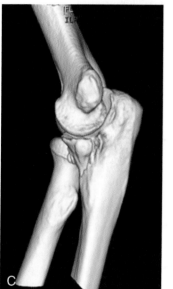
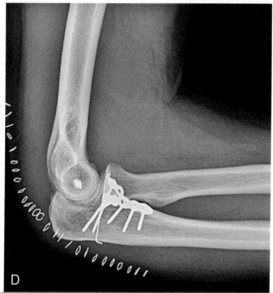
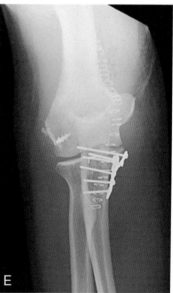

Figure 5 Preoperative radiographs (**A** and **B**) and a three-dimensional CT reconstruction (**C**) of an anteromedial coronoid facet fracture are shown. Because of the large size of the fracture fragment and the associated joint instability, ORIF (**D** and **E**) was accomplished via a flexor carpi ulnaris split approach. A lateral collateral ligament repair was performed for varus posteromedial instability.

joint may subluxate (Figure 5). This malalignment, with the trochlea articulating with the fractured surface of the anteromedial coronoid, will result in accelerated onset of posttraumatic arthritis. Unstable anteromedial coronoid fractures need to be identified early to prevent late instability and degenerative changes.

Typically, AP and lateral elbow radiographs can lead to the diagnosis. If an isolated coronoid fracture is identified without an associated radial head fracture, the possibility of varus posteromedial instability should be considered. At times, the anteromedial facet fracture is difficult to fully identify on radiographs, and the double crescent sign may be the only abnormal finding. In addition, an asymmetric medial joint line on the AP radiograph may offer a clue to this injury. Anteromedial facet fractures are relatively uncommon and accounted for only 17% of the coronoid fractures in one study.[43]

Literature on the treatment and outcomes of anteromedial coronoid facet fractures is scarce. Therefore, surgical indications, approaches, and techniques are still being developed. The current recommendations for the treatment of anteromedial facet fractures are based on expert opinion and small case series.

No studies have evaluated the outcome of nonsurgical treatment specifically. A small series of anteromedial facet fractures included two patients with insufficient fixation of the coronoid fracture, three patients who were

3: Upper Extremity

treated nonsurgically, and four patients in whom the anteromedial facet fracture was not addressed in surgery. Seven of these nine patients had persisting elbow instability (subluxation of the trochlea into the defect) and arthrosis at the time of final follow-up.[44]

ORIF of an anteromedial facet fracture is typically conducted through the floor of the ulnar nerve (splitting between the two heads of the flexor carpi ulnaris). The flexor pronator group is carefully elevated off the ulna from a distal to proximal direction, exposing the sublime tubercle, the coronoid fracture, and the anterior bundle of the MCL. After the anteromedial facet fracture is exposed, it may be stabilized with screws, small plates, or precontoured fracture-specific plates. After fixation of the coronoid, the LCL should be assessed and, if required for stability, repaired.

Monteggia Injuries and Variants

Monteggia fractures were initially described in 1814 as an anterior dislocation of the radial head in association with a fracture of the ulnar shaft. The term Monteggia lesions was coined in 1967 to describe any fracture of the ulna associated with a dislocation of the radiocapitellar joint, and the Bado classification of these injuries was developed. The Jupiter classification expanded the Bado classification to more accurately represent Monteggia injuries in adults.

Generally speaking, Monteggia fractures in adults require surgery. The management of these patients should be aimed at anatomic reduction of the ulnar fracture and recognition and treatment of associated injuries. Initially, the fracture-dislocation should be reduced and stabilized in a long arm splint. A utilitarian midline posterior skin incision is recommended. Anatomic alignment of the ulna is critical to obtain a reduction of the radial head and a stable radiocapitellar joint. Failure to reestablish ulnar geometry can result in persistent subluxation or dislocation of the radial head. Generally, the ulnar fracture is reconstructed from distal to proximal. Repair of the proximal olecranon fragment with the attached triceps may obscure fracture reduction if performed before the articular reconstruction.

The ulna has a complex morphology, and studies have demonstrated that anatomic reconstruction is important.[45,46] If the radiocapitellar joint remains unstable after fixation of the ulnar fracture, the ulnar fracture reduction must be critically assessed to rule out a possible malreduction. Fixation techniques such as double plating, fragment-specific fixation, or precontoured anatomic plates may be required.

Distal Humeral Fractures

Epidemiology

Distal humeral fractures occur in a bimodal age distribution, with an incidence of 5.7 per 100,000 per year.

The most common mechanism of injury is a simple fall from standing height. These fractures occur with an increasing incidence among women older than 60 years. In young adults, such fractures are typically caused by high-energy injuries, such as motor vehicle collisions, falls from height, sports-related injuries, industrial accidents, and firearm-related injuries. In a 2003 series, the most common fracture pattern was extra-articular fracture, which accounted for approximately 40% of the fractures. Bicolumn or complete intra-articular fracture was the second most common fracture pattern, accounting for 37% of the fractures.[47]

Classification

Several classification systems exist to describe distal humeral fractures. The authors prefer the Orthopaedic Trauma Association (OTA)/AO comprehensive classification system. This system classifies distal humeral fractures using an alphanumeric system that assigns the fractures a code beginning with the number 13 and classifies them on the basis of location and the degree of articular involvement.

Assessment

The history should determine the mechanism and the energy level of the injury. In patients with high-energy injuries, systemic injuries and associated fractures must be identified. Pain from polytrauma and alcohol or drug intoxication may make identification of concomitant injuries difficult.

Most patients with distal humeral fractures are elderly (older than 65 years) and should be evaluated for nonmechanical falls, such as those resulting from a cerebrovascular accident, arrhythmias, polypharmacy, or alcoholism. Special attention must be directed toward identifying comorbidities and reversible diseases that may affect treatment recommendations and perioperative risks. A neurologic examination is important and must be documented preoperatively and postoperatively; the authors of one study reported that 26% of the patients with distal humeral fractures had an associated incomplete ulnar nerve neuropathy at the time of presentation.[48]

Standard radiographs of the elbow are usually sufficient for diagnosis, classification, and surgical templating, but CT with three-dimensional reconstruction significantly improves both identification and visualization of fracture patterns. It has been reported that three-dimensional CT improved both the intraobserver and interobserver reliability of the AO classification system.[49]

Treatment
Nonsurgical Treatment
Nonsurgical management of distal humeral fractures in young patients is rarely recommended. In general, nonsurgical management is reserved for elderly, low-demand patients deemed medically unfit to undergo surgery. Patients with nondisplaced fractures may also be treated with a trial of nonsurgical management.

These patients should be followed for the first 3 to 4 weeks with weekly serial radiographs to ensure that displacement or angulation does not occur. Few data are available on the outcomes of nonsurgical management of distal humeral fractures.

Surgical Treatment

Distal humeral fractures are generally complex injuries with associated comminution, osteopenia, bony instability, and soft-tissue injury. The possibility of functional impairment is relatively high when these injuries are treated nonsurgically. Contemporary literature supports improved patient outcomes and lower complication rates when these injuries are treated surgically. ORIF of distal humeral fractures is the preferred treatment. However, open reduction and stable internal fixation may not be attainable in elderly patients with osteopenia, comminution, and significant articular fragmentation or in patients with preexisting conditions of the elbow, such as rheumatoid arthritis. In such patients, total elbow arthroplasty (TEA) has been shown to be a reliable treatment option with good patient outcomes.

Open Reduction and Internal Fixation

Several surgical approaches have been described for exposure and the fixation of distal humeral fractures. The ideal approach to a specific fracture pattern should provide sufficient exposure to allow anatomic reconstruction of the fracture and the application of the required internal fixation with minimal soft-tissue or bony disruption, to allow early mobilization. The selection of a surgical approach depends on multiple factors, including the fracture pattern, the extent of articular involvement, associated soft-tissue injury, rehabilitation protocols, and surgeon preference.

Most complex distal humeral fractures are exposed using a posterior approach. Posterior approaches to the elbow are classified according to how the extensor mechanism is mobilized. Three broad types are (1) the olecranon osteotomy; (2) triceps-disrupting approaches, including reflecting, splitting, or dividing of the triceps; and (3) triceps-on approaches. The olecranon osteotomy provides the best visualization of the articular surface, but it does have complications associated with hardware prominence and nonunion. The triceps-disrupting approaches avoid the complications associated with an olecranon osteotomy; however, they provide less than complete visualization of the articular surface and may have problems with weakness and nonhealing of the triceps. The triceps-on approach, also referred to as the paratricipital approach, provides less visualization of the joint but allows for immediate unprotected mobilization because there is no concern with triceps healing.

The sequence of fracture fixation consists of reconstruction of the articular surface followed by rigid fixation of the articular surface to the humeral shaft. This fixation is achieved by a minimum of two 3.5-mm pelvic reconstruction plates or fracture-specific precontoured plates; the use of thinner plates, such as semitubular plates, is contraindicated. The use of locking systems, although found to be beneficial in biomechanical testing, has not definitively demonstrated clinical superiority.

Controversy surrounds the use of parallel versus orthogonal plate position. In some biomechanical cadaver studies, parallel plating had higher stiffness and ultimate torque in varus and axial/sagittal loading to failure as well as lower screw loosening rates.[50,51] In contrast, other researchers demonstrated no differences.[52]

Recently, a randomized prospective study compared clinical and radiographic outcomes of parallel versus orthogonal plating and reported no significant differences between groups, although the study may have been underpowered.[53] Several studies with various techniques have demonstrated satisfactory clinical and radiographic outcomes following the principles of stable bicolumn internal fixation, anatomic articular reduction, and early mobilization.[54-58]

Total Elbow Arthroplasty

Open reduction and rigid internal fixation of distal humerals fractures is considered the preferred treatment; however, it may not be possible in elderly patients with comminution and osteopenia or in patients with preexisting joint derangements, such as rheumatoid arthritis. Nonsurgical treatment, although appropriate for some elderly patients, often leads to stiffness, nonunion, and unsatisfactory clinical outcome. TEA is a reliable option with good outcomes in patients in whom open reduction and rigid internal fixation cannot be achieved to allow early motion.[59-64]

The authors of a randomized prospective study of elderly patients compared 15 patients who underwent ORIF with 25 patients who underwent TEA at a minimum of 2 years' follow-up.[61] At early follow-up, TEA resulted in a more predictably good functional outcome compared with ORIF. The rates of revision surgery, however, were not statistically different between the groups, with 3 of 25 TEA patients and 4 of 15 ORIF patients requiring revision surgery. These findings, however, should be interpreted with some degree of caution because TEA outcomes will likely deteriorate over time as implant survivorship diminishes.

The authors of a retrospective study compared 9 patients who underwent TEA to 11 patients who underwent ORIF for the treatment of OTA/AO types B and C fractures. At a mean of 15 months' follow-up, no statistically significant differences in clinical outcomes were identified. The authors concluded that implant selection must be based on bone quality, expected outcome, and surgeon experience, and good outcomes may be obtained with either ORIF or TEA.[62]

Complications

Complication rates after the surgical treatment of distal humeral fractures vary from 25% to 48%.[54,59-62] Complications include stiffness, ulnar neuropathy, heterotopic ossification, nonunion, malunion, and wound problems.

Management of the ulnar nerve during exposure and fixation of distal humeral fractures is controversial. In 2012, researchers conducted a retrospective study on the incidence and predisposing factors for the onset of postoperative ulnar neuropathy.[65] In 107 patients with distal humeral fractures, ulnar neuropathy developed in 17 patients (16%). The only risk factor identified was the type of fracture; columnar fractures had a higher incidence of neuropathy compared with capitellar or trochlear fractures. This result was independent of whether the ulnar nerve was transposed. These findings are supported by a 2010 study in which researchers reported that ulnar nerve transposition did not protect from postoperative neuropathy.[66] In 2010, the authors of a multicenter retrospective cohort study compared the incidence of ulnar neuropathy with and without ulnar nerve transposition during ORIF of distal humeral fractures. Patients who underwent ulnar nerve transposition at the time of ORIF had almost four times the incidence of postoperative ulnar neuritis compared with those without ulnar nerve transposition.[67] However, in patients with preoperative ulnar neuropathy, the literature supports intraoperative ulnar nerve anterior transposition.

The rate of postoperative heterotopic ossification after the surgical treatment of distal humeral fractures ranges from 0% to 21%.[54,63,64,68,69] The available literature lacks clear evidence for using pharmacologic prophylaxis for heterotopic ossification.[48,53,70] Radiation therapy for the prophylaxis of heterotopic ossification was, however, shown to have an unacceptably high rate of complications, particularly nonunions.[71]

Capitellar and Trochlear Fractures

Capitellar and trochlear fractures are distinctly different from distal humeral fractures. These fractures do not typically extend proximal to the olecranon fossa or involve the columns. These injuries, however, may be associated with collateral ligament ruptures and fractures of the epicondyles or radial head. These fractures are thought to be the result of coronal shear forces, which cause coronal plane fractures of the anterior distal humeral articular surface.

Isolated fractures of the capitellum are relatively rare, and isolated fractures of the trochlea are even more rare.[72] The reported annual incidence of articular fractures of the distal humerus is 1.5 per 100,000 per year with a marked female predominance.[73] Associated injuries, such as radial head fractures and collateral ligament tears, occur in up to 20% of patients.[73]

Assessment and Classification

Standard elbow radiographs are typically sufficient to diagnose the injury. The authors recommend routine CT, however, because it is better able to identify associated articular comminution, epicondylar involvement, posterior capitellar impression fractures, and the degree of trochlear involvement.

The Hahn-Steinthal or type I fracture involves the capitellar articular surface along with subchondral bone. The Kocher-Lorenz or type II fracture is rare and consists of the capitellar articular surface along with a thin shell of subchondral bone. The authors of one study described capitellar fractures as a spectrum of injuries.[74] They observed that injuries that appeared to be simple capitellar fractures on standard radiographs were often found to be more complex with CT. The authors of another study classified capitellar and trochlear fractures and related fracture complexity to outcome.[72]

Treatment
Nonsurgical Treatment
Nonsurgical management of a displaced articular fracture of the distal humerus in young patients is rarely recommended, and it is generally reserved for patients deemed medically unfit to undergo surgery. Nonsurgical management techniques include above-elbow casting, and collar and cuff treatment with early mobilization also referred to as the "bag of bones" method.

Closed reduction under anesthesia and casting is a described method for the treatment of displaced capitellar fractures. The reduction maneuver involves placing the elbow into full extension and forearm supination, which typically results in reduction of the capitellum. If the capitellum is still displaced, pressure over the capitellum and a varus force to the elbow may assist with the reduction. If the reduction is successful, the elbow is flexed so that the radial head captures the capitellum. Fluoroscopy is used to confirm the reduction. In 2012, researchers reported on seven patients with capitellar fractures who underwent closed reduction and early mobilization at 14 days. All of the fractures healed and had good to excellent outcomes based on the Disabilities of the Arm, Shoulder and Hand score and a subjective rating of patient satisfaction.[75]

Open Reduction and Internal Fixation
ORIF is considered the preferred treatment of most displaced articular fractures of the distal humerus. Rigid fixation allows fracture healing to occur anatomically while permitting early ROM to maximize function. In patients in whom sufficient fracture stability cannot be obtained to allow early motion, anatomic reconstruction of the articular surface and overall elbow alignment take precedence. An anatomically aligned stiff elbow with a healed articular surface can be subsequently managed with contracture release, but a fracture with malunion, hardware failure, articular nonunion, or fragmentation is difficult to manage with revision surgery.

Fractures of the capitellum with or without involvement of the lateral ridge of the trochlea can be approached through a posterior skin incision or a direct lateral skin incision. The fragment is typically anteriorly displaced and is reduced by elbow extension, forearm supination, and application of a gentle varus force. After the fragment has been reduced, ORIF can be accomplished with anterior-to-posterior countersunk screws placed through the articular surface[76] or posterior-to-anterior screws placed retrograde into the fragment from the posterolateral column.[77] The placement of posterior-to-anterior screws has been shown to be biomechanically more stable and has the added clinical benefit of not violating the articular surface.[78] Posterior comminution or impaction of the posterior aspect of the lateral column may prevent anatomic reduction of the capitellum. These impaction fractures may require disimpaction and possibly bone grafting. In patients with severe posterior comminution that may compromise anterior articular fixation, supplemental posterior lateral column plating may be required.[72]

Capitellar fractures that involve a large portion of the trochlea also require anatomic reduction and rigid internal fixation. Typically, these fractures require a greater exposure for ORIF. Options for exposure of associated large trochlear fractures include LCL release, the use of a lateral epicondylar fracture to hinge open the elbow, a medial-sided approach, or an olecranon osteotomy. The authors of a recent biomechanical study examined the importance of the trochlea as an elbow stabilizer.[79] They reported that excision of an irreparable capitellar fracture may be considered if the collateral ligaments are intact; however, excision of some or all of the trochlea should not be performed.

Complications following the surgical management of capitellar and trochlear fractures include nonunion, malunion, osteonecrosis, posttraumatic arthritis, and elbow stiffness.

Olecranon Fractures

Epidemiology

Olecranon fractures represent 10% of all elbow fractures and about 0.9% of all fractures. They typically occur as a result of a fall directly onto the proximal ulna from a standing height. In younger patients, olecranon fractures usually occur secondary to a higher-energy injury. Associated ipsilateral upper extremity injuries occur in 22% of patients, with the most common being an associated radial head fracture (17%). Open olecranon fractures account for approximately 6% of all olecranon fractures.

Assessment and Classification

A standard radiograph is typically all that is required for diagnosis and management. In certain patients with high comminution or associated injuries, a CT scan may be helpful, especially when depressed articular segments are present at the base of the coronoid.

Several classification systems exist to describe olecranon fractures. The authors use the Mayo Classification, which is based on three parameters: elbow instability, fracture comminution, and fracture displacement. Type I fractures are nondisplaced. Type II fractures are displaced, but there is no associated elbow joint subluxation or dislocation, and type III fractures

demonstrate joint instability. A comminution modifier exists for each type: A for noncomminuted fractures and B for comminuted fractures.

Treatment

Nonsurgical management is reasonable for nondisplaced fractures of the olecranon. When nonsurgical management is elected, patients must be followed weekly for the first 3 to 4 weeks to ensure that fracture displacement does not occur. Nonsurgical management generally consists of immobilization in a long arm cast for 1 to 3 weeks followed by protected ROM. In older patients with significant medical comorbidities that preclude surgery, the results of nonsurgical treatment can yield satisfactory results even with the high rate of radiographic pseudarthrosis.

The treatment of choice of most displaced olecranon fractures is ORIF. The goal is to restore articular congruency and extensor mechanism integrity. The fixation construct should be stable enough to provide early functional rehabilitation with minimal need for protective immobilization.

Several fixation methods have been described for the ORIF of olecranon fractures. Tension band wiring with Kirschner wires has been consistently reported as safe and effective. This fixation method, however, is better suited to olecranon fractures with minimal comminution. The authors of a 2012 study reported that K-wires lodged into the anterior cortex of the ulna had a substantially lower rate of proximal migration and resultant gap formation at the fracture site. They also reported a lower rate of radiographic ulnohumeral arthrosis compared with intramedullary wires.[80] Placing K-wires through the anterior cortex of the ulna is not without risks; the authors of a 2011 cadaver study found that the K-wires had mean (standard deviation [SD]) distances of 16 mm (6 mm), 14 mm (5 mm), and 7 mm (4 mm) to the anterior interosseous nerve, the ulnar artery, and the proximal radioulnar joint, respectively. To avoid injury to important anterior structures, the authors recommended withdrawing K-wires a short distance before impacting them under the triceps tendon.[81]

The outcomes of tension band wiring are generally satisfactory, with good to excellent outcomes reported in 75% to 87% of patients. As with all surgical techniques, complications are reported and include hardware irritation, nonunion, malunion, stiffness, arthritis, and the need for revision surgery.

In patients with comminuted and/or unstable fracture patterns and in elderly patients with poor bone quality, plate fixation may be a better fixation option. Traditionally, olecranon fractures were fixed with 3.5-mm reconstruction plates; however, precontoured fracture-specific plates are now ubiquitous. The authors of a 2011 study, in a direct biomechanical comparison of interfragmentary compression achieved by tension band wiring versus plate fixation, found that plates provided significantly higher compression across the entire fracture surface as well as at the articular side

3: Upper Extremity

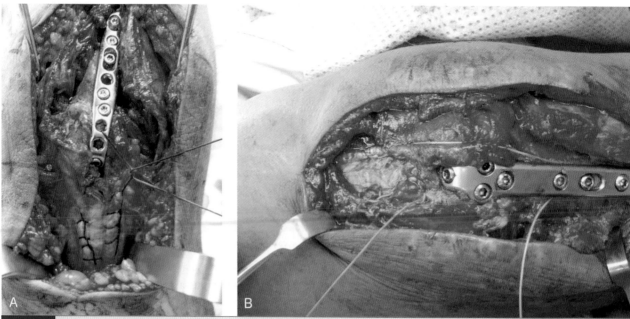

Figure 6 A high-strength fiber-type suture is used to secure the distal triceps tendon in a running locking configuration. The free suture ends are then passed through a hole in the plate (**A**) or under the plate (**B**), tensioned, and then tied, which offloads the olecranon fracture fragments from the pull of the extensor mechanism. The off-loading triceps suture technique is a load-sharing mechanism to decrease distraction forces on olecranon fracture fragments caused by the extensor mechanism. (Reproduced with permission from Izzi J, Athwal GS: An off-loading triceps suture for augmentation of plate fixation in comminuted osteoporotic fractures of the olecranon. *J Orthop Trauma* 2012;26[1]:59-61.)

of the fracture. In addition, the theoretic concept of compression at the articular side of the fracture with a true tension band construct was not found because overall articular-sided compression was reduced with a simulated triceps muscle contraction.[82]

The authors of a 2011 biomechanical study compared five precontoured olecranon plating systems and reported that locking plates and various screw designs offered no advantages in stabilizing osteoporotic olecranon fractures.[83] In addition, the authors of a 2012 study recommended limiting postoperative rehabilitation loads to less than 1.6 kg in an effort to minimize the adverse effects of torsional strains on olecranon healing.[84]

In an effort to decrease fixation failure in highly comminuted osteoporotic olecranon fractures in elderly patients, the authors of a 2012 article described an off-loading triceps suture technique for the augmentation of plate fixation.[85] The technique involves suturing the distal triceps tendon with a high-strength suture in a running locking fashion (**Figure 6**). The suture is then tied to the plate with enough tension to offload the pull of the triceps mechanism on the proximal olecranon fracture fragment.

Although several precontoured plating systems are available, not all are truly anatomic. The authors of a 2010 study reported that 96% of the patients had a sagittal plane angulation of the proximal ulna with a mean of 5.7° and located a mean of 47 mm distal to the olecranon tip. This angulation, referred to as the proximal ulna dorsal angulation, must be anatomically re-

duced and fixed to prevent malunion and potential maltracking of the radiocapitellar joint. Contralateral measurements of the dorsal ulna angulation may be helpful to evaluate the patient's unique anatomy in severely comminuted proximal ulnar fractures.[46]

In a 2012 anatomic study, researchers compared the morphologic features of the proximal ulna to several commercially available precontoured olecranon plates. The authors reported that some plates differed significantly from the normal morphologic features of the proximal ulna. The authors cautioned against using precontoured anatomic plates to obtain a reduction in comminuted fractures because the normal ulnar anatomic variability will not be re-created, leading to subtle malunion.[86]

In various outcome studies, good to excellent outcomes have been reported in 78% to 93% of patients treated with plate fixation.[64,65] Unfortunately, as with tension band wiring, painful and prominent hardware is reported in 20% to 47% of patients.

Finally, the authors of a 2012 study reported the outcomes of 10 patients with displaced olecranon fractures after no treatment or intentional nonsurgical management. At final follow-up, ROM was a mean of 117°, and eight patients declined surgical intervention.[87] The authors concluded that patients with nonunion after a displaced olecranon fracture that was managed nonsurgically have reasonable elbow function and uncommonly request surgical treatment.

Diaphyseal Forearm Fractures

Diaphyseal forearm fractures most commonly occur in younger male patients and are typically caused by high-energy trauma. In elderly patients, they occur as fragility fractures with a fall on the outstretched arm and have a higher incidence in women.

In patients with forearm fractures, neurovascular injury, injury to the interosseous membrane, and forearm compartment syndrome should be ruled out. Adjacent joints, such as the elbow, the distal radioulnar joint, and the proximal radioulnar joint, should be evaluated to recognize special fracture patterns or associated injuries.

Treatment

The treatment of choice in adult patients with diaphyseal forearm fractures is ORIF. Only in very rare, nondisplaced fractures and in patients whose general health is insufficient for surgical treatment, a long arm cast in 90° of elbow flexion in neutral forearm rotation can be applied.

Plate fixation is considered the preferred treatment of both-bone forearm fractures, and overall good results are reported. Several implant choices, such as conventional plates, dynamic compression plates, limited contact compression plates, and locking plates, are available. The current literature lacks good evidence to support one plating technique over another. New locking plate technology, although attractive in theory, has not demonstrated clinical or biomechanical superiority.[88-90]

Regarding implant position and surgical approach, radioulnar synostosis is associated with a single-incision approach. It is theorized that this results from dorsal plate position and the more extensive soft-tissue dissection that occurs when a single-incision approach is used.[91] Recently, the authors of a cadaver study reported that plates placed through a single incision came much closer together during forearm rotation than plates placed through a double-incision approach.[92] A double-incision approach is preferred by the authors for ORIF of both-bone forearm fractures.

Intramedullary nailing is often used in pediatric forearm fractures and has also been reported in adults. The potential advantages of interlocking intramedullary nailing over plate osteosynthesis are less soft-tissue damage and reported shorter surgical times. In general, longer postoperative immobilization times are reported but have not resulted in substantial problems with stiffness of the wrist or elbow.

Early studies of interlocking intramedullary nailing designs show encouraging results,[93] but the levels of evidence are low.[94,95] A recent study[96] showed good results after hybrid fixation with standard plating of the radial fracture and intramedullary nail fixation of the ulna. Further comparative studies are needed before these techniques can be recommended over conventional plate fixation.

Summary

There have been substantial changes to the understanding, evaluation, and treatment of fractures and dislocations of the elbow and forearm. In many cases, standardized treatment protocols have been developed to manage these complex injuries. Advances have been made with new surgical techniques and fracture-specific implants. Future research is required to determine the value of these advances and further investigate complex instability patterns, such as varus posteromedial rotatory instability.

Key Study Points

- Varus posteromedial rotatory instability with an often innocuous-appearing anteromedial coronoid facet fracture must be identified and treated appropriately.

- Nonsurgical management of elbow fractures and dislocations is indicated for elderly, low-demand patients. The role of nonsurgical management in terrible triad injuries and anteromedial coronoid facet fractures requires further investigation.

- TEA is indicated in the management of comminuted osteoporotic fractures of the distal humerus in elderly, low-demand patients.

Annotated References

1. Duckworth AD, Clement ND, Jenkins PJ, Aitken SA, Court-Brown CM, McQueen MM: The epidemiology of radial head and neck fractures. *J Hand Surg Am* 2012; 37(1):112-119.

   This is an epidemiologic investigation of the incidence of radial head and neck fractures in a prospective trauma database over a year. Associated injuries were more common in younger patients with higher-energy injuries. Level of evidence: IV.

2. Rineer CA, Guitton TG, Ring D: Radial head fractures: Loss of cortical contact is associated with concomitant fracture or dislocation. *J Shoulder Elbow Surg* 2010; 19(1):21-25.

   The authors retrospectively evaluated 121 radial head fractures displaced more than 2 mm for loss of cortical contact of at least one fragment and concomitant injuries. Among the group with loss of cortical contact, the likelihood of more complex and concomitant injuries was much higher (91% versus 33%) than in the group with cortical contact between the fragments. Level of evidence: IV.

3. Guitton TG, Ring D; Science of Variation Group: Inter-observer reliability of radial head fracture classification:

Two-dimensional compared with three-dimensional CT. *J Bone Joint Surg Am* 2011;93(21):2015-2021.

In this study, 85 orthopaedic surgeons were randomly assigned to evaluate 12 radial head fractures either by radiographs and two-dimensional CT scans or by radiographs and three-dimensional reconstructions of CT scans for fracture classification, fracture characteristics, and treatment recommendation. There was a small but significant decrease in intraobserver variation of the Broberg and Morrey classification with the addition of advanced imaging. CT allowed visualization of fracture fragments that were too small to repair, determination of the fragment number, and determination of central impaction. No differences were found between the remaining fracture characteristics and the surgeons' treatment recommendations. Level of evidence: I.

4. Chalidis BE, Papadopoulos PP, Sachinis NC, Dimitriou CG: Aspiration alone versus aspiration and bupivacaine injection in the treatment of undisplaced radial head fractures: A prospective randomized study. *J Shoulder Elbow Surg* 2009;18(5):676-679.

5. Akesson T, Herbertsson P, Josefsson PO, Hasserius R, Besjakov J, Karlsson MK: Primary nonoperative treatment of moderately displaced two-part fractures of the radial head. *J Bone Joint Surg Am* 2006;88(9):1909-1914.

6. Paschos NK, Mitsionis GI, Vasiliadis HS, Georgoulis AD: Comparison of early mobilization protocols in radial head fractures. *J Orthop Trauma* 2013;27(3):134-139.

This prospective, randomized trial compared three different rehabilitation protocols after nonsurgical treatment of 180 radial head fractures. The best results were noted in the early and late posttraumatic phase with early ROM exercises. Level of evidence: I.

7. Herbertsson P, Josefsson PO, Hasserius R, Karlsson C, Besjakov J, Karlsson MK: Displaced Mason type I fractures of the radial head and neck in adults: A fifteen- to thirty-three-year follow-up study. *J Shoulder Elbow Surg* 2005;14(1):73-77.

8. Beingessner DM, Dunning CE, Gordon KD, Johnson JA, King GJ: The effect of radial head fracture size on elbow kinematics and stability. *J Orthop Res* 2005;23(1):210-217.

9. Iftimie PP, Calmet Garcia J, de Loyola Garcia Forcada I, Gonzalez Pedrouzo JE, Giné Gomà J: Resection arthroplasty for radial head fractures: Long-term follow-up. *J Shoulder Elbow Surg* 2011;20(1):45-50.

This is a retrospective clinical and radiographic evaluation of 27 patients at a mean follow-up of 16.9 years after radial head excision for a radial head fracture. Good or excellent results were achieved in 96% of the patients; proximal radius migration was observed in 7 of 27 patients. The mean carrying angle of the elbow was increased significantly by 7°. Level of evidence: IV.

10. Antuña SA, Sánchez-Márquez JM, Barco R: Long-term results of radial head resection following isolated radial head fractures in patients younger than forty years old. *J Bone Joint Surg Am* 2010;92(3):558-566.

In this study, 26 patients younger than 40 years at the time of injury with isolated radial head fractures (Mason type II and III) treated with radial head excision were reviewed retrospectively at a minimum follow-up of 15 years. Good or excellent results according to the Mayo Elbow Performance Score were achieved in 92%. The elbow carrying angle was increased, and degenerative radiographic changes occurred in all patients with no clinical correlation. Level of evidence: IV.

11. Karlsson MK, Herbertsson P, Nordqvist A, Hasserius R, Besjakov J, Josefsson PO: Long-term outcome of displaced radial neck fractures in adulthood: 16-21 year follow-up of 5 patients treated with radial head excision. *Acta Orthop* 2009;80(3):368-370.

12. Schiffern A, Bettwieser SP, Porucznik CA, Crim JR, Tashjian RZ: Proximal radial drift following radial head resection. *J Shoulder Elbow Surg* 2011;20(3):426-433.

Thirteen patients who had undergone radial head resection for different injury patterns were retrospectively reviewed clinically and radiographically at a mean follow-up of 72 months. Significant medial and posterior migration of the radial stump as well as degenerative changes in the elbow joint were observed. No correlation between radiographic and clinical outcome was found. Level of evidence: IV.

13. Lindenhovius AL, Felsch Q, Doornberg JN, Ring D, Kloen P: Open reduction and internal fixation compared with excision for unstable displaced fractures of the radial head. *J Hand Surg Am* 2007;32(5):630-636.

14. Ikeda M, Sugiyama K, Kang C, Takagaki T, Oka Y: Comminuted fractures of the radial head: Comparison of resection and internal fixation. *J Bone Joint Surg Am* 2005;87(1):76-84.

15. Ring D, Quintero J, Jupiter JB: Open reduction and internal fixation of fractures of the radial head. *J Bone Joint Surg Am* 2002;84-B(10):1811-1815.

16. Grewal R, MacDermid JC, Faber KJ, Drosdowech DS, King GJ: Comminuted radial head fractures treated with a modular metallic radial head arthroplasty: Study of outcomes. *J Bone Joint Surg Am* 2006;88(10):2192-2200.

17. Dotzis A, Cochu G, Mabit C, Charissoux JL, Arnaud JP: Comminuted fractures of the radial head treated by the Judet floating radial head prosthesis. *J Bone Joint Surg Br* 2006;88-B(6):760-764.

18. Zunkiewicz MR, Clemente JS, Miller MC, Baratz ME, Wysocki RW, Cohen MS: Radial head replacement with a bipolar system: A minimum 2-year follow-up. *J Shoulder Elbow Surg* 2012;21(1):98-104.

This is a retrospective review of 29 patients with a minimum 2-year follow-up after radial head replacement with a bipolar smooth-stem radial head prosthesis. Clinically and radiographically, a stable elbow with slightly decreased ROM compared with the contralateral side was observed. The functional results were superior when the prosthesis was implanted for the treatment of an acute fracture rather than for the treatment of a chronic disorder. Level of evidence: IV.

19. Moon JG, Berglund LJ, Zachary D, An KN, O'Driscoll SW: Radiocapitellar joint stability with bipolar versus monopolar radial head prostheses. *J Shoulder Elbow Surg* 2009;18(5):779-784.

20. Moungondo F, El Kazzi W, van Riet R, Feipel V, Rooze M, Schuind F: Radiocapitellar joint contacts after bipolar radial head arthroplasty. *J Shoulder Elbow Surg* 2010;19(2):230-235.

    In six cadaver specimens, radiocapitellar contact was measured before and after implantation of a bipolar radial head prosthesis (Judet). Contact areas were independent of elbow position; systematic subluxation of the prosthesis over the lateral margin of the trochlea occurred in supination.

21. Flinkkilä T, Kaisto T, Sirniö K, Hyvönen P, Leppilahti J: Short- to mid-term results of metallic press-fit radial head arthroplasty in unstable injuries of the elbow. *J Bone Joint Surg Br* 2012;94(6):805-810.

    This is a retrospective clinical and radiographic review of 37 patients treated with a metallic press-fit radial head prosthesis for traumatic instability of the elbow with radial head fracture at a mean follow-up of 50 months. Loosening of the prosthesis was common, occurring in 12 patients and leading to removal in 9 patients. Functional scores were significantly lower in the affected elbow than in the unaffected elbow. Level of evidence: IV.

22. O'Driscoll SW, Herald JA: Forearm pain associated with loose radial head prostheses. *J Shoulder Elbow Surg* 2012;21(1):92-97.

    This study is a retrospective review of 14 patients undergoing revision of a radial head prosthesis (multiple prosthetic designs) and preoperative forearm pain. Radiographic evidence of loosening of the prosthesis was found in 12 of 14 patients. The authors concluded that in patients with an apparently ingrown prosthesis, forearm pain must be considered as a result of implant loosening, even in the absence of radiographic signs. Level of evidence: IV.

23. Fehringer EV, Burns EM, Knierim A, Sun J, Apker KA, Berg RE: Radiolucencies surrounding a smooth-stemmed radial head component may not correlate with forearm pain or poor elbow function. *J Shoulder Elbow Surg* 2009;18(2):275-278.

24. svan Riet RP, Sanchez-Sotelo J, Morrey BF: Failure of metal radial head replacement. *J Bone Joint Surg Br* 2010;92-B(5):661-667.

    This is a retrospective review of 44 patients undergoing revision surgery for radial head prosthesis failure. Different initial implants and implant designs (monopolar, bipolar, cemented, noncemented) were used in the index surgery. Indications for revision were painful loosening, stiffness, instability, and deep infection. Overlengthen-

ing of the prosthesis was detected in 11 patients. Level of evidence: IV.

25. Doornberg JN, Linzel DS, Zurakowski D, Ring D: Reference points for radial head prosthesis size. *J Hand Surg Am* 2006;31(1):53-57.

26. Rowland AS, Athwal GS, MacDermid JC, King GJ: Lateral ulnohumeral joint space widening is not diagnostic of radial head arthroplasty overstuffing. *J Hand Surg Am* 2007;32(5):637-641.

27. Frank SG, Grewal R, Johnson J, Faber KJ, King GJ, Athwal GS: Determination of correct implant size in radial head arthroplasty to avoid overlengthening. *J Bone Joint Surg Am* 2009;91(7):1738-1746.

28. Athwal GS, Rouleau DM, MacDermid JC, King GJ: Contralateral elbow radiographs can reliably diagnose radial head implant overlengthening. *J Bone Joint Surg Am* 2011;93(14):1339-1346.

    Bilateral elbow radiographs of 50 patients were compared for joint dimensions; no significant side-to-side differences could be detected. Subsequently, different sizes of radial head implants (leading to 0 to 8 mm overlengthening) were inserted into four cadaveric elbows sequentially (120 scenarios). Joint dimension measurements were obtained from standard radiographs and compared with the contralateral, intact specimen radiographs. Successful prediction of implant size within 2 mm based on side-to-side comparison of the joint dimensions was obtained in 87% of the scenarios. Level of evidence: III.

29. Rosenblatt Y, Young C, MacDermid JC, King GJ: Osteotomy of the head of the radius for partial articular malunion. *J Bone Joint Surg Br* 2009;91-B(10):1341-1346.

30. Sabo MT, Shannon H, De Luce S, et al: Elbow kinematics after radiocapitellar arthroplasty. *J Hand Surg Am* 2012;37(5):1024-1032.

    This is a biomechanical evaluation of elbow kinematics before and after insertion of a radiocapitellar arthroplasty and sectioning of the MCL. In the setting of an intact MCL, no differences in kinematics occurred. After secctioning of the MCL, more valgus angulation and more external ulnar rotation in the pronated-valgus loaded position was observed.

31. Stoneback JW, Owens BD, Sykes J, Athwal GS, Pointer L, Wolf JM: Incidence of elbow dislocations in the United States population. *J Bone Joint Surg Am* 2012;94(3):240-245.

    The authors performed database research to examine the incidence of elbow dislocation in the United States. The highest incidence occurred in patients age 10 and 19 years; 44.5% occurred in sports. The incidence of elbow dislocations was estimated to be 5.21 per 100,000 per year. Level of evidence: II.

32. Fitzpatrick MJ, Diltz M, McGarry MH, Lee TQ: A new fracture model for "terrible triad" injuries of the elbow:

Influence of forearm rotation on injury patterns. *J Orthop Trauma* 2012;26(10):591-596.

In this biomechanical study, 14 elbow specimens were tested with axial load to failure, 7 in pronation and 7 in supination. In pronation, a terrible triad injury was observed in 6 of 7 elbows. In supination, 6 of 7 elbows dislocated without fracture; the remaining elbow sustained a terrible triad injury. Lateral ligaments failed first with the ulna in external rotation; medial structures failed first with the ulna in internal rotation.

33. McKee MD, Schemitsch EH, Sala MJ, O'Driscoll SW: The pathoanatomy of lateral ligamentous disruption in complex elbow instability. *J Shoulder Elbow Surg* 2003; 12(4):391-396.

34. Regan W, Morrey B: Fractures of the coronoid process of the ulna. *J Bone Joint Surg Am* 1989;71(9):1348-1354.

35. O'Driscoll SW, Jupiter JB, Cohen MS, Ring D, McKee MD: Difficult elbow fractures: Pearls and pitfalls. *Instr Course Lect* 2003;52:113-134.

36. Guitton TG, Ring D: Nonsurgically treated terrible triad injuries of the elbow: Report of four cases. *J Hand Surg Am* 2010;35(3):464-467.

In this case series, three of four patients with terrible triad injuries showed good results after nonsurgical treatment. The authors concluded that the criteria for a good outcome include small and only minimally displaced radial and coronoid fractures as well as good elbow alignment. Level of evidence: IV.

37. Mathew PK, Athwal GS, King GJ: Terrible triad injury of the elbow: Current concepts. *J Am Acad Orthop Surg* 2009;17(3):137-151.

38. Beingessner DM, Dunning CE, Stacpoole RA, Johnson JA, King GJ: The effect of coronoid fractures on elbow kinematics and stability. *Clin Biomech (Bristol, Avon)* 2007;22(2):183-190.

39. Moon JG, Zobitz ME, An KN, O'Driscoll SW: Optimal screw orientation for fixation of coronoid fractures. *J Orthop Trauma* 2009;23(4):277-280.

40. Garrigues GE, Wray WH III, Lindenhovius AL, Ring DC, Ruch DS: Fixation of the coronoid process in elbow fracture-dislocations. *J Bone Joint Surg Am* 2011; 93(20):1873-1881.

This is a retrospective chart review of 40 patients after surgical treatment of a terrible triad injury with either ORIF (12 patients) for coronoid fracture fixation or the suture lasso technique (28 patients). Intraoperative and postoperative stability was assessed, and the lasso technique showed better results. Hardware failure rates and the prevalence of malunion or nonunion were higher with ORIF. Level of evidence: III.

41. Rodriguez-Martin J, Pretell-Mazzini J, Andres-Esteban EM, Larrainzar-Garijo R: Outcomes after terrible triads of the elbow treated with the current surgical protocols:

A review. *Int Orthop* 2011;35(6):851-860.

This review article analyzes the results in 137 elbow triad injuries of five studies treated using current protocols. These include fixation of the coronoid fracture, repair or replacement of the radial head, and repair of the lateral ligament complex. MCL repair and hinged external fixation was used only in cases with residual instability. Mean flexion ROM was 111.4°, mean overall flexion was 132.5°, and forearm rotation ROM was 135.5°. Even if treatment achieves satisifiying results, complications, including joint stiffness, ulnar nerve symptoms, or posttraumatic arthritis, can occur.

42. Pipicelli JG, Chinchalkar SJ, Grewal R, Athwal GS: Rehabilitation considerations in the management of terrible triad injury to the elbow. *Tech Hand Up Extrem Surg* 2011;15(4):198-208.

This article provides a review of key concepts in postoperative rehabilitation after terrible triad injuries. Level of evidence: III.

43. Adams JE, Sanchez-Sotelo J, Kallina CF IV, Morrey BF, Steinmann SP: Fractures of the coronoid: Morphology based upon computer tomography scanning. *J Shoulder Elbow Surg* 2012;21(6):782-788.

This retrospective analysis of CT scans performed for elbow trauma revealed 52 coronoid fractures over a 2-year period. Five different coronoid fracture patterns were identified: tip (29%), midtransverse (24%), basal (23%), anteromedial (17%), and anterolateral (7%). Good interobserver and intraobserver reliability was shown. Level of evidence: III.

44. Doornberg JN, Ring DC: Fracture of the anteromedial facet of the coronoid process. *J Bone Joint Surg Am* 2006;88(10):2216-2224.

45. Grechenig W, Clement H, Pichler W, Tesch NP, Windisch G: The influence of lateral and anterior angulation of the proximal ulna on the treatment of a Monteggia fracture: An anatomical cadaver study. *J Bone Joint Surg Br* 2007;89-B(6):836-838.

46. Rouleau DM, Faber KJ, Athwal GS: The proximal ulna dorsal angulation: A radiographic study. *J Shoulder Elbow Surg* 2010;19(1):26-30.

In 100 bilateral elbow radiographs, the proximal ulnar dorsal angulation (PUDA) and the olecranon tip-to-apex distance to the PUDA were measured; 96% of the patients had a sagittal plane angulation to the proximal ulna, with a mean of 5.7°. The authors recommended to anatomically reduce and fix the PUDA to prevent malunion and potential maltracking of the radiocapitellar joint.

47. Robinson CM, Hill RM, Jacobs N, Dall G, Court-Brown CM: Adult distal humeral metaphyseal fractures: Epidemiology and results of treatment. *J Orthop Trauma* 2003;17(1):38-47.

48. Gofton WT, Macdermid JC, Patterson SD, Faber KJ, King GJ: Functional outcome of AO type C distal humeral fractures. *J Hand Surg Am* 2003;28(2):294-308.

49. Doornberg J, Lindenhovius A, Kloen P, van Dijk CN, Zurakowski D, Ring D: Two and three-dimensional computed tomography for the classification and management of distal humeral fractures: Evaluation of reliability and diagnostic accuracy. *J Bone Joint Surg Am* 2006;88(8):1795-1801.

50. Zalavras CG, Vercillo MT, Jun BJ, Otarodifard K, Itamura JM, Lee TQ: Biomechanical evaluation of parallel versus orthogonal plate fixation of intra-articular distal humerus fractures. *J Shoulder Elbow Surg* 2011;20(1): 12-20.

    This biomechanical study evaluated the stiffness to cyclic loading, the ultimate torque under loading to failure, and screw loosening of distal humeral fracture fixation in 14 paired human elbow specimens. Parallel plating constructs showed significantly better biomechanical properties compared with orthogonal constructs.

51. Arnander MW, Reeves A, MacLeod IA, Pinto TM, Khaleel A: A biomechanical comparison of plate configuration in distal humerus fractures. *J Orthop Trauma* 2008;22(5):332-336.

52. Koonce RC, Baldini TH, Morgan SJ: Are conventional reconstruction plates equivalent to precontoured locking plates for distal humerus fracture fixation? A biomechanics cadaver study. *Clin Biomech (Bristol, Avon)* 2012;27(7):697-701.

    In this biomechanical study, the authors compared three types of distal humeral fracture fixation for stiffness in sagittal bending, axial compression, and torsion. Thirty distal humeral specimens were stripped of soft tissue, osteotomized, and fixed with either perpendicular nonlocking or perpendicular versus parallel locking plates. No significant differences were found.

53. Shin SJ, Sohn HS, Do NH: A clinical comparison of two different double plating methods for intraarticular distal humerus fractures. *J Shoulder Elbow Surg* 2010;19(1): 2-9.

    In this study, 35 patients with distal, intra-articular humeral fractures were prospectively randomized into two treatment groups: orthogonal plating with either 3.5-mm reconstruction plates or precontoured plates or parallel plating with precontoured plates. All of the implants were made of titanium. No statistically significant differences in outcome were seen, but two nonunions occurred in the orthogonal group. Level of evidence: II.

54. Athwal GS, Hoxie SC, Rispoli DM, Steinmann SP: Precontoured parallel plate fixation of AO/OTA type C distal humerus fractures. *J Orthop Trauma* 2009;23(8): 575-580.

55. Theivendran K, Duggan PJ, Deshmukh SC: Surgical treatment of complex distal humeral fractures: Functional outcome after internal fixation using precontoured anatomic plates. *J Shoulder Elbow Surg* 2010; 19(4):524-532.

    This retrospective case series reviews the results of 16 patients after parallel precontoured locking plate fix-

ation of distal humeral fractures after a mean follow-up of 35 months. Good results in clinical scoring systems with some decrease in grip strength and no nonunions were reported. Level of evidence: IV.

56. Vennettilli M, Athwal GS: Parallel versus orthogonal plating for distal humerus fractures. *J Hand Surg Am* 2012;37(4):819-820.

    Current concepts related to parallel versus orthogonal plating techniques in distal humeral fractures are reviewed. Level of evidence: IV.

57. Erpelding JM, Mailander A, High R, Mormino MA, Fehringer EV: Outcomes following distal humeral fracture fixation with an extensor mechanism-on approach. *J Bone Joint Surg Am* 2012;94(6):548-553.

    This is a retrospective review of 29 patients who underwent ORIF for a distal humeral fracture with a triceps-on approach with either parallel or orthogonal plating. Excellent clinical and functional results were reported, with a median loss of triceps strength of 10%. Level of evidence: IV.

58. Huang JI, Paczas M, Hoyen HA, Vallier HA: Functional outcome after open reduction internal fixation of intra-articular fractures of the distal humerus in the elderly. *J Orthop Trauma* 2011;25(5):259-265.

    This is a retrospective clinical and radiographic review of 14 patients older than 65 years who underwent ORIF for distal humeral fractures. The mean follow-up was 51 months. Reasonable ROM was achieved in the patients with stable fixation and fracture union, but persistent pain was also observed. Level of evidence: IV.

59. Athwal GS, Goetz TJ, Pollock JW, Faber KJ: Prosthetic replacement for distal humerus fractures. *Orthop Clin North Am* 2008;39(2):201-212, vi.

60. Popovic D, King GJ: Fragility fractures of the distal humerus: What is the optimal treatment? *J Bone Joint Surg Br* 2012;94-B(1):16-22.

    This review article discusses the management and current trends in the treatment of fragility fractures of the distal humerus. Surgical fixation and early mobilization is generally the treatment of choice. The relative indications for and results of total elbow replacement versus internal fixation are discussed.

61. McKee MD, Veillette CJ, Hall JA, et al: A multicenter, prospective, randomized, controlled trial of open reduction—internal fixation versus total elbow arthroplasty for displaced intra-articular distal humeral fractures in elderly patients. *J Shoulder Elbow Surg* 2009;18(1):3-12.

62. Egol KA, Tsai P, Vazques O, Tejwani NC: Comparison of functional outcomes of total elbow arthroplasty vs plate fixation for distal humerus fractures in osteoporotic elbows. *Am J Orthop (Belle Mead NJ)* 2011;40(2): 67-71.

    This is a retrospective clinical and radiographic review of 20 patients older than 60 years who were treated with either semiconstrained, cemented TEA (9 patients) or ORIF (11 patients) for distal humeral fractures. One

3: Upper Extremity

asymptomatic nonunion and four radiographic loosenings were observed. No significant difference in functional outcomes was observed. Level of evidence: III.

63. Srinivasan K, Agarwal M, Matthews SJ, Giannoudis PV: Fractures of the distal humerus in the elderly: Is internal fixation the treatment of choice? *Clin Orthop Relat Res* 2005;434:222-230.

64. Zagorski JB, Jennings JJ, Burkhalter WE, Uribe JW: Comminuted intraarticular fractures of the distal humeral condyles: Surgical vs. nonsurgical treatment. *Clin Orthop Relat Res* 1986;202:197-204.

65. Wiggers JK, Brouwer KM, Helmerhorst GT, Ring D: Predictors of diagnosis of ulnar neuropathy after surgically treated distal humerus fractures. *J Hand Surg Am* 2012;37(6):1168-1172.

This retrospective study examined the incidence and predisposing factors for the onset of postoperative ulnar neuropathy. In 107 patients with distal humeral fractures, ulnar neuropathy developed in 17 patients (16%). The only risk factor identified was the type of fracture. This result was independent of possible ulnar nerve transposition. Level of evidence: III.

66. Vazquez O, Rutgers M, Ring DC, Walsh M, Egol KA: Fate of the ulnar nerve after operative fixation of distal humerus fractures. *J Orthop Trauma* 2010;24(7):395-399.

This is a retrospective chart review of ulnar neuropathy in 69 patients undergoing ORIF of distal humeral fractures who had no dysfunction preoperatively. The incidence was 10.1% in the immediate postoperative period and 16% at final follow-up, and no predisposing factors, including surgical treatment, were identified. Level of evidence: IV.

67. Chen RC, Harris DJ, Leduc S, Borrelli JJ Jr, Tornetta P III, Ricci WM: Is ulnar nerve transposition beneficial during open reduction internal fixation of distal humerus fractures? *J Orthop Trauma* 2010;24(7):391-394.

This multicenter retrospective cohort study compared the incidence of ulnar neuropathy with and without ulnar nerve transposition during ORIF of distal humeral fractures. The results indicated that patients who underwent an ulnar nerve transposition at the time of ORIF had almost four times the incidence of postoperative ulnar neuritis than those who did not undergo transposition. Level of evidence: III.

68. Rebuzzi E, Vascellari A, Schiavetti S: The use of parallel pre-contoured plates in the treatment of A and C fractures of the distal humerus. *Musculoskelet Surg* 2010;94(1):9-16.

The authors performed a retrospective review of 13 patients with distal humeral fractures after ORIF with pre-contoured locking plates (7 type A, 6 type C). Excellent results were achieved in 6 of 7 type A patients and 5 of 6 type C patients. No nonunions occurred, but complications were observed in 6 of 13 patients. Level of evidence: IV.

69. Atalar AC, Demirhan M, Salduz A, Kılıçoğlu O, Seyahi A: Functional results of the parallel-plate technique for complex distal humerus fractures. *Acta Orthop Traumatol Turc* 2009;43(1):21-27.

70. Liu JJ, Ruan HJ, Wang JG, Fan CY, Zeng BF: Double-column fixation for type C fractures of the distal humerus in the elderly. *J Shoulder Elbow Surg* 2009;18(4):646-651.

71. Hamid N, Ashraf N, Bosse MJ, et al: Radiation therapy for heterotopic ossification prophylaxis acutely after elbow trauma: A prospective randomized study. *J Bone Joint Surg Am* 2010;92(11):2032-2038.

In a prospective randomized study, patients having ORIF for distal humeral fractures or elbow fracture-dislocation with and without postoperative radiation to prevent heterotopic ossification were compared. The study was terminated prior to completion because of the high number of adverse events: 38% of patients in the radiation group (versus 4% in the nonradiation group) developed nonunions, but no significance in the prevalence of heterotopic ossification could be observed. Level of evidence: I.

72. Dubberley JH, Faber KJ, Macdermid JC, Patterson SD, King GJ: Outcome after open reduction and internal fixation of capitellar and trochlear fractures. *J Bone Joint Surg Am* 2006;88(1):46-54.

73. Watts AC, Morris A, Robinson CM: Fractures of the distal humeral articular surface. *J Bone Joint Surg Br* 2007;89-B(4):510-515.

74. Ring D, Jupiter JB, Gulotta L: Articular fractures of the distal part of the humerus. *J Bone Joint Surg Am* 2003;85(2):232-238.

75. Puloski S, Kemp K, Sheps D, Hildebrand K, Donaghy J: Closed reduction and early mobilization in fractures of the humeral capitellum. *J Orthop Trauma* 2012;26(1):62-65.

This is a case series of seven patients treated with closed reduction, casting, and early mobilization for type I (Hahn-Steinthal) capitellar fractures. All patients achieved bony union and rated their result as excellent (five patients) or good (two patients) with a mean ROM for flexion and extension of 126° and no substantial loss of forearm rotation. Level of evidence: IV.

76. Mighell M, Virani NA, Shannon R, Echols EL Jr, Badman BL, Keating CJ: Large coronal shear fractures of the capitellum and trochlea treated with headless compression screws. *J Shoulder Elbow Surg* 2010;19(1):38-45.

This is a retrospective review of 18 patients with Dubberley type IA (11 patients) or type IIA (7 patients) fractures who underwent ORIF with anterior-to-posterior countersunk screws through the articular surface (mean follow-up, 26 months). Good or excellent results were obtained in 94.4% of the patients, not correlating with the radiographic finding of osteonecrosis (three patients) and osteoarthritis (five patients). Level of evidence: IV.

77. Singh AP, Singh AP, Vaishya R, Jain A, Gulati D: Fractures of capitellum: A review of 14 cases treated by open reduction and internal fixation with Herbert screws. *Int Orthop* 2010;34(6):897-901.

In this retrospective review of 14 patients who underwent ORIF for capitellar fractures (11 patients, all Morrey types) or nonunions (3 patients) with an average follow-up of 4.8 years, all of the patients had a stable, pain-free elbow with a good ROM at final follow-up without radiographic signs of osteonecrosis. Level of evidence: IV.

78. Elkowitz SJ, Polatsch DB, Egol KA, Kummer FJ, Koval KJ: Capitellum fractures: A biomechanical evaluation of three fixation methods. *J Orthop Trauma* 2002;16(7): 503-506.

79. Sabo MT, Fay K, McDonald CP, Ferreira LM, Johnson JA, King GJ: Effect of coronal shear fractures of the distal humerus on elbow kinematics and stability. *J Shoulder Elbow Surg* 2010;19(5):670-680.

This biomechanical investigation of ulnohumeral and radiocapitellar kinematics of eight elbow specimens with sequential resection of capitellar fragments, simulation of coronal shear fractures of the capitellum, and subsequent dynamic testing showed that the capitellum alone does not contribute to elbow stability, whereas the resection of trochlear parts resulted in multiplanar instability.

80. van der Linden SC, van Kampen A, Jaarsma RL: K-wire position in tension-band wiring technique affects stability of wires and long-term outcome in surgical treatment of olecranon fractures. *J Shoulder Elbow Surg* 2012;21(3):405-411.

In this retrospective evaluation of 59 patients with tension-band wiring of olecranal fractures, intramedullary K-wire placement was compared to K-wires that engaged the anterior cortex of the proximal ulna. Bicortical K-wires showed a substantially lower rate of proximal migration and resultant gap formation at the fracture site, resulting in a lower rate of radiographic ulnohumeral arthrosis. Level of evidence: III.

81. Catalano LW III, Crivello K, Lafer MP, Chia B, Barron OA, Glickel SZ: Potential dangers of tension band wiring of olecranon fractures: An anatomic study. *J Hand Surg Am* 2011;36(10):1659-1662.

This cadaveric study examined the proximity of anatomic structures to bicortical K-wires on 15 intact proximal ulnas. The K-wires had mean (SD) distances of 16 mm (6 mm), 14 mm (5 mm), and 7 mm (4 mm) to the anterior interosseous nerve, the ulnar artery, and the proximal radioulnar joint, respectively. The authors recommended withdrawing K-wires before impacting them under the triceps tendon and proposed safe insertion angles.

82. Wilson J, Bajwa A, Kamath V, Rangan A: Biomechanical comparison of interfragmentary compression in transverse fractures of the olecranon. *J Bone Joint Surg Br* 2011;93-B(2):245-250.

This biomechanical study compared interfragmentary compression achieved by tension band wiring versus plate fixation on 10 bone models. Plates provided significantly higher compression across the entire fracture surface as well as at the articular side of the fracture. Overall, articular-sided compression was reduced with a simulated triceps muscle contraction.

83. Edwards SG, Martin BD, Fu RH, et al: Comparison of olecranon plate fixation in osteoporotic bone: Do current technologies and designs make a difference? *J Orthop Trauma* 2011;25(5):306-311.

In this biomechanical cadaver comparative study, the authors tested five precontoured olecranon plating systems in 30 osteoporotic elbows. Advantages from innovations such as locking plates and various screw designs in stabilizing osteoporotic olecranon fractures were not observed.

84. Edwards SG, Martin BD, Fu RH, et al: Quantifying and comparing torsional strains after olecranon plating. *Injury* 2012;43(6):712-717.

The authors performed a biomechanical cadaveric study of torsion in physiologic loading on 50 cadaveric elbows with simulated comminuted olecranon fractures and five different plate systems. Three of five plates allowed less than 1° of torsion up to loading of 1.6 kg; the remaining two plates allowed for consequently higher torsion. Therefore, limiting postoperative rehabilitation loads to 1.6 kg was recommended for all plates.

85. Izzi J, Athwal GS: An off-loading triceps suture for augmentation of plate fixation in comminuted osteoporotic fractures of the olecranon. *J Orthop Trauma* 2012; 26(1):59-61.

This article describes an offloading triceps suture technique. This technique is a load-sharing mechanism to decrease distraction forces caused by the extensor mechanism on comminuted osteopenic olecranon fracture fragments managed with plate fixation. Level of evidence: IV.

86. Puchwein P, Schildhauer TA, Schöffmann S, Heidari N, Windisch G, Pichler W: Three-dimensional morphometry of the proximal ulna: A comparison to currently used anatomically preshaped ulna plates. *J Shoulder Elbow Surg* 2012;21(8):1018-1023.

This CT study examined 40 human elbow specimens. The mean dorsal hook angle of 95.3° and its mean distance from the olecranon tip of 24.7 mm showed significant gender-specific differences (male, 92.2° and 26.1 mm; female, 98.3° and 23.4 mm). The investigated precontoured plates did not offer adequate shapes in most cases, and their use is therefore not routinely recommended to restore proximal ulna anatomy in comminuted fractures.

87. Bruinsma W, Lindenhovius A, McKee M, Athwal GS, Ring D: Non-union of non-operatively treated displaced olecranon fractures. *J Shoulder Elbow Surg* 2012;4: 273-276.

This is a case series of 10 patients (mean age, 59 years) with a nonunion of a displaced fracture of the olecranon. Mean flexion/extension ROM was 117°, and mean forearm rotation ROM was 172°. Two of 10 patients had difficulties in activities of daily life; the remaining 8

3: Upper Extremity

patients declined surgical treatment of the nonunion. Level of evidence: IV.

88. Gardner MJ, Brophy RH, Campbell D, et al: The mechanical behavior of locking compression plates compared with dynamic compression plates in a cadaver radius model. *J Orthop Trauma* 2005;19(9):597-603.

89. Henle P, Ortlieb K, Kuminack K, Mueller CA, Suedkamp NP: Problems of bridging plate fixation for the treatment of forearm shaft fractures with the locking compression plate. *Arch Orthop Trauma Surg* 2011; 131(1):85-91.

    The authors performed a retrospective review of 53 patients who underwent bridging plate fixation with locking compression plates for forearm shaft fractures with a mean follow-up of 23.3 months. Complications at hardware removal occurred in 7 of 10 patients. Clinical and radiologic evaluation showed results that were comparable with those of conventional implants. Level of evidence: IV.

90. Saikia K, Bhuyan S, Bhattacharya T, Borgohain M, Jitesh P, Ahmed F: Internal fixation of fractures of both bones forearm: Comparison of locked compression and limited contact dynamic compression plate. *Indian J Orthop* 2011;45(5):417-421.

    This prospective comparative study compared the clinical, functional, and radiologic outcomes in 36 patients with both-bone forearm fractures treated with either locking compression plates or limited-contact dynamic compression plating. The mean follow-up was 2.1 years. No significant differences in outcomes or complication rates were found. Level of evidence: II.

91. Bauer G, Arand M, Mutschler W: Post-traumatic radioulnar synostosis after forearm fracture osteosynthesis. *Arch Orthop Trauma Surg* 1991;110(3):142-145.

92. Dietz SO, Müller LP, Gercek E, Hartmann F, Rommens PM: Volar and dorsal mid-shaft forearm plating using DCP and LC-DCP: Interference with the interosseous membrane and forearm-kinematics. *Acta Chir Belg* 2010;110(1):60-65.

    This biomechanical study evaluated possible interosseous membrane damage and plate malpositioning in dorsal-sided versus flexor-sided plating for both-bone forearm fractures in 16 human cadavers. The smallest distances of the plates were much smaller with dorsal plating (17.23 mm versus 5.04 mm). The authors conclude that even minimal plate malposition could have a bigger effect in dorsal plating.

93. Lee YH, Lee SK, Chung MS, Baek GH, Gong HS, Kim KH: Interlocking contoured intramedullary nail fixation for selected diaphyseal fractures of the forearm in adults. *J Bone Joint Surg Am* 2008;90(9):1891-1898.

94. Bansal H: Intramedullary fixation of forearm fractures with new locked nail. *Indian J Orthop* 2011;45(5): 410-416.

    This is a retrospective review of 32 patients who underwent intramedullary nailing of both-bone forearm fractures in adolescence with a mean follow-up of 14.1 years. The union rate was 98%. Limitations in ROM occurred in 15.6% of the patients but only in patients younger than 15 years and was not associated with a change in radial bow. Level of evidence: IV.

95. Hong G, Cong-Feng L, Hui-Peng S, Cun-Yi F, Bing-Fang Z: Treatment of diaphyseal forearm nonunions with interlocking intramedullary nails. *Clin Orthop Relat Res* 2006;450:186-192.

96. Behnke NM, Redjal HR, Nguyen VT, Zinar DM: Internal fixation of diaphyseal fractures of the forearm: A retrospective comparison of hybrid fixation versus dual plating. *J Orthop Trauma* 2012;26(11):611-616.

    This is a retrospective evaluation of 56 patients with both-bone forearm fractures with either dual plating (27 patients) or hybrid fixation (intramedullary nailing of the ulna, plating of the radius; 29 patients). Comparable results concerning bony union, complications, and functional outcomes were achieved in both groups. Level of evidence: IV.

3: Upper Extremity

Chapter 30

Elbow Instability and Reconstruction

April D. Armstrong, MD   Anand Murthi, MD

Elbow Arthritis

Osteoarthritis

Symptomatic osteoarthritis of the elbow is relatively rare and affects less than 2% of the population.[1] The average age of presentation is 50 years, with men affected more often than women by a ratio of 4:1. Hand dominance and heavy manual labor are associated with primary elbow osteoarthritis. Osteoarthritis of the elbow is different from osteoarthritis of other joints in that the articular cartilage is relatively preserved and is characterized by peripheral osteophyte formation, capsular contracture, and loose body formation. Rarely, advanced disease presents with joint space narrowing. The periarticular hypertrophic osteophytes act as a mechanical block, restricting flexion and extension end range of motion.

Patients typically present with a loss of terminal extension and painful catching or clicking of the elbow, or sometimes even locking of the elbow. The pain is more pronounced at terminal flexion and extension, and the patient is relatively pain free through the midrange arc of motion. Forearm rotation is relatively preserved until later in the disease process. Ulnar neuropathy may be present in 50% of patients.

Radiographs show typical osteophyte formation at the coronoid process (which extends medially), coronoid fossa, radial head, radial fossa, olecranon tip, and olecranon fossa. Joint space at the ulnohumeral and radiocapitellar joints may be narrowed but relatively preserved. Loose bodies may also be evident. CT may be useful for surgical planning to better assess osteophyte formation (Figure 1).

Nonsurgical treatment includes rest, activity modification to avoid terminal range of motion, medications such as NSAIDs, and possibly joint injections. Surgical indications include pain that has failed to respond to nonsurgical treatment, loss of motion that interferes with activities of daily living, and painful locking or catching of the elbow. Joint-sparing approaches—such as open or arthroscopic débridement with the excision of osteophytes, capsular release, and the removal of loose bodies—are the mainstay of surgical treatment. Interposition arthroplasty and joint arthroplasty are rarely indicated.

The classic open débridement procedure is Outerbridge-Kashiwagi arthroplasty. This procedure requires a posterior approach in which a circular trephine is used to open the olecranon fossa to remove the osteophyte on the tip of the olecranon. The elbow is then maximally flexed to allow for débridement of the coronoid tip, and the anterior joint is swept with a finger for any loose bodies. The limitations of this procedure are that it does not allow for a complete an-

Dr. Armstrong or an immediate family member has received nonincome support (such as equipment or services), commercially derived honoraria, or other non–research-related funding (such as paid travel) from Zimmer and serves as a board member, owner, officer, or committee member of the American Shoulder and Elbow Surgeons. Dr. Murthi or an immediate family member serves as a paid consultant to or is an employee of Zimmer, Ascension, and Arthrex.

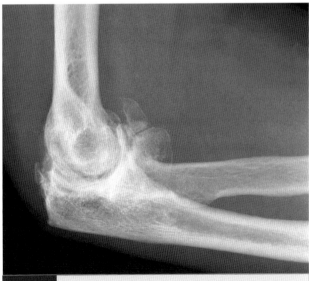

Figure 1   Lateral radiograph of the elbow with typical osteophyte formation. (Reproduced from Armstrong AD: Arthritides of the elbow, in Lieberman JR, ed: *AAOS Comprehensive Orthopaedic Review*. Rosemont, IL, American Academy of Orthopaedic Surgeons, 2009, pp 871-876.)

3: Upper Extremity

terior release; osteophyte removal at the radial fossa, resulting in less increase in flexion; or complete removal of osteophytes in the olecranon fossa, which is more oval in shape with osteophytes along the far medial and lateral columns of the fossa. A column procedure or the ulnohumeral arthroplasty procedure—a formal capsular release—currently is more commonly used to allow for a more thorough débridement.[2-5] Any limited or combined medial, lateral, or posterior approach to effectively remove the osteophytes is acceptable.

The arthroscopic osteocapsular arthroplasty procedure has also evolved, which allows for an extensive débridement of the osteophytes and capsular release. This demanding procedure requires the surgeon to have advanced skills in elbow arthroscopy. The reported short-term results of this procedure have shown 30° to 60° of improvement in arc of motion and patient pain and satisfaction.[6-9] The long-term durability of the procedure is unknown.

A comparison of open and arthroscopic débridement procedures showed that patients who underwent an open approach experienced greater improvement of flexion, whereas patients who underwent an arthroscopic approach experienced greater reduction in pain. No difference was found in terms of the overall perceived effectiveness of the surgery.[10] Regardless of whether the procedure is done open or arthroscopically, ulnar nerve decompression or transposition and release of the posterior bundle of the medial collateral ligament should be considered for patients who have less than 90° to 100° of elbow flexion.[2]

Posttraumatic Arthritis

Often underappreciated, subtle and obvious posttraumatic elbow arthritis remains challenging to treat. Many potential diagnoses exist, including radiocapitellar, ulnohumeral, and combined arthritis that may lead to decline in function after trauma. These arthritic injuries are often delayed in presentation after elbow fractures, especially nonsurgically treated radial head fractures and elbow dislocations with coronoid injuries.

Radiocapitellar arthritis, most commonly identified after elbow trauma, often causes pain with motion and active functional activities. The condition is most commonly seen after nonsurgically treated radial head and/or capitellar fractures. Evaluation consists of a thorough history and examination based on range of motion and stability of the elbow. Therapeutic treatments are based on improving range of motion while decreasing discomfort. Elbow stiffness, a major complaint with these injuries, is often related to extrinsic soft-tissue contractures along with intrinsic bony and/or cartilaginous irregularities to the normal anatomy. Imaging modalities, especially three-dimensional CT, provide an excellent tool for preoperative evaluation.

Various surgical options for radiocapitellar arthritis exist: from débridement to arthroplasty. Because these patients are often young and active with high functional demands, nonarthroplasty alternatives are often the initial treatment choice. Arthroscopic or open os-

teocapsular arthroplasty (usually without radial head excision) offers the advantages of improving motion while sparing the joint surfaces. One study reported on 25 elbows treated successfully with arthroscopic elbow débridement while maintaining the radial head with improvements in pain and function.[7] These patients often did well, especially in the absence of proximal radioulnar joint symptoms or extreme stiffness. In a retrospective study, 36 patients underwent arthroscopic radial head excision and/or ulnohumeral joint débridement. Those undergoing excision alone had greater functional improvements. This finding may have resulted from baseline differences between elbow groups.[11] Disrupting ligamentous/capsular structures with a radial resection may lead to increased ulnohumeral stress and elbow dysfunction. However, intrinsic stiffness and pain from radial head and/or capitellar arthritic malunion will benefit from radial head excision.

Anconeus arthroplasty offers a salvage technique for radiocapitellar arthrosis in the setting of proximal radioulnar disease or axial instability.[12] This interposition resurfacing maintains lateral column length. Concomitant radial head excision and anconeus placement at the radiocapitellar joint may lead to improved function. Functional motion is allowed while the risk of unreliable prosthetic implantation is avoided.

A prospective study of 20 patients with débridement and lateral resurfacing prosthesis revealed improved pain relief, motion, and function with 100% implant survival at a mean of 22.6 months follow-up.[13] This study demonstrated that using a metallic radial head replacement offers an option in chronic arthritis when simple radial head excision may lead to instability or uneven load distribution of the ulnohumeral joint.

Radiocapitellar arthritis with its frequently associated stiffness is a challenging issue. Surgical treatment options are considered when nonsurgical treatment, including medications, corticosteroid injections, and therapy, fail. Arthroscopic and open procedures offer options to improve function while decreasing pain. Joint preservation techniques should be emphasized as primary options.

Ulnohumeral arthritis is more common in younger, higher-demand patients and is also challenging to treat in this population. Joint preservation is crucial because prosthetic replacement has a high failure rate in these posttraumatic conditions.[14] When nonsurgical treatment (corticosteroid injections, therapy, splinting, and anti-inflammatory medications) fails, therapies based on improving motion and recontouring the joint have proven successful. Although elbow fusion is successful for pain relief, the lack of elbow mobility renders this a rarely chosen option. Joint resurfacing with grafts may prove beneficial in the short term while preserving humeral bone stock. Elbow replacement works well for motion and pain relief, but unfortunately it has a high rate of failure and requires revision secondary to prosthetic wear.

Improved motion in posttraumatic ulnohumeral arthritis may be achieved with arthroscopic or open os-

Table 1	

Definition of Larsen Grades

Larsen Grade	Radiographic Findings
1	Osteopenia; no major joint space or bone deformity
2	Osteopenia; mild to moderate joint space narrowing
3	Osteopenia; joint destruction and bone loss with variable cystic formation
4	Osteopenia; severe gross joint destruction with elbow instability

(Adapted from Larsen A, Dale K, Eek M: Radiographic evaluation of rheumatoid arthritis and related conditions by standard reference films. *Acta Radiol Diagn (Stockh)* 1977;18[4]:481-491.)

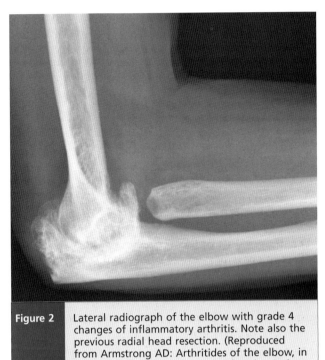

Figure 2	Lateral radiograph of the elbow with grade 4 changes of inflammatory arthritis. Note also the previous radial head resection. (Reproduced from Armstrong AD: Arthritides of the elbow, in Lieberman JR, ed: *AAOS Comprehensive Orthopaedic Review.* Rosemont, IL, American Academy of Orthopaedic Surgeons, 2009, pp 871-876.)

teocapsular arthroplasty.[9] Any opportunity to improve motion while treating both intrinsic and extrinsic etiologies is essential for functional improvement. Laterally or medially based open capsulectomy with joint débridement of the olecranon and coronoid articulations will improve motion while sparing stability.[15] These joint-sparing procedures are effective in patients with mild to moderate arthritis. In patients with severe stiffness, joint resurfacing is often necessary.

In the largest series from the Mayo Clinic, interposition elbow arthroplasty led to satisfactory results in a salvage setting for the younger, high-demand patient. Failure to maintain elbow stability led to poorer results. The advantages included maintenance of humeral bone stock, moderate pain relief, and improved motion. This treatment is relatively contraindicated in the unstable elbow.[16] Revision interposition arthroplasty may also be an option in those requiring high elbow demands and long-term durability.[17]

The final option of ulnohumeral replacement arthroplasty must be considered with caution. Short-term outcomes are good; however, midterm and long-term issues with prosthetic failure can be catastrophic.[14] The failure modes of ulnohumeral replacement arthroplasty include bushing wear, infection, periprosthetic fracture, and component loosening.[14] Surgeons should consider triceps-sparing approaches and unconstrained prosthetic options to promote component longevity. Perhaps options of distal humeral hemiarthroplasty may be advantageous in this select group of patients.[18]

Inflammatory Arthritis
The most common form of inflammatory arthritis of the elbow is rheumatoid arthritis. Typically, patients present early with hand and wrist involvement, and elbow symptoms do not usually present until later in the disease process. Occasionally, the elbow may be the first initial isolated presentation of the disease, but this is atypical. A 61% incidence of radiologic involvement of the elbow in patients with rheumatoid arthritis has been reported.[19]

Pain and loss of motion of the elbow are the initial symptoms caused by the extensive synovitis that develops. If the synovitis persists, a fixed flexion contracture (loss of elbow extension) will develop. On physical examination, evidence of swelling or bogginess of the elbow joint will be seen, particularly in the posterolateral joint. With continued proliferation of the granulation tissue and pannus, the patient will progressively continue to lose elbow range of motion as a result of progressive cartilage destruction and narrowing of the joint space. The continued presence of the erosive pannus eventually will produce cystic changes and bony destruction, leading to attenuation of the soft tissues and gross instability or deformity of the joint. Patients may also present with elbow nodules, olecranon bursitis, and/or ulnar neuropathy.

The Larsen classification[20] is used to grade radiographic changes that develop with elbow rheumatoid arthritis and can also help guide treatment (Table 1). A fifth grade was later added to include elbow ankylosis[21] (Figure 2).

Treatment requires a multidisciplinary approach. A rheumatologist or a primary care practitioner should optimize medical management by using disease-modifying drugs. Tumor necrosis factor inhibitors recently have been used in treatment. A combined drug therapy approach is often used. Joint injections are often used for temporary relief of acute inflammatory exacerbations. Physical and occupational therapists play an important role in educating patients about joint protection, maintaining strength and motion, using resting

3: Upper Extremity

splints, and modifying activity. Surgery is indicated when nonsurgical treatment fails and pain becomes unbearable. Other indications for surgery include a loss of functional range of motion and gross instability of the joint; however, pain is the main indication for surgery. Surgical treatment options are typically synovectomy with or without radial head resection for Larsen grades 1 and 2 and total elbow arthroplasty for Larsen grades 3 and 4.

Elbow synovectomy may be performed either open or arthroscopically. Recently, a meta-analysis was performed to compare open and arthroscopic synovectomy for knees and elbows.[22] Compared with an open approach, arthroscopic synovectomy showed similar pain reduction but more frequent recurrences of synovitis and radiographic progression and a similar decreased risk of future implant replacement.. The presence of advanced preoperative rheumatologic radiographic changes was not an absolute contraindication to surgical synovectomy and did not correlate with worse pain scores or an increased need for subsequent arthroplasty. This suggests that elbow synovectomy can be considered, particularly to delay a total elbow arthroplasty in younger patients with rheumatoid arthritis who have advanced disease. Favorable results following arthroscopic elbow synovectomy with preoperative Larsen grade 1 or 2 radiographic changes have been reported.[23] The goal with either the open or arthroscopic approach is to reduce the synovial tissue to control pain and theoretically slow down further joint destruction. Arthroscopic elbow synovectomy is a challenging procedure because of abundant synovitis, poor visualization, and reduced joint volume. To decrease the risk of neurovascular injury, only an experienced elbow arthroscopist should consider performing arthroscopic synovectomy of the elbow. Radial head resection is considered if there is painful restriction of forearm rotation, but this procedure is contraindicated in patients with medial collateral ligament insufficiency because of the potential for increased valgus instability. More favorable results for elbow synovectomy and radial head resection have been reported when forearm rotation is reduced to less than 50% with no severe restriction in elbow flexion and extension arc (> 60°).[24] Linked total elbow arthroplasty in patients following a previous synovectomy may be associated with a higher complication rate, but it has not been shown to affect the final outcome.[25]

Rheumatoid arthritis is the primary indication for total elbow arthroplasty. The long-term results of total elbow arthroplasty approach that of hip and knee arthroplasty for patients with inflammatory arthritis, with survival rates over 90% at 10 years.[26-28] However, revision rates for total elbow arthroplasty are higher in younger patients. A 22% revision rate has been reported in patients younger than 40 years, with a higher incidence of failure in patients with a preoperative diagnosis of posttraumatic arthritis compared with those patients with inflammatory arthritis.[29]

Total elbow arthroplasty implants are classified as linked, unlinked, and combined. Linked implants are joined together by a sloppy hinge that allows for some varus and valgus laxity during elbow range of motion. In patients with rheumatoid arthritis, the soft tissues are often attenuated, so linked implants are more typically used. Unlinked implants rely on the surrounding soft tissues for stability of the prosthesis. Combined implants have the interchangeable option of linking or unlinking the same implant interface. This is helpful if an unlinked construct is used in a patient and then becomes unstable. The surgeon then has the option to convert the same implant to a linked construct without having to remove the entire implant. A systematic review of the literature to determine the complications associated with modern-day total elbow arthroplasty showed an overall significant complication rate of 24.3 ± 5.8%.[30] The most common complications included implant loosening, instability, deep infection, and intraoperative fracture. Ulnar nerve complications were 2.0 ± 3.3% if the nerve was surgically handled including transposition and 3.2 ± 3.1% if it was not surgically handled. Triceps dehiscence or clinically significant weakness was reported in 1.2 ± 3.3% after triceps reflection in continuity, 1.8 ± 2.6% after triceps splitting approach, and 1.2 ± 2.3% after v-shaped tongue approach. Patients with rheumatoid arthritis have a higher risk for wound complications, and persistent wound drainage has been shown to have a high correlation for deep infection and subsequent implant removal.[31] Image-based navigation techniques for improving total elbow implant alignment are under development.[32,33]

Recurrent Elbow Instability

Valgus Elbow Instability

A medial collateral ligament injury most often develops in patients who participate in repetitive overhead throwing and is most commonly diagnosed in baseball pitchers. The anterior bundle of the medial collateral ligament is the primary valgus stabilizer of the elbow.[34-36] The tensile strength of the anterior bundle of the medial collateral ligament is exceeded during the late cocking and early acceleration phases of throwing.[37,38] It has been reported that professional athletes with a higher pitch velocity are at increased risk for medial collateral ligament injury.[39] A study of 490 baseball players referred for shoulder and elbow rehabilitation for baseball-related injuries showed that high school and collegiate baseball players were more likely to have medial collateral ligament injury or superior labrum anterior to posterior injuries compared with junior players.[40] They also reported that pitchers and outfielders, rather than infielders, as well as taller and heavier players, were also at a greater risk for medial collateral ligament injury.[40]

Athletes with valgus elbow instability typically describe focal pain at the medial aspect of the elbow. They may also describe a distinct event during throwing when they felt a pop. However, the athlete may no-

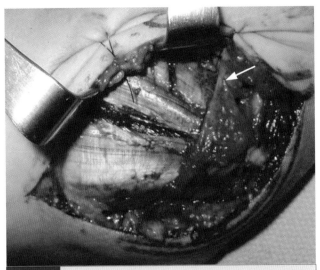

tice only a gradual onset of increased pain and decreased ability to throw with the desired precision and velocity. Occasionally, the athlete may describe transient ulnar nerve symptoms and pain in the posteromedial elbow related to valgus extension overload. Posteromedial elbow impingement was originally understood to occur at lower flexion angles during deceleration or release of the ball secondary to valgus elbow instability.[41,42] A recent biomechanical study proposed that this impingement occurs throughout the entire arc of flexion and coincides with the ulnohumeral chondral injury pattern.[43] The valgus stress test, the milking maneuver, and the moving valgus stress test[44] are commonly used to assess valgus instability. Patients with a positive moving valgus stress test typically describe pain between 70° and 120° of flexion. The physical examination for valgus elbow instability should also include an examination of the patient's ipsilateral shoulder, core strength, and throwing mechanics. A higher

Video 30.1: The Physical Examination of the Cadaver Elbow to Improve Understanding of the Tests. Davide Blonna, MD; Filippo Castoldi, MD: Michele Scelsi, MDi Alessandra Tellini, MD; Andrea Ferro, MD (20.00 min)

incidence of glenohumeral internal rotation deficit has been shown in injured throwers with medial collateral ligament injury compared with uninjured throwers.[45] Imaging studies such as MRI with or without arthro-

gram, valgus stress plain films, and ultrasound may also aid in diagnosis. Thickening of the medial collateral ligament and posteromedial subchondral sclerosis of the trochlea may be normal adaptations of the elbow as a result of throwing.[46] Higher peak internal elbow adduction moments during throwing have been associated with these adaptations.[47] Dynamic ultrasound assessments for diagnosing medial collateral ligament tears are being developed.[48]

The initial treatment of medial collateral ligament injury is dedicated rest and rehabilitation for 3 to 6 months, with treatment focused on improving strength and endurance of the flexor pronator muscles, addressing tightness of the posterior shoulder capsule, and improving core strength and throwing mechanics. If nonsurgical treatment fails and the goal is to resume throwing, then surgical intervention is considered. The classic surgical treatment of a medial collateral ligament injury is ligament reconstruction. A recent biomechanical study simulated two critical phases of throwing and measured contact pressures at the radiocapitellar joint.[49] This study showed that medial collateral ligament reconstruction restored articular pressures of the radiocapitellar joint to within 20% of the intact elbow values. An alternative in younger athletes may be surgical repair of the ligament because there is less attritional change to the ligament.[50] A 91% return to sport at 6 months has been reported for repairs of proximal or distal avulsion injuries in young athletes.

Ligament reconstruction remains the preferred treatment of valgus instability in throwing athletes. Numerous reconstruction techniques have been described. On average, the reported rate of return to sport is 83% and ranges from 68% to 95%.[51] The results for a modified classic figure-of-8 reconstruction technique with subcutaneous ulnar nerve transposition were recently investigated in 942 patients with 2-year follow-up.[52] The rate of return to sport was 83%, with an average time to return to sport of 11.6 months. Complications were mostly related to the ulnar nerve, and the transposition technique was modified with improved results. Open excision of posteromedial osteophytes was required in 34% of the patients. More recent developments in medial collateral ligament reconstruction include a flexor pronator-splitting approach without transposition of the ulnar nerve (**Figure 3**), which has been reported to result in a decreased incidence of ulnar nerve symptoms.[53] A more commonly used technique of reconstruction is the docking technique.[54-56] Single-strand ligament reconstructions are also evolving, and rates for return to sport match those of the two-strand reconstruction techniques.[57] Patients older than 30 years with a combined flexor pronator muscle injury and medial collateral ligament tear are less likely to return to throwing, with only 12.5% returning to sport.[43]

There is growing concern that the incidence of medial collateral ligament injuries is rising, particularly in collegiate and high-school athletes. Prevention is the mainstay of treatment. Published guidelines from the USA Baseball Medical Safety Advisory Committee have

3: Upper Extremity

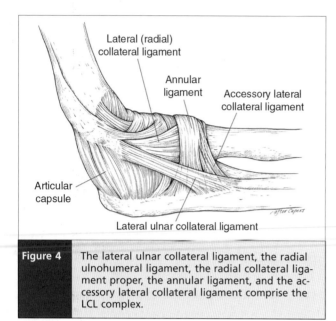

Figure 4 The lateral ulnar collateral ligament, the radial ulnohumeral ligament, the radial collateral ligament proper, the annular ligament, and the accessory lateral collateral ligament comprise the LCL complex.

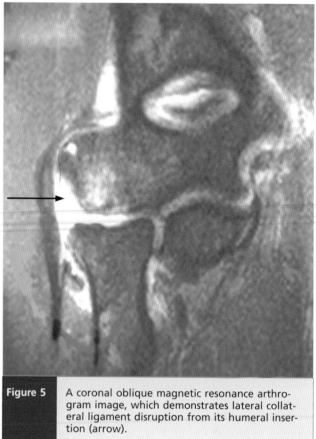

Figure 5 A coronal oblique magnetic resonance arthrogram image, which demonstrates lateral collateral ligament disruption from its humeral insertion (arrow).

been provided.[58] The amount of pitching and fatigue has the strongest correlation with resultant arm injury.[58,59]

Posterolateral Rotatory Elbow Instability

Lateral collateral ligament (LCL) injuries can often be difficult to diagnose and treat. They typically occur as a result of elbow trauma but can also be mistaken for more benign causes of lateral elbow pain. Recent improved understanding of elbow anatomy has allowed better diagnosis and treatment of this complex problem.

Even simple elbow dislocations can lead to chronic LCL attenuation, and complex fracture-dislocations often lead to more obvious LCL disruption and elbow instability. However, chronic, indolent LCL attenuation is much more challenging to diagnose because the signs and symptoms can be subtle. Patients may have received multiple corticosteroid injections[60] or may have undergone multiple lateral-sided surgical procedures, such as lateral epicondylitis débridements and releases, which can lead to iatrogenic LCL disruption.

The LCL is composed of four major components (Figure 4). The lateral ulnohumeral ligament is the most important stabilizer against posterolateral rotatory instability. It inserts distally into the supinator crest of the ulna. The annular ligament hooks around the radial neck and stabilizes the proximal radioulnar joint. The proper radial collateral ligament lies anterior to the radial ulnar collateral ligament and is the primary restraint against varus forces. The final component of the LCL is the accessory LCL. In addition to the LCL, the capsule acts as a static stabilizer, especially with the elbow in extension, and the anconeus and extensors act as dynamic stabilizers.

If the LCL complex is injured, posterolateral rotatory instability can occur. Posterolateral rotatory instability typically occurs with the elbow in supination and

extension with a valgus load, with resulting compression without restraint at the radiocapitellar joint. When compression occurs, the ulnohumeral joint can rotate, causing the radial head to subluxate or dislocate posteriorly. It is not clear whether an isolated injury to the radial ulnar collateral ligament is sufficient to cause posterolateral rotatory instability or if more extensive damage to the lateral ulnar collateral ligament is required.[61]

The diagnosis of posterolateral rotatory instability is challenging. Symptoms range from mild mechanical clicking or popping to frank elbow dislocation. The physical examination findings can be difficult to elicit in the clinic in the awake patient because of guarding. Often, the final diagnosis must be made during an examination with the patient under anesthesia and with the aid of fluoroscopy. The classic test described in the literature is the supine lateral pivot-shift test.[62] The patient is placed supine on the examining table. The elbow is placed in slight flexion and full supination while the examiner applies a valgus load. The radial head can be palpated in its subluxated position. At this point, the entire ulnohumeral joint is subluxated with its associated radioulnar joint. As the elbow is flexed, the radial head and the ulnohumeral joint relocate, and the examiner feels the joint "clunk" back into place. Patients with posterolateral rotatory instability are unable to complete push-ups with their forearm in supination. The chair push-up test forces a patient to push up from

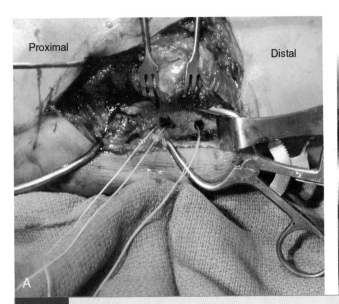
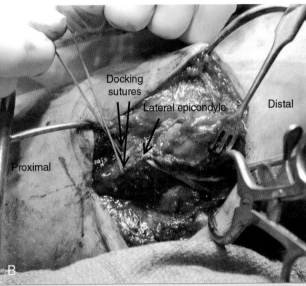

Figure 6 Clinical photographs of the elbow of a 40-year-old right-handed man in whom iatrogenic posterolateral instability developed after a failed arthroscopic lateral epicondylitis release. **A,** Intraoperative view of a lateral ulnar collateral ligament reconstruction using the docking technique. Two 4.0-mm drill holes are shown in the ulna before graft passage with suture shuttle to pass the graft. **B,** The graft has been passed through the ulnar tunnels and "docked" in the single tunnel in the lateral epicondyle. (Courtesy of Columbia University Center for Shoulder, Elbow and Sports Medicine, New York, NY.)

a chair with the forearm in supination. Pain as the elbow extends is a positive test result. The drawer sign is performed with the patient supine on the table. The arm is brought over the patient's head and supinated. The examiner places the index finger under the radial head and the thumb over it. If the examiner can feel the radial head subluxate with a posteriorly directed force, this is a positive test result.

Standard APr and lateral radiographs are usually of little value and may appear normal. Occasionally, a small avulsion fracture off the lateral epicondyle or degenerative changes of the radiocapitellar joint are revealed. Stress radiographs can be helpful and are best obtained with the use of fluoroscopy. Magnetic resonance arthrograms may identify injuries to the LCL complex and/or posterolateral capitellar erosions (Figure 5).

Nonsurgical treatment is based on modifying patient activities and expectations while strengthening the elbow through a stable range of motion. If an LCL injury is identified early (such as in association with simple elbow dislocation), nonsurgical treatment can be attempted. A hinged brace applied with the elbow in pronation for 4 to 6 weeks can prevent chronic instability in some patients.[63] Patients with mild symptoms might benefit from wearing a neoprene sleeve and physical therapy exercises to strengthen their extensors to improve dynamic stability.

Surgical reconstruction techniques are numerous, but all are based on reconstructing the LCL with autograft or allograft between the supinator crest and the inferior/posterior lateral epicondyle. There is no true isometric point for the LCL.[64] These techniques include the figure-of-8 yoke technique, the docking technique

(Figure 6), and split anconeus fascia.[65-67] Direct repair is recommended only in the setting of acute trauma. New arthroscopic techniques aim to plicate the LCL while allowing concomitant treatment of intra-articular pathology, such as the common Osborne-Cotterill capitellar lesion, a predictor of posterolateral rotatory instability.[68,69]

Postoperative rehabilitation is based on a slow progression to full elbow range of motion while gradually progressing from the flexed position to extension and supination. The LCL is stressed in supination, so early maintenance in the pronated position will protect the reconstruction. Strengthening is delayed for a minimum of 6 to 8 weeks until full motion is obtained.

The proper diagnosis of LCL injuries can lead to successful ligament reconstructions. A simple algorithm can be followed to determine the best treatment, and surgeons should be familiar with all of the technique options before performing surgery. Patients with rotatory instability should undergo a trial of nonsurgical treatment focused on elbow strengthening and/or bracing. If this fails, surgical reconstruction can lead to good elbow function and stability.

Summary

Nonarthroplasty surgical treatment options for the treatment of elbow arthritis, in general, include synovectomy, extensive bony and soft-tissue débridements, and interposition arthroplasty. Patient age and the type of arthritic condition are important factors to take into consideration when deciding on treatment plans. Nonarthroplasty surgical treatment is typically considered in younger patients with osteoarthritis, posttraumatic arthritis, and early stages of inflammatory arthritis. Total elbow replacement is generally reserved for individuals with low demand and advanced stages of inflammatory arthritis. Recurrent elbow instability is uncommon. Valgus elbow instability is most common in athletes who participate in repetitive throwing or overhead activities. Medial collateral ligament reconstruction is the treatment of choice when nonsurgical treatment is unsuccessful and the athlete wants to return to throwing sports. Prevention is the mainstay of treatment and should be the focus of future intervention. Posterolateral rotatory instability is typically posttraumatic and is not well tolerated by patients. It does not respond well to nonsurgical treatment and LCL reconstruction is usually necessary to restore elbow stability and function.

Key Study Points

- Nonarthroplasty surgical options should be attempted in young patients with elbow osteoarthritis to avoid early prosthetic failure.

- Linked total elbow arthroplasty remains the surgical procedure of choice in inflammatory arthritis of the elbow in most patients.

- Medial collateral ligament injury is increasingly common in overhead athletes and has led to an epidemic rise in reconstructive surgery to allow these athletes return to prior levels of function.

Annotated References

1. Kozak TK, Adams RA, Morrey BF: Total elbow arthroplasty in primary osteoarthritis of the elbow. *J Arthroplasty* 1998;13(7):837-842.

2. Antuña SA, Morrey BF, Adams RA, O'Driscoll SW: Ulnohumeral arthroplasty for primary degenerative arthritis of the elbow: Long-term outcome and complications. *J Bone Joint Surg Am* 2002;84(12):2168-2173.

3. Phillips NJ, Ali A, Stanley D: Treatment of primary degenerative arthritis of the elbow by ulnohumeral arthroplasty: A long-term follow-up. *J Bone Joint Surg Br* 2003;85(3):347-350.

4. Sarris I, Riano FA, Goebel F, Goitz RJ, Sotereanos DG: Ulnohumeral arthroplasty: Results in primary degenerative arthritis of the elbow. *Clin Orthop Relat Res* 2004; 420:190-193.

5. Tashjian RZ, Wolf JM, Ritter M, Weiss AP, Green A: Functional outcomes and general health status after ulnohumeral arthroplasty for primary degenerative arthritis of the elbow. *J Shoulder Elbow Surg* 2006;15(3): 357-366.

6. Adams JE, Wolff LH III, Merten SM, Steinmann SP: Osteoarthritis of the elbow: Results of arthroscopic osteophyte resection and capsulectomy. *J Shoulder Elbow Surg* 2008;17(1):126-131.

7. Kelly EW, Bryce R, Coghlan J, Bell S: Arthroscopic debridement without radial head excision of the osteoarthritic elbow. *Arthroscopy* 2007;23(2):151-156.

8. Kim SJ, Shin SJ: Arthroscopic treatment for limitation of motion of the elbow. *Clin Orthop Relat Res* 2000; 375:140-148.

9. Krishnan SG, Harkins DC, Pennington SD, Harrison DK, Burkhead WZ: Arthroscopic ulnohumeral arthroplasty for degenerative arthritis of the elbow in patients under fifty years of age. *J Shoulder Elbow Surg* 2007; 16(4):443-448.

10. Cohen AP, Redden JF, Stanley D: Treatment of osteoarthritis of the elbow: A comparison of open and arthroscopic debridement. *Arthroscopy* 2000;16(7):701-706.

11. McLaughlin RE II, Savoie FH III, Field LD, Ramsey JR: Arthroscopic treatment of the arthritic elbow due to primary radiocapitellar arthritis. *Arthroscopy* 2006;22(1): 63-69.

12. Morrey BF, Schneeberger AG: Anconeus arthroplasty: A new technique for reconstruction of the radiocapitellar and/or proximal radioulnar joint. *J Bone Joint Surg Am* 2002;84(11):1960-1969.

13. Shore BJ, Mozzon JB, MacDermid JC, Faber KJ, King GJ: Chronic posttraumatic elbow disorders treated with metallic radial head arthroplasty. *J Bone Joint Surg Am* 2008;90(2):271-280.

14. Throckmorton T, Zarkadas P, Sanchez-Sotelo J, Morrey B: Failure patterns after linked semiconstrained total elbow arthroplasty for posttraumatic arthritis. *J Bone Joint Surg Am* 2010;92(6):1432-1441.

    Semiconstrained elbow replacement leads to relatively early, high failure rates for the treatment of posttraumatic elbow arthritis. Associated high demands placed on the implant may occur. Level of evidence: IV.

15. Hattori Y, Doi K, Sakamoto S, Hoshino S, Dodakundi C: Capsulectomy and debridement for primary osteoarthritis of the elbow through a medial trans-flexor approach. *J Hand Surg Am* 2011;36(10):1652-1658.

    The authors described the medial flexor trans-tendon approach to elbow débridement with good short-term results. Level of evidence: IV.

16. Larson AN, Morrey BF: Interposition arthroplasty with an Achilles tendon allograft as a salvage procedure for the elbow. *J Bone Joint Surg Am* 2008;90(12):2714-2723.

17. Larson AN, Adams RA, Morrey BF: Revision interposition arthroplasty of the elbow. *J Bone Joint Surg Br* 2010;92(9):1273-1277.

    The authors described their results in a limited group of revision interposition allograft arthroplasty for elbow arthritis. Level of evidence: IV.

18. Steinmann SP: Hemiarthroplasty of the ulnohumeral and radiocapitellar joints. *Hand Clin* 2011;27(2):229-232, vi.

    This review discussed the indications and outcomes of the author's use of distal humeral hemiarthroplasty. Level of evidence IV.

19. Lehtinen JT, Kaarela K, Kauppi MJ, Belt EA, Mäenpää HM, Lehto MU: Bone destruction patterns of the rheumatoid elbow: A radiographic assessment of 148 elbows at 15 years. *J Shoulder Elbow Surg* 2002;11(3):253-258.

20. Larsen A, Dale K, Eek M: Radiographic evaluation of rheumatoid arthritis and related conditions by standard reference films. *Acta Radiol Diagn (Stockh)* 1977;18(4):481-491.

21. Connor PM, Morrey BF: Total elbow arthroplasty in patients who have juvenile rheumatoid arthritis. *J Bone Joint Surg Am* 1998;80(5):678-688.

22. Chalmers PN, Sherman SL, Raphael BS, Su EP: Rheumatoid synovectomy: Does the surgical approach matter? *Clin Orthop Relat Res* 2011;469(7):2062-2071.

    The authors performed a meta-analysis of arthroscopic versus open débridement and synovectomy for rheumatoid arthritis. Both surgical approaches showed similar pain relief, but arthroscopic synovectomy may have a higher risk for recurrence. Level of evidence: IV.

23. Horiuchi K, Momohara S, Tomatsu T, Inoue K, Toyama Y: Arthroscopic synovectomy of the elbow in rheumatoid arthritis. *J Bone Joint Surg Am* 2002;84(3):342-347.

24. Gendi NS, Axon JM, Carr AJ, Pile KD, Burge PD, Mowat AG: Synovectomy of the elbow and radial head excision in rheumatoid arthritis: Predictive factors and long-term outcome. *J Bone Joint Surg Br* 1997;79(6):918-923.

25. Whaley A, Morrey BF, Adams R: Total elbow arthroplasty after previous resection of the radial head and synovectomy. *J Bone Joint Surg Br* 2005;87(1):47-53.

26. Fevang BT, Lie SA, Havelin LI, Skredderstuen A, Furnes O: Results after 562 total elbow replacements: A report from the Norwegian Arthroplasty Register. *J Shoulder Elbow Surg* 2009;18(3):449-456.

27. Skyttä ET, Eskelinen A, Paavolainen P, Ikävalko M, Remes V: Total elbow arthroplasty in rheumatoid arthritis: A population-based study from the Finnish Arthroplasty Register. *Acta Orthop* 2009;80(4):472-477.

28. Gill DR, Morrey BF: The Coonrad-Morrey total elbow arthroplasty in patients who have rheumatoid arthritis: A ten to fifteen-year follow-up study. *J Bone Joint Surg Am* 1998;80(9):1327-1335.

29. Celli A, Morrey BF: Total elbow arthroplasty in patients forty years of age or less. *J Bone Joint Surg Am* 2009;91(6):1414-1418.

30. Voloshin I, Schippert DW, Kakar S, Kaye EK, Morrey BF: Complications of total elbow replacement: A systematic review. *J Shoulder Elbow Surg* 2011;20(1):158-168.

    A systematic review of total elbow complications is presented. Level of evidence: IV.

31. Jeon IH, Morrey BF, Anakwenze OA, Tran NV: Incidence and implications of early postoperative wound complications after total elbow arthroplasty. *J Shoulder Elbow Surg* 2011;20(6):857-865.

    The authors studied 97 patients from a group of 1,749 total elbow arthroplasties and found that although the overall incidence of serious wound complications was slightly less than anticipated, significance was considerable, and individuals with rheumatoid arthritis are most likely to have septic complications. Level of evidence: IV.

32. McDonald CP, Johnson JA, Peters TM, King GJ: Image-based navigation improves the positioning of the humeral component in total elbow arthroplasty. *J Shoulder Elbow Surg* 2010;19(4):533-543.

    This article describes improved accuracy of humeral component placement using image-based navigation in cadaveric speciments. Level of evidence: IV.

33. McDonald CP, Peters TM, Johnson JA, King GJ: Stem abutment affects alignment of the humeral component in computer-assisted elbow arthroplasty. *J Shoulder Elbow Surg* 2011;20(6):891-898.

    The authors validated the accuracy of a technique for computer-assisted implant alignment and identified variations in distal humeral morphology that had an effect on this alignment. Level of evidence: IV.

34. Hotchkiss RN, Weiland AJ: Valgus stability of the elbow. *J Orthop Res* 1987;5(3):372-377.

35. Morrey BF, An KN: Articular and ligamentous contributions to the stability of the elbow joint. *Am J Sports Med* 1983;11(5):315-319.

36. Søjbjerg JO, Ovesen J, Nielsen S: Experimental elbow instability after transection of the medial collateral ligament. *Clin Orthop Relat Res* 1987;218:186-190.

37. Dillman CJ, Fleisig GS, Andrews JR: Biomechanics of pitching with emphasis upon shoulder kinematics. *J Orthop Sports Phys Ther* 1993;18(2):402-408.

38. Fleisig GS, Andrews JR, Dillman CJ, Escamilla RF: Kinetics of baseball pitching with implications about in-

jury mechanisms. *Am J Sports Med* 1995;23(2): 233-239.

39. Bushnell BD, Anz AW, Noonan TJ, Torry MR, Hawkins RJ: Association of maximum pitch velocity and elbow injury in professional baseball pitchers. *Am J Sports Med* 2010;38(4):728-732.

    The authors studied 23 professional baseball pitchers and found a significant association between maximum pitch velocity and elbow injury. Level of evidence: IV.

40. Han KJ, Kim YK, Lim SK, Park JY, Oh KS: The effect of physical characteristics and field position on the shoulder and elbow injuries of 490 baseball players: Confirmation of diagnosis by magnetic resonance imaging. *Clin J Sport Med* 2009;19(4):271-276.

41. Ahmad CS, Park MC, Elattrache NS: Elbow medial ulnar collateral ligament insufficiency alters posteromedial olecranon contact. *Am J Sports Med* 2004;32(7): 1607-1612.

42. Kamineni S, ElAttrache NS, O'Driscoll SW, et al: Medial collateral ligament strain with partial posteromedial olecranon resection: A biomechanical study. *J Bone Joint Surg Am* 2004;86(11):2424-2430.

43. Osbahr DC, Dines JS, Breazeale NM, Deng XH, Altchek DW: Ulnohumeral chondral and ligamentous overload: Biomechanical correlation for posteromedial chondromalacia of the elbow in throwing athletes. *Am J Sports Med* 2010;38(12):2535-2541.

    A cadaveric biomechanical model demonstrated that posteromedial overload occurs throughout the arc of motion, not just at end range.

44. O'Driscoll SW, Lawton RL, Smith AM: The "moving valgus stress test" for medial collateral ligament tears of the elbow. *Am J Sports Med* 2005;33(2):231-239.

45. Dines JS, Frank JB, Akerman M, Yocum LA: Glenohumeral internal rotation deficits in baseball players with ulnar collateral ligament insufficiency. *Am J Sports Med* 2009;37(3):566-570.

46. Hurd WJ, Kaufman KR, Murthy NS: Relationship between the medial elbow adduction moment during pitching and ulnar collateral ligament appearance during magnetic resonance imaging evaluation. *Am J Sports Med* 2011;39(6):1233-1237.

    Findings of elbow MRI scans for 20 uninjured asymptomatic high-school baseball pitchers were compared using three-dimensional motion analysis testing. Medial collateral ligament thickening was associated with a higher peak internal elbow adduction moment. Level of evidence: IV.

47. Hurd WJ, Eby S, Kaufman KR, Murthy NS: Magnetic resonance imaging of the throwing elbow in the uninjured, high school-aged baseball pitcher. *Am J Sports Med* 2011;39(4):722-728.

    Twenty-three uninjured, aymptomatic high-school baseball pitchers showed thickening of the anterior band of the medial collateral ligament and posteromedial subchondral sclerosis thatd may be considered normal or warning signs of risk for injury. Level of evidence: IV.

48. Smith W, Hackel JG, Goitz HT, Bouffard JA, Nelson AM: Utilization of sonography and a stress device in the assessment of partial tears of the ulnar collateral ligament in throwers. *Int J Sports Phys Ther* 2011;6(1):45-50.

49. Duggan JP Jr, Osadebe UC, Alexander JW, Noble PC, Lintner DM: The impact of ulnar collateral ligament tear and reconstruction on contact pressures in the lateral compartment of the elbow. *J Shoulder Elbow Surg* 2011;20(2):226-233.

    A biomechanical cadaveric study that showed medial collateral ligament reconstruction restored valgus stability and decreased radiocapitellar contact pressures close to normal levels.

50. Savoie FH III, Trenhaile SW, Roberts J, Field LD, Ramsey JR: Primary repair of ulnar collateral ligament injuries of the elbow in young athletes: A case series of injuries to the proximal and distal ends of the ligament. *Am J Sports Med* 2008;36(6):1066-1072.

51. Vitale MA, Ahmad CS: The outcome of elbow ulnar collateral ligament reconstruction in overhead athletes: A systematic review. *Am J Sports Med* 2008;36(6): 1193-1205.

52. Cain EL Jr, Andrews JR, Dugas JR, et al: Outcome of ulnar collateral ligament reconstruction of the elbow in 1281 athletes: Results in 743 athletes with minimum 2-year follow-up. *Am J Sports Med* 2010;38(12):2426-2434.

    An outcome report for 942 patients, with minimum 2-year follow-up, that had a medial collateral ligament reconstruction using a modified Jobe technique with subcutaneous ulnar nerve transposition is presented. Reported return to sport rate was 83%, average time to competition was 11.6 months, and complications were 16% minor, mostly related to ulnar neuropathy, and 4% major. Level of evidence: IV.

53. Smith GR, Altchek DW, Pagnani MJ, Keeley JR: A muscle-splitting approach to the ulnar collateral ligament of the elbow: Neuroanatomy and operative technique. *Am J Sports Med* 1996;24(5):575-580.

54. Koh JL, Schafer MF, Keuter G, Hsu JE: Ulnar collateral ligament reconstruction in elite throwing athletes. *Arthroscopy* 2006;22(11):1187-1191.

55. Paletta GA Jr, Wright RW: The modified docking procedure for elbow ulnar collateral ligament reconstruction: 2-year follow-up in elite throwers. *Am J Sports Med* 2006;34(10):1594-1598.

56. Rohrbough JT, Altchek DW, Hyman J, Williams RJ III, Botts JD: Medial collateral ligament reconstruction of the elbow using the docking technique. *Am J Sports Med* 2002;30(4):541-548.

57. Dines JS, ElAttrache NS, Conway JE, Smith W, Ahmad CS: Clinical outcomes of the DANE TJ technique to treat ulnar collateral ligament insufficiency of the elbow. *Am J Sports Med* 2007;35(12):2039-2044.

58. Kerut EK, Kerut DG, Fleisig GS, Andrews JR: Prevention of arm injury in youth baseball pitchers. *J La State Med Soc* 2008;160(2):95-98.

59. Dun S, Loftice J, Fleisig GS, Kingsley D, Andrews JR: A biomechanical comparison of youth baseball pitches: Is the curveball potentially harmful? *Am J Sports Med* 2008;36(4):686-692.

60. Kalainov DM, Cohen MS: Posterolateral rotatory instability of the elbow in association with lateral epicondylitis: A report of three cases. *J Bone Joint Surg Am* 2005;87(5):1120-1125.

61. Nestor BJ, O'Driscoll SW, Morrey BF: Ligamentous reconstruction for posterolateral rotatory instability of the elbow. *J Bone Joint Surg Am* 1992;74(8):1235-1241.

62. O'Driscoll SW, Bell DF, Morrey BF: Posterolateral rotatory instability of the elbow. *J Bone Joint Surg Am* 1991;73(3):440-446.

63. Cohen MS, Hastings H II: Acute elbow dislocation: Evaluation and management. *J Am Acad Orthop Surg* 1998;6(1):15-23.

64. Goren D, Budoff JE, Hipp JA: Isometric placement of lateral ulnar collateral ligament reconstructions: A biomechanical study. *Am J Sports Med* 2010;38(1):153-159.

    This biomechanical study suggested that there is no true isometric point for the lateral ulnar collateral ligament both on the humerus and supinator crest.

65. Sanchez-Sotelo J, Morrey BF, O'Driscoll SW: Ligamentous repair and reconstruction for posterolateral rotatory instability of the elbow. *J Bone Joint Surg Br* 2005; 87(1):54-61.

66. Jones KJ, Dodson CC, Osbahr DC, et al: The docking technique for lateral ulnar collateral ligament reconstruction: Surgical technique and clinical outcomes. *J Shoulder Elbow Surg* 2012;21(3):389-395.

    The docking technique is described for lateral ulnar collateral ligament reconstruction with surgical technique and outcomes. Level of evidence: IV.

67. Stein JA, Murthi AM: Posterolateral rotatory instability of the elbow: Our approach. *Oper Tech Orthop* 2009; 19:251-257.

68. Jeon IH, Min WK, Micic ID, Cho HS, Kim PT: Surgical treatment and clinical implication for posterolateral rotatory instability of the elbow: Osborne-Cotterill lesion of the elbow. *J Trauma* 2011;71(3):E45-E49.

    A review of 1,749 procedures showed that the most common postoperative problems were delayed wound healing, drainage, and hematoma. Level of evidence: IV.

69. Savoie FH III, O'Brien MJ, Field LD, Gurley DJ: Arthroscopic and open radial ulnohumeral ligament reconstruction for posterolateral rotatory instability of the elbow. *Clin Sports Med* 2010;29(4):611-618.

    The authors described a successful technique and outcomes for both arthroscopic and open repair/plication of the LCL complex to correct elbow rotatory instability. Level of evidence: IV.

Video Reference

30.1: Blonna D, Castoldi F, Scelsi M, Tellini A, Ferro A: The Physical Examination of the Cadaver Elbow to Improve Understanding of the Tests. Available at http://orthoportal.aaos.org/emedia/singleVideoPlayer.aspx?resource=EMEDIA_OSVL_11_28. Accessed January 15, 2014.

3: Upper Extremity

Chapter 31

Hand and Wrist Trauma

Peter Tang, MD, MPH   Steve K. Lee, MD

Fractures and Dislocations of the Hand

Phalangeal Fractures

Distal phalanx fractures most commonly occur after a crush injury, which leads to a tuft fracture. These injuries often are associated with a nail bed injury and are theoretically open fractures. However, adequate irrigation and débridement can be performed in the emergency department. If a subungual hematoma involving more than 50% of the area of the nail bed is present, a significant nail bed laceration also may be present, and it is generally recommended that the nail plate be removed for repair. However, it is unclear if more damage is possible with nail removal. It is also recommended that after débridement and repair, the nail or foil be placed underneath the nail fold to keep it open, but this has never been proven in the literature to be necessary. If there is significant displacement of a transverse fracture, reduction and Kirschner wire (K-wire) pinning can be performed.

The goals of treatment of middle and proximal phalangeal shaft fractures are to achieve adequate length and alignment, initiate early mobilization, and realize maximum hand function. Nondisplaced, stable fractures can be buddy taped and patients sent to occupational therapy with a certified hand therapist. Strengthening can be started at 4 weeks. Displaced fractures can be reduced. If reduction is successful, displaced fractures can be splinted for 4 weeks, after which the splint is discontinued and therapy started. Unstable injuries with malalignment (> 10° angulation, > 50% overlap of an adjacent digit, and shortening [every millimeter of middle phalanx shortening leads to 10° of distal inter-

phalangeal {DIP} joint extension lag; every millimeter of proximal phalanx shortening leads to 12° of proximal interphalangeal {PIP} joint lag]) may need surgical intervention. The objective is to achieve reduction and stable fixation with the least invasive means to minimize adhesions and stiffness. After closed reduction manually or with tenaculum-type bone clamps, K-wires can be placed in a variety of patterns. The K-wires can be used as joysticks in the fracture fragment to perform the reduction. If closed techniques fail, a small incision can be made to mobilize the fracture. If the reduction is still not successful, a formal open reduction is done, and K-wires or minifragment screws and/or plates can be placed. Motion is started early.

Distal Interphalangeal Joint Injuries

Mallet fingers are injuries of the extensor mechanism of the DIP joint that can involve only the terminal tendon (Doyle Ia) or have a bony fragment (Doyle Ib). Most of these injuries can be treated with splinting in full extension for 6 to 8 weeks with no flexion of the DIP joint. Ideally, the treatment is started immediately, but good outcomes have been reported even with delayed treatment (> 4 weeks).[1] Indications for surgery include open injuries, fractures that involve more than 30% of the joint surface, and joint subluxation (greater joint involvement leads to joint subluxation). Some physicians argue that almost all mallet fractures can be successfully treated nonsurgically. Surgical options include dorsal block splinting (where the DIP joint is flexed and the pin is placed in the head of the middle phalanx, then the joint is extended so that the fracture fragment abuts the pin and is reduced, and then the joint is pinned in extension) or internal fixation with a screw or a plate.

Proximal Interphalangeal Joint Injuries

Any injury to the PIP joint is challenging to treat because of the joint's proclivity to stiffness. Simple dorsal dislocations without fracture are usually stable after they are reduced. Splinting should be limited to a few days duration. Buddy taping can be used in lieu of splinting. Early motion should be initiated with therapy. Despite early motion, a mild residual flexion contracture is common. Volar dislocations need to be evaluated for central slip injury with the Elson test. If the test is positive, full-time PIP joint splinting in full extension is initiated for 6 to 8 weeks along with flexion ex-

Dr. Tang or an immediate family member has received research or institutional support from AxoGen and serves as a board member, owner, officer, or committee member of the American Society for Surgery of the Hand. Dr. Lee or an immediate family member has received royalties from Arthrex; is a member of a speakers' bureau or has made paid presentations on behalf of Arthrex serves as a paid consultant to or is an employee of Arthrex serves as an unpaid consultant to Synthes; has received research or institutional support from Arthrex, Mitek, Integra, and Medartis; and serves as a board member, owner, officer, or committee member of the American Society for Surgery of the Hand.

3: Upper Extremity

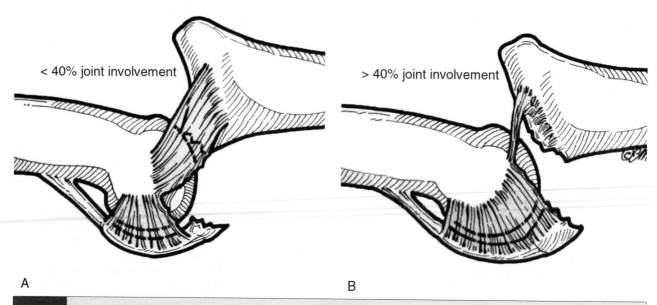

< 40% joint involvement

> 40% joint involvement

A

B

Figure 1 Drawings showing dorsal fracture-dislocations of the PIP joint. **A,** Dorsal fracture-dislocation with less than 40% of the joint involved may have enough collateral ligament attached to the middle phalanx to maintain joint stability. **B,** When more than 40% of the joint is involved, the collateral ligaments are attached to the fracture fragment, rendering the joint unstable. (Copyright Elizabeth Martin, Clarington, PA.)

ercises of the DIP joint. Volar fracture-dislocations of the PIP joint result in fracture of the dorsal, proximal aspect of the middle phalanx, which is the insertion of the central slip. Fixation of the fracture may be performed with percutaneous K-wires or internal fixation.

Dorsal fracture-dislocations of the PIP joint have varying degrees of involvement of the proximal volar aspect of the middle phalanx. If the fracture is a small volar plate avulsion fracture from the middle phalanx, then treatment is the same as for a simple dislocation. If less than 40% of the joint surface is involved, the dorsal portion of the collateral ligaments may be attached to the middle phalanx maintaining joint stability (Figure 1). These can be treated with dorsal block splinting for 3 weeks blocked to within the stable range of motion. Each week, 10° of additional extension are permitted. If more than 40% of the joint surface is involved, most of the collateral ligaments will be attached to the fracture fragment, rendering the joint unstable so that surgical intervention is needed. Also, if more than 40° of flexion is needed to maintain reduction in any injury pattern, surgery is indicated. These injuries are extremely challenging, and there are multiple treatment options.

A new percutaneous, closed reduction technique was described that involves placing K-wires from volar to dorsal.[2] Often, the fracture is comminuted making the stability of any kind of fixation poor. Other surgeons recommend plating through a volar approach,[3,4] but the incision and the exposure may lead to stiffness and scarring. Volar plate arthroplasty can be performed by securing the volar plate to the proximal, volar defect of the middle phalanx after resection of the fracture. Outcomes appear better with this procedure when the in-

jury is treated acutely (< 6 weeks). Hemihamate arthroplasty involves replacing the injured articular surface with part of the hamate. Again, acute injuries have better success than chronic injuries.

Pilon fractures involve complete joint involvement of the proximal middle phalanx, where axial compressive forces cause central joint depression and dorsal and volar fragment displacement. Surgical fixation is almost always necessary, but good outcomes are difficult to achieve. Open reduction and internal fixation (ORIF) is challenging because the fracture fragments are small, and swelling and stiffness from the injury, the incision, and the approach ensue. Another approach is dynamic external fixation, where K-wires and rubber bands or an external fixator is placed, which allows motion while applying traction. The traction allows ligamentotaxis to reduce the fracture; if there is residual fracture malalignment, it can be reduced and held with a K-wire or a screw. The device allows motion so that, theoretically, joint motion may be maintained.

Articular injuries of the proximal phalangeal head are surgically treated if there is articular incongruity of more than 1 mm, finger malalignment, or malrotation. Even initially nondisplaced fractures may be unstable and warrant close follow-up. Closed reduction and percutaneous pinning are attempted first; if not successful, ORIF is then performed.

Metacarpophalangeal Joint Injuries

Metacarpophalangeal (MCP) joint dislocations are relatively uncommon. The dislocation may be simple (closed reduction possible) or complex (requires open treatment). Dorsal dislocations are more common than

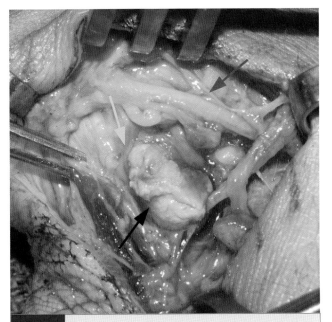

Figure 2 Stener lesion in a left thumb (left is distal, right is proximal) showing the distal ulnar collateral ligament (black arrow) displaced proximal to the adductor aponeurosis (blue arrow). A branch of the superficial radial sensory nerve (red arrow) is seen at the top part of the picture. (Reproduced from Tang P: Collateral ligament injuries of the thumb metacarpophalangeal joint. *J Am Acad Orthop Surg* 2011;19:287-296.)

Volar approach — auxilla digital n. injury

volar dislocations. Dorsal dislocations are caused by a hyperextension injury, and volar dislocations are caused by either a hyperextension or a hyperflexion injury. Simple dislocations can be easily converted to complex injuries if longitudinal traction is used to perform the reduction. Irreducible dorsal dislocations are a result of interposition of the volar plate in the joint or the metacarpal head buttonholing between the flexor tendons and the radial lumbrical. Irreducible volar dislocations are caused by interposed dorsal capsule, the distal insertion of the volar plate, and/or the collaterals. After reduction is obtained, the collateral ligaments should be evaluated to determine if rupture has occurred and whether repair is needed.

The ulnar and radial collateral ligaments of the thumb MCP joint are the primary stabilizers of the joint.[5] Injuries to these structures can be easily missed in the emergency department. Complete ulnar collateral ligament tears are diagnosed by more than 30° to 35° of thumb MCP joint angulation, or more than 10° to 15° compared with the contralateral side, with radial stress of the proximal phalanx with the metacarpal held stable. These parameters are also applied to radial collateral injuries but with stress in the ulnar direction. Complete tears on the ulnar side commonly have a Stener lesion (**Figure 2**), where the distal ligament is displaced superficial and proximal to the adductor aponeurosis, which is thought to prohibit the ligament's proper healing to its insertion. This situation rarely occurs on the radial side. Partial injuries can be splinted, whereas complete tears are usually repaired surgically. Suture anchors are the contemporary choice for fixation of the ligament to bone. When the tissue to be repaired in the chronic injury is of poor quality, ligament reconstruction with palmaris longus has been described.

Metacarpal Fractures

Metacarpal neck fractures should undergo reduction when angulation exceeds 10° in the index, 20° in the middle, 30° in the ring, and 40° to 50° in the small fingers. Patients who undergo reduction should be placed in a molded three-point hand splint to be worn for 4 weeks. Stable patterns can be treated with a removable splint, buddy taping, or an elastic bandage. If closed reduction is not successful, using K-wires to joystick the distal head and neck or levering the fracture site may be helpful. If these procedures fail, open reduction supplemented with pinning or plating to maintain the reduction may be attempted.

Metacarpal shaft fractures that are malaligned should undergo closed reduction and placement of a molded splint for 4 weeks. Indications for surgery include open fractures, multitrauma, multiple adjacent metacarpal fractures, finger malrotation (5° of malrotation can cause 1.5 cm of digital overlap), any apex dorsal angulation of the index and middle metacarpal, dorsal angulation of greater than 20° for the ring metacarpal and greater than 30° for the small metacarpal. For every 2 mm of shortening, there is 7° of MCP joint lag, but this is usually well tolerated because hyperextension is most often found at the MCP joint. In terms of fixation, the options include percutaneous K-wires, intramedullary K-wires, interosseous wiring, plating, and external fixation.[6]

Carpometacarpal Joint Injuries

Carpometacarpal (CMC) joint injuries are uncommon and constitute less than 1% of wrist and hand injuries. These joints derive their stability from the joint articulation (concave on the metacarpal side and convex on the distal carpal side) and the volar, dorsal, and intermetacarpal ligaments. The third CMC joint is most stable because its articulation is more proximal to the rest (keystone). Going from a radial to an ulnar direction, the CMC articular surface is flatter, which leads to less stability and more mobility to allow the small and ringer fingers to rotate toward the thumb. This decreased stability predisposes the more ulnar joints to injury. These injuries may be subtle and require a high index of suspicion for diagnosis. Substantial swelling of the hand and abnormal appearance on plain radiographs at the level of the CMC joint are signs of this injury. A CT scan may be needed to diagnose and/or delineate this injury. A pure dislocation can occur, but small fractures of the carpal bones are often seen. Closed reduction and percutaneous pinning with 0.062-inch K-wires is performed, with wire removal at 4 to 6 weeks. When the reduction cannot be confirmed radiographically, or cannot be achieved, open reduction is required. Small associated carpal fractures can usually be treated nonsurgically but may warrant fixation if large enough.

Bennett injuries describe a fracture-subluxation of the thumb metacarpal.[7,8] The "constant fragment" is the small articular fracture that maintains its anatomic location as a result of the attachment of the anterior oblique ligament. The rest of the metacarpal is displaced radially, proximally, and in supination because of the forces of the adductor pollicis and the abductor pollicis longus. The goals of treatment are reduction of the joint and articular congruity. Stability usually cannot be maintained with closed reduction alone. If intervention is early, closed reduction can result in fracture and articular surface reduction; 0.062-inch K-wires can then be placed to maintain the reduction for 6 weeks. If fracture reduction is not adequate, open reduction may be needed.

Rolando fractures are Y- or T-type fracture patterns of the base of the thumb metacarpal. Because of comminution, this injury can be challenging to treat. If the fragments are large enough, open reduction with internal or K-wire fixation may be performed. For comminuted patterns, distraction and ligamentotaxis may be of benefit. Distraction may be maintained by external fixation or pinning the thumb to the index metacarpal. As in Bennett fractures, the quality of the reduction may not correlate with symptoms.

Fracture and Dislocation of the Wrist

Carpal Fractures and Nonunion
Acute Fractures
The most common carpal fracture is of the scaphoid bone. It occurs most commonly in men approximately 20 to 40 years of age, usually from a fall onto an outstretched hand. Scaphoid fractures are particularly important for two reasons. First, the scaphoid is the link between the proximal and distal carpal rows; with intrascaphoid instability, the carpus may collapse, leading to a pattern of arthrosis known as scaphoid nonunion advanced collapse (SNAC).[9] The second aspect of scaphoid fractures is that they are prone to nonunion because of the retrograde blood supply. The more proximal the fracture, the more likely it is to develop a nonunion.

Several scaphoid fracture classifications exist, but the most useful method is simply to classify by location: waist (most common, 70%), proximal pole (20%), and distal pole (10%). Distal pole fractures usually are treated with a thumb spica splint or cast. Proximal pole fractures are unstable and require surgical stabilization. Nondisplaced waist fractures may be treated with or without surgery. A randomized controlled study showed that surgical treatment returned an active-duty military population of patients back to work earlier, but the overall rate of union was unchanged.[10] For nonsurgical treatment, use of a long versus short arm cast is controversial. Fractures have been shown to heal faster with a long arm-thumb spica cast.[11]

If surgery is elected, the approach is based on fracture location and surgeon preference. For a proximal pole fracture, a dorsal approach is preferable because it allows precise reduction and fixation of the smaller proximal fragment back to the remainder of the scaphoid. A small incision with retraction of the tendons out of the paths of the guidewire, drill, and headless compression screw is recommended to avoid tendon injury. Waist fractures can be treated with either dorsal or volar approaches. The advantage of the dorsal approach is that a cannulated screw may be placed down the long axis of the scaphoid. The disadvantage is that the wrist must be flexed to gain access to the scaphoid entry point and must remain flexed until the guidewire is removed, which makes fluoroscopy more challenging. For the volar approach, the wrist is extended maximally to move the trapezium out of the path of the scaphoid entry point, and part of the trapezium may need to be resected for better screw placement. This also reduces a flexed scaphoid. The hardware can be placed in a percutaneous manner because there are no tendons or other structures crossing the entry point. The disadvantage is that the true anatomic axis is difficult to achieve from this approach. For a proximal waist fracture, fewer screw threads can cross into the proximal fragment, and displacement may occur. The benefits of oblique fluoroscopic images to assess implant placement from the volar approach and thereby prevent intra-articular screw penetration have been shown.[12] With appropriate fixation methods, healing rates have been reported as high as 100%[10,13] (Table 1). Other carpal fractures are much less common, but all other bones may be injured.[14]

Nonunion
Some patients with scaphoid nonunions present with a remote history of a fall believed to be a sprain and for which there was no medical treatment. Other patients have had previous treatment. Overall nonunion rates are approximately 10% to 15% in treated scaphoid fractures.[13] Osteonecrosis more commonly occurs in proximal pole nonunions and can be as high as 30%. Scaphoid nonunion is usually treated with bone grafting and fixation. One study has shown that established unstable nonunions should be treated with screw fixation and wedge grafting.[15] In addition, a vascularized graft may be preferable for patients with osteonecrosis of the proximal fragment or with a previously failed surgery. The medial femoral condyle free-tissue transfer has been advocated for the treatment of scaphoid nonunions with humpback deformity and osteonecrosis.[16] In a comparison of the medial femoral condyle versus the 1,2 supraretinacular artery vascularized bone graft, the medial femoral condyle graft had superior results (Table 2).

Nonunions of other carpal bones are rare. Nonunions of the hook of the hamate and trapezial ridge, when symptomatic, are treated with excision of the fragment.

Table 1

Treatment of Acute Scaphoid Fractures

Acute Scaphoid Fracture Type	Treatment
Stable fractures, nondisplaced	
Tubercle fracture	Thumb spica cast or splint for 4 to 6 weeks
Distal third fracture and/or incomplete fracture	Thumb spica cast for 6 to 8 weeks
Nondisplaced waist fracture	Short or long thumb spica cast for at least 6 weeks until radiography or CT confirms healing, especially for sedentary or low-demand patients or patients with a preference for nonsurgical treatment
	Percutaneous or open internal fixation, especially for active and young manual workers, athletes, patients with high-demand occupations, or patients with a preference for early range of motion
Proximal pole fracture, nondisplaced	Percutaneous or open internal fixation
Unstable fractures (displacement > 1 mm, lateral interscaphoid angle > 35°, bone loss or comminution, perilunate fracture-dislocation)	Dorsal percutaneous or open screw fixation

(Adapted from Geissler WB, Adams JE, Bindra RR, Lanzinger WD, Slutsky DJ: Scaphoid fractures: What's hot, what's not. *Instr Course Lect* 2012;61:71-84.)

Table 2

Treatment of Scaphoid Nonunions

Type of Scaphoid Nonunion	Treatment
Delayed union	Percutaneous or open rigid fixation with a headless compression screw
Established (fibrous or sclerotic) nonunion	Curettage of nonunion, autografting, and fixation (dorsal approach for proximal fracture, volar for distal fracture)
Humpback nonunion, waist	Volar approach and corticocancellous wedge graft
Proximal pole nonunion, nonischemic	Dorsal approach; percutaneous or open bone grafting and fixation with headless screw; consider stabilizing distal scaphoid to capitate with headless screw or K-wire or stabilize proximal fragment between lunate and scaphoid waist with headless screw or K-wire
Avascular nonunion, waist or proximal pole	Consider vascularized bone graft: dorsal or volar approach

K-wire = Kirschner wire.
(Adapted from Geissler WB, Adams JE, Bindra RR, Lanzinger WD, Slutsky DJ: Scaphoid fractures: What's hot, what's not. *Instr Course Lect* 2012;61:71-84.)

Carpal Instability

Scapholunate Dissociation

The scapholunate complex is the most common ligament complex injured in the wrist. The spectrum of injury ranges from partial ligament tears to arthrosis (scapholunate advanced collapse [SLAC] wrist)[17] (Table 3). The history usually includes a fall onto an outstretched hand, the pertinent physical examination findings are tenderness over the scapholunate joint and a positive scaphoid shift test (Watson maneuver). With complete tears the classic drive-through sign can be observed during arthroscopy.

SLAC wrist findings include pain and swelling over the radioscaphoid joint. Treatment ranges from arthroscopic débridement, scapholunate pinning, and thermal

Video 31.1: The Drive-Through Sign. Melvin P. Rosenwasser, MD (0.46 min). This video demonstrates the drive-through sign during wrist arthroscopy, whereby the arthroscope can be "driven through" the space between the scaphoid and the lunate when there is a complete scapholunate ligament tear. The scope moves from the radiocarpal joint into the midcarpal joint, and the capitate can be seen.

3: Upper Extremity

Table 3

Stages of Scapholunate Instability

			Stage		
	I. Occult	II. Dynamic	III. Scapholunate Dissociation	IV. Dorsal Intercalated Segment Instability	V. Scapholunate Advanced Collapse
Injured ligaments	Partial SLIL	Incompetent or complete SLIL; partial volar extrinsics	Complete SLIL, volar or dorsal extrinsics	Complete SLIL volar extrinsics; secondary changes in RL, ST, DIC ligaments	As in stage IV
Radiographs	Normal	Usually normal	SL gap ≥ 3 mm; RS angle ≥ 60°	SL angle ≥ 70° SL gap ≥ 3 mm RL ≥ 15° CL ≥ 15°	I. Styloid DJD II. RS DJD III. CL DJD IV. Pancarpal DJD
Stress radiographs	Normal; abnormal fluoroscopy	Abnormal	Grossly abnormal	Unnecessary	Unnecessary
Treatment	Pinning or capsulodesis or thermal shrinkage	SLIL repair with capsulodesis	SLIL repair with capsulodesis, triligament reconstruction or RASL	Reducible: triligament reconstruction or RASL Fixed: intercarpal fusion	Scaphoid excision, intercarpal fusion, PRC, arthrodesis, or total wrist replacement

CL = capiltolunate; DIC = dorsal intercarpal ligament; DJD = degenerative joint disease; RL = radiolunate; RS = radioscaphoid; SL = scapholunate; SLIL = scapholunate interosseous ligament; ST = scaphotrapezoid; RASL = reduction and association of the scaphoid and lunate; PRC = proximal row carpectomy.
(Adapted with permission from Kuo CE, Wolfe SW: Scapholunate instability: Current concepts in diagnosis and management. *J Hand Surg Am* 2008;33[6]:998-1013.)

shrinkage for low-grade injuries to repair and capsulodesis for acute and dynamic injuries. For static injuries, the treatment remains elusive and includes capsulodesis, tenodesis, and screw placement between the scaphoid and the lunate (reduction and association of the scaphoid and lunate).[18] Treatment of SLAC wrist includes scaphoid excision four-bone fusion (SEFBF) or proximal row carpectomy (PRC), depending on what joints are preserved, the patient's age, and surgeon preference. In a comparison of SEFBF and PRC, the flexion-extension arc was 81° following PRC (62% of contralateral) and 80° following SEFBF (58% of contralateral). Grip strength averaged 71% for the PRC group compared with 79% for the SEFBF group. Pain relief was similar using a variety of measures, and patient satisfaction was equivalent.[19] It has been shown that PRC in patients younger than 35 years is not as successful as in older patients.[20] Techniques for gaining fusion in SEFBF vary and include K-wires, headless compression screws, staples, and circular plates.

Lunate and Perilunate Dislocations

Lunate and perilunate dislocations are relatively uncommon and occur after high-energy trauma such as a fall from a height and motor vehicle collisions. The Mayfield classification has been used to describe perilunate injuries starting from the scapholunate joint (stage I); to the midcarpal joint (stage II); to the lunotriquetral joint (stage III), to the "spilled teacup," where the lunate is completely extruded from the lunate fossa (stage IV, lunate dislocation). Expeditious treatment is imperative, first with a closed reduction in the emergency department using sedation, hematoma block, fingertrap distraction, and manipulation. Median nerve compression is common; if it is not resolved after reduction, decompression is required. ORIF of perilunate injuries is the standard of care with dorsal or dorsal/volar approaches (Figure 3). Regarding outcomes, a review of the literature showed flexion/extension arcs of 70% of the contralateral side and grip strength 80% of the contralateral side. Pain was mild to moderate, intermittent, and activity related. Medium- and long-term studies demonstrate radiographic evidence of midcarpal and radiocarpal arthrosis, although this does not correlate with functional outcomes.[21]

Distal Radius Fractures

Distal radius fractures are the most common fracture of the upper extremity. The goal of treatment is to achieve a painless, mobile, durable wrist and upper extremity with the least morbid means in the shortest period of

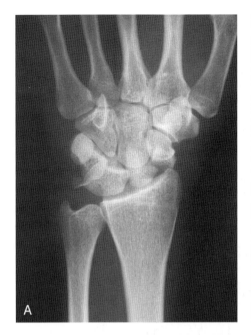

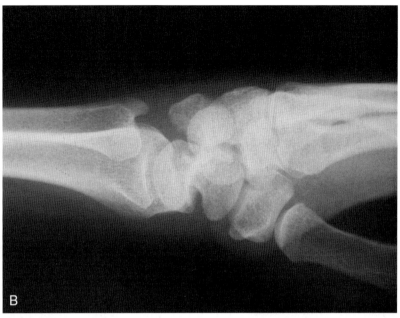

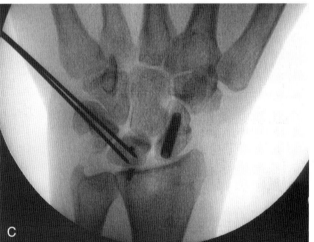

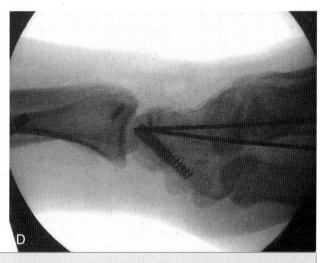

Figure 3 A, PA radiograph of a wrist showing transcaphoid perilunate Mayfield type III dislocation. B, Lateral radiograph of a wrist showing transsscaphoid perilunate Mayfield type III dislocation with the entire carpus dislocated dorsal to the lunate. C, Fluoroscopic PA image of the wrist after open reduction and internal fixation with a headless screw for the scaphoid fracture, K-wire pinning of the lunotriquetral joint, and repair of the dorsal radioulnar ligament with suture anchors. D, Fluoroscopic lateral image of the wrist after open reduction internal fixation. (Courtesy of Steve K. Lee, MD, New York, NY.)

time. Plain radiographs are included in the workup; except for articular shear fractures (volar or dorsal Barton) and nondisplaced fractures, the initial management includes a closed reduction with a hematoma block with or without sedation. Surgery is indicated for open fractures, unstable fractures, and in the setting of multitrauma. Indications for unstable distal radius fractures are controversial. Older patients may be able to tolerate more radiographic malalignment; one study found equal outcomes between surgical and nonsurgical patients 65 years and older.[22] An American Academy of Orthopaedic Surgeons (AAOS) workgroup gave a moderate strength recommendation that surgery is suggested for fractures with postreduction radial short-

ening >3 mm, dorsal tilt > 10°, or intra-articular displacement or stepoff >2 mm.[23] A recent development is the AAOS's Appropriate Use Criteria on the treatment of distal radius fractures, which rates the options as appropriate, may be appropriate, or rarely appropriate, for 216 patient scenarios composed of factors that clinicians use to determine treatment, including fracture type, mechanism of injury, functional demands, American Society of Anesthesiology status, and associated injuries. The Appropriate Use Criteria can be found on the AAOS website (www.aaos.org/auc) or as a web-based application (http://aaos.webauthor.com/go/auc).

Surgical options include closed reduction and pinning with K-wires; external fixation with or without K-wires; internal fixation with nonlocking or locking dorsal, volar, or radial column plates; and intramedullary implants.[24,25] Despite a lack of definitive evidence to prove superior results, internal fixation with locking volar plates is becoming the most popular surgical treatment of choice.[26] One study found that internal fixation led to better grip strength and range of motion at 1 year, and there were fewer malunions than with external fixation.[27] A 2011 study found that malunion after a distal radius fracture was associated with higher arm-related disability regardless of age.[28] Because it is accepted that internal fixation gives better radiologic outcomes, it could be inferred from these two studies that internal fixation will result in better functional outcomes. Furthermore, in a randomized treatment study of locking volar plates, augmented external fixation, and radial column plates, better Disabilities of the Arm, Shoulder and Hand (DASH) scores were noted in the locking volar plate group in the first 3 months after surgery, but at 1 year, the DASH scores, grip strength, and range of motion were equal among the three groups.[29]

Ulnar styloid fractures are commonly associated with distal radius fractures, and the appropriate treatment was controversial. According to two studies, the presence of an ulnar styloid fracture or an ulnar styloid nonunion had no effect on wrist functional outcomes or distal radioulnar joint (DRUJ) stability when a volar locking plate was used.[30,31] The current trend is to refrain from treating ulnar styloid fractures.

In terms of hardware options for locking volar plates, there was no difference in using all distal locking screws versus a distal hybrid (locking and nonlocking screws) construct.[32] In a comparison of four versus seven locking screws in the distal plate, no statistical difference in stiffness and load to failure was found.[33] A 2012 study found that a dorsal rim fracture does not affect outcomes after volar plate fixation.[34] Also, there has been concern that the volar approach with the violation of the pronator would lead to weakness in pronation, but this was not found to be the case after volar plating in one study.[35]

Distal Radioulnar Joint

The DRUJ is a diarthrodial articulation that consists of the ulnar head and the sigmoid notch of the radius. It serves as a pivot for forearm pronation and supination so that the radius can rotate around the stable ulna unit. The osseous anatomy affords little stability. The major static stabilizer is the triangular fibrocartilage complex (TFCC), which consists of the triangular fibrocartilaginous proper (the articular disk), the palmar and dorsal radioulnar ligaments, the meniscal homolog, the ulnar collateral ligament, and the subsheath of the extensor carpi ulnaris. Patients with TFCC injuries without frank DRUJ dislocation can have pain, weakness and, less likely, instability. The Palmer classification is most commonly used; type 1 is traumatic, and type 2 is degenerative. Traumatic injuries most often occur after a twisting injury of the wrist. They can initially be treated nonsurgically with wrist splinting, NSAIDs, or steroid injections. Patients with persistent symptoms may benefit from arthroscopic repair or débridement. Arthroscopic outside-in capsule to articular disk repairs were beneficial in tears of the superficial TFCC fibers when the deep fibers to the fovea were intact.[36] The Palmer 1B subgroup, which consists of ulnar-sided TFCC avulsion with or without styloid fracture, does not make the distinction between tears of the superficial fibers or the deep fibers.

Simple dislocations are most often amenable to closed reduction and splinting in the position of stability for 4 to 6 weeks. Most dislocations are dorsal (by convention in the direction in which the ulnar head goes) and can be held stable in supination. Conversely, volar dislocations are splinted in pronation. If the reduction is not possible by closed means, soft-tissue interposition of the extensor carpi ulnaris tendon or sheath should be suspected, and open reduction is necessary.

DRUJ injuries often occur with other bony injuries such as fractures of the distal radius, as reviewed in the previous section. DRUJ injuries associated with a radial shaft fracture are termed a Galeazzi fracture-dislocation. A higher association of DRUJ involvement when the fracture was within 7.5 cm of the lunate fossa has been described.[37] It is unclear whether immobilization in a particular position is beneficial after treatment of a Galeazzi fracture. A small study (n = 10) found no advantage of 4 weeks of immobilization in supination compared with 2 weeks of immobilization in neutral position after surgically treated shaft fractures with a stable DRUJ.[38]

Soft-Tissue Injuries

Extensor Tendon Injuries

Extensor tendon injuries are relatively common because the dorsum of the hand is exposed to the environment. Extensor tendon zones are numbered as zones I, III, and V at the DIP, PIP, and MCP joints, respectively. Treatment is based on location; sharp lacerations are repaired acutely or subacutely. A recent biomechanical study showed that the running interlocking horizontal mattress technique had superior biomechanical characteristics compared with the augmented Becker or the modified Bunnell repairs[39] (Figure 4).

Flexor Tendon Injuries

The treatment of flexor tendon injuries is controversial; however, evidence-based protocols do exist. Early motion following surgery is preferable and leads to increased tendon strength and decreased tendon adhesions. A four-strand repair as a core suture is the minimal requirement for a controlled active motion protocol. The circumferential suture method adds strength and helps improve the morphology of the repair site for best gliding in the repair site.[40] If repair of the flexor digitorum superficialis in addition to the

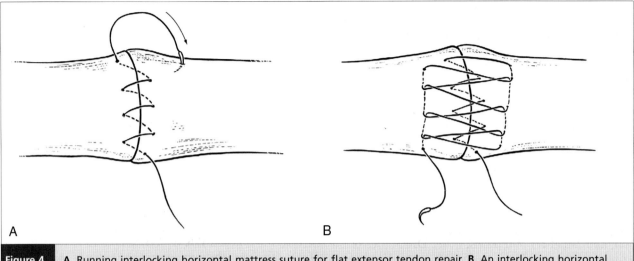

Figure 4   **A,** Running interlocking horizontal mattress suture for flat extensor tendon repair. **B,** An interlocking horizontal mattress suture completes the running interlocking horizontal mattress suture. (Reproduced with permission from Lee SK, Dubey A, Kim BH, Zingman A, Landa J, Paksima N: A biomechanical study of extensor tendon repair methods: Introduction to the running-interlocking horizontal mattress extensor tendon repair technique. *J Hand Surg Am* 2010;35[1]:19-23.)

flexor digitorum profundus is too bulky, then resection of one flexor digitorum superficialis slip decreases gliding resistance.[41]

Nerve Injuries

Nerve injuries are common and can range from brachial plexus injuries to digital nerve lacerations. Regarding brachial plexus reconstruction, one of the major advances has been in the area of nerve transfer.[42] One of the key transfers is the double fascicular transfer, in which fascicles of the ulnar and median nerves are transferred to the nerves to the biceps and brachialis muscles to recover elbow flexion.[43,44] Another key transfer is the spinal accessory nerve to the suprascapular nerve combined with the triceps branch to axillary nerve transfer for shoulder reanimation.[45] Nerve conduits are gaining popularity, and collagen conduits were recently found to be effective for gaps of up to 2 cm for digital nerves.[46] A new alternative is decellularized nerve allografts, which have been effective for treating 2-cm sensory nerve defects in the hand.[47] However, nerve autografts continue to be the gold standard to span nerve defects of motor and mixed nerves, but have associated morbidity and limitations.

High-Pressure Injection Injuries

High-pressure injection injuries are potentially devastating injuries that may lead to amputation in 30% of patients.[48] The injection site is often innocuous and may lead to misdiagnosis and delay in treatment. The nondominant index finger is most often involved. Radiographs may be helpful in determining the extent of injury by air or fat planes or when the material itself is radiopaque. Injury is caused by the physical trauma of the high-pressure injection (with higher pressures caus-

ing more damage), the substance that is injected, and the amount injected. Organic solvents, such as paint thinner, oil-based paint, diesel fuel, jet fuel, and oil, are the most caustic agents that incite a significant inflammatory response that leads to vasospasm and tissue necrosis. Grease, chlorofluorocarbon, and water-based paints are relatively less caustic, whereas water and air are the least caustic. Less severe injuries can be treated nonsurgically with intravenous antibiotics, elevation, observation, and early motion.

Injection with caustic agents constitutes a surgical emergency. One study found that surgery within 6 hours of the injury led to amputation 40% of the time, compared with 57% when surgery was delayed more than 6 hours.[48] Débridement allows decompression of the digit or the hand, removal of some of the material (it is often impossible to remove it all), and resection of nonviable tissue. The use of an additional solvent to clean organic compound injections is contraindicated because it may cause additional damage. Positive cultures do not seem to affect outcomes, and it is unclear if the use of steroids improves outcomes.

Digital Replantation

The frequency of digital replantation in the United States is on the decline because of improved safety with work tools and stricter indications for surgery. Indications still include multiple digits, all thumb injuries, any digit in a child, and amputations in flexor tendon zone I. Relative contraindications are a single digit in zone II, a mangled amputated part, and other comorbidities that make surgery unsafe. Current practices for anticoagulation include no anticoagulation, aspirin, intravenous heparin, low-molecular-weight heparin (LMWH), intravenous dextran, direct heparin applica-

3: Upper Extremity

tion, warfarin, and leech therapy. Evidence regarding best efficacy is lacking.[49]

Hand Replantation

Hand transplantation programs are increasingly being established at medical centers. The procedure entails transplanting a composite (skin, muscle, tendon, nerve, artery, or vein) tissue allograft. These programs require a true multidisciplinary approach with hand surgeons, transplant immunologists, hand therapists, psychiatrists, medical specialists, anesthesiologists, and others. Success depends on proper patient selection, a well-performed surgery, intensive rehabilitation, long-term immunosuppression that prevents rejection with low side effects, and continuous monitoring for rejection.[50] It is questioned whether this procedure is affordable in the current healthcare environment and whether it is necessary given the risks of long-term immunosuppression because it is a life-enhancing, not life-saving, procedure.[51] However, encouraging results have been reported with this procedure.

Summary

Hand and wrist trauma can be challenging because of injuries of more than one system, for example, musculoskeletal (bone, joint, tendon, ligament), nervous, vascular, and skin/soft tissue. Those who treat these conditions must address all injured aspects of the extremity and provide the appropriate treatment as well as tailored postoperative care and rehabilitation. The tolerance for deficits is low, especially in the finger. As in all orthopaedic disciplines, more research is needed in hand and wrist trauma. However, there have been some advances in this field that have affected the management of these injuries.

Key Study Points

- Current studies support no surgical intervention for ulnar styloid fractures during surgical treatment of distal radius fractures because the presence of ulnar styloid fractures and nonunions does not appear to affect outcomes.

- Patients age 65 years and older may not benefit from the surgical treatment of distal radius fractures because equal outcomes have been found between these patients treated surgically and nonsurgically.

- Digital nerve injuries with up to a 2-cm gap can be effectively repaired with nerve conduits; acellular nerve allograft may be a viable option for the same nerve defect length.

Annotated References

1. Smit JM, Beets MR, Zeebregts CJ, Rood A, Welters CF: Treatment options for mallet finger: A review. *Plast Reconstr Surg* 2010;126(5):1624-1629.

   This review states that splinting appears to be effective in uncomplicated and complicated cases of mallet finger. Equal results have been reported for early and delayed splinting therapy. Cases that do not do well with splint therapy are best treated surgically.

2. Vitale MA, White NJ, Strauch RJ: A percutaneous technique to treat unstable dorsal fracture-dislocations of the proximal interphalangeal joint. *J Hand Surg Am* 2011;36(9):1453-1459.

   This study reviewed six patients with unstable dorsal fracture-dislocations of the PIP joint treated with a new percutaneous technique. Level of evidence: IV.

3. Ikeda M, Kobayashi Y, Saito I, Ishii T, Shimizu A, Oka Y: Open reduction and internal fixation for dorsal fracture dislocations of the proximal interphalangeal joint using a miniplate. *Tech Hand Up Extrem Surg* 2011; 15(4):219-224.

   This study reviewed 19 dorsal fracture-dislocations. Active PIP motion averaged 85°. Level of evidence: IV.

4. Cheah AE, Tan DM, Chong AK, Chew WY: Volar plating for unstable proximal interphalangeal joint dorsal fracture-dislocations. *J Hand Surg Am* 2012;37(1): 28-33.

   This study reviewed 13 cases of dorsal fracture-dislocations treated with a volar plate. The authors found good objective and subjective outcomes, but there was a 39% complication rate. Level of evidence: IV.

5. Tang P: Collateral ligament injuries of the thumb metacarpophalangeal joint. *J Am Acad Orthop Surg* 2011; 19(5):287-296.

   The author reviewed the history and treatment of ulnar and radial collateral ligament injuries the thumb. Surgery is indicated for MCP radial deviation (for the ulnar collateral ligament) and ulnar deviation (for the radial collateral ligament) greater than 30° to 35° or 15° greater than the contralateral side.

6. Ochman S, Doht S, Paletta J, Langer M, Raschke MJ, Meffert RH: Comparison between locking and nonlocking plates for fixation of metacarpal fractures in an animal model. *J Hand Surg Am* 2010;35(4):597-603.

   Monocortical locking plates were found to be stronger than nonlocking bicortical plates, although this was not statistically significant.

7. Huang JI, Fernandez DL: Fractures of the base of the thumb metacarpal. *Instr Course Lect* 2010;59:343-356.

   The authors reviewed fractures of the base of the thumb metacarpal.

8. Brownlie C, Anderson D: Bennett fracture dislocation: Review and management. *Aust Fam Physician* 2011;

40(6):394-396.

A current review of the literature on Bennett fracture-dislocation is presented. Inadequate treatment leads to osteoarthritis, weakness, and/or loss of function of the first CMC joint. The key to a successful outcome is adequate reduction and maintenance of the reduction.

9. Vender MI, Watson HK, Wiener BD, Black DM: Degenerative change in symptomatic scaphoid nonunion. *J Hand Surg Am* 1987;12(4):514-519.

10. Bond CD, Shin AY, McBride MT, Dao KD: Percutaneous screw fixation or cast immobilization for nondisplaced scaphoid fractures. *J Bone Joint Surg Am* 2001; 83(4):483-488.

11. Gellman H, Caputo RJ, Carter V, Aboulafia A, McKay M: Comparison of short and long thumb-spica casts for non-displaced fractures of the carpal scaphoid. *J Bone Joint Surg Am* 1989;71(3):354-357.

12. Kim RY, Lijten EC, Strauch RJ: Pronated oblique view in assessing proximal scaphoid articular cannulated screw penetration. *J Hand Surg Am* 2008;33(8):1274-1277.

13. Geissler WB, Adams JE, Bindra RR, Lanzinger WD, Slutsky DJ: Scaphoid fractures: What's hot, what's not. *J Bone Joint Surg Am* 2012;94(2):169-181.

This review of scaphoid fractures discusses the latest treatment of acute scaphoid fractures and scaphoid nonunions.

14. Vigler M, Aviles A, Lee SK: Carpal fractures excluding the scaphoid. *Hand Clin* 2006;22(4):501-516, abstract vii.

15. Merrell GA, Wolfe SW, Slade JF III: Treatment of scaphoid nonunions: Quantitative meta-analysis of the literature. *J Hand Surg Am* 2002;27(4):685-691.

16. Jones DB Jr, Bürger H, Bishop AT, Shin AY: Treatment of scaphoid waist nonunions with an avascular proximal pole and carpal collapse: A comparison of two vascularized bone grafts. *J Bone Joint Surg Am* 2008; 90(12):2616-2625.

17. Kuo CE, Wolfe SW: Scapholunate instability: Current concepts in diagnosis and management. *J Hand Surg Am* 2008;33(6):998-1013.

18. Rosenwasser MP, Miyasajsa KC, Strauch RJ: The RASL procedure: Reduction and association of the scaphoid and lunate using the Herbert screw. *Tech Hand Up Extrem Surg* 1997;1(4):263-272.

19. Cohen MS, Kozin SH: Degenerative arthritis of the wrist: Proximal row carpectomy versus scaphoid excision and four-corner arthrodesis. *J Hand Surg Am* 2001;26(1):94-104.

20. Stern PJ, Agabegi SS, Kiefhaber TR, Didonna ML:

Proximal row carpectomy. *J Bone Joint Surg Am* 2005; 87(pt 2, suppl 1):166-174.

21. Stanbury SJ, Elfar JC: Perilunate dislocation and perilunate fracture-dislocation. *J Am Acad Orthop Surg* 2011;19(9):554-562.

This article reviews dorsal, volar, and pilon proximal interphalangeal joint fracture-dislocation patterns. The authors state that an acceptable outcome depends on achieving a well-aligned joint, reestablishing normal joint kinematics, and restoring motion. Anatomic articular reduction is desirable but not absolutely necessary for a good outcome.

22. Arora R, Lutz M, Deml C, Krappinger D, Haug L, Gabl M: A prospective randomized trial comparing nonoperative treatment with volar locking plate fixation for displaced and unstable distal radial fractures in patients sixty-five years of age and older. *J Bone Joint Surg Am* 2011;93(23):2146-2153.

This study found at 12 months' follow-up examination that the range of motion, the level of pain, and the Patient-Rated Wrist Evaluation and DASH scores were not different between the surgical and nonsurgical treatment groups. Patients in the surgical treatment group had better grip strength for the entire time period of the study. Level of evidence: I.

23. Lichtman DM, Bindra RR, Boyer MI, et al: Treatment of distal radius fractures. *J Am Acad Orthop Surg* 2010; 18(3):180-189.

An AAOS workgroup's guideline on the treatment of distal radius fractures is presented. Surgical fixation is recommended for postreduction radial shortening greater than 3 mm, dorsal tilt greater than 10°, or intra-articular displacement or stepoff greater than 2 mm. They also recommend rigid immobilization rather than removable splints for nonsurgical treatment, beginning early wrist motion following stable fixation, and adjuvant treatment with vitamin C to prevent disproportionate pain.

24. Nishiwaki M, Tazaki K, Shimizu H, Ilyas AM: Prospective study of distal radial fractures treated with an intramedullary nail. *J Bone Joint Surg Am* 2011;93(15): 1436-1441.

This prospective study found that intramedullary nailing can be safe and effective. At 1 year, range of motion compared with the contralateral side was 95% for flexion and extension, and grip strength was 96%. The modified Mayo wrist score was excellent in 20 patients and good in 9 patients. The mean DASH score was 4.8. Level of evidence: IV.

25. Tan V, Bratchenko W, Nourbakhsh A, Capo J: Comparative analysis of intramedullary nail fixation versus casting for treatment of distal radius fractures. *J Hand Surg Am* 2012;37(3):460-468, e1.

Intramedullary nail fixation, compared with casting, results in less functional disability in the early and 1-year follow-up evaluation for unstable extra-articular or simple intra-articular distal radius fractures. Level of evidence: II.

3: Upper Extremity

26. Chung KC, Shauver MJ, Yin H: The relationship between ASSH membership and the treatment of distal radius fracture in the United States Medicare population. *J Hand Surg Am* 2011;36(8):1288-1293.

    This therapeutic study found that Medicare beneficiaries who were treated by American Society for Surgery of the Hand member surgeons receive internal fixation at a significantly higher rate than do patients of other physicians. Level of evidence: II.

27. Abramo A, Kopylov P, Geijer M, Tägil M: Open reduction and internal fixation compared to closed reduction and external fixation in distal radial fractures: A randomized study of 50 patients. *Acta Orthop* 2009;80(4): 478-485.

28. Brogren E, Hofer M, Petranek M, Wagner P, Dahlin LB, Atroshi I: Relationship between distal radius fracture malunion and arm-related disability: A prospective population-based cohort study with 1-year follow-up. *BMC Musculoskelet Disord* 2011;12:9.

    This prospective study found that malunion after a distal radius fracture was associated with higher arm-related disability regardless of age. Level of evidence: II.

29. Wei DH, Raizman NM, Bottino CJ, Jobin CM, Strauch RJ, Rosenwasser MP: Unstable distal radial fractures treated with external fixation, a radial column plate, or a volar plate: A prospective randomized trial. *J Bone Joint Surg Am* 2009;91(7):1568-1577.

30. Kim JK, Koh YD, Do NH: Should an ulnar styloid fracture be fixed following volar plate fixation of a distal radial fracture? *J Bone Joint Surg Am* 2010;92(1):1-6.

    This prognostic study found that an accompanying ulnar styloid fracture in patients with stable fixation of a distal radius fracture had no apparent adverse effects on wrist function or stability of the DRUJ. Level of evidence: II.

31. Kim JK, Yun YH, Kim DJ, Yun GU: Comparison of united and nonunited fractures of the ulnar styloid following volar-plate fixation of distal radius fractures. *Injury* 2011;42(4):371-375.

    This observational study found that ulnar styloid nonunion does not appear to affect wrist functional outcomes, ulnar-sided wrist pain, or DRUJ stability, at least when a distal radius fracture is treated by open reduction and volar plate fixation. Level of evidence: III.

32. Sokol SC, Amanatullah DF, Curtiss S, Szabo RM: Biomechanical properties of volar hybrid and locked plate fixation in distal radius fractures. *J Hand Surg Am* 2011;36(4):591-597.

    This study found that the biomechanical properties were similar between all distal locking screws versus distal hybrid (locking and nonlocking) constructs in locked plates.

33. Moss DP, Means KR Jr, Parks BG, Forthman CL: A biomechanical comparison of volar locked plating of intra-articular distal radius fractures: Use of 4 versus 7 screws for distal fixation. *J Hand Surg Am* 2011; 36(12):1907-1911.

    This biomechanical cadaver study found increased stiffness and higher failure load in fractures fixed distally with seven locking screws; the results were not statistically significant compared with fractures fixed with only four screws.

34. Kim JK, Cho SW: The effects of a displaced dorsal rim fracture on outcomes after volar plate fixation of a distal radius fracture. *Injury* 2012;43(2):143-146.

    This case-control study found no significant difference in wrist function or wrist pain between patients who had a displaced (> 2 mm) dorsal rim fracture and those without a dorsal rim fracture. Level of evidence: III.

35. Chirpaz-Cerbat JM, Ruatti S, Houillon C, Ionescu S: Dorsally displaced distal radius fractures treated by fixed-angle volar plating: Grip and pronosupination strength recovery. A prospective study. *Orthop Traumatol Surg Res* 2011;97(5):465-470.

    This prospective study evaluated whether violation of the pronator quadratus with repair in the setting of a fixed-angle palmar plate affected pronation strength. They found good recovery of grip, pronation, and supination strength. Level of evidence: IV.

36. Wysocki RW, Richard MJ, Crowe MM, Leversedge FJ, Ruch DS: Arthroscopic treatment of peripheral triangular fibrocartilage complex tears with the deep fibers intact. *J Hand Surg Am* 2012;37(3):509-516.

    The authors of this study found improvement in pain and function with outside-in repair of the articular disk back to the ulnar capsule for tears of the superficial fibers with the deep fibers intact. Return to sports was variable and appeared worse for those who bear weight through the hands. Level of evidence: IV.

37. Rettig ME, Raskin KB: Galeazzi fracture-dislocation: A new treatment-oriented classification. *J Hand Surg Am* 2001;26(2):228-235.

38. Park MJ, Pappas N, Steinberg DR, Bozentka DJ: Immobilization in supination versus neutral following surgical treatment of Galeazzi fracture-dislocations in adults: Case series. *J Hand Surg Am* 2012;37(3):528-531.

    The authors of this study found, in the setting of surgically treated radial shaft fractures with internal fixation with no treatment of the DRUJ in the setting of the Galeazzi fracture-dislocations, no advantage of splinting in supination for 4 weeks over splinting in neutral for 2 weeks. However, the study had only five patients in each group. Level of evidence: III.

39. Lee SK, Dubey A, Kim BH, Zingman A, Landa J, Paksima N: A biomechanical study of extensor tendon repair methods: Introduction to the running-interlocking horizontal mattress extensor tendon repair technique. *J Hand Surg Am* 2010;35(1):19-23.

    In a biomechanical study, a new tendon repair method for flat extensor tendons was compared with two other previously reported methods. The new running interlocking horizontal mattress method has superior biomechanical characteristics.

40. Lee SK, Goldstein RY, Zingman A, Terranova C, Nasser P, Hausman MR: The effects of core suture purchase on the biomechanical characteristics of a multistrand locking flexor tendon repair: A cadaveric study. *J Hand Surg Am* 2010;35(7):1165-1171.

The authors of this biomechanical study investigated the effect of suture purchase on biomechanical characteristics for the combination repair method cross-locked cruciate–interlocking horizontal mattress method. Ten-millimeter suture purchase is optimal with 90 N 2-mm gap resistance and 111 N ultimate strength.

41. Paillard PJ, Amadio PC, Zhao C, Zobitz ME, An KN: Pulley plasty versus resection of one slip of the flexor digitorum superficialis after repair of both flexor tendons in zone II: A biomechanical study. *J Bone Joint Surg Am* 2002;84(11):2039-2045.

42. Lee SK, Wolfe SW: Nerve transfers for the upper extremity: New horizons in nerve reconstruction. *J Am Acad Orthop Surg* 2012;20(8):506-517.

Nerve transfers have had a positive effect on brachial plexus and complex nerve reconstruction. Advantages of nerve transfers include shortened nerve regeneration distance, selective motor or sensory donor transfers, and the lack of need for nerve grafts. Expendable donor nervers are transferred to denervated nerves with the goal of functional recovery. Transfers may be subdivided into intraplexal, extraplexal, and distal types.

43. Liverneaux PA, Diaz LC, Beaulieu JY, Durand S, Oberlin C: Preliminary results of double nerve transfer to restore elbow flexion in upper type brachial plexus palsies. *Plast Reconstr Surg* 2006;117(3):915-919.

44. Ray WZ, Pet MA, Yee A, Mackinnon SE: Double fascicular nerve transfer to the biceps and brachialis muscles after brachial plexus injury: Clinical outcomes in a series of 29 cases. *J Neurosurg* 2011;114(6):1520-1528.

The efficacy of the groundbreaking nerve transfer set to achieve elbow flexion was demonstrated. Twenty-eight of 29 patients achieved M3 or better elbow flexion, and 23 of 29 achieved M4 or better elbow flexion. Level of evidence: IV.

45. Leechavengvongs S, Witoonchart K, Uerpairojkit C, Thuvasethakul P: Nerve transfer to deltoid muscle using the nerve to the long head of the triceps, part II: A report of 7 cases. *J Hand Surg Am* 2003;28(4):633-638.

46. Taras JS, Jacoby SM, Lincoski CJ: Reconstruction of digital nerves with collagen conduits. *J Hand Surg Am* 2011;36(9):1441-1446.

A clinical series demonstrating efficacy of collagen conduits for digital nerve reconstruction with gaps less than 2 cm is presented. Level of evidence: IV.

47. Karabekmez FE, Duymaz A, Moran SL: Early clinical outcomes with the use of decellularized nerve allograft for repair of sensory defects within the hand. *Hand (NY)* 2009;4(3):245-249.

48. Hogan CJ, Ruland RT: High-pressure injection injuries to the upper extremity: A review of the literature. *J Orthop Trauma* 2006;20(7):503-511.

49. Buckley T, Hammert WC: Anticoagulation following digital replantation. *J Hand Surg Am* 2011;36(8):1374-1376.

The authors reviewed anticoagulation treatment after digital replantation. For the article's theoretic case of the young patient after two-digit replantation, the authors recommended 325 mg of aspirin daily and LMWH for deep vein thrombosis prophylaxis. If during the surgery there were vascular difficulties (thrombosis, revision of an anastomosis), then they used intravenous heparin to be switched to warfarin or LMWH for a total of 30 days after surgery.

50. Shores JT, Imbriglia JE, Lee WP: The current state of hand transplantation. *J Hand Surg Am* 2011;36(11):1862-1867.

Hand transplantation findings in 2011 were reviewed. Success requires a multidisciplinary approach as well as proper patient selection, a technically sound procedure, appropriate rehabilitation, and an immunotherapy protocol that prevents rejection and has low morbidity.

51. Chang J, Mathes DW: Ethical, financial, and policy considerations in hand transplantation. *Hand Clin* 2011;27(4):553-560, xi.

The nonmedical aspects of hand transplantation were reviewed. Ethical debate continues regarding the risks and benefits of this nonlifesaving procedure. Clinicians, patients, and society must agree whether hand transplantation is ethical and affordable. If a decision is made to perform hand transplantation, the procedure must be performed at a dedicated center.

Video Reference

31.1: Rosenwasser MP: Video. *The Drive-Through Sign.* New York, NY, 2013.

Chapter 32

Hand and Wrist Reconstruction

Michael V. Birman, MD   Robert J. Strauch, MD

Osteoarthritis

Thumb Carpometacarpal Joint

Arthritis at the carpometacarpal (CMC) joint of the thumb is the second most common location for arthritis in the hand, after the distal interphalangeal (DIP) joint. The Eaton-Glickel (Littler) classification of arthritis at the thumb CMC joint is commonly used to characterize the degree of arthritis. However, because of moderate interobserver reliability[1] and a lack of correlation of clinical symptoms to the extent of radiographic arthritis, a complete evaluation of the individual patient is necessary to guide treatment of this condition. Primary patient complaints include pain localizing to the base of the thumb and difficulty with activities that require thumb pinch or grip. The key findings on examination are a positive grind test and focal tenderness at the thumb CMC joint, which must be differentiated from pain localizing to the first dorsal compartment (de Quervain tenosynovitis) or the scaphotrapezial trapezoid (STT) joint. The basis of subluxation of the thumb CMC joint as degenerative changes progress is a failure of the ligamentous supports of the joint in addition to bony derangement. Historically, the key stabilizer for the joint had been considered the anterior oblique (or volar beak) ligament; however, a recent study has demonstrated the importance of the dorsoradial ligament as the primary ligamentous stabilizer.[2]

Initial treatment is generally nonsurgical, which includes NSAIDs, activity modification, splints, and corticosteroid injections. Hyaluronic acid injections may be considered as an off-label use, but a prospective, randomized, double-blind study evaluating hyaluronic acid, steroid, and placebo injections for thumb CMC arthritis found no statistically significant differences among these agents.[3]

A wide variety of surgical options have been described, often correlated with the stages of the Eaton-Glickel classification. The surgical treatment options for Eaton stage I (widening of the joint) include ligament reconstruction or metacarpal extension osteotomy. The next two stages, II and III, are characterized by progressive narrowing of the joint space, increasing osteophytes, sclerosis, and subluxation of the joint. The addition of arthritis at the STT joint characterizes stage IV. Trapeziectomy (partial or complete), with or without ligament reconstruction and tendon interposition, is typically performed for stages III and IV. Trapeziometacarpal arthrodesis is uncommonly performed but may be considered for a young manual laborer (younger than 40 years). Arthrodesis has the potential downside of nonunion and progressive degeneration of the STT joint, in addition to difficulty reaching into pants and coat pockets because of a lack of flexion and rotation at the trapeziometacarpal joint. There is a lack of evidence that any additional steps beyond trapeziectomy (**Figure 1**) improve patient outcomes; nevertheless, ligament reconstruction and tendon interposition is favored by many surgeons.[4,5] Most commonly, the flexor carpi radialis or the abductor pollicis longus are used for suspension, and the rest of the harvested tendon is used for interposition. Some surgeons prefer the wide variety of nonautogenous options that are available for interposition, but many of these nonautogenous materials have demonstrated significant complications without a well-defined benefit.[6] The presence of

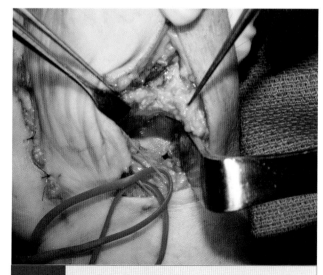

| Figure 1 | Intraoperative photograph of the defect remaining following surgical excision of the trapezium. |

Dr. Strauch or an immediate family member serves as a board member, owner, officer, or committee member of the American Society for Surgery of the Hand. Neither Dr. Birman nor any immediate family member has received anything of value from or has stock or stock options held in a commercial company or institution related directly or indirectly to the subject of this chapter.

3: Upper Extremity

arthritis at the STT joint leads many surgeons to perform a complete rather than a partial trapeziectomy, whereas others believe that an asymptomatic but arthritic STT joint does not mandate complete trapeziectomy.[7] Concomitant painful arthritis of the thumb metacarpophalangeal (MCP) joint is best treated by arthrodesis; a hyperextensible but nonarthritic MCP joint should be treated at the time of CMC arthroplasty. Soft-tissue stabilization, such as volar capsulodesis or advancement of the intrinsic muscles,[8,9] may suffice for mild to moderate hyperextension (< 45°), but severe MCP hyperextension may require arthrodesis. Untreated thumb MCP joint hyperextension results in flexion at the CMC joint with pinch, which may compromise the CMC arthroplasty.

Scaphotrapezial Trapezoid Joint

Arthritis of the STT joint often occurs concomitantly with arthritis of the trapeziometacarpal joint. In this setting, arthritis at the STT joint is treated with complete resection of the trapezium, along with additional excision of the proximal 2 mm of the trapezoid if indicated by intraoperative findings of STT arthritis. Symptomatic isolated arthritis of the STT joint may be managed with an algorithm that progresses from NSAIDs, splints, and corticosteroid injections to surgical STT excisional arthroplasty (excision of the distal pole of the scaphoid) or STT arthrodesis. In isolated STT arthritis, some patients have a dorsal intercalated segment instability (DISI) deformity, which in this setting represents a nondissociative midcarpal instability pattern with extension of both the scaphoid and the lunate, a normal scapholunate angle, and no radiographic scapholunate widening. A preexisting DISI deformity may be exacerbated in this setting if distal pole scaphoid excision is performed.[10]

Metacarpophalangeal Joint

MCP joint arthritis is more common in the thumb than the fingers. The etiology for the arthritis may be degenerative, traumatic, inflammatory, or crystalline. Thumb MCP joint motion normally varies widely between individuals, with a range from 0° to a 180° arc. Arthrodesis for painful arthritis of the thumb MCP joint is the procedure of choice, with a fusion angle ranging from 5° to 15° of flexion. By contrast, for the other fingers, where rheumatoid arthritis is the more common etiology, arthroplasty is favored over arthrodesis. In the setting of rheumatoid arthritis, if ulnar drift is present, it must be corrected with intrinsic releases and realignment of the extensor mechanism. Arthroplasty options include silicone implants and unconstrained surface replacement (pyrolytic carbon and metal-on-polyethylene) implants. The surface replacement implants require adequate bone stock, minimal deformity, and good soft tissues; otherwise, a silicone implant is the preferred option. Although the short-term results of silicone implants show high patient satisfaction and reported function, long-term follow-up studies have reported high rates of implant fracture and recurrence of

deformity.[11-14] In osteoarthritis and early rheumatoid arthritis, unconstrained surface replacement implants may be considered, but long-term outcome studies are not available.

Proximal and Distal Interphalangeal Joints

Osteoarthritis of the proximal interphalangeal (PIP) joint and the DIP joint is common. On the dorsum of the DIP joints, the development of an overlying mucous cyst may require treatment if symptomatic; surgery must include débridement of the DIP joint osteophytes. Whether the etiology of the PIP joint arthritis is degenerative or inflammatory, surgical treatment options include arthrodesis versus arthroplasty. Arthroplasty is traditionally favored for the middle and ring fingers, and arthrodesis is used for the index and sometimes the small fingers. Arthrodesis is recommended for the index finger because of the importance of joint stability for coronal-plane pinch (or key pinch) activities. PIP joint arthrodesis is classically positioned at 30° to 45° of flexion, with greater degrees of flexion in the ulnar digits. Similar to the MCP joint, arthroplasty options include silicone implants and surface replacement implants, such as metal-on-polyethylene and pyrolytic carbon. Long-term studies of silicone implants found good pain relief and relatively low revision rates despite implant fractures and failure to make lasting significant gains in range of motion.[15] Follow-up periods for surface replacement arthroplasty are still shorter than for silicone implants; revision surgery may be required for complications including dislocation, extensor lag, implant fracture, and joint contracture. A randomized, controlled, multicenter trial comparing three types of implants (titanium-polyethylene, pyrocarbon, and silicone) concluded that although surface replacement arthroplasty devices showed a tendency for temporary superior maximum postoperative range of motion, they had markedly higher postoperative complication and explantation rates compared with silicone.[16] Symptomatic advanced arthritis of the DIP joint is treated with arthrodesis, in neutral to slight flexion.

Posttraumatic Arthritis of the Wrist

Scapholunate Advanced Collapse Wrist

Scapholunate advanced collapse (SLAC) wrist characterizes the most common pattern of wrist arthritis. It is traditionally associated with long-standing disruption of the scapholunate ligament that may result from trauma, crystalline synovitis, or genetics. Asymptomatic bilateral SLAC wrist has been shown to exist without antecedent trauma.[17,18] Although the specific natural history and progression of arthritis is controversial, a significant percentage of patients with SLAC wrist can be classified according to the stages of the disease process described by Watson and Ballet.[19] Stage I SLAC wrist is characterized by degenerative changes localizing to the joint space between the radial styloid and the scaphoid. Stage II SLAC wrist describes disease progression to involve the proximal radioscaphoid joint. The final stage described by Watson and Ballet is stage III SLAC wrist, which is characterized by progression of arthritis to the capitolunate joint space. The radiolunate joint is usually spared. Some authors also include a stage IV, which describes pancarpal arthritis. Patients may present with wrist joint effusion, dorsal radial wrist swelling, tenderness at the radioscaphoid joint, and decreased wrist range of motion.

Nonsurgical management of SLAC wrist includes splints, injections, and therapeutic modalities. When nonsurgical modalities fail, the surgical options for symptomatic SLAC wrist range from arthroscopy, wrist denervation, radial styloidectomy, and proximal row carpectomy (PRC) to partial or total wrist arthrodesis. For pancarpal arthritis, total wrist arthroplasty is an option, although long-term clinical studies for the specific indication of SLAC wrist have not been performed. Wrist arthroscopy for débridement with arthroscopic or open radial styloidectomy is a promising—but little studied—technique for early or advanced stage SLAC wrist.[20] Several authors have reported the results of partial and complete wrist denervation for wrist arthritis, with a small subset of these patients having SLAC wrists. Denervation can offer partial or complete pain relief while maintaining wrist motion and avoiding hardware or fusion; however, the results are not universally successful, particularly when satisfaction and pain relief rates are compared with those of PRC or partial wrist arthrodesis.[17,21]

Although partially dictated by surgeon preference and patient characteristics, the decision to perform a PRC as opposed to a four-corner arthrodesis depends on relatively well-preserved capitate articular cartilage. The condition of the capitate head articular surface may be evaluated on radiographs, on MRI, or more definitively by wrist arthroscopy or direct visual inspection. If little or no wear is present on the capitate head, PRC may be considered; significant wear usually precludes PRC, but the extent of maintained cartilage required for successful PRC is unknown. To proceed with PRC when there is some damage on the capitate, some surgeons may use soft-tissue interposition or resurface focal lesions on the capitate.[22]

Comparison studies of PRC and four-corner arthrodesis in the literature show minimal differences in outcomes of pain relief, grip strength, and subjective measures. Some authors favor PRC because it avoids potential complications from hardware, nonunion, and malposition of the lunate, which in a four-corner arthrodesis should be positioned in neutral to slight flexion to avoid limiting motion as a result of impingement. In a systematic review of outcomes, the authors concluded that PRC may provide better postoperative range of movement and lacks the potential complications specific to four-corner arthrodesis.[23] However, in a study with a minimum 10-year follow-up of PRC, four failures were reported in a group of 22 wrists; all four were in patients who were 35 years or younger at the time of the index procedure.[24] The evidence comparing the two techniques was summarized in another

study.[25] Both procedures are comparable in successfully decreasing pain in approximately 85% of patients and improving grip strength to about 80% of the contralateral side. An average flexion-extension arc of 75° to 80° can be expected, but it is usually 10° less for four-corner arthrodesis than PRC. The risk of conversion to total wrist arthrodesis for both procedures is equal, approximately 5%. The risk of subsequent osteoarthritis is significantly higher in patients who undergo PRC, but it is generally asymptomatic, and symptoms do not correlate with radiographic joint space narrowing.

Scaphoid Nonunion Advanced Collapse Wrist

An untreated scaphoid nonunion can lead to progressive arthritic change in the wrist, a pattern termed scaphoid nonunion advanced collapse (SNAC). Staging for SNAC wrist is analogous to SLAC wrist with the exception that the surface between the proximal scaphoid fragment and the distal radius is spared. In early SNAC wrist, the scaphoid nonunion can be repaired, with a radial styloidectomy performed concomitantly to treat the first stage of arthritic wear at the styloid. In the absence of arthritic changes at the capitolunate joint and generally when at least half of the scaphoid can be retained, excision of the nonunited distal scaphoid pole is an option for radioscaphoid pain as a result of chronic SNAC wrist. A study of 13 patients who underwent this procedure concluded that it can provide pain relief and increase range of motion.[26] As SNAC wrist progresses, salvage procedures as described for SLAC wrist can be considered.

Distal Radioulnar Joint

Arthritis at the distal radioulnar joint (DRUJ) may be caused by posttraumatic, degenerative, or inflammatory etiologies. Nonsurgical treatment includes rest, splinting, and a corticosteroid injection, which may be beneficial for diagnostic and/or therapeutic purposes. If nonsurgical treatment fails, the surgical treatment options include hemiresection of the ulnar head with or without soft-tissue interposition (Bowers hemiresection interposition arthroplasty or the Watson matched distal ulna resection), resection of the entire ulnar head (Darrach procedure), arthrodesis of the DRUJ with resection of a portion of the ulnar proximal to the sigmoid notch (Sauve-Kapandji procedure), or, more recently, implant arthroplasty. In the setting of a stable DRUJ with intact triangular fibrocartilage complex (TFCC), hemiresection has the theoretic but unproven advantage of maintaining the attachment for the TFCC at the DRUJ, although radioulnar convergence can still occur. Concern about instability of the distal ulna and convergence of the distal radius and ulna following a Darrach procedure leads some surgeons to favor it only in the older, low-demand patient, particularly in the setting of rheumatoid arthritis, although the procedure can be successful in posttraumatic cases. Implant arthroplasty is still in the early stages of development, but several reports of short- and intermediate-term follow-up are available. A recent 10-year follow-up of one design

3: Upper Extremity

Table 1

Lichtman Classification of Kienböck Disease

Radiographic Stage	Description
I	Normal radiographs; low signal on MRI, possible linear or compression fracture
II	Radiographic lunate sclerosis without collapse
IIIA	Lunate collapse without scaphoid rotation
IIIB	Lunate collapse with rotatory scaphoid deformity
IV	Radiocarpal and/or midcarpal arthrosis

found improved pain and outcome scores but no significant improvement in forearm rotation and wrist function; there was 83% implant survival at 6 years, and 30% of the patients required additional surgery most often for instability.[27] Implant arthroplasty for the DRUJ has potential, but its indications and designs are still being studied, and long-term studies are still needed to fully assess both clinical outcomes and complication or failure rates.

Kienböck Disease

Kienböck disease is characterized by osteonecrosis of the carpal lunate bone, resulting in sclerosis, fragmentation, and collapse of the lunate. Thought to be the result of a combination of vascular, mechanical, and systemic factors, the etiology and the natural history of the disease process is still unclear. Patients may present with reports of wrist pain, decreased wrist range of motion, and swelling (indicative of synovitis) over the dorsum of the wrist. The radiographic patterns are described by the Lichtman classification, which is presented in Table 1, representing the progression from MRI signal changes to lunate collapse and carpal arthritis. Radiographs are adequate for assessing advanced disease, but the early stages are best evaluated with MRI, particularly in differentiating the disease from ulnocarpal impaction where focal, rather than diffuse, changes are seen in the lunate. The staging helps guide treatment, as does additional consideration of the ulnar variance. Although commonly associated with an ulnar negative variance, Kienböck disease is also seen in the setting of ulnar neutral or positive variance.

Treatment is initially nonsurgical, consisting of observation, immobilization, and activity modification. The surgical treatments of Kienböck disease are myriad, with most surgical series describing adequate pain relief. The surgical treatment options include joint leveling procedures (radial shortening or osteotomy), partial wrist fusions (STT, scaphocapitate, capitohamate), capitate shortening, vascularized bone grafting, and core decompression procedures of the radius, the ulna, or the lunate bones. Other described procedures include lunate excision with tendon ball interposition, PRC, and wrist fusion. A systematic review of the literature evaluated the various treatments of both the early and late stages of Kienböck disease and concluded that no specific treatment proved superior.[28] The most common and well-studied procedure for Kienböck disease with ulnar minus variance is radial shortening osteotomy for stages I to IIIB.

Ulnar Wrist Pain

Differential of Ulnar Wrist Pain

The evaluation of ulnar wrist pain involves careful clinical examination of the relevant anatomy, including the TFCC, the lunotriquetral (LT) ligament, the extensor and flexor carpi ulnaris tendons, and the relevant bony articulations (ulnocarpal, pisotriquetral, LT, and distal radioulnar). The common causes of ulnar wrist pain include ulnar styloid fracture, TFCC injury, extensor carpi ulnaris tendinitis, LT injury, ulnocarpal impaction, and pisotriquetral arthritis.

Triangular Fibrocartilage Complex

The TFCC stabilizes the ulnar carpus and the DRUJ. Both traumatic and degenerative conditions can affect the TFCC, leading to ulnar wrist pain. Tenderness localizes to the ulnar fovea, which has been found to be both a sensitive and a specific sign of TFCC pathology.[29] In addition to standard radiographs of the wrist, including a neutral rotation PA view, a grip PA view in pronation (pronation maximizes the ulnar variance) helps assess for dynamic ulnar impaction. MRI and magnetic resonance arthrography (MRA) are the most useful advanced imaging modalities for TFCC injuries, with high sensitivity and specificity for central TFCC tears but notably lower for peripheral TFCC lesions and LT ligament tears. A meta-analysis of MRI and MRA evaluation of full-thickness TFCC tears concluded that MRA was superior to MRI; sensitivity and specificity were 0.75 and 0.81, respectively, for MRI, versus 0.84 and 0.95, respectively, for MRA.[30] In addition, there is an advantage to using greater field strength magnets to improve the diagnostic sensitivity, specificity, and accuracy in detecting TFCC tears.[30]

Table 2 presents the Palmer classification, whereby tears are categorized into traumatic and degenerative variants. Degenerative tears, or class II, are subclassified by the degree of ligamentous and articular damage. They are associated with ulnocarpal impaction secondary to ulnar positive variance, and treatment of ulnar length is required. Traumatic tears are further classified by the location of the tear; the most common class is IA, which corresponds to a central tear. Treatment begins with nonsurgical measures, including initial immobilization. The best type of immobilization, whether a short arm splint, a short arm cast, or a Munster splint, is not clear from the literature. Some patients will improve with immobilization; the authors of a 2010 study

Table 2

Palmer Classification of TFCC Injuries

Type	Description
I	**Traumatic Tears**
IA	Central TFCC tear
IB	Peripheral tear at base of ulnar styloid
IC	TFCC disruption from the ulnar extrinsic ligaments
ID	Detachment of the TFCC from the sigmoid notch of the distal radius
II	**Degenerative Tears**
IIA	TFCC wear without perforation or chondromalacia
IIB	TFCC wear with chondromalacia of the lunate or the ulna
IIC	Perforation of the TFCC with lunate chondromalacia
IID	TFCC perforation with ulna and/or lunate chondromalacia and LT ligament injury without carpal instability
IIE	TFCC perforation with arthritic changes involving the ulna and the lunate; LT ligament injury

TFCC = triangular fibrocartilage complex, LT = lunotriquetral.

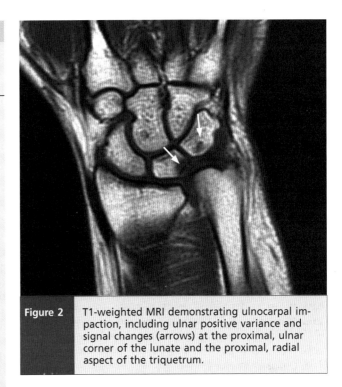

Figure 2 T1-weighted MRI demonstrating ulnocarpal impaction, including ulnar positive variance and signal changes (arrows) at the proximal, ulnar corner of the lunate and the proximal, radial aspect of the triquetrum.

found that 48 of 84 patients (57%) with a clinical diagnosis of TFCC injury who were immobilized in a short arm cast or a splint for 4 weeks improved and did not require surgical intervention.[31] Therapeutic modalities and a corticosteroid injection may be helpful as part of a treatment algorithm. Patients in whom nonsurgical treatment has failed may consider surgical treatment. As the vascular supply to the TFCC extends only to the peripheral 10% to 40% of the structure, leaving the remainder avascular, central tears are débrided rather than repaired. In contrast, peripheral ulnar tears may be amenable to repair. A variety of open, inside-out, outside-in, and all-inside repair techniques have been described.

Ulnocarpal Impaction

Ulnocarpal impaction, or chronic overload of the ulnocarpal joint, may be congenital or acquired. The key risk factor for this condition is positive ulnar variance, which overloads the ulnocarpal joint. In addition to static and dynamic radiographs, an MRI finding of signal changes at the proximal, ulnar corner of the lunate; the proximal, radial aspect of the triquetrum; and the distal, radial corner of the ulnar head are important clues to diagnosing impaction (Figure 2). Signal changes may progress to sclerosis and subchondral cysts in these areas. Initial nonsurgical treatment includes immobilization, activity modification (for example, avoid ulnar deviation), NSAIDs, and corticosteroid injections. The surgical options involve unloading procedures, such as an ulnar shortening osteotomy or a wafer procedure, or arthroscopic or open procedures.

The primary limitation of the wafer procedure is that a central TFCC tear either must be present or created if the procedure is done arthroscopically, and the procedure can theoretically alter joint contours and reduce contact areas at the DRUJ by shortening the proximal-distal amount of ulnar head cartilage. An ulnar shortening osteotomy may be complicated by delayed healing or nonunion, along with the potential need for hardware removal. In comparison studies, pain relief and function between arthroscopic wafer and ulnar shortening osteotomy are similar at final follow-up; however, some authors have highlighted a lower rate of tendinitis and secondary procedures, as well as avoiding the risk of nonunion, as the rationale for favoring the wafer procedure.[32]

Dupuytren Disease

Dupuytren disease is clinically characterized by the development of pathologic nodules and cords in the palm and fingers, potentially leading to progressive flexion contracture of the MCP and/or PIP joints of the fingers. Nodules rarely require treatment, although some patients may report painful nodules and/or cords; these often eventually become nonpainful; however, surgical treatment of these nodules may be considered when they cause pain for 1 year or longer.[33] Classic indications for surgical treatment of MCP and PIP flexion contractures are greater than 30° at the MCP joint or greater than 0° to 20° at the PIP joint, often characterized by an inability to place the hand flat on a table (tabletop test). However, these parameters must be considered in light of the patient's goals, activities, and limitations, as well as his or her age and comorbidities.

hand. Provocative maneuvers compress the nerve at the various described sites of compression of pronator syndrome; these tests include resisted pronation with the forearm in neutral and elbow in extension, resisted contraction of the flexor digitorum superficialis (FDS) to the middle finger, and resisted elbow flexion with the forearm in supination. Electrodiagnostic tests are usually negative but can be helpful in excluding other sites of compression. Nonsurgical treatment is preferred and may include NSAIDs, splinting, and activity modification. Decompression of the median nerve in the proximal forearm may be considered if prolonged nonsurgical treatment fails or if a space-occupying lesion is present. The success rates of treatment are difficult to estimate because the literature is limited to a few relatively small retrospective case series.

Anterior Interosseous Nerve Syndrome

The anterior interosseous nerve (AIN) is a motor-only nerve that innervates the flexor pollicis longus (FPL), the flexor digitorum profundus (FDP) to the index and middle fingers, and the pronator quadratus. The presentation may range from weakness to paralysis of these muscles, sometimes as an incomplete palsy. AIN palsy may theoretically be the result of compression of the AIN or the median nerve proper; however, an important differential diagnosis is Parsonage-Turner syndrome, also known as brachial neuritis or neuralgic amyotrophy, which may present with isolated AIN palsy. Electrodiagnostic tests can be helpful to evaluate for a site of compression. The mixing of these various etiologies for AIN syndrome may contribute to some of the differing recommendations for treatment. It is generally accepted that there is a high likelihood that AIN palsy will resolve with expectant treatment, and the literature includes cases where full recovery occurs even after as much as 1 year after the onset of symptoms. Surgical decompression of the AIN can be successful but should generally be considered only after a failure of nonsurgical treatment after 6 to 9 months; whether surgical decompression accelerates the resolution of symptoms is controversial.

Ulnar Nerve Compression
Cubital Tunnel Syndrome

Compression of the ulnar nerve most commonly occurs at the elbow. Specific sites of compression are listed in Table 3. Patients may present with paresthesias in the ulnar distribution of the hand, including the dorsal sensory branch (unlike when compression is present at the Guyon canal), weakness and atrophy of the intrinsic hand muscles, and sometimes with medial elbow pain that may radiate to the hand. Provocative tests include the Tinel and flexion-pressure tests; flexion-pressure tests are 98% sensitive and 95% specific when elbow flexion and direct pressure on the nerve is performed in combination for 1 minute.[51] Progressive atrophy of the intrinsic muscles can lead to clawing of the small and ring fingers. Among many well-described characteristic findings of advanced ulnar nerve compression, two of the most commonly mentioned include the Froment sign (compensation for weak key pinch by flexion of the thumb interphalangeal [IP] joint) and the Wartenberg sign (ulnar deviation and weak adduction of the small finger as a result of unopposed extensor digit minimi [EDM]). As in CTS, the opinions of various authors differ on the utility of electrodiagnostic studies for cubital tunnel syndrome, but they can be generally helpful to confirm the diagnosis, assess its severity, localize compression, and evaluate for other sites of compression.

Initial treatment, particularly when the symptoms are intermittent or mild, includes activity modification, avoiding direct pressure on the cubital tunnel and limiting elbow hyperflexion, and nighttime elbow extension splinting (at 45° of flexion). A randomized controlled trial demonstrated that patients with mild or moderate symptoms who are informed of the causes of cubital tunnel syndrome and how to avoid provocation can have a good prognosis (89.5% improved at follow-up) regardless of whether or not night splinting or nerve gliding exercises are added to the treatment regimen.[52] When nonsurgical treatment fails or if muscle denervation is present, surgical treatment is indicated. Surgical options include in situ decompression (open or endoscopic), medial epicondylectomy, subcutaneous transposition, intramuscular transposition, or submuscular transposition. In general, comparison studies, including several randomized controlled trials, have found that these various techniques all can be equally effective.[53,54] Therefore, the literature supports in situ decompression for most cases; exceptions to this include the posttraumatic elbow with stiffness and scarring. If transposition is performed, the simplest technique of subcutaneous transposition is usually reasonable, although some surgeons prefer intramuscular or submuscular transposition. Failures most commonly may be caused by incomplete release, including failing to release all potential sites of compression, or perineural scarring. In addition, injury to a medial antebrachial cutaneous (MABC) branch during the surgical approach can cause a painful neuroma. Depending on the suspected cause of failure, revision cubital tunnel decompression is performed with a technique different from the index procedure, with special attention paid to neuromas of the MABC nerve.

Ulnar Tunnel Syndrome (Guyon Canal)

Compression of the ulnar nerve infrequently occurs at the wrist. Three anatomic zones have been described, and the etiologies and the symptoms help localize the site of compression within the canal. A variety of specific etiologies may cause compression within specific zones of the Guyon canal, including ganglia and other space-occupying lesions, thrombosis and pseudoaneurysms, anomalous muscles, acute trauma (especially hook of hamate fractures and nonunions), repetitive trauma (possibly in the setting of hypothenar hammer syndrome), or prolonged compression (handlebar palsy in bikers). The suspected etiology helps direct advanced imaging studies, including CT, MRI, and vascular studies. Surgical treatment when indicated requires exploration and release of the entire Guyon canal.

Radial Nerve Compression

Posterior Interosseous Nerve Syndrome

The motor branch of the radial nerve in the forearm, the posterior interosseous nerve (PIN), may be compressed at multiple sites in the forearm. The resulting syndrome is characterized by weakness in the muscles innervated by the PIN, which includes all the wrist and finger extensors, except the extensor carpi radialis longus (ECRL) and the brachioradialis. Potential sites of compression are summarized in Table 3. Physical examination and electrodiagnostic testing, typically positive, are useful for making the diagnosis. Extensor tendon rupture or subluxation of the extensor digitorum communis may mimic a partial PIN palsy and should be considered in the differential diagnosis. Except in the setting of a space-occupying lesion, management is initially nonsurgical and can include splinting, stretching, and activity modification. Surgical release of the potential sites of compression of the PIN may be considered if nonsurgical management fails. The timing of surgical intervention is poorly established, and a large variability in the success of surgical treatment is reported.

Radial Tunnel Syndrome

Radial tunnel syndrome is a controversial diagnosis, and some authors dispute its existence. Pain is described in the lateral aspect of the proximal forearm. Theoretically, this pain may occur concomitantly with lateral epicondylitis, but it likewise must be differentiated from lateral epicondylitis. Symptoms may be provoked by a combination of elbow extension, forearm pronation, and wrist flexion, which places traction on the radial nerve; other maneuvers have also been described to exacerbate the symptoms. Electrodiagnostic testing is typically negative. Treatment is primarily nonsurgical; if activity modification fails, an injection of corticosteroid and local anesthetic may be attempted. If prolonged nonsurgical treatment fails, surgical release of the PIN at all sites of compression may be considered.

Wartenberg Syndrome

The superficial radial nerve may become entrapped between the brachioradialis and the ECRL in the distal forearm, a condition termed Wartenberg syndrome or cheiralgia paresthetica. The etiologies include blunt trauma or compression as a result of a wristband or handcuffs. Symptoms include pain and paresthesias radiating from the dorsal-radial forearm to the dorsum of the thumb and the index finger. A positive Tinel sign on examination is helpful for diagnosis. Symptoms may be exacerbated by maneuvers that also elicit pain in de Quervain tenosynovitis, which must be differentiated (although it may be present concomitantly). Treatment involves splinting and activity modification (such as removal of a wristwatch), splinting, possible local corticosteroid injections, and rarely surgical release when nonsurgical treatment fails.

Tendon Transfers

Principles of Tendon Transfer

In the setting of an irrecoverable nerve deficit or musculotendinous injury leading to functional deficits in the upper extremity, tendon transfers allow restoration of key functions. Eight well-established principles facilitate successful tendon transfers.

1. **Supple joints:** Prior to a tendon transfer, the joints that will be moved must be supple with passive range of motion maximized.

2. **Tissue equilibrium:** The soft tissues should be at equilibrium, with the surrounding soft tissue and bone healed and any scarring matured to minimize potential for adhesions.

3. **One tendon, one function:** A tendon transfer should be designed to restore only one function because splitting the transfer will compromise function by halting motion at the shorter excursion.

4. **Straight line of pull:** A straight line will maximize the force that can be generated.

5. **Similar excursion:** The excursion of the donor must be adequate to allow function similar to the recipient.

6. **Similar strength:** The relative strength of the donor and the recipient should be similar.

7. **Expendable donor:** The selected donor should not compromise existing function.

8. **Synergistic transfer:** For example, wrist flexion is accompanied by finger extension, making transfer of the flexor carpi radialis (FCR) muscle or the flexor carpi ulnaris (FCU) muscle to the extensor digitorum communis muscle a synergistic transfer that requires little retraining.

Table 4 summarizes the functions that are lost in specific palsies, and the common tendon transfer options available to restore these functions. In addition to tendon transfer selection, setting the proper tension on the transfer must be considered. Postoperative rehabilitation is an important aspect of the process, and the patient's motivation to comply with the postoperative protocols must be assessed before surgery.

Radial Nerve Palsy

Radial nerve palsy is the most common indication for tendon transfer in the upper extremity. Low radial nerve palsy involves the PIN alone, whereas a high radial nerve palsy involves the entire radial nerve, typically at or proximal to the elbow. Low radial nerve palsy is characterized by deficits of thumb extension and finger MCP joint extension as well as radial deviation with wrist extension because of preservation of the ECRL/extensor carpi radialis brevis (ECRB) and absent extensor carpi ulnaris. Nonsurgical management includes range-of-motion exercises and static and dynamic splinting, all

3: Upper Extremity

Table 4

Tendon Transfers for Nerve Palsies

Palsies	Deficits	Tendon Transfers
Low radial nerve	Thumb extension	PL to EPL; FDS ring to EPL if no PL
	Finger extension	FCR (Brand) or FCU (Jones) or FDS (Boyes) to extensor digitorum communis
High radial nerve	Wrist extension	Pronator teres to ECRB
Low median nerve	Thumb opposition	EIP to abductor pollicis brevis FDS ring finger to abductor pollicis brevis (Boyes) Abductor digiti minimi to abductor pollicis brevis (Huber) PL to abductor pollicis brevis (Camitz)
High median nerve	Thumb flexion	Brachioradialis to flexor pollicis longus
	Index and long finger flexion	Side-to-side transfer of FDP ring and small to FDP index and long
Low ulnar nerve	Key pinch	ECRB (Smith) or FDS ring to adductor pollicis
	Clawing	Capsulodesis (if Bouvier test okay); If Bouvier test fails or power needed, FDS or ECRL or ECRB as two- or four-tailed grafts to radial lateral bands of the small and ring, or all digits
	Abduction of small finger	Ulnar insertion of EDM to radial collateral ligament or A1 pulley of small finger
High ulnar nerve	Loss of ring and small FDP	Side-to-side transfer of FDP ring and small to FDP index and long

FDS = flexor digitorum superficialis; FDP = flexor digitorum profundus; ECRL = extensor carpi radialis longus; ECRB = extensor carpi radialis brevis; PL = palmaris longus; EPL = extensor pollicis longus; FCR = flexor carpi radialis; FCU = flexor carpi ulnaris; EIP = extensor indicis proprius; EDM = extensor digiti minimi.

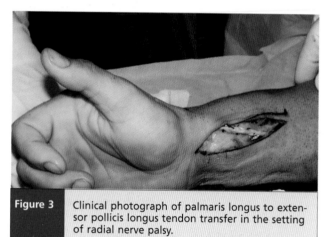

Figure 3   Clinical photograph of palmaris longus to extensor pollicis longus tendon transfer in the setting of radial nerve palsy.

with the goal of preventing contractures and maintaining range of motion during nerve recovery or in preparation for tendon transfer surgery. Three primary combinations of tendon transfers for radial nerve palsy have been described in Table 4; all involve pronator teres to ECRB to restore wrist extension. Commonly, the palmaris longus is transferred to the extensor pollicis longus for thumb extension (Figure 3).

Median Nerve Palsy

Low median nerve palsy is the second most common reason for tendon transfer in the upper extremity. Loss of sensation in the distribution of the median nerve can affect patient function; in the absence of sensory recov-

ery, the benefit of a tendon transfer restoring function may be limited.

Low median nerve palsies affect the thenar muscles and are characterized by loss of thumb opposition as a result of loss of function of the abductor pollicis brevis, which is the primary muscle for the important function of thumb opposition. When this deficit affects patient function, a variety of tendon transfers may be considered to restore thumb opposition. Described tendon transfers to restore opposition include palmaris longus, flexor digitorum superficialis, extensor indicis proprius (EIP), ECRL, extensor carpi ulnaris, EDM, and abductor digiti minimi. The four most classically described opponensplasties are presented in Table 4. One of the common indications for opponensplasty is advanced CTS with loss of opposition as a result of atrophy of the thenar muscles. Although the Camitz transfer using the palmaris longus has been popularized in this setting, other reported tendon transfers may be selected with equal or even greater success. The Huber transfer is specifically used in the setting of congenital hypoplastic thumb because it provides an additional benefit of increasing the thenar muscle bulk while restoring opposition.

High median nerve palsy leads to loss of thumb, index finger, and middle finger flexion, as well as pronator quadratus as a result of loss of anterior interosseous nerve innervation. The FCR, FDS, and pronator teres are also nonfunctional with a complete median nerve lesion at or above the elbow. Thumb opposition is restored by transfer of the EIP or another similar opponensplasty. The additional loss of thumb IP joint flexion may be restored by transferring the brachioradialis to the FPL. Loss of index and middle finger flexion can be restored by side-to-side transfer of the FDP of the ring and small fingers to the index and middle fingers. Loss of FDS function to the ring and small fingers and FCR function is functionally minimized because of retained FDP function to these digits and FCU function for wrist flexion. In addition, loss of forearm pronation can be addressed by rerouting the biceps around the radius to convert it from a supinator into a pronator.

Ulnar Nerve Palsy

Ulnar nerve palsy can significantly affect function, particularly as a result of loss of key pinch, and can affect hand appearance because of progressive clawing and intrinsic muscle atrophy. Key pinch is lost because of paralysis of the adductor pollicis and first dorsal interosseous muscles; patients compensate for this by using the extensor pollicis longus to adduct the thumb and the FPL to flex the thumb IP joint to the index finger. Clawing of the ring and small finger in ulnar nerve palsy is the result of intrinsic paralysis; preservation of lumbrical function to the index and middle finger prevents clawing of these fingers in isolated ulnar nerve palsy. The abducted posture of the small finger is a result of loss of function of the palmar interosseous and unopposed function of the EDM. In addition, hand function is affected because of an inability to coordinate MCP joint flexion with IP flexion; this leads to a phenomenon termed roll-up flexion, whereby the ability to pick up small objects is impaired. In high ulnar nerve palsy, the loss of the FDP to the small and ring fingers leads to less visible clawing.

When recovery is not expected, tendon transfers can restore function and correct the clawing deformity. The Bouvier maneuver (performed by preventing MCP extension and asking the patient to extend his or her fingers where an inability to extend the IP joint indicates an incompetent or attenuated extensor mechanism) is an important preoperative examination because it predicts whether a static or dynamic procedure will be required to alleviate clawing. Restoration of key, or lateral, pinch is most commonly done by transferring the ECRB, elongated with a tendon graft, to the adductor insertion to improve pinch power. In high ulnar nerve palsy, loss of IP joint flexion of the ring and small fingers can be restored by side-to-side transfer of the median-innervated FDP tendons of the index and middle fingers.

Combined Nerve Palsies

When nerve palsies are combined, fewer tendon transfer options to restore function are available. The most common combination is low median and low ulnar nerve palsies, followed by combined high median and high ulnar nerve palsies. By prioritizing functional losses and adhering to the principles of tendon transfers, the surgeon may develop a surgical plan to best restore a patient's function. The effect of sensory losses in these combined palsies must also be considered, and techniques using nerve transfers or neurovascular cutaneous flaps are growing.

Summary

The treatment of hand and wrist arthritis begins with nonsurgical modalities. Persistent symptoms may be an indication for surgical treatment specific to the joint, often including arthroplasty versus arthrodesis. SLAC and SNAC wrist surgical options include partial arthrodesis or PRC, both yielding similar outcomes. No treatment for Kienböck disease has proved superior. Less invasive treatment options including percutaneous aponeurotomy and collagenase injections have gained popularity recently for treatment of Dupuytren contractures, but their role and safety when compared with open surgical treatment still requires further investigation. A firm knowledge of sites of compression of the peripheral nerves helps guide treatment of upper extremity neuropathies. Finally, tendon transfers can successfully restore lost function after nerve injury with a clear understanding of the well-established principles for selecting the donor musculotendinous unit.

Key Study Points

- For thumb CMC arthritis, no additional surgical steps beyond excision of the trapezium have led to improved patient outcomes.

- No treatment has proven superior in addressing early or late stages of Kienböck disease.

- Collagenase injection to rupture the cords causing Dupuytren contracture is a promising option for a subset of these patients.

Annotated References

1. Spaans AJ, van Laarhoven CM, Schuurman AH, van Minnen LP: Interobserver agreement of the Eaton-Littler classification system and treatment strategy of thumb carpometacarpal joint osteoarthritis. *J Hand Surg Am* 2011;36(9):1467-1470.

   Five musculoskeletal radiologists and eight hand surgeons were presented 40 cases of thumb CMC arthritis and asked to stage the radiographs. Only moderate interobserver agreement was shown. Level of evidence:III.

2. Lin JD, Karl JW, Strauch RJ: Trapeziometacarpal joint stability: The evolving importance of the dorsal ligaments. *Clin Orthop Relat Res* 2013; Epub ahead of print.

   The authors conducted a systematic review of the literature to examine the evidence for the contribution of specific ligaments to the stability of the trapeziometacarpal joint. They concluded that there is increasing evidence for the dorsoradial ligament being the primary stabilizer of the joint. Level of evidence: IV.

3. Heyworth BE, Lee JH, Kim PD, Lipton CB, Strauch RJ, Rosenwasser MP: Hylan versus corticosteroid versus

38. Chen NC, Shauver MJ, Chung KC: Cost-effectiveness of open partial fasciectomy, needle aponeurotomy, and collagenase injection for dupuytren contracture. *J Hand Surg Am* 2011;36(11):1826-1834, e32.

  The study is a cost-utility analysis to compare three treatments of Dupuytren contracture: traditional fasciectomy, needle aponeurotomy, and collagenase injection. Level of evidence: II.

39. Rahr L, Søndergaard P, Bisgaard T, Baad-Hansen T: Percutaneous needle fasciotomy for primary Dupuytren's contracture. *J Hand Surg Eur Vol* 2011;36(7):548-552.

  The authors present 2-year follow-up data for 92 patients who underwent percutaneous needle aponeurotomy for Dupuytren contracture. Level of evidence: IV.

40. van Rijssen AL, ter Linden H, Werker PM: Five-year results of a randomized clinical trial on treatment in Dupuytren's disease: Percutaneous needle fasciotomy versus limited fasciectomy. *Plast Reconstr Surg* 2012;129(2):469-477.

  One-hundred fifteen hands were randomized to percutaneous aponeurotomy and limited fasciectomy. Five-year follow-up results were reported. Significantly more frequent and rapid recurrence was seen with percutaneous aponeurotomy. Level of evidence: II.

41. Becker GW, Davis TR: The outcome of surgical treatments for primary Dupuytren's disease—a systematic review. *J Hand Surg Eur Vol* 2010;35(8):623-626.

  The authors systematically reviewed the Dupuytren literature to evaluate rates of recurrence, complications, and strength of evidence for specific procedures.

42. Crean SM, Gerber RA, Le Graverand MP, Boyd DM, Cappelleri JC: The efficacy and the safety of fasciectomy and fasciotomy for Dupuytren's contracture in European patients: A structured review of published studies. *J Hand Surg Eur Vol* 2011;36(5):396-407.

  The authors assessed the efficacy and safety of fasciectomy and percutaneous aponeurotomy in 48 published studies of European patients with Dupuytren contracture.

43. Denkler K: Surgical complications associated with fasciectomy for Dupuytren's disease: A 20-year review of the English literature. *Eplasty* 2010;10:e15.

  The author reviewed the literature on fasciectomy for primary and recurrent Dupuytren disease over a 10-year period. A list of complications and the frequency of these complications was compiled. Level of evidence: IV.

44. Shiri R, Miranda H, Heliövaara M, Viikari-Juntura E: Physical work load factors and carpal tunnel syndrome: A population-based study. *Occup Environ Med* 2009;66(6):368-373.

45. Palmer KT, Harris EC, Coggon D: Carpal tunnel syndrome and its relation to occupation: A systematic literature review. *Occup Med (Lond)* 2007;57(1):57-66.

46. Graham B: The value added by electrodiagnostic testing in the diagnosis of carpal tunnel syndrome. *J Bone Joint Surg Am* 2008;90(12):2587-2593.

47. Tai TW, Wu CY, Su FC, Chern TC, Jou IM: Ultrasonography for diagnosing carpal tunnel syndrome: A meta-analysis of diagnostic test accuracy. *Ultrasound Med Biol* 2012;38(7):1121-1128.

  The authors performed a meta-analysis examining ultrasound measurements for CTS. From 28 studies, they concluded that a cross-sectional area at the carpal tunnel inlet of greater than or equal to 9 mm is the best single diagnostic criterion.

48. Page MJ, Massy-Westropp N, O'Connor D, Pitt V: Splinting for carpal tunnel syndrome. *Cochrane Database Syst Rev* 2012;7:CD010003.

  This Cochrane review compared the effectiveness of splinting for CTS with no treatment or another nonsurgical intervention. Level of evidence: II.

49. Marshall S, Tardif G, Ashworth N: Local corticosteroid injection for carpal tunnel syndrome. *Cochrane Database Syst Rev* 2007;2:CD001554.

50. Burke FD, Wilgis EF, Dubin NH, Bradley MJ, Sinha S: Relationship between the duration and severity of symptoms and the outcome of carpal tunnel surgery. *J Hand Surg Am* 2006;31(9):1478-1482.

51. Novak CB, Lee GW, Mackinnon SE, Lay L: Provocative testing for cubital tunnel syndrome. *J Hand Surg Am* 1994;19(5):817-820.

52. Svernlöv B, Larsson M, Rehn K, Adolfsson L: Conservative treatment of the cubital tunnel syndrome. *J Hand Surg Eur Vol* 2009;34(2):201-207.

53. Caliandro P, La Torre G, Padua R, Giannini F, Padua L: Treatment for ulnar neuropathy at the elbow. *Cochrane Database Syst Rev* 2012;7:CD006839.

  This Cochrane review included six randomized controlled trials that met inclusion criteria to examine nonsurgical and surgical treatment of cubital tunnel syndrome. They concluded that simple decompression and decompression with transposition are equally effective in idiopathic ulnar neuropathy at the elbow. Level of evidence: I.

54. Zlowodzki M, Chan S, Bhandari M, Kalliainen L, Schubert W: Anterior transposition compared with simple decompression for treatment of cubital tunnel syndrome: A meta-analysis of randomized, controlled trials. *J Bone Joint Surg Am* 2007;89(12):2591-2598.

Video Reference

32.1: Birman MV, Tang P: Video. *Dupuytren Contracture Manipulation. Parts I and II*. Arlington Heights, IL, 2013.

Section 4

Lower Extremity

SECTION EDITOR:

Frank A. Liporace, MD

Chapter 33

Fractures of the Pelvis and the Acetabulum

Berton R. Moed, MD   Mark C. Reilly, MD

Introduction

Injuries to the pelvic ring and the acetabulum commonly occur as a result of high-energy blunt trauma caused by motor vehicle collisions or falls from heights. Consequently, they are often accompanied by additional musculoskeletal and other system injuries and are associated with relatively high rates of morbidity and mortality. Before the 1980s, these injuries were treated mainly by nonsurgical means with generally unsatisfactory results. With the advent of more aggressive treatment, patient care and outcomes dramatically improved. However, patients continue to die from pelvic ring injuries, and those with pelvic and acetabular fractures continue to have difficulty attaining a functional level approximating their preinjury status.[1-3]

Pelvic Fractures

Anatomy and Basic Biomechanics of the Pelvic Ring

The pelvis is a ring structure composed of the articulations of three bones (the sacrum and the left and right innominate bones) and their connecting ligamentous structures. The pelvic ring has no inherent bony stability; its integrity is completely dependent on the strength of the connecting ligaments.[2] Anteriorly, the innominate bones articulate with each other through fibrocartilage surrounded by a series of thin ligaments forming the pubic symphysis. Posteriorly, the left and right sacroiliac joints are formed by the articulation of the respective innominate bone with the sacrum, which is stabilized by the anterior sacroiliac ligament, the posterior sacroiliac ligament, and the interosseous ligament (the strongest in the body). Two additional ligaments,

---

the sacrospinous and the sacrotuberous, support the pelvic floor and are believed to be important contributors to pelvic ring stability.[2] With the pelvis loaded in a double-leg stance, there are tensile forces anteriorly and compressive forces at the posterior pelvis; when the pelvis is loaded in a sitting position or in a single-leg stance, there are compressive forces anteriorly and tensile forces posteriorly.[2] Although the posterior ligaments are most important in maintaining stability, the anterior structures are also important. In a double-leg stance, 60% of stability comes from the posterior structures, but 40% comes from the anterior structures.[2] This information is important when determining appropriate fixation constructs for repair of the disrupted pelvic ring.

The anterior sacroiliac and sacrospinous ligaments generally resist horizontal (transverse) plane rotational forces, and the posterior sacroiliac, interosseous, and sacrotuberous ligaments resist shearing (translational) forces. The pubic symphyseal structures, along with the pubic rami, act as a strut to prevent anterior collapse during weight bearing and resist rotational forces.[2] However, it has been difficult to determine the specific contributions of particular ligamentous structures because their analysis is dependent on how the pelvis is loaded and the order in which the structures are cut.[2] For example, the actual contributions of the sacrospinous and sacrotuberous ligaments to pelvic ring stability may be minimal.

Force Patterns of Injury

The major directions of force acting alone or in combination on the pelvic ring are anteroposterior compression (APC), lateral compression (LC), and vertical shear (VS). APC forces cause external rotation of the injured hemipelvis. The APC force disrupts an anterior ring structure (that is, pubic symphysis and/or rami) and, subsequently, the pelvic floor and anterior sacroiliac ligament(s), creating a rotationally unstable pelvis. At this point of injury, the pelvis may "open like a book" either unilaterally or bilaterally, but it will not translate vertically. With continuation of this force, disruption of the remaining posterior ligamentous structures can occur, which causes the pelvis to be completely unstable, allowing cephalad and translational displacement. An LC force applied to the ilium

Table 1

Tile/Pennal Classification

Type A: Stable Injuries

A1: Avulsion fractures not involving the pelvic ring

A2: Iliac wing fractures or minimally displaced fractures of the ring

A3: Transverse fractures of the coccyx and the sacrum

Type B: Rotationally Unstable, Vertically Stable (Partially Stable) Injuries

B1: Open-book injury (external rotational instability)

B2: Lateral compression injury

B3: Bilateral type B injuries

Type C: Rotationally and Vertically Unstable (Vertical Shear)

C1: Unilateral

C2: Bilateral; one side type C, the other type B

C3: Bilateral; both sides type C

(Adapted with permission from Tile M: Pelvic ring fractures: should they be fixed? *J Bone Joint Surg Br* 1988;70:1-12; and Tile M: Classification, in Tile M, ed: *Fractures of the Pelvis and Acetabulum*, ed 2. Baltimore, MD, Williams and Wilkins, 1995, pp 66-101.)

produces an internal rotation injury of the hemipelvis. A pure LC force vector causes compression of the posterior pelvic ring structures so that although the bone fractures, the surrounding soft tissues can remain intact. The accompanying anterior ring injury may be ipsilateral or contralateral to the posterior injury, involve the rami bilaterally, disrupt the pubic symphysis, or include any combination thereof. The magnitude of internal rotational deformity and the extent of rotational instability depends on injury sustained by the posterior sacroiliac complex. A bony injury through cancellous sacral bone may be impacted, resulting in an internally rotated and deformed but stable hemipelvis. An LC bony injury through the posterior ilium may be both internally rotated and rotationally unstable. A continuing LC force carried across the midline can result in an APC-type injury to the contralateral hemipelvis. Although LC injuries do not typically translate vertically, the internal rotation of the hemipelvis is often accompanied by hemipelvis flexion and adduction. This may result in a limb-length discrepancy as the center of rotation of the ipsilateral hip joint is moved proximally. VS injuries result from a shearing force, coursing in the vertical plane perpendicular to the main posterior bony trabecular pattern, as in a fall from a height. This VS force causes gross disruption of the soft tissues and marked displacement of bony structures. The posterior injury can occur through the sacrum, the sacroiliac joint, the ilium, or any combination thereof. Similarly, the anterior lesion can occur through any of the anterior structures. With complete disruption of the posterior sacroiliac complex, the hemipelvis becomes globally unstable and can translate in any plane.

Classification

The extent of injury to the pelvis depends on several factors, including the magnitude, the direction, and the location of the injuring force. Because the pelvis is a ring structure, an injury to one area must be accompanied by a second injury elsewhere in the ring. Because of the structural anatomy of the pelvis and the understanding that the force of injury can occur in directions other than pure APC, LC, and VS, various systems have been developed to classify pelvic ring disruptions. The two main classification systems (Tile/Pennal and Young-Burgess) are based on the magnitude and the direction of the applied injuring force. In the Tile/Pennal classification, which evolved over time, the disruptions are based on the LC, APC, and VS force vectors with the addition of a stability component, described as (A) stable, (B) stable vertically but unstable rotationally, and (C) unstable both rotationally and vertically (Table 1). In the Young-Burgess classification, subsets of LC and APC injury were added to quantify the amount of applied force, and a fourth category (combined mechanical injury) was added to allow for pathology that cannot be strictly categorized as occurring from APC, LC, or VS directions (Table 2). The main goal was to create a system of pattern recognition to enable treating physicians to better identify frequently missed lesions, have a predictive index for associated injuries and related resuscitative requirements, and reduce morbidity and mortality by selecting the most appropriate treatment. Unfortunately, the prognostic value of the classified injury pattern to reliably identify specific associated diagnoses, treatments, and outcomes has not proved consistent for any classification.[4,5]

The AO/Orthopaedic Trauma Association (OTA) classification is now the commonly used system.[6] It is mainly derived from the method developed by Title and Pennal, using the type A, B, and C stability groupings but incorporating aspects of the Young-Burgess classification in its subgroup and qualification sections. Type A injuries do not compromise the integrity of the posterior arch, such as iliac wing fractures or transverse fractures of the sacrum and the coccyx. Type B injuries involve incomplete disruption of the posterior arch, creating a pelvic ring that is partially stable (rotationally unstable but vertically stable). These rotational injuries are either external rotation injuries attributable to APC forces (type 61-B1) or internal rotation injuries resulting from LC forces (type B2). Type 61-B3 injuries are bilateral, having a B1 or B2 on each side. Type 61-C injuries, of which there are many subcategories, involve complete disruption of the posterior arch, creating a pelvic ring that is globally unstable, and can translate in any plane. Unfortunately, none of these classifications is all-encompassing. For example, LC pelvic fractures represent a heterogeneous group of injuries for which the classification systems do not provide an adequate description and are poorly suited to help guide treatment.[7]

Table 2

Young-Burgess Classification

APC Injuries

I: Slight opening of the pubic symphysis and the anterior aspect of the sacroiliac joint

II: Symphyseal diastasis or anterior ring fracture with a widened anterior aspect of the sacroiliac joint

III: Symphyseal diastasis or anterior ring fracture with complete sacroiliac joint disruption but no vertical displacement

LC Injuries

I: Anterior ring fracture with a sacral compression fracture on the side of impact

II: Anterior ring fracture with a crescent (iliac wing) fracture on the side of impact

III: LC-I or LC-II on the side of impact with a contralateral open book (APC) injury

VS Injury

Symphyseal diastasis or anterior ring fracture with vertical displacement anteriorly and posteriorly through the sacroiliac joint, iliac wing, or the sacrum

CM Injury

Combination of other injury patterns: LC/VS or LC/APC

APC = anteroposterior compression; LC = lateral compression; VS = vertical shear; CM = combined mechanical.
(Adapted with permission from Burgess AR, Eastridge BJ, Young JWR, et al: Pelvic ring disruptions: Effective classification system and treatment protocols. *J Trauma* 1990;30:848-856.)

Initial Evaluation and Management

With the possible exception of pelvic insufficiency fractures, a pelvic fracture serves as a marker of high-energy injury commonly associated with other severe injuries and extra-pelvic hemorrhage (chest, 15%; intra-abdominal, 32%; long bones, 40%), which can confound the initial workup.[8] The mortality rate is highest in patients with type C fractures.[9] It is also higher in patients with nonisolated pelvic fractures.[9] It is important for each institution treating pelvic fractures to have practice guidelines that have been shown to reduce mortality.[8] Furthermore, surgeon exposure to pelvic injuries with life-threatening hemorrhage is decreasing, limiting the training opportunities necessary to prepare surgeons for rare but highly demanding emergency situations.[10] Although multifactorial, this decrease is related to an overall reduction in the number of severe pelvic ring injuries, improved prehospital care, and a reduction in the number of associated injuries. Initial data suggest that a novel pelvic emergency simulator (or a device similar to it) can be used to train surgeons to reduce blood loss in severe pelvic ring injuries.[10]

For patients with a pelvic ring fracture (as in all trauma patients), the Advanced Trauma Life Support protocol should be followed. An AP radiograph may be obtained during the evaluation sequence. When a patient is found to have a pelvic ring injury, specific protocols for initial evaluation and treatment should be followed. Pertinent information in the patient history includes the magnitude and the direction of injury, which can be helpful to identify potential associated orthopaedic and nonorthopaedic injuries, as well as the type of pelvic injury. The most common injuries associated with pelvic fractures are chest injury, long-bone

fractures, head injury, intra-abdominal injury (spleen, liver, bladder, and urethra), spine fractures, and lumbosacral plexus injuries.[11]

A complete physical examination is important for patients with an injured pelvic ring. A visual inspection should be performed to assess for open wounds, soft-tissue degloving (Morel-Lavalee lesion), and signs of urologic injury (blood at the urethra meatus or perineal or scrotal ecchymosis). The examination should be as complete as possible to identify and document any neurologic injury, such as a lumbosacral plexopathy. Any lack of function should be noted and not merely attributed to a patient's pain or inattentiveness. If an alert patient (Glasgow Coma Scale score higher than 13) does not report pelvic pain or palpable tenderness, he or she likely did not sustain an unstable pelvic fracture.[12] However, the converse is not necessarily true.[12] Although pain on posterior palpation of the sacrum and the sacroiliac joint is indicative of an injury to the posterior ring, it is not specifically indicative of an unstable pelvic ring injury, but it does merit further evaluation.[12] Suspected pelvic ring deformity is an unreliable indicator of an unstable pelvic ring injury.[12] A stress examination of the pelvis in an awake patient in the acute setting is also unreliable and not indicated.[12] However, a stress examination under general anesthesia can be beneficial to diagnose the severity of injury and choose appropriate treatment.[13,14]

Patients presenting with an unstable pelvic ring injury and hemodynamic instability require temporary stabilization of the pelvis. Although emergency fixation devices, such as the pelvic C-clamp and the anterior external fixator frame, continue to have their place in the treating physician's armamentarium, circumferential compression using an ordinary sheet or a commercially available pelvic binder has become the mainstay of acute treatment.[15] Commercially available pelvic circumferential compression devices have demonstrated sufficient reduction in partially stable and unstable pelvic fractures without incurring the adverse risk of inducing additional deformity.[16] However, circumferential pelvic binding is a temporizing measure and should be followed by definitive pelvic ring fixation, as needed, which may be preceded by interim interventions such as external fixation or skeletal traction.

After the initial resuscitation is completed, additional studies, including pelvic inlet and outlet radiographic views and CT, are obtained to further define the pelvic ring injury. Ideal inlet and outlet views have been variously described, most commonly as being directed 45° caudally and 45° cranially, respectively, from the AP view.[17] Although these are orthogonal views, they may not be in the best plane to evaluate a pelvic injury because of variability in lumbopelvic anatomy. Recent studies indicate that initial screening inlet and outlet radiographs are best made at 25° and 60°, respectively, to provide better visualization of the clinically relevant posterior osseous pelvic anatomy.[17,18]

Open Fractures

Open pelvic fractures account for approximately 3% of all pelvic fractures. They usually result from blunt, high-energy trauma and are among the most devastating injuries in musculoskeletal trauma, requiring a multidisciplinary approach. Historically, mortality rates were reported in the 50% range. However, more recently, likely because of aggressive multidisciplinary protocols, mortality rates have dropped to below 30%.[19] Management includes aggressive treatment of associated soft-tissue injuries with early administration of broad-spectrum antibiotics and wound débridement. Although there have been conflicting reports on the need for a diverting colostomy, the consensus is that selective diversion based on wound location (that is, rectal and perineal) reduces infective complications and subsequent mortality in patients with open pelvic fractures.[19] Nonetheless, infection rates are high, with or without fecal diversion, if the rectal area is injured. If a diverting colostomy is used, the location of the stoma should be carefully considered to avoid compromising potential subsequent orthopaedic procedures. Wound care is facilitated when the pelvis is stabilized, and this may be the most important aspect of treatment.

Open pelvic fractures sustained as the result of a civilian gunshot wound represent a much different situation. Emergent surgery for vascular, visceral, and urogenital injuries is often required. However, pelvic ring instability is rare, and the orthopaedic complication rate is low.[20]

Definitive Treatment

Subsequent to the initial evaluation and treatment phase, the definitive treatment of a pelvic ring injury is based on the classification, as determined from radiographic studies and other examinations. Injuries that are stable to physiologic stress do not require surgical

intervention. In general, nonsurgical treatment is indicated for the following: all type A injuries, pubic symphyseal disruptions with a diastasis less than 2.5 cm (APC-I in the Young-Burgess classification) and impacted sacral fractures and other stable LC injuries without major deformity (cephalad displacement or internal malrotation).

Surgical intervention is indicated for unstable type B and C injuries. Type B1 (open-book) injuries have been defined as those with a pubic symphyseal diastasis of more than 2.5 cm, indicating associated disruption of the sacrospinous, sacrotuberous, and anterior sacroiliac ligaments; however, because of variations in pelvic morphology, there is doubt that this absolute criterion applies in all cases.[21] Type B2 (LC) injuries present a more ambiguous situation. The indications for reduction include an internal rotation deformity causing a loss of ipsilateral lower extremity external rotation past neutral, a limb-length discrepancy exceeding 1 to 1.5 cm, symphyseal disruption with overlapping pubic bodies, and malalignment causing dyspareunia resulting from bony perineal protrusion or sitting imbalance. The indicators of instability include bilateral pubic rami fractures, complete comminuted fractures of the sacrum, and crescent fractures.[7,22] Type C pelvic injuries with posterior displacement of 1 or more are completely unstable and require fixation. As noted previously, when in doubt, a stress examination under anesthesia may prove helpful in differentiating stable from unstable injuries.[7,13,14]

Fixation of Pelvic Ring Injuries
Type B1 Injuries (Pubic Symphyseal Disruptions: APC-II)

External fixation can be used for the definitive treatment of type B1 injuries; however, plate fixation is biomechanically more stable.[2] The posterior addition of an iliosacral screw does not provide substantial additional stability.[23] A plating configuration with at least two points of fixation on each side of the symphysis is more stable than a two-hole plate construct and may result in lower rates of malunion.[24] Biplanar or dual plating does not appear to offer any advantage over a single plate. In addition, locked plating has been shown to have no advantage over standard internal fixation constructs.[25,26] Fixation failure with recurrent widening of the pubic space is common after plating of the pubic symphysis for traumatic diastasis.[27,28] However, this late plate fixation failure is not clinically important.[28] Nonetheless, patients should be advised of the common occurrence of radiographic failure and small likelihood of the need for revision surgery.[27,28]

Type B2.1 Injuries (LC-I)

As noted earlier, B2.1 (LC-I) injuries represent a heterogeneous group of injuries. In general, reduction and fixation of the anterior ring is sufficient. If the anterior lesion is through the pubic symphysis, symphyseal plating is preferred. For rami fractures, spanning external fixation (**Figure 1**) can be used to distract and fix

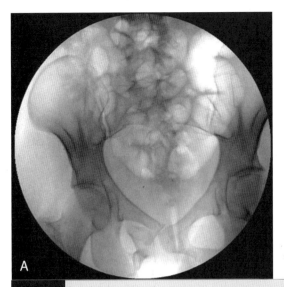
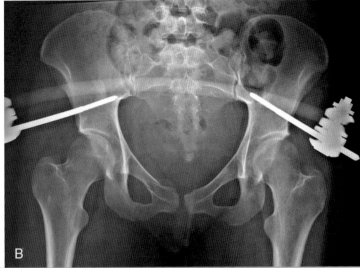

Figure 1 Imaging studies from a 21-year-old woman who sustained a lateral compression injury in a motor vehicle collision. **A,** Intraoperative radiograph showing fractures of the superior and inferior rami on the right with substantial internal rotation of the hemipelvis. **B,** Postoperative radiograph after distraction external fixator placement.

the internally rotated hemipelvis. For this purpose, the placement of external fixation pins no smaller than 5 mm in diameter at the supra-acetabular level is a preferred technique.[29] The stabilization of rami fractures also can be accomplished by direct plate fixation. Alternatively, a superior pubic ramus fracture can be fixed using an intramedullary screw placed in either an antegrade or a retrograde fashion.[30] Elderly women are at risk for fixation failure with this technique, with loss of reduction more common in fractures medial to the lateral border of the obturator foramen.[30]

Although fixation of the anterior ring is believed sufficient to address type B2.1 injuries, the heterogeneity of the spectrum of injury, concern regarding disimpaction of the sacral fracture during reduction of the hemipelvic internal malrotation, and the possibility of misdiagnosis of an actual type C injury has led many surgeons to add stabilization of the posterior ring to the type B2 fixation construct.[5,28] Fixation of the posterior ring component only has also been recommended.[31] Further study is needed to define the indications for posterior ring fixation in these injuries.

Type B2.2 and B2.3 Injuries (Crescent and Iliac Wing Fractures: LC-II)

Type B2.2 and B2.3 injuries represent fracture/dislocations of the sacroiliac joint caused by an LC force vector. As such, the posterior sacroiliac and interosseous ligaments remain attached to the crescent fracture fragment. The pelvic floor and the sacrospinous and sacrotuberous ligaments are not damaged. If sufficient ligamentous stability remains intact, fixation of this fracture fragment to the remainder of the ilium should restore the posterior tension band and rotational stability. With this injury, as opposed to type B2.1, fixation is directed to the posterior lesion. After open reduction through a posterior approach, standard

fixation consists of lag screws inserted from posterior to anterior across the fracture and into the iliac wing fragment. Antiglide plates, which may be placed on the outer table across the fracture, with one plate located superiorly just beneath the iliac crest and the second plate located inferiorly, often are necessary to control fracture obliquity and the tendency to redisplace (**Figure 2**).

If the LC force also causes an anterior compression fracture of the sacrum, fixation of the crescent fracture alone may not suffice. Depending on the amount of anterior sacral impaction and the type of anterior ring injury, the fixed ilium can internally malrotate to a position against the impacted sacrum. In this situation, supplemental anterior fixation may be warranted. Posterior fracture lines have a small intact posterior superior iliac spine fragment and may be treated similarly to a pure ligamentous dislocation of the sacroiliac joint with fixation crossing the joint. Anterior fractures with a large intact posterior superior iliac spine fragment are often treated similarly to pure ilium fractures with interfragmentary screw and plate fixation.[2]

A percutaneous technique has been described for the fixation of type B2.2 and B2.3 injuries, which uses screws placed from the anterior inferior iliac spine toward the posterior inferior iliac spine. A supplemental iliosacral screw is added for those with a small crescent fracture fragment. However, this technique does not appear to be in general use.

Type C Injuries (VS: APC-III)

Type C pelvic injuries are completely unstable because of disruption of the posterior sacroiliac complex, and they require fixation. Reduction of the displacement often requires a great deal of force. Many injury-specific reduction clamps and standard reduction maneuvers have been described for the open reduction of posterior

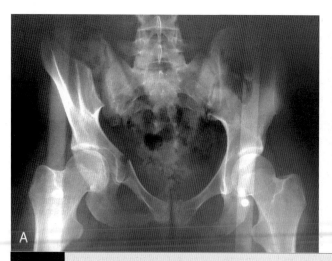
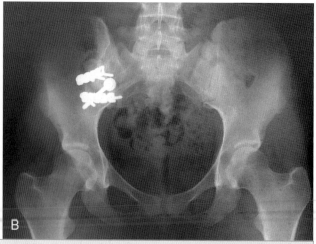

Figure 2   **A,** AP injury radiograph showing a type B2.2 pelvic ring disruption. **B,** Two-year follow-up AP radiograph. (Copyright Berton R. Moed, MD, St. Louis, MO.)

injuries.[2] More recently, studies have described rigidly stabilizing patients to the operating room table using some form of table-skeletal fixation to obtain either open or closed reductions.[32,33] The type of fixation construct is dictated by the location of the posterior injury; however, iliosacral screw fixation is most commonly used. Iliosacral screw placement using standard techniques without neurodiagnostic monitoring is associated with a low rate of neurologic complications (0% in one study).[34] If iliosacral screw fixation is used, two screws are preferable to single-screw fixation.[2] This second screw can be placed in either the S1 or the S2 body. In addition, fixation of the anterior ring injury improves the stability of the construct.[2]

Sacroiliac Joint Dislocations

Fixation can be accomplished with plating using an anterior surgical approach or with iliosacral screws inserted percutaneously or after an open surgical reduction. Iliosacral screw fixation is most commonly used and is inserted into the body of S1 perpendicular to the sacroiliac joint line, coursing in an anterior superior direction to avoid the S1 neural canal. Partially threaded screws allow compression of the joint as the screw is tightened, and the use of a washer resists the screw head being pulled through the lateral ilium. If a screw inserted in the S2 body is used, its pathway is perpendicular to the sagittal axis of the sacrum and not typically perpendicular to the sacroiliac joint surfaces (**Figure 3**).

Sacral Fractures

Sacral fractures may occur in three zones relative to the position of the neural foramina. Zone I is lateral to the foramina, zone II is the region of the neural foramina, and zone III is the region medial to the neural foramina. Neurologic deficits are more common in zone II and III fractures. The fixation of type C sacral fractures is commonly achieved using iliosacral screws, which, if

possible, are inserted perpendicular to the fracture line. Anatomic fracture reduction is important to improve fracture stability and increase the diameter of the safe corridor for iliosacral screw placement. Cranial displacement exceeding 5 mm substantially decreases the space available for iliosacral screw placement. When cranial displacement exceeds 10 mm, iliosacral screw fixation may not be technically possible.

There are some controversies concerning iliosacral screw fixation of sacral fractures. These mainly involve whether or how the fracture should be compressed to enhance the stability of the fixation construct, the related use of fully threaded versus partially threaded

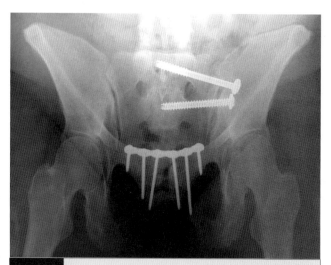

Figure 3   Posterior cephalad radiograph after fixation in a 53-year-old obese woman who sustained a type C injury in a motor vehicle collision. The radiograph shows the obliquely oriented, partially threaded screw inserted into S1 and the screw inserted into the body of S2 oriented perpendicular to the sagittal axis of the sacrum as a second point of fixation. (Copyright Berton R. Moed, MD, St. Louis, MO.)

screws, and the necessary length of the screw(s). In any case, vertical sacral fractures fixed percutaneously with iliosacral screws appear to pose a risk for fixation failure. This may be related to inadequate compression of the fracture fragments because of the concern that compression of zone II fractures places the nerve roots exiting the foramina at risk for iatrogenic injury. Other possibilities are inaccurate reduction, limited screw purchase in the sacrum, preexisting osteopenic bone, the need for longer (transsacral) screws, or the general limitations of the technique. Recent biomechanical and clinical studies suggest that transsacral fixation of one type or another may provide significant improvement over the standard iliosacral construct.[35-37] Further study is warranted; although some have advocated for spinopelvic fixation for comminuted sacral fractures, this construct has many known drawbacks, such as prominent and symptomatic hardware, delayed union and nonunion, lumbosacral scoliosis, the need for eventual removal, and a reported relatively high iatrogenic rate (13%) of nerve root injury.[38] Consequently, selective use of this technique is recommended when reliable iliosacral or transsacral screw fixation cannot be achieved.[38,39]

U-Shaped Sacral Fractures and Spinopelvic Dissociation

U-shaped sacral fractures (consisting of bilateral vertical fracture lines through the sacral foramina and a transverse fracture line separating the upper and lower sacral segments) cause spino-pelvic dissociation but may not result in instability of the pelvic ring. Variations in the fracture may produce H or Y patterns, which consist of a U-shaped unstable lumbar upper sacral fracture fragment and an unstable pelvic ring disruption.[36] These fractures are not easily classified or clearly described and are best understood through an approach incorporating multiple classification systems. U-shaped fractures are sacral zone III injuries (described in the literature) and have been subclassified and further modified by various researchers. These patients often present with neurologic injury. When present, a vertical sacral fracture component may indicate an associated type B or C pelvic ring injury.

Fixation of these injuries with long iliosacral or transsacral screws is possible but best reserved for noncomminuted fractures in which spinopelvic displacement is minimal.[40] For patients with more unstable displaced and comminuted fractures, lumbopelvic fixation is indicated.[39,41] The indications for surgical decompression of lower sacral nerve root injuries in association with these fractures remain undefined.[41]

Percutaneous Versus Open Reduction and Fixation

Infection is one of the major complications of open reduction and fixation of the posterior pelvic ring, occurring in 14% of patients in one series.[42] A major risk factor for infection is performance of open surgery through a compromised soft-tissue envelope; percutaneous treatment has been shown to minimize the risk for infection.[42] However, a recent report with a large study group of 236 patients with type C pelvic fractures found a surgical site infection in only eight patients (3.4%).[43] Percutaneous treatment mandates that an adequate closed reduction be achieved before screw placement. With proper patient selection and surgical technique, open reduction should pose minimal risk for catastrophic wound complications or high infection rates identified by others reporting on smaller series of patients.[43]

New Fixation Techniques

The advent of an internal anterior fixator (INFIX) allows for definitive anterior pelvic stabilization without the complications of an external fixator.[44] It consists of single supra-acetabular pedicle screws placed on either side and connected with a subcutaneous rod. Application of the INFIX is an elective surgical procedure and is contraindicated in patients who are hemodynamically unstable.[44] In one study, INFIX was associated with high rates of union for anterior injury in unstable pelvic fractures; patients were able to sit, stand, and ambulate without difficulty and demonstrated an acceptably low complication rate.[45] A second surgical procedure is required for device removal.

Another study described a minimally invasive alternative to the anterior external fixator: anterior pelvic bridge plating using either locking reconstruction plates and screws or an occipitocervical fusion plate-rod hybrid implant with pedicle screws for fixation.[46,47] The initial limited clinical experience was encouraging, showing a lower wound complication rate and fewer surgical site symptoms while maintaining a reduction equal to external fixation.[46] Although not necessarily new, renewed interest in transsacral fixation through the S1 or the S2 body with or without a locking nut (Figure 4) offers the potential for improved fixation in complex fractures and osteopenic bone using open or percutaneous techniques.[35-37]

Outcomes

Currently, radiographic measurement is the most commonly used outcome tool.[48] Conventional wisdom states that functional outcomes are related to fracture reduction. However, outcome studies based on the quality of pelvic fracture reduction are hampered by the fact that these radiographic measurements have been taken using largely unstandardized and universally untested techniques.[48] Clearly, better methods are needed. It is believed that functional outcomes are worst for type C injuries, followed by type B1, and is best for type B2.[2] However, unstable B2 pelvic ring injuries also have resulted in persistent disability based on validated outcome measurements.[49] Nonetheless, it is clear that a displaced pelvic ring disruption results in long-term functional impairment and pain in most patients.[2] High rates of sexual and urinary dysfunction have been reported, even in the absence of obvious genitourinary injury.[50-52] However, overall functional outcomes are dependent on many factors and have been

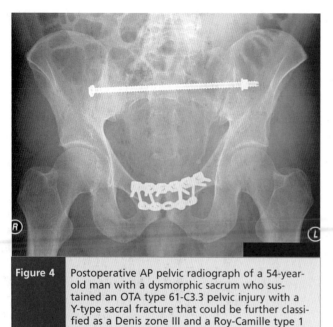

Figure 4 Postoperative AP pelvic radiograph of a 54-year-old man with a dysmorphic sacrum who sustained an OTA type 61-C3.3 pelvic injury with a Y-type sacral fracture that could be further classified as a Denis zone III and a Roy-Camille type 1 after reduction and placement of a locked transsacral screw for the bilateral sacral fractures and plate fixation of the symphysis pubis dislocation.

difficult to ascertain. A recent systematic literature review indicates that existing literature is inadequate to inform surgeons or patients in a meaningful way about the functional outcomes of these fractures.[53]

Acetabular Fractures

Anatomy and Stability of the Acetabulum

The goal of treating an acetabular fracture is to restore the congruity and stability of the hip joint. Acetabular fracture treatment is based on a thorough understanding of the anatomy of the innominate bone, which is formed as a condensation of the pubis, ischium, and ilium at the acetabular triradiate cartilage. Ossification of the acetabulum starts around puberty and is completed at the time of skeletal maturity. The articular surface of the acetabulum can be visualized as being supported between an inverted Y formed by two columns of bone, one anterior and the other posterior.[54]. The anterior column refers to the anterior half of the iliac wing that is contiguous with the pelvic brim to the superior pubic ramus and also includes the anterior half of the acetabular articular surface; the posterior column begins at the superior aspect of the greater sciatic notch and is contiguous with the greater and lesser sciatic notches inferiorly and includes the ischial tuberosity.[54] The anterior and posterior walls of the acetabulum are components of the respective columns. After bony injury, the stability of the hip joint is determined by the amount of remaining intact acetabulum. Therefore, displaced acetabulum fractures often have a concomitant dislocation of the femoral head.[54,55]

Mechanisms of Injury and Associated Injuries

Acetabular fractures occur from impact of the femoral head into the acetabular articular surface. This force to the femoral head may be applied via the greater trochanter (along the axis of the femoral neck) or from anywhere along the long axis of the femoral shaft.[56] The pattern of the fracture depends on the position of the hip at the time of impact, along with the location and the direction of the applied force.[54] The extent of fracture displacement, fracture comminution, and articular impaction depends on the amount of applied force and the strength of the underlying bone. Therefore, patients with osteopenic bone can sustain severely comminuted fractures despite experiencing a relatively low-energy injury.[57] These relatively low-energy injuries usually produce isolated fracture trauma, whereas high-energy injuries are often associated with additional skeletal or other system trauma.

In one study, a lower extremity fracture was found to be the most commonly associated injury (36%), followed by injuries to the lungs, the retroperitoneum, and the upper extremities, respectively (ranging from 21% to 26%).[58] Other injuries occurred, in decreasing order, to the bowel, kidney, vascular system, bladder, spleen, liver, brain, and spine (ranging from 2% to 16%). This is consistent with previous studies.[54,55] Nerve injury occurs in more than 10% of cases.[54,55] In addition, even isolated fractures of the acetabulum often necessitate blood replacement, reportedly 35% of the time in one series.[59] Therefore, even in patients with an apparent isolated injury, the initial evaluation must be detailed and part of a well-organized, overall approach.

Radiographic Imaging

In 1964, researchers recognized that the plane of the ilium is approximately 90° to the plane of the obturator foramen, and both of these structures are oriented roughly 45° to the frontal plane.[56] Accurate interpretation of plain radiographs results from correlation of the normal anatomy of the innominate bone with the pertinent radiographic landmarks seen on each view of the pelvis. Based on the bony morphology, the AP view and two 45° oblique (obturator and iliac) views of the pelvis are used to study the radiographic anatomy of the acetabulum. The current classification of acetabular fractures is directly derived from this original work.[54,56] This fracture analysis was expanded to include preoperative two-dimensional CT.[54,60] Subsequent advances in CT technology, such as three-dimensional volume-rendered CT and CT-derived reconstructed radiographs, have improved the information provided by two-dimensional images and offer promise.[60] However, further study is needed to validate the clinical usefulness of this methodology. Currently, these newer imaging studies should be considered to augment, not replace, the three plain radiographic projections (**Figure 5**).

The AP view shows six basic radiographic landmarks[54] (**Figure 6**). The iliopectineal line is the major

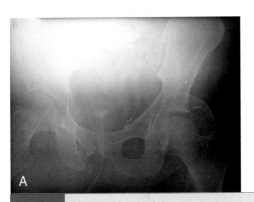
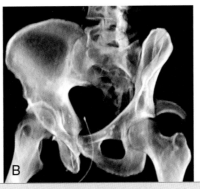
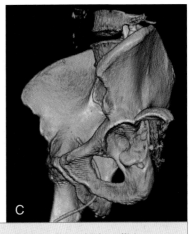

Figure 5 Imaging studies of an obese 57-year-old man who sustained an acetabular fracture in a motor vehicle collision. **A,** After several attempts, this obturator oblique radiograph was considered to be the best obtainable. **B,** The obturator oblique CT-generated radiograph obtained on the day of injury using the shaded opaque volume-rendering technique. **C,** Selected three-dimensional CT using the volume-rendering technique. (Copyright Berton R. Moed, MD, St. Louis, MO.)

4: Lower Extremity

landmark of the anterior column. The ilioischial line, extending from the posterosuperior greater sciatic notch to the ischial tuberosity, generally is considered a radiographic landmark of the posterior column.[54] The radiographic U, or teardrop, consists of a lateral and a medial limb; the lateral limb represents the inferior aspect of the anterior wall of the acetabulum, and the medial limb is formed by the obturator canal and the anteroinferior portion of the quadrilateral surface. The dense line of the superior articular surface of the acetabulum on the AP view is known as the roof; it results from the tangency of the x-ray beam to the subchondral bone in the superior acetabulum. The anterior and posterior rims of the acetabulum represent, respectively, the peripheral contours of the anterior and posterior walls of the acetabulum.

An obturator oblique radiograph is taken with a patient placed so the injured hemipelvis is rotated 45° toward the x-ray beam. This view shows the obturator foramen in its largest dimension and profiles the anterior column. The iliopectineal line has the same relationship to the pelvic brim as on the AP radiograph. The posterior rim of the acetabulum is best seen in this view, as is a fracture involving the posterior wall. The iliac oblique radiograph is taken with the patient placed so that the injured hemipelvis is rotated 45° away from the x-ray beam. This view shows the iliac wing in its largest dimension and profiles the greater and lesser sciatic notches and the anterior rim of the acetabulum. Involvement of the posterior column often can best be seen on this view, along with fractures of the anterior column traversing the iliac wing.

The CT scan is an essential adjunct to the three radiographic projections to further define the fracture pattern and assess for associated bony injuries.[54,60] Two-dimensional axial CT images are superior to plain radiographs in showing the extent and location of acetabular wall fractures, the presence of intra-articular free fragments or injury to the femoral head, impacted

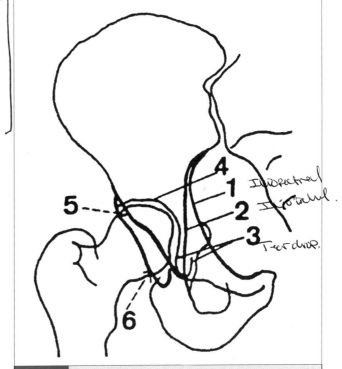

Figure 6 Schematic diagram showing the six acetabular landmarks seen on an AP radiograph: iliopectineal line (1), ilioischial line (2), U or teardrop (3), roof (4), anterior rim (5), and posterior rim (6). (Reproduced from Templeman D, Olson S, Moed BR, Duwelius P, Matta JM: Surgical treatment of acetabular fractures. *Instr Course Lect* 1999;48:481-496.)

fragments at the fracture margins, the orientation of the fracture lines, the presence of any additional fracture lines (such as the vertical portion of a T-shaped fracture), the rotation of fracture fragments, and the

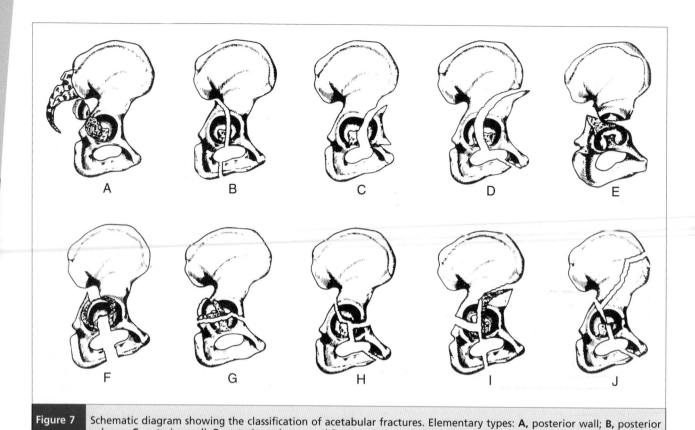

Figure 7 Schematic diagram showing the classification of acetabular fractures. Elementary types: **A**, posterior wall; **B**, posterior column; **C**, anterior wall; **D**, anterior column; and **E**, transverse. Associated types: **F**, posterior column plus posterior wall; **G**, transverse plus posterior wall; **H**, T-shaped; **I**, anterior column plus posterior hemitransverse; and **J**, both-column. (Reproduced from Moed BR, Dickson KF, Kregor PJ, Reilly MC, Vrahas MS: Surgical treatment of acetabular fractures. *Instr Course Lect* 2010;59:481-502.)

status of the posterior pelvic ring. The orientation of one or more fracture lines can help distinguish among the fracture types.

Classification

The AO and OTA comprehensive fracture classifications use a basic alphanumeric system to codify the acetabular fracture classification developed by Judet and Letournel and offer no clinical advantage.[6,54,56] The so-called Letournel acetabular fracture classification is preferred internationally by most treating surgeons and is based on the anatomy of the fracture pattern. It has 10 categories, including 5 elementary and 5 associated patterns[61] (Figure 7). With 10 main fracture types in the classification used to describe a spectrum of injury, however, many transitional fracture configurations do not exactly fit a specific category. For example, the anterior morphologic equivalent of a posterior wall fracture not involving the pelvic brim was not formally described by Letournel and Judet. This extremely rare injury has been subsequently recognized, but controversy exists whether it is best classified as a variant anterior wall fracture or a posterior wall fracture. It has been shown that the Letournel classification can be used reliably as a guide for the treatment of acetabular fractures by orthopaedic trauma surgeons.[60] The use of an algorithm for classifying acetabular fractures may

prove helpful for those with less experience treating these injuries.[62]

Initial Evaluation and Management

The patient history is often helpful, especially when determining the specific cause of injury. In most cases, a patient with a fracture of the acetabulum has sustained high-energy trauma, and these patients often have an associated injury that must be identified during the initial workup. A detailed physical examination is a necessity. The soft tissues should be carefully evaluated. Local closed degloving soft-tissue injuries (the Morel-Lavallee lesion) can harbor pathogenic bacteria and lead to wound breakdown and deep infection. Débridement followed by delayed wound closure and, subsequently, delayed fracture fixation may be required.[54] More recently, a percutaneous method of débridement has been described. Currently, the appropriate treatment method must be individualized and left to the judgment of the treating physician. Open wounds usually necessitate débridement followed by delayed wound closure. Acetabular fractures are often associated with hip dislocation, and posterior wall fractures are common.[54,55,63] Shortening of the entire limb likely is present if the hip is dislocated; however, limb shortening of 1 or 2 cm is often difficult to determine in this clinical setting.[63-65] The physical findings regarding limb

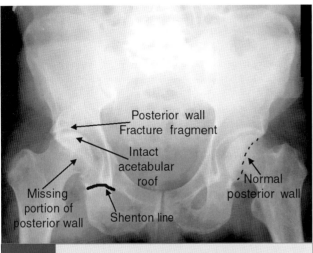

Figure 8 AP radiograph showing a dislocated hip on the right with the hip in neutral position. Signs of a posterior hip dislocation present on this radiograph include a break in the Shenton line, proximal migration of the lesser trochanter, relatively smaller size of the affected femoral head (closer to the x-ray cassette), and a bony double density above the femoral head, which is caused by the displaced posterior wall fragment that often sits atop the dislocated femoral head and can give the appearance of a normal joint space, potentially resulting in a misdiagnosis. (Copyright Berton R. Moed, MD, St. Louis, MO.)

position commonly ascribed to a posterior dislocation of the hip (flexion, adduction, and internal rotation of the hip with a shortened lower extremity) may not be present because a large posterior wall fracture fragment allows the femoral head to dislocate directly posterior without forcing the proximal femur into this expected abnormal position[63-65] (**Figure 8**). Therefore, the treating physician must have a high level of suspicion for this condition. A complete and clearly documented neurologic examination is important both for patient prognosis and to address medicolegal concerns. Neurologic injury involving the ipsilateral lower extremity occurs in more than 10% of patients with acetabular fractures, and sciatic nerve injury is the most common type.[54,63] Other peripheral nerves, such as the femoral, obturator, and superior gluteal nerves, also may be injured.[54]

In contradistinction to the situation with an unstable pelvic ring injury, a closed fracture of the acetabulum is rarely associated with severe bleeding and hypotensive shock. Although vascular injury may occur, such as the superior gluteal artery lacerated by fracture displacement in the greater sciatic notch, this is an infrequent occurrence. Although patients with an acetabular fracture may require blood transfusion, this is not typically associated with a vascular injury.[64]

Initial management depends on the specific fracture pattern, the amount of fracture displacement, and the relative stability and congruency of the hip joint. Dislocation of the femoral head can be diagnosed on the initial AP radiograph (**Figure 8**). Prompt reduction is required, especially in the case of a posterior wall fracture because the rate of osteonecrosis may significantly increase if reduction is not performed within 12 hours of the injury.[63-65] Patients with an acetabular fracture may not need skeletal traction. However, there are notable situations in which skeletal traction is either mandatory or desirable. Unstable fracture-dislocations necessitate skeletal traction after reduction to prevent recurrent dislocation. When hip stability is in doubt, it is prudent to use traction pending further evaluation. Preoperative skeletal traction is also important to prevent further femoral head articular surface damage from abrasion by the raw acetabular bony fracture surfaces and may occasionally improve fracture position.

Indications for emergency surgery are uncommon and include situations such as recurrent hip dislocation despite traction, irreducible hip dislocation, and open fractures. Acetabular fractures caused by gunshots are a special category of injury. Emergent surgery is often required for vascular, visceral, and urogenital injuries.[20,66] Compared with the situation for gunshot wounds to the pelvis, gunshot wounds to the acetabulum are often catastrophic injuries, with a high complication rate and poor functional outcomes.[66] In one recent study of 39 gunshot wounds to the acetabulum, injury to the bowel along with an associated fracture pattern was found to correlate with deep infection and poor outcome.[66] Generally, surgical fixation of an acetabular fracture is not an emergency and usually is delayed for several days to allow for stabilization of a patient's general status and preoperative planning. According to conventional wisdom, undergoing this surgery within the first 24 hours of injury puts patients at risk for increased blood loss. However, a 2013 study indicates that posterior wall fractures might be a subset of acetabular fractures and can be treated immediately without increased risk for excessive blood loss.[67] In any case, an inordinate delay in time to surgery has been shown to be an important predictor of radiologic and clinical outcome.[54,68] In one study, a good-to-excellent clinical outcome was more likely when surgery was performed within 15 days for elementary fractures and 10 days for associated types.[68]

Definitive Treatment

A stable acetabular fracture that does not involve the superior acetabular dome and has a congruent hip joint generally can be treated nonsurgically. Various methods have been used to determine stability. Roof arc measurements can be made to determine whether the remaining intact acetabulum is sufficient to maintain a stable and congruous relationship with the femoral head. The roof arc is measured on each of the three radiographic views with the leg out of traction. The roof arc is the angle created by a vertical line drawn through the center of the femoral head, and a second line is drawn from the center of the femoral head to the fracture location at the articular surface on each standard view. It is generally accepted that fractures with a medial roof arc angle exceeding 45°, an anterior roof arc

4: Lower Extremity

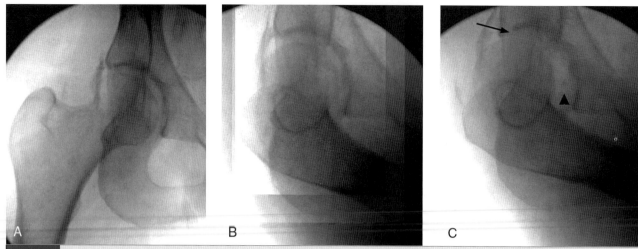

Figure 9   Fluoroscopic views showing the dynamic examination under anesthesia. **A,** The intraoperative obturator oblique fluoroscopic view with the hip in full extension shows a located and congruent hip joint. **B,** The intraoperative obturator oblique fluoroscopic view with the hip in neutral rotation and flexed to approximately 90° shows a located and a congruent hip joint. **C,** The intraoperative obturator oblique fluoroscopic view with the hip in neutral rotation and flexed to approximately 90° with axial load applied shows gross subluxation with loss of hip joint parallelism and joint congruency (arrow) and gross enlargement of the medial clear space (arrowhead). (Reproduced with permission from Moed BR, Ajibade DA, Israel H: Computed tomography as a predictor of hip stability status in posterior wall fractures of the acetabulum. *J Orthop Trauma* 2009;23:7-15.)

angle exceeding 25°, and a posterior roof arc angle exceeding 70° have sufficient intact acetabulum for nonsurgical treatment. However, a 2012 biomechanical study suggests that with the acetabulum subjected to sit-to-stand loading rather than single–leg-stance loading, the critical angles are substantially higher.[69] The clinical implications of these findings are yet to be determined. In any case, roof arc measurements are not applicable to both-column fractures and fractures of the posterior wall. For both-column fractures, there is no intact portion of the acetabulum to measure. Displaced both-column fractures of the acetabulum may be considered for nonsurgical management in the presence of secondary congruence, which is defined as congruency between the femoral head and the displaced acetabular articular fragments without skeletal traction being applied.[54]

For fractures of the posterior wall, there is no method for interpreting routine static imaging studies to reliably determine hip stability status in all cases.[70-72] Using two-dimensional CT to measure posterior wall size, fractures involving more than 50% of the articular surface reliably may be considered unstable; however, fractures involving between 20% and 50% of the surface are indeterminate.[70,71] Although it previously was believed that fractures involving less than 20% of the posterior wall are stable, it has been shown that hip instability can be present in a small percentage of these cases.[71] A history of an associated hip dislocation is not a reliable indicator of persistent hip instability.[72] Although further study is needed, it appears that a specifically described dynamic stress examination under anesthesia is a diagnostic study that can define hip stability status and the need for surgical intervention of fractures of the posterior wall[72] (Figure 9).

Surgical Approaches
Standard Surgical Approaches
The standard surgical approaches to the acetabulum as described by Letournel and Judet are the Kocher-Langenbeck, ilioinguinal, iliofemoral, and extended iliofemoral.[54] The surgical approach usually is dictated by the location of the major fracture displacement and is selected with the expectation that it will allow for entire fracture reduction and fixation (Table 3). The three nonextensile approaches rely on indirect manipulation for reduction of any fracture lines that traverse the opposite column. The extended iliofemoral approach allows almost complete direct access to all aspects of the acetabulum. It most often is used for delayed treatment of an associated fracture type in which fracture healing precludes indirect manipulation. However, alternative approaches have been proposed that may offer important advantages over these standard methods.

The Modified Gibson Approach and the Trochanteric Flip Osteotomy
The modified Gibson approach differs from the Kocher-Langenbeck approach in that the interval between the gluteus maximus and tensor fasciae lata muscles is developed rather than splitting the gluteus maximus muscle.[73] In this way, the neurovascular supply to the anterior portion of the gluteus maximus muscle is not at risk. Other advantages include improved anterosuperior access and a more cosmetically appealing incision, especially in female patients who are obese. A trochanteric flip osteotomy, in which the abductor and vastus lateralis muscle insertions remain attached to the trochanteric fragment, can be combined with either the modified Gibson approach or the Kocher-Langenbeck

Table 3

Acetabular Fracture Patterns and Preferred Standard Surgical Approaches

Fracture Type	Potential Standard Surgical Approach for Each Fracture Pattern				
	Kocher-Langenbeck	Ilioinguinal	Iliofemoral	Combined	Extended Iliofemoral
Elementary					
Posterior wall	X				
Posterior column	X				
Anterior wall		X	X		
Anterior column		X	X		
Transverse infra/juxtatectal	X	X			
Transverse transtectal	X				X
Associated					
Posterior column + wall	X				
Anterior + posterior hemitransverse		X		X	X
Transverse infra/juxtatectal + posterior wall	X				
Transverse transtectal + posterior wall	X				X
T-shaped infra/juxtatectal	X			X	
T-shaped transtectal				X	**X**
Both-column		X		X	X

Note: "X" in bold denotes the most preferred approach.

approach.[74] Further anterosuperior exposure is facilitated, as well as intraoperative dislocation of the femoral head for inspection of the joint.

Modified Stoppa Approach

The modified Stoppa intrapelvic approach is an alternative to the ilioinguinal approach.[75] It was described in the treatment of anterior wall, anterior column, transverse, T-shaped, anterior column/wall-plus-posterior hemitransverse, and both-column fractures but it initially was only infrequently combined with the lateral window of the ilioinguinal approach.[76] More recently, as its utility has been more fully appreciated, it is commonly used in conjunction with the lateral window.[75,77] In one series, this combination was required in 34 of 57 patients (60%) for fracture reduction and/or fixation placement.[75] At another center reporting on a small number of patients (17), the addition of the lateral window became standard.[77] The modified Stoppa approach offers improved exposure of the quadrilateral surface and the posterior column, making it useful for fractures that require buttress plating of the quadrilateral surface while minimizing the use of the "middle window" of the ilioinguinal approach.[78,79]

Fixation Options

Fracture reduction is the most difficult and critical element of a surgical procedure. There are many published texts that deal with the specifics of this important aspect.[54,64] The fracture usually is fixed with 3.5-mm hardware; however, smaller screw sizes often are needed for the fixation of a posterior wall or an osteochondral fracture fragment.[54,63,64] The standard fracture fixation constructs (**Figure 10**) often must be modified to accommodate individual fracture morphology. Recently, a safe zone was identified to assist in avoiding intra-articular screw placement when using the ilioinguinal or modified Stoppa approach.[80] Locking plates have been advocated for use in many areas of the skeletal system, and a biomechanical study in a transverse acetabular fracture model has shown these constructs to be as strong as conventional plating in combination with an interfragmentary screw.[81] However, clinical evidence for its advantages in acetabular fracture surgery remains limited.[82]

Percutaneous Techniques

Percutaneous fixation with or without closed reduction has been proposed to prevent potential fracture displacement. It also has been used in elderly patients with displaced acetabular fractures for whom a malreduction might have less severe implications, for simple

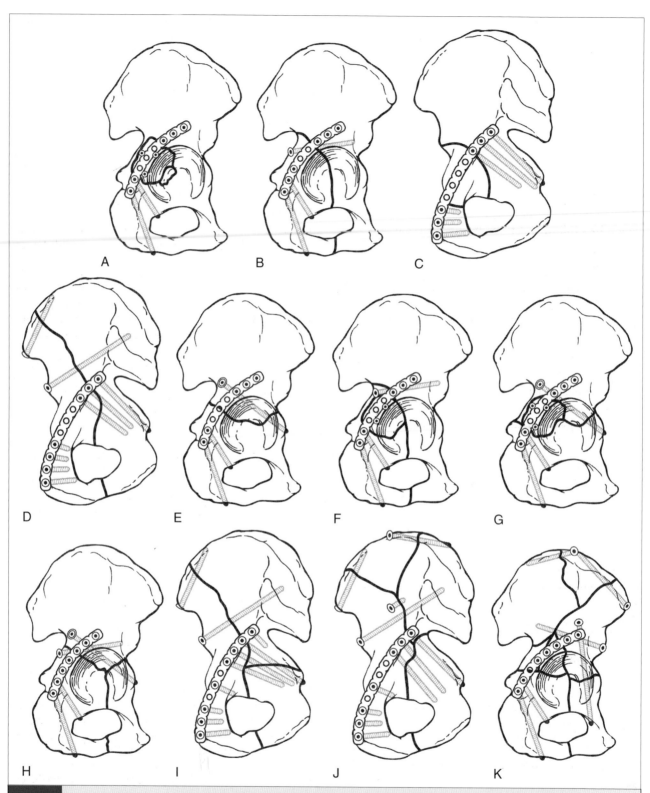

Figure 10 Schematic diagrams showing the 10 acetabular fracture types, with typical fixation constructs. (**A** through **E** show elementary types; **F** through **K** show associated types.) **A,** Multifragmented posterior wall fracture with intra-articular comminution; **B,** posterior column fracture; **C,** anterior wall fracture; **D,** high anterior column fracture; **E,** juxtatectal transverse fracture; **F,** posterior column plus posterior wall fracture; **G,** transverse plus posterior wall fracture; **H,** T-shaped fracture; **I,** anterior column plus posterior hemitransverse fracture; **J,** both-column fracture with the ilioinguinal approach used; **K,** both-column fracture with posterior column comminution with the extended iliofemoral approach used. (Copyright Berton R. Moed, MD, St. Louis, MO.)

fractures with minimal displacements, and for patients who are morbidly obese. It has been used as an adjunct to standard open reduction and internal fixation techniques, in conjunction with limited open surgery as a staging procedure for total hip arthroplasty (THA), and in young patients with severe injuries that preclude formal open reduction and internal fixation. In general, evidence to support all of these indications is limited. However, evidence is mounting in support of treatment for elderly patients (defined as those at least 60 years of age) using minimally invasive reduction and percutaneous fixation.[83,84] In one study of 75 fractures, rates of conversion to THA were comparable to open treatment, and soft tissues were preserved for future surgery.[83] In a follow-up study including 36 patients, functional outcomes and the conversion rate to THA were not significantly different when compared with published series of patients treated with formal open reduction and internal fixation.[84] These results may be influenced by finding that anatomic reduction may not be necessary to attain a good functional outcome for acetabular fractures in elderly patients.[85]

Percutaneous fixation requires adherence to specific described techniques.[83] Determining the appropriate size of the screws to be inserted in the posterior and anterior columns is an important aspect. Insertion in the anterior column of 3.5- to 4.5-mm screws can be accommodated in most if not all patients. In a study using three-dimensional modeling of CT images of 82 adult patients, a difference was found between men and women, with the anterior column accommodating screw diameters ranging from 6.9 to 10.8 mm in men and 5.6 to 10.0 mm in women.[86] Another study found the anterior column capable of accommodating screw diameters ranging from 5.0 mm to 7.3 mm, and the posterior column capable of accommodating screw diameters ranging from 9.4 to 13.3 mm.[87] Both studies indicated that the size of the screws used for percutaneous column fixation should not be based solely on the measurement of cross-sectional diameter, and virtual three-dimensional reconstructions might be useful in preoperative planning.

Acute THA

There has been an increase in the age of patients presenting with displaced acetabular fractures, including an increasing incidence in those who are older than 60 years.[88] These older patients sustain fractures associated with poor outcomes, including impaction of the weight-bearing acetabular roof, a femoral head articular injury, and multifragmentary posterior wall fractures.[63,88] Outcomes for THA after nonsurgical treatment or failed open reduction and internal fixation of acetabular fractures have been inferior when compared with outcomes after primary THA for nontraumatic conditions. Improved results have been reported more recently, however.[89] Consequently, the indications for primary acute arthroplasty remain uncertain. Problems associated with the use of a two-incision technique (that is, anterior for fracture fixation followed by posterior for arthroplasty) include high rates of blood transfusion, lengthy anesthetic times, and various technical difficulties.[90] It appears that the results are improved with a single-incision approach.[90,91] However, postoperative component dislocation remains problematic.[90,91]

Outcomes

Acetabular fracture treatment outcomes are dependent on how the outcomes are measured. The clinical outcomes, as measured using hip function and radiographic scores, are directly related to the accuracy of fracture reduction.[54,55,63] Using the modified rating scale of Merle d'Aubigné and Postel, which is the most commonly used acetabular fracture clinical hip score, good-to-excellent long-term clinical results should be expected in 75% to 81% of patients.[54,55,63] Studies using functional outcome instruments, such as the Musculoskeletal Function Assessment as the evaluative measure of health status, paint a very different picture. In one study of 150 patients with acetabular fractures treated surgically and evaluated using the Musculoskeletal Function Assessment, complete recovery was uncommon, with residual functional deficits involving wide-ranging aspects of everyday living that do not necessarily have an obvious direct connection to hip function.[92] Other investigators have reported similar findings.[65,93] In a 2012 study, investigators from Sweden using the Medical Outcomes Study 36-Item Short Form (SF-36) and Life Satisfaction-11 to evaluate quality of life in 136 patients treated surgically and followed for at least 2 years, found that although the SF-36 outcomes keep improving in the physical domains over a 2-year period, the outcome scores are below normal values.[3] However, patients with anatomic reduction scored better than those with residual displacement of at least 2 mm. In addition, life satisfaction plateaued at 6 months and generally was lower than normal.[3]

Today's outcomes are evaluated using a very different measure: survivorship of the hip using conversion to THA or hip fusion as an indirect indication of the development of posttraumatic osteoarthritis.[83,94] From a total of 1,208 hips treated by open reduction and internal fixation, evaluation of the 816 hips available for follow-up showed a cumulative survivorship of 79% at 20 years.[94] The factors that were predictive of the need for early conversion to THA were (1) age older than 40 years, (2) anterior dislocation, (3) femoral head cartilage lesion, (4) involvement of the posterior wall, (5) marginal impaction, (6) initial displacement of at least 20 mm, (7) nonanatomic reduction, (8) postoperative incongruence of the acetabular roof, and (9) the use of the extended iliofemoral approach.[94] Using the available data, a normogram was constructed to help select patients who could potentially benefit from acute primary THA by predicting the need for a THA by 2 years after open reduction and internal fixation.[94] Other investigators reported cumulative survivorship of 65% at 11.9 years of follow-up in patients age 60 and older who underwent percutaneous reduction and fixation.[83]

Summary

Injuries to the pelvic ring and the acetabulum represent a heterogeneous group of high-energy injuries. Although these injuries are relatively infrequent, the potential for significant morbidity and mortality and the relative unfamiliarity of most surgeons with these injuries leads to a high degree of anxiety related to their treatment. A careful review of appropriate imaging studies and an understanding of the complex three-dimensional anatomy of the pelvis is necessary for surgeons to maximize the functional recovery of their patients. Surgeons must be familiar with multiple reduction techniques and fixation strategies to successfully treat these difficult injury patterns.

Key Study Points

- Surgical intervention is recommended for all unstable type B and C pelvic ring injuries.

- For an acetabular fracture to be amenable to nonsurgical management, the hip must remain congruent on all three standard plain radiographs of the acetabulum.

- Anatomic reduction of an acetabular fracture correlates with improved radiographic and functional outcomes at long-term follow-up.

Annotated References

1. Pohlemann T, Stengel D, Tosounidis G, et al: Survival trends and predictors of mortality in severe pelvic trauma: Estimates from the German Pelvic Trauma Registry Initiative. *Injury* 2011;42(10):997-1002.

   Researchers studying 5,014 pelvic trauma cases found that in contrast to an overall decline in trauma mortality, complex pelvic ring injuries remain associated with a significant risk of death. All-cause in-hospital mortality declined from 8% in 1991 to 5% in 2006. Level of evidence: IV.

2. Tile M, Helfet DL, Kellam JF, eds: *Fractures of the Pelvis and Acetabulum*, ed 3. Philadelphia, PA, Lippincott Williams & Wilkins, 2003, pp 409-416.

3. Borg T, Berg P, Larsson S: Quality of life after operative fixation of displaced acetabular fractures. *J Orthop Trauma* 2012;26(8):445-450.

   Quality of life was evaluated in 136 patients followed up for 2 years via the SF-36 and Life Satisfaction-11. Investigators found that although quality of life improved over a 2-year period, it remained lower than the norm, and anatomic reduction resulted in better outcomes. Level of evidence: IV.

4. Manson T, O'Toole RV, Whitney A, Duggan B, Sciadini M, Nascone J: Young-Burgess classification of pelvic ring fractures: Does it predict mortality, transfusion requirements, and non-orthopaedic injuries? *J Orthop Trauma* 2010;24(10):603-609.

   Mortality, transfusion requirements, and nonorthopaedic injuries were measured. The results indicated that the Young-Burgess fracture pattern probably does not predict mortality very well. There were few significant differences in nonorthopaedic injuries between fracture types, and transfusion requirements were less numerous than in the original series. Level of evidence: IV.

5. Furey AJ, O'Toole RV, Nascone JW, Copeland CE, Turen C, Sciadini MF: Surgeon variability in the treatment of pelvic ring injuries. *Orthopedics* 2010;33(10):714.

   Agreement among surgeons was investigated regarding the relationship between injury type and treatment plan in 89 pelvic injuries using the Young-Burgess and Tile/Pennal classification systems. Finding only moderate levels of agreement, the investigators question the usefulness of the two classification systems.

6. Marsh JL, Slongo TF, Agel J, et al: Fracture and dislocation classification compendium—2007: Orthopaedic Trauma Association Classification, Database and Outcomes Committee. *J Orthop Trauma* 2007;21(10, suppl):S1-S133.

7. Weaver MJ, Bruinsma W, Toney E, Dafford E, Vrahas MS: What are the patterns of injury and displacement seen in lateral compression pelvic fractures? *Clin Orthop Relat Res* 2012;470(8):2104-2110.

   In 318 LC fractures retrospectively reviewed, LC injuries, especially LCI, were found to be a heterogeneous group with a wide range of fracture patterns. Those with more complex sacral fractures or crescent fractures or bilateral pubic rami fractures had higher degrees of initial displacement. Level of evidence: IV.

8. White CE, Hsu JR, Holcomb JB: Haemodynamically unstable pelvic fractures. *Injury* 2009;40(10):1023-1030.

9. Holstein JH, Culemann U, Pohlemann T; Working Group Mortality in Pelvic Fracture Patients: What are predictors of mortality in patients with pelvic fractures? *Clin Orthop Relat Res* 2012;470(8):2090-2097.

   Data from 2004 to 2011 on 5,340 patients from the German Pelvic Trauma Registry showed that 4% died a median of 2 days after trauma. Nonsurvivors had more complex pelvic injuries (32% versus 8%), had fewer isolated pelvic ring fractures (13% versus 49%), had major hemorrhage, and were male (56%). Level of evidence: III.

10. Pohlemann T, Culemann U, Holstein JH: Initial experience using a pelvic emergency simulator to train reduction in blood loss. *Clin Orthop Relat Res* 2012;470(8):2098-2103.

    Investigators developed a novel pelvic emergency simulator and found that it can be used as a tool to train surgeons to reduce blood loss in severe pelvic ring injuries.

11. Demetriades D, Karaiskakis M, Toutouzas K, Alo K, Velmahos G, Chan L: Pelvic fractures: Epidemiology and predictors of associated abdominal injuries and outcomes. *J Am Coll Surg* 2002;195(1):1-10.

12. Shlamovitz GZ, Mower WR, Bergman J, et al: How (un)useful is the pelvic ring stability examination in diagnosing mechanically unstable pelvic fractures in blunt trauma patients? *J Trauma* 2009;66(3):815-820.

13. Suzuki T, Morgan SJ, Smith WR, Stahel PF, Flierl MA, Hak DJ: Stress radiograph to detect true extent of symphyseal disruption in presumed anteroposterior compression type I pelvic injuries. *J Trauma* 2010;69(4):880-885.

    Stress radiographs under general anesthesia were performed on 22 patients with symphyseal diastasis of at least 1.0 cm but less than 2.5 cm on AP radiographs or CT images. This examination was found to be beneficial in diagnosing the severity of injury and choosing appropriate treatment.

14. Sagi HC, Coniglione FM, Stanford JH: Examination under anesthetic for occult pelvic ring instability. *J Orthop Trauma* 2011;25(9):529-536.

    In their study of 62 patients, investigators found that performing an examination under anesthesia with dynamic stress fluoroscopy revealed occult instability in 50% of presumed APC-I injuries, 39% of APC-II injuries, and 37% of LC-I injuries.

15. Spanjersberg WR, Knops SP, Schep NW, van Lieshout EM, Patka P, Schipper IB: Effectiveness and complications of pelvic circumferential compression devices in patients with unstable pelvic fractures: A systematic review of literature. *Injury* 2009;40(10):1031-1035.

16. Knops SP, Schep NW, Spoor CW, et al: Comparison of three different pelvic circumferential compression devices: A biomechanical cadaver study. *J Bone Joint Surg Am* 2011;93(3):230-240.

    In a biomechanical cadaver study, three devices were evaluated: the pelvic binder, the SAM Pelvic Sling (SAM Medical Products), and the T-POD (PYNG Medical). All three provided sufficient reduction in partially stable and unstable (Tile/Pennal type B1 and C) pelvic fractures. No undesirable overreduction was noted.

17. Ricci WM, Mamczak C, Tynan M, Streubel P, Gardner M: Pelvic inlet and outlet radiographs redefined. *J Bone Joint Surg Am* 2010;92(10):1947-1953.

    Using sagittal reconstructions, the inlet and outlet angles were quantified in 68 patients without pelvic ring injury who had routine CT scans. The investigators found that screening inlet and outlet radiographs at 25° and 60°, respectively, provide accurate views of the relevant posterior pelvic anatomy.

18. Graves ML, Routt ML Jr: Iliosacral screw placement: Are uniplanar changes realistic based on standard fluoroscopic imaging? *J Trauma* 2011;71(1):204-208.

    In 10 consecutive patients, the perpendicular angles required to achieve the ideal inlet and outlet views were measured intraoperatively. The average tilt required for the inlet view was 25° (range, 21° to 33°) and 42° (range, 30° to 50°) for the outlet. These views never created an orthogonal system.

19. Dong JL, Zhou DS: Management and outcome of open pelvic fractures: A retrospective study of 41 cases. *Injury* 2011;42(10):1003-1007.

    A retrospective review of 41 patients from 2001 to 2010 revealed that despite treatment advances, the mortality rate remained at 24% (10 of 41). Multivariate analysis showed that a Revised Trauma Score of 8 or lower was independently associated with both overall mortality and late mortality.

20. Bartkiw MJ, Sethi A, Coniglione F, et al: Civilian gunshot wounds of the hip and pelvis. *J Orthop Trauma* 2010;24(10):645-652.

    In 42 patients with gunshot wound fractures of the hip and pelvis, nonorthopaedic injuries included 15 bowel perforations, 7 vessel lacerations, and 2 urogenital injuries that required surgery. All fractures healed, and none was associated with pelvic ring instability or chronic osteomyelitis.

21. Doro CJ, Forward DP, Kim H, et al: Does 2.5 cm of symphyseal widening differentiate anteroposterior compression I from anteroposterior compression II pelvic ring injuries? *J Orthop Trauma* 2010;24(10):610-615.

    Using cadaver human pelves, investigators could not confirm 2.5 cm of symphyseal diastasis as differentiating between stable and unstable injuries. The data support that anterior sacroiliac ligament disruption likely exists for diastasis exceeding 4.5 cm and is unlikely when diastasis is less than 1.8 cm.

22. Bruce B, Reilly M, Sims S: OTA highlight paper predicting future displacement of nonoperatively managed lateral compression sacral fractures: Can it be done? *J Orthop Trauma* 2011;25(9):523-527.

    Of 117 Young-Burgess LC-I or OTA 61-B2.1 fractures, 19% (23 of 117) displaced. Incomplete sacral fractures with ipsilateral rami fractures are unlikely to displace. Those with a complete sacral fracture and bilateral rami fractures displace at a significantly higher rate.

23. Van Loon P, Kuhn S, Hofmann A, Hessmann MH, Rommens PM: Radiological analysis, operative management and functional outcome of open book pelvic lesions: A 13-year cohort study. *Injury* 2011;42(10):1012-1019.

    In a series of 38 patients with presumed type B1 injuries, 9 were treated using supplemental iliosacral screw fixation. The investigators could not determine the need for this posterior fixation, and the functional outcomes for these patients were worse.

24. Sagi HC, Papp S: Comparative radiographic and clinical outcome of two-hole and multi-hole symphyseal plating. *J Orthop Trauma* 2008;22(6):373-378.

25. Grimshaw CS, Bledsoe JG, Moed BR: Locked versus standard unlocked plating of the pubic symphysis: A ca-

daver biomechanical study. *J Orthop Trauma* 2012; 26(7):402-406.

Fixation with six-hole locked and unlocked symphyseal plates was compared using cadaver pelves to simulate a bilateral rotationally unstable open book (OTA 61-B3.1) injury. Minor loss of reduction was evident in all pelves regardless of fixation, and locked plating did not offer any advantage.

26. Moed BR, Grimshaw CS, Segina DN: Failure of locked design-specific plate fixation of the pubic symphysis: A report of six cases. *J Orthop Trauma* 2012;26(7): e71-e75.

Six cases with failed stainless-steel design-specific locked symphyseal plates were evaluated. The failure mechanisms included those seen with conventional uniplanar fixation, as well as those common to locked plating. It was concluded that indications for these implants remain to be determined. Level of evidence: IV.

27. Collinge C,, Archdeacon MT, Dulaney-Cripe E, Moed BR: Radiographic changes of implant failure after plating for pubic symphysis diastasis: An underappreciated reality? *Clin Orthop Relat Res* 2012;470(8):2148-2153.

Of 127 patients with OTA 61-B or 61-C injuries and minimum follow-up of 6 months, symphyseal fixation failure occurred in 95 (75%), with widening of the symphyseal space in 84 (88%). Only one patient required revision surgery. The investigators concluded that symphyseal widening can be expected and may represent a benign condition as motion is restored. However, patients should be counseled regarding the high rate of radiographic failure and small likelihood of revision surgery. Level of evidence: IV.

28. Morris SA, Loveridge J, Smart DK, Ward AJ, Chesser TJ: Is fixation failure after plate fixation of the symphysis pubis clinically important? *Clin Orthop Relat Res* 2012;470(8):2154-2160.

Among 148 patients followed for a minimum of 12 months who were treated with symphyseal plate fixation, hardware breakage occurred in 63 patients (43%), of which 61 were asymptomatic. The investigators concluded that the high rate of late symphyseal plate fixation failure is not clinically important.

29. Archdeacon MT, Arebi S, Le TT, Wirth R, Kebel R, Thakore M: Orthogonal pin construct versus parallel uniplanar pin constructs for pelvic external fixation: A biomechanical assessment of stiffness and strength. *J Orthop Trauma* 2009;23(2):100-105.

30. Starr AJ, Nakatani T, Reinert CM, Cederberg K: Superior pubic ramus fractures fixed with percutaneous screws: What predicts fixation failure? *J Orthop Trauma* 2008;22(2):81-87.

31. Osterhoff G, Ossendorf C, Wanner GA, Simmen H-P, Werner CM: Posterior screw fixation in rotationally unstable pelvic ring injuries. *Injury* 2011;42(10):992-996.

32. Lefaivre KA, Starr AJ, Reinert CM: Reduction of displaced pelvic ring disruptions using a pelvic reduction frame. *J Orthop Trauma* 2009;23(4):299-308.

33. Matta JM, Yerasimides JG: Table-skeletal fixation as an adjunct to pelvic ring reduction. *J Orthop Trauma* 2007;21(9):647-656.

34. Gardner MJ, Farrell ED, Nork SE, Segina DN, Routt ML Jr: Percutaneous placement of iliosacral screws without electrodiagnostic monitoring. *J Trauma* 2009; 66(5):1411-1415.

35. Gardner MJ, Routt ML Jr: Transiliac-transsacral screws for posterior pelvic stabilization. *J Orthop Trauma* 2011;25(6):378-384.

In a "technical trick" article, the authors show the technique to insert screws from the injured hemipelvis' ilium, coursing through the sacral body and exiting the contralateral iliac cortical bone for use in difficult situations (such as marked comminution or osteopenia) when standard iliosacral screws may provide inadequate fixation and lead to reduction loss.

36. Moed BR, Whiting DR: Locked transsacral screw fixation of bilateral injuries of the posterior pelvic ring: Initial clinical series. *J Orthop Trauma* 2010;24(10): 616-621.

The authors describe the use of a transsacral screw with a novel locking capability in 10 patients with bilateral posterior injury. Fixation failure did not occur, and satisfactory reduction was maintained in all cases. Additional suggested indications included situations in which routine transsacral screw fixation might otherwise be considered. Level of evidence: IV.

37. Tabaie SA, Bledsoe JG, Moed BR: Biomechanical comparison of standard iliosacral screw fixation to transsacral locked screw fixation in a type C zone II pelvic fracture model. *J Orthop Trauma* 2013;27(9):521-526.

A type C injury was created in cadaver pelves with vertical osteotomies through zone II of the sacrum and the ipsilateral pubic rami. The sacrum was reduced, maintaining a 2-mm fracture gap, and fixed with an iliosacral screw plus either a locked transsacral screw or another iliosacral screw. In biomechanical testing, the transsacral construct performed significantly better. Level of evidence: IV.

38. Sagi HC, Militano U, Caron T, Lindvall E: A comprehensive analysis with minimum 1-year follow-up of vertically unstable transforaminal sacral fractures treated with triangular osteosynthesis. *J Orthop Trauma* 2009; 23(5):313-321.

39. Jones CB, Sietsema DL, Hoffmann MF: Can lumbopelvic fixation salvage unstable complex sacral fractures? *Clin Orthop Relat Res* 2012;470(8):2132-2141.

In a study of 15 patients, it was found that complex posterior pelvic ring injuries of the sacrum not amenable to traditional fixation options can be salvaged with lumbopelvic fixation. Prominent hardware resulted in more pain. However, hardware prominence and associated pain are markedly reduced with screw head recession. Level of evidence: IV.

40. Conflitti JM, Graves ML, Chip Routt ML Jr: Radiographic quantification and analysis of dysmorphic upper sacral osseous anatomy and associated iliosacral screw insertions. *J Orthop Trauma* 2010;24(10):630-636.

When evaluating 24 patients, investigators found that the S2 segment provides a larger site for screw insertion, and longer screws are possible when compared with solutions for dysmorphic sacrums. The S2 screw pathway was perpendicular to the sagittal axis, so screws could traverse S2 from one posterior ilium to the other. Level of evidence: IV.

41. Schildhauer TA, Bellabarba C, Nork SE, Barei DP, Routt ML Jr, Chapman JR: Decompression and lumbopelvic fixation for sacral fracture-dislocations with spino-pelvic dissociation. *J Orthop Trauma* 2006;20(7):447-457.

42. Keating JF, Werier J, Blachut P, Broekhuyse H, Meek RN, O'Brien PJ: Early fixation of the vertically unstable pelvis: The role of iliosacral screw fixation of the posterior lesion. *J Orthop Trauma* 1999;13(2):107-113.

43. Stover MD, Sims S, Matta J: What is the infection rate of the posterior approach to type C pelvic injuries? *Clin Orthop Relat Res* 2012;470(8):2142-2147.

In a retrospective review of 236 patients treated with a posterior approach at six institutions, surgical site infections occurred in 3.4% of patients (8 of 236). No patient required soft-tissue reconstruction. The investigators concluded that with proper patient selection and surgical technique, the risk for catastrophic wound complications or high infection rates as reported by others should be minimal. Level of evidence: IV.

44. Vaidya R, Colen R, Vigdorchik J, Tonnos F, Sethi A: Treatment of unstable pelvic ring injuries with an internal anterior fixator and posterior fixation: Initial clinical series. *J Orthop Trauma* 2012;26(1):1-8.

The investigators present a novel device (an anterior subcutaneous internal fixator) using supra-acetabular spinal pedicle screws and a subcutaneous connecting rod. In 24 patients, all fractures healed without significant reduction loss. There were no infections, delayed unions, or nonunions. However, a second surgical procedure is required to remove the device. Level of evidence: IV.

45. Vaidya R, Kubiak EN, Bergin PF, et al: Complications of anterior subcutaneous internal fixation for unstable pelvis fractures: A multicenter study. *Clin Orthop Relat Res* 2012;470(8):2124-2131.

In a follow-up multicenter study of the anterior subcutaneous internal fixator, investigators reviewed 91 patients from four level I trauma centers who were followed for at least 6 months. Injuries healed without loss of reduction in 89 patients. Complications included six early revisions resulting from technical error and three infections. Irritation of the lateral femoral cutaneous nerve was reported in 27 patients and resolved in all but 1. Asymptomatic heterotopic ossification around the implants occurred in 32 patients. Level of evidence: IV.

46. Cole PA, Gauger EM, Anavian J, Ly TV, Morgan RA, Heddings AA: Anterior pelvic external fixator versus subcutaneous internal fixator in the treatment of anterior ring pelvic fractures. *J Orthop Trauma* 2012;26(5):269-277.

The investigators present a new minimally invasive technique, the anterior pelvic bridge, which is a percutaneous method for fixing the anterior pelvis through limited incisions over the iliac crest(s) and pubic symphysis. In a retrospective study of 48 patients, this technique was compared with anterior pelvic external fixation. The bridge method demonstrated a lower wound complication rate and associated morbidity and fewer surgical site symptoms while maintaining equivalent reduction. Level of evidence: III.

47. Hiesterman TG, Hill BW, Cole PA: Surgical technique: A percutaneous method of subcutaneous fixation for the anterior pelvic ring. The pelvic bridge. *Clin Orthop Relat Res* 2012;470(8):2116-2123.

In a limited prospective study of the anterior pelvic bridge in 11 patients, this new method was compared with external fixation, and there were minimal problems in either group. The surgical technique is more completely described, and a newly developed "plate-rod fixator" is shown. Level of evidence: II.

48. Lefaivre KA, Slobogean G, Starr AJ, Guy P, O'brien PJ, Macadam SA: Methodology and interpretation of radiographic outcomes in surgically treated pelvic fractures: A systematic review. *J Orthop Trauma* 2012;26(8):474-481.

A systematic review of the available literature was performed using all major databases to evaluate previously described methods for the measurement and interpretation of radiographic outcomes of surgical treated pelvic fractures. The findings revealed that reporting of radiographic outcomes has been done using largely unstandardized and universally untested measurement techniques. The interpretations of these measurements are also inconsistent and untested. Future research is needed in this area.

49. Hoffmann MF, Jones CB, Sietsema DL: Persistent impairment after surgically treated lateral compression pelvic injury. *Clin Orthop Relat Res* 2012;470(8):2161-2172.

Using the Short Musculoskeletal Function Assessment functional outcome measure, persistent disability was found despite near-anatomic fracture reduction in a retrospective review of 119 patients followed for at least 12 months. The investigators concluded that patients with these injuries should be counseled concerning the possibility of persistent disability. Level of evidence: IV.

50. Odutola AA, Sabri O, Halliday R, Chesser TJ, Ward AJ: High rates of sexual and urinary dysfunction after surgically treated displaced pelvic ring injuries. *Clin Orthop Relat Res* 2012;470(8):2173-2184.

In a retrospective study of patients evaluated by mailed questionnaire, new sexual dysfunction occurred in 43% of the responding patients (61 of 143) and urinary dysfunction in 41% of responding patients (61 of 150). Neither new sexual nor urinary dysfunction was associ-

39. Barton TM, Gleeson R, Topliss C, Greenwood R, Harries WJ, Chesser TJ: A comparison of the long gamma nail with the sliding hip screw for the treatment of AO/OTA 31-A2 fractures of the proximal part of the femur: A prospective randomized trial. *J Bone Joint Surg Am* 2010;92(4):792-798.

This prospective randomized controlled trial compared treatment of AO/OTA 31-A2 fractures with an SHS versus a long gamma nail. The authors found no difference in reoperation rates within the first year. All hardware failures correlated with tip-apex distance. No differences were found in mortality rates, hospital length of stay, transfusion requirements, or other secondary outcome measures. Level of evidence: I.

40. Anglen JO, Weinstein JN; American Board of Orthopaedic Surgery Research Committee: Nail or plate fixation of intertrochanteric hip fractures: Changing pattern of practice. A review of the American Board of Orthopaedic Surgery Database. *J Bone Joint Surg Am* 2008; 90(4):700-707.

41. Baumgaertner MR, Curtin SL, Lindskog DM, Keggi JM: The value of the tip-apex distance in predicting failure of fixation of peritrochanteric fractures of the hip. *J Bone Joint Surg Am* 1995;77(7):1058-1064.

42. Kuzyk PR, Zdero R, Shah S, Olsen M, Waddell JP, Schemitsch EH: Femoral head lag screw position for cephalomedullary nails: A biomechanical analysis. *J Orthop Trauma* 2012;26(7):414-421.

A biomechanical analysis of cephalomedullary nail lag screw position within the femoral head in a unstable pertrochanteric femoral fracture model is presented. Inferior lag screw placement on the AP radiograph coupled with central placement on the lateral produced the highest axial and torsional stiffness.

43. Roberts JW, Libet LA, Wolinsky PR: Who is in danger? Impingement and penetration of the anterior cortex of the distal femur during intramedullary nailing of proximal femur fractures: Preoperatively measurable risk factors. *J Trauma Acute Care Surg* 2012;73(1):249-254.

The authors presented a retrospective review of 150 patients with proximal femoral fractures treated with intramedullary nailing. Patients were assessed for risk factors leading to anterior cortical impingement or penetration. Patients with shorter stature and increased femoral bow and more posterior starting points were more likely to have anterior cortical impingement or penetration. Level of evidence: IV.

44. Kim TY, Ha YC, Kang BJ, Lee YK, Koo KH: Does early administration of bisphosphonate affect fracture healing in patients with intertrochanteric fractures? *J Bone Joint Surg Br* 2012;94-B(7):956-960.

The authors presented a retrospective, randomized, multicenter trial of 90 intertrochanteric hip fracture patients to determine the effects of postfracture bisphophonate treatment timing on healing and complication rates. Postfracture treatment was initiated at one week, one month, or three months after surgery. There was no difference in rate of healing, functional outcomes, or the incidence of complications. Level of evidence: II.

45. Mortazavi SM, RGreenky M, Bican O, Kane P, Parvizi J, Hozack WJ: Total hip arthroplasty after prior surgical treatment of hip fracture is it always challenging? *J Arthroplasty* 2012;27(1):31-36.

This study compared salvage total hip arthroplasty in patients with internal fixation of previous femoral neck and intertrochanteric fractures. Salvage of intertrochanteric fractures was more technically demanding with greater intraoperative blood loss, surgical time, and the need for trochanteric osteotomy and revision femoral components. Level of evidence: III.

46. Stewart NA, Chantrey J, Blankley SJ, Boulton C, Moran CG: Predictors of 5 year survival following hip fracture. *Injury* 2011;42(11):1253-1256.

The authors reported the results of their prospective cohort study of 2640 patients with hip fractures in the geriatric population. Increased survival rates at 5 years were shown in patients younger than 80 years, having Abbreviated Mental Test Scores greater than or equal to 7 of 10, independent mobility status, and living in own home at time of admission. Level of evidence: III.

47. Moran CG, Wenn RT, Sikand M, Taylor AM: Early mortality after hip fracture: Is delay before surgery important? *J Bone Joint Surg Am* 2005;87(3):483-489.

48. Cornwall R, Gilbert MS, Koval KJ, Strauss E, Siu AL: Functional outcomes and mortality vary among different types of hip fractures: A function of patient characteristics. *Clin Orthop Relat Res* 2004;425:64-71.

49. Holt G, Smith R, Duncan K, Hutchison JD, Gregori A: Epidemiology and outcome after hip fracture in the under 65s—evidence from the Scottish Hip Fracture Audit. *Injury* 2008;39(10):1175-1181.

50. Söderqvist A, Miedel R, Ponzer S, Tidermark J: The influence of cognitive function on outcome after a hip fracture. *J Bone Joint Surg Am* 2006;88(10):2115-2123.

51. Robinson CM, Houshian S, Khan LA: Trochanteric-entry long cephalomedullary nailing of subtrochanteric fractures caused by low-energy trauma. *J Bone Joint Surg Am* 2005;87(10):2217-2226.

52. Ekström W, Németh G, Samnegård E, Dalen N, Tidermark J: Quality of life after a subtrochanteric fracture: A prospective cohort study on 87 elderly patients. *Injury* 2009;40(4):371-376.

53. Ostrum RF, Marcantonio A, Marburger R: A critical analysis of the eccentric starting point for trochanteric intramedullary femoral nailing. *J Orthop Trauma* 2005; 19(10):681-686.

54. Russell TA, Mir HR, Stoneback J, Cohen J, Downs B: Avoidance of malreduction of proximal femoral shaft fractures with the use of a minimally invasive nail insertion technique (MINIT). *J Orthop Trauma* 2008;22(6):391-398.

4: Lower Extremity

55. Afsari A, Liporace F, Lindvall E, Infante A Jr, Sagi HC, Haidukewych GJ: Clamp-assisted reduction of high subtrochanteric fractures of the femur. *J Bone Joint Surg Am* 2009;91(8):1913-1918.

56. Kuzyk PR, Bhandari M, McKee MD, Russell TA, Schemitsch EH: Intramedullary versus extramedullary fixation for subtrochanteric femur fractures. *J Orthop Trauma* 2009;23(6):465-470.

57. Forward DP, Doro CJ, O'Toole RV, et al: A biomechanical comparison of a locking plate, a nail, and a 95° angled blade plate for fixation of subtrochanteric femoral fractures. *J Orthop Trauma* 2012;26(6):334-340.

   The authors presented a biomechancal study of a locking plate, a cephalomedullary nail, and 95°-angled blade plate fixation in a subtrochanteric femoral fracture model. The authors found the cephalomedullary nail to be biomechanically superior to other constructs, withstanding significantly more cycles, failing at higher force, and withstanding greater loads. Level of evidence: V.

58. Lee PC, Hsieh PH, Yu SW, Shiao CW, Kao HK, Wu CC: Biologic plating versus intramedullary nailing for comminuted subtrochanteric fractures in young adults: A prospective, randomized study of 66 cases. *J Trauma* 2007;63(6):1283-1291.

59. Afsari A, Liporace F, Lindvall E, Infante A Jr, Sagi HC, Haidukewych GJ: Clamp-assisted reduction of high subtrochanteric fractures of the femur: Surgical technique. *J Bone Joint Surg Am* 2010;92(suppl 1, pt 2):217-225.

   The authors described their surgical technique using a percutaneously placed clamp to assist in the reduction of subtrochanteric femoral fractures during reaming and intramedullary nail fixation. Level of evidence: V.

60. Kennedy MT, Mitra A, Hierlihy TG, Harty JA, Reidy D, Dolan M: Subtrochanteric hip fractures treated with cerclage cables and long cephalomedullary nails: A review of 17 consecutive cases over 2 years. *Injury* 2011; 42(11):1317-1321.

   The authors reviewed 17 patients with subtrochanteric femoral fractures treated with open reduction and stabilization with cerclage cables during intramedullary nailing. Sixteen patients were available for follow-up; 15 healed uneventfully, with 1 nonunion reported. Level of evidence: IV.

61. Ekman EF: The role of the orthopaedic surgeon in minimizing mortality and morbidity associated with fragility fractures. *J Am Acad Orthop Surg* 2010;18(5): 278-285.

   This review article covers evaluation of the osteoporotic patient from the perspective of the orthopaedic surgeon's practice. Assessment of fracture risk, reduction of risk, medical treatments, and fragility fracture follow-up are discussed.

Chapter 35

Hip and Pelvic Reconstruction and Arthroplasty

Adam Sassoon, MD   George J. Haidukewych, MD

4: Lower Extremity

Introduction

Degenerative changes of the hip and the pelvis are the result of congenital and acquired deformities, trauma, osteonecrosis, and arthritis. This chapter reviews hip and pelvic reconstruction strategies that address these processes. Failed reconstructive efforts, their workup, and advanced revision techniques also are discussed.

Congenital and Acquired Deformities

Femoroacetabular Impingement

Background

Femoroacetabular impingement (FAI) occurs as the result of abnormal contact between the femoral neck and the acetabular rim. Contact forces may be increased when morphologic variations or posttraumatic deformities are present on either side of the joint. Increased demand related to hip range of motion (required for activities such as martial arts, gymnastics, and ballet) may aggravate abnormal hip mechanics and precipitate symptoms of FAI. These forces result in labral shearing and cartilage degeneration, which have been implicated in accelerating osteoarthritis.

Bony deformity contributing to FAI can be classified as cam, pincer, or combined (Figures 1 and 2). Cam deformities feature a bony prominence at the femoral head-neck junction that abuts the acetabular rim during flexion and internal rotation. Cam lesions commonly arise de novo, following trauma, or as the result of a healed slipped capital femoral epiphysis. Pincer-

type impingement results from acetabular overcoverage, which vilifies the acetabular rim as the source of bony abutment. Combined deformities may involve

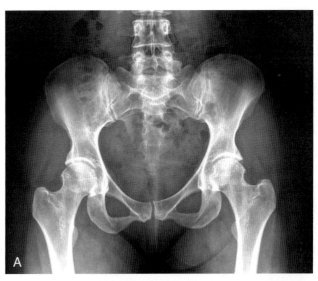

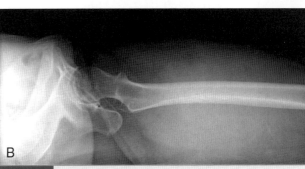

Figure 1   AP (**A**) and lateral (**B**) radiographs of the pelvis of a 33-year-old woman with mostly pincer-type FAI of the left hip, with coxa profunda involving sourcil. The lateral cross-table radiograph depicts the typical "coup-contrecoup" lesion, with narrowing of the posterior acetabular cartilage. (Reproduced from Sierra RJ, Della Valle CJ: Hip and Pelvic reconstruction and arthroplasty, in Flynn JM (ed): *Orthopaedic Knowledge Update*, ed 10. Rosemont, IL, American Academy of Orthopaedic Surgeons, pp 413-430.)

Dr. Haidukewych or an immediate family member has received royalties from DePuy; serves as a paid consultant to or is an employee of Smith & Nephew and Synthes; has stock or stock options held in Orthopediatrics and the Institute for Better Bone Health; and serves as a board member, owner, officer, or committee member of the American Academy of Orthopaedic Surgeons. Neither Dr. Sassoon nor any immediate family member has received anything of value from or has stock or stock options held in a commercial company or institution related directly or indirectly to the subject of this chapter.

simultaneous pathology on both sides of the hip joint or, possibly, changes over time as a result of a primary cam or pincer lesion.

Video 35.1: Physical Evaluation of Hip Pain in Non/Prearthritic Patient and Athlete. Allston J. Stubbs, MD; Adam William Anz, MD; Benjamin L. Long, MD; John Frino, MD; Stephanie Cheetham, MD (18.05 min)

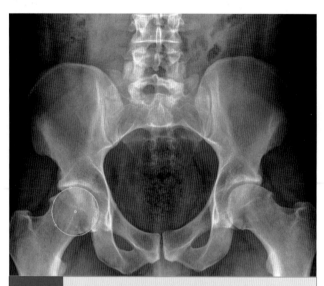

Figure 2 AP radiograph of the pelvis of a 27-year-old man with advanced cam-type FAI. The patient has asphericity of the femoral head depicted by extension of the lateral aspect of the femoral head outside the white circle. (Reproduced from Sierra RJ, Della Valle CJ: Hip and Pelvic reconstruction and arthroplasty, in Flynn JM (ed): *Orthopaedic Knowledge Update*, ed 10. Rosemont, IL, American Academy of Orthopaedic Surgeons, pp 413-430.)

Evaluation

The clinical evaluation of FAI begins with a thorough history, during which patients are prompted to describe any activity-related pain centered in the groin. Limits in passive range of motion of 105° of flexion or less and internal rotation of 15° or less with the hip in flexion are commonly noted. An anterior impingement test that places the hip in flexion, adduction, and internal rotation often can re-create activity-related pain symptoms.

Radiographic evaluation often demonstrates a classic cam lesion at the head-neck junction in femoral-sided impingement. Correlation with both the history and the physical examination is important when evaluating cam lesions because they have been noted in asymptomatic patients. Pincer impingement is associated with radiographic signs of anterior overcoverage, including a lateral center-edge (LCE) angle of more than 40°, an acetabular index (AI) less than 0°, a positive crossover sign, or a positive posterior wall sign.[1-3] Coxa profunda, previously thought to be pathognomonic for pincer-type impingement, recently has been proven independent from other indices of acetabular overcoverage and should not be relied on as a sole diagnostic criterion for FAI[4] (Table 1).

MRI and magnetic resonance arthrography (MRA) have been used as adjunctive tools in detecting labral and articular cartilage pathology and in the setting of FAI (Figure 3). However, these costly tests should be used with caution and only on a confirmatory basis because the incidence of asymptomatic labral tears is significant. Recent data have shown that MRA has only fair interobserver reliability and a poor negative predictive value of 13% to 19%.[5]

Treatment

The treatment of FAI encompasses a spectrum of options that vary depending on the severity of symptoms, the findings on imaging, and patient demands and expectations. Nonsurgical options, such as activity modification and anti-inflammatory medications, can be explored. After nonsurgical measures have been exhausted or deemed ineffective, surgical measures should be considered. Arthroscopic procedures, including osteoplasty, labral débridement, and labral detachment with rim trimming and refixation, have been de-

Table 1

Definitions of Radiographic Measurements Obtained in Patients With Structural Abnormalities Related to Femoroacetabular Impingement

Coxa profunda	When the floor of the fossa acetabuli touches the ilioischial line.
Protrusio acetabulum	When the femoral head overlaps the ilioischial spine medially.
Aspheric head	When the epiphysis of the head protrudes laterally out of the circle around the head.
Pistol grip	Lateral contour of the femoral head extends into a convex shape to the base of the neck.
Double contour sign	Ossification of the rim caused by bone apposition resulting in a double projection of the anterior and posterior walls.

(Reproduced from Sierra RJ, Della Valle CJ: Hip and Pelvic reconstruction and arthroplasty, in Flynn JM (ed): *Orthopaedic Knowledge Update*, ed 10. Rosemont, IL, American Academy of Orthopaedic Surgeons, pp 413-430.)

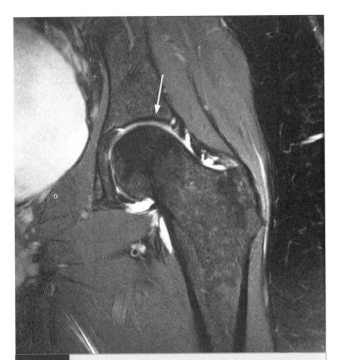

Figure 3 T2-weighted MRI with gadolinium shows an anterior-superior labral tear (arrow), seen as an increase in signal intensity that extends to the articular surface. (Reproduced from Sierra RJ, Della Valle CJ: Hip and Pelvic reconstruction and arthroplasty, in Flynn JM (ed): *Orthopaedic Knowledge Update*, ed 10. Rosemont, IL, American Academy of Orthopaedic Surgeons, pp 413-430.)

Video 35.2: 23-Point Arthroscopic Examination of the Hip. James L. Bond, MD; Carlos Guanche, MD (13.26 min)

scribed.[6] A study comparing labral débridement with refixation at 3.5 years' follow-up demonstrated that both groups showed improvement based on subjective outcome measures; however, only 68% of the patients who underwent labral débridement had good to excellent results, whereas 92% of the patients had good to excellent results with labral refixation.[7]

Arthroscopic labral refixation is influenced by two factors: the location of the labral pathology and the amount and the quality of the remaining labral tissue. Open surgical procedures to treat FAI have been used to address the arthroscopic limitations of acetabular visualization. A direct anterior approach can be used to treat FAI, and data support improvement and return to sports for athletes. Direct anterior approaches, however, offer only limited visualization of some acetabular lesions (depending on their location). Direct anterior approaches also may cause neuropraxic complications. Combined arthroscopic and limited open approaches have been investigated and showed promising results in

both Harris hip scores and radiographic parameters at 2-year follow-up.[8]

Although further research is needed to determine the most effective surgical strategy to address FAI, the current preferred treatment remains surgical dislocation of the hip with an open osteoplasty and labral treatment as indicated. This option provides the best visualization and versatility for managing a wide variety of anatomic deformities and, in the proper hands, often takes less time than arthroscopic treatment. Midterm results of surgical hip dislocation indicate that 82% of patients are satisfied or very satisfied with their results, and 83% of patients rate their hip function as near-normal or normal.[9] This study also indicated that 3% of patients undergoing a surgical dislocation underwent a total hip arthroplasty (THA) during the follow-up period, and that the predictors of a poor outcome were older age, female sex, low body mass index, and residual full-thickness cartilage defects.[9] Surgical dislocation also provides an opportunity to reconstruct a labrum using the ligamentum teres in cases for which remaining tissue is deficient—a technique that demonstrated subjective improvement at 2-year follow-up in 75% of patients.[10] Moreover, surgical dislocation has been shown in a multicenter study to be a safe procedure with a low complication rate. In 334 cases, the procedure did not result in femoral head osteonecrosis or a femoral neck fracture.[11]

Developmental Dysplasia of the Hip
Background
Developmental dysplasia of the hip (DDH) results from acetabular undercoverage of the femoral head during osseous maturation. The decreased joint conformity leads to elevated contact forces over a smaller surface area. Abnormal motion of the femoral head relative to the acetabulum may also induce labral pathology; for example, abnormal joint kinematics and related sequelae contribute to early-onset osteoarthritis. DDH has been classified according to the severity of hip subluxation relative to overall pelvic height and, more qualitatively, as a dysplastic hip, low dislocation, or high dislocation depending on the location of the functional femoropelvic articulation.

Evaluation
Patients with DDH typically describe a history of groin pain that increases with activity. They also may note mechanical symptoms that may be related to concurrent labral pathology. In contrast to patients with FAI, patients with DDH are not classically limited in their passive range of motion but may demonstrate a positive impingement sign if labral damage has occurred or there is anterior apprehension. In patients with advanced disease, abductor dysfunction and a Trendelenburg gait may be observed.

The radiographic evaluation of patients with DDH will demonstrate a lateralized femoral head and acetabular undercoverage (**Figure 4**). There is also increased anteversion of both the acetabulum and the femur. The

4: Lower Extremity

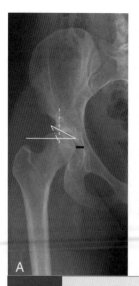
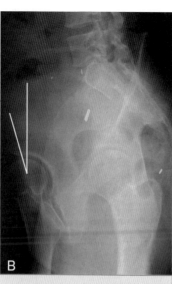

Figure 4 **A,** The right side of an AP pelvic radiograph showing the radiographic measurements used for hip dysplasia. The dashed line denotes the anterior center edge angle. The solid white line denotes the acetabular index. The black line denotes the medial clear space. **B,** A false-profile view showing measurement of the anterior center edge angle. (Reproduced from Sierra RJ, Della Valle CJ: Hip and Pelvic reconstruction and arthroplasty, in Flynn JM (ed): *Orthopaedic Knowledge Update*, ed 10. Rosemont, IL, American Academy of Orthopaedic Surgeons, pp 413-430.)

Table 2

Radiographic Measurements Obtained in Patients With Hip Dysplasia

Lateral center edge angle	
> 25°	Normal
Between 20° and 25°	Borderline
< 20°	Hip dysplasia
Acetabular index	
to 10°	Normal
> 10°	Hip dysplasia
Femoral extrusion index	
> 25%	Hip dysplasia
False profile view (anterior center edge angle)	
> 25°	Normal
< 20°	Hip dysplasia
Between 20° and 25°	Borderline

(Reproduced from Sierra RJ, Della Valle CJ: Hip and Pelvic reconstruction and arthroplasty, in Flynn JM (ed): Orthopaedic Knowledge Update, ed 10. Rosemont, IL, American Academy of Orthopaedic Surgeons, pp 413-430.)

LCE angle in patients with DDH is usually less than 25°,[12] and the AI is more than 10° (Table 2).[2] A break in the Shenton line that is larger than 5 mm also indicates DDH and is associated with excellent intra- and interobserver reliability, with a sensitivity and a specificity of 83% and 98%, respectively.[13] Femoral head sphericity is also important to note on radiographs because this plays a role in the treatment algorithm for DDH.

MRI is a valuable adjunctive imaging modality in DDH because it can help define any labral pathology and assess the articular cartilage condition. T2 mapping of the articular surface can detect cartilage disruption and delamination. Delayed gadolinium-enhanced MRI of cartilage is useful in the earlier stages of cartilage degeneration because it can detect changes in charge density within articular cartilage and correspond to changes in proteoglycan content. Appreciation of the cartilage in patients with DDH is paramount when deciding on and predicting the success of nonarthroplasty treatment options.

Treatment (Nonarthroplasty Options)

Treatment of DDH in the skeletally mature patient depends on the patient's age, pain, activity level, and expectations. The sphericity of the femoral head and the condition of the articular cartilage also can dictate available options. "Out of round" femoral heads and full-thickness cartilage defects portend a poor outcome with nonarthroplasty treatment modalities.

Patients younger than 35 years with round femoral heads and intact articular cartilage demonstrated on MRI or plain radiographs (Tönnis grades 0 and 1) are the best candidates for nonarthroplasty treatment in the form of a Bernese periacetabular osteotomy (PAO). Before surgical intervention, a radiograph obtained in maximum abduction should demonstrate restoration of acetabular coverage with preservation of the joint space. Bernese PAOs are contraindicated in patients who are younger than 11 years secondary to the risk of incurring a significant growth disturbance.

The Bernese PAO, originally described in 1988,[14] represents a powerful tool in pelvic correction because it is positioned close to the joint. The primary corrections associated with this procedure include improvement of acetabular coverage via adduction, medialization of the hip center, and retroversion of the hip socket via extension. The osteotomy is relatively stable and requires minimal instrumentation because the posterior column remains intact. Pelvic dimensions remain largely unaltered, preserving the option for vaginal childbirth.[15]

Bernese PAOs have been shown to restore hip biomechanics by increasing the load-bearing surface of the joint to within a normal range, and, in general, most patients demonstrate improved outcome measures. In patients with Tönnis grades 0 and 1 changes, the long-term results reveal a survivorship of 75% at 20 years.[16] Patients with more severe arthrosis, however, demonstrated only a 13% survivorship at 20 years.

Arthroplasty Treatment

Many patients with DDH will require a THA. Arthroplasty in the setting of DDH involves a special set of technical considerations related to the acetabular and femoral deformities observed in DDH. Alternative bearing surfaces should be considered secondary to

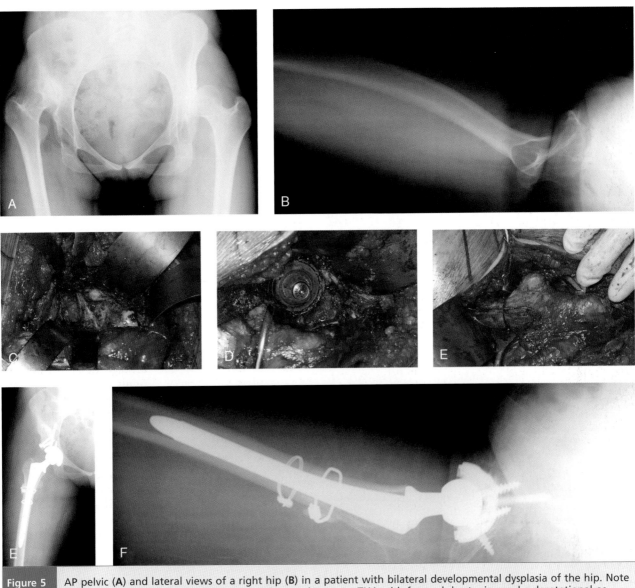

Figure 5 AP pelvic (**A**) and lateral views of a right hip (**B**) in a patient with bilateral developmental dysplasia of the hip. Note the high dislocation on the right. This patient underwent a THA with femoral shortening and a derotational osteotomy. Intraoperative photographs reveal the overgrown true acetabulum (**C**), where the hip center was eventually restored (**D**). Vertical scoring of the femur was used to accurately assess the amount of rotational correction achieved via the femoral osteotomy (**E**). Postoperative AP (**F**) and lateral radiographs (**G**) showing the augmentation of the acetabular bone stock with a femoral head autograph and fixation of the femoral osteotomy. Note the restoration of the anatomic hip center. (Courtesy of Robert Trousdale, MD, Mayo Clinic, Rochester, MN.)

younger patient age (often encountered among patients with DDH who need joint arthroplasty).

Acetabular deformity in DDH leads to bone stock deficiencies anterosuperiorly and superolaterally. In cases of high hip dislocation, the true acetabulum can be difficult to identify and prepare. It is preferable to place the acetabular component in an anatomic position; previous work has demonstrated an unacceptably high rate of loosening with superior placement.[17] Measures to augment acetabular component coverage using autograft from the resected femoral head (thereby avoiding superior component placement or component medialization) have been described and demonstrate graft survival at 11 years.[18]

Femoral deformity in the form of excessive anteversion, coxa valga, and metaphyseal-diaphyseal mismatch often are encountered during THA in patients with DDH. Appropriate preoperative assessment can help plan for these occurrences, and stem modularity has proven to be a valuable tool in dealing with technical challenges. In addition, femoral length may need to be adjusted in cases of high hip dislocation or Crowe type IV dysplasia to avoid injury to the sciatic nerve. When a femoral lengthening of 3 to 4 cm is expected, a subtrochanteric osteotomy can be performed at the time of THA, and excellent results at 5-year follow-up can be expected[19] (Figure 5).

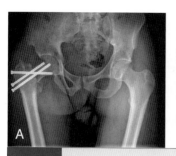
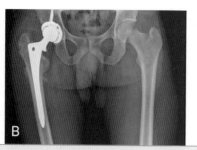
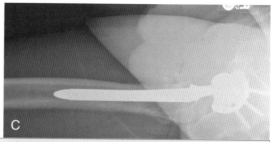

Figure 6   **A,** Preoperative AP pelvic radiograph of a patient with a basicervical femoral nonunion. The patient was treated successfully with a THA using a fully coated, diaphyseal-engaging, cylindrical stem, as shown in the postoperative radiographs (**B** and **C**).

Posttraumatic Arthropathy

Background

Failed open reduction and internal fixation (ORIF) of femoral neck, intertrochanteric, and acetabular fractures often necessitates reconstructive salvage surgery that involves arthroplasty. This is especially true in patients older than 45 years, in those with underlying inflammatory arthritis, and in settings involving acetabular cartilage loss or derangement. These patients require special technical considerations secondary to their acquired/iatrogenic deformity, the presence of hardware, and (often) suboptimal bone quality.

Evaluation

Patients who have failed ORIF of the intracapsular femur or the acetabulum should undergo a workup for an infectious etiology of their nonunion in the form of a physical examination and laboratory testing that includes a complete blood count (CBC) with differential, erythrocyte sedimentation rate (ESR), and C-reactive protein (CRP) level. Patients may undergo additional testing, including an ultrasound or fluoroscopic-guided hip aspiration. Aspiration samples must be sent for a CBC with differential as well as gram stain and cultures. Tissue should be obtained at the time of surgical intervention and sent for pathology and culture. If pathology reveals acute inflammation, reconstructive arthroplasty should be aborted and staged with hardware removal, antibiotic spacer placement, and intravenous antibiotic therapy.

A nutritional and metabolic workup should be initiated to help direct future attempts at salvage. Nutritional deficiencies can influence wound healing over prostheses and may play a role in impaired osseous ingrowth into uncemented components. Once identified, metabolic disorders can be appropriately addressed, which may decrease the risk for future periprosthetic or remote fractures.

Radiographic evaluation is critical in planning the reconstruction of failed internal fixation about the hip. Broken hardware may complicate surgical intervention, and appropriate retrieval sets should be available. Furthermore, after the hardware is removed, stress risers are created and should be appropriately bypassed by new components; the relationship between the extent of hardware removed and the length of the selected prosthesis must be fully elucidated for the treating surgeon. Abnormalities in femoral version, offset, and bone loss also should be appreciated, as these may dictate approach and implant selection. Nonunited acetabular fractures may not be able to support a socket component without revision fixation or the use of a cup cage, which necessitates appropriate instrumentation and planning.

Technical Pearls and Results

Femoral neck fracture nonunions may be addressed with hemiarthroplasty or THA. It is the opinion of the authors that most cases should be treated with a THA secondary to the reliability of pain relief. If a patient is experiencing cognitive decline or is inactive with intact acetabular cartilage, hemiarthroplasty may be an appropriate option. At the time of surgery, the acetabulum should be critically assessed because hardware cutout can damage the articular surface and mandate a THA. Disuse osteopenia may be encountered during acetabular preparation and component placement, so great care should be exercised to avoid overreaming or pelvic penetration. If soft bone is discovered, screw augmentation of cup fixation should be performed.

THA in the setting of femoral neck nonunion is associated with a higher rate of dislocation and superficial infections than primary THA in the setting of a femoral neck fracture.[20] One long-term study employing Charnley hip arthroplasty components in the treatment of femoral neck nonunions noted 93% and 76% survivorship at 10 and 20 years, respectively.[21] In this series, 4.5% of the patients had recurrent dislocation.[21] The use of uncemented components, larger head sizes, lipped liners, and dual-mobility bearing surfaces may lead to improved results in this population, but this has yet to be substantiated in the literature (**Figure 6**).

THA in the setting of intertrochanteric nonunion can be technically challenging secondary to a malunited trochanter preventing entry into the intramedullary canal. Shaping the bone with a high-speed burr can facilitate a path for reamers and the final component without completely compromising the trochanter or necessitating a trochanteric advancement. Femoral geometry alterations to version also may necessitate either a cemented implant

Table 3

Risk Factors Associated With the Development of Osteonecrosis of the Femoral Head

Dysbaric (Caisson disease)

Gaucher disease

Sickle cell disease

Pancreatitis

Steroid use

Alcohol use

Vascular insult

Subacute bacterial endocarditis

Disseminated intravascular coagulation

Polycythemia rubra vera

Systemic lupus erythematosus

Polyarteritis nodosa

Rheumatoid arthritis

Giant cell arteritis

Sarcoid metabolic diabetes

Hyperuricemia

Blood lipid disorders

Idiopathic causes

(Reproduced from Sierra RJ, Della Valle CJ: Hip and Pelvic reconstruction and arthroplasty, in Flynn JM (ed): *Orthopaedic Knowledge Update*, ed 10. Rosemont, IL, American Academy of Orthopaedic Surgeons, pp 413-430.)

Table 4

The Steinberg Classification for Staging Osteonecrosis of the Femoral Head

Stage	Description
0	Normal or nondiagnostic radiograph, bone scan, and MRI
I[a]	Normal radiograph, abnormal bone scan, and/or MRI
II[a]	Abnormal radiograph showing cystic and sclerotic changes in the femoral head
III[a]	Subchondral collapse producing a crescent sign
IV[a]	Flattening of the femoral head
V[a]	Joint narrowing with or without acetabular involvement
VI	Advanced degenerative changes

[a]The extent or grade of involvement should also be indicated as A, mild; B, moderate; or C, severe
(Reproduced from Sierra RJ, Della Valle CJ: Hip and Pelvic reconstruction and arthroplasty, in Flynn JM (ed): *Orthopaedic Knowledge Update*, ed 10. Rosemont, IL, American Academy of Orthopaedic Surgeons, pp 413-430.)

4: Lower Extremity

that can be used to "cheat" the given anatomy (using a smaller component and rotating it within a cement mantle to a desired version), or a modular stem that can allow version variability. Calcar replacement stems may be required at the calcar level to address bone loss. Commonly, the metaphyseal bone has been violated to an extent, which precludes the placement of a standard prosthesis. Longer stems should be used to bypass femoral stress risers created by previous hardware by at least two cortical diameters. In a series of 59 arthroplasty procedures used to treat intertrochanteric nonunions, a standard stem was used in only 15% of the cases; this study also demonstrated a reliable improvement in patient symptoms and mobility.[22]

THA performed after failed acetabular ORIF also has provided reliable functional improvement and pain relief. Surgeons must be prepared to deal with broken hardware, bony defects, and heterotopic bone in these challenging reconstructions. In a series of 33 patients, one study noted no or minimal pain at final follow-up between 10 and 16 years with the use of uncemented components.[23] Three patients in this study required a revision of their cup secondary to osteolysis (two stable and one loose), whereas another patient's cup was revised because of loosening and instability.[23] Of note, these data were collected before the introduction of highly cross-linked polyethylene, which likely would represent an improvement over these outcomes, consid-

ering that most reported failures were related to particle-wear-induced osteolysis.

Osteonecrosis

Background

Vascular insult to the femoral head can lead to collapse of the articular surface, an asymmetric femoral head, and resultant coxarthrosis. This disorder generally occurs in patients younger than 50 years who are undergoing a THA. Osteonecrosis is the second most common surgical indication, occurring in 29% of patients.[24] The underlying cause of vascular compromise can involve multitude conditions and risk factors, most notably trauma, steroid use, alcohol use, sickle cell disease, HIV, and idiopathic causes (Table 3). A genetic predisposition to osteonecrosis has also been postulated.

Osteonecrosis of the femoral head has been classified according to multiple systems. The Arlet-Ficat classification scheme uses a qualitative assessment of radiographs,[25] whereas the Steinberg system combines radiographic and MRI findings in an attempt to quantify the percentage of head involvement[26] (Table 4). The International Classification System combines size and location of a lesion in relation to the weight-bearing area of the femoral head.[27]

Evaluation

Osteonecrosis can be difficult to identify secondary to a lack of findings on imaging. A strong clinical suspicion can be gathered from the history and the physical examination. Patients usually report deep groin or buttock pain that may radiate down to or present solely in the knee. Active and passive range of motion usually will generate pain, and the patient may walk with an antalgic or an avoidance gait.

AP views of the pelvis and the affected hip should be obtained, as well as frog-leg and cross-table lateral views. Radiographs may not demonstrate osseous changes, in which case an MRI scan should be obtained because this imaging modality has been shown to be 98% sensitive and specific in detecting osteonecrosis. Imaging studies are important to elucidate the diagnosis and determine osteonecrosis prognosis. Previous work has demonstrated that lesions comprising less than 15% of the femoral head will remain relatively quiescent, and in the setting of Ficat stage I or II disease will only necessitate THA in less than 10% of cases.[28] MRI measurement of the involved portion of the femoral head also has been validated as a predictor of future collapse.[29] Arc angles measuring the necrotic head segment visualized on two radiographic views have demonstrated prognostic value for determining outcomes after exercising nonarthroplasty treatment options.

After a diagnosis of osteonecrosis has been established, it is important to obtain contralateral hip imaging because bilateral presentation is common. The contralateral hip, even if affected, often is asymptomatic on discovery. A 2010 study demonstrated that most of these asymptomatic lesions will progress to collapse if left untreated.[30]

Treatment Options and Results

Regardless of the osteonecrosis classification system used, the distinctive feature in the spectrum of pathogenesis is collapse of the femoral head. Prior to collapse, head-preserving options can be used with favorable results. Following collapse, however, these options become limited, and their efficacy is dramatically reduced.

Precollapse treatment options include nonsurgical modalities, core decompression, core decompression with bone marrow grafting, vascularized bone grafting, and osteotomy. Nonsurgical treatment of osteonecrosis, such as protected weight bearing, bisphosphonates, and hyperbaric oxygen, have been investigated; however, these treatment modalities should be reserved for patients who are otherwise poor surgical candidates because they are less successful than surgical methods.

Core decompression has been demonstrated as an improvement over nonsurgical treatment, with a success rate of 84% in patients with Ficat stage 1 disease and 65% in patients with Ficat stage 2 disease.[31] Autologous bone marrow transplantation has become a common adjunct to core decompression. A series reporting on 145 hips with Ficat stage 1 disease with 7-year average follow-up demonstrated a THA-free survivorship among 94% of the patients who underwent THA.[32] This study also analyzed the colony-forming unit capabilities of the transplanted bone marrow autograft and determined a correlation with a successful result.[32]

Because osteonecrosis often affects the anterosuperior portion of the femoral head, rotational osteotomies have been used to offload the necrotic lesion. Although early results were encouraging and demonstrated good-to-excellent results in 79% of patients,[33] these results were not reproduced in later studies. Free vascularized bone grafting also is a surgical option in both precollapse and postcollapse disease; however, survivorship of this procedure free from revision in the postcollapse patient cohort was only 65% at 5 years.[34] Proponents of this technique contend that it is the best head-preserving option in advanced disease and can serve to delay hip replacement in this often-young population.

After collapse, THA remains the mainstay in the treatment of osteonecrosis, with excellent midterm results. THA provides reliable improvement of symptoms and has been shown to be associated with up to 98% survival at 10 years.[35] Other arthroplasty options include hemiarthroplasty, hemi resurfacing, and total resurfacing. A prospective study comparing bipolar hemiarthroplasty and THA demonstrated improved outcomes with THA.[36] Total hip resurfacing, while touted as a bone-preserving surgery, incurs additional risk via the introduction of a metal-on-metal (MoM) bearing surface. With the advent and the increased use of highly cross-linked polyethylene, newer data on patients treated with THA and this bearing surface may suggest improved survivorship when compared with other historical series; however, this has yet to be substantiated in the literature.

Arthritis of the Hip

Prevalence and Impact

Arthritis is the most common cause of adult disability in the United States,[37] and in 2005 more than 20% of adults self-reported the condition as physician-diagnosed.[38] In 2009, arthritis was the fourth-leading cause of hospitalization in the United States.[37] Arthritis is more commonly seen in women and less frequently encountered in people of Hispanic origin.[38] Joint pain led to activity limitations in more than 40% of the patients with physician-diagnosed arthritis[37]—a figure expected to increase substantially by 2030.[39] Cost of arthritis-related care in 2003 totaled $128 billion.[37]

Workup

Patients with arthritis of the hip commonly present with activity-related pain centered in their groin and buttock that is insidious in onset. They will often note difficulty walking long distances, donning and doffing footwear, and getting into and out of vehicles. Patients also may present with a chief report of knee pain, which is referred via a branch of the obturator nerve. In light of the origin of pain, anyone presenting to a clinic with knee pain must undergo a radiographic examination of the ipsilateral hip. Patients may have pain over their greater trochanter and may walk with a limp. A limb-length discrepancy may be noted as erosion into the articular cartilage and eburnation of sub-chondral bone and may lead to limb shortening of the affected side. Patients with long-standing arthritis will usually have an external rotation contracture with painful and limited internal rotation on physical examination.

Radiographic evaluation of the hip is of paramount importance, and both AP and lateral views of the affected side should be obtained with an AP view of the pelvis. Additional views of the entire femur or full-length standing views also may be helpful if other deformities warrant their procurement. The classic radiographic signs of coxarthrosis include joint space narrowing, osteophyte formation, subchondral sclerosis, and cystic changes, which are collectively included in the classification schema of Tönnis (Table 5).

Treatment Algorithm

If the history, the physical examination, and radiographic images support a diagnosis of coxarthrosis, nonsurgical and surgical treatment algorithms consisting of weight loss, activity modification, anti-inflammatory medication, and gentle hip abductor strengthening exercises should be used. If these modalities fail or a patient believes his or her quality of life remains impaired, surgical intervention may be considered after a detailed discussion regarding the expectations and activity demands. Temporizing intra-articular injections of the hip should be avoided because the beneficial effect is less predictable and usually shorter lived compared with that of knee injections. An intra-articular steroid injection also may place a patient at increased risk for a periprosthetic infection if performed within 2 months of the definitive arthroplasty procedure.[40]

Primary THA

Approach Update

The direct anterior approach for primary THA has gained in popularity in recent years because clinical data support a low risk for postoperative dislocation,[41] and laboratory data indicate that this approach is less traumatic to hip musculature.[42] Mixed results regarding the learning curve and early postoperative complication rates are associated with this approach, however. A near twofold increase in surgical time and blood loss was noted in a matched cohort study comparing 46 patients undergoing THA with either a direct anterior or posterolateral approach.[43] Component positioning and hospital stay were equivalent in both groups; however, early complication rates were higher in those in whom the direct anterior approach was used. No learning effect was noted for these 46 patients. Another study, however, reported improvement during the first 40 cases.[44] Perioperative complication rates comparable to a less invasive lateral approach were reported in a 2009 study during the learning curve period.[45] The functional results based on gait analysis did not demon-

Table 5	
Classification of Osteoarthritis as Described by Tönnis	
Grade	**Description**
Grade 0	No signs of OA
Grade 1	Increased sclerosis of the head and acetabulum
Grade 2	Small cysts in the head or acetabulum, moderate joint space narrowing, moderate loss of head sphericity
Grade 3	Large cysts in head or acetabulum, severe joint space narrowing or obliteration, severe deformity of the femoral head, evidence of necrosis

(Reproduced from Sierra RJ, Della Valle CJ: Hip and Pelvic reconstruction and arthroplasty, in Flynn JM (ed): *Orthopaedic Knowledge Update*, ed 10. Rosemont, IL, American Academy of Orthopaedic Surgeons, pp 413-430.)

strate an advantage of the direct anterior approach over the posterolateral or direct lateral approaches.[46,47]

Femoral Component Options

A variety of femoral component design options are available for cemented and uncemented implantation techniques. Despite European registry data indicating improved survivorship with cemented implants,[48,49] uncemented femoral components predominate the North American market. Cementless implants are advantageous in that surgical time is decreased, they are technically less demanding, and cement removal is not required after an infection is treated. British registry data indicate higher mortality with cemented femoral components.[48]

Most uncemented primary femoral stems were either proximally treated, tapered, metaphyseal engaging, or extensively coated cylindrical diaphyseal engaging components. Tapered components have shown 95.5% survivorship at 20 years,[50] whereas cylindrical components have demonstrated 97.5% survivorship at 15 years.[51] Recently, interest in shorter, broach-only, flat-wedge, taper designs has grown because of their ease of instrumentation, avoidance of diaphyseal deformity, and ability to be implanted through smaller incisions. The flat-wedge design is associated with fewer intraoperative complications during insertion and a survivorship of 99.8% at 8.9 years.[52]

Modular components have been used in both primary and revision settings with encouraging results. Modularity offers the ability to fine-tune version, offset, and length more effectively than nonmodular stems; however, these components introduce unique complications, including junctional fatigue failure, fretting, and corrosion. Recent designs have moved the modular junction proximal to the neck cut in an effort to combine the advantages of modularity with traditional metaphyseal-engaging, primary stem geometry. Concerns regarding the increased risk of fracture through this proximal modular junction have been raised in recent case reports, especially when long femoral necks, large femoral heads, and patients who are obese are involved.[53] Some designs have demonstrated metal debris generated from taper wear at the modular junction; however, further follow-up is required before the significance of these findings can be concluded.

Hip resurfacing arthroplasty (HRA) has been popularized as a bone-conserving option that facilitates a higher level of postoperative activity. HRA also introduces unique complications, including the possibility of femoral neck fracture and MoM-related failure modes. A recent comprehensive review of the literature demonstrated an overall revision rate of 3.5% of all HRAs, with survivorship rates ranging between 86% and 100% at between 0.6 and 10.5 years' follow-up.[54] Sex differences exist with regard to HRA survivorship; a 10-year follow-up study demonstrated a 95% survivorship in men but a 74% survivorship in women.[55] The authors of this study concluded that HRA should be abandoned in women. Data from the Australian registry indicate that in patients younger than 55 years, those who underwent HRA needed revision more frequently than those who had THA. Moreover, return to activity following arthroplasty procedures has been shown to be more closely related to patient-specific factors rather than implant characteristics.[56] Clear advantages of HRA over THA in young patients have not been proven, which evokes growing concern regarding MoM bearings; consequently, the use of HRA has decreased dramatically in the United States.

Acetabular Component Options

Although cemented acetabular components demonstrate good results at 20 years, recent registry data indicate improved survivorship using uncemented components.[57] Uncemented acetabular reconstruction is favored in North America and offers the advantages of decreased surgical time and technical demand when compared with cemented arthroplasty. Most uncemented components are modular; however, monoblock designs exist and perform well.[58] An analysis of multiple uncemented acetabular designs indicated improved performance of titanium wire and mesh-backed components versus beaded and hydroxyapatite-coated components.[59] Most second-decade failures of uncemented acetabular components are attributed to wear-induced osteolysis and aseptic loosening. It is hoped that improvements in bearing surfaces will address these failures and improve future performance.

Bearing Surface Options

Osteolysis, secondary to wear-related polyethylene debris, leads to component loosening and revision arthroplasty. Highly cross-linked polyethylene was developed to mitigate this problem. The results of a prospective, double-blinded, controlled trial revealed that highly cross-linked polyethylene possesses improved in vivo wear resistance when compared with conventional polyethylene at 5-year follow-up.[60] Hard-on-hard bearing surfaces, such as ceramic and cobalt-chromium, have been investigated as alternative solutions, especially for younger patients. Although both options help avoid polyethylene debris, they have their inherent risks. Although ceramic-on-ceramic bearings offer the only bearing surface that shows a complete absence of wear-induced osteolysis at 20-year follow-up,[61] they can fail disastrously if a fracture occurs. Squeaking also has been reported as a reason for revision in certain instances. MoM bearing surfaces have been implicated as the cause of failure secondary to metal ion-induced pseudotumor and aseptic lymphocytic vasculitis-associated lesions (ALVALs).[62] A review of the literature demonstrated a likelihood of revision when an MoM bearing surface is used and found that this risk increased in THA when using larger head diameters.[63] A ceramic-on-highly-cross-linked polyethylene bearing couple provides an attractive option for young, active patients by decreasing the risk for component fracture and squeaking while improving wear characteristics.

Deep Vein Thrombosis Prophylaxis

The American Academy of Orthopaedic Surgeons has published clinical guidelines on the prevention of venous thromboembolic disease, which are available at http://www.aaos.org/research/guidelines/VTE/VTE_guideline.asp.

Failed Hip Arthroplasty

Background

THA can fail for a variety of reasons, and understanding the cause of failure is of primary importance so that the failure can be addressed with the appropriate revision strategies. Common modes of failure include infection, loosening, instability, and periprosthetic fracture. Unique modes of failure observed in MoM bearing surfaces will be addressed in this section because these failures have increased in frequency.

Clinical Evaluation

Patients presenting with a history of painful hip arthroplasty should undergo a thorough history and physical examination. The key signs to elucidate from the history include absence of pain relief following the initial procedure, prolonged wound healing, the need for antibiotics or other procedures related to wound problems, persistent drainage, or a history of prolonged limitations on weight-bearing status. A history of dislocations, mechanical symptoms of locking or catching, and squeaking also should be ascertained. An understanding of comorbid conditions or habits that might lead to perioperative complications, such as smoking, diabetes, steroid use, or coagulopathy, should be gathered. A physical examination should document gait, length discrepancies, abductor strength, range of motion, and any localized tenderness or masses. The skin should be closely examined for evidence of sinus tracts, poor wound healing, or venous stasis.

Radiographs should be scrutinized for current component positioning, mechanical failure, periprosthetic fracture, and available bone stock. The component interface should be critically evaluated for signs of loosening. Component migration also should be investigated if serial radiographs are available. Dedicated Judet views should be obtained if pelvic discontinuity is suspected. CT may also help determine the extent of bone loss or osteolysis in the revision setting.

Baseline laboratory studies, including a CBC with differential, ESR, and CRP level, should be obtained. If inflammatory markers are elevated, an aspiration of the hip under ultrasound or fluoroscopic guidance is warranted and should be obtained. Nucleated cell counts higher than 1,700 or a neutrophil percentage exceeding 65% is strongly suggestive of a periprosthetic infection.[64]

Periprosthetic Infection

After discovery, a periprosthetic infection can be treated with an irrigation, débridement, liner exchange, single-stage revision, or two-stage resection and reimplantation following a course of intravenous antibiotics. The type of treatment is usually dictated by the timing of presentation in relation to the onset of symptoms and the causative organism. Acute infections may respond to an irrigation and débridement with a bearing exchange. Chronic infections are generally treated with a staged approach in North America, with mid- to long-term survivorship free from reinfection in as many as 93% of cases.[65] This study also highlighted the importance of achieving stable component fixation; mechanical failure rates were noted to be higher than those of reinfection. Another study noted a recurrence of infection in 26% of patients after a two-stage approach, and the risk factors for failure included a poor host and resistant organisms.[66]

Instability

Recurrent instability has been established as the most common reason for revision hip arthroplasty.[67] Instability following THA may result from malpositioned components, sequelae of infection, or poor abductor tension. The cause of instability should be determined because it will dictate treatment. Acetabular components should be placed in approximately 40° to 45° of abduction and 15° to 20° of anteversion; however, the combined anteversion of both components must be considered to optimize hip stability. These requirements may be altered if abnormal pelvic tilt and incidence is encountered, as is seen in patients who have undergone lumbar and lumbosacral fusion. Weakened abductors that have been damaged iatrogenically during multiple approaches to the hip with poor soft-tissue management or in instances of greater trochanteric fractures should be identified, and the need for trochanteric advancement or abductor reconstruction assessed. In cases in which abductor function cannot be restored, constrained liners provide an alternative means to achieve hip stability. If constrained liners are used, the surgeon must be aware of the additional strain placed on the bone component interface and should augment cup fixation with additional screws.

Interest has surged regarding acetabular components that employ a dual-mobility design. These components, which have been used in Europe for two decades, pair a large polyethylene head with a cobalt-chromium liner. A smaller head is snap fit within the polyethylene head. This construct creates a larger articulating surface, providing for an improved head-to-neck ratio and greater jump distance. The results of dual mobility components used in the setting of recurrent instability were reviewed by investigators who noted that in three European studies with between 4 and 8 years of follow-up, future dislocation was prevented in 95% to 98% of the patients.[68] An additional advantage of the dual-mobility concept is that theoretically it places less force on the acetabular component than a constrained device; however, this has yet to be proven in clinical studies.

Aseptic Loosening and Osteolysis

Researchers have extensively classified bone loss encountered in the acetabulum and the femur during revision THA.[69,70] Acetabular defects can be more broadly characterized as contained, segmental, or involving a pelvic discontinuity. Contained defects usually can be successfully managed with impaction of cancellous allograft or a bone substitute and large hemispherical cups. Segmental defects can be successfully managed with large hemispherical cups with multiple screws, assuming an ingrowth surface in contact with at least 50% of surface contact with bone is achieved. Tricortical iliac crest autograft or bulk allograft can be fixed with screws to the remaining acetabulum and reamed if insufficient contact and implant instability is noted. Pelvic discontinuity can be managed through a variety of techniques. Stable distraction can be accomplished by using a large acetabular component, the affected column can be plated before acetabular component placement, and a cup-cage construct or a custom triphlange component can be used (**Figure 7**). The technique used depends on the relative stability of the pelvis, the size of the associated bone defect, and surgeon preference.

Femoral bone loss assessment should focus on the portion of bone that remains relatively intact because this will refine a surgeon's revision fixation options. In most cases, the metaphysis has been violated and will not impart reliable stability to a revision implant. Consequently, extensively coated cylindrical stems and modular tapered stems are preferentially used because they achieve their fixation in the diaphysis. In a recent study comparing these two stem designs in the revision setting, the modular tapered stems were associated with better outcome scores, fewer intraoperative fractures, and restored femoral anatomy more accurately than cylindrical stems.[71] Other techniques used include impaction grafting with cemented stem allograft-prosthetic composites and intussusception grafting; however, these options involve considerable technical mastery. Proxi-

4: Lower Extremity

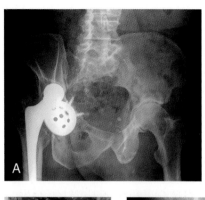
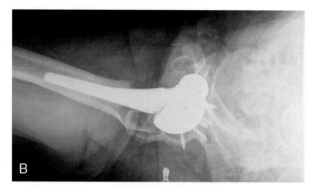
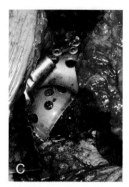

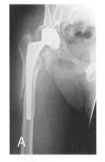
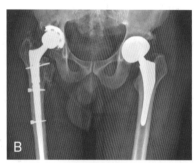
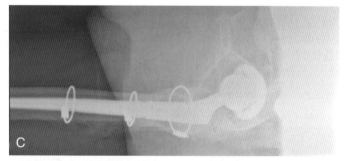

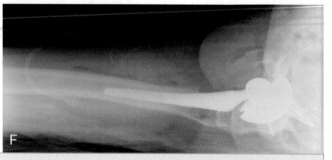

Figure 7 Preoperative oblique (**A**) and lateral (**B**) views of a right THA, which failed secondary to osteolysis and aseptic loosening, with eventual cup migration and dislocation. Intraoperative photographs (**C** and **D**) demonstrate the cup-cage construct that was used to achieve stable fixation of the revision acetabular component shown in the postoperative radiographs (**E** and **F**). (Courtesy of David Lewallen, MD, Mayo Clinic, Rochester, MN.)

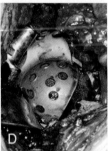
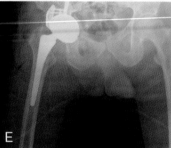

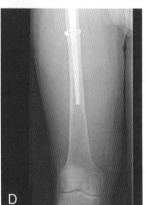
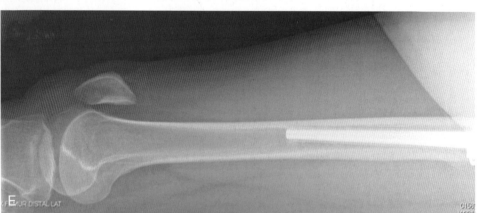

Figure 8 **A,** AP radiograph of a right THA demonstrating a Vancouver B2 periprosthetic fracture in the setting of osteolysis. Note the asymmetric wear of the acetabular liner. This patient was successfully treated with a femoral component revision using a modular tapered stem that bypassed the fracture. Bone grafting through the acetabular component and liner exchange also was performed (**B** through **E**).

mal femoral replacement and total femur arthroplasty also can be used in salvage situations.

Periprosthetic Fractures

Periprosthetic fractures can be classified according to the Vancouver classification system. Fractures with an associated loose stem are classified as Vancouver B2 and B3 fractures, and those in which the stem remains well fixed to host bone are Vancouver B1 fractures. Fractures with stable stems can be managed with ORIF, but a loose stem demands revision. Good results have been observed with treatment that includes cortical on-lay struts and plating around stable stems.[72] One study, however, demonstrated fewer complications when Vancouver B1 fractures were treated with implant revision.[73] Early weight bearing associated with fixing B1 fractures through component revision has been shown to lead to decreased perioperative mortality.[74] Mid- to long-term results following the treatment of periprosthetic fractures with component revision using a variety of components demonstrated a 90% survivorship at 5 years and a 79% survivorship at 10 years.[75] The primary reason for component failure in this setting was mechanical loosening. A recent study of 32 Vancouver B2 and B3 fractures managed solely with modular, tapered, fluted stems revealed fracture healing in all instances and no cases of stem subsidence at short-term follow-up (**Figure 8**). Bony ingrowth was observed in 28 cases, and a stable fibrous ingrowth occurred in 4 cases.[76]

MoM Failure

MoM hip arthroplasties are subject to the traditional modes of failure seen with other bearing surfaces and also pose their own unique means of failure. Ten of the first 37 MoM hips revised at the Mayo Clinic developed metal hypersensitivity reactions, with 8 of those demonstrating histologic evidence of ALVAL.[77] Successful treatment of a painful MoM hip arthroplasty begins with an appropriate workup. In general, asymptomatic, well-functioning MoM bearings with normal radiographic findings can be followed annually without additional intervention. Vigilance should be maintained during follow-up for signs or symptoms indicating a decline in function or increased pain. Serum cobalt and chromium levels should be obtained as a baseline, even in asymptomatic patients. Future symptomatic decline correlating with a rise in serum ions may guide treatment. Furthermore, elevated serum ion levels (> 5 µg/L) were associ-

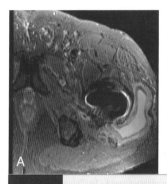
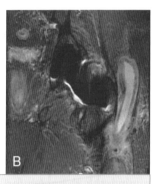

Figure 9 Axial (**A**) and coronal (**B**) T2-weighted MRIs demonstrating a pseudotumor about a metal-on-metal THA. Note the involvement of the hip abductor musculature. (Courtesy of Robert Trousdale, MD, Mayo Clinic, Rochester, MN.)

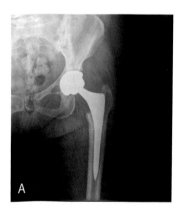
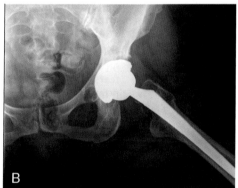
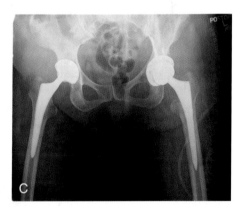
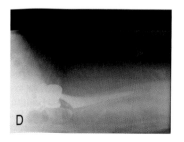
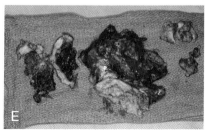

Figure 10 **A** and **B**, AP and lateral radiographs, respectively, of a painful MoM THA for which revision of the acetabular component was performed and conversion to a metal-on-polyethylene bearing couple occurred (**C** and **D**). **E**, The pseudotumor that was resected at the time of revision. (Courtesy of Robert Trousdale, MD, Mayo Clinic, Rochester, MN.)

of open femoral shaft fractures. *J Orthop Trauma* 2010; 24(11):677-682.

Ninety patients with open femoral fractures treated with RGN were retrospectively identified using trauma databases from four level I trauma centers. The author found only one case of a septic knee associated with RGN. Level of evidence: IV.

26. Becher S, Ziran B: Retrograde IM nailing of open femoral shaft fractures: A retrospective case series. *J Trauma Acute Care Surg* 2012;72(3):696-698.

This is a retrospective review of 35 open femoral fractures treated with RGN. The authors demonstrated a 97% union rate and a 6% deep infection rate with no cases of septic knee. A 6% rate of arthrofibrosis requiring operative treatment was reported. Level of evidence: IV.

27. Halvorson JJ, Barnett M, Jackson B, Birkedal JP: Risk of septic knee following retrograde IM nailing of open and closed femur fractures. *J Orthop Surg Res* 2012; 7:7.

Within a single institution, 143 closed femoral fractures, 38 open femoral fractures, and 4 closed fractures with traumatic knee arthrotomy were retrospectively identified. All fractures were treated with RGN, and no postoperative septic knees were identified. Level of evidence: IV.

28. El Moumni M, Schraven P, ten Duis HJ, Wendt K: Persistent knee complaints after retrograde unreamed nailing of femoral shaft fractures. *Acta Orthop Belg* 2010; 76(2):219-225.

This retrospective review of 75 patients with femoral fractures treated with RGN highlighted the high incidence of persistent knee pain following treatment. Younger age was associated with a higher risk for knee pain, but symptoms improved in all patients after removing the distal interlocking screws of the nail. Level of evidence: IV.

29. Daglar B, Gungor E, Delialioglu OM, et al: Comparison of knee function after antegrade and retrograde IM nailing for diaphyseal femoral fractures: Results of isokinetic evaluation. *J Orthop Trauma* 2009;23(9): 640-644.

30. Watson JT, Moed BR: Ipsilateral femoral neck and shaft fractures: Complications and their treatment. *Clin Orthop Relat Res* 2002;399:78-86.

31. Bedi A, Karunakar MA, Caron T, Sanders RW, Haidukewych GJ: Accuracy of reduction of ipsilateral femoral neck and shaft fractures—an analysis of various internal fixation strategies. *J Orthop Trauma* 2009;23(4): 249-253.

32. Nork SE, Agel J, Russell GV, Mills WJ, Holt S, Routt ML Jr: Mortality after reamed IM nailing of bilateral femur fractures. *Clin Orthop Relat Res* 2003;415: 272-278.

33. Cannada LK, Taghizadeh S, Murali J, Obremskey WT, DeCook C, Bosse MJ: Retrograde IM nailing in treatment of bilateral femur fractures. *J Orthop Trauma* 2008;22(8):530-534.

34. Stavlas P, Giannoudis PV: Bilateral femoral fractures: Does IM nailing increase systemic complications and mortality rates? *Injury* 2009;40(11):1125-1128.

35. Hartsock LA, Barfield WR, Kokko KP, et al: Randomized prospective clinical trial comparing reamer irrigator aspirator (RIA) to standard (SR) in both minimally injured and multiply injured patients with closed femoral shaft fractures treated with reamed IM nailing (IMN). *Injury* 2010;41(suppl 2):S94-S98.

This prospective RCT compared the inflammatory response of 20 patients with femoral shaft fractures treated with IM nailing using either standard or RIA reaming. Measurements of the inflammatory mediators IL-6 and IL-10 postoperatively indicated a potential protective effect of RIA reaming. Level of evidence: I.

36. Husebye EE, Opdahl H, Røise O, Aspelin T, Lyberg T: Coagulation, fibrinolysis and cytokine responses to IM nailing of the femur: An experimental study in pigs comparing traditional reaming and reaming with a one-step reamer-irrigator-aspirator system. *Injury* 2011; 42(7):630-637.

This is an animal study using a pig model that compared the inflammatory responses induced by RIA reaming and standard reaming. Standard reaming was shown to induce greater procedure-related coagulation and fibrinolytic responses as well as significantly higher IL-6 levels than RIA. Level of evidence: II.

37. Husebye EE, Lyberg T, Opdahl H, Laurvik H, Røise O: Cardiopulmonary response to reamed IM nailing of the femur comparing traditional reaming with a one-step reamer-irrigator-aspirator reaming system: An experimental study in pigs. *J Trauma* 2010;69(4):E6-E14.

This is a second animal study investigating the pulmonary effects of standard versus RIA reaming. The RIA group showed lower numbers of embolisms per square centimeter of lung area than the standard reaming group. Level of evidence: II.

38. Volgas DA, Burch T, Stannard JP, Ellis T, Bilotta J, Alonso JE: Fat embolus in femur fractures: A comparison of two reaming systems. *Injury* 2010;41(suppl 2): S90-S93.

This prospective RCT compared the embolic load delivered to the right atrium in two groups of patients with femoral fractures treated with either standard or RIA reaming. A transesophageal echocardiogram demonstrated a significantly decreased amount of fat emboli delivered to the cardiopulmonary system with RIA reaming. Level of evidence: II.

39. Streubel PN, Desai P, Suk M: Comparison of RIA and conventional reamed nailing for treatment of femur shaft fractures. *Injury* 2010;41(suppl 2):S51-S56.

This retrospective trial comparing conventional and RIA reaming in 156 patients with femoral fractures failed to demonstrate a statistical difference with regard to pulmonary complications, healing rates, or death. There was a trend toward delayed healing in the RIA group. Level I

40. Kanakaris NK, Morell D, Gudipati S, Britten S, Giannoudis PV: Reaming Irrigator Aspirator system: Early experience of its multipurpose use. *Injury* 2011; 42(suppl 4):S28-S34.

This case series demonstrates multiple clinical uses for the RIA system, including the treatment of femoral fractures, débridement for cases of osteomyelitis, and obtaining morcellized bone graft.

41. Zalavras CG, Sirkin M: Treatment of long bone IM infection using the RIA for removal of infected tissue: Indications, method and clinical results. *Injury* 2010; 41(suppl 2):S43-S47.

This technique paper and case series describes the use of the RIA system for the treatment of osteomyelitis in 11 patients.

42. Bellapianta J, Gerdeman A, Sharan A, Lozman J: Use of the reamer irrigator aspirator for the treatment of a 20-year recurrent osteomyelitis of a healed femur fracture. *J Orthop Trauma* 2007;21(5):343-346.

43. Hüfner T, Citak M, Suero EM, et al: Femoral malrotation after unreamed IM nailing: An evaluation of influencing operative factors. *J Orthop Trauma* 2011;25(4): 224-227.

A retrospective chart review identified 82 patients with femoral fractures who were treated with either antegrade or retrograde unreamed nailing without the use of a fracture table. All patients had been evaluated with postoperative CT scans to determine any rotational malunion. They found that there was a 22% incidence of more than 15° of rotational malalignment. Both comminution and surgery time of day correlated with an increased severity of malrotation.

44. Vaidya R, Anderson B, Elbanna A, Colen R, Hoard D, Sethi A: CT scanogram for limb length discrepancy in comminuted femoral shaft fractures following IM nailing. *Injury* 2012;43(7):1176-1181.

Postoperative CT scanograms were believed to be excellent tools to evaluate for leg length inequality in Winquist III or IV femoral fractures treated with IM nailing. Incidentally, it was found that the majority of these patients had unequal uninjured tibias, which complicated the determination of the overall amount of correction required. Only 10% had equal tibias. Level of evidence: III.

45. Lindsey JD, Krieg JC: Femoral malrotation following IM nail fixation. *J Am Acad Orthop Surg* 2011;19(1): 17-26.

This review article discusses rotational malalignment of femoral fractures treated with IM nailing. Prevention, evaluation, and surgical options are presented.

46. Langer JS, Gardner MJ, Ricci WM: The cortical step sign as a tool for assessing and correcting rotational deformity in femoral shaft fractures. *J Orthop Trauma* 2010;24(2):82-88.

This article discusses the use of the cortical step sign as a method to assess and correct for potential rotational deformities of femoral fractures during surgical stabilization. If any incongruity of cortical widths exists on either side of a fracture, there should be concern for rotational malalignment. However, the sign did not help determine the direction of malrotation (internal or external).

47. Phillips JR, Trezies AJ, Davis TR: Long-term follow-up of femoral shaft fracture: Relevance of malunion and malalignment for the development of knee arthritis. *Injury* 2011;42(2):156-161.

There is uncertainty regarding the long-term effects of femoral malalignment on adjacent joints. In a cohort group of patients treated for a femoral shaft fracture with a median follow-up of 22 years, no association between malunion and knee arthritis could be shown. Level of evidence: II.

48. Gelalis ID, Politis AN, Arnaoutoglou CM, et al: Diagnostic and treatment modalities in nonunions of the femoral shaft: A review. *Injury* 2012;43(7):980-988.

This is a review of the treatment options for femoral shaft nonunions. Diagnosis and classification are also discussed. Level of evidence: V.

49. Hakeos WM, Richards JE, Obremskey WT: Plate fixation of femoral nonunions over an IM nail with autogenous bone grafting. *J Orthop Trauma* 2011;25(2): 84-89.

A small series of patients with diaphyseal femoral fracture nonunions was treated with plate fixation and autogenous bone grafting. The nonunion site was débrided, and the previously placed intramedullary nail was retained. Immediate weight bearing was allowed. All patients experienced healing. Level of evidence: IV.

50. Park J, Kim SG, Yoon HK, Yang KH: The treatment of nonisthmal femoral shaft nonunions with intramedullary nail exchange versus augmentation plating. *J Orthop Trauma* 2010;24(2):89-94.

Eighteen patients with nonisthmal femoral nonunions were treated either with an exchange nail (7 patients) or plating with autogenous bone grafting (11 patients). Only two of the seven nonunions treated with exchange nails went on to union, compared with 100% union in the augmentation plating group. Level of evidence: III.

51. Giannoudis PV, Kanakaris NK, Dimitriou R, Gill I, Kolimarala V, Montgomery RJ: The synergistic effect of autograft and BMP-7 in the treatment of atrophic nonunions. *Clin Orthop Relat Res* 2009;467(12):3239-3248.

52. Kanakaris NK, Lasanianos N, Calori GM, et al: Application of bone morphogenetic proteins to femoral nonunions: A 4-year multicentre experience. *Injury* 2009; 40(suppl 3):S54-S61.

53. Kammerlander C, Riedmüller P, Gosch M, et al: Functional outcome and mortality in geriatric distal femoral fractures. *Injury* 2012;43(7):1096-1101.

This article documents the poor functional long-term outcome of elderly patients with distal femoral fractures in a small group of patients. They were also found to have a higher perioperative risk of dying in the hospital when compared with hip fracture patients.

54. Baker BJ, Escobedo EM, Nork SE, Henley MB: Hoffa fracture: A common association with high-energy supracondylar fractures of the distal femur. *AJR Am J Roentgenol* 2002;178(4):994.

55. Garnavos C, Lygdas P, Lasanianos NG: Retrograde nailing and compression bolts in the treatment of type C distal femoral fractures. *Injury* 2012;43(7):1170-1175.

    The authors report their use of RGN combined with an independent compression bolt in the treatment of type C distal femoral fractures. They reported a 100% union rate with excellent range of motion. Patient outcomes were also assessed with the New Oxford Knee score with a mean of 42.05 (out of 48). Level of evidence: IV.

56. Lujan TJ, Henderson CE, Madey SM, Fitzpatrick DC, Marsh JL, Bottlang M: Locked plating of distal femur fractures leads to inconsistent and asymmetric callus formation. *J Orthop Trauma* 2010;24(3):156-162.

    In a retrospective cohort study, radiographs of patients treated for distal femoral fractures with periarticular locking plates were evaluated for periosteal callus size. An asymmetric pattern of callus formation was detected, with the medial cortex having significantly more callus (64%) than the anterior or posterior cortices. In addition, titanium plates were found to have more callus than stainless steel plates at all time points. The plating systems differed in terms of screw fixation, which should also be taken into consideration. Level of evidence: III.

57. Doornink J, Fitzpatrick DC, Madey SM, Bottlang M: Far cortical locking enables flexible fixation with periarticular locking plates. *J Orthop Trauma* 2011; 25(suppl 1):S29-S34.

    This biomechanical study evaluated the effect of a new type of screw, the far cortical locking screw, on the construct stiffness of periarticular distal femoral plates. These screws lock into the plate and the far cortex only. The shaft diameter is reduced, allowing for elastic flexion. The use of these screws led to reduced stiffness and generated parallel interfragmentary motion while retaining the strength of the overall construct.

58. Beingessner D, Moon E, Barei D, Morshed S: Biomechanical analysis of the less invasive stabilization system for mechanically unstable fractures of the distal femur: Comparison of titanium versus stainless steel and bicortical versus unicortical fixation. *J Trauma* 2011;71(3): 620-624.

    This biomechanical study evaluated three different LISS plate constructs. Stainless steel and titanium plates using unicortical screws and a stainless steel LISS using bicortical screws had similar biomechanical profiles.

59. Collinge CA, Gardner MJ, Crist BD: Pitfalls in the application of distal femur plates for fractures. *J Orthop Trauma* 2011;25(11):695-706.

    This is an excellent overview of the pitfalls that occur when treating distal femoral fractures. Various tricks and tips are outlined to help orthopaedic surgeons manage these challenging fractures. Level of evidence: V.

60. Buckley R, Mohanty K, Malish D: Lower limb malrotation following MIPO technique of distal femoral and proximal tibial fractures. *Injury* 2011;42(2):194-199.

    Minimally invasive plate osteosynthesis was found to have a much higher incidence of malrotation than previously reported. In a small prospective cohort of patients treated for either a proximal tibial fracture or distal femoral fracture, there was a 50% and 38.5% incidence of malrotation, respectively. Statistical significance was achieved for the femur for differences in mean measures between the operative and uninjured sides. Level of evidence: III.

61. Henderson CE, Kuhl LL, Fitzpatrick DC, Marsh JL: Locking plates for distal femur fractures: Is there a problem with fracture healing? *J Orthop Trauma* 2011; 25(suppl 1):S8-S14.

    This review article looks at the literature regarding distal femoral fracture treatment. Fifteen articles and three abstracts were included. Complications regarding healing requiring revisions ranged from 0 to 32% and included nonunions, delayed unions, and implant failures. Level of evidence: III.

62. Firoozabadi R, McDonald E, Nguyen TQ, Buckley JM, Kandemir U: Does plugging unused combination screw holes improve the fatigue life of fixation with locking plates in comminuted supracondylar fractures of the femur? *J Bone Joint Surg Br* 2012;94(2):241-248.

    The failure of distal femoral locking plates often has occurred through the unfilled holes adjacent to the comminuted fracture site. To decrease the failure rate of the implant, a biomechanical study was performed to evaluate the effect of screw plugs placed into these empty holes. The use of these plugs did not improve the in vitro fatigue life of the plate.

Chapter 37

Tibial Plateau Fractures and Extensor Mechanism Injuries

William M. Ricci, MD   Samir Mehta, MD

4: Lower Extremity

Tibial Plateau Fractures

Tibial plateau fractures involve the articular surface of the proximal tibia and represent a diverse group of fractures spanning a large spectrum of severity. Simple injuries resulting from low-energy mechanisms are straightforward to treat and have predictably excellent outcomes. Complex fractures or fracture-dislocation patterns resulting from high-energy trauma present treatment challenges and can leave patients with substantial functional deficits. Accordingly, the optimal treatment of tibial plateau fractures takes many forms. Nonsurgical and multiple surgical fracture management methods are potentially applicable. A clearly defined diagnosis is critical to determine the most appropriate treatment method. Multiple imaging modalities and requisite clinical experience that prepare surgeons to recognize associated soft-tissue injuries about the knee may be required to appreciate all of the subtle aspects of any given tibial plateau fracture.

Low-energy fractures pose minimal risk for associated soft-tissue disruptions. High-energy tibial plateau fractures, however, can be associated with myriad associated conditions, such as ligamentous injury, cartilage damage, compartment syndrome, and vascular compromise, which lead to poor functional outcomes and

threaten limb viability.[1,2] Careful attention to the general principles of fracture care is paramount to ensure the patients with tibial plateau fractures have optimal outcomes.

Evaluation

Mechanism of Injury and Associated Injuries

Tibial plateau fractures can result from low-energy mechanisms, such as a fall from a standing height. These fractures typically occur in elderly patients or younger patients with poor bone quality. These low-energy mechanisms typically impart varus or valgus stress to the knee with some degree of axial load, resulting in unicondylar fractures—most commonly to the lateral plateau—that are related to the normal valgus alignment of the knee and the propensity for directional forces from the lateral side. Associated soft-tissue injuries about the knee resulting from low-energy lateral plateau fractures can include medial collateral ligament sprains (the midclavicular line acts as a tether during valgus loads) and meniscal tears when split or depressed fractures are widely displaced. A depression of at least 8 mm is associated with a 53% incidence of a lateral meniscal tear, and split widening of at least 8 mm is associated with a 73% incidence of a lateral meniscal tear. A depression of at least 10 mm is associated with an eight-fold increased risk for a lateral meniscal tear.[3,4]

High-energy mechanisms have a predominance of axial load and result in an entirely different set of tibial plateau fracture patterns and much more severe soft-tissue injury versus those seen with low-energy fractures. Motor and recreational vehicle and motorcycle collisions, as well as sporting injuries and falls from heights, can cause high-energy tibial plateau fractures and most commonly occur in younger patients.[2,5] In contrast with low-energy injuries, high-energy fractures are more likely to be bicondylar and associated with soft-tissue injuries. Partial or complete collateral ligament, cruciate ligament, or meniscal tears are commonly associated with tibial plateau fractures, especially those associated with high-energy mechanisms. MRI scans and arthroscopic evaluations indicate that the frequency of soft-tissue injuries with tibial plateau fractures is in the range of 40% to 80%.[1,6-8] Ultimately, it is important to distinguish knee instability attributable to bone deformity from instability related to

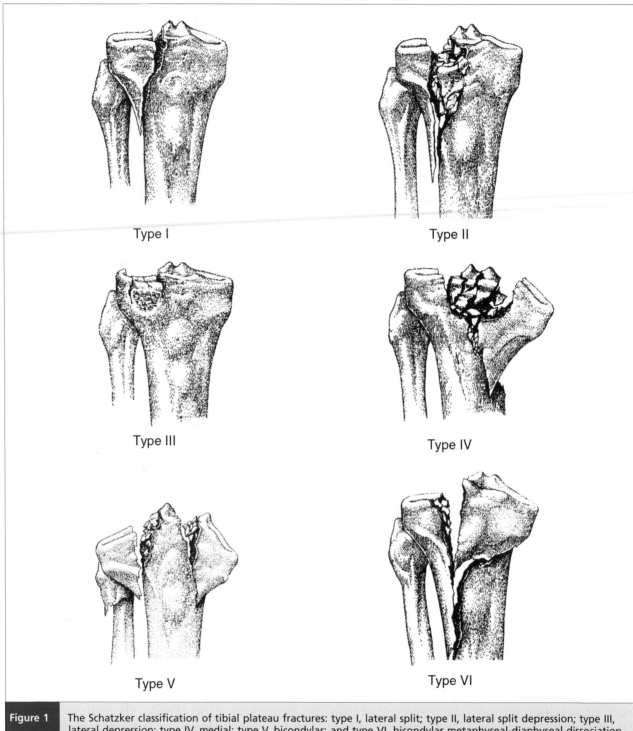

Type I

Type II

Type III

Type IV

Type V

Type VI

Figure 1   The Schatzker classification of tibial plateau fractures: type I, lateral split; type II, lateral split depression; type III, lateral depression; type IV, medial; type V, bicondylar; and type VI, bicondylar metaphyseal-diaphyseal dissociation. (Reproduced from Sirkin MS: Fractures of the tibial plateau, in Kellam JF, Fischer TJ, Tornetta P III, Bosse MJ, Harris MB, eds: *Orthopaedic Knowledge Update: Trauma*, ed 2. Rosemont, IL, American Academy of Orthopaedic Surgeons, 2000, pp 167-175.)

ligamentous laxity with a physical examination after bone reconstruction or an MRI scan.

Compartment syndrome and vascular injury, each a potentially devastating injury, should be considered while evaluating patients with tibial plateau fractures because compartment syndrome may be present in as many as 10% of patients with these fractures and in up to 30% of patients with Schatzker VI patterns[9] (Figure 1). Even when recognized and treated appropriately, the presence of these injuries substantially increases the complexity of treatment and may lead to poor functional outcomes.[10]

History and Physical Examination

The pertinent history associated with tibial plateau fractures starts with the mechanism and a determination of the relative energy. Innocuous-appearing mechanisms, such as noncontact sporting injuries, can result in high-energy injury patterns. Therefore, the mechanism history is important, and the radiographic personality of the fracture will help guide the index of suspicion for associated injuries that can accompany high-energy injuries. General baseline functional status, baseline knee function, and any history of prior knee injuries and surgeries help guide both prognosis and treatment.

The physical examination of a patient with a tibial plateau fracture is important to elucidate associated injuries about and distant to the knee. Inspecting the soft-tissue envelope about the knee helps determine the timing of surgical treatment and the need for staged treatments. Open fractures are treated expeditiously; closed, low-energy fractures without severe soft-tissue swelling can be treated acutely or in a delayed fashion; and closed, high-energy injuries with substantial soft-tissue swelling are treated definitively in a delayed fashion after initial stabilization with a splint or a spanning external fixator. A thorough neurovascular examination focuses on potential injury to the peroneal nerve and the potential for vascular compromise. The common peroneal nerve as it courses around the head of the fibula is at potential risk for injury. Vascular compromise can result from complete transection, most commonly in association with a knee dislocation at the level of the popliteal artery or at the trifurcation, or from more subtle arterial injuries such as intimal tears. Because incomplete injuries can thrombose and progress to a completely dysvascular limb, it is important to identify subtle injuries acutely. A deviation from symmetric distal pulses between injured and uninjured limbs warrants an ankle-brachial index (ABI) measurement. An ABI lower than 0.9 may warrant more detailed vascular studies.[11] Related to the abundant muscular envelope surrounding the proximal tibia, compartment syndrome is considered for patients with tibial plateau fractures, especially those with high-energy injuries.

Imaging

The radiographic examination for patients with suspected tibial plateau fractures begins with AP and lateral radiographs of the knee. Oblique views are useful to identify occult fractures but are of little value otherwise. CT scans, particularly sagittal and coronal reconstructions, are useful to clarify the fracture pattern, identify the degree and the location of articular depressions, and help plan surgical approaches and fixation strategies.[12] MRI, which may be a useful adjunct with which to diagnose occult fractures and identify cartilage and ligament injures about the knee, also can potentially refine surgical decision making.[13] CT and MRI are most useful when limb alignment and knee joint congruity are optimally restored; consequently, these studies are deferred until provisional stabilization is completed either with splint immobilization or, if indicated, after external fixation.

Classification

The Schatzker classification, the most commonly applied classification scheme for tibial plateau fractures, has six types:[14]

- Schatzker type I: Lateral split
- Schatzker type II: Lateral split depression
- Schatzker type III: Lateral depression
- Schatzker type IV: Medial
- Schatzker type V: Bicondylar
- Schatzker type VI: Bicondylar metaphyseal-diaphyseal dissociation

Lateral fractures are typically the result of low-energy mechanisms. Pure lateral split fractures (type I) usually occur in younger patients with good bone quality. Lateral split depression fractures (type II) are the most common, and pure lateral depression fractures (type III) are the most rare. MRI studies show nondisplaced split components associated with most pure depression-type fractures diagnosed with plain radiography.[8] Fractures involving the medial plateau, especially those with bicondylar dissociation of the metaphysis from the diaphysis (type VI), are generally the result of high-energy mechanisms. All pure medial fractures are grouped into the type IV pattern; however, there are common variations seen with medial fractures. The posterior-medial type has a coronal fracture through the weight-bearing articular surface, whereas the weight-bearing medial plafond remains intact with total medial condylar fractures. Distinguishing the bicondylar fracture (type V) from a bicondylar metaphyseal-diaphyseal dissociation (type VI) can be difficult. An inexperienced evaluator often points to the continuity of minute central portions of the tibial spine, as shown in **Figure 1**,[14] to distinguish between type V and type VI fractures. In contrast, a more experienced evaluator takes into consideration the fracture personality rather than relying on strict definitions. In general, fractures amenable to medial and lateral buttress plating act like bicondylar (type V) patterns (**Figure 2**), and those that require more stout forms of fixation, such as lateral locked plating with or without supplemental medial fixation, act like bicondylar dissociation patterns (type VI) (**Figure 3**).

A deficiency of the Schatzker classification scheme is that it does not account for knee subluxation or dislocation and the commonly associated coronal oblique fracture planes. A common fracture pattern includes lateral subluxation of the tibia relative to the femoral condyle with a coronal posterior-medial fracture with or without an associated lateral fracture. Failure to identify such joint disruption can lead to treatment that focuses on reestablishing the alignment of the joint fragments relative to the shaft of the tibia but does not restore joint congruity (**Figure 4**).

Although the Schatzker system remains the most commonly used in clinical practice, the Orthopaedic

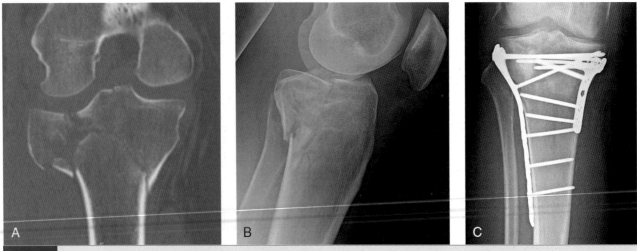

Figure 2 A, A CT coronal reconstruction depicting a bicondylar (Schatzker type V) fracture. B, A lateral radiograph of a type V fracture with a coronal posterior medial component. C, An AP postoperative radiograph after medial and lateral plating.

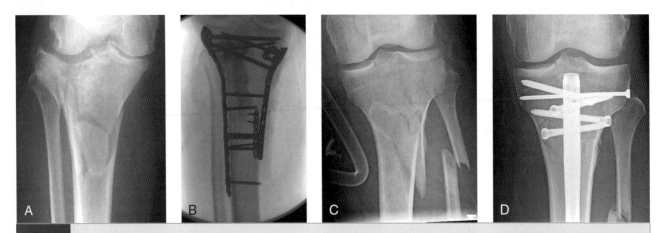

Figure 3 AP radiographs of two different bicondylar tibial plateau fractures with metaphyseal-diaphyseal dissociation (Schatzker type VI; A and C), one treated with plating and a ceramic bone void filler (B), and the other treated with an intramedullary nail with a lag screw across the articular split (D).

Trauma Association (OTA) classification is more comprehensive.[15] The numeric portion of the OTA classification of tibial plateau fractures is 41, with the 4 indicating the bone (tibia) and the 1 indicating the portion of the bone (proximal). The alphabetic portion of the classification—A, B, or C—differs depending on the fracture type: type A fractures are extra-articular; type B fractures are partial articular; and type C fractures are complete articular. Each category has many additional alphanumeric subtypes that are generally most useful for the purpose of research.

Treatment

Nonsurgical Treatment
Nondisplaced tibial plateau fractures and displaced fractures may be treated nonsurgically for very–low-demand patients or those who cannot tolerate surgery. The authors' protocol for nonsurgical treatment typically consists of bracing with either a hinged knee brace or a knee immobilizer and approximately 4 to 8 weeks of protected weight bearing. No weight bearing or only toe-touch weight bearing during the first 4 weeks is followed by variable progression during the next 4 weeks based on clinical and radiographic evidence of healing. Surveillance radiographs taken at weekly and then biweekly intervals are useful to rule out secondary displacement. Because of the varus moment about the knee, progressive secondary displacement of nondisplaced and minimally displaced medial tibial plateau fractures is not uncommon. In such cases, a low threshold for surgical intervention is prudent to avoid unacceptable varus alignment at the time of ultimate healing.

The threshold of displacement that should be the limit for nonsurgical management is controversial. Given the protective effects of the menisci, the knee joint is relatively tolerant of articular incongruity—more so for the lateral side than the medial side. Lateral articular step-off seen with split-type fractures of several millimeters may be well tolerated, especially in lower-demand patients. Lateral depression up to 10 mm also may be well tolerated from the perspective of joint arthrosis. Progressive symptomatic arthritis of the knee is unusual; however, large lateral depressions, particularly depressions that encompass the entire lateral joint, can lead to symptomatic joint instability in the coronal plane and objectionable valgus deformity.[5]

A decision in favor of nonsurgical management of tibial plateau fractures must be individualized, not based on a predetermined threshold of displacement in millimeters. The basis for decision making should take into account fracture displacement, fracture location, the propensity for secondary displacement, the risk of joint arthrosis, instability, and deformity. Of course, patient-specific factors, such as surgical risk, functional demands, expectations, and desires, are primarily considered.

Surgical Treatment

In a general sense, patients with tibial plateau fractures who likely will not fare well with nonsurgical treatment are most likely to benefit from surgical intervention, assuming they are fit to undergo an operation. Displaced bicondylar and shaft dissociation patterns, medial fractures with more than a couple of millimeters of displacement, and any pattern that includes joint subluxation are indications for surgical management. Lateral fractures with a displaced split component, a large depression, or valgus alignment or instability also meet surgical indications.

After surgical management is chosen, decisions must be made regarding the timing of surgery (soon after presentation or delayed) and the staging strategy (definitive surgery in one stage or provisional external fixation followed by planned staged definitive fixation). The condition of the surrounding soft tissues and the presence or the absence of compartment syndrome or vascular compromise strongly influence these decisions.[16]

Provisional Management

During the interval between presentation and surgical intervention, regardless of whether the first surgery will be definitive or provisional, the fracture is immobilized with either a long leg splint or a brace (hinged knee brace or immobilizer). Low-energy lateral injuries with minimal soft-tissue swelling are the subset most amenable to bracing. The convenience of a brace to allow removal for bathing and its relative light weight are the main factors supporting this method. Any fracture with substantial soft-tissue swelling, a highly unstable injury pattern, or joint subluxation is best managed with a long leg splint at this juncture. Bracing in these situations does not provide sufficient immobilization to stabilize the fracture, and insufficient stabilization can lead to discomfort and persistent swelling.

Patients with soft-tissue swelling that precludes immediate internal fixation are candidates for provisional

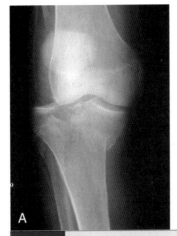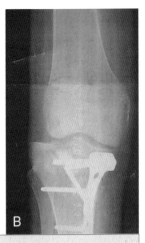

Figure 4 **A,** An AP radiograph shows a lateral tibial plateau fracture with lateral subluxation of the tibia relative to the femoral condyles. **B,** A postoperative AP radiograph shows adequate fracture fixation but failure to reduce the joint subluxation.

external fixation.[16] However, not all patients meeting these criteria are treated with external fixation. Those with axially stable patterns, unicondylar fractures, and no substantial joint subluxation are optimally managed with a long leg splint before definitive surgery. Indications for provisional external fixation include substantial soft-tissue swelling associated with axial or joint instability when compartment syndrome or vascular injuries are present. The primary goals of external fixation are to restore limb length, achieve accurate fracture alignment and joint congruity to result in appropriate soft-tissue relationships, and protect the articular surface from further injury. This allows definitive fixation to occur without the need to correct deformities resisted by contracted soft tissues. A realigned and stabilized limb also provides for optimal secondary imaging and patient comfort. Provisional external fixation for tibial plateau fractures is not without potential problems and disadvantages. The requirement for additional surgery, the potential for pin site infection, and the cost of required implants add risk and expense.

Provisional External Fixation Technique

The principles of provisional external fixation call for adequate but not necessarily maximal stability and the placement of half pins outside the zone of injury, future implants, and incisions. To best anticipate needs that may evolve with advancing age, it is useful to diagram predicted future incisions. Typically, two pins are placed in the femur and two in the tibia. The trajectories of the femoral pins are either lateral-to-medial or anterior-to-posterior. Laterally oriented pins placed just anterior to the intermuscular septum theoretically reduce binding of the quadriceps, while anterior pins may provide improved stability by virtue of being coplanar with knee-joint motion. Both techniques are commonly used and are equally acceptable. Distal pins are typically placed through the crest of the tibia or the subcutaneous medial surface. Heat generation during pin placement should be minimized to avoid necrosis of the adjacent bone and soft tissues, especially the skin over the subcutaneous border of the tibia. Predrilling of diaphyseal bone and liberal use of cooling irrigation are useful in this regard. The femoral and tibial pins are connected with bars and clamps, with care being taken to avoid interference by the clamps with postoperative imaging of the fracture and knee joint. Length restoration without overdistraction and fracture and joint alignment are achieved with traction and manual manipulations.

Definitive Surgical Management

The diversity of injury patterns seen with tibial plateau fractures necessitates an equally diverse array of internal fixation constructs for consideration. Pure lateral fractures are generally treated with laterally based plates and screws. Pure medial fractures are generally treated with medially based implants, but effective stabilization can sometimes be accomplished with lateral locked plates.[17] Bicondylar fractures can be treated with lateral locked plates alone or with lateral and medial plates. Adjunctive bone void fillers are commonly used for filling subchondral defects. Meniscal tears can be identified by direct vision via a submeniscal arthrotomy or arthroscopy. If present, these tears should be repaired. The benefit of acute ligament reconstruction for fracture-dislocation patterns remains controversial.

Technique for Open Reduction and Internal Fixation of Lateral Tibial Plateau Fractures

Open reduction and internal fixation (ORIF) principles and techniques for lateral tibial plateau fractures, Schatzker types I to III, are similar. The patient position is supine, with a leg positioner beneath the affected limb to allow unencumbered lateral radiographs. The surgical approach is through a curvilinear incision centered over the Gerdy tubercle. The fascia is divided parallel to the skin incision, with care taken to avoid devitalizing the subcutaneous fat. The anterior compartment muscles are elevated from the proximal tibia. A submeniscal arthrotomy is used in nearly all cases unless there is MRI evidence to confirm an intact lateral meniscus and the fracture does not involve the weight-bearing portion of the lateral plateau. Visualization of the meniscus and the joint is greatly facilitated by using a femoral distractor with one half pin placed in the distal femur and the other in the mid tibia. Split fractures can be hinged open (generally with a posterior-based hinge) to provide access to the joint. Even fractures without a displaced split fracture are often managed by completing or creating a split with an osteotome because the visualization that accompanies this approach cannot be equaled with a submeniscal arthrotomy alone. Using a metaphyseal window for the placement of tamps to aid in articular reduction is another strategy. Regardless of the method, the goal is anatomic reduction of the articular surface, reduction of the nonarticular shell of lateral bone, and restoration of the normal condylar slope and width (alterations to the condylar slope and width are easily overlooked because they are often subtle). A large periarticular reduction clamp or lag screws are useful to narrow a widened plateau. Contralateral radiographs of the uninjured knee are helpful to avoid overcorrections and re-create normal anatomy.

After reduction and provisional fixation are accomplished, fixation of lateral fractures is relatively straightforward and various configurations can be equally effective. Split fragments are secured with a buttress plate and nonlocked screws just distal to the apex, with lag screws through the fragment. Subchondral screws are used to support previously depressed articular fragments. Multiple methods of subchondral support may be used with success (**Figure 5**). Either locked or unlocked screws through a lateral plate or independent of a lateral plate are acceptable (**Figure 5, B**). When good medial bone quality is present, locked screws through a plate do not provide substantial advantage. Unicondylar oblique locked screws can be useful to position screws very close to the subchondral bone, however. Residual subchondral defects are often filled with bone void fillers (**Figure 5, B and C**). Many ceramic formulations are commercially available with different compressive strengths, biologic properties, and resorption rates. This class of bone graft substitutes appears to provide better support for articular reduction and minimizes secondary subsidence better than autograft and allograft.[18,19]

Technique for ORIF of Medial Tibial Plateau Fractures

Isolated medial fractures are treated similar to isolated lateral fractures, but with some important distinctions. Medial tibial plateau fractures typically have a split pattern involving the entire medial plateau, or they are partially articular involving the posterior medial portion of the medial plateau. The posterior medial pattern is in a coronal oblique plane with the fracture traversing the articular surface. Depressed medial patterns are uncommon. Direct visualization of the medial articular surface is difficult; consequently, judgment of articular reduction often is indirect via a combination of fluoroscopy and direct visualization of cortical fracture lines. The surgical approach for medial tibial plateau fractures is posterior medial. The pes anserine tendons are identified and retracted, and the posterior compartment musculature is elevated to expose the fracture. The medial collateral ligament is also preserved and provides a barrier to direct medial exposure. A combination of valgus stress, applied manually or with a femoral distractor, and reduction clamps aid in reduction. After reduction is accomplished, split fragments are secured with a buttress plate and nonlocked screws just distal to the apex, with lag screws through the fragment. Modifications of posterior approaches may be helpful in select situations.[20,21]

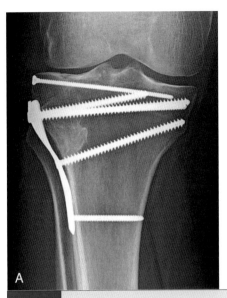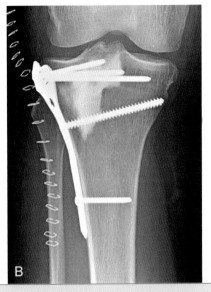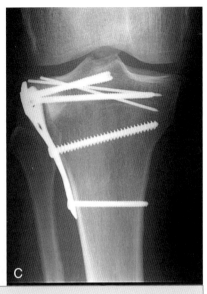

Figure 5 AP radiographs showing various forms of treatment of lateral tibial plateau fractures. **A,** A lateral plate with an independent subchondral screw. **B,** A lateral plate with oblique subchondral locking screws and a ceramic bone void filler. **C,** A lateral plate with adjunctive buried Kirschner wires and ceramic bone void filler.

Technique for ORIF of Bicondylar Tibial Plateau Fractures

Bicondylar fractures vary in pattern and severity. Bicondylar fractures without metaphyseal dissociation (Schatzker type V injuries) are generally amenable to medial and lateral buttress plating (**Figure 2**). The orientation of the articular fragments relative to each other and the shaft should be restored. Recent investigations have called attention to the relative sagittal plane alignment of each condyle. In bicondylar injuries, the medial and lateral plateaus are typically angulated more than 5° from the normal anatomic posterior slope, with the lateral plateau flexed more than the medial plateau.[22] Restoration of normal slope of both condyles may be required independently. Fixation of the medial condyle with a lateral locking plate and locking screws is a reasonable alternative to dual-plate constructs under certain circumstances.[23] Large medial fragments that can be captured by multiple locked screws can be adequately stabilized in this fashion. Fixation of incomplete or comminuted medial fragments, particularly the commonly encountered posterior medial coronal fracture, should be approached from the lateral side with great caution. Clinical and biomechanical investigations support dual plates, lateral and posterior medial, for these patterns.[2,24,25]

Intramedullary Nailing and External Fixation of Tibial Plateau Fractures

Intramedullary (IM) nailing (**Figure 3**) and circular external fixation are reasonable alternatives to ORIF for bicondylar patterns with metaphyseal dissociation, reasonably large condylar fragments, and simple articular components. For IM nailing, the articular fragments typically are reduced and fixed with screws before nailing. The screws used for articular fixation must be placed out of the path for the nail, usually proximal and posterior within the articular fragment. After fixation of the articular block is completed, all of the inherent challenges of nailing extra-articular proximal tibial fractures must be addressed. Extension and valgus deformities are common unless an optimal starting point and trajectory are identified. The semiextended technique combined with an intra-articular approach and the use of blocking screws and reduction plates is a commonly used technical modification that has proven useful to help obtain and maintain satisfactory reduction of nailed proximal tibial fractures.[26-29]

External fixation, when used for the definitive management of tibial plateau fractures, usually takes the form of fine-wire circular fixation and is often combined with limited internal fixation.[30,31] This method of treatment is most often chosen when soft-tissue considerations, such as recalcitrant swelling, traumatic wounds, and wounds related to compartment syndrome, preclude internal fixation. Hybrid fixation—circular attachments to the proximal fragment and half pin attachments (without circular rings) to the distal fragments—has been replaced by constructs with circular attachments both proximally and distally. These frames provide more symmetric loading of the fracture than hybrid frames and provide for more reliable healing. Securing the frame proximally is the most substantial technical challenge because of the small size of the proximal fragments, fracture lines, and the proximity of the joint capsule reflections. Typically, three tensioned wires are placed in various planes and spaced away from the joint to minimize the risk for septic arthritis if the joint capsule is penetrated.[32-34] Distal fixation may be accomplished with half pins, tensioned wires, or a combination of both attached to a circular ring. The proximal and distal rings are connected with four rods or six struts. When limb alignment is easily accomplished, nonadjustable connecting rods may be sufficient. If correction is required, a frame using adjustable struts is advantageous.

Outcomes

Lateral Tibial Plateau Fractures

As described in literature dating back to Schatzker's original report,[14] lateral tibial plateau fractures, particularly split types without substantial depression, have consistently been associated with the best outcomes of any type of tibial plateau fracture. These types of fractures also are associated with the lowest incidence of secondary arthritis, especially when the lateral meniscus is preserved.[35] Lateral fractures with depression also have been associated with good results when knee stability is preserved and subsidence of the lateral plateau is avoided.[36]

Medial and Bicondylar Tibial Plateau Fractures

There is scant literature scrutinizing the outcomes of pure medial tibial plateau fractures. Lateral locked plating of medial fractures was recently supported in a 2012 study of 13 patients.[17] The high frequency of articular displacement exceeding 2 mm (5 of 13 patients) is a shortcoming of this technique and a reason for the trend away from this method in favor of medial buttress plating for these injuries. The literature indicates that patients with high-energy bicondylar tibial plateau fractures have worse functional outcomes than those with unicondylar injuries.[36] These patients often have significant residual dysfunction compared with patients representing normative data, with leisure, employment, and movement Musculoskeletal Functional Assessment domains displaying the worst scores.[2]

Complications

Secondary loss of reduction is among the most common complications potentially controlled by the surgeon. In one study, subsidence of depressed lateral plateau fractures was shown to occur in 9 of 21 patients, although the methods used to support the lateral articular surface were not discussed in detail.[37] In a randomized trial comparing autologous bone graft with a ceramic cement to fill subchondral voids, at least 2 mm of subsidence was identified in 30% of patients in the autogenous group, compared with 9% of those in the ceramic group.[19] Split fractures rarely displace if treated with buttress plating. In contrast, posterior medial split fractures treated with lateral locking plates alone were recently found to displace in 14% of cases and have a statistically significant higher magnitude of varus displacement when treated with lateral locked plating compared with dual plating.[38] Infectious complications related to dual plating via dual incisions are relatively low: 8.4% in a series of 83 patients in which the presence of a dysvascular limb requiring vascular reconstruction was statistically associated with a deep wound infection.[24] This is in stark contrast to an infection rate of 87.5% with dual plating via single incisions

in a midline approach.[39] Compartment syndrome is seen in about 15% of patients with bicondylar fractures;[24] in this subset of patients, it is associated with a high rate of subsequent deep infection (23%).[40]

Extensor Mechanism Injuries

Extensor mechanism injuries (including injuries to the quadriceps tendon, the patella, and/or the patellar tendon) occur frequently and result from excessive tension through the extensor mechanism or via a direct blow. Extensor mechanism injuries can lead to stiffness, extension weakness, and patellofemoral arthritis. Nondisplaced fractures or partial tendon injuries with an intact extensor mechanism may be successfully treated nonsurgically. Surgical treatment is recommended for injuries that result in an inability to perform a straight leg raise or fractures demonstrating more than 2 to 3 mm of step-off and 1 to 4 mm of displacement. Early primary repair of a torn tendon or anatomic reduction and fixation with a tension band technique for patellar fractures is associated with the best outcomes.

Evaluation

Biomechanics of the Extensor Mechanism

The knee extensor mechanism generates torque and keeps the body upright against gravity. The patella acts as a pulley, shifting the pull of the quadriceps tendon anteriorly, thus increasing the moment arm of the quadriceps tendon by up to 30%.[41] Loading patterns about the extensor mechanism are complex. In addition to the quadriceps tendon loading the patella in tension, knee flexion results in compressive forces along the posterior patella. In addition, three-point bending stresses are created within the patella during flexion. A tremendous amount of force per unit area is transferred to the patellar tendon. Maximal tensile forces through the quadriceps and patellar tendons have been recorded as high as 3200 N and 2800 N, respectively. Activities such as stair climbing and squatting can generate patellofemoral compressive forces exceeding seven times body weight and anterior patellar surface strains approaching values that result in fracture.[42,43]

Mechanism of Injury

Ruptures of the quadriceps tendon or the patellar tendon typically occur through indirect forces across the knee.[42] Fractures of the patella may occur through direct or indirect forces, with the type of force leading to predictable fracture patterns.[42,43] Direct forces refer to a direct blow to the anterior knee, often resulting from a fall or a dashboard injury. This mechanism causes the patella to fail in compression as it is driven into the distal femur, resulting in comminuted or stellate fracture patterns. Although more than one half of these fractures will be nondisplaced with the extensor mechanism remaining intact, substantial chondral damage or osteochondral fractures may occur. The quadriceps tendon, the patellar tendon, or the patella more commonly fail in tension as indirect force across the knee joint results in either failure of the patella (as a result of the pull of the extensor mechanism) or failure at the superior or inferior bone-tendon junction.[41] Typically, this occurs from rapid knee flexion against a fully contracted quadriceps tendon. The force often continues beyond the quadriceps tendon, the patella, or the patellar tendon, extending transversely through the retinaculum to result in displacement and loss of active knee extension.

History and Physical Examination

The evaluation of a patient with knee pain who cannot perform a straight leg raise should begin with a detailed history and physical examination. The diagnostic triad, which is composed of pain, an inability to actively extend the knee, and a gap usually is present. A history of a direct blow to the knee or eccentric loading should raise suspicion for a patellar fracture or other extensor mechanism injury. Patients who are older than 40 years are at risk for a rupture of the quadriceps tendon, and those who are younger than 40 years are at risk for a patellar tendon rupture. Associated injuries, such as femoral neck fractures, posterior wall acetabular fractures, and knee dislocations, should be suspected in association with high-energy dashboard mechanisms. Additional soft-tissue injuries may include the cruciates and the menisci.

A knee examination begins with inspection of the soft-tissue envelope. Suspected open injuries are best evaluated with a saline load test performed with 150 mL of sterile saline.[44] In closed extensor mechanism injuries, further inspection and palpation will often reveal a hemarthrosis, pain with palpation, and a palpable defect. The continuity of the extensor mechanism can be evaluated with a straight leg raise. If pain is present, aspiration of the hemarthrosis and injection of local anesthetic may allow patients to attempt this maneuver. An inability to perform a straight leg raise or maintain an extended position with the leg is indicative of an extensor mechanism injury. Patients may be able to perform a partial straight leg raise but still have an extensor lag as a result of injury to the extensor mechanism with an intact retinaculum. An extensor lag exceeding 5° to 10° may affect clinical outcomes.

Both the quadriceps tendon and the patellar tendon can sustain and maintain their integrity despite supraphysiologic loads. As such, rupture of the quadriceps tendon or the patellar tendon requires a weakened tendon. Therefore, aside from indirect loading, other factors may make the tendon susceptible to rupture. In fact, approximately one third of patients presenting with bilateral spontaneous quadriceps rupture and 20% of those with unilateral quadriceps tendon rupture have a systemic medical condition that may accelerate degeneration of the healthy tendon. Nearly 90% of patients with patellar tendon ruptures have an underlying metabolic abnormality affecting their tendon.[45]

Imaging

Standard AP and lateral views of the knee should be obtained. Because of superimposition of the patella on the femoral condyles, the AP view may be difficult to interpret. A lateral radiograph is useful in the setting of transverse fracture patterns to assess displacement and articular congruity. In soft-tissue injuries of the knee, the lateral view may show patella alta or patella baja, indicating a patellar tendon or quadriceps tendon rupture, respectively. Axial radiographs are of limited utility with the exception of visualizing vertical fracture patterns of the patella. Advanced imaging techniques such as arthrography, CT, MRI, and bone scans are rarely indicated for isolated acute patellar fractures. CT may be helpful in defining fracture fragments in a comminuted or stellate pattern, but the significance in influencing preoperative plans or treatment has not been shown. For soft-tissue extensor mechanism injuries, MRI can confirm a complete versus partial tendon rupture. Routine use of MRI for the diagnosis of extensor mechanism injuries is not recommended because that clinical examination and history are specific.[45] More recently, ultrasound has been used to assess both the quadriceps and patellar tendons; however, the use of ultrasound is highly dependent on technician skill as well as the radiologist's interpretation of the imaging.

Classification

Patellar fractures may be classified as displaced (step-off less than 2 to 3 mm and fracture gap less than 1 to 4 mm) or nondisplaced, which often dictates treatment. However, more commonly, fractures of the patella are classified descriptively according to the fracture pattern, which may offer some information regarding mechanism but does not direct treatment. The OTA classification system is based on the degree of articular involvement and the number of fracture fragments; however, the clinical utility of this classification remains uncertain.[15]

Treatment

The goals of treatment include restoration of the extensor mechanism (the ability to do a straight leg raise). When patellar fractures are present, articular congruency should be maintained, and every effort should be made to preserve as much patellar bone as possible.

Nonsurgical Treatment

Nonsurgical treatment is indicated in patients who have an intact extensor mechanism as defined by the ability to perform or maintain a straight leg raise. In patients with a fracture of the patella, nonsurgical treatment should be considered with a clinically intact extensor mechanism and minimal step-off (less than 2 to 3 mm) and/or fracture displacement (less than 1 to 4 mm). Two different treatment regimens are associated with successful results. One study retrospectively reviewed 40 nonsurgically treated patients with intact extensor mechanisms. Patients were treated with a long leg splint for several days, followed by partial weight bearing and physiotherapy. Using this protocol, 80% of the patients were pain free, and 90% had full range of motion at an average follow-up of 30.5 months.[46] In a large series, patients with an intact extensor mechanism, less than 3 mm of articular step-off, and less than 4 mm of fracture widening were treated with plaster immobilization for a mean of 4 weeks.[47] Good or excellent outcomes were reported in 98% of the fractures (210/212) at a mean of 9 years of follow-up. Current protocols use early weight bearing as tolerated and straight leg raises in a hinged knee brace locked in extension, with active and active-assisted range of motion beginning at 1 to 2 weeks and resistance exercises added at 6 weeks. Radiographs are obtained 1 week after motion is allowed to evaluate for displacement.

Surgical Treatment of Quadriceps and Patellar Tendon Ruptures

An incompetent extensor mechanism is the most common indication for surgery. Surgery should be performed within 2 weeks to limit retraction or fibrous degenerative changes of the tendon. The tendon can be exposed through many incisions; however, a longitudinal midline extensile incision centered over the tendon is preferred, with full medial and lateral flaps for access to the tendon, the patella, and the retinaculum. Midsubstance ruptures can be treated with an end-to-end primary repair if sufficient tendon exists proximally and distally. Ruptures at or near the osseotendinous junction, the most common site of injury, may be repaired through drill holes in the patella. Two heavy, nonabsorbable sutures are placed in a locked, running (Krakow or Bunnell) arrangement through the end of the tendon, leaving four loose strands free at the distal stump. The superior or inferior pole of the patella is débrided, and the anatomic insertion of the tendon is roughened to obtain a fresh cancellous bed that will allow tendon-to-bone healing. Three 2-mm drill holes are made parallel to each other and the longitudinal axis of the patella. Using a Keith needle, a Beath pin, or a Hewson suture passer, the free ends of the sutures are passed through the holes and tied with the knee in full extension. Suture anchors have been used in place of drill holes, with good results. The retinacular sutures are tied, although some surgeons prefer to leave the lateral retinaculum open to function as a release. The knee is taken through a 0° to 90° range of motion to ensure proper patellar tracking and observe tension on the repair. Augmentation usually is not necessary but may be done with wire or Mersilene tape if the repair appears to be tenuous.

Neglected or chronic rupture of the quadriceps and patellar tendons presents a difficult problem in terms of reconstruction. The reported results of delayed surgical management (longer than 6 weeks) are generally less satisfactory than results after the treatment of acute tears. When the tendon ends can be approximated, repair may be done as described for acute tears. However, a large defect between the two ends of the tendon may occur, preventing tendon apposition. Augmentation with allograft or autograft tendon may be necessary, along with possible advancement of the tendon; however, the results from delayed treatment are inferior to those associated with acute management regardless of salvage technique.

Surgical Treatment of Patellar Fractures

Patellar fractures with an incompetent extensor mechanism require fixation. In some cases, despite active knee extension, fracture separation exceeding 1 to 4 mm or step-off more than 2 to 3 mm may be relative indications for surgical treatment. Residual fracture displacement of 1 mm or more is associated with thigh atrophy and pain. Additional surgical indications include intra-articular loose bodies and osteochondral fractures.

Open Reduction and Internal Fixation

ORIF is the preferred method of treatment of nearly all displaced patellar fractures. The techniques and the materials used for patellar fixation have evolved significantly; however, the goals of restoration of normal anatomy and extensor function remain.

Similar to quadriceps and patellar tendon ruptures, patellar fractures can be exposed through several types of incisions, but a longitudinal midline extensile incision centered over the patella is preferred. For transverse fracture treatment, full-thickness medial and lateral flaps allow access to retinacular tears, and reduction of the joint surface is confirmed with palpation. One group of investigators advocated a lateral parapatellar arthrotomy with internal rotation of the patella to 90° for direct visual reduction of comminuted fractures.[48] Transverse incisions generally should be avoided because they compromise approaches for future knee procedures.

Tension band wiring commonly has been used for the treatment of patellar fractures and works by converting the anterior tension forces produced by the extensor mechanism and knee flexion into compression forces at the articular surface. Numerous techniques have been described. Early techniques such as the standard tension band and the modified anterior tension band (MATB) were modified so that the MATB used longitudinal Kirschner wires (K-wires) and 18-gauge stainless steel wire in a figure-of-8 pattern looped over the anterior patella. This construct traditionally has been the most widely accepted method of fixation for transverse and comminuted patellar fractures. Over the years, many of these techniques underwent biomechanical testing. Magnusson wiring and MATB wiring permitted less fracture fragment separation than circumferential wiring or standard tension band wiring in a cadaver model.[49] Repair of the retinacular defect was found to contribute to the overall stability of the construct. With the addition of a cerclage wire to the MATB, increased compressive strain was shown in a transverse fracture model.[50] In a cadaver model, it was demonstrated that screw fixation alone was adequate for the treatment of transverse fractures with good

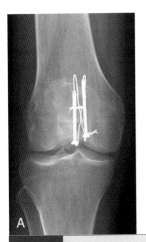 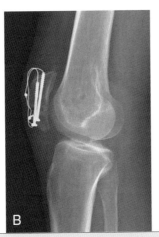 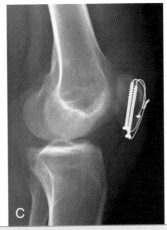 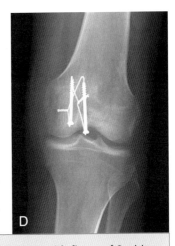

Figure 6 AP (**A**) and lateral (**B**) knee radiographs of an attempted modified tension band technique with figure-of-8 wiring. Numerous technical deficiencies are noted, including screws placed too close together in the coronal plane and not parallel to the joint in the sagittal plane. Each wire is not apposed to bone. Lateral (**C**) and AP (**D**) knee radiographs depicting appropriate fixation using the modified anterior tension band technique.

bone stock; however, the MATB performed better for fractures with comminution or osteopenia.[50] In addition, it was found that simple wiring techniques, such as the Magnusson and Lotke longitudinal anterior band techniques, may not allow sufficient fixation for early activity.

Screws (instead of longitudinal K-wires) in the MATB construct lead to improved biomechanical performance. Screws provide increased rigidity over K-wires throughout knee range of motion and also provide resistance against tensile loading when the knee is in full extension. One study used a cadaver model to show that the MATB technique with cancellous screws performed better than the MATB technique with K-wires.[51] However, in the clinical setting, it is often difficult to place the tension band wires around the tips and heads of screws. A revised method in which a figure-of-8 tension band wire is passed through parallel cannulated screws was devised to circumvent this difficulty (**Figure 6**). A second study that used a cadaver fracture model found that tension band wiring through parallel 4.0-mm cannulated lag screws leads to improved stability over all previous techniques.[52]

Alternative Tension Band Techniques and Materials

Because of the difficulty in manipulating stainless steel wire and revision surgery rates secondary to painful hardware or wire migration, techniques using wire alternatives have been investigated. One study compared 1-mm stainless steel wire to 1-mm stainless steel braided cable fastened with a crimping tool in cadaveric specimens.[53] For noncomminuted, transverse fractures, braided cable was superior to monofilament wire and performed more predictably in cyclic loading.[53] Series also have been reported using minifragment plates to augment fixation of comminuted patellar fractures, and use of this technique is increasing as a primary fixation method.[54]

Partial Patellectomy and the Treatment of Inferior Pole Fractures

A partial patellectomy was developed as an alternative to total patellectomy and has been described in the treatment of various fracture patterns.[48,55,56] Through retention of a portion of the patella, partial patellectomy is thought to preserve some of the patellar moment arm and improve strength. One study reported the results of 40 patients with displaced transverse or comminuted fractures treated with a partial patellectomy and reapproximation of the patellar tendon or the quadriceps tendon to the articular edge of the remaining patella.[55] At an average of 8.4 years, good or excellent results were experienced by 78% of the patients, and mean quadriceps tendon strength of the contralateral extremity was 85%.[55] It was concluded that a partial patellectomy can be an effective treatment for selected patellar fractures. Another study found that poor outcomes could be expected with partial patellectomy involving more than 40% of the patella.[48] A cadaver study conducted 12 years later evaluated the effect of patellectomy size and the location of tendon reattachment on patellofemoral contact patterns and stresses.[56] It was demonstrated that patellofemoral contact stress increased as the size of the discarded portion of the patella increased.

A partial patellectomy is indicated most often for the treatment of comminuted fractures of the inferior patellar pole. Some fractures involving the inferior pole may be effectively treated as patellar tendon avulsions with fragment excision and tendon reattachment via suture and transosseous tunnels or suture anchors. Cerclage reinforcement of the repair with a heavy suture or wire passed through the quadriceps tendon and a tibial tubercle bone tunnel also has been described.[45] Newer methods of fracture fixation have been described in an effort to preserve patellar bone and allow for early range of motion.[57]

4: Lower Extremity

Total Patellectomy

As knowledge of knee biomechanics improves and internal fixation techniques are refined, the indications for total patellectomy have diminished. A total patellectomy may result in upwards of a 49% decrease in quadriceps strength. In addition, few excellent clinical outcomes have been observed with total patellectomy. As a result, every attempt to retain all, or even a portion, of the patella should be made. Total patellectomy may be indicated in rare cases of failed internal fixation, infection, tumor, or patellofemoral arthritis. When total patellectomy is performed, consideration should be given to advancement of the vastus medialis obliquus over a longitudinally closed defect because this technique has demonstrated improved strength and outcomes compared with a standard total patellectomy.[48,55]

Postoperative Rehabilitation

After repair, the knee is placed into a knee immobilizer for 48 hours, after which the wound is checked and drains (if used) are discontinued. Isometric quadriceps- and hamstring-strengthening exercises begin nearly immediately after surgery. Active flexion and passive extension of the knee are initiated 2 weeks after surgery, starting at 0 to 45° and advancing 30° per week. Active knee extension is permitted at 3 weeks after surgery. Toe-touch weight bearing is initiated immediately after surgery and is advanced to full weight bearing without crutches within 2 weeks. Early range of motion should be employed; however, no difference in range of motion was found between early range of motion and immobilization in a study of 53 ruptures.[57] The brace is removed after 6 weeks or when the patient has good quadriceps muscle control and can perform a straight leg raise. Good range of motion should be achieved by 12 to 16 weeks after repair or fixation.

Outcomes

Most patients who undergo primary repair or fixation of soft-tissue extensor mechanism injuries in a timely fashion achieve nearly full return of knee motion and quadriceps tendon strength. Persistent quadriceps tendon atrophy commonly occurs but tends not to affect the return of strength. The only factor that appears to correlate with clinical outcome is the timing of the repair.

However, outcomes after patellar fracture fixation do not mimic those experienced after soft-tissue repairs. One series reported that Knee Injury and Osteoarthritis Outcome scores for patellar fractures were significantly lower than for normalized knees.[57] In addition, more than 50% of the patients in this series required hardware removal, had significant difficulty achieving full range of motion, and experienced limitations in maximal strength.[57]

The treatment of extensor mechanism injuries is associated with complications inherent to the injury and specific to the treatment. Symptomatic hardware problems are among the most frequently encountered complications in patellar fracture treatment, with reported rates ranging between 0 and 60%, which often necessitates hardware removal.[58,59] Hardware failure occurs infrequently. However, wire migration into the popliteal fossa and the right ventricle has been reported secondary to late hardware failure.[58]

Knee stiffness is known to complicate extensor mechanism injuries.[59] Many authors advocate early range of motion; however, this has not been proven to mitigate this complication. Others report immobilization duration does not affect stiffness, and the cause of stiffness remains unclear. Significant knee extensor weakness has been observed with total or partial patellectomy. Nonunion appears to be quite rare in the modern treatment of closed fractures; most recent series report a nonunion rate of 1% or lower.[57,58] Deep infection in the treatment of extensor mechanism injuries occurs rarely (0 to 5%). The rates of radiographic osteoarthritis are rarely reported in the literature. Although extensor mechanism injuries have been associated with increased rates of patellofemoral osteoarthritis, the correlation to type of injury and fixation strategy has not been defined.

Summary

Injuries about the knee, including fracture of the tibial plateau and disruption of the extensor mechanism, can have a dramatic effect on lower extremity function. Restoration of the articular congruity and alignment after tibial plateau fractures is essential. Furthermore, assessment of the soft tissue is critical to prevent complications such as instability, vascular injury, or compartment syndrome. Having an intact extensor mechanism is essential for knee function, with particular attention to active knee extension. Restoration of the quadriceps tendon or the patellar tendon with early primary repair is critical. Similarly, adequate fixation of the patella is essential to allow for bony healing in the presence of a fracture. Although patients may develop hardware-related complications or posttraumatic arthritis, physical therapy will often help restore range of motion and function to the limb.

Key Study Points

- Maintaining alignment with respect to varus and valgus and restoration of the articular surface are critical in the management of tibial plateau fractures, particularly bicondylar injuries.

- Soft-tissue injuries are common in combination with tibial plateau fractures, with particular attention on the menisci, ligaments, and vascular structures.

- Extensor mechanism injuries resulting in loss of active extension should be treated surgically in nearly every clinical scenario to restore function.

Annotated References

1. Stannard JP, Lopez R, Volgas D: Soft tissue injury of the knee after tibial plateau fractures. *J Knee Surg* 2010; 23(4):187-192.

   Knee MRI was used to evaluate 103 patients with tibial plateau fractures attributable to high-energy mechanisms. Seventy-three patients had torn at least one major ligament group, and 55 patients tore multiple ligaments. Level of evidence: II.

2. Barei DP, Nork SE, Mills WJ, Coles CP, Henley MB, Benirschke SK: Functional outcomes of severe bicondylar tibial plateau fractures treated with dual incisions and medial and lateral plates. *J Bone Joint Surg Am* 2006;88(8):1713-1721.

3. Ringus VM, Lemley FR, Hubbard DF, Wearden S, Jones DL: Lateral tibial plateau fracture depression as a predictor of lateral meniscus pathology. *Orthopedics* 2010;33(2):80-84.

   Eighty-five patients who sustained a lateral tibial plateau fracture and underwent ORIF were reviewed. Patients with at least 10 mm of depression had an eightfold increased risk for a lateral meniscus tear compared with those with less than 10 mm of depression. Patients younger than 48 years had a fourfold increased risk for a lateral meniscus tear. Level of evidence: IV.

4. Gardner MJ, Yacoubian S, Geller D, et al: Prediction of soft-tissue injuries in Schatzker II tibial plateau fractures based on measurements of plain radiographs. *J Trauma* 2006;60(2):319-324.

5. Marsh JL, Smith ST, Do TT: External fixation and limited internal fixation for complex fractures of the tibial plateau. *J Bone Joint Surg Am* 1995;77(5):661-673.

6. Abdel-Hamid MZ, Chang CH, Chan YS, et al: Arthroscopic evaluation of soft tissue injuries in tibial plateau fractures: Retrospective analysis of 98 cases. *Arthroscopy* 2006;22(6):669-675.

7. Shepherd L, Abdollahi K, Lee J, Vangsness CT Jr: The prevalence of soft tissue injuries in nonoperative tibial plateau fractures as determined by magnetic resonance imaging. *J Orthop Trauma* 2002;16(9):628-631.

8. Gardner MJ, Yacoubian S, Geller D, et al: The incidence of soft tissue injury in operative tibial plateau fractures: A magnetic resonance imaging analysis of 103 patients. *J Orthop Trauma* 2005;19(2):79-84.

9. Chang YH, Tu YK, Yeh WL, Hsu RW: Tibial plateau fracture with compartment syndrome: A complication of higher incidence in Taiwan. *Chang Gung Med J* 2000;23(3):149-155.

10. Crist BD, Della Rocca GJ, Stannard JP: Compartment syndrome surgical management techniques associated with tibial plateau fractures. *J Knee Surg* 2010; 23(1):3-7.

    This technique article discusses one- and two-incision fasciotomy surgical techniques and the surgical decision making and technique modifications to use when there is an associated tibial plateau fracture. Level of evidence: IV.

11. Levy BA, Zlowodzki MP, Graves M, Cole PA: Screening for extremity arterial injury with the arterial pressure index. *Am J Emerg Med* 2005;23(5):689-695.

12. Chan PS, Klimkiewicz JJ, Luchetti WT, et al: Impact of CT scan on treatment plan and fracture classification of tibial plateau fractures. *J Orthop Trauma* 1997;11(7): 484-489.

13. Yacoubian SV, Nevins RT, Sallis JG, Potter HG, Lorich DG: Impact of MRI on treatment plan and fracture classification of tibial plateau fractures. *J Orthop Trauma* 2002;16(9):632-637.

14. Schatzker J, McBroom R, Bruce D: The tibial plateau fracture: The Toronto experience 1968-1975. *Clin Orthop Relat Res* 1979;138:94-104.

15. Marsh JL, Slongo TF, Agel J, et al: Fracture and dislocation classification compendium—2007: Orthopaedic Trauma Association classification, database and outcomes committee. *J Orthop Trauma* 2007;21(suppl 10): S1-S133.

16. Egol KA, Tejwani NC, Capla EL, Wolinsky PL, Koval KJ: Staged management of high-energy proximal tibia fractures (OTA types 41): The results of a prospective, standardized protocol. *J Orthop Trauma* 2005;19(7): 448-456.

17. Ehlinger M, Rahme M, Moor BK, et al: Reliability of locked plating in tibial plateau fractures with a medial component. *Orthop Traumatol Surg Res* 2012;98(2): 173-179.

    Twenty patients were managed for tibial plateau fractures with a medial component with a single lateral anatomically contoured locking compression plate with or without additional isolated screws. A single lateral locked plate ensured the stable reduction of tibial plateau fractures with a medial component. Level of evidence: IV.

18. Bajammal SS, Zlowodzki M, Lelwica A, et al: The use of calcium phosphate bone cement in fracture treatment: A meta-analysis of randomized trials. *J Bone Joint Surg Am* 2008;90(6):1186-1196.

19. Russell TA, Leighton RK; Alpha-BSM Tibial Plateau Fracture Study Group: Comparison of autogenous bone graft and endothermic calcium phosphate cement for defect augmentation in tibial plateau fractures: A multicenter, prospective, randomized study. *J Bone Joint Surg Am* 2008;90(10):2057-2061.

20. Fakler JK, Ryzewicz M, Hartshorn C, Morgan SJ, Stahel PF, Smith WR: Optimizing the management of Moore type I postero-medial split fracture dislocations

4: Lower Extremity

of the tibial head: Description of the Lobenhoffer approach. *J Orthop Trauma* 2007;21(5):330-336.

21. Carlson DA: Posterior bicondylar tibial plateau fractures. *J Orthop Trauma* 2005;19(2):73-78.

22. Streubel PN, Glasgow D, Wong A, Barei DP, Ricci WM, Gardner MJ: Sagittal plane deformity in bicondylar tibial plateau fractures. *J Orthop Trauma* 2011;25(9):560-565.

    Considerable sagittal plane deformity exists in the majority of bicondylar tibial plateau fractures. The lateral plateau has a higher propensity for sagittal angulation and tends to have increased posterior slope. The identification of this deformity allows for accurate preoperative planning and specific reduction maneuvers to restore anatomic alignment. Level of evidence: III.

23. Ricci WM, Rudzki JR, Borrelli J Jr: Treatment of complex proximal tibia fractures with the less invasive skeletal stabilization system. *J Orthop Trauma* 2004;18(8):521-527.

24. Barei DP, Nork SE, Mills WJ, Henley MB, Benirschke SK: Complications associated with internal fixation of high-energy bicondylar tibial plateau fractures utilizing a two-incision technique. *J Orthop Trauma* 2004;18(10):649-657.

25. Higgins TF, Klatt J, Bachus KN: Biomechanical analysis of bicondylar tibial plateau fixation: How does lateral locking plate fixation compare to dual plate fixation? *J Orthop Trauma* 2007;21(5):301-306.

26. Lindvall E, Sanders R, Dipasquale T, Herscovici D, Haidukewych G, Sagi C: Intramedullary nailing versus percutaneous locked plating of extra-articular proximal tibial fractures: Comparison of 56 cases. *J Orthop Trauma* 2009;23(7):485-492.

27. Nork SE, Barei DB, Schrick JL: Intramedullary nailing of proximal quarter tibia fractures. *Orthopaedic Trauma Association Annual Meeting Proceedings*. October 12, 2002, pp 161-162.

28. Ricci WM, O'Boyle M, Borrelli J, Bellabarba C, Sanders R: Fractures of the proximal third of the tibial shaft treated with intramedullary nails and blocking screws. *J Orthop Trauma* 2001;15(4):264-270.

29. Tornetta P III, Collins E: Semiextended position of intramedullary nailing of the proximal tibia. *Clin Orthop Relat Res* 1996;328:185-189.

30. Canadian Orthopaedic Trauma Society: Open reduction and internal fixation compared with circular fixator application for bicondylar tibial plateau fractures: Results of a multicenter, prospective, randomized clinical trial. *J Bone Joint Surg Am* 2006;88(12):2613-2623.

31. Katsenis D, Dendrinos G, Kouris A, Savas N, Schoinochoritis N, Pogiatzis K: Combination of fine wire fixation and limited internal fixation for high-energy tibial plateau fractures: Functional results at minimum 5-year follow-up. *J Orthop Trauma* 2009;23(7):493-501.

32. Hutson JJ Jr, Zych GA: Infections in periarticular fractures of the lower extremity treated with tensioned wire hybrid fixators. *J Orthop Trauma* 1998;12(3):214-218.

33. Hyman J, Moore T: Anatomy of the distal knee joint and pyarthrosis following external fixation. *J Orthop Trauma* 1999;13(4):241-246.

34. DeCoster TA, Crawford MK, Kraut MA: Safe extracapsular placement of proximal tibia transfixation pins. *J Orthop Trauma* 1999;13(4):236-240.

35. Honkonen SE: Degenerative arthritis after tibial plateau fractures. *J Orthop Trauma* 1995;9(4):273-277.

36. Rademakers MV, Kerkhoffs GM, Sierevelt IN, Raaymakers EL, Marti RK: Operative treatment of 109 tibial plateau fractures: Five- to 27-year follow-up results. *J Orthop Trauma* 2007;21(1):5-10.

37. Ali AM, El-Shafie M, Willett KM: Failure of fixation of tibial plateau fractures. *J Orthop Trauma* 2002;16(5):323-329.

38. Weaver MJ, Harris MB, Strom AC, et al: Fracture pattern and fixation type related to loss of reduction in bicondylar tibial plateau fractures. *Injury* 2012;43(6):864-869.

    When lateral locked plating was used in the presence of a medial coronal fracture line, there was a significantly higher rate of subsidence (median 2.0°) compared with use in patients with no medial fracture line ($P = 0.002$). Patients with coronal fracture lines treated with dual plating had significantly less loss of reduction than those treated with lateral locked plating ($P = 0.01$). Level of evidence: III.

39. Young MJ, Barrack RL: Complications of internal fixation of tibial plateau fractures. *Orthop Rev* 1994;23(2):149-154.

40. Zura RD, Adams SB Jr, Jeray KJ, et al: Timing of definitive fixation of severe tibial plateau fractures with compartment syndrome does not have an effect on the rate of infection. *J Trauma* 2010;69(6):1523-1526.

    This study demonstrated no statistical difference in the rate of infection when tibial plateau fractures with four-compartment fasciotomies were treated with ORIF before fasciotomy closure, at fasciotomy closure, or after fasciotomy closure. Level of evidence: IV.

41. Kaufer H: Mechanical function of the patella. *J Bone Joint Surg Am* 1971;53(8):1551-1560.

42. Huberti HH, Hayes WC, Stone JL, Shybut GT: Force ratios in the quadriceps tendon and ligamentum patellae. *J Orthop Res* 1984;2(1):49-54.

43. Carpenter JE, Kasman R, Matthews LS: Fractures of the patella. *Instr Course Lect* 1994;43:97-108.

44. Nord RM, Quach T, Walsh M, Pereira D, Tejwani NC: Detection of traumatic arthrotomy of the knee using the saline solution load test. *J Bone Joint Surg Am* 2009; 91(1):66-70.

45. Matava MJ: Patellar tendon ruptures. *J Am Acad Orthop Surg* 1996;4(6):287-296.

46. Braun W, Wiedemann M, Rüter A, Kundel K, Kolbinger S: Indications and results of nonoperative treatment of patellar fractures. *Clin Orthop Relat Res* 1993;289: 197-201.

47. Boström A: Fracture of the patella: A study of 422 patellar fractures. *Acta Orthop Scand Suppl* 1972;143: 1-80.

48. Böstman O, Kiviluoto O, Nirhamo J: Comminuted displaced fractures of the patella. *Injury* 1981;13(3): 196-202.

49. Weber MJ, Janecki CJ, McLeod P, Nelson CL, Thompson JA: Efficacy of various forms of fixation of transverse fractures of the patella. *J Bone Joint Surg Am* 1980;62(2):215-220.

50. Benjamin J, Bried J, Dohm M, McMurtry M: Biomechanical evaluation of various forms of fixation of transverse patellar fractures. *J Orthop Trauma* 1987; 1(3):219-222.

51. Burvant JG, Thomas KA, Alexander R, Harris MB: Evaluation of methods of internal fixation of transverse patella fractures: A biomechanical study. *J Orthop Trauma* 1994;8(2):147-153.

52. Carpenter JE, Kasman RA, Patel N, Lee ML, Goldstein SA: Biomechanical evaluation of current patella fracture fixation techniques. *J Orthop Trauma* 1997;11(5): 351-356.

53. Scilaris TA, Grantham JL, Prayson MJ, Marshall MP, Hamilton JJ, Williams JL: Biomechanical comparison of fixation methods in transverse patella fractures. *J Orthop Trauma* 1998;12(5):356-359.

54. Matejcić A, Puljiz Z, Elabjer E, Bekavac-Beslin M, Ledinsky M: Multifragment fracture of the patellar apex: Basket plate osteosynthesis compared with partial patellectomy. *Arch Orthop Trauma Surg* 2008;128(4): 403-408.

55. Tang SC: Results of treatment of displaced patellar fractures by partial patellectomy. *J Bone Joint Surg Am* 1991;73(8):1273-1274.

56. Marder RA, Swanson TV, Sharkey NA, Duwelius PJ: Effects of partial patellectomy and reattachment of the patellar tendon on patellofemoral contact areas and pressures. *J Bone Joint Surg Am* 1993;75(1):35-45.

57. LeBrun CT, Langford JR, Sagi HC: Functional outcomes after operatively treated patella fractures. *J Orthop Trauma* 2012;26(7):422-426.

    In the largest series examining the outcomes of patients after the fixation of patellar fractures, the authors report significant deficits in knee outcome scores, range of motion, and strength in the leg. Hardware removal rates are at least 50% of higher. Level of evidence: IV.

58. Biddau F, Fioriti M, Benelli G: Migration of a broken cerclage wire from the patella into the heart: A case report. *J Bone Joint Surg Am* 2006;88(9):2057-2059.

59. Smith ST, Cramer KE, Karges DE, Watson JT, Moed BR: Early complications in the operative treatment of patella fractures. *J Orthop Trauma* 1997;11(3): 183-187.

4: Lower Extremity

Chapter 38

Soft-Tissue Injuries About the Knee

Robin M. Gehrmann, MD   Guillem Gonzalez-Lomas, MD

Anterior Cruciate Ligament Injuries

In the United States, approximately 150,000 anterior cruciate ligament (ACL) injuries occur annually, making this injury one of the most common athletic knee injuries. The emotional, economic, and overall healthcare costs of ACL injuries warrant research on reconstruction and injury prevention.

Anatomy and Function

The primary function of the ACL is to prevent anterior translation of the tibia relative to the femur. It also plays a secondary role in controlling internal rotation of the tibia. Anatomically, the ACL consists of two bundles—anteromedial (AM) and posterolateral (PL)—which are named after their tibial insertions. The bundles are separated on the femur by a bony prominence known as the lateral bifurcate ridge (Figure 1).

The AM bundle is maximally taut between 45° and 60°, whereas the PL bundle is tight in extension.[1] The AM bundle appears to control anterior translation, whereas the PL bundle has an important role in rotatory stability and anterior motion.

Mechanism of Injury and Diagnosis

Injury to the ACL typically occurs as the result of a noncontact deceleration mechanism, which usually involves landing on a flat foot, often in valgus and hyperextension. The diagnosis of an ACL tear is made clinically by history and physical examination and can be confirmed with MRI. The Lachman and anterior drawer tests are more sensitive indicators of AP laxity, whereas the pivot-shift test is an indicator of rotatory instability.

Surgical Management

Anteroposterior stability after reconstruction has not always correlated with successful outcomes. After successful reconstructions, radiographic degenerative changes developed in 79% of patients.[2] In a meta-analysis of ACL reconstructions, approximately 33%

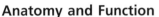

Video 38.1: Lachman and Anterior Drawer Test. Robin M. Gehrmann, MD (0.46 min)

Video 38.2: Pivot Shift. Robin M. Gehrmann, MD (0.44 min)

and 41% of the reconstructions were reported as normal based on International Knee Documentation Committee (IKDC) scores.[3]

These less-than-ideal outcomes have prompted further investigation into the importance of rotational stability in ACL reconstructions.

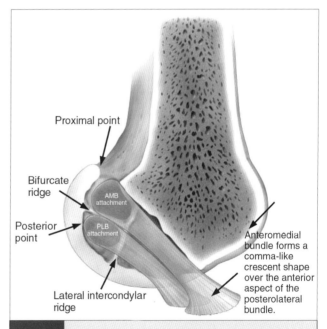

| Figure 1 | Illustration of a left lateral knee in extension showing the relationship between the anteromedial and posterolateral bundles (AMB, PLB) to pertinent bony landmarks. (Reproduced with permission from Ziegler C, Pietrini S, Westerhaus B, et al: Arthroscopically pertinent landmarks for tunnel positioning in single-bundle and double-bundle anterior cruciate ligament reconstructions. *Am J Sports Med* 2011;39:743-752.) |

4: Lower Extremity

Table 1

Relative Load to Failure of Various ACL Grafts

Graft Type	Relative Load to Failure
Native ACL	2160 N
10-mm bone-patellar tendon autograft	2977 N
Quadrupled hamstring tendon autograft	4090 N
Quadriceps tendon autograft	2352 N

ACL = anterior cruciate ligament.

Tunnel Placement

The concept of anatomic ACL reconstructions, applied to either single- or double-bundle reconstructions, has been proposed to improve kinematics in the postoperative knee. The term anatomic reconstruction refers to tunnel placement in the native femoral and tibial attachment sites of the ACL.[1] In a patient with a large anatomic footprint, this may be best achieved with a double-bundle reconstruction, whereas in smaller patients, an anatomically placed single bundle may achieve the same result. Arthroscopic transtibial techniques facilitate femoral tunnel drilling but limit the location of drilling on the lateral wall, often creating a more vertical graft with less rotational stability. To achieve more anatomic femoral tunnel positions, techniques such as medial portal drilling have been devised.

Although biomechanical evidence exists to suggest that double-bundle reconstructions result in better restoration of intact knee stability than nonanatomic single-bundle reconstructions, there is little evidence to confirm that this translates into clinical differences.[4] Similarly, there is no evidence that double-bundle reconstructions clinically outperform anatomic single-bundle reconstructions.[5]

Graft Choices

Another important factor in ACL reconstruction is the type of graft to use. Graft choices can be broadly classified as autograft and allograft tissue. Autograft options include hamstring tendon, bone-patellar tendon-bone, and quadriceps tendon. Relative loads to failure are described in Table 1. The gold standard for many years has been the patellar tendon autograft; clinical studies, however, have not found statistically significant differences in outcomes among these grafts.

Another increasingly popular graft choice is allograft tissue. Allografts allow for faster surgical procedures, less postoperative pain, no donor site morbidity, and more rapid return to activities of daily living. The disadvantages include the risk of disease transmission and, in some series, higher failure rates. In an in vivo sheep model, it was noted that recellularization and revascularization were significantly less in allograft versus autograft tissue. However, when irradiated and chemi-cally processed grafts were excluded, the failure rates were no longer significantly different between the autograft and allograft groups.[6] The authors concluded that slower rehabilitation earlier during the postoperative period might be preferable if an allograft is used, thus decreasing the potential failure rate.[7]

The Female Athlete and ACL Injuries

Over the past 30 years, there has been a significant increase in young women participating in sports at the high school and collegiate levels. Women currently have a fourfold to sixfold increased risk of ACL injury compared with their male counterparts. The reason for this difference is multifactorial. Various physiologic and anatomic factors, such as increased Q angle, valgus leg alignment, the hormonal influences of estrogen, the anatomic size of the ACL itself, notch width, and increased joint laxity have been implicated.[8] Sex-specific neuromuscular differences, which include an increased quadriceps-hamstrings ratio in females and landing patterns on a more extended knee with greater hip adduction moments, have also been cited. This latter group of differences has been the focus of ACL injury prevention programs, which have demonstrated success in reducing the incidence of ACL injury in female athletes.[8]

Medial-Sided Knee Injuries

Anatomy and Function

The medial knee ligaments are the most frequently injured knee ligaments, with a reported incidence of 24 per 100,000 per year in the United States.[9,10] The major functional medial-sided ligamentous structures include the superficial medial collateral ligament (MCL), the posterior oblique ligament (POL), and the deep MCL (Figure 2). The superficial MCL is the primary restraint to valgus at 30°. The POL resists valgus and external rotation with the knee between 0 and 30° of flexion.[11]

Imaging

Valgus stress radiographs can help quantify the medial joint line opening.[12] MRI can identify torn ligaments, with an accuracy of close to 90%. Trabecular bone bruises, typically in the lateral compartment, have been found in up to 45% of patients with MCL injuries.[13]

Prophylactic Bracing

Prophylactic brace use in athletics is controversial. Although biomechanical data[14] have demonstrated that most braces provide 20% to 30% increased MCL strain relief, their use may affect performance.[15]

Nonsurgical Treatment

The rich blood supply to the MCL and its extrasynovial location allow grade I and II injuries to respond fairly reliably to nonsurgical treatment that includes early controlled motion and protected weight bearing. Long-term immobilization is detrimental to collagen integrity and

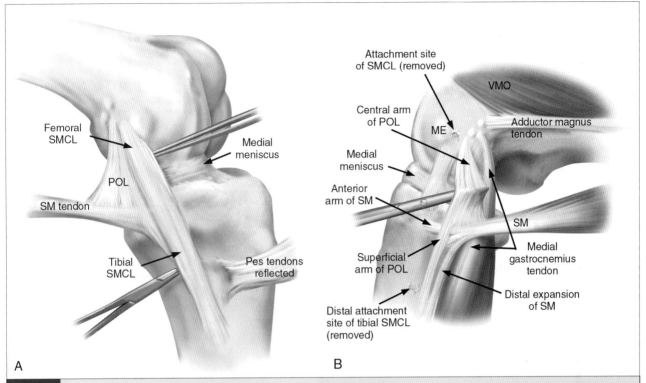

A   B

Figure 2	The major medial-sided structures include the superficial medial collateral ligament (SMCL), the posterior oblique ligament (POL), and the deep medial collateral ligament. ME = medial epicondyle; SM = semimembranosus; VMO = vastus medialis obliquus muscle. (Reproduced with permission from LaPrade RF, Engebretsen AH, Ly TV, Johansen S, Wentorf FA, Engbretsen L: The anatomy of the medial part of the knee. *J Bone Joint Surg Am* 2007;89[9]:2000-2010.)

should be avoided. Rupture at either attachment site may take longer to heal than a midsubstance tear.[16] Although nonsurgical treatment of grade I and II injuries has been validated, treatment of isolated grade III injuries remains controversial. Several studies have demonstrated good results and return to previous level of activity with non-surgical treatment.[17] Nevertheless, several investigators have pointed out residual laxity and an increased risk of osteoarthritis in nonsurgically treated, isolated MCL injuries.[18,19] Indications for acute repair or reconstruction of grade III tears include superficial MCL avulsions off the tibia with interposed pes anserinus tendons (similar to a Stener lesion), residual pain and instability after non-surgical treatment, and multiligament knee injuries, specifically ACL/MCL injuries.

Surgical Treatment

Surgical treatment options include direct repair of the injured structures, primary repair with augmentation, and reconstruction of either the superficial MCL and POL or the superficial MCL alone (**Figure 3**). In patients with chronic injuries, reconstruction has been shown to more reliably restore stability. Posteromedial capsular shift also should be considered in cases of chronic POL deficiency. Biomechanical studies have shown that combined superficial MCL/POL reconstructions restore knee stability most closely to normal values, but these findings still lack clinical validation.[20,21]

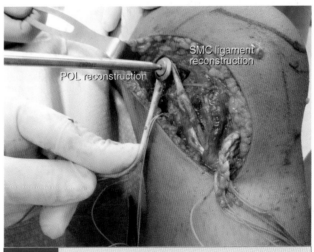

Figure 3	Clinical photograph showing medial collateral ligament (MCL) reconstruction of both the superficial MCL and the posterior oblique ligament (POL) using semitendinosus (ST) autograft. The superficial MCL arm has been created by leaving the ST attached to the pes insertion. The ST is then secured to the medial epicondyle with a post and washer, with the knee in valgus at 30° flexion. The POL arm will be then secured to the proximal posterior tibia (at the semimembranosus insertion) with another post and washer.

4: Lower Extremity

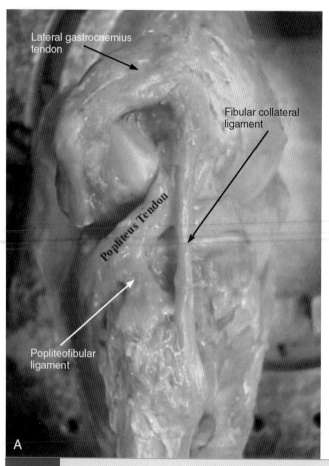

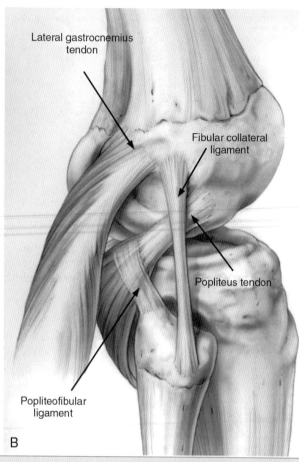

Figure 4   Photograph (**A**) and illustration (**B**) demonstrating the isolated fibular collateral ligament and the gastrocnemius tendon (lateral view). (Adapted with permission from LaPrade R, Thuan V, Wentorf F, Engebratson L: The posterolateral attachments of the knee. *Am J Sports Med* 2003;31[6]:854-860.)

Combined ACL and MCL Injuries

Biomechanical data suggest that there are increased forces across an ACL graft in an MCL-deficient knee.[10] Clinically, patients with combined injury who undergo ACL reconstruction alone have greater laxity.[22,23] One protocol for the management of these combined injuries consists of preoperative rehabilitation to restore range of motion and strength while the MCL is given a chance to heal. Any residual intraoperative valgus laxity at the time of ACL reconstruction is addressed at that time.

Lateral-Sided Knee Injuries

Anatomy and Function

The complex anatomy of the lateral side of the knee has been the object of study for decades. The role of the posterolateral corner (PLC) is to resist varus, external tibial rotation, and posterior tibial translation. Although the PLC has many components, restoration of varus and external rotation stability ultimately depends on the integrity of four main structures: the fibular collateral ligament (FCL), the popliteus tendon, the popliteofibular ligament, and the lateral capsule (Figure 4).

Diagnosis

Because of the intricate anatomy and function of the lateral knee structures, injuries can be missed if the knee is not carefully examined. Signs of injury can be identified manually by physical examination, with the use of stress radiography, and on arthroscopic inspection. On physical examination, asymmetric varus stress testing in 30° is indicative of a lateral collateral ligament injury. Rotational assessment is done using the dial test and the posterolateral drawer test.

 Video 38.3: Posterolateral Drawer Test. Robin M. Gehrmann, MD (0.35 min)

External rotation recurvatum testing that is positive and demonstrates a hyperextension deformity indicates severe injury to the posterior capsule in addition to the PLC structures. In cases of acute injuries, patients may guard the extremity too much to make these physical examination tests meaningful. Examination under anesthesia in these patients can help determine the severity of instability as well as the clinical significance of associated MRI findings.

Video 38.4: Posterior Cruciate Ligament, Lateral Collateral Ligament, and Posterolateral Corner Examination. Robin M. Gehrmann, MD (0.43 min)

Varus stress radiographs that demonstrate increased lateral compartment opening by 2.7 mm are consistent with an isolated FCL injury, whereas an increase of 4 mm or more indicates a grade III PLC injury.[24]

Arthroscopic evaluation of knees with complex ligamentous injuries also can aid in the diagnosis. If there is greater than 1 cm of lateral compartment opening when a varus stress is applied, a PLC injury should be suspected (**Figure 5**).

Treatment

The treatment of lateral-sided knee injuries depends on the associated injuries and the degree or grade of ligamentous injury. Isolated grade I and II injuries to the lateral collateral ligament or the PLC usually can be treated nonsurgically with bracing, protected weight bearing, and gradual progression of strengthening and motion. Return to full activity typically occurs between 3 and 4 months. Grade III injuries are usually treated surgically. Anatomic FCL reconstruction using semitendinosus grafts demonstrated improved patient outcomes.[25]

For grade III PLC injuries, the evidence supports surgical management. Acute repair is no longer the preferred treatment. In one study, acute repairs within 3 weeks of injury had a 37% failure rate versus 9% in a delayed reconstruction group.[26] Another study saw similar results with a 40% failure rate in the repair group compared with 6% in the reconstruction group.[27] A combination of acute repair of avulsed structures, reconstruction of midsubstance injuries, and concurrent cruciate reconstruction seems to provide the most reliable results.[28] Care must be taken to repair acute capsular avulsions or address redundant tissue with a posterolateral capsular shift in chronic cases. Augmentation of primary repairs with allograft reconstruction may potentially improve surgical success rates.

Posterior Cruciate Ligament Injuries

Anatomy and Function

The posterior cruciate ligament (PCL) is an intra-articular, extrasynovial structure composed of two major bundles: a smaller posteromedial bundle and a larger anterolateral bundle. The bundles are named after their footprint locations on the femur (posterior or anterior) and on the tibia (medial or lateral).

Overall, the PCL femoral footprint is broad and vertical, and its center is approximately 1 cm proximal to

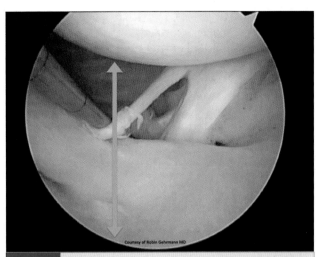

| Figure 5 | Arthroscopic drive-through sign view of a widened lateral compartment with evidence of injury/ longitudinal tearing of the popliteus tendon. (Courtesy of Robin M. Gehrman, MD, Warren, NJ.) |

Video 38.5: Lateral and Posterolateral Anatomy. Eric William Fester, MD; Justin P. Strickland, MD; Frank R. Noyes, MD (22.15 min)

the distal articular surface. On the tibia, both bundles insert approximately 1.0 to 1.5 cm distal to the joint line.[29] In addition, two meniscofemoral ligaments, of which one or both exist in 90% of the population, accompany the PCL.

The PCL is the primary restraint to posterior tibial translation. Because of the anterolateral bundle's greater load to failure and stiffness, surgeons have focused on restoring it during single-bundle PCL reconstruction. Both bundles are nonisometric and participate in resisting posterior translation at different knee angles.[30]

Mechanism of Injury

The standard mechanism of injury of the PCL is a posterior load to the tibia that can occur during dashboard injuries, contact sports, or a fall onto a flexed knee, especially when the foot is in plantar flexion. Higher energy injuries combining posterior and rotational forces can result in multiligament injuries that include the PCL.

Physical Examination

Several maneuvers can help identify PCL deficiency. The posterior drawer test is the most accurate test for PCL injury (grades 1 through 3). A grade 3 test, with the medial tibial plateau posterior to the medial femoral condyle, may denote an injury to the PLC corner.[31] Other important tests include the quadriceps active test, the reverse pivot-shift test, the posterolateral drawer test, and the dial test.

Table 2

Modified Schenk Classification of Knee Dislocations[a]

Classification		Injury
KD I		Cruciate intact (PCL intact most often)
KD II		Bicruciate injury with intact collateral ligaments
KD III		Bicruciate injury (+) collateral
KD III	M	Bicruciate injury (+) medial structures
KD III	L	Bicruciate injury (+) lateral structrues
KD IV		All four ligaments involved
KD V		Two or more injured ligaments (+) periarticular fracture

[a]The C (arterial injury) and N (nerve injury) classifications can be added to any injury listed.

Video 38.6: Posterior Drawer and Quadriceps Active Test. Robin M. Gehrmann, MD (0.41 min)

Radiographic Evaluation

Radiographic evaluation should include standard knee films and MRI to reveal concomitant injuries. Stress radiographs can further help grade the injury. Bone scans can be useful in patients with chronic PCL injuries with pain and disability. These patients typically have medial and patellofemoral compartment degenerative changes.

Nonsurgical Treatment

Several studies have confirmed that PCL tears can heal, although with elongation, possibly because of the ligament's extrasynovial location. Nonsurgical treatment is indicated for isolated grade 1 and 2 PCL injuries. Patients are treated with a period of immobilization followed by range of motion, quadriceps strengthening, and avoidance of active hamstring strengthening for approximately 4 weeks. Grade 3 PCL injuries are more controversial, and concomitant PLC damage must be ruled out.

Surgical Treatment

Bone Avulsion

Fixation of an avulsion fragment can be accomplished either with screws or suture fixation. The surgical approaches include an open posterior approach, with the patient in the prone position, or an arthroscopic approach.

Single-Bundle Reconstruction

On the femoral side, studies have shown that tunnel placement either in the anterolateral or the central aspect of the native femoral PCL footprint most closely approximates forces across the graft.[32]

Several tibial fixation techniques have been investigated. Transtibial fixation can create a 90° "killer" turn as the graft exits the tibia posteriorly, leading to elongation and failure.[33] Rasping the anterior edge of the tunnel, aperture fixation, and backup screw and washer fixation have been shown to decrease elongation.[34] The tibial inlay technique avoids the killer turn and generates lower anteroposterior laxity.[33] However, it requires an open approach with its associated possible complications.

Single- Versus Double-Bundle Reconstruction

PCL reconstruction using either a single-bundle or a double-bundle technique continues to generate controversy. There appears to be a theoretic advantage to reconstructing both bundles based on several biomechanical studies,[35,36] demonstrating it may more closely approximate the biomechanical properties of the intact PCL. Clinically, multiple studies have concluded that there are no reproducible significant differences between single- and double-bundle reconstructions both in the context of multiligament[37] and isolated PCL injuries.

Clinical Outcomes

Overall, PCL reconstructions appear to improve function from preoperative levels, although the return to previous level of activity is less reliable.[38,39] Patients can expect to regain one grade from the posterior drawer test.[40] Nevertheless, normal stability is not reproduced nor does reconstruction appear to prevent the onset of osteoarthritis.

Knee Dislocations

Any knee with complete disruption of two or more ligaments should be thought of as a knee dislocation until proven otherwise. Knee dislocations have a high incidence of associated limb-threatening injuries. These injuries include popliteal artery injuries, with a reported incidence of 23% to 32% after a dislocation,[41] and common peroneal nerve injuries, with a 25% incidence. Fewer than 50% of those with peroneal nerve injuries regain significant neurologic function.[42] Knee dislocations were first classified based on the direction of the injury. Unfortunately, many dislocations will spontaneously reduce, making this system less clinically meaningful. These injuries are classified anatomically in the Schenk knee dislocation classification[43] based on the injured ligaments. This classification system is best used during examination under anesthesia (Table 2). Dislocations can also be classified as acute, less than 3 weeks; subacute, 3 weeks to 3 months; and chronic, greater than 3 months. Although knee dislocations are typically thought of as high-velocity injuries, collision sports such as football can also produce a subset of injuries described as low-velocity knee dislocations, which can also have associated neurovascular injuries.[44] Recently, another cohort of patients with ultralow-velocity knee dislocations has been described.[45] These

Table 3

Incidence of Associated Injuries in Knee Dislocations

Type of Injury	Incidence
High-Velocity Dislocation	
Arterial injury	14% to 65%
Neuologic injuries	20% to 30%
Associated fractures	50% to 60%
Life-threatening injuries	27%
Low-Velocity Dislocation	
Vascular injury	5% to 15%
Neurologic injury	< 5%
Meniscal injury	20%
Ultralow-Velocity Dislocation	
Vascular injury	41%
Neurologic injury	41%

patients typically are morbidly obese (average body mass index of approximately 48) yet sustain knee dislocations after a seemingly trivial traumatic event. Interestingly, the associated incidence of neurovascular injuries in this group parallels that of high-velocity dislocations (Table 3). These patients can be challenging to treat because of their complex injuries, multiple comorbidities, and large body habitus.

Initial Treatment

The initial evaluation of a knee dislocation should be focused on the vascular status of the limb. It has been demonstrated that physical examination is not sufficient in suspected knee dislocations.[46] The author of one study concluded that an ankle-brachial index great than or equal to 0.9 indicated no risk of major arterial injury, but serial vascular examinations over 24 hours were recommended to detect delayed thrombosis.[47] An ankle-brachial index less than 0.9 mandates further investigation. The choice of which modality to use depends on the vascular status of the limb and available services at each institution. If indicated, intraoperative angiography is recommended because it allows immediate treatment of the vascular injury.

After the neurovascular status is assessed and stabilized, physical examination findings should be supplemented with radiographs and MRI to help demonstrate associated injuries.

Surgical Treatment

Treatment can be categorized into acute, subacute, and delayed intervention. Acute management should be performed for knees with vascular injuries, open or irreducible dislocations, open fractures, or gross instability. Subacute intervention can be implemented for lateral-sided ligamentous injuries or concomitant neurologic injuries. Treatment can often be delayed for medial-sided knee injuries, allowing healing and return of motion before surgical treatment is begun.

Because of the high-energy mechanism associated with many of these injuries, some dislocations may have other life- or limb-threatening pathology that will dictate surgical timing. Although there is no consensus on the ideal treatment algorithm, it appears that surgical intervention within 3 weeks provides better functional outcomes than those treated later or nonsurgically.[48]

Rehabilitation of these injuries should be tailored to the individual injury. It can be expected that return to high-level sports is not likely in this population, although it is not impossible.

Meniscal Injury

Arthroscopic partial meniscectomy is one of the most common orthopaedic procedures performed in the United States and the most common Current Procedural Terminology code presented by American Board of Orthopaedic Surgery Part II applicants. Because of its ubiquity, there is considerable interest in meniscal injury, the effects of partial meniscectomy, and meniscal preservation techniques.

Anatomy and Function

The menisci have several important roles in knee function. They enhance congruity between tibial and femoral articular surfaces, facilitating tibiofemoral load transmission and shock absorption. They also aid in joint lubrication and act as secondary stabilizers of the knee.[49] The medial meniscus resists anterior translation in the ACL-deficient knee as replicated by the Lachman test. The lateral meniscus also plays an important role in resisting anterior translation in the ACL-deficient knee during the pivot shift (combined valgus and rotatory loads) maneuver.[50]

The blood supply to the menisci originates from branches of the medial and lateral geniculate arteries. These arteries supply the peripheral 10% to 30% of the medial meniscus and 10% to 25% of the lateral meniscus.

Treatment

Meniscal tears have been classified by tear pattern, location, vascularity, and chronicity. All of these variables affect treatment options. In general, older (> 50 years), more sedentary patients with nonacute tears are more likely to respond to nonsurgical treatment; a repaired tear in this population is less likely to heal because of its complex, degenerative nature. If the tear remains symptomatic, meniscectomy is the preferred treatment. Good candidates for repair are typically younger (30 years or younger) and have an acute injury that creates a noncomplex, vertical tear pattern that is peripheral in location (Figure 6). Studies of failures of meniscal repair for bucket-handle tears have shown that

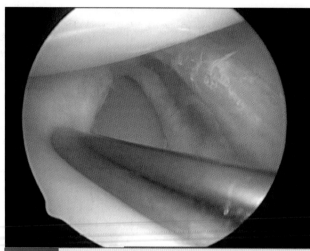

Figure 6 Arthroscopic view of an acute vertical longitudinal tear in a medial meniscus demonstrating the vascularized peripheral portion of the meniscus (to the right of the pointer). (Courtesy of Robin M. Gehrman, MD, Warren, NJ.)

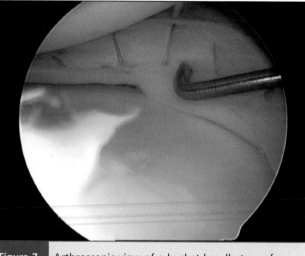

Figure 7 Arthroscopic view of a bucket-handle tear of a medial meniscus repaired with multiple inside-out vertical mattress sutures. (Courtesy of Robin M. Gehrmann, MD, Warren, NJ.)

80% of the meniscal repair failures were in tears with a degenerative component.[51] Associated ACL reconstruction also appears to enhance the healing response, presumably from the release of marrow that occurs during tunnel drilling.

Rim width is indicative of vascularity and healing potential. It has been shown that 80% of tears heal with a rim width of 0 to 1 mm, and only 33% healed when the rim was larger than 3 mm.[52] Surgical treatment is used for patients who are refractory to nonsurgical treatment. Several studies highlight the importance of meniscal repair over meniscectomy. Lower incidences of osteoarthritic progression and higher return to preinjury activity level are seen with repairs versus meniscectomy.[53,54]

Video 38.7: Diagnostic Arthroscopic Knee Examination. Randy R. Clark, MD; Mark H. Getelman, MD (9.29 min)

Meniscal root tears are injuries that may frequently be missed but have significant consequences if left untreated. Biomechanical studies have indicated that meniscal root injury can cause loss of the ability to absorb hoop stresses and biomechanical overload of the joint. Repair seems to restore contact pressures comparable to those of the control knee.[55]

Repair can be performed one of three ways: inside-out, outside-in, or all inside. The gold standard has been inside-out with a vertical mattress suture configuration (Figure 7). The technique used is largely determined by surgeon comfort level and tear location. The posterior portion of the meniscus can be repaired reli-

ably with an inside-out technique; as the tear becomes more anterior, an outside-in approach is needed. Modern all-inside devices have made it possible to place vertical mattress sutures, which seem to have healing rates similar to the classic inside-out techniques; however, more implant-related complications were observed.[56]

After meniscectomy in a physiologically younger (30 years or younger), active patient, persistent pain and effusions can ensue. In these patients, meniscal transplantation has been shown to significantly reduce pain, decrease activity-related effusions, and improve function in patients with a prior meniscectomy.[57] Because of the close proximity of the anterior and posterior horns of the lateral meniscus, transplantation is usually with a single bony bridge housing both horns, whereas the medial meniscus is typically transplanted with two separate bone plugs for the anterior and posterior horns. Suture-only techniques demonstrate a higher rate of meniscal extrusion and graft tears compared with methods that incorporate bony fixation methods.[58]

Rehabilitation

Rehabilitation after repair or transplantation has not been standardized but often involves protected weight bearing and limited range of motion to eliminate shear forces on the repair. Motion greater than 90° is usually started after 4 to 6 weeks, with return to full unrestricted activity between 4 and 6 months. Accelerated rehabilitation programs allow immediate unrestricted weight bearing in full extension based on the premise that hoop stresses are created and aid in reduction of the meniscal repair.[59] Radial tears that are repaired require a period of 6 weeks or more of no weight bearing. The postoperative management will also depend on associated pathology and its treatment.

Table 4

ICRS Cartilage Grading

Lesion Grade	Lesion Depth	Classification	Description
0	Normal	A	Soft indentation
1	Superficial	B	Superficial fissures and cracks
2	< 50%		Abnormal
3	> 50%	A	> 50% cartilage depth
		B	To calcific layer
		C	To subchondral bone
		D	Blisters
4	Through subchondral bone	A	Through subchondral bone but not full diameter
		B	Through subchondral bone and full diameter

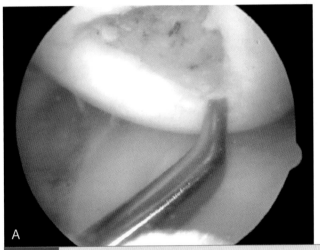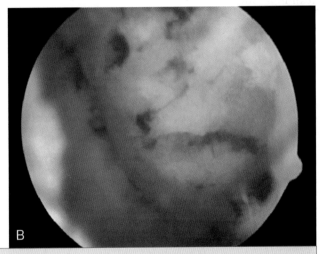

Figure 8   Arthroscopic views of the microfracture technique. **A,** Vertical walls are created with a curet, and the calcific layer is removed. A specialized awl is used to make 2- to 3-mm deep perforations 3 to 4 mm apart. **B,** Marrow contents begin to emerge from the perforations to create a "super clot."

Articular Cartilage

Cartilage Injury

The current management of articular cartilage injuries must consider the size and extent of the lesion, any associated injuries to the menisci or ligaments, and the patient's current activity and and functional goals. The Outerbridge Classification and, more recently, the International Cartilage Repair Society classification have been used to grade cartilage lesions (Table 4). Of all imaging modalities, MRI best assesses the quality of articular cartilage. Newer biochemical MRI techniques, such as T2 mapping, T1rho, sodium MRI, and (delayed gadolinium-enhanced MRI of cartilage (dGEMRIC), show promise in detecting subtler and earlier changes in the microstructure of articular cartilage.[60]

After a partial-thickness injury, proteoglycan loss, increased water content, and decreased cartilage stiffness cause subchondral bone stiffness to increase and leads to further chondral degeneration.[61] Full-thickness lesions that penetrate the subchondral bone, however, lead to an egress of marrow stem cells and growth factors, including transforming growth factor-beta, insulin-like growth factor, fibroblast growth factor, and complementary DNA, which can initiate a healing response. After an initial hematoma is formed, stem cell migration and eventually synthesis of type I collagen follows, producing fibrocartilage.

Nonsurgical Treatment

The goal of nonsurgical treatment of chondral injuries is to ameliorate symptoms, not restore chondral integrity. NSAIDs and disease-modifying osteoarthritis drugs used judiciously, intra-articular hyaluronic acid, physical therapy, muscle strengthening, gait training, taping, and appropriate bracing can provide effective symptom relief.

Surgical Treatment

Good outcomes in surgically treated full-thickness chondral lesions can be optimized by careful patient se-

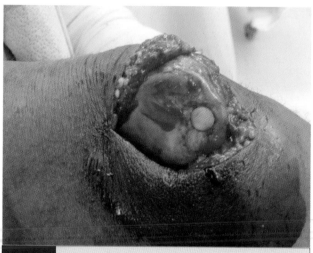

Figure 9 Clinical photograph of two osteochondral autograft system plugs placed in a defect in the medial patellar facet. The plugs were harvested from the nonarticulating portion of the medial trochlea.

lection. Patients should be younger than 50 years; have a stable knee, with preoperative or concurrent reconstruction performed as necessary; have a stable neutral tracking extensor mechanism and mechanical axis alignment; and have intact menisci (with concurrent meniscal allograft performed as necessary). Single femoral condyle or patellar defects with no kissing lesions on the opposite chondral surface are more amenable to successful treatment. The defect should not be part of more global arthritis or associated with inflammatory arthritis.

To stratify patients accordingly, current strategies have been grouped into palliative, reparative, and restorative techniques.[62] Palliative management includes arthroscopic débridement and is indicated for low-demand patients with small lesion sizes for temporary relief.

Microfracture is the most commonly used reparative marrow stimulation technique. By creating evenly spaced perforations in the subchondral bone, stem cells and growth factors are released, forming a fibrin superclot and eventually leading to the production of fibrocartilage (**Figure 8**). A recent large literature review demonstrated clear acute improvement in knee function at 2 years but inconsistent improvement after more than 2 years. More successful outcomes seem to occur with contained, small (< 2 cm²), unipolar, single compartment, full-thickness lesions, in individuals younger than 35 years and thin patients (body mass index < 30 kg/m²).[63,64]

Restorative techniques attempt to fill the chondral defect with hyaline or hyaline-like cartilage. These techniques include autologous chondrocyte implantation (ACI), osteochondral autograft system (OATS) (**Figure 9**), osteochondral allograft transplantation, and newer techniques such as minced juvenile cartilage allograft or autograft transplantation.

Comparative Studies

Several studies have compared the different chondral defect management procedures. A recent level I prospective randomized clinical trial[65] comparing ACI and mosaicplasty with a minimum 10-year follow-up found better functional outcomes in patients with ACI.

ACI has not yet shown definitive superiority over microfracture. Similar satisfactory results were found in both ACI and microfracture groups at 2 years.[66]

Osteochondral autografts have been compared with microfracture. One randomized, placebo-controlled study in athletes found good to excellent results in 96% of patients treated with OATS compared with 52% treated with microfracture.[67]

For full-thickness chondral knee injuries, microfracture is still regarded as the first line treatment, although its effectiveness appears to wane with time. In young athletes, OATS treatment may yield improved longer term results.

Patellar Instability

Epidemiology

Patellofemoral instability can occur from acute trauma, including a direct blow, or from a seemingly low-energy, noncontact, indirect pivoting event with valgus and lower limb external rotation. As with the shoulder, the cause of patellar instability lies on a spectrum between a traumatic event and underlying baseline laxity. Redislocation occurs more commonly in younger patients, females, and patients with a family history of patellar instability.

Anatomy and Pathophysiology

Patellar stability results from a complex interplay of dynamic muscular restraints, static soft-tissue restraints, bony morphology, and lower limb alignment. Four structural components play a role in maintaining the patella. First, the quadriceps, specifically the vastus medialis obliquus, provides active control. Second, the medial patellofemoral ligament (MPFL) and medial retinaculum provide static soft-tissue restraints to lateral translation, up to 50% of the restraining force to lateral patellar translation in extension.[68] Third, the patellofemoral joint geometry governs stability after the patella has engaged the trochlear groove at approximately 30° of flexion. The osseous features that have been found to predispose to recurrent patellar instability include patellar tilt, patella alta, lateral trochlear dysplasia (classified using the Dejour and Le Coultre classification system)[69] (**Figure 10**), and increased tibial tubercle–trochlear groove (TT-TG) distances. Fourth, increased overall lower limb alignment as defined by a larger Q angle increases the laterally directed force vector on the patella.

Physical Examination

A hemarthrosis should be aspirated to assess range of motion and ensure that there is no block, possibly from

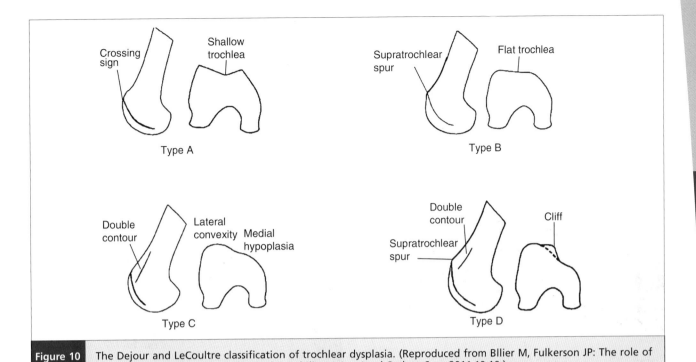

Figure 10 The Dejour and LeCoultre classification of trochlear dysplasia. (Reproduced from Bllier M, Fulkerson JP: The role of trochlear dysplasia in patellofemoral instability. *J Am Acad Orthop Surg* 2011;19:10.)

an osteochondral loose body. The J sign and patellar apprehension indicate an incompetent MPFL. The recently proposed moving patellar apprehension test has high sensitivity and specificity.[70] Patellar tilt should also be evaluated. It is important to stress that a tight lateral retinaculum alone does not cause patellar instability. There must be incompetent medial structures to produce instability.

 Video 38.8: Patellar J Sign. Robin M. Gehrmann, MD (0.32 min)

Imaging

Patellar instability is a clinical, not a radiographic, diagnosis. Nevertheless, imaging can be helpful to clarify etiology. Merchant radiographs will show patellar tilt and lateral trochlear shape. Patella height is assessed on a lateral radiograph with the knee at 30° of flexion. Of all patellar height indices, the Blackburne-Peel ratio appears to have the least interobserver variability[71] (**Figure 11**). The lateral radiograph also can show a crossing sign and a supratrochlear spur, both indicative of trochlear dysplasia (**Figure 12**). CT and MRI have also been used effectively in cases of patellar instability, especially for TT-TG measurements[72] (**Figure 13**).

Treatment Options
Nonsurgical
The management of primary patellar dislocations remains controversial. Typically, first-line treatment in-

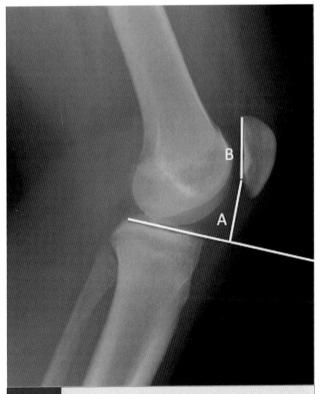

Figure 11 Radiograph showing the Blackburne-Peel ratio. Line A is measured from the distal aspect of the patellar articular surface to a point perpendicular to a line drawn along the tibial plateau. Line B is the length of the patellar articular surface. The normal A/B ratio is 0.8. A ratio greater than 1.0 indicates patella alta. The knee should ideally be flexed 30°.

4: Lower Extremity

4: Lower Extremity

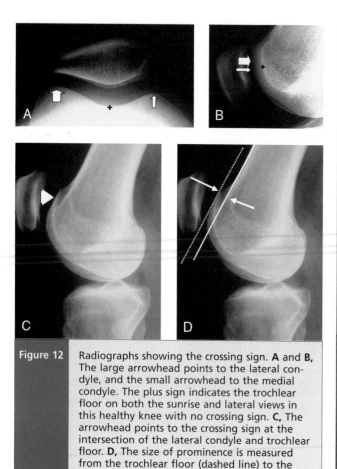

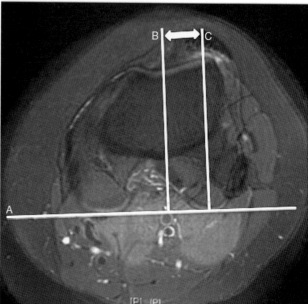

Figure 12 Radiographs showing the crossing sign. **A** and **B,** The large arrowhead points to the lateral condyle, and the small arrowhead to the medial condyle. The plus sign indicates the trochlear floor on both the sunrise and lateral views in this healthy knee with no crossing sign. **C,** The arrowhead points to the crossing sign at the intersection of the lateral condyle and trochlear floor. **D,** The size of prominence is measured from the trochlear floor (dashed line) to the solid line extending from the anterior femoral cortex. (Reproduced with permission from Fithian DC, Nyret PO, Elvire S: Patellar instability: The Lyon experience. *Curr Orthop Pract* 2008;19:328-338.)

Figure 13 Tibial tubercle–trochlear groove (TT-TG) distance assessed using MRI T2 sequence. A line (A) is drawn connecting the posterior aspect of the femoral condyles on the first image, an axial cut with the most pronounced trochlear sulcus. A line (B) is then drawn perpendicular to the posterior condylar line, through the nadir of the sulcus. The axial cut with the most anteriorly prominent tibial tubercle is then superimposed on the first image. A line (C) is drawn perpendicular to the posterior condylar line and through the most anterior aspect of the tubercle. This line is parallel to the line through the sulcus. The distance between the two parallel lines (B and C) is measured. A distance greater than 25 mm in the setting of instability is an indication for a tubercle osteotomy and medialization. The goal of surgery is to restore the distance to 10 to 12 mm. The TT-TG distance does not appear to increase with age.

corporates a brief period of immobilization (3 to 6 weeks) followed by physical therapy. Mobilizing the knee too soon generated a three times higher risk of re-dislocation than when patients were immobilized for 6 weeks, although longer immobilization increases the risk of stiffness.[73] Indications for surgical management include persistent instability, osteochondral or chondral fractures, and when a complete avulsion is seen on MRI or if surgery is planned anyway to remove a loose body.

Surgical

Considerations in surgical management for instability include the following points: First, lateral release in isolation should be routinely avoided and performed only in the context of an MPFL reconstruction to address residual patellar issues such as tilt. Second, trochlear osteoplasties should be performed sparingly because there is a high risk of osteochondral fracture or future arthritis. Third, distal realignment procedures in patients with elevated TT-TG distances greater than 20 mm or patella alta[74] can be effective for good long-term knee

function. Preexisting medial or superior patellar facet chondrosis is a contraindication because of potential overload in these areas after the osteotomy. Fourth, surgical procedures on skeletally immature patients should be performed judiciously because of a dearth of evidence-based studies. Fifth, MPFL reconstruction (**Figure 14**) should be performed so as to place the graft as isometrically as possible.[75] Anisometric placement has been implicated in abnormally large patellofemoral forces, leading to pain and chondral deterioration and even overt failure.

Clinical Outcomes

Overall, the recurrence rate for nonsurgical treatment is approximately 13% to 52%; for surgical stabilization, it is between 10% and 30%.[76] Although surgical stabilization does decrease the recurrence rate, it has not been shown to reduce the incidence of osteoarthritis.[76]

Anterior Knee Pain

Pathophysiology

Anterior knee pain can arise from the soft tissues around the knee, overloaded subchondral bone, or chondral injury. The fat pad and synovial tissues seem to have greater pain sensitivity than other knee structures[77] and because of the presence of free nerve endings and the nociceptive transmitters substance P and calcitonin gene-related peptide.[78] Recent evidence points to the importance of evaluating the knee within the context of the entire lower extremity. One prospective study identified predisposing factors, including decreased quadriceps and gastrocnemius flexibility, increased vastus medialis obliquus reflex response time, delayed vastus medialis obliquus firing compared with the vastus lateralis, decreased explosive strength, and ligamentous laxity.[79]

Nonsurgical Treatment

Immobilization or extended rest should be avoided because it may result in deconditioning that can delay symptom relief. One randomized study found that both closed chain and open chain overall lower extremity strengthening improved pain relief and return to function. Studies support quadriceps, gluteal and hip abductor strengthening, patellar taping, and hip and hamstring stretching.[80]

Surgical Treatment

Surgical management for anterior knee pain should be focused on a specific etiology if one can be identified. Surgery is rarely indicated.

Summary

Knee injuries continue to be a major source of disability, especially with the increased young male and female athletic population. Techniques in ligament reconstruction are focusing on more anatomic reconstructive procedures, with an emphasis on both primary repair and augmentation of multiligamentous injuries. Meniscal injuries have been shown to demonstrate improved long-term results when they are repaired rather than resected, although no clear advantage is seen in any single repair technique. Treatment options for full-thickness articular cartilage defects are regarded as palliative, reparative, and restorative. The goal is to create hyaline cartilage, and although success in this area has been limited, microfracture still appears to be a good first-line treatment, showing results similar to ACI in the intermediate term. In young athletic patients, OATS may show longer term good results. Patellar instability treatment should focus on appropriate rehabilitation followed by repair or reconstruction of soft-tissue injuries and osseous malalignment when necessary. The role of surgical intervention is limited in most cases of anterior knee pain, unless a specific cause can be identified.

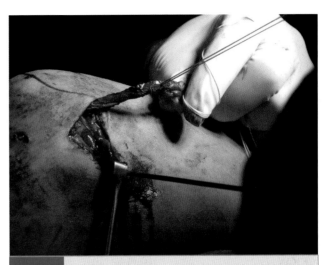

Figure 14 Clinical photograph showing medial patellofemoral ligament reconstruction. A semitendinosus autograft has been placed in a bone tunnel at the proximal one third–distal two thirds junction of the patella. Isometry is tested, and it is tensioned before insertion just anterior to the medial epicondyle (shown by a Kirschner wire.) Optimal femoral tunnel placement has been shown to be 10 mm distal and 5 mm posterior to the adductor tubercle. Tensioning the graft with the knee flexed to 60° and the patella solidly ensconced in the trochlear groove ensures that the graft is not overtightened.

Key Study Points

- Double-bundle ACL reconstruction has been shown to restore biomechanical knee stability better than nonanatomic single-bundle reconstructions but has not shown any significant improvement in clinical outcomes at this time.

- The treatment of multiligamentous knee injuries appears to demonstrate better results with a combination of acute repair of injured structures in addition to reconstruction or augmentation of those structures that are not amenable to repair.

- For patellar dislocations, indications for surgical management include persistent instability, osteochondral or chondral fractures, and when a complete avulsion is seen on MRI or if surgery is planned anyway to remove a loose body. Lateral release is not indicated in isolation for patellar instability. Surgery for anterior knee pain is rarely indicated unless a specific etiology can be isolated.

Annotated References

1. Kawaguchi Y, Kondo E, Kitamura N, Kai S, Inoue M, Yasuda K: Comparisons of femoral tunnel enlargement in 169 patients between single-bundle and anatomic double-bundle anterior cruciate ligament reconstructions with hamstring tendon grafts. *Knee Surg Sports Traumatol Arthrosc* 2011;19(8):1249-1257.

Seventy-two patients who underwent single-bundle hamstring ACL reconstructions were compared with 97 patients who underwent double-bundle hamstring ACL reconstructions to assess the effects of reconstruction type on tunnel enlargement. The incidence and the degree of tunnel enlargement were both significantly less in the double-bundle group 2 years after surgery. Level of evidence: II.

2. Salmon LJ, Russell VJ, Refshauge K, et al: Long-term outcome of endoscopic anterior cruciate ligament reconstruction with patellar tendon autograft: Minimum 13-year review. *Am J Sports Med* 2006;34(5):721-732.

3. Biau DJ, Tournoux C, Katsahian S, Schranz P, Nizard R: ACL reconstruction: A meta-analysis of functional scores. *Clin Orthop Relat Res* 2007;458:180-187.

4. Meredick RB, Vance KJ, Appleby D, Lubowitz JH: Outcome of single-bundle versus double-bundle reconstruction of the anterior cruciate ligament: A meta-analysis. *Am J Sports Med* 2008;36(7):1414-1421.

5. Hussein M, van Eck CF, Cretnik A, Dinevski D, Fu FH: Individualized anterior cruciate ligament surgery: A prospective study comparing anatomic single- and double-bundle reconstruction. *Am J Sports Med* 2012;40(8):1781-1788.

Patients were divided into anatomic single-bundle and anatomic double-bundle ACL reconstructions based on the size of tibial ACL footprint (less than 16 mm = single bundle, > 16 mm = double bundle) All grafts were autograft hamstrings fixed with suspensory fixation on the femur and biointerference screws on the tibia. No significant differences were noted in the groups for Lysholm and IKDC scores or anterior tibial translation and pivot-shift testing. Level of evidence: II.

6. Krych AJ, Jackson JD, Hoskin TL, Dahm DL: A meta-analysis of patellar tendon autograft versus patellar tendon allograft in anterior cruciate ligament reconstruction. *Arthroscopy* 2008;24(3):292-298.

7. Dustmann M, Schmidt T, Gangey I, Unterhauser FN, Weiler A, Scheffler SU: The extracellular remodeling of free-soft-tissue autografts and allografts for reconstruction of the anterior cruciate ligament: A comparison study in a sheep model. *Knee Surg Sports Traumatol Arthrosc* 2008;16(4):360-369.

8. Hewett TE, Ford KR, Myer GD: Anterior cruciate ligament injuries in female athletes: Part 2. A meta-analysis of neuromuscular interventions aimed at injury prevention. *Am J Sports Med* 2006;34(3):490-498.

9. Daniel D, Pedowitz RA, O'Connor JJ, Akeson WH: *Daniel's Knee Injuries: Ligament and Cartilage Structure, Function, Injury and Repair*, ed 2. Philadelphia, PA, Lippincott Williams and Wilkins, 2003.

10. Matsumoto H, Suda Y, Otani T, Niki Y, Seedhom BB, Fujikawa K: Roles of the anterior cruciate ligament and the medial collateral ligament in preventing valgus instability. *J Orthop Sci* 2001;6(1):28-32.

11. Wijdicks CA, Griffith CJ, LaPrade RF, et al: Radiographic identification of the primary medial knee structures. *J Bone Joint Surg Am* 2009;91(3):521-529.

12. Laprade RF, Bernhardson AS, Griffith CJ, Macalena JA, Wijdicks CA: Correlation of valgus stress radiographs with medial knee ligament injuries: An in vitro biomechanical study. *Am J Sports Med* 2010;38(2):330-338.

Valgus stress radiographs documented the amount of medial compartment gapping after MCL knee injuries in a controlled laboratory study. Isolated superficial MCL injuries produced gapping of 1.7 mm and 3.2 mm at 0° and 20° of flexion, respectively, whereas complete MCL injuries produced gapping of 6.5 mm and 9.8 mm at 0° and 20°, respectively.

13. Miller MD, Osborne JR, Gordon WT, Hinkin DT, Brinker MR: The natural history of bone bruises: A prospective study of magnetic resonance imaging-detected trabecular microfractures in patients with isolated medial collateral ligament injuries. *Am J Sports Med* 1998;26(1):15-19.

14. Brown TD, Van Hoeck JE, Brand RA: Laboratory evaluation of prophylactic knee brace performance under dynamic valgus loading using a surrogate leg model. *Clin Sports Med* 1990;9(4):751-762.

15. Najibi S, Albright JP: The use of knee braces, part 1: Prophylactic knee braces in contact sports. *Am J Sports Med* 2005;33(4):602-611.

16. Frank CB, Loitz BJ, Shrive NG: Injury location affects ligament healing: A morphologic and mechanical study of the healing rabbit medial collateral ligament. *Acta Orthop Scand* 1995;66(5):455-462.

17. Indelicato PA, Hermansdorfer J, Huegel M: Nonoperative management of complete tears of the medial collateral ligament of the knee in intercollegiate football players. *Clin Orthop Relat Res* 1990;256:174-177.

18. Reider B, Sathy MR, Talkington J, Blyznak N, Kollias S: Treatment of isolated medial collateral ligament injuries in athletes with early functional rehabilitation: A five-year follow-up study. *Am J Sports Med* 1994;22(4):470-477.

19. Kannus P: Long-term results of conservatively treated medial collateral ligament injuries of the knee joint. *Clin Orthop Relat Res* 1988;226:103-112.

20. Laprade RF, Wijdicks CA: The management of injuries to the medial side of the knee. *J Orthop Sports Phys Ther* 2012;42(3):221-233.

Surgical and nonsurgical options for the treatment of MCL knee injuries are discussed. A thorough knowledge of anatomy is necessary for surgical intervention. Most acute grade III injuries will heal after a nonsurgical rehabilitation program.

21. Laprade RF, Wijdicks CA: Surgical technique: Development of an anatomic medial knee reconstruction. *Clin*

Orthop Relat Res 2012;470(3):806-814.

Twenty-eight patients were followed prospectively for a minimum of 6 months to evaluate an anatomic MCL reconstruction. Preoperative medial compartment gapping (mean, 6.2 mm) was reduced after the reconstruction (mean, 1.3 mm). IKDC subjective scores improved from an average of 43.5 preoperatively to 76.2 postoperatively. Level of evidence: III.

22. Zaffagnini S, Bignozzi S, Martelli S, Lopomo N, Marcacci M: Does ACL reconstruction restore knee stability in combined lesions? An in vivo study. *Clin Orthop Relat Res* 2007;454:95-99.

23. Halinen J, Lindahl J, Hirvensalo E, Santavirta S: Operative and nonoperative treatments of medial collateral ligament rupture with early anterior cruciate ligament reconstruction: A prospective randomized study. *Am J Sports Med* 2006;34(7):1134-1140.

24. LaPrade RF, Heikes C, Bakker AJ, Jakobsen RB: The reproducibility and repeatability of varus stress radiographs in the assessment of isolated fibular collateral ligament and grade-III posterolateral knee injuries: An in vitro biomechanical study. *J Bone Joint Surg Am* 2008;90(10):2069-2076.

25. LaPrade RF, Spiridonov SI, Coobs BR, Ruckert PR, Griffith CJ: Fibular collateral ligament anatomical reconstructions: A prospective outcomes study. *Am J Sports Med* 2010;38(10):2005-2011.

Twenty patients underwent anatomic LCL reconstruction using semitendinosus graft for isolated grade III LCL injuries. At an average of 2 years after surgery, 16 patients were available for follow-up. All patients had significant improvements in IKDC, Cincinnati scores, and varus stress radiographs when compared with preoperative values. Level of evidence: IV.

26. Stannard JP, Brown SL, Farris RC, McGwin G Jr, Volgas DA: The posterolateral corner of the knee: Repair versus reconstruction. *Am J Sports Med* 2005;33(6):881-888.

27. Levy BA, Dajani KA, Morgan JA, Shah JP, Dahm DL, Stuart MJ: Repair versus reconstruction of the fibular collateral ligament and posterolateral corner in the multiligament-injured knee. *Am J Sports Med* 2010;38(4):804-809.

Acute repair of the FCL/PLC with delayed cruciate reconstruction was compared with single-stage multiligament reconstruction. The repair/staged group included 10 knees, and the reconstruction group 18 knees. Repair failed in 40% of the repair group versus 6% of the reconstruction group. This demonstrated a statistically significant higher rate of failure for repair compared with reconstruction of the FCL/PLC. Level of evidence: III.

28. Geeslin AG, LaPrade RF: Outcomes of treatment of acute grade-III isolated and combined posterolateral knee injuries: A prospective case series and surgical technique. *J Bone Joint Surg Am* 2011;93(18):1672-1683.

This study reports on the surgical treatment of acute grade III posterolateral knee injuries treated within 6 weeks of injury. All patients had an anatomic repair and/or reconstruction of the PLC with acute repair of avulsed structures or reconstruction of midsubstance tears and concurrent reconstruction of any cruciate ligament tears. This resulted in significantly improved objective stability and subjective IKDC and Cincinnati outcome scores. Level of evidence: IV.

29. Edwards A, Bull AM, Amis AA: The attachments of the fiber bundles of the posterior cruciate ligament: An anatomic study. *Arthroscopy* 2007;23(3):284-290.

30. Ahmad CS, Cohen ZA, Levine WN, Gardner TR, Ateshian GA, Mow VC: Codominance of the individual posterior cruciate ligament bundles: An analysis of bundle lengths and orientation. *Am J Sports Med* 2003; 31(2):221-225.

31. Sekiya JK, Whiddon DR, Zehms CT, Miller MD: A clinically relevant assessment of posterior cruciate ligament and posterolateral corner injuries: Evaluation of isolated and combined deficiency. *J Bone Joint Surg Am* 2008;90(8):1621-1627.

32. Markolf KL, Zemanovic JR, McAllister DR: Cyclic loading of posterior cruciate ligament replacements fixed with tibial tunnel and tibial inlay methods. *J Bone Joint Surg Am* 2002;84(4):518-524.

33. Bergfeld JA, McAllister DR, Parker RD, Valdevit AD, Kambic HE: A biomechanical comparison of posterior cruciate ligament reconstruction techniques. *Am J Sports Med* 2001;29(2):129-136.

34. Margheritini F, Rihn JA, Mauro CS, Stabile KJ, Woo SL, Harner CD: Biomechanics of initial tibial fixation in posterior cruciate ligament reconstruction. *Arthroscopy* 2005;21(10):1164-1171.

35. Race A, Amis AA: PCL reconstruction: In vitro biomechanical comparison of 'isometric' versus single and double-bundled 'anatomic' grafts. *J Bone Joint Surg Br* 1998;80(1):173-179.

36. Harner CD, Janaushek MA, Kanamori A, Yagi M, Vogrin TM, Woo SL: Biomechanical analysis of a double-bundle posterior cruciate ligament reconstruction. *Am J Sports Med* 2000;28(2):144-151.

37. Fanelli GC, Beck JD, Edson CJ: Single compared to double-bundle PCL reconstruction using allograft tissue. *J Knee Surg* 2012;25(1):59-64.

Single-bundle PCL reconstructions with Achilles allograft were comparable to double-bundle PCL reconstructions with Achilles allograft (AL bundle) and tibialis anterior (PM bundle) when evaluated with stress radiography, arthrometer measurements, and knee ligament rating scales.

38. Kim YM, Lee CA, Matava MJ: Clinical results of arthroscopic single-bundle transtibial posterior cruciate ligament reconstruction: A systematic review. *Am J Sports Med* 2011;39(2):425-434.

4: Lower Extremity

Arthroscopic single-bundle transtibial PCL reconstruction improves posterior knee laxity by one grade but does not reliably restore normal knee stability. There is a postoperative rate of normal or nearly normal outcomes of 75%. Degenerative osteoarthritis is not prevented by PCL reconstruction.

39. Hammoud S, Reinhardt KR, Marx RG: Outcomes of posterior cruciate ligament treatment: A review of the evidence. *Sports Med Arthrosc* 2010;18(4):280-291.

    This systemic review included 21 studies of isolated PCL reconstructions and 10 studies of combined PCL reconstructions. The rate of overall graft failure was 11.6%. Return to preinjury activity in the combined PCL studies ranged from 19% to 68%. In the isolated PCL studies, these values were 50% to 82%. Of the patients in the combined PCL studies, 36% to 70% had a normal posterior drawer test at final follow-up.

40. Voos JE, Mauro CS, Wente T, Warren RF, Wickiewicz TL: Posterior cruciate ligament: Anatomy, biomechanics, and outcomes. *Am J Sports Med* 2012;40(1):222-231.

    This review article documents recent evidence and controversies involving PCL reconstructions. Double-bundle PCL reconstructions may restore better knee biomechanics, but clinical outcome differences between these and single-bundle reconstructions have not been found. Tibial inlay techniques may decrease the graft elongation because of the killer turn of the transtibial technique.

41. Johnson ME, Foster L, DeLee JC: Neurologic and vascular injuries associated with knee ligament injuries. *Am J Sports Med* 2008;36(12):2448-2462.

42. Niall DM, Nutton RW, Keating JF: Palsy of the common peroneal nerve after traumatic dislocation of the knee. *J Bone Joint Surg Br* 2005;87(5):664-667.

43. Schenck RC Jr, Hunter RE, Ostrum RF, Perry CR: Knee dislocations. *Instr Course Lect* 1999;48:515-522.

44. Shelbourne KD, Porter DA, Clingman JA, McCarroll JR, Rettig AC: Low-velocity knee dislocation. *Orthop Rev* 1991;20(11):995-1004.

45. Azar FM, Brandt JC, Miller RH III, Phillips BB: Ultra-low-velocity knee dislocations. *Am J Sports Med* 2011;39(10):2170-2174.

    A subset of patients (average body mass index = 48 g [greater than 40 is severe obesity]) was identified with ultralow velocity knee dislocations that occurred while stepping off a curb or stair or simply falling while walking. Of 17 patients, neurologic injuries occurred in 7 and popliteal injuries in 7. All patients underwent closed reduction and stabilization; ligament reconstructions were done in 8, vascular repairs in 7. Above-knee amputations were required in 2, and 1 died from cardiac arrest. Neurovascular injuries were frequent in these ultralow velocity dislocations in patients who are severely obese. Surgical ligament reconstruction appears to improve outcomes. Level of evidence: IV.

46. McDonough EB Jr, Wojtys EM: Multiligamentous injuries of the knee and associated vascular injuries. *Am J Sports Med* 2009;37(1):156-159.

47. Mills WJ, Barei DP, McNair P: The value of the ankle-brachial index for diagnosing arterial injury after knee dislocation: A prospective study. *J Trauma* 2004;56(6):1261-1265.

48. Levy BA, Dajani KA, Whelan DB, et al: Decision making in the multiligament-injured knee: An evidence-based systematic review. *Arthroscopy* 2009;25(4):430-438.

49. Maffulli N, Longo UG, Campi S, Denaro V: Meniscal tears. *Open Access J Sports Med* 2010;1:45-54.

    Long-term studies show that virtually all meniscectomized knees develop arthritic changes with time. Meniscectomy has shown good short-term results, but over time radiographic signs of arthritis occur. Meniscal repair has shown improved long-term results, and techniques have evolved from open to arthroscopic techniques that include inside-out, outside-in, and all-inside. Patients who are symptomatic after complete or subtotal meniscectomy appear to benefit from meniscal transplantation.

50. Musahl V, Citak M, O'Loughlin PF, Choi D, Bedi A, Pearle AD: The effect of medial versus lateral meniscectomy on the stability of the anterior cruciate ligament-deficient knee. *Am J Sports Med* 2010;38(8):1591-1597.

    This cadaver study examined the stabilizing effects of the medial and lateral menisci on ACL-deficient knees. It was noted that although the medial meniscus is a critical secondary stabilizer to anteriorly directed forces during Lachman examination, the lateral meniscus appears to be a more important restraint to anterior tibial translation during combined valgus and rotatory loads during a pivot shift maneuver.

51. Shelbourne KD, Carr DR: Meniscal repair compared with meniscectomy for bucket-handle medial meniscal tears in anterior cruciate ligament-reconstructed knees. *Am J Sports Med* 2003;31(5):718-723.

52. Johnson MJ, Lucas GL, Dusek JK, Henning CE: Isolated arthroscopic meniscal repair: A long-term outcome study (more than 10 years). *Am J Sports Med* 1999;27(1):44-49.

53. Brophy RH, Wright RW, David TS, et al: Association between previous meniscal surgery and the incidence of chondral lesions at revision anterior cruciate ligament reconstruction. *Am J Sports Med* 2012;40(4):808-814.

    Data from a multicenter cohort were reviewed for patients undergoing revision ACL reconstruction. Knees that had prior meniscal repair or partial meniscectomy were compared with those with no prior meniscal pathology for evidence of chondrosis in the compartments where the meniscal pathology was noted. After adjusting for age, there was no difference between knees without previous meniscal surgery and knees with previous meniscal repair. Previous partial meniscectomy was associated with a higher rate of chondrosis in the same compartment compared with knees without prior meniscal surgery. Level of evidence: II.

54. Stein T, Mehling AP, Welsch F, von Eisenhart-Rothe R, Jäger A: Long-term outcome after arthroscopic meniscal repair versus arthroscopic partial meniscectomy for traumatic meniscal tears. *Am J Sports Med* 2010;38(8): 1542-1548.

Eighty-one patients were retrospectively reviewed after meniscal surgery to compare meniscal repair versus partial meniscectomy and the effects on radiographic signs of osteoarthritis and sports activity. In the meniscal repair group (N = 42) at long-term follow-up, 80.8% showed no osteoarthritic progression; in the partial meniscectomy group (N = 39), only 40.4% showed no progression. The athletes showed a significant loss in sports activity in the meniscectomy group compared with the meniscal repair group. Level of evidence: III.

55. Marzo JM, Gurske-DePerio J: Effects of medial meniscus posterior horn avulsion and repair on tibiofemoral contact area and peak contact pressure with clinical implications. *Am J Sports Med* 2009;37(1):124-129.

56. Grant JA, Wilde J, Miller BS, Bedi A: Comparison of inside-out and all-inside techniques for the repair of isolated meniscal tears: A systematic review. *Am J Sports Med* 2012;40(2):459-468.

This study sought to compare healing rates for all-inside and inside-out meniscal repair techniques for unstable peripheral longitudinal meniscal tears. A systematic review of the literature was performed, and it was noted that the clinical failure rate for inside-out repairs was 17% versus 19% for all-inside repairs. Subjective outcomes were not significantly different between the groups. More nerve symptoms were associated with the inside-out repair, and more implant-related complications were seen with the all-inside technique.

57. LaPrade RF, Wills NJ, Spiridonov SI, Perkinson S: A prospective outcomes study of meniscal allograft transplantation. *Am J Sports Med* 2010;38(9):1804-1812.

Forty patients (mean age, 25 years) underwent meniscal transplantation. After mean final follow-up of 2.5 years, IKDC and Cincinnati knee scores improved significantly. Five patients sustained tears of their meniscal transplant and underwent partial meniscectomy of the graft. The results confirm that meniscal transplantation significantly reduces pain, decreases activity-related effusions, and improves function in patients with a prior meniscectomy. The long-term chondroprotective effects remain unknown. Level of evidence: IV.

58. Abat F, Gelber PE, Erquicia JI, Pelfort X, Gonzalez-Lucena G, Monllau JC: Suture-only fixation technique leads to a higher degree of extrusion than bony fixation in meniscal allograft transplantation. *Am J Sports Med* 2012;40(7):1591-1596.

Meniscal transplants were performed: 33 with a suture-only technique and 55 with bone-plug methods. A higher percentage of extruded meniscal tissue was found in the suture-only group. No association was found between the degree of extrusion and the functional score. Graft tears were seen in 21.4% of the suture-only group

versus 7.3% in the bone-plug fixation group. It appears that the fixation of meniscal allografts leads to less graft extrusion and fewer graft tears at an average of 40 months. Level of evidence: II.

59. Shelbourne KD, Patel DV, Adsit WS, Porter DA: Rehabilitation after meniscal repair. *Clin Sports Med* 1996; 15(3):595-612.

60. Jazrawi LM, Alaia MJ, Chang G, Fitzgerald EF, Recht MP: Advances in magnetic resonance imaging of articular cartilage. *J Am Acad Orthop Surg* 2011;19(7): 420-429.

This review article summarized the use of MRI for diagnosis and the assessment of chondral injuries. T2 mapping, T1rho, sodium MRI, and dGEMRIC are discussed.

61. Pearle AD, Warren RF, Rodeo SA: Basic science of articular cartilage and osteoarthritis. *Clin Sports Med* 2005; 24(1):1-12.

62. Tetteh ES, Bajaj S, Ghodadra NS: Basic science and surgical treatment options for articular cartilage injuries of the knee. *J Orthop Sports Phys Ther* 2012;42(3): 243-253.

This review article explains various modalities and techniques for the treatment of articular cartilage injuries of the knee. The basic science involving cartilage homeostasis and injury as well as indications for the various palliative, reparative, and restorative joint preservation techniques are reviewed.

63. Steadman JR, Briggs KK, Rodrigo JJ, Kocher MS, Gill TJ, Rodkey WG: Outcomes of microfracture for traumatic chondral defects of the knee: Average 11-year follow-up. *Arthroscopy* 2003;19(5):477-484.

64. Mithoefer K, Williams RJ III, Warren RF, et al: The microfracture technique for the treatment of articular cartilage lesions in the knee: A prospective cohort study. *J Bone Joint Surg Am* 2005;87(9):1911-1920.

65. Bentley G, Biant LC, Vijayan S, Macmull S, Skinner JA, Carrington RW: Minimum ten-year results of a prospective randomised study of autologous chondrocyte implantation versus mosaicplasty for symptomatic articular cartilage lesions of the knee. *J Bone Joint Surg Br* 2012;94(4):504-509.

One hundred patients were followed for a minimum of 10 years to compare ACI with mosaicplasty for the treatment of knee articular cartilage defects. Failure rates were 17% in the ACI group and 55% in the mosaicplasty group. The defects were very large: 440 mm in the ACI group and 399 mm in the mosaicplasty group.

66. Van Assche D, Staes F, Van Caspel D, et al: Autologous chondrocyte implantation versus microfracture for knee cartilage injury: A prospective randomized trial, with 2-year follow-up. *Knee Surg Sports Traumatol Arthrosc* 2010;18(4):486-495.

Thirty-four patients who underwent ACI were compared with 33 patients who underwent microfracture over a 2-year follow-up period. Initial recovery at 9 and

4: Lower Extremity

12 months was slower in the ACI group. At 2 years, functional outcomes were similar in the microfracture and ACI groups.

67. Gudas R, Kalesinskas RJ, Kimtys V, et al: A prospective randomized clinical study of mosaic osteochondral autologous transplantation versus microfracture for the treatment of osteochondral defects in the knee joint in young athletes. *Arthroscopy* 2005;21(9):1066-1075.

68. Conlan T, Garth WP Jr, Lemons JE: Evaluation of the medial soft-tissue restraints of the extensor mechanism of the knee. *J Bone Joint Surg Am* 1993;75(5):682-693.

69. Dejour D, Le Coultre B: Osteotomies in patello-femoral instabilities. *Sports Med Arthrosc* 2007;15(1):39-46.

70. Ahmad R, Kumar GS, Katam K, Dunlop D, Pozo JL: Significance of a "hot patella" in total knee replacement without primary patellar resurfacing. *Knee* 2009;16(5):337-340.

71. Seil R, Müller B, Georg T, Kohn D, Rupp S: Reliability and interobserver variability in radiological patellar height ratios. *Knee Surg Sports Traumatol Arthrosc* 2000;8(4):231-236.

72. Balcarek P, Jung K, Frosch KH, Stürmer KM: Value of the tibial tuberosity-trochlear groove distance in patellar instability in the young athlete. *Am J Sports Med* 2011; 39(8):1756-1761.

One hundred nine young athletes with lateral patellar instability were compared with 136 control patients in terms of TT-TG distance and history of patellar dislocation. Young athletes demonstrated an association with increased TT-TG distance with patellar dislocation; this distance was, on average, 4 mm larger in patients with patellar dislocation.

73. Jain NP, Khan N, Fithian DC: A treatment algorithm for primary patellar dislocations. *Sports Health* 2011; 3(2):170-174.

This review article summarized identification and management of primary patellar dislocations. First-time dislocations should be treated conservatively unless there is a displaced osteochondral piece.

74. Mayer C, Magnussen RA, Servien E, et al: Patellar tendon tenodesis in association with tibial tubercle distalization for the treatment of episodic patellar dislocation with patella alta. *Am J Sports Med* 2012;40(2):346-351.

The authors found that patellar tendon tenodesis and tibial tubercle distalization lead to normal patellar tendon length, a stable patellofemoral joint, and good knee function. Level of evidence: IV.

75. Smirk C, Morris H: The anatomy and reconstruction of the medial patellofemoral ligament. *Knee* 2003;10(3):221-227.

76. Andrish J: The management of recurrent patellar dislocation. *Orthop Clin North Am* 2008;39(3):313-327, vi.

77. Dye SF, Vaupel GL, Dye CC: Conscious neurosensory mapping of the internal structures of the human knee without intraarticular anesthesia. *Am J Sports Med* 1998;26(6):773-777.

78. Sanchis-Alfonso V, Roselló-Sastre E, Monteagudo-Castro C, Esquerdo J: Quantitative analysis of nerve changes in the lateral retinaculum in patients with isolated symptomatic patellofemoral malalignment: A preliminary study. *Am J Sports Med* 1998;26(5):703-709.

79. Witvrouw E, Lysens R, Bellemans J, Cambier D, Vanderstraeten G: Intrinsic risk factors for the development of anterior knee pain in an athletic population: A two-year prospective study. *Am J Sports Med* 2000; 28(4):480-489.

80. Fukuda TY, Rossetto FM, Magalhães E, Bryk FF, Lucareli PR, de Almeida Aparecida Carvalho N: Short-term effects of hip abductors and lateral rotators strengthening in females with patellofemoral pain syndrome: A randomized controlled clinical trial. *J Orthop Sports Phys Ther* 2010;40(11):736-742.

Seventy sedentary women were distributed randomly into a conventional knee exercise group, a knee and hip abductor and external rotator strengthening group, and a group that did not receive treatment. Hip abductor and external rotator muscle strengthening was effective in improving pain in sedentary women with patellofemoral pain syndrome, but this finding was significant only with pain going down stairs. Level of evidence: III.

Video References

38.1: Gehrmann RM: Video. *Lachman and Anterior Drawer Test*. Newark, NJ, 2013.

38.2: Gehrmann RM: Video. *Pivot Shift*. Newark, NJ, 2013.

38.3: Gehrmann RM: Video. *Posterolateral Drawer Test*. Newark, NJ, 2013.

38.4: Gehrmann RM: Video. *Posterior Cruciate Ligament, Lateral Collateral Ligament, and Posterolateral Corner Examination*. Newark, NJ, 2013.

38.5: Fester EW, Strickland JP, Noyes FR: Video. *Lateral and Posterolateral Knee Anatomy*. Available at http://orthoportal.aaos.org/emedia/singleVideoPlayer.aspx?resource=EMEDIA_OSVL_09_06. Accessed January 15, 2014.

38.6: Gehrmann RM: Video. *Posterior Drawer and Quadriceps Active Test*. Newark, NJ, 2013.

38.7: Clark RR, Getelman MH: Video. *Diagnostic Arthroscopic Knee Examination*. Available at http://orthoportal.aaos.org/emedia/singleVideoPlayer.aspx?resource=EMEDIA_OSVL_12_27. Accessed January 15, 2014.

38.8: Gehrmann RM: Video. *Patellar J Sign*. Newark, NJ, 2013.

Chapter 39

Bone Loss

J. Tracy Watson, MD   Iain McFadyen, MBChB, FRCS (Tr&Orth)   Joshua Langford, MD

4: Lower Extremity

Introduction

The treatment of segmental bone loss occurring as the result of acute trauma has traditionally been a complex surgical problem. Numerous procedures have been devised to reconstitute bone stock, obtain fracture union, and provide a stable functional limb.[1-4]

What constitutes a critical-sized defect varies with the anatomic location of the defect as well as the state of the soft tissues surrounding it. General guidelines for a critical defect size that have been suggested in the literature include a defect length greater than 2 cm and greater than 50% loss of bone circumference.[1]

For successful limb reconstitution to occur, two factors must always be present or provided for during the reconstructive effort. First, a competent biologic stimulus must be present or provided for (osteoblasts and viable cellular elements, vascularized fibrous tissue, and a healthy soft-tissue envelope). The inability of the traumatized soft tissues to proceed with centrifugal revascularization is a primary factor in the development of nonunions or the failure of graft materials.[5] The second requirement for successful limb reconstruction is mechanical stability. Inadequate fixation techniques, which allow excessive motion at the fracture site, in conjunction with compromised biology can contribute to the development of nonunion and subsequent failure.

Applied biologic stimuli are numerous and most traditionally have included open autogenous bone grafting,[3,4] intramedullary reaming, vascularized free-tissue transfers (muscle and bone), and distraction osteogenesis techniques.[2,6,7] Other modalities that may provide a biologic "jump start" include electrical stimulation and ultrasound application.[8,9] The injection or the implantation of bone growth factors and autogenous cellular grafts has been shown to augment healing in both animal and human nonunion studies.[10] Newer composite bone grafting techniques,[11] in conjunction with the development of vascularized soft-tissue envelopes, the Masquelet technique,[12-14] and titanium segmental bone replacement, have shown early success in reconstructing chronic segmental bone loss.

Mechanical stability can be achieved through many modalities. Tension band plating has been used for defect management in periarticular locations or in situations where a significant deformity accompanies the defect. This method also has been used to bridge the defect in situations of metaphyseal bone loss bridging the shaft and articular regions, allowing for metadiaphyseal grafting. Intramedullary nails, as well as external fixation, are also excellent means of achieving stability and have the additional benefit of fostering weight bearing with accompanying cyclic loading, which acts as a stimulus to propagate the fracture healing cascade involving both biomechanical and bioelectric factors.[2,6] This chapter discusses the current technologies available for reconstructing segmental bone loss in the context of concomitant fixation methodologies and orthobiologic augmentation.

Clinical Evaluation and Biology of the Defect

Bone loss, which may be accompanied by significant deformity or limb-length discrepancy, makes acute correction challenging. In addition, the fracture site may be so exceptionally stiff that acute correction using simple plating or nailing procedures may require extensive exposures and lead to significant associated morbidity. The invasive nature of open plating may compromise vascularity surrounding the fracture site, and reactivation of the infection is possible.

In general, as the magnitude of the skeletal defect increases, the viability and the competency of the soft-tissue envelope decreases; thus, these situations are more likely to be managed with external fixation techniques, specifically bone transport. In cases of infected defects, draining sinuses with atrophic and scarred soft tissues are often present at the defect site. Consider-

Dr. Watson or an immediate family member has received royalties from Biomet, DePuy, and Smith & Nephew; is a member of a speakers' bureau or has made paid presentations on behalf of Medtronic and Stryker; serves as a paid consultant to or is an employee of Bioventus and Smith & Nephew; serves as an unpaid consultant to Accelalox and Ellipse; and serves as a board member, owner, officer, or committee member of the Orthopaedic Trauma Association. Dr. McFadyen or an immediate family member is a member of a speakers' bureau or has made paid presentations on behalf of Smith & Nephew and Synthes. Dr. Langford or an immediate family member serves as a paid consultant to or is an employee of Stryker and has stock or stock options held in the Institute for Better Bone Health, LLC.

Table 1

Average Volumes of Bone Graft Obtained by Site

Harvest Site	Average Graft Obtained
Anterior iliac crest	30 mL
Greater trochanter	40 mL
Posterior iliac crest	40 mL
RIA femoral shaft	40 to 90 mL

RIA = reamer irrigator aspirator.

ation of these issues helps determine the extent of nonviable tissue débridement necessary to obtain healthy vascular tissue.

MRI can be helpful to determine the extent of marrow dysvascularity found in a proposed transport segment if bone transport is being considered or at the defect site if direct grafting onto the defect is the treatment option being considered. In addition, arteriography may be useful to determine distal vascularity (blush) with regard to proposed docking segment viability as well as soft-tissue viability. In cases where microvascular techniques, such as a vascularized free fibula, are being considered, CT angiography is essential not only to determine the ability to provide adequate flow to the graft but also evaluate the recipient host bed.[15]

In many instances, these skeletal defects occur in concert with soft-tissue deficits. A competent soft-tissue envelope is required to begin the reconstruction phase. For acute or chronic bone loss, it is advantageous to avoid local rotational flaps because the rotated muscle is often involved in the previous zone of injury, and thus performing a rotational myoplasty may further damage a compromised muscle. Ultimately, the additional vascularity supplied by this compromised muscle may be of minimal value. The use of free-tissue transfer helps provide a well-vascularized tissue bed through which any of the grafting methodologies can be performed.

Autogenous Bone Grafting

Direct bone grafting into the segmental defect through an open exposure continues to be the mainstay for smaller critical-sized defects less than 3 to 4 cm.[2,4] In the case of a tibial defect, a posterolateral approach has been used to accomplish a tibia pro fibula technique to bypass the defect region and has historically demonstrated excellent rates of union.[3,4] Fresh cancellous autograft provides the quickest and most reliable type of bone graft. Its open structure allows rapid revascularization; a 5-mm graft may be totally revascularized in 20 to 25 days. It is estimated that approximately 30 mL of graft can reliably be harvested from an anterior iliac

crest.[16] However, many other sites of harvest have been described, differing only in the amount of graft obtained from each harvest site (Table 1). Recent literature has demonstrated histologic differences between iliac crest and tibial bone graft, suggesting superiority of the iliac crest in terms of osteogenic and hematopoietic progenitor cell content.[17] Studies document success rates approaching 100% for subcritical-sized defects (1- to 2-cm defects) requiring 20 mL or less of autograft.[2,4]

There are many issues regarding autogenous iliac crest bone graft (AICBG) because of the limited quantity available and the reported rates of postoperative pain from the graft harvest site.[18,19] Substantial rates of complications related to the harvest site have been reported.[17,18] It has been thought that this technique is restricted to short defects—in the range of 4 to 6 cm. Numerous studies report favorable union results for critical-sized defects up to 4 cm. However, in many of these studies, multiple graft procedures were required to achieve solid union.[2-4]

The ability to obtain substantial amounts of autogenous graft material would appear to be an advantage for the treatment of critical-sized defects. The reamer irrigator aspirator (RIA; Synthes) offers a technique to achieve substantial amounts of graft volumes for the treatment of larger segmental defects. The medullary canal of the femur or the tibia is reamed with a device designed to collect the reamings and deliver them for potential grafting procedures.[20,21] Variable amounts of harvested graft have been reported in the literature and range from 30 to 90 mL. A recent comparison between a historical control group using anterior iliac harvesting (40 patients) versus a study group using femoral shaft RIA harvesting (41 patients) documented 25 to 75 mL of harvested RIA graft (average, 40.3 mL).[20] The authors reported a favorable union rate with RIA bone grafting (37 of 41 patients) versus AICBG (32 of 40 patients), although it was not statistically significant. There were significantly lower postoperative harvest site pain scores from the RIA group versus the AICBG group at 48 hours, 48 hours to 3 months, and greater than 3 months (P = 0.001, 0.001, and 0.004, respectively). There were two complications related to the graft harvest site in the RIA group (one perforation of the distal anterior femoral cortex treated conservatively and one excessive reaming of the femoral neck treated with prophylactic cannulated screws) versus 12 harvest site complications in the AICBG group (3 infections, 1 hematoma, and 8 patients with numbness). This study had several limitations, including the concurrent use of bone morphogenetic protein-2 (BMP-2) in most cases. This somewhat limits the ability to draw strong conclusions regarding the relative efficacy of RIA bone graft versus AICBG from this study.[20]

A recent study reported on the treatment of 20 bone defects ranging from 2 to 14.5 cm (average = 6.6 cm) using RIA bone graft.[22] Eighteen of the 20 patients were initially treated with an antibiotic cement spacer using the Masquelet technique (discussed in the following section). The average graft volume obtained using

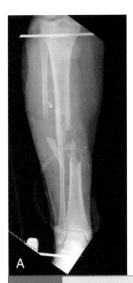
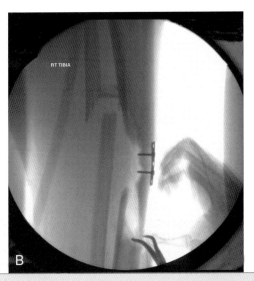
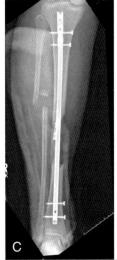
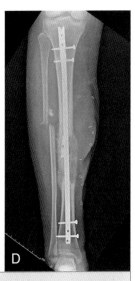

Figure 1   **A,** An open tibial shaft fracture with nearly complete segmental bone loss and temporized with a spanning external fixator to allow for the zone of injury to declare itself prior to definitive stabilization. **B,** At the time of definitive intramedullary nailing and flap wound closure, the resultant defect was noted to be nearly 5 cm with minimal bayonet apposition. The small plate was used to achieve a single intact cortex to facilitate grafting. RIA bone harvest from the femur plus allograft augmentation was used as a graft material at 6 weeks post flap. Final AP **C** and lateral **D,** follow-up views at 7 months after the graft demonstrating incorporation of the graft and reestablishment of the cortices.

the RIA was 64 mL. Seventeen of the 20 bone defects ultimately healed, although 7 of these required repeat surgery. The authors reported no significant complications related to the bone graft harvest site[18,22] (Figure 1).

Multiple reports of post-RIA iatrogenic fractures have recently been reported and are mostly attributed to the technical aspects of harvesting as a result of aggressive eccentric reaming.[23] Thus, the surgeon must be aware of this potential complication and avoid eccentric placement of the reaming guidewire and proceed with caution.

Numerous basic science studies have demonstrated the biologic potential of RIA bone graft. Investigators have documented elevated amounts of osteoinductive growth factors[24-27] and osteoprogenitor and endothelial progenitor cell types[26,28] compared with AICBG. Although the early evidence regarding RIA bone grafting is encouraging, there is currently a lack of high-level comparative evidence.

Masquelet Technique (Membrane-Directed Bone Formation)

Recently, antibiotic spacers have been used to induce a well-vascularized pseudomembrane in preparation for the bone grafting of critical-sized defects. The original clinical series was first published in English in 2003.[14] A two-stage technique for the treatment of long-bone defects was described that involved the formation of an induced membrane around a cement spacer. The spacer was removed at a second stage and replaced with AICBG. A series of 35 patients treated with this tech-

nique for bone defects ranging from 5 to 25 cm was discussed. Thirty-one of the 35 patients (89%) experienced healing of their bone defects. Four patients sustained late fractures through the grafted defect after it was considered healed. These fractures healed with cast immobilization in all cases. It was proposed that the cement spacer maintained the space for bone reconstruction and formed a synovium-like membrane that prevented graft resorption and also favored vascularization and corticalization of the graft.

Other authors have reported impressive results when performing this two-stage reconstructive procedure.[12,13,29] Following the development of a healthy, biologically competent wound, an antibiotic spacer is placed into the defect cavity and closed either by primary wound closure or soft-tissue flap procedures. A tubular pseudomembrane is allowed to develop surrounding the spacer. Following complete wound healing, the antibiotic spacer is carefully removed, preserving and maintaining the defect cavity and the surrounding membrane. Traditional cancellous autografting was then placed directly into the tubularized membrane. Rapid reconstitution of the defect then occurred, with improved consolidation times and improved rates of union compared with historic rates of bone grafting large segmental defects (Figure 2). Other authors have demonstrated similar improved union rates grafting into the composite grafts of these membranes, such as demineralized bone matrix (DBM) plus BMP adjuvants, vascularized free fibula grafts, and RIA-derived grafts.[30-33]

Defects treated with this methodology have ranged in size from 3 to 25 cm. The improved graft performance is thought to be caused by the induced mem-

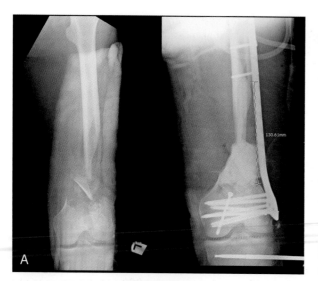
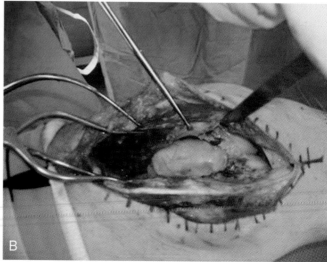
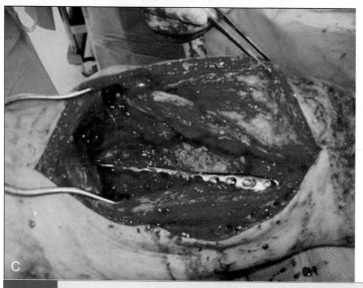
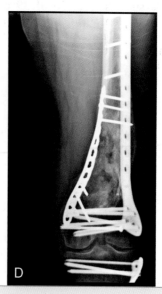

Figure 2 **A,** Injury and postoperative radiographs of a severe open distal femoral fracture with 13 cm of metadiaphyseal bone loss. At the time of definitive closure, a stemmed antibiotic spacer was implanted to maintain length and develop a Masquelet membrane. At 10 weeks after spacer insertion, a second surgery removed the spacer (**B**), and an 80 mL RIA graft was inserted into the pseudomembrane with an adjunctive medial plate (**C**). **D,** Radiograph showing healing of the massive defect after 1 year.

brane's ability to secrete various endogenous growth factors, including vascular endothelial growth factor (VEGF), transforming growth factor–β1 (TGF-β1), and BMP-2.[12,13,34-37] These induced membranes have also been shown to favor the differentiation of human marrow stromal cells into an osteoblastic lineage.[35-37] Thus, the graft site is providing the ideal local environment for the rapid differentiation of a host of graft materials, assuming a threshold of colony-forming cells is present in the graft material.[10] This innovation gives rise to the idea of using a combination approach for restoring these large segmental defects.

Osteobiologics and Defect Augmentation

The emergence of orthobiologics holds great promise for large skeletal defects. The ability to augment large defects with applied growth factor adjuvants to reduce prolonged consolidation times is an attractive alternative to other treatment strategies. In an effort to augment the limited quantities of autograft or avoid autograft, the concept of composite grafting is now achieving favorable results for the treatment of subcritical- and critical-sized defects (1 to 4 cm or less).

Bone marrow aspirate concentrate (BMAC) contains a viable population of osteoprogenitor cells capable of participating in osteogenesis.[10] This material has been combined with multiple adjuvants (composites) that serve as osteoconductive carriers to deliver these osteogenic marrow elements. Basic science and clinical series document the various carriers as effective and include DBM, collagen sponges, calcium ceramics, and titanium cages.[10,11,38]

DBM is formed by acid extraction of the mineralized extracellular matrix of allograft bone. In theory, the noncollagenous proteins, including osteoinductive proteins such as the BMPs, remain viable, but its osteoinductivity is relatively limited and highly variable among the different preparations and donors. DBM is highly osteoconductive because of its particulate nature and presents a large surface area and three-dimensional architecture to serve as a site of cellular attachment. DBM combined with BMAC has been shown to have results comparable to AICBG for the treatment of subcritical-sized nonunion defects. One study reported on the use of BMAC in combination with DBM as a composite graft for the treatment of osseous defects in 39 patients.[39] A 77% success rate (30 of 39 patients) was reported overall in terms of osseous union, although the results were less impressive in the subgroup of patients with nonunion (61% union rate).

A composite graft using BMAC combined with a collagen sponge or porous hydroxyapatite granules as a scaffold has reported encouraging results in a prospective clinical trial.[40] The authors reported on 39 bone defects (ranging in size from 0.54 cm³ to 151.2 cm³) treated with BMAC/scaffold combined with AICBG. Thirty-six of the 39 defects (92%) healed following treatment, with no significant complications reported. Confounding the results was the fact that AICBG was also added to the composite graft. However, basic science studies have demonstrated efficacy when using BMAC-loaded alloplastic graft materials ($CaPO_4$) and a variety of porous calcium-based conductive substrates.[38]

One study showed excellent rates of union using iliac aspirate concentrates combined with and without DBM for the treatment of nonunion defects up to 2 to 3 cm.[10] Excellent results were dependent on achieving a threshold number of colony-forming units in the composite graft to achieve union in these subcritical-sized defects. This technique holds promise for the future as the ability to collect and concentrate autogenous cellular elements improves.[10] Simple application of aspirate alone has demonstrated mixed results in uncontrolled case series. It is clear that a threshold concentration of these bone-forming cells is the critical factor.[10]

A multifactorial approach is being exploited by investigators and combines titanium cages with various mixtures of autograft, DBM, and allograft bone for the reconstruction of large segmental defects.[41] The basic technique requires that the defect tract be completely viable with competent soft tissues and have no evidence of deep infection. These defects are usually stabilized initially with external fixation until the rigid wound requirements have been met. During a second-stage procedure, the defect is then reconstructed by placing a titanium cage into the defect. The cage is loaded with a combination of various grafting materials, including autograft, DBM, and allograft or combinations of these materials. The cage/limb composite is then stabilized by many standard techniques, most commonly an intramedullary rod. Plates and external fixation also have been reported as adjuvants providing the necessary mechanical stability until these cage/graft composites unite. Multiple studies report excellent rates of union and the restoration of limb function for treating a host of long-bone defects, including tibial, humeral, and femoral segmental defects up to 15 cm.[11,41]

To avoid a second surgical exposure and the need for secondary graft procedures, the use of inductive proteins has demonstrated encouraging results for the reconstruction of segmental defects. The implantation of BMP-2 combined with allograft compared with autograft for the treatment of acute segmental defects was investigated in a prospective, randomized controlled trial of 30 patients with tibial diaphyseal bone defects.[42] The average defect size was 4 cm (range, 1 to 7 cm). At 12-month follow-up, 80% of the patients (12 of 15 patients) in the AICBG group and 87% of the patients (13 of 15 patients) in the allograft/recombinant human BMP-2 (rhBMP-2) group experienced healing without reintervention ($P = 0.2$). There were no significant differences in complication rates or functional outcomes between the two groups. This study suggests that rhBMP-2/allograft is safe and as effective as traditional autogenous bone grafting for the treatment of tibial fractures associated with extensive traumatic diaphyseal bone loss.

Currently, only rhBMP-7 (osteogenic protein-1) is approved for the treatment of chronic nonunion for patients in whom previous autogenous bone grafting has failed (approved under FDA Humanitarian Device Exemption). The FDA has approved the use of rhBMP-2 only for anterior lumbar interbody spine fusions and acute, open tibial fractures treated with an intramedullary nail. The use of rhBMP-2 combined with allograft for the treatment of bone defects currently represents an off-label use.

Free-Tissue Transfer

For massive defects, vascularized fibular grafts have been shown to bridge extended defects. Vascularized fibular grafts have been shown as an effective means of treating destructive osteomyelitis and infected nonunions for defects greater than 8 to 10 cm. The vascularized fibula graft was first used to restore integrity in a tibial defect. Since then, it has become the most commonly used free bone graft for diaphyseal defects because of its length and relative donor site morbidity compared with a vascularized iliac crest harvest or other composite vascularized bone or muscle graft harvest sites. The indications have been extended to defect management in the humerus as well as the femoral shaft. In cases of large defects (> 8 cm), many authors consider it the treatment of choice, particularly in sites with poor host bed vascularity. However, these patients must be protected for prolonged periods of time following healing of the grafts because remodeling is very

4: Lower Extremity

slow and these grafts have shown a tendency to stress fracture. This technique requires a specialized skill set, requires a large amount of hospital resources, can have a relatively high failure rate of the vascular anastomosis, and is associated with relative harvest site morbidity. Because of these disadvantages, these techniques have been combined with distraction techniques in an effort to overcome the slow remodeling times for larger free fibular grafts.[43]

Bone Transport

When considering bone transport for segmental bone loss, it is paramount to determine if a biologically sound healing environment can be achieved at both the site of the proposed corticotomy and the docking sites. The success of both corticotomy and solid docking involves well-vascularized segments of bone and soft tissue. If soft-tissue incompetence (dysvascularity) is present at the proposed corticotomy site, the production of healthy regenerate may be in question.[2,6] Associated soft-tissue compromise may be coexistent elsewhere in the limb, which may involve the site of the proposed corticotomy.

Solid healing of the docking site requires all of the biologic components necessary to heal what is equivalent to an acute fracture. If the docking fragments are excessively mobile, the moving bone ends will traumatize the local blood supply. Thus, the influence of a stable mechanical environment facilitates docking site union. The hallmark of these events is the inflammatory phase of fracture healing that promotes the revascularization process. This area must be manipulated to provide the appropriate vascular response either thru aggressive débridement or soft-tissue coverage techniques.

If distraction techniques are being considered, the question of indolent infection may still be an issue. Every effort should be made to remove any devitalized bone and necrotic soft tissue. This may appear to involve unnecessary trips to the operating room; however, the most common failure of bone transport is indolent or delayed presentation of infection at the docking site. Thus, a staged approach has resulted in a significant improvement in rates of union.[2,6,43] If infection is not in question, reconstruction can begin immediately without the intermediate débridement stage.

Transport Methodology

Acute or gradual shortening offers advantages over transport in patients with vascular insufficiency; a single-vessel leg with free vascularized tissue transfer is more challenging. Patients with a systemic small vessel disease process (diabetes, severe peripheral vascular disease, or a connective tissue disorder) are also candidates for shortening strategies.

Analysis of multiple large transport case series reveals an algorithm for the application of these techniques depending on the size of the defects to be treated (Level III and IV evidence). Segmental defects of up to 5 cm are best treated by initial shortening followed by callus distraction.[7,43,44] Bony defects from 5 to 12 cm are best treated by segmental transport while maintaining limb length.[2,6,7,43,45] Defects larger than 12 cm are best treated by reconstruction with a vascularized free fibula graft combined with transport and lengthening.[2,6,7,43,44,46]

Shortening acutely can be accomplished safely for defects up to 3 to 4 cm in the tibia and the humerus.[7,43,46] More shortening can be tolerated acutely in a femoral defect up to 5 to 7 cm. In some situations, it is advantageous to decrease the transport distance and thus time in the frame. Shortening aids in soft-tissue coverage by decreasing tension and gaps in the open wound; this approach combined with negative pressure dressings may allow wounds to be closed by delayed primary closure or healed by secondary intention or simple skin grafting.

Acute shortening more than 4 cm can cause the development of tortuous vasculature and actually produces a low flow state with detrimental consequences.[6,43,44] Open soft-tissue wounds, when acutely compressed, can become notably bunched and dysvascular with the development of significant edema and the possibility of additional tissue necrosis and infection. More than 4 cm may be safely accomplished in the femur; however, similar problems with wound edema and bunching may occur.

If a chronic soft-tissue defect is larger than can safely be closed acutely following resection, or if the patient is not a candidate for free-flap soft-tissue augmentation, a gradual shortening can accomplish the same goals. Shortening at a rate of 5 mm per day in divided doses will rapidly oppose the skeletal defect as well as avoid the detrimental soft-tissue consequences and vascular element kinking of acute defect compression.

Massive defects greater than 8 to 10 cm are candidates for combined treatment options. The success of massive transport is directly proportional to the number of complications associated with these rigorous reconstructions. It is recommended that combination methodologies be initiated with great caution, in cases where all transport parameters are optimized, for example, intact vascularity, small vessel disease, and intact soft-tissue sleeve. Acutely shortening the defect can reduce the transport time required to achieve docking. After docking is accomplished, straightforward lengthening can then be performed.

The development of a tabularized transport envelope is helpful to avoid deviation of the transport segment and allow for unencumbered transport. An antibiotic spacer is placed into the proposed transport tract at the time of wound closure or free-flap coverage.[43,44,46] This method is very similar to the Masquelet technique, allowing the development of a well-circumscribed soft-tissue sleeve through which the transport segment can occur. After soft-tissue healing (flap healing) has been accomplished, the transport can be initiated 6 to 8 weeks after wound closure (Figure 3).

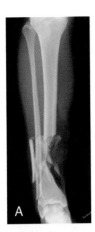

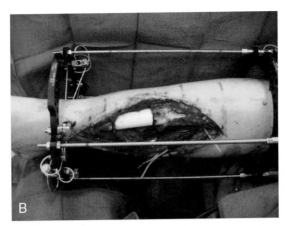

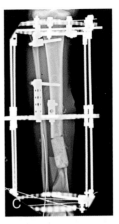

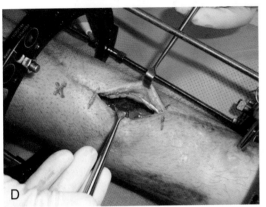

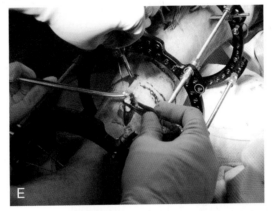

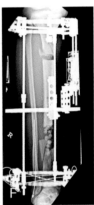

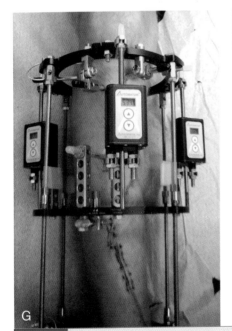

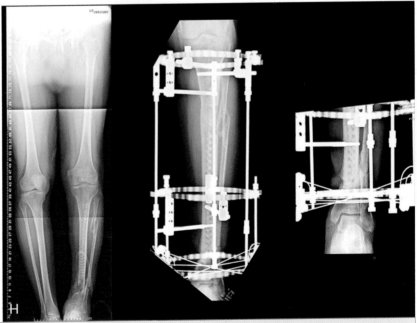

Figure 3 Radiographs and clinical photographs of transport. **A,** Injury with significant bone and soft-tissue loss. Multiple débridements were required to achieve a biologically stable wound. **B** and **C,** An antibiotic spacer spans the defect at the time of composite free-flap coverage to induce the development of a Masquelet membrane. **D** and **E,** Following flap maturation, the antibiotic spacer is carefully removed (note the thickened pseudomembrane) and preserved. A small chain of antibiotic beads is then placed into the defect to maintain the transport tract integrity. **F** and **G,** Bone transport is initiated using auto distracters, compressing the antibiotic beads at the docking site. Prior to docking, the beads are removed, and a small autograft implanted to augment rapid healing of the docking site. **H,** Similar infected defect undergoing segmental transport. The docking site was grafted to help achieve rapid consolidation. Regenerate and docking site consolidation viewed immediately prior to frame removal.

4: Lower Extremity

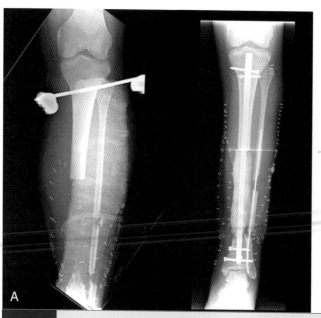
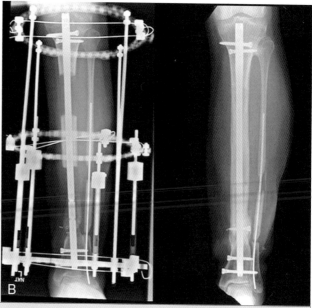

Figure 4 **A,** A severe open tibial shaft fracture requiring multiple débridements. Stabilization was facilitated with an intramedullary nail and at time of free-flap coverage, and an antibiotic spacer was placed into the defect to encourage the formation of a Masquelet membrane. **B,** Segmental bone transport was initiated over the intramedullary nail with fixator assistance. The nail provides excellent support to slowly developing regenerate and facilitates docking site union. The docking site required bone grafting to achieve solid union of this 18-cm regenerate. (Case courtesy of Hank Hutchinson, MD, Tallahassee, FL.)

At the time of the secondary procedure, the antibiotic spacer is removed and a solitary chain of antibiotic cement beads is placed into the defect. The beads provide and maintain a potential space or fibrous tunnel through which the transport segment will travel and prevent invagination of the intact soft-tissue envelope into the transport tract. Also, the well-vascularized Masquelet transport sleeve facilitates the healing of the docking site. Bone transport is continued until the antibiotic beads have been compressed to approximately the width of one bead. At this time, the patient is returned to surgery, and the docking site is exposed to remove the antibiotic beads. A high-speed burr is used to freshen the docking site to ensure maximal cortical contact, and grafting of the docking site is then performed. AICBG as well as numerous alloplastic materials have been used to augment and aid in the rapid consolidation of the docking site. Docking site augmentation has been shown to decrease the overall rate of nonunion and decrease frame time[2,6,43,44,46-48] (**Figure 3**).

The lengthening process can be halted in patients who may experience frame fatigue during prolonged bone transport. This will allow the lengthened regenerate to consolidate, with the only morbidity being a short functional limb.

Alternatively, after stable limb healing (shortening) has been achieved, delayed lengthening can reestablish limb length. Straightforward lengthening can now be accomplished by newer techniques, such as rapid lengthening over an intramedullary nail (**Figure 4**). In addition, distraction rates can be augmented and complications moderated using autodistractor devices that eliminate patient-directed adjustments.[7,47,49] Patients have been able to achieve a rapid lengthening, decreasing the overall time in the external device. These devices may also decrease the discomfort associated with traditional lengthening techniques. Similar results are also being reported with internal lengthening nails. These intramedullary devices distract the limb segment with limb rotation or by internal servomotors, and no external distraction device is required.

Bifocal and trifocal strategies, such as double-level transport combined with acute shortening, can be used.[43,44,46] A secondary limb lengthening over intramedullary devices for a significant defect may be performed after the first procedure.

Transport over nails has also been used for larger defects in both tibial and femoral deficiencies.[43,47,49] A similar approach uses transport under a minimally invasive percutaneous plate osteotomy bridge, which provides stability after the segment is transported and allows earlier frame removal.[48] New frame constructs using fewer Schanz pins have decreased frame complexity and have contributed to increased patient comfort as well as decreased transport complications related to pins and wires.[2,6,43,44,46,49] These hybrid transports using internal and external fixation combinations have limited applicability, and the published results are limited at best. Thus, the use of these transports should be performed with great caution and under ideal circumstances.

In cases of extremely long transports, the docking site usually heals long before consolidation of the regenerate occurs. Inadequate regenerate may result in late deformation and regenerate collapse of the limb. Frame removal should not occur until the regenerate has matured. Electrical stimulation and ultrasound have been used with encouraging results to help speed the consolidation of these very extensive regenerate segments.[8] Percutaneous augmentation of regenerate using various orthobiologic adjuvants is demonstrating encouraging results in decreasing consolidation intervals before frame removal.[44,46,49] In select cases, autogenous grafting may assist in the consolidation of a marginal regenerate.

Free vascularized fibula combined with acute shortening and bone transport has also been reported as a methodology to reduce the substantial frame time required for massive bone defect reconstruction of femoral, tibial, and humeral defects.[7,49] Transverse ipsilateral fibular transport has been reported for the reconstruction of massive tibial defects. Commonly this involves the transport of the entire fibula transversely into the tibial defect. Precise frame orientation must be assured, such that the fibula correctly "docks" at either end of the defect. A variation of fibular transfer is the split fibular transfer, in which the inner one half of the fibula is transported into the tibial defect site.[49] These procedures are technically demanding, and with the development of membrane-directed bone formation techniques as well as advances in osteobiologics, they are no longer popular and used primarily for rare indications, such as a final limb salvage attempt.

Summary

As limb salvage techniques have improved, the need to address increasingly larger defects has become critical. It is apparent that there is a limit to the size defect that can be managed with autogenous grafting methodologies alone. Contemporary management now occurs though a combination of techniques that can be used for the treatment of these defects. The use of antibiotic spacer-induced membranes combined with transport techniques, free-tissue transfer, the application of unique biomaterials, and the use of orthobiologic graft substitutes now makes the routine salvage of massive skeletal defects a reality. Although these treatment options have been described and reported in the literature, a high level of comparative evidence to guide decision making is lacking. Large-scale multicenter trials are necessary to develop these guidelines.

Key Study Points

- RIA harvested graft is equal to if not superior to AICBG in terms of the osteoinductive growth factors present and the amount of osteoprogenitor cells or endothelial progenitor cells found in the graft.

- Masquelet grafting techniques require the development of a highly vascularized pseudomembrane with which to graft into after removal of the antibiotic spacer.

- No orthobiologic adjuvant (graft substitute) has been shown to be superior to autogenous cancellous autograft.

Annotated References

1. Keating JF, Simpson AH, Robinson CM: The management of fractures with bone loss. *J Bone Joint Surg Br* 2005;87(2):142-150.

2. Watson JT, Anders M, Moed BR: Management strategies for bone loss in tibial shaft fractures. *Clin Orthop Relat Res* 1995;315:138-152.

3. Reckling FW, Waters CH III: Treatment of non-unions of fractures of the tibial diaphysis by posterolateral cortical cancellous bone-grafting. *J Bone Joint Surg Am* 1980;62(6):936-941.

4. Christian EP, Bosse MJ, Robb G: Reconstruction of large diaphyseal defects, without free fibular transfer, in Grade-IIIB tibial fractures. *J Bone Joint Surg Am* 1989;71(7):994-1004.

5. Rhinelander FW: The normal microcirculation of diaphyseal cortex and its response to fracture. *J Bone Joint Surg Am* 1968;50(4):784-800.

6. Paley D, Catagni MA, Argnani F, Villa A, Benedetti GB, Cattaneo R: Ilizarov treatment of tibial nonunions with bone loss. *Clin Orthop Relat Res* 1989;241:146-165.

7. Mekhail AO, Abraham E, Gruber B, Gonzalez M: Bone transport in the management of posttraumatic bone defects in the lower extremity. *J Trauma* 2004;56(2):368-378.

8. Gold SM, Wasserman R: Preliminary results of tibial bone transports with pulsed low intensity ultrasound (Exogen). *J Orthop Trauma* 2005;19(1):10-16.

9. Brighton CT, Shaman P, Heppenstall RB, Esterhai JL Jr, Pollack SR, Friedenberg ZB: Tibial nonunion treated with direct current, capacitive coupling, or bone graft. *Clin Orthop Relat Res* 1995;321:223-234.

10. Hernigou P, Poignard A, Beaujean F, Rouard H: Percutaneous autologous bone-marrow grafting for nonunions:

Influence of the number and concentration of progenitor cells. *J Bone Joint Surg Am* 2005;87(7):1430-1437.

11. Lindsey RW, Wood GW, Sadasivian KK, Stubbs HA, Block JE: Grafting long bone fractures with demineralized bone matrix putty enriched with bone marrow: Pilot findings. *Orthopedics* 2006;29(10):939-941.

12. Pelissier P, Martin D, Baudet J, Lepreux S, Masquelet AC: Behaviour of cancellous bone graft placed in induced membranes. *Br J Plast Surg* 2002;55(7):596-598.

13. Masquelet AC, Begue T: The concept of induced membrane for reconstruction of long bone defects. *Orthop Clin North Am* 2010;41(1):27-37.

    An induced membrane could be used to prevent resorption of the graft and to secrete growth factors, and appears as a biologic chamber. Level of evidence: V.

14. Masquelet AC: Muscle reconstruction in reconstructive surgery: Soft tissue repair and long bone reconstruction. *Langenbecks Arch Surg* 2003;388(5):344-346.

15. Bishop JA, Palanca AA, Bellino MJ, Lowenberg DW: Assessment of compromised fracture healing. *J Am Acad Orthop Surg* 2012;20(5):273-282.

    This review article highlighted the evaluation of fracture union and local blood flow. Level of evidence: V.

16. Sen MK, Miclau T: Autologous iliac crest bone graft: Should it still be the gold standard for treating nonunions? *Injury* 2007;38(suppl 1):S75-S80.

17. Chiodo CP, Hahne J, Wilson MG, Glowacki J: Histological differences in iliac and tibial bone graft. *Foot Ankle Int* 2010;31(5):418-422.

    Iliac crest and tibial cancellous grafts were examined histologically. All iliac grafts contained active hematopoietic marrow. The medullary space of tibial grafts contained fat and little hematopoietic marrow. This raises questions about the cellular contributions of different sources of bone graft. Level of evidence: IV.

18. Goulet JA, Senunas LE, DeSilva GL, Greenfield ML: Autogenous iliac crest bone graft: Complications and functional assessment. *Clin Orthop Relat Res* 1997; 339:76-81.

19. Loeffler BJ, Kellam JF, Sims SH, Bosse MJ: Prospective observational study of donor-site morbidity following anterior iliac crest bone-grafting in orthopaedic trauma reconstruction patients. *J Bone Joint Surg Am* 2012; 94(18):1649-1654.

    A prospective observational study of 92 patients undergoing anterior iliac crest bone graft harvest is presented. Substantial, persistent pain from the donor site was seen in only 2% of the patients. Level of evidence: II.

20. Belthur MV, Conway JD, Jindal G, Ranade A, Herzenberg JE: Bone graft harvest using a new intramedullary system. *Clin Orthop Relat Res* 2008;466(12):2973-2980.

21. Kobbe P, Tarkin IS, Frink M, Pape HC: Voluminous bone graft harvesting of the femoral marrow cavity for autologous transplantation: An indication for the "Reamer-Irrigator-Aspirator-" (RIA-) technique. *Unfallchirurg* 2008;111(6):469-472.

22. McCall TA, Brokaw DS, Jelen BA, et al: Treatment of large segmental bone defects with reamer-irrigator-aspirator bone graft: Technique and case series. *Orthop Clin North Am* 2010;41(1):63-73.

    The RIA technique allows access to a large volume of cancellous bone graft, and the average graft volume obtained using the RIA was 64 mL. The average defect size treated was 6.6 cm. Seventeen of the 20 bone defects ultimately healed. Level of evidence: IV.

23. Lowe JA, Della Rocca GJ, Murtha Y, et al: Complications associated with negative pressure reaming for harvesting autologous bone graft: A case series. *J Orthop Trauma* 2010;24(1):46-52.

    This technique has reported events associated with reaming and the fracture of donor femurs, which were all attributed to technical error. To avoid such issues, surgeons should assess the cortical diameters of the harvest site, monitor intraoperative reaming, and avoid harvesting in patients with osteoporosis or osteopenia. Level of evidence: IV.

24. Schmidmaier G, Herrmann S, Green J, et al: Quantitative assessment of growth factors in reaming aspirate, iliac crest, and platelet preparation. *Bone* 2006;39(5): 1156-1163.

25. Sagi HC, Young ML, Gerstenfeld L, Einhorn TA, Tornetta P: Qualitative and quantitative differences between bone graft obtained from the medullary canal (with a Reamer/Irrigator/Aspirator) and the iliac crest of the same patient. *J Bone Joint Surg Am* 2012;94(23): 2128-2135.

    Both AICBG and a graft obtained with RIA were harvested from 10 patients. Debris from RIA possessed a similar transcriptional profile to AICBG for genes known to act in the early stages of bone repair and formation. Level of evidence: IV.

26. Cox G, McGonagle D, Boxall SA, Buckley CT, Jones E, Giannoudis PV: The use of the reamer-irrigator-aspirator to harvest mesenchymal stem cells. *J Bone Joint Surg Br* 2011;93(4):517-524.

    The authors of this basic science study looked at the effluent water that passes through the filter. They showed that in addition to the reamings collected, the waste water was a potent source of mesenchymal stem cells. Level of evidence: IV.

27. Stannard JP, Sathy AK, Moeinpour F, Stewart RL, Volgas DA: Quantitative analysis of growth factors from a second filter using the Reamer-Irrigator-Aspirator system: Description of a novel technique. *Orthop Clin North Am* 2010;41(1):95-98.

    The authors demonstrated that the effluent water from the RIA has potent growth factors and using a second filter with beta-tricalcium phosphate can act as a graft extender when bathed in the effluent water. Level of evidence: IV.

28. Henrich D, Seebach C, Sterlepper E, Tauchmann C, Marzi I, Frank J: RIA reamings and hip aspirate: A comparative evaluation of osteoprogenitor and endothelial progenitor cells. *Injury* 2010;41(suppl 2):S62-S68.

    RIA aspirate was collected from 26 patients undergoing nailing of femoral fractures. Iliac crest aspirate was collected from 38 patients undergoing bone grafts. The concentration of mesenchymal stem cells and endothelial progenitor cells was assessed. RIA contained significantly higher CD34+ progenitor cells, mesenchymal stem cells, and early endothelial progenitor cells. Level of evidence: III.

29. Karger C, Kishi T, Schneider L, Fitoussi F, Masquelet AC; French Society of Orthopaedic Surgery and Traumatology (SoFCOT): Treatment of posttraumatic bone defects by the induced membrane technique. *Orthop Traumatol Surg Res* 2012;98(1):97-102.

    Eighty-four posttraumatic defects were studied retrospectively. Union was obtained in 90% of the cases; however, a mean of 6.11 interventions was necessary to obtain union. Level of evidence: III.

30. Donegan DJ, Scolaro J, Matuszewski PE, Mehta S: Staged bone grafting following placement of an antibiotic spacer block for the management of segmental long bone defects. *Orthopedics* 2011;34(11):e730-e735.

    This technique of staged bone grafting following the placement of an antibiotic spacer was used to successfully manage defects ranging from 4 to 15 cm. Osseous consolidation and full weight bearing was achieved in 10 of 11 patients. Level of evidence: IV.

31. Stafford PR, Norris BL: Reamer-irrigator-aspirator bone graft and bi Masquelet technique for segmental bone defect nonunions: A review of 25 cases. *Injury* 2010; 41(suppl 2):S72-S77.

    Twenty-five patients with 27 segmental bone loss nonunions were evaluated. The average deficit size was 5.8 cm in length (range, 1 to 25 cm). At 6 months and 1 year after surgery, 70% and 90% of the nonunions were healed clinically and radiographically, respectively. Level of evidence: IV.

32. Pelissier P, Boireau P, Martin D, Baudet J: Bone reconstruction of the lower extremity: Complications and outcomes. *Plast Reconstr Surg* 2003;111(7):2223-2229.

33. Huffman LK, Harris JG, Suk M: Using the bi-Masquelet technique and reamer-irrigator-aspirator for posttraumatic foot reconstruction. *Foot Ankle Int* 2009; 30(9):895-899.

34. Taylor BC, French BG, Fowler TT, Russell J, Poka A: Induced membrane technique for reconstruction to manage bone loss. *J Am Acad Orthop Surg* 2012;20(3): 142-150.

    A review article on the principles and the application of the induced membrane technique is presented. Level of evidence: V.

35. Pelissier P, Masquelet AC, Bareille R, Pelissier SM, Amedee J: Induced membranes secrete growth factors including vascular and osteoinductive factors and could stimulate bone regeneration. *J Orthop Res* 2004;22(1): 73-79.

36. Viateau V, Guillemin G, Bousson V, et al: Long-bone critical-size defects treated with tissue-engineered grafts: A study on sheep. *J Orthop Res* 2007;25(6):741-749.

37. Gruber HE, Riley FE, Hoelscher GL, et al: Osteogenic and chondrogenic potential of biomembrane cells from the PMMA-segmental defect rat model. *J Orthop Res* 2012;30(8):1198-1212.

    Biomembranes harvested from rat segmental defects were evaluated. Molecular analysis of biomembrane cells versus control periosteum showed significant upregulation of key genes functioning in mesenchymal stem cell differentiation and proliferation. The biomembrane demonstrates a pluripotent stem cell population. Level of evidence: IV.

38. Guda T, Walker JA, Singleton BM, et al: Guided bone regeneration in long-bone defects with a structural hydroxyapatite graft and collagen membrane. *Tissue Eng Part A* 2013;19(17-18):1879-1888.

    In a rabbit defect, a composite collagen membrane/porous hydroxyapatite bone graft was evaluated. This study indicates that using a collagen membrane with a hydroxyapatite structural graft provides benefits for bone tissue regeneration in terms of early graft integration. Level of evidence: IV.

39. Tiedeman JJ, Garvin KL, Kile TA, Connolly JF: The role of a composite, demineralized bone matrix and bone marrow in the treatment of osseous defects. *Orthopedics* 1995;18(12):1153-1158.

40. Jäger M, Herten M, Fochtmann U, et al: Bridging the gap: Bone marrow aspiration concentrate reduces autologous bone grafting in osseous defects. *J Orthop Res* 2011;29(2):173-180.

    Thirty-nine patients with bone defects were treated with BMAC plus collagen sponge (12 patients) and with hydroxyapatite; (27 patients). Clinical and radiographic findings were completed. BMAC combined with hydroxyapatite can reduce the time to healing compared with BMAC combined with collagen sponge. Level of evidence: III.

41. Cobos JA, Lindsey RW, Gugala Z: The cylindrical titanium mesh cage for treatment of a long bone segmental defect: Description of a new technique and report of two cases. *J Orthop Trauma* 2000;14(1):54-59.

42. Jones AL, Bucholz RW, Bosse MJ, et al: Recombinant human BMP-2 and allograft compared with autogenous bone graft for reconstruction fo diaphyseal tibial fractures with cortical defects: A randomized, controlled trial. *J Bone Joint Surg Am* 2006;88(7):1431-1441.

43. Robert Rozbruch S, Weitzman AM, Tracey Watson J, Freudigman P, Katz HV, Ilizarov S: Simultaneous treat-

4: Lower Extremity

ment of tibial bone and soft-tissue defects with the Ilizarov method. *J Orthop Trauma* 2006;20(3):197-205.

44. Mahaluxmivala J, Nadarajah R, Allen PW, Hill RA: Ilizarov external fixator: Acute shortening and lengthening versus bone transport in the management of tibial non-unions. *Injury* 2005;36(5):662-668.

45. Guerreschi F, Azzam W, Camagni M, Lovisetti L, Catagni MA: Tetrafocal bone transport of the tibia with circular external fixation: A case report. *J Bone Joint Surg Am* 2010;92(1):190-195.

   A case report describing proximal and distal transport via two corticotomies from one small ring of viable mid shaft bone is presented. Level of evidence: IV.

46. Lowenberg DW, Feibel RJ, Louie KW, Eshima I: Combined muscle flap and Ilizarov reconstruction for bone and soft tissue defects. *Clin Orthop Relat Res* 1996; 332:37-51.

47. Oh CW, Song HR, Roh JY, et al: Bone transport over an intramedullary nail for reconstruction of long bone defects in tibia. *Arch Orthop Trauma Surg* 2008;128(8): 801-808.

48. Girard PJ, Kuhn KM, Bailey JR, Lynott JA, Mazurek MT: Bone transport combined with locking bridge plate fixation for the treatment of tibial segmental defects: A report of two cases. *J Orthop Trauma* 2013;27(9):e220-e226.

   The treatment of large tibial bone defects using locked bridge plating and bone transport with a monolateral external fixation frame is described. The complications were minimal, and all patients healed. This technique offers an alternative to standard ring fixator bone transport. Level of evidence: IV.

49. Rozbruch SR, Ilizarov S: *Limb Lengthening and Reconstructive Surgery*. New York, NY, Informa Healthcare, 2012.

   Multiple adjuvants are reviewed for augmentation of the regenerate and docking sites. Modalities such as autodistractors, percutaneously applied orthobiologic adjuvants, ultrasound augmentation, and free tissue transfer in combination with bone transport are discussed. All of these materials and techniques have been combined to facilitate earlier regenerate consolidation and limit total frame time in patients undergoing bone transport procedures. Level of evidence: V.

Chapter 40

Soft-Tissue Coverage Options in the Lower Extremity

John T. Capo, MD

Principles of Soft-Tissue Injury

Open soft-tissue injuries often accompany fractures of the lower extremity. The energy required to create these injuries may simultaneously disrupt the soft-tissue envelope. Soft-tissue defects can be created by a variety of mechanisms, including open fractures from blunt trauma with an inside-out mechanism; penetrating injuries from assault or missile injury; an infectious process that creates soft-tissue defects; and tumorous conditions that require excision of the mass and result in a soft-tissue defect.

Initial Management of Open Injuries

The proper initial management of open fractures is essential and perhaps the most critical portion of these cases. All nonviable tissue should be removed, and the bony injury should be stabilized. The bony stabilization may be provisional or definitive. The advantage of definitive fixation is that the overall alignment is established, and the soft-tissue envelope can be set accordingly. In addition, there will be no further traction on the neurovascular structures. In contrast, the advantages of provisional fixation, such as an external fixator, are that a more thorough, repeat débridement is possible. Regardless of the type of early bony treatment, it is essential that there is good communication between the orthopaedist and the surgeon performing the reconstructive procedure.

Adjuvant Therapy

Adjuvant therapy currently being used for treating open wounds includes negative pressure wound therapy

Dr. Capo or an immediate family member has received royalties from Wright Medical Technology is a member of a speakers' bureau or has made paid presentations on behalf of Integra Life Sciences; and serves as a paid consultant to or is an employee of Synthes and Wright Medical Technology.

(NPWT) and bead pouch therapy. These methods are helpful but do not replace the essential technique of sharp débridement of contaminated and nonviable tissue. These adjuvant techniques are effective when the wound requires repeat débridement or as a temporizing measure when soft-tissue coverage is mandated. NPWT decreases tissue edema and promotes microvascularization and granulation tissue.[1-3] If after initial débridement the wound is open, some type of sealed dressing coverage is required. Standard moist, wet-to-dry, or nonadherent dressings are not adequate because desiccation of the tissue can occur. These dressings also make the wound susceptible to infection if periodic opening and inspection are required. The advantage of NPWT or a bead pouch is that the wound is sealed and will stay sterile and moist. If the wound requires further débridement, can undergo staged closure, or requires only a skin graft, then NPWT treatment is more appropriate.[4,5] In addition, even if the wound can be closed but is somewhat tenuous, a vacuum-assisted closure (VAC) dressing applied directly to the incision has proven to be helpful.[6-8] VAC dressings also may decrease the extent of soft-tissue coverage required on the soft-tissue reconstructive ladder.[9-11]

Bead pouch application involves thorough débridement of the wound, followed by the placement of antibiotic impregnated methyl methacrylate beads and then sealing of the wound with an iodophor-impregnated adhesive dressing (**Figure 1**). The effectiveness of antibiotic-impregnated cement beads, calcium sulfate, or other bone grafts has been demonstrated.[12-14] The sealing effect of the bead pouch localizes the antibiotic delivery and aids in increasing the tissue levels in the open wound. Local antibiotic delivery systems should not be combined with a VAC dressing because this may lower the level of local antibiotics.[15,16]

A bead pouch dressing is effective in two main situations: (1) when the wound is extremely contaminated or previously infected and requires a high dose of local antibiotics and (2) when the wound has been rendered surgically "clean" and now is awaiting flap coverage. If the wound is ready for soft-tissue coverage, a bead pouch is ideal because the wound is sealed, the tissue stays viable, and procedures, such as an arteriogram can be performed with it in place. In addition, the pouch can be left in place for several days while the coordination of surgical services for flap coverage is determined.

Characteristics of the Lesion

When the soft-tissue has been débrided and the wound has been stabilized, the exact characteristics of the defect should be analyzed. The critical factors are the surface area (a × b in centimeters), the depth of the wound, anatomic location, and what anatomic structures are within the bed of the wound (bone, tendon, or muscle). The depth of the wound also is important

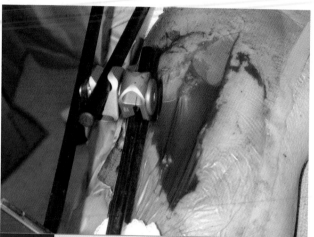

| Figure 1 | Photograph showing an open proximal tibia fracture spanned with an external fixator and covered with a bead pouch. Note that the soft tissue is covered with a blood/fluid layer and thus does not desiccate. (Copyright John T. Capo, MD, Hoboken, NJ.) |

when selecting an appropriate coverage technique. Deeply concave wounds benefit from muscle coverage for durability and an aesthetically appealing result. In general, wounds with viable muscle exposed can be covered with some type of skin graft, whereas wounds with bone or tendon exposed require vascularized tissue.[17,18] This vascularized tissue may be a fasciocutaneous flap that contains its own skin component or a muscle flap that requires subsequent skin grafting. A general overview of the indications for various flaps used in the lower extremity is presented in Table 1. If a later skin graft is required, this is typically done 3 to 5 days after flap coverage to allow better monitoring of the flap for pulses and viability without overlying skin; it also minimizes the chance of losing the skin graft by ensuring that the flap is viable.

Timing of Soft-Tissue Coverage

The timing of soft-tissue coverage should be expeditious and appropriate. The previously quoted window of 72 hours is based on old literature[19] and has recently been dispelled.[20] Using the techniques of VAC and bead-pouch dressing have allowed the coverage time of these wounds to be extended to a more appropriate time point.[21] A bead pouch can be left in place for 3 to 5 days in preparation for free-flap coverage. Recent studies have shown that successful wound coverage after VAC dressing can be safely done 5 to 10 days after injury. The rates of infection and flap survival are similar to procedures done earlier.[22,23] A larger multicenter study showed that timely coverage is needed, which averaged 5.7 days in their patients, with acceptable rates of infection and bony union.[24] Typically, these wounds are covered 5 to 10 days after the original injury.

Table 1

Exposed Tissue

Anatomic Location	Muscle	Tendon	Bone	
			Small/Superficial Wound	Large/Deep Wound
Thigh	STSG	DRM and STSG	Biceps femoris rotation flap, NPWT, STSG	FVMF, STSG
Knee	STSG	DRM and STSG	Medial or lateral gastrocnemius, STSG	FVMF and STSG, ALTF
Proximal tibia	STSG	DRM and STSG	Medial or lateral gastrocnemius, STSG	Medial or lateral gastrocnemius, STSG
Midtibia	STSG	Sural fasciocutaneous rotation flap	Soleus rotation flap, STSG	FVMF and STSG, ALTF
Distal tibia	STSG	Sural fasciocutaneous rotation flap	Sural fasciocutaneous rotation flap	FVMF and STSG, ALTF
Foot and ankle	STSG or FTSG	DRM and STSG	Sural fasciocutaneous rotation flap	FVMF and STSG, ALTF

STSG = split-thickness skin graft; NPWT = negative pressure wound therapy; FVMF = free vascularized muscle flap; ALTF = anterolateral thigh flap; FTSG = full-thickness skin graft. DRM = dermal replacement matrix.

Soft-Tissue Defects About the Distal Femur, Knee, and Proximal Tibia

Open wounds about the knee and the proximal tibia typically occur after tibial plateau fractures and infections or wound problems after total knee arthroplasty.[25] The problematic areas are the patella and the medial tibial plateau because of their subcutaneous position. This also makes skin grafting uncommon in these areas. An extremely versatile coverage option is the gastrocnemius vascularized rotational muscle flap. Either the medial or the lateral gastrocnemius can be used, but the medial side is more commonly used (**Figure 2**) because the medial tibia more often has soft-tissue problems, and the medial head of the gastrocnemius is broader and longer.[26] The lateral head must course over the fibula and the peroneal nerve when transposed, thus limiting its coverage options.

When wounds are more proximal in the distal femur, rotation flaps such as a biceps femoris rotation flap may be appropriate. This flap involves detaching the distal biceps tendon and rotating the muscle over the open area. After a rotation flap has stabilized, continued VAC treatment is sometimes helpful to create a more homogeneous tissue bed for skin grafting (**Figure 3**). A free flap is required for very large defects; a latissimus flap can be used if muscle bulk is required or an anterolateral fascial flap if thinner coverage is desired.[27]

Middle Third Open Tibial Wounds

Open middle third tibial fractures are usually caused by motor vehicle crashes and falls from a height. The crest of the tibial shaft becomes subcutaneous at its proximal third and remains that way distally to the ankle. In particular, the medial surface of the tibia is covered by only a thin soft-tissue layer of subcutaneous tissue and skin.

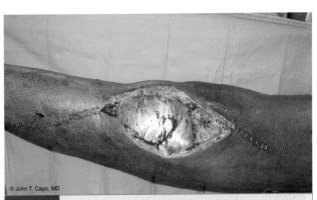

| Figure 2 | Photograph showing a wound over a medial tibial plateau fracture that is adequately covered with a medial gastrocnemius rotation flap. The flap is ready for split-thickness skin grafting. (Copyright John T. Capo, MD, Hoboken, NJ.) |

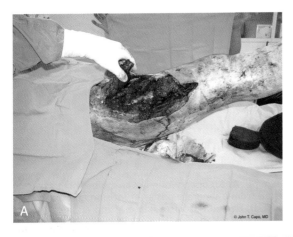

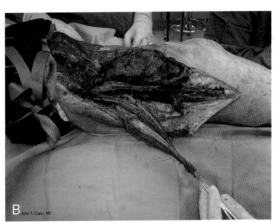

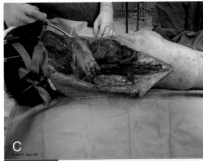

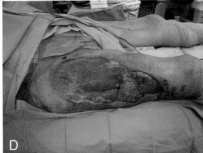

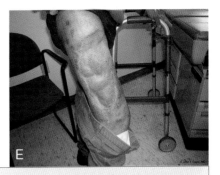

| Figure 3 | Photographs showing treatment of an open femoral shaft fracture. **A,** The fracture is covered with a biceps femoris rotational muscle flap. **B** and **C,** The biceps is released distally and rotated over the anteriorly exposed femoral bone. **D,** The wound then underwent additional VAC treatment to make the wound more homogeneous. **E,** Final result after skin grafting and 6 weeks after muscle flap coverage. (Copyright John T. Capo, MD, Hoboken, NJ.) |

4: Lower Extremity

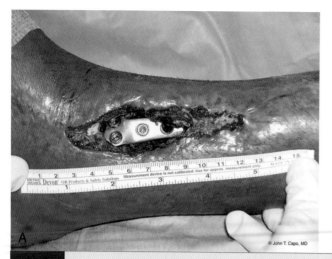
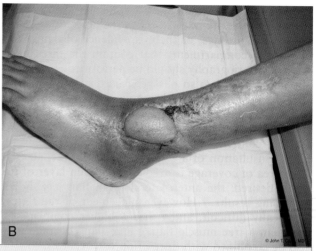

Figure 7 Photographs showing a lateral ankle defect. **A,** Lateral ankle defect and exposed tibial plate. **B,** A sural fasciocutaneous flap was harvested from the posterior calf and rotated laterally to cover the ankle defect. The intervening skin bridge was divided, and the pedicle was covered with a skin graft. (Copyright John T. Capo, MD, Hoboken, NJ.)

placed noninnervated and thus will atrophy over time. A smaller muscle that may be more appropriately size matched for small defects is the serratus anterior muscle flap, which is thinner than a rectus abdominis or latissimus muscle. The size of the flap available is approximately 5 × 7 cm. However, the dissection for the harvest is technically difficult, and care needs to be taken to remove only the lower three or four slips of the serratus to avoid the complication of scapular winging. The flap also can be combined with a portion of a rib if bony reconstruction is required.[35]

An alternative to a free muscle flap in this area is one of the various fasciocutaneous rotation flaps that are available.[36,37] A particularly useful flap that can cover areas around the distal tibia is the distally based lateral sural fasciocutaneous flap,[38,39] which relies on accompanying vessels to the sural nerve and has a pivot point 4 cm proximal to the distal fibula, midway between the Achilles and peroneal tendons. The flap can be taken up to 10 × 7 cm and is centered at the distal split of the gastrocnemius muscle. The donor site is partially closed, and the resulting defect is covered with a split-thickness skin graft. If a smaller flap is taken (5 × 3 cm), the donor site can be closed primarily. The flap can be rotated anteriorly or posteriorly. A drawback associated with this flap is that the sural nerve must be sacrificed, although most patients do not report major sensory deficits.

Foot and Ankle Soft-Tissue Defects

The foot and ankle present unique issues for soft-tissue coverage because there are many subcutaneous bony and tendinous structures, and coverage tissue must be thin and pliable to allow shoe wear. The heel pad is a unique load-bearing structure that poses specific challenges for the reconstructive surgeon. Insufficient cushion with resulting pain and frequent skin breakdown can lead to ambulation difficulties, infection, and the subsequent need for amputation. Flaps that are advantageous for foot and ankle coverage include the sural fasciocutaneous flap,[40] the tensor fascia-lata flap, and a combination of biologic coverage and skin grafting.

The sural fasciocutaneous flap is harvested by first starting 4 cm proximal to the tip of the distal fibula and then elevating all of the fascia between the Achilles and peroneal tendons. This fascial sleeve contains the sural nerve and its accompanying vascular plexus, which contain a distinct sural artery and vein. The required defect is mapped using a paper template, and the flap is centered over the two heads of the gastrocnemius muscle. It can be extended a few additional centimeters proximally, only if clearly necessary, because this portion has a random blood supply and is less reliable. The flap contains the deep fascia, subcutaneous fat, and skin over the gastrocnemius muscle, whereas the pedicle is the fascial sleeve containing the neurovascular structures. The sural nerve, artery, and vein are divided proximally. The proximal sural nerve should be retracted into the wound, divided sharply, and allowed to retract under the muscle bellies to minimize the chance of subsequent neuroma formation.

The sural flap can be rotated laterally to cover defects of the lateral ankle, such as an exposed lateral plate on the distal tibia (**Figure 7**). The pedicle can be tunneled through the associated skin bridge; alternatively, the skin bridge can be divided, then the pedicle is covered with a skin graft. The advantage of dividing any soft-tissue bridge is that any areas of compression will be removed. The flap also can be rotated posteriorly or anteriorly to reach the medial ankle. Another ideal area for coverage is the lateral heel with wound problems after surgical fixation of a calcaneal fracture.

If lower-profile coverage is desired (less than the sural fasciocutaneous flap can provide), the flap can be modified. The sural flap can be taken as an adipose-fascial flap alone. The donor site is marked out for the

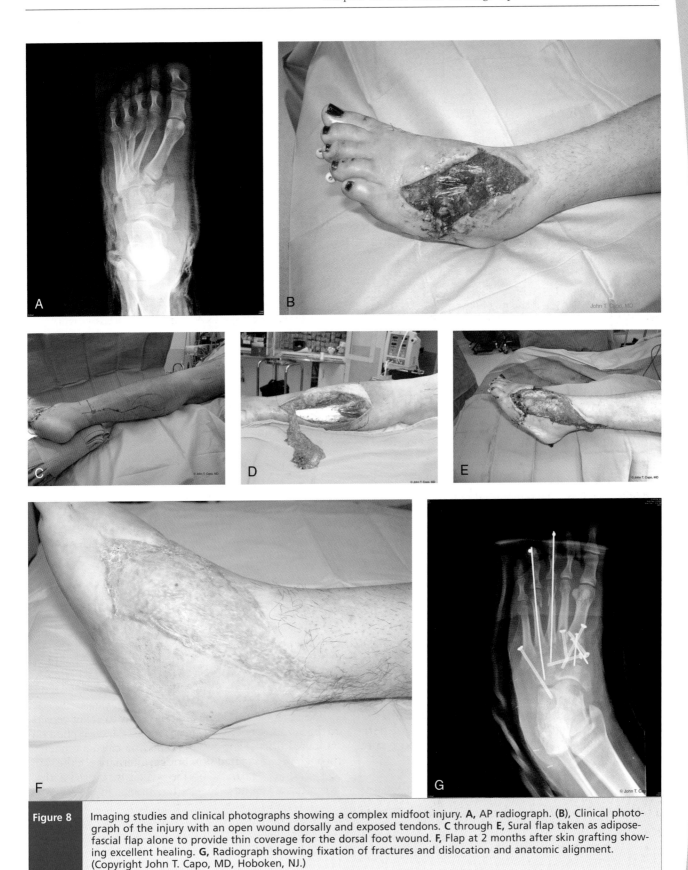

Figure 8 Imaging studies and clinical photographs showing a complex midfoot injury. **A,** AP radiograph. **(B),** Clinical photograph of the injury with an open wound dorsally and exposed tendons. **C** through **E,** Sural flap taken as adipose-fascial flap alone to provide thin coverage for the dorsal foot wound. **F,** Flap at 2 months after skin grafting showing excellent healing. **G,** Radiograph showing fixation of fractures and dislocation and anatomic alignment. (Copyright John T. Capo, MD, Hoboken, NJ.)

appropriate defect, but the skin is incised longitudinally, and the flap is taken as only the subcutaneous fat and deep fascia. The flap can be rotated in a manner resembling the page of a book; thus, the fascia will be-

4: Lower Extremity

come superficial and receive the skin graft. The advantages of this technique is that the pedicle is not twisted and the flap is extremely thin. This flap modification is ideal for defects over the dorsum of the foot (**Figure 8**).

New Biologics for Wound Coverage

A variety of skin graft substitutes are currently available and include dermal replacement matrices (DRMs) composed mostly of collagen, processed skin xenografts, and biologic matrices derived from porcine small intestinal submucosa. Currently available is a bilayer membrane that is made of collagen derived from bovine tendons and chondroitin-6 sulfate. It is a three-dimensional matrix that allows for neovascularization, with the patients' own cells migrating into the substance. It is covered with a silicone outer sheet that can be sutured to the wound edges and effectively seals the wound. It can be placed over vascularized tissue, including muscle, bleeding bone, or paratenon. Small areas of nonvascularized tissue, such as nerves and tendons, also may be covered.[41] A split-thickness skin graft is applied to the DRM following the removal of the silicone layer 2 to 3 weeks after application. Topical negative pressure has been shown to accelerate tissue ingrowth and decrease the incorporation time for the dermal graft.[42]

DRM has been used extensively in burn patients, where significant wound coverage is often necessary.[43,44] Theoretically, the neodermis that forms minimizes fibroblast formation and results in less adhesions to the underlying structures and may promote better tendon gliding.[45] The wound bed should be free of any signs of infection before the placement of any biologic skin substitute. Use of this DRM has shown promise and good results in the hand and upper extremity.[46,47]

Also commercially available is a processed dermal porcine xenograft. It can be stored at room temperature and has a shelf life of about 18 months.[47] Although this graft does not become vascularized, it can promote epithelialization by acting as an epidermal barrier. One study reported that this material used in burn patients resulted in decreased hospital stays.[48] This biologic dressing serves as a temporary covering that minimizes the need for dressing changes. Wounds treated with this material subsequently require covering with a split-thickness skin graft.

A third product is a biologic matrix derived from porcine small intestinal submucosa; it has a 2-year shelf life and is indicated for the management of open wounds. The material can be applied in the operating room or in the outpatient setting and sometimes requires multiple applications. It can eventually result in wound healing by itself or may require coverage with a skin graft. Published results on the clinical use of this material are limited.[49,50]

Summary

Open wounds of the lower extremity pose real problems for patients and great surgical challenges. The particular treatment chosen should minimize patient morbidity while providing appropriate treatment. The available treatment choices range from delayed closure to free microvascular tissue transfer. New biologic materials have lowered morbidity compared with complex reconstructive options. Although these new off-the-shelf products are helpful, the principles of soft-tissue débridement and coverage with healthy, durable tissue must be followed.

Key Study Points

- The most important aspect of open fracture treatment is timely and adequate débridement. All nonviable tissue should be removed. Large articular fragments that are critical for joint stability and essential neurovascular structures are exceptions to the rule of discarding all tissue without soft-tissue attachments.

- Close communication between the orthopaedic trauma surgeon and the microvascular reconstructive surgeon is critical for successful outcomes. Early visualization and exploration of the wound by the soft-tissue surgeon will allow for an expedited plan for coverage.

- The addition of novel rotational and perforator flaps, as well as new off-the-shelf biologic products, has aided in the coverage of difficult wounds. These techniques are particularly helpful in wounds of the distal tibia, foot, and ankle, where low-profile coverage is desired.

Annotated References

1. Pollak AN: Use of negative pressure wound therapy with reticulated open cell foam for lower extremity trauma. *J Orthop Trauma* 2008;22(10, suppl):S142-S145.

2. Herscovici D Jr, Sanders RW, Scaduto JM, Infante A, DiPasquale T: Vacuum-assisted wound closure (VAC therapy) for the management of patients with high-energy soft tissue injuries. *J Orthop Trauma* 2003;17(10):683-688.

3. Labler L, Rancan M, Mica L, Härter L, Mihic-Probst D, Keel M: Vacuum-assisted closure therapy increases local interleukin-8 and vascular endothelial growth factor levels in traumatic wounds. *J Trauma* 2009;66(3):749-757.

4. Friedrich JB, Katolik LI, Hanel DP: Reconstruction of soft-tissue injury associated with lower extremity fracture. *J Am Acad Orthop Surg* 2011;19(2):81-90.

   This review article describes the reconstructive ladder that should be followed for coverage of soft-tissue defects. Clear images and an outstanding diagram of the sural flap are presented. Level of evidence: V.

5. Bollero D, Carnino R, Risso D, Gangemi EN, Stella M: Acute complex traumas of the lower limbs: A modern reconstructive approach with negative pressure therapy. *Wound Repair Regen* 2007;15(4):589-594.

6. Stannard JP, Gabriel A, Lehner B: Use of negative pressure wound therapy over clean, closed surgical incisions. *Int Wound J* 2012;9(suppl 1):32-39.

   This review article discusses different types of therapy, including NPWT, for surgical wounds. The literature is reviewed, and the author's clinical experience is shared. Several specific clinical cases showing the use of NPWT over closed incisions are illustrated. Level of evidence: V.

7. Stannard JP, Robinson JT, Anderson ER, McGwin G Jr, Volgas DA, Alonso JE: Negative pressure wound therapy to treat hematomas and surgical incisions following high-energy trauma. *J Trauma* 2006;60(6):1301-1306.

8. Reddix RN Jr, Leng XI, Woodall J, Jackson B, Dedmond B, Webb LX: The effect of incisional negative pressure therapy on wound complications after acetabular fracture surgery. *J Surg Orthop Adv* 2010;19(2):91-97.

   This study evaluated 301 patients who underwent surgical treatment of acetabular fractures. There was a significant difference in infection rate between the 235 patients treated with an incisional VAC (1.3%) and the 66 patients treated without NPWT (6.1%). Level of evidence: III.

9. Rinker B, Amspacher JC, Wilson PC, Vasconez HC: Subatmospheric pressure dressing as a bridge to free tissue transfer in the treatment of open tibia fractures. *Plast Reconstr Surg* 2008;121(5):1664-1673.

10. Dedmond BT, Kortesis B, Punger K, et al: The use of negative-pressure wound therapy (NPWT) in the temporary treatment of soft-tissue injuries associated with high-energy open tibial shaft fractures. *J Orthop Trauma* 2007;21(1):11-17.

11. Dedmond BT, Kortesis B, Punger K, et al: Subatmospheric pressure dressings in the temporary treatment of soft tissue injuries associated with type III open tibial shaft fractures in children. *J Pediatr Orthop* 2006;26(6):728-732.

12. Decoster TA, Bozorgnia S: Antibiotic beads. *J Am Acad Orthop Surg* 2008;16(11):674-678.

13. Thomas DB, Brooks DE, Bice TG, DeJong ES, Lonergan KT, Wenke JC: Tobramycin-impregnated calcium sulfate prevents infection in contaminated wounds. *Clin Orthop Relat Res* 2005;441:366-371.

14. Beardmore AA, Brooks DE, Wenke JC, Thomas DB: Effectiveness of local antibiotic delivery with an osteoinductive and osteoconductive bone-graft substitute. *J Bone Joint Surg Am* 2005;87(1):107-112.

15. Stinner DJ, Hsu JR, Wenke JC: Negative pressure wound therapy reduces the effectiveness of traditional local antibiotic depot in a large complex musculoskeletal wound animal model. *J Orthop Trauma* 2012;26(9):512-518.

   The effectiveness of a bead pouch was compared with antibiotic beads with NPWT in a goat model. The animals were inoculated with *Staphylococcus aureus* and divided into the two treatment arms. The wounds in the antibiotic bead pouch group had a sixfold less bacteria count than the augmented NPWT group (P = 0.01). Level of evidence: I.

16. Large TM, Douglas G, Erickson G, Grayson JK: Effect of negative pressure wound therapy on the elution of antibiotics from polymethylmethacrylate beads in a porcine simulated open femur fracture model. *J Orthop Trauma* 2012;26(9):506-511.

   In a pig model, polymethyl methacrylate beads with vancomycin and tobramycin were covered with NPWT directly or over closed or open fascia. The NPWT group did not decrease local antibiotic concentrations but did decrease the total amount of eluted antibiotics locally available when the fascia was left open. Level of evidence: I.

17. Levin LS: Principles of definitive soft tissue coverage with flaps. *J Orthop Trauma* 2008;22(10, suppl):S161-S166.

18. Tielinen L, Lindahl JE, Tukiainen EJ: Acute unreamed intramedullary nailing and soft tissue reconstruction with muscle flaps for the treatment of severe open tibial shaft fractures. *Injury* 2007;38(8):906-912.

19. Godina M: Early microsurgical reconstruction of complex trauma of the extremities. *Plast Reconstr Surg* 1986;78(3):285-292.

20. Karanas YL, Nigriny J, Chang J: The timing of microsurgical reconstruction in lower extremity trauma. *Microsurgery* 2008;28(8):632-634.

21. Parrett BM, Matros E, Pribaz JJ, Orgill DP: Lower extremity trauma: Trends in the management of soft-tissue reconstruction of open tibia-fibula fractures. *Plast Reconstr Surg* 2006;117(4):1315-1324.

22. Steiert AE, Gohritz A, Schreiber TC, Krettek C, Vogt PM: Delayed flap coverage of open extremity fractures after previous vacuum-assisted closure (VAC) therapy: Worse or worth? *J Plast Reconstr Aesthet Surg* 2009;62(5):675-683.

23. Hou Z, Irgit K, Strohecker KA, et al: Delayed flap reconstruction with vacuum-assisted closure management of the open IIIB tibial fracture. *J Trauma* 2011;71(6):1705-1708.

This retrospective clinical study evaluated 32 patients with type IIIB open tibial fractures initially treated with NPWT. Of the total number of patients, 27 underwent rotational muscle flap, and 4 had free muscle flaps. There was a high complication rate in this study, with nine patients requiring below-knee amputation. The authors found an increased rate of infection in those patients who had more than 7 days from the time of injury to flap coverage. Level of evidence: III.

24. Pollak AN, Jones AL, Castillo RC, Bosse MJ, MacKenzie EJ; LEAP Study Group: The relationship between time to surgical debridement and incidence of infection after open high-energy lower extremity trauma. *J Bone Joint Surg Am* 2010;92(1):7-15.

This large multicenter study comes from the Lower Extremity Amputation Prevention group and studied 315 patients with severe high-energy trauma. The treatment protocol included aggressive débridement, antibiotic administration, fracture stabilization, and timely soft-tissue coverage. The only factor that had a significant effect on the infection rate was the time between injury and admission to the definitive trauma center. Level of evidence: III.

25. Cetrulo CL Jr, Shiba T, Friel MT, et al: Management of exposed total knee prostheses with microvascular tissue transfer. *Microsurgery* 2008;28(8):617-622.

26. Veber M, Vaz G, Braye F, et al: Anatomical study of the medial gastrocnemius muscle flap: A quantitative assessment of the arc of rotation. *Plast Reconstr Surg* 2011;128(1):181-187.

This cadaver study evaluated the arc of rotation of the medial gastrocnemius-soleus complex flap from the tibial tuberosity to the distal flap segment. The addition of dissection around the pes anserinus and the medial condyle increased the arc of rotation by a minimum of 7%. Level of evidence: V.

27. Hong JP, Shin HW, Kim JJ, Wei FC, Chung YK: The use of anterolateral thigh perforator flaps in chronic osteomyelitis of the lower extremity. *Plast Reconstr Surg* 2005;115(1):142-147.

28. Hyodo I, Nakayama B, Takahashi M, Toriyama K, Kamei Y, Torii S: The gastrocnemius with soleus bi-muscle flap. *Br J Plast Surg* 2004;57(1):77-82.

29. Hammert WC, Minarchek J, Trzeciak MA: Free-flap reconstruction of traumatic lower extremity wounds. *Am J Orthop (Belle Mead NJ)* 2000;29(9, suppl):22-26.

30. Sadove R, Merrell JC: The split rectus abdominis free muscle transfer. *Ann Plast Surg* 1987;18(2):179-181.

31. Rodriguez ED, Bluebond-Langner R, Copeland C, Grim TN, Singh NK, Scalea T: Functional outcomes of posttraumatic lower limb salvage: A pilot study of anterolateral thigh perforator flaps versus muscle flaps. *J Trauma* 2009;66(5):1311-1314.

32. Demirtas Y, Kelahmetoglu O, Cifci M, Tayfur V, Demir A, Guneren E: Comparison of free anterolateral thigh flaps and free muscle-musculocutaneous flaps in soft tissue reconstruction of lower extremity. *Microsurgery* 2010;30(1):24-31.

Fifty-three patients whose skin and soft tissue of the lower extremities had been reconstructed were divided into two groups: a perforator flap group, reconstructed using an anterolateral thigh (ALT) fasciocutaneous free flap (23 cases), and a musculocutaneous group, either latissimus dorsi or rectus abdominis free flaps (30 cases). Complete flap survival was 78.3%, with four total and one partial flap loss in the ALT group, and 90.0%, with one total and two partial failures in the muscle flap group. Level of evidence: III.

33. Chim H, Sontich JK, Kaufman BR: Free tissue transfer with distraction osteogenesis is effective for limb salvage of the infected traumatized lower extremity. *Plast Reconstr Surg* 2011;127(6):2364-2372.

The authors discussed a retrospective series of 28 patients in whom massive bone loss required bone transport. Free-tissue transfer was used either before transport was initiated or after docking, with good clinical results. Level of evidence: IV.

34. Kiyokawa K, Tanaka S, Kiduka Y, Inoue Y, Yamauchi T, Tai Y: Reconstruction of the form and function of lateral malleolus and ankle joint. *J Reconstr Microsurg* 2005;21(6):371-376.

35. Lin CH, Yazar S: Revisiting the serratus anterior rib flap for composite tibial defects. *Plast Reconstr Surg* 2004;114(7):1871-1877.

36. Parrett BM, Winograd JM, Lin SJ, Borud LJ, Taghinia A, Lee BT: The posterior tibial artery perforator flap: an alternative to free-flap closure in the comorbid patient. *J Reconstr Microsurg* 2009;25(2):105-109.

37. Parrett BM, Talbot SG, Pribaz JJ, Lee BT: A review of local and regional flaps for distal leg reconstruction. *J Reconstr Microsurg* 2009;25(7):445-455.

38. Parrett BM, Pribaz JJ, Matros E, Przylecki W, Sampson CE, Orgill DP: Risk analysis for the reverse sural fasciocutaneous flap in distal leg reconstruction. *Plast Reconstr Surg* 2009;123(5):1499-1504.

39. Cho AB, Pohl PH, Ruggiero GM, Aita MA, Mattar TG, Fukushima WY: The proximally designed sural flap based on the accompanying artery of the lesser saphenous vein. *J Reconstr Microsurg* 2010;26(8):501-508.

The authors investigated a variant of the sural flap by maintaining the lesser saphenous vein and artery in this more proximally based flap. This variant had a higher flap survival rate (100% versus 83%) but also a higher complication rate (43% versus 33%) than the standard sural fasciocutaneous flap. This modified sural flap was found to easily reach the anterior aspect of the tibia in its middle and distal thirds. Level of evidence: III.

40. Köse R, Mordeniz C, Şanli C: Use of expanded reverse sural artery flap in lower extremity reconstruction. *J Foot Ankle Surg* 2011;50(6):695-698.

Ten patients with defects about the foot and ankle underwent successful wound coverage with a two-stage procedure involving the sural fasciocutaneous flap and a tissue expander. This technique successfully increased the size of the wound that could be covered by the sural flap. Level of evidence: IV.

41. Shores JT, Hiersche M, Gabriel A, Gupta S: Tendon coverage using an artificial skin substitute. *J Plast Reconstr Aesthet Surg* 2012;65(11):1544-1550.

The authors reported the results of using a DRM for soft-tissue reconstruction overlying tendons with loss of paratenon in upper and lower extremity soft-tissue defects. Forty-two patients (35 men and 7 women) with exposed tendons as a result of trauma (37), cancer excision (2), or chronic wounds (3) underwent reconstruction. All of the patients experienced healing, with an average split-thickness skin graft take rate of 92.5% and an average range of motion of 91.2% ± 6.5 (range, 80% to 100%). Level of evidence: IV.

42. Moiemen NS, Yarrow J, Kamel D, Kearns D, Mendonca D: Topical negative pressure therapy: Does it accelerate neovascularisation within the dermal regeneration template, Integra? A prospective histological in vivo study. *Burns* 2010;36(6):764-768.

Eight patients underwent application of a DRM combined with NPWT for wound reconstructions. Serial biopsies were taken at days 7, 14, 21, and 28 and showed progressive revascularization. This combination therapy is recommended to reduce shear forces, minimize seroma, and improve patient tolerance. Level of evidence: IV.

43. Heitland A, Piatkowski A, Noah EM, Pallua N: Update on the use of collagen/glycosaminoglycate skin substitute: Six years of experiences with artificial skin in 15 German burn centers. *Burns* 2004;30(5):471-475.

44. Lou RB, Hickerson WL: The use of skin substitutes in hand burns. *Hand Clin* 2009;25(4):497-509.

45. Carothers JT, Brigman BE, Lawson RD, Rizzo M: Stacking of a dermal regeneration template for reconstruction of a soft-tissue defect after tumor excision from the palm of the hand: A case report. *J Hand Surg Am* 2005;30(6):1322-1326.

46. Herlin C, Louhaem D, Bigorre M, Dimeglio A, Captier G: Use of Integra in a paediatric upper extremity degloving injury. *J Hand Surg Eur Vol* 2007;32(2):179-184.

47. Jung JJ, Woo AS, Borschel GH: The use of Integra® bilaminar dermal regeneration template in apert syndactyly reconstruction: A novel alternative to simplify care and improve outcomes. *J Plast Reconstr Aesthet Surg* 2012;65(1):118-121.

This case report described bilateral central syndactyly separation and covering. One side was treated with a standard groin flap and the other side with a DRM. Both sides had similar functional outcomes, but the groin flap required debulking, and the DRM was easier. Level of evidence: V.

48. Still J, Donker K, Law E, Thiruvaiyaru D: A program to decrease hospital stay in acute burn patients. *Burns* 1997;23(6):498-500.

49. Bello YM, Falabella AF, Eaglstein WH: Tissue-engineered skin: Current status in wound healing. *Am J Clin Dermatol* 2001;2(5):305-313.

50. MacLeod TM, Sarathchandra P, Williams G, Sanders R, Green CJ: Evaluation of a porcine origin acellular dermal matrix and small intestinal submucosa as dermal replacements in preventing secondary skin graft contraction. *Burns* 2004;30(5):431-437.

4: Lower Extremity

Chapter 41

Knee Reconstruction and Replacement

Brett R. Levine, MD, MS   Frank A. Liporace, MD

Clinical Assessment

Knee pain is an exceedingly common diagnosis. In obtaining a thorough history, it is important to ascertain if the patient experiences mechanical symptoms, has had recurrent falls or instability, or recalls knee problems as a child. The severity of pain and impairment must be taken into account when setting expectations for treatment to allow for appropriate levels of patient satisfaction.[1-3]

Self-administered quality-of-life questionnaires are crucial tools for assessing the effect of knee injuries and/or arthritis and the effectiveness of subsequent treatments. These assessments include the Oxford Knee Score, Knee Society Score (KSS; the new and old versions), the Western Ontario and McMaster Universities Osteoarthritis Index (WOMAC), the Medical Outcomes Study 36-Item Short Form (SF-36), the Knee Injury and Osteoarthritis Outcome Score (KOOS), and the European Quality of Life Questionnaire (EQ-5D).[4] Treatment recommendations and guidelines using evidence-based medicine are available to help counsel patients and provide cost-effective management of knee pain, injuries, and arthritic conditions.[5-7]

Dr. Levine or an immediate family member serves as a paid consultant to or is an employee of DePuy, Johnson & Johnson, and Zimmer; has received research or institutional support from Biomet and Zimmer; and serves as a board member, owner, officer, or committee member of the American Academy of Orthopaedic Surgeons. Dr. Liporace or an immediate family member has received royalties from DePuy and Biomet; is a member of a speakers' bureau or has made paid presentations on behalf of DePuy, Synthes, Smith & Nephew, Stryker, and Medtronic; serves as a paid consultant to or is an employee of DePuy, Medtronic, Synthes, Smith & Nephew, and Stryker; serves as an unpaid consultant to AO; and has received research or institutional support from Synthes, Smith & Nephew, and Acumed.

Physical Examination

Observing patients as they enter the examination room can lead to a quick assessment of their overall status and yield significant information; these findings include antalgic gait (decreased stance phase on the affected limb), Trendelenburg gait (hip conditions), steppage gait (evidence of foot drop, neurologic disorder), or a crouched gait (related to hamstring tightness or knee flexion contractures). A thorough examination requires complete exposure of the lower extremity to be examined.

The knee soft-tissue envelope should be inspected for prior surgical scars, effusion, and skin lesions. A detailed examination includes range of motion, ligamentous stress testing, joint line palpation, and assessment of all adjacent joints (particularly the hip, because pathology can lead to referred knee pain). Notation of flexion contracture, extensor lag, and pain as well as comparison with the contralateral limb are critical for assessing a native or a replaced knee.

Radiographic Evaluation

Based on examination findings, certain screening imaging studies may be considered: degenerative knee series (AP, 45° weight-bearing, lateral, and Merchant views). Standing views offer the best assessment of joint space deterioration and alignment. Additional plain radiographic tests include oblique views, full leg-length radiographs (mechanical axis), and stress radiographs. When the aforementioned evaluations do not provide a consistent diagnosis, advanced imaging studies may be indicated.

MRI is a sensitive tool for detecting intra-articular pathology, yet it is often overused. Articular cartilage injuries, meniscal pathology, ligamentous injuries, and tumors can be identified with various levels of accuracy. In addition, metal-artifact reduction sequences (MARS) can be ordered to help identify soft-tissue injuries adjacent to metallic implants.[8] These sequences involve two recently developed three-dimensional MRI techniques that allow for good peri-implant visualization by correcting for the metal artifact using slice encoding for metal artifact correction (SEMAC) or

Table 1

Nonpharmacologic and Pharmacologic Modalities to Treat Symptomatic Knee Pain

Nonpharmacologic Modalities	Pharmacologic Modalities
Weight loss	Nutriceuticals
Aerobic (low-impact) or aquatic exercises	Glucosamine and chondroitin sulfate
Shoe inserts	Vitamin-based treatments
Medial wedge for valgus knees	NSAIDs
Subtalar strapped lateral inserts for varus knees	Oral
Patella taping	Topical
Assistive devices (cane, crutches, walker)	Tramadol
Hot/cold therapy	Acetaminophen
Unloader braces	Injections
Psychosocial Interventions	Corticosteroids
	Viscosupplementation
	Platelet-rich plasma
	Opioids (try to avoid)
	Local anesthetic patches or creams

multi-acquisition variable-resonance image combination (MAVRIC).[8]

Nonsurgical Treatment

The modalities available to treat symptomatic knee pain have evolved substantially over the past decade, and nonpharmacologic modalities are strongly recommended for managing osteoarthritis (OA) of the knee[5,9] (Table 1). Nonsupportive braces and wraps can provide an element of hydraulic support and are a common self-employed form of treatment. More robust braces help unload the medial or lateral sides of the knee; however, data to support their efficacy are weak, and long-term utilization and compliance have recently been called into question.[9]

Agents such as glucosamine and chondroitin sulfate are generally well tolerated and are frequently used with variable levels of efficacy and incomplete understanding of their mode of action.[10] Other pharmacologic modalities conditionally recommended for OA management include acetaminophen, oral and topical NSAIDs, and tramadol. However, concerns about cardiac events, kidney damage, and peptic ulcers have limited the long-term use of NSAIDs. Similarly, liver disease and damage have also limited the use of acetaminophen. Intra-articular corticosteroid injections are generally well tolerated and have been shown to have outcomes similar to joint lavage in regard to efficacy and safety. Viscosupplementation injections are available in various regimens and may provide some symptomatic relief in OA of the knee, with the highest molecular weight formularies having the best results. Platelet-rich plasma preparations have been trialed, and preliminary data suggest some efficacy in managing OA

knee pain.[11] For patients with more severe cases and who are not surgical candidates and have had an inadequate response to initial therapies, opioids, pain medications, and duloxetine may be used for pain management.[5]

Joint-Preserving Surgery

Arthroscopy

Arthroscopic management of the arthritic knee has been a controversial subject since the 2002 publication of a randomized comparison of arthroscopic lavage showing only nominal benefit.[12] Recently, it appears that the number of knee arthroscopies to treat OA is decreasing during surgeons' board collection periods, which may represent a trend to a more judicious use of this procedure.[13] Pathologic mechanical symptoms from loose bodies, meniscal tears, and unstable cartilaginous flaps can be adequately treated with knee arthroscopy. It appears that the success of these procedures is limited and should not routinely be used for treating knee OA.[14]

Osteotomy

After a traumatic knee injury, to avoid arthroplasty, or for a deformity greater than 15°, osteotomy of the proximal tibia or the distal femur may be indicated. A preoperative complete radiographic knee series should be obtained for evaluation and templating. A CT scan may also be helpful in select cases.

For symptomatic treatment, osteotomy should be reserved for the younger patient with single-compartment degeneration and angular malalignment. This procedure also can be useful in conjunction with osteochondral grafting. Contraindications include tricompartmental OA, patellofemoral OA, inflammatory arthritis, knee range of motion (ROM) less than 120°, flexion contracture greater than 5°, and age older than 60 years.[15]

Femoral

A distal femoral valgus osteotomy (medial closing wedge or lateral opening wedge) is performed for lateral compartment disease secondary to varus malunion or valgus malalignment. Without malunion of the distal femur and the presence of a postligamentous injury or with isolated medial compartment disease, varus is usually treated with a proximal tibial osteotomy.[16]

Tibial

Young patients with isolated medial compartment degenerative joint disease can be treated with either a medial opening wedge or a lateral closing wedge tibial osteotomy. Contraindications include flexion contracture, less than 90° of flexion, ligamentous instability, and inflammatory arthritis. The closing wedge osteotomy has three potential drawbacks: limb shortening, extensive surgical dissection, and the need for a fibular osteotomy. A medial opening wedge osteotomy requires bone

Table 2

Outcomes of the Most Recent Studies on Closing and Opening Wedge High Tibial Osteotomy

Study	Technique	No. of Knees	Mean Follow-up in Years (Range)	Results
Papachristou et al[18]	Closing wedge	44	10 (5-17)	80% survivorship at 10 years of follow-up, 66% at 15 years, and greater than 52.8% at 17 years
Fletcher et al[19]	Closing wedge	372	18 (12-28)	85% survivorship at 20 years
Gstöttner et al[20]	Closing wedge	134	12.4 (1-25)	94% survivorship at 5 years of follow-up, 79.9% at 10 years, 65.5% at 15 years, and 54.1% at 18 years
Akizuki et al[21]	Closing wedge	118	16.4 (16-20)	97.6% survivorship at 10 years, 90.4% at 15 years
Kolb et al[22]	Opening wedge	51	4.3	Hospital for Special Surgery score was excellent in 57% of patients, good in 24%, fair in 8%, and poor in 10%
Saragaglia et al[23]	Opening wedge	124	10	88.8% survivorship at 5 years, 74% at 10 years
DeMeo et al[24]	Opening wedge	20	8.3	70% survivorship at 8 years

(Reproduced from Rossi R, Bonasia DE, Amendola A: The role of high tibial osteotomy in the varus knee. *J Am Acad Orthop Surg* 2011;19[10]:590-599.)

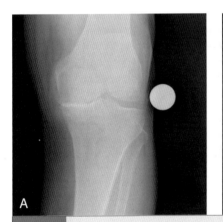
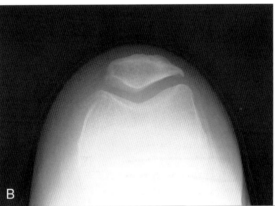
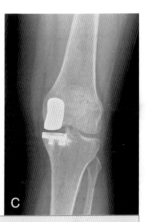

Figure 1 Preoperative AP (**A**) and Merchant (**B**) radiographs of isolated medial compartment degenerative joint disease. **C**, Postoperative AP radiograph of a successful medial unicompartmental knee arthroplasty at 4-year follow-up.

graft, has weight-bearing restrictions, and has a higher risk of nonunion.[17] Good to excellent results have been reported for both osteotomy methods[18-24] (Table 2). Concerns of technical challenges (difficult exposure) during postosteotomy total knee arthroplasty (TKA) may arise if overcorrection occurs during the index procedure.

Arthroplasty Options

Currently available arthroplasty options include unicompartmental knee arthroplasty (UKA, medial or lateral), patellofemoral arthroplasty (PFA), bicompartmental arthroplasty, or TKA. TKA implants typically have had good success and endure for 15 to 20 years. Recently, UKAs have shown slightly inferior survival rates, and certain bicompartmental options have been

recalled for catastrophic component failure. Arthroplasty procedures should be delayed as long as possible, preferably until at least 60 years of age.

Unicompartmental Knee Arthroplasty

When OA affects only one compartment of the knee, it is possible to resurface only the diseased area (Figure 1). Improved surgical techniques and increased patient demands have led to a current resurgence of UKA. Although it is generally accepted that TKA has a better long-term survival than UKA, recent reports have described 10-year survival rates of 80.2% to 98%.[17,25,26]

High levels of success can be achieved with stringent indications, including isolated single compartment pain and radiographic disease. More global disease is associated with persistent discomfort and higher rates of revision. Accepted contraindications to UKA include inflammatory arthritis, large fixed deformities,

4: Lower Extremity

tricompartmental/bicompartmental disease, ligamentous laxity, anterior cruciate ligament (ACL) deficiency (recently called into question),[27] and a prior meniscectomy in the contralateral compartment. Alternatively, the classic indications for UKA involved patients older than 60 years with low-demand levels, weight less than 180 lb (body mass index [BMI] < 35),[28] flexion contracture less than 10°, varus deformity less than 10°, or valgus deformity less than 15°.

The advantages of UKA over TKA include minimal bone loss, the preservation of ligamentous structures, faster recovery, fewer short-term complications, lower costs, decreased length of hospitalization, better ROM, and high satisfaction rates.[29] There does not appear to be a risk for patella baja compared with a tibial osteotomy, making future surgical approaches easier. Many comparison studies have been performed and corroborate the aforementioned findings with the general consensus of better long-term survivorship of TKA. Conversely, in comparing UKA to a high tibial osteotomy (HTO), it appears that better long-term outcomes are found with UKA. HTO has a higher reoperation rate, wound complications, neurovascular injury, and lower levels of pain relief at 12- to 17-year follow-up. The results of UKA after a prior HTO are relatively poor, with an almost 30% revision rate.[30]

The keys to success with UKA include minimal bony resection, restoration of a near-neutral coronal and sagittal alignment, and adequate component fixation. Current reports show that UKA provides better functional recovery than TKA and can be performed medially or laterally with equal success.[31,32] The growing popularity of UKA has led to expanding indications, including tolerance for asymptomatic radiographic findings of patellofemoral degenerative changes.[33] Lateral subluxation of the patella cannot be disregarded and is better treated with TKA.[34] Other modern techniques that are available, with limited peer-reviewed literature, include navigation, custom cutting guides, and robot-assisted surgery.

Mobile and fixed-bearing options are available for UKA with mid- and long-term follow-up available for both.[35] In vitro assessment of UKA designs has shown decreased wear rates with fixed-bearing and medial-sided implants and were lower under all conditions compared with mobile and lateral components.[35,36] Mobile-bearing UKAs were found to have better kinematics and lower rates of radiolucencies but similar knee function compared with fixed-bearing components at 2-year follow-up. Specific long-term failure modes have been elucidated for these components at an average of 17 years of follow-up, including aseptic loosening, dislocation, and arthritis progression for mobile-bearing implants and wear and arthritis progression for fixed-bearing designs.[37]

UKA revision is typically related to one of the following mechanisms of failure: wear (12%), loosening (45%), subsidence (3.6%), arthritis progression (15%), infection (1.9%), technical problems (11.5%—patella impingement and bearing dislocation), or unexplained pain (5.5%).[38] Current data support the following parameters as indicators for UKA infection: greater than 27 mm/hour for erythrocyte sedimentation rate (ESR), 14 mg/L for C-reactive protein (CRP), 6200/µL synovial fluid white blood cell count (WBC), and 60% polymorphonuclear leukocytes on the differential.[39] With modern insertion techniques for UKA, conversion to TKA can be quite successful, with rates similar to those of primary TKA for OA.[40] Conversion should be performed with care, and revision TKA techniques should be used when necessary.[41]

Patellofemoral Arthroplasty

Patellofemoral OA is a common finding, reportedly occurring in up to 24% of adults older than 50 years, with a higher prevalence in women.[42] Trauma, trochlear deformities, abnormal patellar tilt, and obesity have been implicated in the development of isolated patellofemoral OA. When nonsurgical treatment has been deemed ineffective, nonarthroplasty options for treating isolated patellofemoral OA include soft-tissue realignment (tubercle transfer and lateral release),[43] autologous chondrocyte implantation for focal chondral defects,[44] arthroscopy, and patellectomy. When nonsurgical and less conservative measures are unsuccessful, it is reasonable to consider arthroplasty options, such as PFA or TKA.

The most common mechanisms for PFA failure are loosening and OA progression to the tibiofemoral articulation.[45] Correlations have been found between OA progression and high BMI, patella alta/baja, and intraoperative tibiofemoral articular surface damage. Alternative early implant designs have had a greater level of success, with 10-year and 20-year survivorship of 84% and 69%, respectively.[45]

Greater levels of success have been reported with modern implant designs, with a 5-year survival rate of 95.8%, with revision as the end point. Similar data have been reproduced at other centers, with 95% and 88% survival rates at 5 and 7 years, respectively.[46] OA progression may be somewhat predicted based on the status of the tibiofemoral joint articular surface when visualized intraoperatively. PFA has been reported to be more successful in cases of trochlear dysplasia and malalignment compared with primary patellofemoral OA. It has been reported that TKA for isolated patellofemoral OA has better results than PFA and results similar to that for tricompartmental disease at an average 7-year follow-up.[47]

Total Knee Arthroplasty

TKA is the final common pathway for end-stage degenerative joint disease and is an elective procedure that should be reserved for when nonsurgical management fails. The three key elements to determine if a patient is an acceptable candidate include (1) history, physical examination, and radiographic findings consistent with end-stage OA, along with debilitating pain and functional limitations in performing activities of daily living; (2) symptoms refractory to nonsurgical measures; and (3) medical and mental health status compatible with tolerating the stresses of surgery and postoperative recovery.

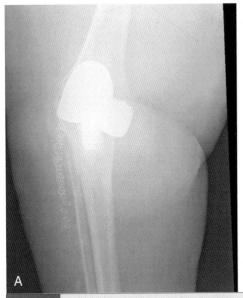
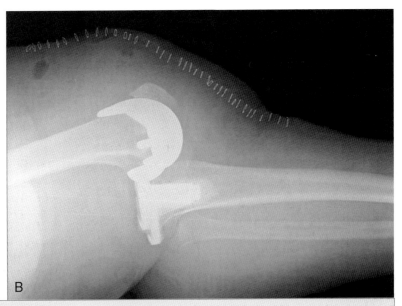

Figure 2 **A,** Radiograph showing ligamentous instability secondary to medial collateral ligament rupture in a morbidly obese patient (BMI, 61). Revision total knee arthroplasty was performed because of gross recurrent dislocation. **B,** Lateral radiograph of the knee before revision surgery.

Factors Affecting Outcomes

Excellent survivorship has been reported following TKA, with greater than 90% at 10 years, 80% at 15 years, and 75% at 20 years. Specific issues that affect the outcome of TKA can be categorized into patient-related factors and implant design. Patient factors include age, sex, expectations, and primary diagnosis. Those younger than 55 years will likely require multiple surgical procedures when a TKA is performed.[48] However, younger age should not be considered an absolute contraindication because reports have shown acceptable results at 5 to 10 years in patients younger than 55 years.[46,49] In addition, patients older than 70 years have an associated increase in long-term survival rates. In isolation, advancing age should not be considered a contraindication to TKA.

Although women typically present with worse preoperative physical function, they tend to recover faster and achieve the same degree of functional improvement as men.[50-52] Long-term survivorship is better for women than men after TKA, yet they tend to have final pain scores that are less favorable.

Preoperative patient expectations can affect the overall outcome of TKA. A recent study has shown that the fulfillment of expectations correlates highly with patient satisfaction.[53] By targeting behavioral outcome expectancies and addressing concerns with pain, it may be possible to improve surgical outcomes.[54] The primary diagnosis of OA portends an adverse effect on the survivorship of TKA components compared with those with rheumatoid arthritis.

Obesity

Surgical concerns for patients who are obese include an increased complexity of the procedure and the possibility of component malalignment because of difficulty with visualizing the external landmarks. Greater risks of perioperative complications also have been reported, including wound healing, superficial infections, and medial collateral ligament (MCL) injuries (**Figure 2**). It is important to counsel patients who are morbidly obese on these increased risks, particularly infection with reports of rates as high as 4.66%.[55] Clinical studies have revealed mixed outcomes with TKA in patients who are morbidly obese, with some reporting significant improvements in pain relief and function, whereas others report lower satisfaction rates and ROM.[56-58] Most agree that, if applicable, preoperative weight loss is favored before moving forward with TKA.

Diabetes Mellitus

Patients with diabetes undergoing TKA require more detailed counseling on associated risk stratification. Diabetes itself is known to modulate immune function, leading to abnormal neutrophil and monocyte activity and an increased potential for infection. Complications are more common in the early postoperative period in these patients and include a higher rate of wound complications, deep infections, urinary tract infections, and increased length of hospital stay. Deep infection rates of 3.4% to 7% have been reported in patients with diabetes compared with typical rates of approximately 1% in the general, healthy population without diabetes.[59,60] Hemoglobin A1c (HBA1c) has not been shown to be a reliable predictor of risk for infection after joint arthroplasty.[59] Another study found diabetes mellitus and morning postoperative hyperglymecia (blood glucose

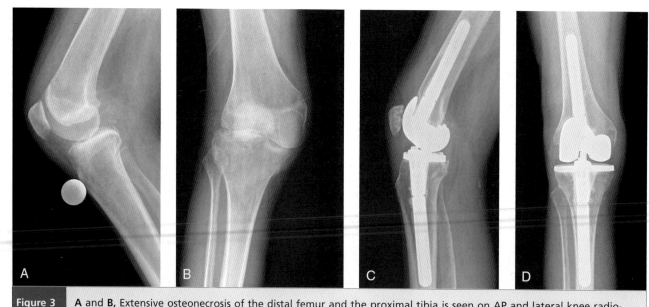

Figure 3 **A** and **B**, Extensive osteonecrosis of the distal femur and the proximal tibia is seen on AP and lateral knee radiographs, respectively. **C** and **D**, AP and lateral radiographs, respectively, depict the complex reconstruction that was required using revision style implants to offset the encountered bony defects.

level greater than 200 mg/dL) were predictors for deep infection following TKA.[61] This concept suggests that perioperative blood glucose may be the crucial factor in predicting complications. Even in patients without diabetes, those with postoperative day 1 blood glucose levels greater than 140 mg/dL were three times more likely to develop an infection. Uncontrolled diabetes has been implicated in significantly higher rates of stroke, urinary tract infection, ileus, postoperative hemorrhage, wound infection, and death.[61] Long-term data suggest that patients with diabetes mellitus will experience a worse outcome after TKA compared with an age- and BMI- matched cohort without diabetes.[62]

Osteonecrosis

Osteonecrosis sometimes occurs in the knee and often affects younger patients (younger than 45 years and more common in males) with a history of chronic corticosteroid use, alcoholism, sickle cell anemia, and organ transplant (**Figure 3**). Secondary osteonecrosis often involves both femoral condyles, and up to 80% of patients may have bilateral disease and/or another joint involved.[63] The diagnosis typically is confirmed on standard radiographs; however, MRI can be used to assess the extent of osteonecrosis in the knee. Nonsurgical treatment should be initiated first, followed by attempts at joint preservation via core decompression-type techniques, arthroscopy, osteotomy, and bone grafting.[63] Spontaneous osteonecrosis of the knee (the more common form in older patients and often in the medial femoral condyle based on a single nutrient vessel and watershed area) and postarthroscopy osteonecrosis can be treated with similar techniques and are often successful with nonsurgical management when diagnosed and treated early.

TKA in these patients can be more challenging because of poor-quality bone and secondary comorbidi-

ties. With appropriate indications, UKA can be successful in limited cases of localized disease.[64] In cases with more extensive osteonecrosis, TKA has been reported to provide excellent results with modern implants and augment options (**Figure 3**). Historical studies have shown a lower rate of success in osteonecrosis cases versus what has been reported with TKA for primary OA.

Hemophilic Arthropathy

Hemophilia is an inherited disease (sex-linked, recessive) that can lead to degenerative joint disease because of repeated intra-articular hemorrhage and a cycle of chronic synovitis and inflammation. Approximately 15% of patients with hemophilia (factor VIII deficiency) will develop an antibody to replacement factors, which play a role in preparation before any surgical interventions.[65] When TKA is indicated, to safely intervene it is important to maintain factor levels of greater than 60% just before an operation and then sustain levels at 30% to 60% for 2 weeks postoperatively.[65]

Concerns regarding arthrofibrosis and associated medical comorbidities (immunosuppression/HIV) are important considerations to keep in mind because infection and manipulation under anesthesia (MUA) rates are higher in this patient population. In addition, survivorship rates and ROM are lower for patients with hemophilic arthropathy compared with those being treated for primary OA.[66] Infection is a long-term issue because of the need for transfusions and concomitant medical conditions.

TKA After Tibial Plateau Fractures

It has been suggested that the most important factor to long-term success in the treatment of a patient with a

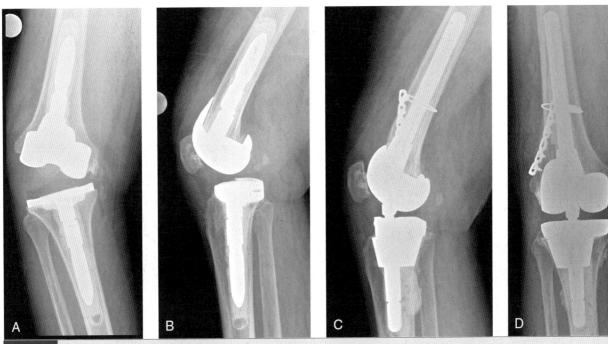

| Figure 4 | AP (**A**) and lateral radiographs (**B** and **C**) of a knee in which a flexion-extension imbalance and a contracted medial side led to instability and recurrent effusions. The flexion-extension mismatch was corrected with a hinged prosthesis (**D**). |

tibial plateau fracture may be mechanical axis alignment.[67] Other factors to consider in the prognosis of patients with tibial plateau fractures include meniscal integrity, ligamentous laxity, and residual articular depression.[67,68] When nonsurgical treatment of symptomatic posttraumatic arthritis has failed, TKA may be indicated. Preoperative considerations include the need for a complete workup to rule out infection.

In cases of TKA after a tibial plateau fracture, preoperative mechanical axis radiographs should be reviewed, and stems and augments should be available for bypassing areas of incomplete union or prior comminution. Based on the competency of the remaining collateral ligaments, semiconstrained/high-post tibia polyethylene and hinged arthroplasty options should be available. Acute arthroplasty at the time of injury has not yielded consistent results and has had a higher complication rate compared with elective TKA.[69]

Surgical Considerations

In arthroplasty procedures, it is important to restore the natural mechanical axis, maintain good component-bone fixation, and achieve appropriate ligamentous balance. Precise cuts are critical, and limited (minimally invasive) exposure may compromise this accuracy, leading to component malpositioning and difficulty with soft-tissue balancing.[70,71] Bone cuts can be achieved with intramedullary, extramedullary, and custom cutting guides and/or computer navigation with acceptable levels of accuracy and success.[72,73] Ulti-

mately an equal determinant for a successful outcome is the attention to detail in soft-tissue balancing while minimizing the level of constraint inherent to the components. Appropriate osseous and soft-tissue technique should reestablish nearly normal kinematics with a medial pivot during midflexion and bicondylar posterior rollback with deep knee flexion.[74]

Ligamentous balancing in TKA centers around the critical nature of obtaining symmetric and equal tibiofemoral gaps in both flexion and extension. Inadequate balance can lead to gap mismatches and problems with ROM, stability, recurrent effusions, and stiffness (**Figure 4**). Typically, resections are based on a measured resection technique (replace what is cut), a gap balance technique (cuts based on tibial and soft-tissue tensioning), or a combined approach. Computer-assisted techniques are available to assist in balancing flexion and extension gaps, with encouraging early results using either balancing philosophies.[75,76] Poor gap balancing can lead to midflexion instability, which has recently been shown to be independent of component design and more related to unrecognized ligament laxity.[77]

Femoral rotation directly affects the flexion gap because the native tibia is typically sloped in 3° of varus, yet it is routinely cut perpendicular to its long axis. Therefore, the posterior femoral condylar resection should re-create a rectangular gap that matches that of the knee in extension. Femoral rotation can be based on anatomic landmarks or established off the initial cut surface of the tibia, with subsequent appropriate soft-tissue releases. Studies have shown equivalent outcomes and success using either technique.[78] Anatomic land-

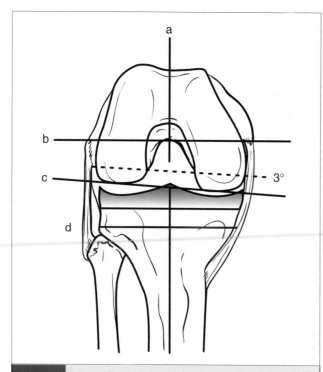

Figure 5 Drawing showing the means to determine external rotation of the femur using various landmarks. a = AP axis; b = epicondylar axis; c = posterior condylar axis; d = tibial cut surface. (Reproduced from Fromison MI: Knee reconstruction and replacement, in Vaccaro AR, ed: *Orthopaedic Knowledge Update*, ed 8. Rosemont, IL, American Academy of Orthopaedic Surgeons, 2008, pp 457-470.)

marks include the epicondylar axis, the Whiteside line, or a line 3° to 5° externally rotated from the posterior condylar axis[79,80] (Figure 5).

Posterior Cruciate Ligament Management

There are three ways to manage the posterior cruciate ligament (PCL) in TKA: retention, sacrifice, and substitution. TKA components have yielded excellent clinical and radiographic outcomes using each design at long-term follow-up. Despite the lack of a consensus, a contemporary database review found a higher survivorship rate (90% versus 77%) at 15-year follow-up in cruciate-retaining (CR) versus posterior-stabilized (PS) TKA, respectively.[81]

PCL-retaining TKA proponents cite physiologic femoral rollback, enhanced joint line restoration, reduced bony resections, less force transfer to the tibial baseplate, and improved proprioception of the intact ligament as advantages for this design. Ligamentous balancing is critical to long-term success; if the PCL is too tight, excessive rollback and anterior tibial liftoff can occur. This in turn leads to asymmetric posterior tibial wear, femoral subluxation/dislocation, and periarticular osteolysis. Conversely, if the PCL is excessively recessed, then early or late failure may occur and lead to flexion instability, knee effusion, and pain with loading

of the flexed knee. Other concerns stem from kinematic studies showing that the PCL may not function in a physiologic manner with paradoxical anterior sliding of the femoral condyles with increasing knee flexion and less femoral rollback.[74]

The PCL also can be sacrificed during TKA and either substituted with a cam-post mechanism or managed with more conforming polyethylene options to direct femoral rollback. Historically, better ROM has been described because of the consistent femoral rollback of a cam-post mechanism; however, this has continued to be a topic of debate.[82-84] The cam-post mechanism is susceptible to dislocation ("jumping the post"), albeit a rare complication occurring in less than 0.5% of cases. The jump height is related to the clearance required for the cam to dislocate over the tibial post and varies among knee systems. Ultracongruent designs achieve a similar level of directed rollback without a cam-post substitution mechanism. These devices also may be subject to dislocation at a lower rate as the elevated areas are further away from the midline.

An additional concern with the substituting design remains the potential for post impingement, polyethylene wear, and fracture.[85] Varus-valgus instability can lead to post wear, increased polyethylene debris, and osteolysis. Anterior post fracture may occur with knee hyperextension, when the femoral component is placed in flexion, or with excessive posterior tibial slope.[86] Such impingement concerns can lead to early aseptic loosening and osteolysis. Although reports suggest improvements with modern implants and cross-linked polyethylene, these factors highlight the need for accurate component placement and ligamentous balancing in TKA.[87]

Fixation

Cemented fixation using polymethyl methacrylate (PMMA) is the gold standard in TKA, with fewer than 10% of surgeons choosing cementless knee designs.[88] Recent efforts have focused on improving porous coatings, strengthening implants, and enhancing the knee kinematics used in cementless knee technology to avoid the need for additional fixation points afforded by adjunctive stems, screws, and pegs. Screws have been implicated in transferring polyethylene debris toward the tibial metaphysis as well as providing a source of metallic debris secondary to fretting. Strategies using highly porous metals with low moduli of elasticity have been used to highlight the potential benefits of cementless TKA, which include a simplified surgical procedure, bone conservation, biologic fixation, reduced potential for third-body wear, and decreased surgical time.[89]

A stronger emphasis on proper surgical techniques and more reliable instrumentation has led to a resurgence in cementless TKA. Excellent results have been reported, with a recent study describing equal survivorship and outcomes in bilateral TKAs, with one implanted with cementless implants and the other cemented components of a similar design.[90,91] Hybrid fixation with cementless femoral components and cemented tibial components has yielded mixed results, as have reverse hybrid constructs. Historically, cementless TKA was considered to be a procedure better suited for CR designs because the stress from the cam-post interaction was thought to lead to early micromotion and tibial component failure. A recent study has questioned this validity, reporting excellent early results of cementless PS TKA.[89] Ultimately, bone quality, implant design, and surgical technique greatly affect the success of cementless TKA; therefore, identifying appropriate candidates may improve overall outcomes.[91]

Modularity: Mobile Versus Fixed Bearing

Modular tibial baseplates have become increasingly popular because they provide the ability to transfer stress more evenly to the proximal tibial bone while allowing greater intraoperative flexibility in regard to the level of constraint and polyethylene thickness. In addition modularity affords the possibility of a relatively simple revision procedure in the setting of articular wear and well-fixed components. However, the addition of another surface opens up the possibility of backside or nonarticular surface wear as well as locking mechanism failure. Modern designs have led to stronger, more secure locking mechanisms as well as the consideration of the potential benefits in polishing tibial baseplates.

In removing all elements of modularity, monoblock TKA components are available and include all-polyethylene and porous tantalum tibias. Registry data have reported greater than 98% survival of all-polyethylene tibial components at 14 years in patients older than 75 years.[92] This represented approximately $700 per case savings on implant costs. Alternatively, porous tantalum monoblock components are typically inserted using a cementless technique and have good early results reported in several series.[93,94] However, concerns regarding implant cost, the potential for component failure, and the short follow-up period remain.

Mobile-bearing TKAs have been developed to address issues with backside wear.[95] With these devices, the articular surface is highly conforming, which translates into higher contact areas and lower contact stresses. At long-term follow-up, there has been equivalent survivorship between fixed-bearing and mobile-bearing TKA.[96] There are several unique potential complications with these devices, including component dislocation/spin out and soft-tissue impingement.

Patellar Management

Patellar resurfacing in primary TKA is a controversial topic. Anterior knee pain and patellofemoral complications are a common source of dysfunction regardless of whether the patella is resurfaced primarily. Studies have not been conclusive as to which technique provides better results because several reports support both sides of the argument.[97,98] The quality and the quantity of remaining patella cartilage has not been shown to be a predictor of failure in unresurfaced patellae.

Table 3

Host Factors Associated With an Increased Risk of Postoperative Infection

Malnutrition
  Albumin < 3.5 g/dL
  Total lymphocyte count < 1,500 cells/mm^3

Smoking

Alcoholism

Prior open surgical procedures

Multiple blood transfusions

Corticosteroid use

Rheumatoid arthritis

Immunosuppression
  Disease-related
  Medication-related

Morbid obesity

Urinary tract infection

Diabetes mellitus

Addressing anterior knee pain following TKA is a complex issue and may involve many factors, including maltracking, component malrotation, soft-tissue impingement, bursitis, and complex regional pain syndrome. A positive bone scan for a "hot" patella has been suggested as a reason for conversion to a resurfaced patella. However, revision to resurface the patella has been met with limited success; only 50% to 65% of patients experience pain improvement that meet their expectations.[99,100] Complications associated with patellar resurfacing including patellar fracture, component loosening, and osteonecrosis.

Complications

Infection

Prosthetic infection is a devastating and life-changing complication best managed with preventive measures. Preoperative modalities include advance cutaneous disinfection protocols and preoperative screening for colonization of *Staphylococcus aureus* species.[101,102] In addition, prophylactic antibiotics should be initiated within 1 hour of the surgical incision and continued for 24 hours postoperatively. Routine prophylaxis typically consists of cephalosporin medications, with clindamycin being reserved for those with β-lactam allergies and vancomycin for those in which the preoperative screening has identified colonization with *Staphylococcus* species.[103] Table 3 lists the host risk factors associated with an increased risk for infection.[104]

For patients presenting with late postoperative pain and/or wound drainage, diagnostic clinical practice guidelines have been published by The American Academy of Orthopaedic Surgeons (AAOS).[105] The diagnosis

4: Lower Extremity

of infection is typically based on the history and physical examinations, laboratory data (ESR and CRP), and aspiration results (WBC count, polymorphonuclear leuckocyte percentage, and cultures) preoperatively. Additional tools used in the diagnosis of infection include WBC-labeled bone scans, leukocyte esterase strips, interleukin-6 blood levels, and positron emission tomography scans. Current research is focused on detecting infection at the microbiology level with various assays as well as developing rapid testing for methicillin-resistant *S aureus* and resistant bacterial infections.

Venous Thromboembolism

Although there is a general consensus that some form of prophylaxis should be administered, a uniform protocol and optimal regimens have been long debated. Recent clinical practice guidelines have been established by the AAOS with a consensus on early mobilization of arthroplasty patients, and, in the absence of bleeding concerns, chemoprophylaxis with adjunctive mechanical compression devices should be prescribed.[106] Although there is support for multiple modalities in preventing deep vein thrombosis (DVT) and pulmonary embolism, concerns arise for achieving the appropriate balance between adequate prophylaxis and potential bleeding complications.[107] Currently accepted pharmacologic options are presented in the AAOS practice guidelines. In those patients unable to receive chemical or mechanical prophylaxis, an inferior vena cava filter should be considered. Furthermore, those patients with a history of a previous venous thromboembolic event require more aggressive prophylaxis with consideration for filter placement and a hematology workup preoperatively.

Ligamentous Injury

Ligamentous injury may occur intraoperatively or can be related to postoperative trauma. The MCL is crucial to the normal function of the knee; an MCL injury can lead to accelerated wear and failure. When the MCL is injured during the course of the procedure, appropriate management involves either conversion to a more constrained prosthesis or direct repair/reattachment of the damaged ligament with bracing for 6 weeks.[108-110] There is some evidence that direct repair may be more successful in CR TKAs because the PCL provides secondary stability to the knee medially.[108,109] Overall, successful outcomes with motion and knee scores similar to uncomplicated TKAs can be expected when an MCL injury is recognized and managed appropriately.

However, extensor mechanism disruption is one of the most devastating complications that can occur during a TKA. Disturbance of the extensor mechanism can occur in one of three locations: the quadriceps tendon, the patella, or the patellar tendon. With quadriceps and patellar tendon injuries, primary surgical repair has failed to provide satisfactory results. Reports have described improved success rates with adjunct fixation to the standard suture fixation through transosseous tun-nels using local tendon autograft, allograft, or cerclage wires. Prolonged immobilization is usually necessary after repair, and long-term ROM may be compromised. In cases of delayed diagnosis, chronic extensor mechanism dysfunction or failure of a prior repair, extensor mechanism allograft reconstruction may be necessary. Most often either a fresh frozen Achilles tendon allograft or complete extensor mechanism allograft is used for the reconstruction.[111,112] Alternatively, a recent description using a synthetic mesh in reconstructing the extensor mechanism has reported satisfactory early results and represents a cost-effective option without the possibility for graft disease transmission.[113]

Arthrofibrosis

Most often, the etiology of knee stiffness is multifactorial, with causes including inadequate physical therapy, poor pain control or tolerance, complex regional pain syndrome, technical errors, infection, increased likelihood of arthrofibrosis, heterotopic ossification, and muscle spasm. The patient's preoperative motion is the greatest predictor of possible postoperative ROM. When arthrofibrosis is diagnosed early, MUA may be performed with aggressive physical therapy. MUA is recommended during the first 6 weeks after surgery but may be performed in the first 12 weeks and more reliably restores knee flexion than extension. Late management of knee stiffness with MUA is associated with a greater risk of periprosthetic fracture. To minimize the risk of fracture, some advocate using arthroscopic lysis of adhesions with concomitant MUA for patients more than 3 months after surgery. Dynamic bracing may play a role in progressively stretching the knee, but it should be reserved for compliant patients with a good pain tolerance. Modern techniques, including better pain management and tunneled/extended indwelling epidural catheters, have provided excellent results in restoring motion without the revision surgery. When surgical correction is required to manage malalignment, oversized components, or malposition, revision results are satisfactory. Despite substantial gains in ROM, revision surgery for knee arthrofibrosis is fraught with complications, with rates reported as high as 49%.[114]

Neurovascular Injury

Nerve injury after TKA is a relatively uncommon complication (0.3% to 1.3%). The peroneal nerve is most often affected because it is tethered at the level of the fibula head and is susceptible to stretch injury. Table 4 lists the factors that increase the relative risk of peroneal nerve injury. Patients with only a partial initial injury or deficit have a better prognosis for recovery. Traditionally, if a palsy is recognized in the immediate postoperative period, knee flexion and removal of the dressing are suggested to ease tension on the nerve. In patients in whom function has not returned, favorable results have been reported with peroneal nerve decompression.[115]

Vascular injury during TKA is an uncommon (< 0.25%) albeit serious complication.[116] Knee flexion moves the popliteal artery posteriorly, although this averages only 9 mm from the posterior tibial plateau to the vascular bundle in the fossa. The artery typically lies anterior to the vein in knee flexion and thus is more susceptible to injury. Common pathology associated with a popliteal artery injury includes intraoperative hemorrhage, arterial thrombosis formation, pseudoaneurysm, and arteriovenous fistula formation.[117] Most injuries require consultation for vascular surgery and repair or vessel reconstruction.

Periprosthetic Fractures

Periprosthetic fractures have a reported incidence of 0.3% to 5.5% after primary TKA and up to 30% after revision TKA.[117-119] Supracondylar femoral fractures are the most common type, with an incidence of 0.3% to 2.5% for primary TKA and 1.6% to 38% for revision TKA.[117,118] Periprosthetic tibial fractures occur less commonly, with the Mayo Clinic database reporting an incidence of 0.1% intraoperative and 0.4% postoperative fractures, with a higher incidence following revision TKA.[120] Periprosthetic fractures of the patella (0.68% incidence) occur in knees with and without patellar resurfacing, but there is an increase in frequency in knees without patellar resurfacing.[121] Fractures of the patella have a sixfold greater risk of occurrence after revision TKA.[122] Most periprosthetic fractures are the result of low-energy injuries, with only approximately 10% caused by high-energy mechanisms.

Multiple predisposing risk factors for periprosthetic fractures have been identified. Metabolic issues, such as osteoporosis and rheumatoid arthritis, are known risk factors for the development of periprosthetic fractures adjacent to a TKA. One study showed decreased periprosthetic bone loss in patients undergoing TKA treated with concomitant bisphosphonate therapy.[123] The surgical technique, specifically, notching of the anterior distal femur, has been implicated. Some studies have shown that anterior distal femoral notching is a risk factor, and others have shown no clinical correlation. A large clinical series of 660 patients undergoing TKA revealed that only 2 of 180 patients who had anterior femoral notching sustained a fracture.[118]

Periprosthetic fractures about a TKA are classified based on anatomic location and component involvement. A classification system that lends itself to treatment regimens has been created[124] (Table 5). Similarly, periprosthetic tibial fractures are often stratified using the Mayo Classification System[125] (Figure 6). This system is based on the location of the fracture, component stability, and intraoperative occurrence.

Periprosthetic patellar fractures have been classified based on disruption of the extensor mechanism, component stability, and bone stock. A classification system that would help guide treatment has been proposed[121] (Table 6).

As with other periprosthetic fractures, implants that are loose require revision. Fractures about a stable femoral component typically are treated with intramedullary nailing or laterally based locked plating. Nailing has been demonstrated to be superior to locked plating biomechanically in a cadaver model of periprosthetic fractures of the distal femur.[126] One disadvantage is that retrograde nailing can be performed only in TKA with an open box, and adequate distal bone stock must be present for distal fixation. In addition, the location of the box can alter the starting point of the retrograde nail, leading to sagittal plane deformity. High union rates, satisfactory functional outcomes, and low revision rates have been demonstrated.[127] Occasionally, an-

---

Table 4

Risk Factors Associated With an Increased Risk for Peroneal Nerve Injury During Total Knee Arthroplasty

Fixed preoperative deformities
    Fixed valgus (3% to 4% incidence)
    Fixed valgus with flexion contracture
    Flexion contracture greater than 60° (up to 8% incidence)

Prior HTO

History of lumbar laminectomy

Tourniquet time > 2 hours

Dressing applied to tightly

Epidural anesthesia

HTO = high tibial osteotomy

Table 5

The Mayo Clinic Comprehensive Classification System for Periprosthetic Femoral Fractures

Type	Fracture Reducible	Bone Stock in Distal Fragment	Component Well Positioned and Well Fixed	Treatment
IA	Yes	Good	Yes	Conservative
IB	No	Good	Yes	Surgical fixation
II	Yes/No	Good	No	Revision with long stem component
III	Yes/No	Poor	No	Prosthetic replacement

(Adapted from Kim KI, Egol KA, Hozack WJ, Parvizi J: Periprosthetic fractures after total knee arthroplasties. *Clin Orthop Relat Res* 2006;446:167-175.)

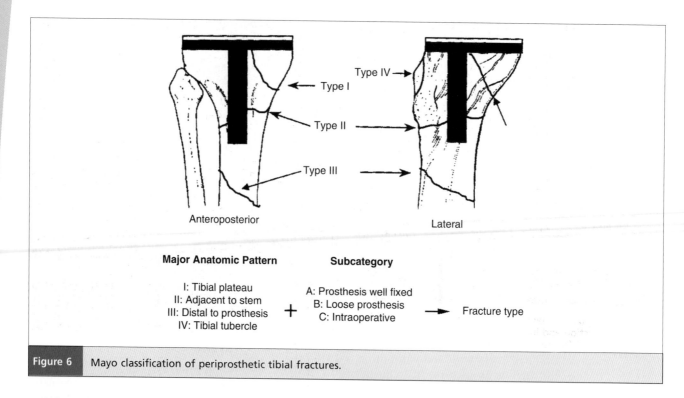

Figure 6 | Mayo classification of periprosthetic tibial fractures.

Table 6

Mayo Clinic Classification System for Periprosthetic Patellar Fractures After Total Knee Arthroplasty

Type of Fracture	Characteristics
I	Stable implant, intact extensor mechanism
II	Disrupted extensor mechanism
IIIa	Loose patellar component, reasonable bone stock
IIIb	Loose patellar component, poor bone stock

(Reproduced with permission from Ortiguera CJ, Berry DJ: Patellar fracture after total knee arthroplasty. *J Bone Joint Surg Am* 2002;84:532-540.)

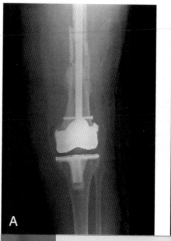
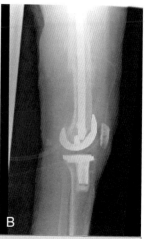

Figure 7 | AP (**A**) and lateral (**B**) radiographs showing retrograde nailing of a periprosthetic femoral fracture after total knee arthroplasty.

tegrade femoral nailing can be used for periprosthetic distal femoral fractures if there is a long distal segment to provide stable fracture fixation (Figure 7).

The advantages of locked plating include multiple fixed-angle points of fixation, increased biomechanical strength, and insertion with minimally invasive techniques.[128] It is crucial to avoid malalignment, typically valgus and hyperextension of the distal fragment. Multiple studies have reported a high union rate with locked plating for periprosthetic fractures.[129,130] Few studies have directly compared locked plating to retrograde nailing. Because of the lack of good evidence, it is difficult to decide on the best treatment option. The authors of a 2010 study described a salvage technique combining retrograde intramedullary nailing aug-

mented with PMMA cement; all patients had an uncomplicated recovery and achieved preinjury functional status within 4 months.[131] Therefore, nailed cementoplasty is a reasonable option when standard retrograde nailing or plating alone is inadequate in the severely medically ill patient.

When periprosthetic fractures of the distal femur coincide with a loose component, revision arthroplasty is the treatment of choice. Prosthetic revision options include standard revision components, distal femoral replacement, or an allograft-prosthetic composite. If prosthetic revision stemmed components are the treatment, the stem should bypass the fracture by at least

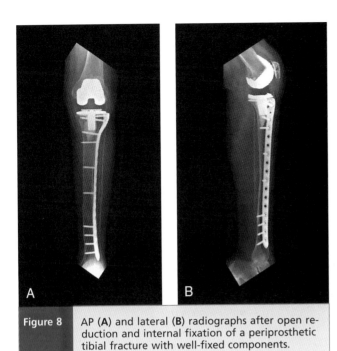

Figure 8   AP (**A**) and lateral (**B**) radiographs after open reduction and internal fixation of a periprosthetic tibial fracture with well-fixed components.

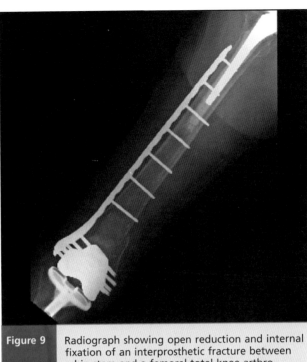

Figure 9   Radiograph showing open reduction and internal fixation of an interprosthetic fracture between a hip stem and a femoral total knee arthroplasty component.

two cortical diameters. In elderly, low-demand patients, a distal femoral replacement has been effective.[132]

Periprosthetic fractures of the tibia are rare but follow the same general principles used for managing femoral fractures. It is imperative to obtain a mechanical axis series as part of the radiographic workup. Fractures about the tibial plateau-implant interface (type I) typically require a revision because the tibial component is usually loose and/or in varus malalignment.[133] The associated bone defect in the tibial plateau requires augmentation either with metallic blocks or allograft. Fractures adjacent to the stem (type II) can be treated nonsurgically if the component is stable. If the tibial component is loose, however, revision surgery using a long-stemmed component bypassing the fracture by at least two cortical diameters is necessary.[133] Type III fractures are distal to the stem and rarely affect implant stability and can be treated with fracture reduction with or without internal fixation (Figure 8). Type IV fractures involving the tibial tubercle are extremely rare and are treated with open reduction and internal fixation (ORIF) and bone grafting of any osteolytic defects.

Periprosthetic patellar fractures are treated based on the integrity of the extensor mechanism. Surgery has a high rate of complications and therefore is discouraged unless the the extensor mechanism is disrupted or the patellar component is loose.[121,134,135] The treatment of choice for type I fractures is nonsurgical if the patellar implant and extensor mechanism are intact. Nonsurgical treatment of type I fractures has a high success rate.[121]

Type II fractures involve a disrupted extensor mechanism. Typical fixation techniques for patellar fractures are difficult because of the patellar component and cement. Fixation strategies often require a circumferential cerclage wire instead of a tension band construct. If the displaced fragment is small or irreparable to the body

of the patella, excision of the fragment with primary soft-tissue repair can be performed.[136] Type III fractures involve a loose component with an intact extensor mechanism. Surgical management involves patelloplasty with component revision versus component removal, depending on the remaining bone stock. If the bone stock is inadequate, then patellar component removal with patelloplasty or complete patellectomy is recommended. One study described a porous tantalum patella for marked patella bone loss during revision TKA, with good or excellent results in 17 of 20 patients (requires at least some remaining bone for a successful outcome).[137]

Interprosthetic Fractures

Interprosthetic fractures between a total hip arthroplasty (THA) and a TKA (Figure 9) or a TKA and ORIF proximally presents a unique challenge. In general, the fixation devices should be long and span both prostheses to avoid stress risers. A recent study reported on 20 consecutive patients with interprosthetic fractures treated with a surgical protocol of plate fixation that spanned the entire interprosthetic zone without the use of supplemental bone grafts. All of the fractures healed after the index procedure.[138] Fractures between a TKA and ORIF proximally are treated in a similar manner; however, the proximal fixation often must be removed and the defect filled with bone cement to augment screw fixation above the previous device.

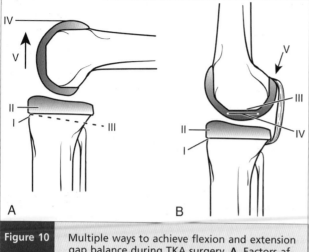

Figure 10 Multiple ways to achieve flexion and extension gap balance during TKA surgery. **A**, Factors affecting the flexion space. I, tibial resection level; II, polyethylene thickness; III, tibial slope; IV, AP dimension of the femoral component; V, AP placement of the femoral component. **B**, Factors affecting the extension space. I, tibial resection level; II, polyethylene thickness; III, distal femoral resection; IV, distal femoral augments; V, posterior capsule. (Reproduced from Froimson MI: Knee reconstruction and replacement, in Vaccaro AR, ed: *Orthopaedic Knowledge Update*, ed 8. Rosemont, IL, American Academy of Orthopaedic Surgeons, 2005, pp 457-470.)

Revision Total Knee Arthroplasty

Evaluation of the Painful TKA

To perform revision TKA with a high level of success, it is important to establish a thorough and accurate diagnosis for the etiology of failure. An initial evaluation starts with a history and physical examination to rule out intrinsic and extrinsic sources of pain. A normal knee examination should prompt assessment of adjacent joints and the lumbar spine. Radiographic evaluation should include preoperative radiographs and serial films from immediately after surgery to the latest follow-up. When extrinsic sources of pain are present, standard hip and/or lumbar spine radiographs and the physical examination should be reviewed before initiating treatment.

Although a painful TKA may have many potential etiologies responsible for the patient's dysfunction, infection must always be ruled out. Screening laboratory tests should include the ESR and CRP level. When either or both of these values are elevated, knee aspiration is recommended. Exact WBC count guidelines are debatable, with values greater than 1,100 to 3,000 cells/μL and neutrophil differential counts greater than 65% considered positive for infection.[139] Further modalities used to establish a source for TKA pain include technetium bone scans, MARS, CT scans, fluoroscopy, and diagnostic local anesthetic injections.

Preoperative Planning

Revision surgery for TKA can be technically challenging and is often affected by factors not necessarily present during primary procedures. Despite advances to manage bone defects and robust revision knee systems, the complication rate may be as high as 25%. Overall higher rates of infection, extensor mechanism dysfunction, stiffness, aseptic loosening, periprosthetic fracture, wound complications, and instability may occur with revision surgery.

Before surgery, it is important to identify what components are present, their sizes, the level of constraint, and the surgical approaches previously used. When vertical incisions are present, it is best to follow the most lateral incision that will provide adequate exposure to perform the surgery. Transverse incisions can be crossed at right angles; when in doubt, plastic surgery consultation can be considered to assess for potential soft-tissue procedures. Bone defects are typically classified using the Anderson Orthopaedic Research Institute classification system,[140] and the deficits anticipated after component removal as well as the fact that defects are often more extensive intraoperatively than they appear on radiographs should be taken into account. Ligamentous stability testing will afford insight regarding the level of constraint that may be necessary to balance the knee.

Maintaining and/or restoring the appropriate joint line level are vital elements to the success of revision TKA surgery. Helpful landmarks include the lateral epicondyle (2.5 cm from the joint line), the medial epicondyle (3 cm from the joint line), and the fibula head (1.5 to 2 cm distal to the joint line). Appropriate gap balancing and options for adjusting the flexion and extension gaps independently are critical for good outcomes and minimizing the level of TKA constraint. Joint line elevation will result in patella baja and limited knee flexion, whereas depression can lead to patella alta and possible maltracking. Addressing flexion and extension gap mismatch may be done with the strategies depicted in **Figure 10**.

In general, it is important to address three areas of fixation for revision TKA: epiphysis (bone surface), metaphysis, and diaphysis. Fixation in these locations leads to a successful revision procedure and may allow for better management of the stress applied to more highly constrained constructs. Epiphyseal fixation is often achieved with cement pressurized into the bone surfaces. Metaphyseal fixation can be achieved with cementless sleeves or cones that not only fill defects but also add biologic fixation to the revision knee system. Diaphyseal fixation can be obtained using press-fit or fully cemented stems with equal levels of success.

Partial Versus Full Revision

Isolated polyethylene liner exchange can be a successful means for TKA revision in cases of well-fixed components with articular surface wear and peri-implant osteolysis. Modular components afford the ability to perform a limited revision with component retention;

however, reports have shown a surprisingly high rate (30% to 40%) of early failure.[141-143] It is important to assess for malalignment, balance deficits too great to overcome with isolated liner exchange, and ligamentous tension predisposing to wear and component failure. Based on these concerns, isolated polyethylene liner revision should be reserved for carefully selected cases, and bone grafting of lytic lesions should occur concomitantly. Common modes of failure include infection, recurrent instability, stiffness, and polyethylene wear. Additional concerns for backside wear and surface damage have called into question isolated liner exchange in revision TKA.

Isolated patella revision has been met with poor results and a high rate of reoperation.[143] Similar overall results have been reported with isolated tibial or femoral component revision. However, in certain cases, such as isolated femoral internal rotation, a single component revision may lead to successful results.[144] Selective component retention in TKA does have a role in certain cases in which a correctable deformity is recognized and the retained components are well fixed and aligned.

Patella Management in Revision Surgery

Management of the patella in revision TKA surgery can be quite difficult because poor bone stock, osteonecrosis, maltracking, and improperly positioned/rotated femoral and tibial components can lead to early failure. Restoring patellar thickness leads to improved biomechanics of the extensor mechanism and is a goal of revision TKA surgery. In select cases, the bone quality and quantity are insufficient for resurfacing, and options such as débridement and the retention of the patellar bone fragment or patellectomy are options. In these cases, extensor lag and weakness is often prevalent because of insufficient patellar height.

In patients with adequate bone stock, restoration of patellar height using standard resurfacing is the first choice of treatment. When bone stock is insufficient, the following options exist: (1) a porous tantalum salvage patella (requires a viable bone fragment), (2) bone grafting of the residual patella and local soft tissue to cover or an artificial material to secure the pocket, (3) gull-wing osteotomy, and (4) extensor mechanism allograft. The results with each option have been encouraging when used under the appropriate indications.[137,145,146]

Management of Bone Defects

Osteolysis, component loosening, cement extraction, and excessive resections can lead to substantial bone loss that requires reconstruction at the time of revision. Preoperative preparation for the worst scenario with allograft, augments, cones or sleeves, and stems is imperative. Contained defects can be managed with metallic augments, bone graft, cement (when < 5 mm) or cones or sleeves. These adjuncts typically are supplemental stem fixation to offload the periarticular reconstruction. Segmental defects can be managed with structural allograft or porous cones or sleeves. Grafting options

and metallic bone graft substitutes can fill combined defects and are fixed with screws to the host bone and bypassed with stem fixation distally. Impaction grafting with or without metallic mesh can transition uncontained defects into contained defects. Larger defects may require allograft prosthetic composites or megaprostheses for reconstruction. Success has been reported for the various techniques to manage bone defects; however, the greater the defect and extent of reconstruction, the greater the risk for perioperative complications and failure.[140,147,148]

Summary

Knee pain and injuries are common findings in orthopaedics. Appropriate diagnosis is crucial to determine the correct treatment. Nonsurgical measures, while often controversial regarding efficacy, should be exhausted prior to surgical intervention. Further joint preservation techniques should be assessed early and for younger patients because arthroplasty is typically reserved for older patients (at least 60 years of age). Perioperative management of surgical patients is critical to optimize outcomes and lower revision and complication rates. Despite a heightened awareness of complication prevention, infection, and venous thromboembolic events, periprosthetic fractures can occur. Classification and treatment algorithms exist for periprosthetic fractures about TKA components with similar goals of restoring motion, reducing pain, and establishing a stable knee joint. Revision TKA should be reserved to manage a specific finding (loosening, infection, or malrotation) with the goals being to restore the anatomic joint line, provide stable implants, and restore normal knee kinematics and alignment. In general, when these classic principles of knee surgery are followed, the outcomes are typically satisfactory.

Key Study Points

- The utility of nonsurgical management of knee pain should be understood for various conditions to include the indications for, success rates, and the limitations for each modality.

- The general principles of TKA must be completely comprehended, including joint line restoration (gap balancing versus measured resection techniques), kinematics (CR versus PS TKAs), mechanical alignment, component fixation (cemented versus cementless), and bearings (fixed versus mobile).

- Periprosthetic fractures are common, and management includes the fixation of fractures with stable implants, revision for loose components, and oncology/megaprostheses for salvage procedures.

- Revision TKA can be successful if the appropriate diagnosis is identified preoperatively and then corrected during the procedure. It is important to follow a standard workup for a painful TKA and always rule out infection.

Annotated References

1. Matsuda S, Kawahara S, Okazaki K, Tashiro Y, Iwamoto Y: Postoperative alignment and ROM affect patient satisfaction after TKA. *Clin Orthop Relat Res* 2013;471(1):127-133.

   A retrospective review of 500 TKAs at a minimum of 2-year follow-up showed on survey answers that better range of motion and avoiding varus malalignment was important for patient satisfaction and in meeting expectations postoperatively. Level of evidence: IV.

2. Culliton SE, Bryant DM, Overend TJ, MacDonald SJ, Chesworth BM: The relationship between expectations and satisfaction in patients undergoing primary total knee arthroplasty. *J Arthroplasty* 2012;27(3):490-492.

   A literature review was performed to include five studies regarding patient satisfaction and expectations after TKA. Postoperative satisfaction ratings correlated with how closely postoperative expectations were met after TKA. The authors recommended preoperative patient education for managing expectations. Level of evidence: IV.

3. Greene KA, Harwin SF: Maximizing patient satisfaction and functional results after total knee arthroplasty. *J Knee Surg* 2011;24(1):19-24.

   This review article presents modern means of maximizing patient satisfaction, including patient education, less invasive surgery, improved prostheses, aggressive rehabilitation, and multimodal pain management. Level of evidence: V.

4. Noble PC, Scuderi GR, Brekke AC, et al: Development of a new Knee Society scoring system. *Clin Orthop Relat Res* 2012;470(1):20-32.

   The introduction of a new knee scoring system is described to include a more comprehensive survey of activities and function. The study compared and validated the new Knee Society scoring system compared with previously validated outcome measures, such as the KOOS, and the SF-12 score. Level of evidence: IV.

5. Hochberg MC, Altman RD, April KT, et al: American College of Rheumatology 2012 recommendations for the use of nonpharmacologic and pharmacologic therapies in osteoarthritis of the hand, hip, and knee. *Arthritis Care Res (Hoboken)* 2012;64(4):465-474.

   A systematic evidence-based review described recommendations for the management of OA. Strong recommendations were given for exercise and weight loss. Conditional recommendations were given to a wide array of pharmacologic regimens (NSAIDs, acetaminophen, tramadol, and injections) and nonpharmacologic modalities (shoe inserts, walking aids, thermal agents, and psychosocial interventions). Level of evidence: III.

6. Zhang W, Moskowitz RW, Nuki G, et al: OARSI recommendations for the management of hip and knee osteoarthritis: Part II. OARSI evidence-based, expert consensus guidelines. *Osteoarthritis Cartilage* 2008;16(2):137-162.

7. Zhang W, Nuki G, Moskowitz RW, et al: OARSI recommendations for the management of hip and knee osteoarthritis: Part III. Changes in evidence following systematic cumulative update of research published through January 2009. *Osteoarthritis Cartilage* 2010;18(4):476-499.

   A systematic review was performed to update numerous modalities for the management of hip and knee OA. The authors found that standard modalities, such as oral and topical NSAIDs and corticosteroid injections, have not had much change in their risk benefit profile. However, for several other modalities, substantial literature has been published annually that affects the risk-benefit ratio for these modalities. Level of evidence: III.

8. Chen CA, Chen W, Goodman SB, et al: New MR imaging methods for metallic implants in the knee: Artifact correction and clinical impact. *J Magn Reson Imaging* 2011;33(5):1121-1127.

   Fourteen volunteers with TKAs underwent MRI scans using SEMAC, MAVRIC, and two-dimensional fast spin-echo to assess the diagnostic abilities of these tests. After a thorough review, it was concluded that SEMAC and MAVRIC correct for metal artifact and provide high-resolution images. Level of evidence: II.

9. Wilson B, Rankin H, Barnes CL: Long-term results of an unloader brace in patients with unicompartmental knee osteoarthritis. *Orthopedics* 2011;34(8):e334-e337.

   This study had an average of 11.2 years follow-up of 30 patients prospectively enrolled to use an unloader brace for unicompartmental knee degenerative joint disease. Twenty-four patients were available for survey follow-up, with 58.6% having undergone a knee arthroplasty procedure at a mean of 3.9 years from their initial evaluation. At 2.7-year follow-up, 35% had discontinued use of the brace; at the latest follow-up, no patients were using the brace. It was concluded that unloader braces provide short-term pain relief and improved function, yet most will subsequently undergo a knee arthroplasty procedure. Level of evidence: IV.

10. Lapane KL, Sands MR, Yang S, McAlindon TE, Eaton CB: Use of complementary and alternative medicine among patients with radiographic-confirmed knee osteoarthritis. *Osteoarthritis Cartilage* 2012;20(1):22-28.

The authors surveyed 2679 patients and found 47% used some form of complementary and alternative medicine in managing their OA symptoms. The overall benefits in symptom treatment and delaying the progression of degenerative joint disease are unproven at this time. Level of evidence: IV.

11. Spaková T, Rosocha J, Lacko M, Harvanová D, Gharaibeh A: Treatment of knee joint osteoarthritis with autologous platelet-rich plasma in comparison with hyaluronic acid. *Am J Phys Med Rehabil* 2012; 91(5):411-417.

In a prospective, controlled cohort study, the authors enrolled 120 patients with radiographic grade 1, 2, or 3 OA. WOMAC and Numeric Rating Scale scores were significantly higher for those in the platelet-rich plasma injection group versus those with a series of three hyaluronic acid injections at 3- and 6-month follow-up. Level of evidence: II.

12. Moseley JB, O'Malley K, Petersen NJ, et al: A controlled trial of arthroscopic surgery for osteoarthritis of the knee. *N Engl J Med* 2002;347(2):81-88.

13. Potts A, Harrast JJ, Harner CD, Miniaci A, Jones MH: Practice patterns for arthroscopy of osteoarthritis of the knee in the United States. *Am J Sports Med* 2012;40(6): 1247-1251.

The authors performed a descriptive epidemiologic study in reviewing the American Board of Orthopaedic Surgery database. Arthroscopic procedures were reported to decline from a peak in 2001 (1,621 cases) to 2009 (966 cases). It appears that during the board collection period, the number of arthroscopy procedures has significantly decreased from 2.36 to 1.40 cases per surgeon, which may be related to the publication of an article documenting minimal efficacy of this procedure. Level of evidence: V.

14. Rönn K, Reischl N, Gautier E, Jacobi M: Current surgical treatment of knee osteoarthritis. *Arthritis* 2011; 2011(2011):454873.

The surgical options for the management of OA, ranging from arthroscopic to arthroplasty and osteotomy procedures, are discussed. Level of evidence: V.

15. Gross AE, Shasha N, Aubin P: Long-term followup of the use of fresh osteochondral allografts for posttraumatic knee defects. *Clin Orthop Relat Res* 2005;435: 79-87.

16. Bedi A, Haidukewych GJ: Management of the posttraumatic arthritic knee. *J Am Acad Orthop Surg* 2009; 17(2):88-101.

17. Spahn G, Hofmann GO, von Engelhardt LV, Li M, Neubauer H, Klinger HM: The impact of a high tibial valgus osteotomy and unicondylar medial arthroplasty on the treatment for knee osteoarthritis: A meta-analysis. *Knee Surg Sports Traumatol Arthrosc* 2013; 21(1):96-112.

Forty-six studies on valgus HTO versus 43 studies on medial UKA were selected for a full literature review. The mean survival time to TKA for valgus HTO was 9.7 years compared with UKA at 9.2 years. However, the clinical outcome was significantly better for medial UKA at 5- to 12-year follow-up, with overall similar complication rates between the two procedures. Level of evidence: II.

18. Papachristou G, Plessas S, Sourlas J, Levidiotis C, Chronopoulos E, Papachristou C: Deterioration of long-term results following high tibial osteotomy in patients under 60 years of age. *Int Orthop* 2006;30(5): 403-408.

19. Fletcher X, Parratte S, Aubaniac JM, Argenson JN: A 12-28-year followup study of closing wedge high tibial osteotomy. *Clin Orthop Relat Res* 2006;452:91-96.

20. Gstöttner M, Pedross F, Liebensteiner M, Bach C: Long-term outcome after high tibial osteotomy. *Arch Orthop Trauma Surg* 2008;128(1):111-115.

21. Akizuki S, Shibakawa A, Takizawa T, Yamazaki I, Horiuchi H: The long-term outcome of high tibial osteotomy: A ten- to 20-year follow-up. *J Bone Joint Surg Br* 2008;90(5):592-596.

22. Kolb W, Guhlmann H, Windisch C, Kolb K, Koller G, Grützner P: Opening-wedge high tibial osteotomy with a locked low-profile plate. *J Bone Joint Surg Am* 2009; 91(11):2581-2588.

23. Saragaglia D, Blaysat M, Imman D, Mercier N: Outcome of opening wedge high tibial osteotomy augmented with a Biosorb® wedge and fixed with a plate and screws in 124 patients with a mean of ten years follow-up. *Int Orthop* 2011;35(8):1151-1156.

The authors evaluated the long-term results of an opening wedge HTO and the tolerance and the integration of a Biosorb wedge.

24. DeMeo PJ, Johnson EM, Chiang PP, Flamm AM, Miller MC: Midterm follow-up of opening-wedge high tibial osteotomy. *Am J Sports Med* 2010;38(10):2077-2084.

A medial opening-wedge HTO is recommended for young patients with varus alignment and medial compartment arthritis. The procedure allows patients to remain active and delays progression to TKA. Level of evidence: IV.

25. Hcyse TJ, Khefacha A, Peersman G, Cartier P: Survivorship of UKA in the middle-aged. *Knee* 2012;19(5): 585-591.

Two hundred twenty-three UKAs in patients younger than 60 years followed for an average of 10.8 years were retrospectively reviewed. Implant survival was 94.3% for the study with survivorship of the entire cohort being 93.5% at 10 years. It was concluded that UKA can be performed successfully in a younger patient population. Level of evidence: IV.

26. Koskinen E, Paavolainen P, Eskelinen A, Pulkkinen P, Remes V: Unicondylar knee replacement for primary osteoarthritis: A prospective follow-up study of 1,819 patients from the Finnish Arthroplasty Register. *Acta Orthop* 2007;78(1):128-135.

27. Boissonneault A, Pandit H, Pegg E, et al: No difference in survivorship after unicompartmental knee arthroplasty with or without an intact anterior cruciate ligament. *Knee Surg Sports Traumatol Arthrosc* 2012;Jul:11.

   In a retrospective review, 42 patients with an ACL deficient knee and a medial UKA were compared to a similar cohort having an intact ACL and UKA. No clinical or survivorship differences were noted at a mean 5-year follow-up. Level of evidence: III.

28. Bonutti PM, Goddard MS, Zywiel MG, Khanuja HS, Johnson AJ, Mont MA: Outcomes of unicompartmental knee arthroplasty stratified by body mass index. *J Arthroplasty* 2011;26(8):1149-1153.

   Patients with a BMI greater than 35 kg/m^2 (40 knees) were compared with those with a BMI less than 35 kg/m^2 (40 knees). Five obese patients required revision and prompted the authors to suggest caution in performing TKA in patients with a high BMI. Level of evidence: III.

29. Noticewala MS, Geller JA, Lee JH, Macaulay W: Unicompartmental knee arthroplasty relieves pain and improves function more than total knee arthroplasty. *J Arthroplasty* 2012;27(8, suppl):99-105.

   Seventy UKAs and 128 TKAs were included in a prospective data study. The overall results and improvements in clinical scores were greater for the UKA cohort than the TKA cohort at a mean follow-up of 3 and 2.9 years, respectively. Level of evidence: III.

30. Rees JL, Price AJ, Lynskey TG, Svärd UC, Dodd CA, Murray DW: Medial unicompartmental arthroplasty after failed high tibial osteotomy. *J Bone Joint Surg Br* 2001;83(7):1034-1036.

31. Willis-Owen CA, Brust K, Alsop H, Miraldo M, Cobb JP: Unicondylar knee arthroplasty in the UK National Health Service: An analysis of candidacy, outcome and cost efficacy. *Knee* 2009;16(6):473-478.

32. Berend KR, Kolczun MC II, George JW Jr, Lombardi AV Jr: Lateral unicompartmental knee arthroplasty through a lateral parapatellar approach has high early survivorship. *Clin Orthop Relat Res* 2012;470(1): 77-83.

   A retrospective review of 93 patients (100 lateral UKAs) at a mean follow-up of 39 months was conducted. The average ROM was 124°, and excellent function was reported with only three reoperations (one revision to TKA). Level of evidence: IV.

33. Berend KR, Lombardi AV Jr, Morris MJ, Hurst JM, Kavolus JJ: Does preoperative patellofemoral joint state affect medial unicompartmental arthroplasty survival? *Orthopedics* 2011;34(9):e494-e496.

   Six hundred thirty-eight UKAs were evaluated, and evidence of patellofemoral degenerative joint disease was graded by the modified Altman classification at 1- to 7-year follow-up. There were 17 overall revisions with a 97.9% survivorship in knees with patellofemoral degenerative joint disease and 93.8% in those without. There were no revisions for anterior knee pain or the progression of patellofemoral arthritis. Level of evidence: IV.

34. Munk S, Odgaard A, Madsen F, et al: Preoperative lateral subluxation of the patella is a predictor of poor early outcome of Oxford phase-III medial unicompartmental knee arthroplasty. *Acta Orthop* 2011;82(5): 582-588.

   A multicenter study reviewed 260 medial Oxford UKAs with 1-year follow-up. Ninety percent were satisfied with the surgery, and it was found that lateral subluxation of the patella was a predictor of poor outcome. Level of evidence: IV.

35. Whittaker JP, Naudie DD, McAuley JP, McCalden RW, MacDonald SJ, Bourne RB: Does bearing design influence midterm survivorship of unicompartmental arthroplasty? *Clin Orthop Relat Res* 2010;468(1):73-81.

   One hundred seventy-nine patients with 229 medial UKAs (79 mobile and 150 fixed bearings) were retrospectively reviewed with a mean 3.6-year follow-up. Revision for the mobile-bearing group was 9% at 2.6-year follow-up and 15% at 6.9-year follow-up with a fixed-bearing design. With an end point of revision, the 5-year survival rates were 88% and 96% for mobile and fixed bearings, respectively. Level of evidence: III.

36. Burton A, Williams S, Brockett CL, Fisher J: In vitro comparison of fixed- and mobile meniscal-bearing unicondylar knee arthroplasties: Effect of design, kinematics, and condylar liftoff. *J Arthroplasty* 2012;27(8): 1452-1459.

   This investigation reviewed the kinematics and femoral liftoff with mobile- and fixed-bearing UKAs. They found lower wear with the fixed bearings and the medial side articular surface. Femoral liftoff resulted in greater wear on the medial side by reduced wear in lateral UKAs.

37. Parratte S, Pauly V, Aubaniac JM, Argenson JN: No long-term difference between fixed and mobile medial unicompartmental arthroplasty. *Clin Orthop Relat Res* 2012;470(1):61-68.

   Seventy-nine fixed-bearing UKAs and 77 mobile-bearing components were retrospectively reviewed. The minimal follow-up was 15 years with a 15% versus 12% revision rate for mobile and fixed bearings, respectively. Alignment overcorrection and peri-implant radiolucencies were higher in the mobile-bearing group (69% versus 24%). Level of evidence: III.

38. Epinette JA, Brunschweiler B, Mertl P, Mole D, Cazenave A; French Society for Hip and Knee: Unicompartmental knee arthroplasty modes of failure: wear is not

the main reason for failure: A multicentre study of 418 failed knees. *Orthop Traumatol Surg Res* 2012;98(6, suppl):S124-S130.

This multicenter study reviewed failed UKAs to determine the etiology of failure and the prevalence of these complications. The authors found that 48.5% of the revisions occurred within 5 years of the initial procedure. Loosening (45%), OA progression (15%), wear (12%), technical problems (11.5%), and infection (1.9%) were the most common indications for revision surgery. Level of evidence: IV.

39. Society of Unicondylar Research and Continuing Education: Diagnosis of periprosthetic joint infection after unicompartmental knee arthroplasty. *J Arthroplasty* 2012;27(8, suppl):46-50.

A retrospective multicenter study was performed to determine the utility of cell counts and laboratories in diagnosing a periprosthetic infection. The optimal cutoffs were ESR, 27 mm/h; CRP, 14 mg/L; and 6,200/μL WBC count; and 60% polymorphonuclear leukocytes on the differential. Level of evidence: V.

40. O'Donnell TM, Abouazza O, Neil MJ: Revision of minimal resection resurfacing unicondylar knee arthroplasty to total knee arthroplasty: Results compared with primary total knee arthroplasty. *J Arthroplasty* 2013; 28(1):33-39.

Fifty-five patients were matched for comparison of minimal resection UKA versus TKA. The most common reason for failure was tibial baseplate subsidence (58%), with revision occurring at approximately 39.2 months after surgery. Revision of these minimal resection UKAs afforded similar outcomes as primary TKA. Level of evidence: III.

41. Springer BD, Scott RD, Thornhill TS: Conversion of failed unicompartmental knee arthroplasty to TKA. *Clin Orthop Relat Res* 2006;446:214-220.

42. Davies AP, Vince AS, Shepstone L, Donell ST, Glasgow MM: The radiologic prevalence of patellofemoral osteoarthritis. *Clin Orthop Relat Res* 2002;402:206-212.

43. Fulkerson JP: Alternatives to patellofemoral arthroplasty. *Clin Orthop Relat Res* 2005;436:76-80.

44. Minas T, Bryant T: The role of autologous chondrocyte implantation in the patellofemoral joint. *Clin Orthop Relat Res* 2005;436:30-39.

45. van Jonbergen HP, Werkman DM, Barnaart LF, van Kampen A: Long-term outcomes of patellofemoral arthroplasty. *J Arthroplasty* 2010;25(7):1066-1071.

At a mean of 13.3-year follow-up, 185 PFAs were reviewed. Survivorship calculations yielded 84% and 69% success at 10 and 20 years, respectively. The rate of revision in patients who are obese was higher than in the nonobese population. Level of evidence: IV.

46. Mont MA, Johnson AJ, Naziri Q, Kolisek FR, Leadbetter WB: Patellofemoral arthroplasty: 7-year mean follow-up. *J Arthroplasty* 2012;27(3):358-361.

The authors reviewed 43 PFAs at an average of 7-years' follow-up. Five-year survivorship was reported to be 95%. Level of evidence: IV.

47. Meding JB, Wing JT, Keating EM, Ritter MA: Total knee arthroplasty for isolated patellofemoral arthritis in younger patients. *Clin Orthop Relat Res* 2007;464:78-82.

48. Odland AN, Callaghan JJ, Liu SS, Wells CW: Wear and lysis is the problem in modular TKA in the young OA patient at 10 years. *Clin Orthop Relat Res* 2011;469(1): 41-47.

This is a retrospective review of 67 knees with a CR (CR; 27%) or PS (PS; 73%) TKA, implanted with a modular tibial baseplate. At a mean follow-up, of 12.4 years, 10 patients had died, 2 were lost to follow-up, and 10 underwent revision for loosening and/or osteolysis. Sixty-five percent were still performing moderate labor or sporting activities. Level of evidence: IV.

49. Keenan AC, Wood AM, Arthur CA, Jenkins PJ, Brenkel IJ, Walmsley PJ: Ten-year survival of cemented total knee replacement in patients aged less than 55 years. *J Bone Joint Surg Br* 2012;94(7):928-931.

One hundred ninety-nine patients were available for follow-up comparing those 55 years or older and those weighing less than 55 kg. Ten-year survival rates of 98.2% with revision as an end point were recorded. The results were similar in both cohorts, and the authors concluded that TKA should not be withheld from patients based on chronological age. Level of evidence: III.

50. O'Connor MI: Implant survival, knee function, and pain relief after TKA: Are there differences between men and women? *Clin Orthop Relat Res* 2011;469(7): 1846-1851.

The literature was reviewed regarding the effect of outcomes in TKA based on sex. Men are more likely to have a higher rate of revision than women. Although similar score results were found among both groups, women often start lower and end lower in regard to KSS. Level of evidence: V.

51. Liebs TR, Herzberg W, Roth-Kroeger AM, Rüther W, Hassenpflug J: Women recover faster than men after standard knee arthroplasty. *Clin Orthop Relat Res* 2011;469(10):2855-2865.

This multicenter study retrospectively reviewed data from a prospective database of three randomized controlled trials evaluating rehabilitation measures after a unisex TKA. They found that in 141 men versus 353 women, the latter recover faster after TKA. Despite greater functional limitations initially, women had better WOMAC function scores at 3- and 6-month follow-up. However, the function scores were not ultimately different between the sexes at 12 and 24 months. Level of evidence: III.

52. MacDonald SJ, Charron KD, Bourne RB, Naudie DD, McCalden RW, Rorabeck CH: The John Insall Award: Gender-specific total knee replacement. Prospectively collected clinical outcomes. *Clin Orthop Relat Res* 2008;466(11):2612-2616.

4: Lower Extremity

53. Scott CE, Bugler KE, Clement ND, MacDonald D, Howie CR, Biant LC: Patient expectations of arthroplasty of the hip and knee. *J Bone Joint Surg Br* 2012; 94-B(7):974-981.

Patient expectations were surveyed prospectively in a cohort of 346 THAs and 323 TKAs. In both groups, improved mobility and a reduction in daytime pain were the most important expectations. Males, younger patients, and poor Oxford scores predicted a higher level of preoperative expectations. THA met the important expectations, whereas TKA fell short in kneeling, squatting, and stair climbing. Satisfaction levels correlated highly with the ability to meet patients' expectations. Level of evidence: III.

54. Sullivan M, Tanzer M, Reardon G, Amirault D, Dunbar M, Stanish W: The role of presurgical expectancies in predicting pain and function one year following total knee arthroplasty. *Pain* 2011;152(10):2287-2293.

This prospective study assessed the value of response expectancies and behavioral outcomes in 120 patients at 12-month follow-up after a primary TKA. Analysis found that pain catastrophizing, pain-related fear of motion, and depression predicted increased pain and reduced function at follow-up. As a result, they suggest that interventions regarding behavioral outcome expectancies and pain might improve postoperative outcomes. Level of evidence: IV.

55. Jämsen E, Nevalainen P, Eskelinen A, Huotari K, Kalliovalkama J, Moilanen T: Obesity, diabetes, and preoperative hyperglycemia as predictors of periprosthetic joint infection: A single-center analysis of 7181 primary hip and knee replacements for osteoarthritis. *J Bone Joint Surg Am* 2012;94(14):e101.

A single-center series of 7,181 primary THAs and TKAs were analyzed to identify periprosthetic infections and correlated with the diagnosis of diabetes from the registers of the Social Insurance Institution of Finland. They found that diabetes (0.37% versus 2.6%), morbid obesity (0.37% versus 4.66%), and a combination of diabetes-morbid obesity (0.37% versus 9.8%) in the same patient increased the risk of infection after both hip and knee replacements. Of note, the type of diabetes did not correlate with the infection rate. Level of evidence: III.

56. Järvenpää J, Kettunen J, Soininvaara T, Miettinen H, Kröger H: Obesity has a negative impact on clinical outcome after total knee arthroplasty. *Scand J Surg* 2012; 101(3):198-203.

The authors divided patients undergoing TKA into obese (BMI > 30), and nonobese (BMI < 30) groups. Patients who were not obese had a better percentage improvement in their KSS, ROM, and physical function. They concluded that obesity had a negative effect on TKA surgery. Level of evidence: III.

57. Mulhall KJ, Ghomrawi HM, Mihalko W, Cui Q, Saleh KJ: Adverse effects of increased body mass index and weight on survivorship of total knee arthroplasty and subsequent outcomes of revision TKA. *J Knee Surg* 2007;20(3):199-204.

58. Mont MA, Mathur SK, Krackow KA, Loewy JW, Hungerford DS: Cementless total knee arthroplasty in obese patients: A comparison with a matched control group. *J Arthroplasty* 1996;11(2):153-156.

59. Iorio R, Williams KM, Marcantonio AJ, Specht LM, Tilzey JF, Healy WL: Diabetes mellitus, hemoglobin A1C, and the incidence of total joint arthroplasty infection. *J Arthroplasty* 2012;27(5):726-729, e1.

A single institution reviewed 4,241 primary or revision hip and knee arthroplasties to assess preoperative HbA1c values. Twelve infections (3.43%) occurred in patients with diabetes and 34 (0.87%) in patients without diabetes. Patients with diabetes and infection had an average HbA1c of 7.2% compared with 6.92% in the noninfected cohort. Although patients with diabetes were found to have a higher rate of complications, the use of HbA1c levels to predict infection is not reliable. Level of evidence: IV.

60. Malinzak RA, Ritter MA, Berend ME, Meding JB, Olberding EM, Davis KE: Morbidly obese, diabetic, younger, and unilateral joint arthroplasty patients have elevated total joint arthroplasty infection rates. *J Arthroplasty* 2009;24(6, suppl):84-88.

61. Mraovic B, Suh D, Jacovides C, Parvizi J: Perioperative hyperglycemia and postoperative infection after lower limb arthroplasty. *J Diabetes Sci Technol* 2011;5(2): 412-418.

An institutional database was evaluated to find two groups of patients after primary THA or TKA. One hundred one patients with infections and 1,847 patients without infections were identified. The percentage of patients with diabetes was 22% and 9% in the infected and noninfected cohorts, respectively. Elevated blood glucose preoperatively and postoperatively increased the risk of infection, with hyperglycemia greater than 200 mg/dL doubling the risk for infection. Overall, diabetes mellitus and postoperative hyperglycema are predictors for prosthetic infection. Level of evidence: IV.

62. Robertson F, Geddes J, Ridley D, McLeod G, Cheng K: Patients with Type 2 diabetes mellitus have a worse functional outcome post knee arthroplasty: A matched cohort study. *Knee* 2012;19(4):286-289.

Matched cohorts of 367 TKAs with and without diabetes were examined at 1, 5, and 10 years postoperatively. Despite a high level of patient satisfaction, the diagnosis of diabetes was associated with a lower maximal flexion angle, total ROM, and KSS at 1 year. By 10 years, a greater degree of fixed flexion was found in the diabetic group. Level of evidence: III.

63. Mont MA, Marker DR, Zywiel MG, Carrino JA: Osteonecrosis of the knee and related conditions. *J Am Acad Orthop Surg* 2011;19(8):482-494.

Osteonecrosis of the knee, including diagnosis, pathophysiology, pathogenesis, and etiology of the three forms of the disease, is comprehensively reviewed. Level of evidence: V.

64. Bruni D, Iacono F, Raspugli G, Zaffagnini S, Marcacci M: Is unicompartmental arthroplasty an accept-

able option for spontaneous osteonecrosis of the knee? *Clin Orthop Relat Res* 2012;470(5):1442-1451.

Eighty-four patients with spontaneous osteonecrosis of the knee were retrospectively reviewed after a medial UKA. The mean follow-up was 98 months, and the 10-year survivorship was reported at 89%. Subsidence and aseptic loosening of the tibia were the most common causes for revision. If isolated to a single condyle, spontaneous osteonecrosis may be an indication for UKA. Level of evidence: IV.

65. Luck JV Jr, Silva M, Rodriguez-Merchan EC, Ghalambor N, Zahiri CA, Finn RS: Hemophilic arthropathy. *J Am Acad Orthop Surg* 2004;12(4):234-245.

66. Zingg PO, Fucentese SF, Lutz W, Brand B, Mamisch N, Koch PP: Haemophilic knee arthropathy: Long-term outcome after total knee replacement. *Knee Surg Sports Traumatol Arthrosc* 2012;Feb:1.

The authors reported on 34 of the possible 43 patients they operated on for hemophilic arthropathy. At a mean follow-up of 9.6 years, 94% reported good or excellent results, and there were two infections and three component revisions. Overall survivorship for infection and component revision was reported to be 90% and 86%, respectively. Level of evidence: IV.

67. Rademakers MV, Kerkhoffs GM, Sierevelt IN, Raaymakers EL, Marti RK: Operative treatment of 109 tibial plateau fractures: Five- to 27-year follow-up results. *J Orthop Trauma* 2007;21(1):5-10.

68. Stevens DG, Beharry R, McKee MD, Waddell JP, Schemitsch EH: The long-term functional outcome of operatively treated tibial plateau fractures. *J Orthop Trauma* 2001;15(5):312-320.

69. Vermeire J, Scheerlinck T: Early primary total knee replacement for complex proximal tibia fractures in elderly and osteoarthritic patients. *Acta Orthop Belg* 2010;76(6):785-793.

Twelve patients with a TKA after a prior complex proximal tibial fracture were retrospectively reviewed. The mean age was 73 years, and all patients were treated within 3 weeks of the injury. Most of the patients (7/11) had an excellent result, and there were no reported revisions. One patient died as a result of unrelated conditions. Level of evidence: IV.

70. Lin WP, Lin J, Horng LC, Chang SM, Jiang CC: Quadriceps-sparing, minimal-incision total knee arthroplasty: A comparative study. *J Arthroplasty* 2009;24(7):1024-1032.

71. Matsumoto T, Muratsu H, Kubo S, et al: Soft tissue balance measurement in minimal incision surgery compared to conventional total knee arthroplasty. *Knee Surg Sports Traumatol Arthrosc* 2011;19(6):880-886.

Fifty TKAs were evenly split between minimally invasive TKA versus conventional TKA to treat varus OA. They found that minimally invasive TKA may lead to ligament imbalance because the component gap was larger in the small incision group. In addition, the varus angle was greater in the minimally invasive group throughout the arc of motion. Level of evidence: III.

72. Boonen B, Schotanus MG, Kort NP: Preliminary experience with the patient-specific templating total knee arthroplasty. *Acta Orthop* 2012;83(4):387-393.

This was a case-control study on the use of patient-specific guides versus traditional intramedullary alignment guides. Surgery time was 10 minutes shorter, and 60 cc less blood loss was found with the patient-specific guides versus intramedullary aligned TKAs. There was an improved overall accuracy of alignment but a high fraction of outliers in the custom guide cohort, stemming the suggestion for a future randomized controlled trial. Level of evidence: III.

73. Meding JB, Berend ME, Ritter MA, Galley MR, Malinzak RA: Intramedullary vs extramedullary femoral alignment guides: A 15-year follow-up of survivorship. *J Arthroplasty* 2011;26(4):591-595.

The results for intramedullary (4,993 TKAs) versus extramedullary (1,733 TKAs) guides for TKA were reviewed, and 15-year survivorship was the same for both techniques. The mean tibiofemoral angle was more accurate with intramedullary (4.6° of valgus) compared with extramedullary (5.1° of valgus) guides. Overall alignment was not as precise with the extramedullary method. Level of evidence: III.

74. Horiuchi H, Akizuki S, Tomita T, Sugamoto K, Yamazaki T, Shimizu N: In vivo kinematic analysis of cruciate-retaining total knee arthroplasty during weight-bearing and non-weight-bearing deep knee bending. *J Arthroplasty* 2012;27(6):1196-1202.

Fluoroscopic imaging was used to assess in vivo knee kinematics of cruciate-retaining TKAs during weight bearing and non–weight-bearing deep knee bending. In the weight-bearing mode, knees displayed bicondylar rollback and a central pivot point. Without the load of a patient's body weight, there was initial anterior motion followed by femoral rollback.

75. Pang HN, Yeo SJ, Chong HC, Chin PL, Ong J, Lo NN: Computer-assisted gap balancing technique improves outcome in total knee arthroplasty, compared with conventional measured resection technique. *Knee Surg Sports Traumatol Arthrosc* 2011;19(9):1496-1503.

This prospective, randomized study assessed the differences between a conventional measured resection technique versus a computer-assisted gap balancing method. The latter group demonstrated significantly better limb alignment, whereas the measured resection technique resulted in a greater number of flexion contractures greater than 5° and anterior tibial translation greater than 5 mm. Overall better functional scores were reported for the computer-assisted gap balancing method, which is thought to be related to more precise soft-tissue balancing and restoration of the natural mechanical axis. Level of evidence: I.

76. Tigani D, Sabbioni G, Ben Ayad R, Filanti M, Rani N, Del Piccolo N: Comparison between two computer-assisted total knee arthroplasty: Gap-balancing versus

measured resection technique. *Knee Surg Sports Traumatol Arthrosc* 2010;18(10):1304-1310.

The two different methods were compared in 126 patients prospectively to examine joint line maintenance, limb alignment, and component position. It was concluded that surgeons should use the method withn which they are most comfortable. However, the measured resection technique resulted in less reduction in the postoperative joint line level. Level of evidence: III.

77. Stoddard JE, Deehan DJ, Bull AM, McCaskie AW, Amis AA: The kinematics and stability of single-radius versus multi-radius femoral components related to mid-range instability after TKA. *J Orthop Res* 2013;31(1):53-58.

An in vitro kinematic analysis of native knees was compared to multi- and single-radius TKA designs. Both knees functioned in a biomechanically similar manner and were inferior compared with the native knee. Anterior laxity was greater, particularly with the knee moving toward extension, but there were no differences beyond 30° of flexion. The authors concluded that mid-range instability may be related to unrecognized ligamentous laxity intraoperatively, not the component design.

78. Luyckx T, Peeters T, Vandenneucker H, Victor J, Bellemans J: Is adapted measured resection superior to gap-balancing in determining femoral component rotation in total knee replacement? *J Bone Joint Surg Br* 2012;94-B(9):1271-1276.

This prospective study compared gap-balancing (n = 48) versus measured resection (n = 48) in regard to component alignment and rotation in 96 TKAs. External rotation of the femoral component was similar between the two groups based on the transepicondylar axis. There was a nonsignificant trend toward slight greater external rotation in the gap-balancing method, 2.4° versus 1.7°. Level of evidence: III.

79. Chon JG, Sun DH, Jung JY, Kim TI, Jang SW: Rotational alignment of femoral component for minimal medial collateral ligament release in total knee arthroplasty. *Knee Surg Relat Res* 2011;23(3):153-158.

Seventy-two TKAs with a minimal MCL release were compared to 61 knees without OA using a CT scan of the knee in 90° of flexion. The authors found that the average rotation angle of the femoral component in conjunction with a minimal medial release was external rotation of 5.6° from the posterior condylar axis and 2° from the Whiteside line. The smaller the femoral component, the greater the need for more external rotation than average; the opposite held true for larger implants to create an ideal rectangular flexion gap. Level of evidence: III.

80. Wraighte PJ, Sikand M, Livesley PJ: Intra- and inter-observer variation during femoral jig rotational alignment in knee arthroplasty. *Arch Orthop Trauma Surg* 2011;131(9):1283-1286.

Eight surgeons determined external rotation of the femur on six cadaver femoral bone casts using the epicondylar axis and the posterior femoral condyles. This was compared to the Whiteside line, and they found no significant differences between the referencing techniques.

81. Abdel MP, Morrey ME, Jensen MR, Morrey BF: Increased long-term survival of posterior cruciate-retaining versus posterior cruciate-stabilizing total knee replacements. *J Bone Joint Surg Am* 2011;93(22):2072-2078.

A retrospective, single-center database review was conducted to compare the long-term survivorship of CR versus PS TKAs. There were 8,117 TKAS (5,389 CR and 2,728 PS) identified over a 10-year period. The overall survivorship at 15 years was 90% for CR TKAs versus 77% for PS TKAs. This difference was retained even after adjusting for age, sex, preoperative diagnosis, and initial deformity. Level of evidence: IV.

82. Kolisek FR, McGrath MS, Marker DR, et al: Posterior-stabilized versus posterior cruciate ligament-retaining total knee arthroplasty. *Iowa Orthop J* 2009;29:23-27.

83. Chaudhary R, Beaupré LA, Johnston DW: Knee range of motion during the first two years after use of posterior cruciate-stabilizing or posterior cruciate-retaining total knee prostheses: A randomized clinical trial. *J Bone Joint Surg Am* 2008;90(12):2579-2586.

84. Kim YH, Choi Y, Kim JS: Range of motion of standard and high-flexion posterior cruciate-retaining total knee prostheses: A prospective randomized study. *J Bone Joint Surg Am* 2009;91(8):1874-1881.

85. Hanson GR, Suggs JF, Kwon YM, Freiberg AA, Li G: In vivo anterior tibial post contact after posterior stabilizing total knee arthroplasty. *J Orthop Res* 2007;25(11):1447-1453.

86. Clarke HD, Math KR, Scuderi GR: Polyethylene post failure in posterior stabilized total knee arthroplasty. *J Arthroplasty* 2004;19(5):652-657.

87. Stoller AP, Johnson TS, Popoola OO, Humphrey SM, Blanchard CR: Highly crosslinked polyethylene in posterior-stabilized total knee arthroplasty: In vitro performance evaluation of wear, delamination, and tibial post durability. *J Arthroplasty* 2011;26(3):483-491.

Tibial post durability was tested in this knee simulator study in both standard and highly cross-linked polyethylene. Wear volume was reduced by 67% to 75% for aged highly cross-linked polyethylene compared with aged standard polyethylene. Tibial post durability was reportedly better in the cross-linked group compared with the traditional polyethylene group.

88. Berry TR, Witcher C, Holt NL, Plotnikoff RC: A qualitative examination of perceptions of physical activity guidelines and preferences for format. *Health Promot Pract* 2010;11(6):908-916.

This is a descriptive study of data collected from 22 patients in five focus groups. The authors found that there was little awareness among the participants of Canada's Physical Activity Guide, and the current format they were using was unappealing.

89. Harwin SF, Kester MA, Malkani AL, Manley MT: Excellent fixation achieved with cementless posteriorly stabilized total knee arthroplasty. *J Arthroplasty* 2013; 28(1):7-13.

A consecutive series of 114 cementless TKAs performed with single-radius PS components was evaluated at a mean of 36 months after surgery. No evidence of stress shielding, osteolysis, or loosening was noted in this cohort. Level of evidence: IV.

90. Park JW, Kim YH: Simultaneous cemented and cementless total knee replacement in the same patients: A prospective comparison of long-term outcomes using an identical design of NexGen prosthesis. *J Bone Joint Surg Br* 2011;93-B(11):1479-1486.

A prospective, randomized trial compared identical cemented and cementless TKA prostheses. Bilateral TKAs were performed in 50 patients (100 knees), with one side cemented and the other cementless, with a mean follow-up of 13.6 years. Radiologic parameters, ROM, and satisfaction were similar in both groups. Survivorship was 100% for the femoral components and 100% versus 98% for the cemented and cementless tibias, respectively. Level of evidence: I.

91. Hofmann AA, Evanich JD, Ferguson RP, Camargo MP: Ten- to 14-year clinical followup of the cementless Natural Knee system. *Clin Orthop Relat Res* 2001;388: 85-94.

92. Gioe TJ, Sinner P, Mehle S, Ma W, Killeen KK: Excellent survival of all-polyethylene tibial components in a community joint registry. *Clin Orthop Relat Res* 2007; 464:88-92.

93. Kamath AF, Lee GC, Sheth NP, Nelson CL, Garino JP, Israelite CL: Prospective results of uncemented tantalum monoblock tibia in total knee arthroplasty: Minimum 5-year follow-up in patients younger than 55 years. *J Arthroplasty* 2011;26(8):1390-1395.

A comparison study between 100 cementless monoblock tantalum tibial components and 312 cemented controls was performed in patients younger than 55 years. A PS TKA was performed, and no difference was found in blood loss, complication rates, or cost. At a minimum of 5 years, porous tantalum components performed well with a shorter surgical time. Level of evidence: III.

94. Unger AS, Duggan JP: Midterm results of a porous tantalum monoblock tibia component: Clinical and radiographic results of 108 knees. *J Arthroplasty* 2011;26(6): 855-860.

At an average of 4.5-year follow-up, 108 monoblock tantalum tibial components were evaluated, with 105 excellent and 3 poor results. No tibial revisions or osteolysis was reported. Level of evidence: IV.

95. Callaghan JJ, Wells CW, Liu SS, Goetz DD, Johnston RC: Cemented rotating-platform total knee replacement: A concise follow-up, at a minimum of twenty years, of a previous report. *J Bone Joint Surg Am* 2010; 92(7):1635-1639.

This study is a follow-up of a previous cohort with 20-year follow-up. Twenty patients were alive from the original 119-person cohort. No revisions were performed since the 15-year follow-up report. Osteolysis was found and increased with longer duration of the implants despite excellent long-term results. Level of evidence: IV.

96. Kim YH, Kim JS, Choe JW, Kim HJ: Long-term comparison of fixed-bearing and mobile-bearing total knee replacements in patients younger than fifty-one years of age with osteoarthritis. *J Bone Joint Surg Am* 2012; 94(10):866-873.

One hundred eight patients were prospectively enrolled to receive a fixed-bearing and a mobile-bearing TKA as part of a bilateral TKA procedure. At mean of 16. 8-year follow-up, there were no differences in ROM and Knee Society clinical or functional scores. Survivorship was reported as 95% in the fixed-bearing knees and 97% for the mobile-bearing devices. Level of evidence:II.

97. Burnett RS, Haydon CM, Rorabeck CH, Bourne RB: Patella resurfacing versus nonresurfacing in total knee arthroplasty: Results of a randomized controlled clinical trial at a minimum of 10 years' followup. *Clin Orthop Relat Res* 2004;428:12-25.

98. Waters TS, Bentley G: Patellar resurfacing in total knee arthroplasty: A prospective, randomized study. *J Bone Joint Surg Am* 2003;85(2):212-217.

99. Garcia RM, Kraay MJ, Goldberg VM: Isolated resurfacing of the previously unresurfaced patella total knee arthroplasty. *J Arthroplasty* 2010;25(5):754-758.

Seventeen patellar resurfacing procedures were performed, and outcomes followed as part of a revision TKA. No further revisions were performed at 47-month follow-up. Forty-seven percent of patients were still symptomatic and 53% were asymptomatic. Surgery was well tolerated, but the results were not as good as expected. Level of evidence: IV.

100. Correia J, Sieder M, Kendoff D, et al: Secondary patellar resurfacing after primary bicondylar knee arthroplasty did not meet patients' expectations. *Open Orthop J* 2012;6:414-418.

Forty-six patients were evaluated with a secondary resurfacing of the patella after TKA. About one half of the patients had no resolution of their symptoms, and an improvement in ROM was found in 56.5% of the patients. Level of evidence: IV.

101. Zywiel MG, Daley JA, Delanois RE, Naziri Q, Johnson AJ, Mont MA: Advance pre-operative chlorhexidine reduces the incidence of surgical site infections in knee arthroplasty. *Int Orthop* 2011;35(7):1001-1006.

The use of an advance cutaneous disinfection protocol was evaluated to assess the effect on the overall number of deep infections. A chlorhexidene gluconate-impregnated cloth was used the night before and the morning of surgery to disinfect the surgical site. The protocol was correctly followed in 15% of 912 TKAs with a lower incidence of infection (0% versus 3%) found in those completing the preoperative surgical washes. Level of evidence: IV.

4: Lower Extremity

102. Rao N, Cannella BA, Crossett LS, Yates AJ Jr, McGough RL III, Hamilton CW: Preoperative screening/decolonization for Staphylococcus aureus to prevent orthopedic surgical site infection: Prospective cohort study with 2-year follow-up. *J Arthroplasty* 2011;26(8):1501-1507.

Preoperative screening and subsequent selective decolonization was assessed at 2-year follow-up. There were 2,284 controls, and the authors found 25% of 1,285 patients were nasal carriers for *Staphylococcus aureus*. Overall surgical site infection rates reduced from 3.7% to 1.2% when screening and selective intervention protocols were followed. Level of evidence: II.

103. Prokuski L: Prophylactic antibiotics in orthopaedic surgery. *J Am Acad Orthop Surg* 2008;16(5):283-293.

104. Garvin KL, Konigsberg BS: Infection following total knee arthroplasty: Prevention and management. *J Bone Joint Surg Am* 2011;93(12):1167-1175.

The principles of prevention and management of prosthetic infection following TKA were reviewed. Level of evidence: V.

105. Parvizi J, Della Valle CJ: AAOS clinical practice guideline: Diagnosis and treatment of periprosthetic joint infections of the hip and knee. *J Am Acad Orthop Surg* 2010;18(12):771-772.

Clinical practice guidelines were developed for the diagnosis and the treatment of periprosthetic joint infections in the hip and the knee. Level of evidence: III.

106. Mont MA, Jacobs JJ: AAOS clinical practice guideline: Preventing venous thromboembolic disease in patients undergoing elective hip and knee arthroplasty. *J Am Acad Orthop Surg* 2011;19(12):777-778.

AAOS guidelines for clinical practice are reviewed in regard to venous thromboembolism prophylaxis in elective THA and TKA. Level of evidence: III.

107. Kakkos SK, Warwick D, Nicolaides AN, Stansby GP, Tsolakis IA: Combined (mechanical and pharmacological) modalities for the prevention of venous thromboembolism in joint replacement surgery. *J Bone Joint Surg Br* 2012;94(6):729-734.

A meta-analysis of six studies including 1,399 patients was conducted to assess the efficacy of mechanical compression and pharmacologic thromboprophylaxis. DVT rates were reduced from 18.7% to 3.7% with anticoagulation alone in TKA. In THA, there was a non-significant reduction in DVT with mechanical compression alone and a significant difference with anticoagulation and mechanical compression. Combined modalities are currently recommended by the authors. Level of evidence: II.

108. Lee GC, Lotke PA: Management of intraoperative medial collateral ligament injury during TKA. *Clin Orthop Relat Res* 2011;469(1):64-68.

A retrospective review of 1,650 primary TKAs was performed to find iatrogenic MCL injuries. Thirty-seven (2.2%) were found to have intraoperative injury to the MCL. In 14, the MCL was repaired; in 30, in-creased prosthetic constraint was used. At an average follow-up of 54 months, there was good success in the patients treated with increased constraint (Knee Society function and pain scores increased to 83 and 88, respectively). Level of evidence: IV.

109. Leopold SS, McStay C, Klafeta K, Jacobs JJ, Berger RA, Rosenberg AG: Primary repair of intraoperative disruption of the medial collateral ligament during total knee arthroplasty. *J Bone Joint Surg Am* 2001; 83(1):86-91.

110. Stephens S, Politi J, Backes J, Czaplicki T: Repair of medial collateral ligament injury during total knee arthoplasty. *Orthopedics* 2012;35(2):e154-e159.

A series of patients with an intraoperative rupture of the MCL treated with direct repair and no change in implant constraint or postoperative protocols was reviewed over a 5-year period. The average BMI was 43.3, and all nine patients were satisfied with the procedure. Outcomes showed average Knee Society pain scores of 91.5 and functional scores of 73.3. Level of evidence: IV.

111. Springer BD, Della Valle CJ: Extensor mechanism allograft reconstruction after total knee arthroplasty. *J Arthroplasty* 2008;23(7, suppl):35-38.

112. Malhotra R, Garg B, Logani V, Bhan S: Management of extensor mechanism deficit as a consequence of patellar tendon loss in total knee arthroplasty: A new surgical technique. *J Arthroplasty* 2008;23(8):1146-1151.

113. Browne JA, Hanssen AD: Reconstruction of patellar tendon disruption after total knee arthroplasty: Results of a new technique utilizing synthetic mesh. *J Bone Joint Surg Am* 2011;93(12):1137-1143.

Thirteen consecutive patients with extensor mechanism reconstruction using a knitted monofilament polypropylene graft were retrospectively reviewed. At a mean of 42 months follow-up, there were three failures and one with infection and subsequent arthrodesis. The other nine had an extensor lag less than 10° and a mean flexion of 103°. The mesh is significantly less expensive than a complete extensor mechanism allograft. Level of evidence: IV.

114. Hartman CW, Ting NT, Moric M, Berger RA, Rosenberg AG, Della Valle CJ: Revision total knee arthroplasty for stiffness. *J Arthroplasty* 2010;25(6, suppl): 62-66.

Thirty-five patients who underwent revision TKA for knee stiffness were retrospectively reviewed. The authors found, at a mean of 54.5 months, the mean arc of motion improved by 44.5°.However, 49% required further intervention for stiffness or sustained a complication. Revision can lead to reasonable improvement but at the cost of a significant complication rate. Level of evidence: IV.

115. Mont MA, Dellon AL, Chen F, Hungerford MW, Krackow KA, Hungerford DS: The operative treatment of peroneal nerve palsy. *J Bone Joint Surg Am* 1996;78(6):863-869.

116. Pal A, Clarke JM, Cameron AE: Case series and literature review: Popliteal artery injury following total knee replacement. *Int J Surg* 2010;8(6):430-435.

Popliteal injury after TKA was reviewed in a nine-patient case series. The authors found three intraoperative hemorrhages, two arterial thrombi, three pseudo-aneurysms, and one arteriovenous fistula. They concluded that the incidence has remained steady with this complication, and ongoing awareness and early diagnosis are crucial in recognizing this complication. Level of evidence: IV.

117. Healy WL, Siliski JM, Incavo SJ: Operative treatment of distal femoral fractures proximal to total knee replacements. *J Bone Joint Surg Am* 1993;75(1):27-34.

118. Ritter MA, Faris PM, Keating EM: Anterior femoral notching and ipsilateral supracondylar femur fracture in total knee arthroplasty. *J Arthroplasty* 1988;3(2):185-187.

119. Figgie MP, Goldberg VM, Figgie HE III, Sobel M: The results of treatment of supracondylar fracture above total knee arthroplasty. *J Arthroplasty* 1990;5(3):267-276.

120. Felix NA, Stuart MJ, Hanssen AD: Periprosthetic fractures of the tibia associated with total knee arthroplasty. *Clin Orthop Relat Res* 1997;345:113-124.

121. Ortiguera CJ, Berry DJ: Patellar fracture after total knee arthroplasty. *J Bone Joint Surg Am* 2002;84(4):532-540.

122. Grace JN, Sim FH: Fracture of the patella after total knee arthroplasty. *Clin Orthop Relat Res* 1988;230:168-175.

123. Wang CJ, Wang JW, Ko JY, Weng LH, Huang CC: Three-year changes in bone mineral density around the knee after a six-month course of oral alendronate following total knee arthroplasty: A prospective, randomized study. *J Bone Joint Surg Am* 2006;88(2):267-272.

124. Kim KI, Egol KA, Hozack WJ, Parvizi J: Periprosthetic fractures after total knee arthroplasties. *Clin Orthop Relat Res* 2006;446:167-175.

125. Stuart MJ, Hanssen AD: Total knee arthroplasty: Periprosthetic tibial fractures. *Orthop Clin North Am* 1999;30(2):279-286.

126. Bong MR, Egol KA, Koval KJ, et al: Comparison of the LISS and a retrograde-inserted supracondylar intramedullary nail for fixation of a periprosthetic distal femur fracture proximal to a total knee arthroplasty. *J Arthroplasty* 2002;17(7):876-881.

127. Chettiar K, Jackson MP, Brewin J, Dass D, Butler-Manuel PA: Supracondylar periprosthetic femoral fractures following total knee arthroplasty: Treatment with a retrograde intramedullary nail. *Int Orthop* 2009;33(4):981-985.

128. Nauth A, Ristevski B, Bégué T, Schemitsch EH: Periprosthetic distal femur fractures: Current concepts. *J Orthop Trauma* 2011;25(suppl 2):S82-S85.

Treatment options for periprosthetic distal femoral fractures, with particular attention focused on displaced fractures with stable implants, were comprehensively reviewed. Level of evidence: V.

129. Kolb W, Guhlmann H, Windisch C, Marx F, Koller H, Kolb K: Fixation of periprosthetic femur fractures above total knee arthroplasty with the less invasive stabilization system: A midterm follow-up study. *J Trauma* 2010;69(3):670-676.

A consecutive series of 23 patients treated with a LISS plate for a periprosthetic femoral fracture about a TKA was retrospectively reviewed. Nineteen patients were available for follow-up at 46 months. All fractures healed at 14 weeks, and no bone graft was required. One patient had 7° of varus, and the mean knee ROM was 102°. There were no nonunions or infections. Level of evidence: IV.

130. Streubel PN, Gardner MJ, Morshed S, Collinge CA, Gallagher B, Ricci WM: Are extreme distal periprosthetic supracondylar fractures of the femur too distal to fix using a lateral locked plate? *J Bone Joint Surg Br* 2010;92-B(4):527-534.

A retrospective, multicenter study involving 89 patients with lateral locked plating of a supracondylar femoral fracture is presented. Of 61 patients available for follow-up, there were two patient groups: those with fractures located proximally (28) and those with fractures that extended distal to the proximal border of the femoral component (33). The authors found similar results between the two types of fractures treated with the same lateral plating technique. Level of evidence: IV.

131. Bobak P, Polyzois I, Graham S, Gamie Z, Tsiridis E: Nailed cementoplasty: A salvage technique for Rorabeck type II periprosthetic fractures in octogenarians. *J Arthroplasty* 2010;25(6):939-944.

Five patients were treated with retrograde nailing augmented with PMMA and followed for a median of 12 months. All patients had an uncomplicated recovery and return to their preinjury level of function within 4 months. This cementoplasty technique is an adequate salvage procedure in octogenarians who cannot withstand a lengthy surgical procedure. Level of evidence: IV.

132. Berend KR, Lombardi AV Jr: Distal femoral replacement in nontumor cases with severe bone loss and instability. *Clin Orthop Relat Res* 2009;467(2):485-492.

133. Rand JA, Coventry MB: Stress fractures after total knee arthroplasty. *J Bone Joint Surg Am* 1980;62(2):226-233.

134. Parvizi J, Kim KI, Oliashirazi A, Ong A, Sharkey PF: Periprosthetic patellar fractures. *Clin Orthop Relat Res* 2006;446:161-166.

135. Sheth NP, Pedowitz DI, Lonner JH: Periprosthetic patellar fractures. *J Bone Joint Surg Am* 2007;89(10): 2285-2296.

136. Della Valle CJ, Haidukewych GJ, Callaghan JJ: Periprosthetic fractures of the hip and knee: A problem on the rise but better solutions. *Instr Course Lect* 2010;59:563-575.

   The principles of treatment of periprosthetic fractures about THA and TKA components are discussed in a review article. Level of evidence: V.

137. Nelson CL, Lonner JH, Lahiji A, Kim J, Lotke PA: Use of a trabecular metal patella for marked patella bone loss during revision total knee arthroplasty. *J Arthroplasty* 2003;18(7, suppl 1):37-41.

138. Mamczak CN, Gardner MJ, Bolhofner B, Borrelli J Jr, Streubel PN, Ricci WM: Interprosthetic femoral fractures. *J Orthop Trauma* 2010;24(12):740-744.

   Twenty-six interprosthetic femoral fractures were retrospectively reviewed. Six fractures were excluded for lack of appropriate follow-up. The remaining 20 fractures all healed with an average time to weight bearing as tolerated of 13 weeks. There were three malunions and two cases of painful implants. It is important to span the entire interprosthetic zone to eliminate additional stress risers. Level of evidence: IV.

139. Della Valle C, Parvizi J, Bauer TW, et al: Diagnosis of periprosthetic joint infections of the hip and knee. *J Am Acad Orthop Surg* 2010;18(12):760-770. An AAOS workgroup evaluated the available literature to determine the utility of diagnostic modalities for determining periprosthetic infection in hips and knees. They found that 10 of the 15 recommendations have strong or moderate evidence to support their use. Level of evidence: III.

140. Engh GA, Ammeen DJ: Bone loss with revision total knee arthroplasty: Defect classification and alternatives for reconstruction. *Instr Course Lect* 1999;48: 167-175.

141. Baker RP, Masri BA, Greidanus NV, Garbuz DS: Outcome after isolated polyethylene tibial insert exchange in revision total knee arthroplasty. *J Arthroplasty* 2013;28(1):1-6.

   Forty-five knees that had an isolated tibial insert exchange for a failed TKA with a minimum of two years of follow-up were retrospectively reviewed. Nine percent of these knees required a subsequent revision. It was concluded that appropriately selected patients can do well after an isolated liner exchange. Level of evidence: IV.

142. Babis GC, Trousdale RT, Morrey BF: The effectiveness of isolated tibial insert exchange in revision total knee arthroplasty. *J Bone Joint Surg Am* 2002;84(1):64-68.

143. Engh CA Jr, Parks NL, Engh GA: Polyethylene quality affects revision knee liner exchange survivorship. *Clin Orthop Relat Res* 2012;470(1):193-198.

   This is a retrospective evaluation of 135 TKAs in which peri-implant osteolysis was thought to have contributed to the need for revision. At a mean follow-up of 6.2 years, 15 patients were lost to follow-up. Five-year survivorship was similar for those who underwent an isolated polyethylene change, a single component revision, or a full revision in the setting of well-placed and appropriately aligned implants. Level of evidence: IV.

144. Pietsch M, Hofmann S: Early revision for isolated internal malrotation of the femoral component in total knee arthroplasty. *Knee Surg Sports Traumatol Arthrosc* 2012;20(6):1057-1063.

   A prospective study including 72 patients screened with a CT scan found that 14 had isolated internal rotation of the femoral component. These 14 underwent revision surgery within 3 years of the index procedure and were followed for a mean of 57 months. The authors completed revision surgery with a condylar constrained implant and PS polyethylene with good success. They concluded that correction of isolated internal malroation of greater than or equal to 4° improves patient outcomes. Level of evidence: IV.

145. Patil N, Lee K, Huddleston JI, Harris AH, Goodman SB: Patellar management in revision total knee arthroplasty: Is patellar resurfacing a better option? *J Arthroplasty* 2010;25(4):589-593.

   Patients undergoing patellar resurfacing (13), retention of the patellar component (22), or patelloplasty (11) at the time of revision TKA were prospectively evaluated. There were no differences among the groups, and it was concluded that individualized care results in successful outcomes. Level of evidence: III.

146. Maheshwari AV, Tsailas PG, Ranawat AS, Ranawat CS: How to address the patella in revision total knee arthroplasty. *Knee* 2009;16(2):92-97.

147. Haidukewych GJ, Hanssen A, Jones RD: Metaphyseal fixation in revision total knee arthroplasty: Indications and techniques. *J Am Acad Orthop Surg* 2011;19(6): 311-318.

   The authors present indications and technique and describe the use of various options for obtaining metaphyseal in revision TKA. Level of evidence: V.

148. Rossi R, Bonasia DE, Amendola A: The role of high tibial osteotomy in the varus knee. *J Am Acad Orthop Surg* 2011;19(10):590-599.

   The technique, clinical indications, and results regarding HTO of the varus knee are reviewed in full detail. Level of evidence: V.

Chapter 42

Tibial Shaft Fractures

Gillian Soles, MD   Philip Wolinsky, MD

Introduction

Fractures of the tibial shaft are common, with a reported annual incidence in the United Sates of 492,000 fractures.[1] Males are more commonly affected than females, and the highest incidence occurs in young men 15 to 19 years of age.[2] There is a bimodal distribution of these fractures, and the second peak occurs for men and women older than 80 years and is attributed to osteoporosis.[2]

The evaluation of a patient with a tibial shaft fracture includes a clinical and radiographic examination to identify any associated injuries. The initial evaluation begins with airway, breathing, and circulation (ABCs), as well as a primary survey of the patient. The history will identify the mechanism of injury. Most fractures occur as a result of motor vehicle crashes, direct blows, falls, sports injuries, and gunshot injuries. The physical examination will demonstrate pain, swelling, and deformity of the affected limb. A thorough circumferential examination of the limb must be performed to look for abrasions and/or open wounds; a careful neurovascular examination should also be performed. The radiographic evaluation should include AP and lateral views of the knee; full-length AP and lateral views of the tibia and the fibula; and AP, lateral, and mortise views of the ankle. Fractures with potential intra-articular extension of proximal or distal fracture lines and those with ipsilateral tibial plateau and ankle fractures require CT to clearly delineate the extent of injury. Following the initial clinical and radiographic workup, treatment options can be formulated.

Dr. Wolinsky or an immediate family member is a member of a speakers' bureau or has made paid presentations on behalf of Zimmer; serves as a paid consultant to or is an employee of Biomet and Zimmer; and serves as a board member, owner, officer, or committee member of the Orthopaedic Trauma Association, the American Academy of Orthopaedic Surgeons, and the American Orthopaedic Association. Neither Dr. Soles nor any immediate family member has received anything of value from or has stock or stock options held in a commercial company or institution related directly or indirectly to the subject of this chapter.

Compartment Syndrome

The most common cause of compartment syndrome is a fracture of the tibial diaphysis.[3] A careful clinical examination should be performed for all patients with tibial shaft fractures to check for the presence of compartment syndrome; these patients should also be monitored closely to ensure that compartment syndrome does not develop. There are currently no tests available to directly measure ischemia of the involved tissues. The clinical signs of compartment syndrome are pain out of proportion to the injury (frequently pain that is initially well controlled and then escalates), pain with passive stretch of the muscles in the involved compartment, and paresthesias.[4] These symptoms are early clinical signs of tissue ischemia and present before irreversible tissue damage that may result in paralysis, pallor, and pulselessness. In an awake, alert patient, the diagnosis of compartment syndrome is made based on clinical signs and symptoms.

For patients who are unable to communicate or cooperate with a clinical examination, including those who are obtunded, sedated, or intubated, intracompartmental pressures can be measured. The diagnosis of compartment syndrome is made when the intracompartmental pressure rises to within 30 mm Hg of the diastolic blood pressure, representing a delta P (diastolic blood pressure – compartment pressure) less than 30 mm Hg.[4] One study reported on 164 patients with acute compartment syndrome, 36% of which occurred after a closed tibial diaphyseal fracture.[3] Most of these patients were young males, with an average age of 30 years. The diagnosis was made clinically or by using compartment pressure monitoring with a differential of less than 30 mm Hg between tissue pressures and the diastolic blood pressure, prompting an emergent fasciotomy. It is now generally accepted that a delta P of less than 30 mm Hg is indicative of acute compartment syndrome and inadequate tissue perfusion.[4]

Another study demonstrated that the intraoperative diastolic blood pressure is significantly lower (on average, 18 mm Hg) than the preoperative or postoperative diastolic blood pressure, and the preoperative diastolic blood pressure is a good indicator of what the postoperative diastolic pressure will be.[5] The authors caution that using intraoperative blood pressures to calculate the delta P may be misleading. They recommend using the preoperative diastolic blood pressure to calculate the delta P intraoperatively.

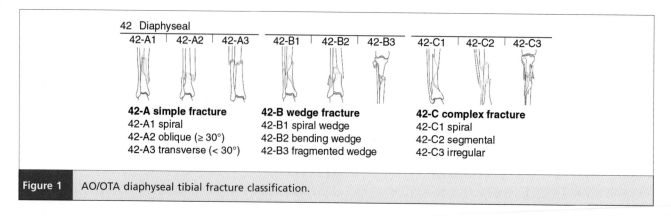

42 Diaphyseal

| 42-A1 | 42-A2 | 42-A3 | 42-B1 | 42-B2 | 42-B3 | 42-C1 | 42-C2 | 42-C3 |

42-A simple fracture
42-A1 spiral
42-A2 oblique (≥ 30°)
42-A3 transverse (< 30°)

42-B wedge fracture
42-B1 spiral wedge
42-B2 bending wedge
42-B3 fragmented wedge

42-C complex fracture
42-C1 spiral
42-C2 segmental
42-C3 irregular

Figure 1 AO/OTA diaphyseal tibial fracture classification.

Table 1

Tscherne Classification

Fracture Grade	Characteristics
0	Minimal soft-tissue injury; typically associated with a simple fracture pattern secondary to an indirect force
1	Superficial abrasions or contusions apparent; may range from a mild to moderately severe fracture pattern
2	Include deep contaminated abrasions associated with localized skin or muscle contusions; severe fracture pattern and impending compartment syndrome
3	Extensive skin contusions or crush with significant underlying muscle damage, compartment syndrome, and severe fracture pattern

(Adapted from Crist BD, Banerjee R: Tibial shaft fractures, in Flynn JM, ed: *Orthopaedic Knowledge Update*, ed 10. Rosemont, IL, American Academy of Orthopaedic Surgeons, 2011, pp 479-491.)

A recent study found that the costs of acute compartment syndrome are substantial, including increases in the length of stay and hospital charges.[6] A cohort of 46 patients with isolated tibial shaft fractures was retrospectively reviewed. Acute compartment syndrome that required a fasciotomy and one to two additional surgeries developed in five patients with closed fractures. Of the remaining 41 patients, 12 had an open fracture and 29 had closed fractures. Patients with medical comorbidities or social issues that could have led to an increased length of stay and/or increased costs were excluded. The authors found that the mean hospital length of stay for the 41 patients without compartment syndrome was 3 days compared with 9 days for the 5 patients with compartment syndrome. The hospital charges were also substantially increased, from $23,800 for the patients without compartment syndrome to $49,700 for the patients with compartment syndrome.

Although it is known that patients with closed diaphyseal tibial fractures that result from a high-energy mechanism of injury are at risk for the development of compartment syndrome, recent data indicate that patients who sustain low-energy tibial fractures during an athletic competition also are at an increased risk for the development of acute compartment syndrome. A retrospective review of 626 consecutive tibial fractures reported a 5.4% incidence of compartment syndrome. It is important to note that patients who sustained tibia fractures while participating in sports such as soccer or football accounted for 25% of the total cases of compartment syndrome despite representing only 3.1% of the total fractures.[7] The authors recommended close monitoring and a high clinical suspicion for compartment syndrome for tibial fractures sustained during athletic competition.

After a patient receives a diagnosis of compartment syndrome, an emergent four-compartment fasciotomy is performed. The complications of missed compartment syndrome, including infections, contractures, and amputation, can be devastating.

Classifications

Tibial shaft fractures are classified descriptively and by the comprehensive AO/Orthopaedic Trauma Association (OTA) system; the associated soft-tissue injuries for closed and open fractures also can be classified. The AO/OTA classification designates tibial diaphyseal fractures by the number 42, with types, groups, and subgroups based on fracture characteristics, the presence or absence of an associated fibular fracture, and whether it is at the same or a different level of the tibial fracture (**Figure 1**). The Tscherne classification[8,9] is used to quantify the extent of soft-tissue injury in closed fractures (**Table 1**), whereas the Gustilo and Anderson classification[10,11] is applied to open fractures (**Table 2**).

Table 2

Gustilo and Anderson Classification

Fracture Type	Characteristics
I	Wounds less than 1 cm; minimal contamination and soft-tissue injury; simple fracture pattern
II	Wounds 1 to 10 cm; moderate comminution and contamination
IIIA	Minimal periosteal stripping and soft-tissue coverage required
IIIB	Significant periosteal stripping at the fracture site; soft-tissue coverage required
IIIC	Indicates an associated repairable vascular injury

(Reproduced from Crist BD, Banerjee R: Tibial shaft fractures, in Flynn JM, ed: *Orthopaedic Knowledge Update*, ed 10. Rosemont, IL, American Academy of Orthopaedic Surgeons, 2011, pp 479-491.)

Treatment Options

Tibial shaft fractures can be treated with nonsurgical or surgical management, and complications occur regardless of the treatment method. Nonsurgical treatment consists of closed reduction followed by casting and then functional bracing with early weight bearing. Surgical treatment options include external fixation, intramedullary nailing, and open reduction and internal fixation (ORIF).

Nonsurgical Treatment

The indications and contraindications for nonsurgical treatment are not universally agreed upon. In general, nonsurgical treatment is indicated for low-energy, nondisplaced or minimally displaced stable fracture patterns or for patients with multiple medical comorbidities and/or low functional demands. The contraindications to closed treatment include the inability to obtain or maintain a closed reduction within acceptable parameters, high-energy or unstable fracture patterns, associated moderate to severe soft-tissue injuries, open fractures, compartment syndrome, an ipsilateral femoral fracture (floating knee), or a vascular and/or nerve injury that requires repair. An intact fibula is a relative contraindication secondary to the increased risk of developing a varus angular deformity. The complications of nonsurgical treatment include a higher risk of nonunion, malunion, and hindfoot stiffness.

Functional bracing of tibial fractures is an effective nonsurgical treatment method that involves casting followed by early functional bracing with weight bearing. Therefore, it is effective only for more stable fracture patterns. The initial management is a closed reduction and placement into a long leg (toe to groin) cast for 2 to 6 weeks, followed by transition to a patellar tendon-bearing cast or a functional brace. Small corrections to alignment and rotation can be performed at the time of recasting or bracing; however, it is recommended that satisfactory length, alignment, and rotation be achieved at the time of the initial closed reduction and manipulation. The patient is encouraged to begin progressive weight bearing as tolerated while the brace is worn, except in cases with proximal or distal intra-articular fracture extension. By 6 weeks, the leg is placed in a functional brace, and full mobility of the knee and the ankle and unrestricted weight bearing are allowed. The brace can be removed when radiographs demonstrate bridging callus across the fracture site.

The results of nonsurgical management using functional bracing have shown the best results when used for low-energy, axially stable, closed, diaphyseal tibial fractures with acceptable initial length, alignment, and rotation. Acceptable alignment is defined as less than 5° of varus or valgus angulation, less than 10° of sagittal plane angulation, greater than 50% cortical apposition, less than 1cm of shortening, and less than 10° to 15° of rotational malalignment.[12]

The largest series of nonsurgical treatment of tibial shaft fractures enrolled 1,000 consecutive closed diaphyseal tibial fractures.[13] Patients were selected for functional bracing if they had axially stable fracture patterns and more than 15 mm of initial shortening. Initial management was closed reduction and placement in a long leg cast followed by application of a functional brace at an average of 3.7 weeks. Clinical and radiographic follow-up was performed at 1-month intervals until healing occurred, which was defined as the absence of pain or motion at the fracture site with pain-free weight bearing and evidence of bridging callus on radiographs. Shortening at healing ranged from 0 to 25 mm; 95% of the patients healed with less than 12 mm of shortening. One third of the patients healed with no frontal plane angulation. Of the remaining two thirds of the patients, 48% healed in varus ranging from 1° to 30°, and 95% healed with less than or equal to 8° of varus. Nineteen percent healed in valgus that ranged from 0° to 12°; 95% healed with less than or equal to 5°. Forty-one percent of the patients healed without any sagittal plane angulation. Procurvatum was observed in 29% of the patients, with a range of 0° to 20°, and 95% healed with less than or equal to 6°. Recurvatum was observed in 30% of the patients, with a range of 0° to 12°, and 95% healed with less than or equal to 7° of deformity. Healing was reported at an average of 18.1 weeks, and the rate of nonunion was 1.1%.

No comparative studies on nonsurgical treatment versus intramedullary nailing or ORIF have been recently published. Older published data[14,15] demonstrated that surgical treatment with an intramedullary nail or ORIF had a more rapid time to union, improved functional results, and less angular deformity or shortening compared with nonsurgical treatment.

Surgical Treatment

External Fixation

External fixation is currently used for tibial shaft fractures as a method of damage control surgery for patients in extremis and/or for patients with fractures with extensive injury to the soft tissues before definitive stabilization. Nonspanning or spanning uniplanar frames placed in a near-far configuration provide relative stability and allow for the management of soft-tissue wounds, the treatment of open fractures, and mobilization of the patient. Definitive treatment of acute tibial fractures with external fixation is usually reserved for highly contaminated open fractures and massive bone loss.

External fixation applied as a temporary measure can safely be transitioned to definitive intramedullary nailing. Previous work demonstrated an improved union rate and better return to function for patients treated with an intramedullary nail after external fixation when compared with those treated in a cast after external fixation.[16] Current evidence shows that there is an average infection rate of 9% and a 90% union rate when intramedullary nailing follows external fixation.[17] The duration of external fixation and the time interval between removal of the external fixator and insertion of an intramedullary nail and the infection risk was also assessed in this systematic review. A shorter duration of external fixation resulted in an 83% risk reduction for infection compared with a longer duration of more than 28 days. A shorter time interval to conversion of less than 14 days also resulted in a reduction in risk for infection.

Intramedullary Nailing

Intramedullary nailing with a statically locked nail is the preferred treatment of most tibial shaft fractures, but the reamed versus unreamed nailing controversy remains unresolved. The Study to Prospectively Evaluate Reamed Intramedullary Nails in Patients with Tibial Fractures (SPRINT)[18] is the largest study to date that compares reamed to unreamed intramedullary nails. This multicenter, blinded, randomized trial of 1,319 adult patients with closed and open tibial shaft fractures compared treatment with reamed and unreamed nails to determine if there was a difference in the reoperation or complication rate. Reoperation within 6 months for nonunion was not permitted per study protocol; however, this stipulation was adhered to in only 55% of the cases. Perioperative care was standardized, and outcomes were assessed at hospital discharge, 2 weeks, 6 weeks, 3 months, 6 months, 9 months, and 1 year postoperatively to identify reoperations and adverse events. At 1 year postoperatively, the primary outcomes recorded were bone grafting, im-

plant exchange, and dynamization for patients with fracture gaps smaller than 1 cm. The trial demonstrated a trend toward a benefit of reaming for closed fractures and no significant differences for the treatment of open fractures. The authors suggested that delaying a reoperation for a nonunion for up to 6 months after the initial procedure might decrease the rate of reoperations.

A recent prospective randomized trial of 100 patients with closed fractures of the tibia compared standard reaming with minimal reaming.[19] The tibias in the standard reaming group were reamed to 12 mm, and an 11-mm nail was inserted. The tibias in the minimal reaming group were reamed to 10 mm, and a 9-mm nail was inserted. Postoperative follow-up was performed at 4, 8, 12, 16, 26, and 52 weeks. Multiple parameters were assessed, including rate of healing, infection, compartment syndrome, return to sport and work activities, and implant failure. A trend toward a faster union time, a lower reoperation rate to achieve union, and earlier return to sport and work activities was noted in the standard reaming group. No statistically significant differences were detected between the two groups.

Retropatellar Nailing Techniques

Alternate nail insertion sites and techniques have been developed recently to address some of the challenges associated with intramedullary nailing of tibial shaft fractures. Standard nail insertion techniques involve either a parapatellar or a patellar tendon-splitting approach, which requires placing the knee in hyperflexion. When used for proximal metaphyseal fractures, this technique may result in malalignment, typically with valgus and apex anterior angulation. The semiextended approach is an alternative and is performed with the knee in approximately 15° of flexion. An open medial parapatellar arthrotomy with lateral subluxation of the patella is performed for instrumentation and nail insertion. All 25 patients with proximal tibial shaft fractures in a study for whom this technique was used had less than 5° of anterior angulation.[20] This technique neutralizes the extension force of the patellar tendon and makes imaging easier.

More recently, a retropatellar portal was described as an alternative site for nail insertion, and a cadaver study was performed using a proximal tibial fracture model.[21,22] The retropatellar technique is performed with the knee in extension, and instrumentation and nail insertion are performed using a quadriceps tendon-splitting approach, with an incision placed superior to the patella. The authors reported that a radiographically correct and anatomically safe start site could be obtained and noted that further clinical investigation is needed.

Fracture Reduction Techniques for Intramedullary Nail/Angularly Stable Intramedullary Nail Locking Bolts

The use of reduction aids, including the application of an external fixator or a femoral distractor, unicortical plates, and blocking screws, as well as technical modifications of intramedullary nails, have improved the ability to obtain and maintain fracture alignment and the stability of the fracture/implant constructs. Blocking screws have been studied extensively and have been shown to assist in obtaining and maintaining alignment for proximal third fractures[23] and improve stability and alignment for proximal and distal metaphyseal fractures.[24]

Open Reduction and Internal Fixation

Plate fixation of tibial shaft fractures can be performed using either direct or indirect reduction techniques and has evolved from dynamic compression plates to limited contact dynamic compression plates and locking plate constructs. The surgical approaches used for plate applications changed based on the poor results of early studies where open acute approaches were used for ORIF and demonstrated high rates of infection, soft-tissue complications, and nonunion, particularly for open fractures.[25] These high infection rates likely were the result of iatrogenic soft-tissue damage and periosteal stripping that resulted from using these extensive open approaches.

A recent biomechanical study of extra-articular distal tibial fractures compared standard plating, locked plating, intramedullary nailing, and angularly stable intramedullary nailing using an axially unstable tibial fracture with an intact fibula model.[26] The authors found that both intramedullary nailing and locked plating provided stable fixation, but intramedullary nailing demonstrated the greatest stiffness, load to failure, and failure energy. In general, plate fixation is not the preferred fixation technique for the treatment of closed diaphyseal tibial shaft fractures, except for skeletally immature patients, patients with tibial canals that are too small to accommodate the smallest diameter intramedullary nail, periprosthetic fractures, and fractures with proximal or distal intra-articular extension.

Proximal Third and Distal Third Fractures

Proximal third and distal third fractures of the tibia and fractures with intra-articular extension have been treated with external fixation, intramedullary nailing, ORIF, or a combination of these techniques. These fracture patterns have presented difficulties for reduction and fixation, and studies have focused on resolving the challenges presented by these fractures.

Proximal third fractures are subject to the deforming forces of the patellar tendon and the pes anserinus. These forces combined with inaccurate starting points and nail trajectories have led to a high incidence of deformity when intramedullary nails are used to stabilize these fractures. Nailing with the knee in extension, the use of a femoral distractor or an external fixator, the insertion of Poller/blocking screws, and the use of provisional or supplementary plate fixation all are options. These techniques were summarized in a recent publication that focused on the use of intramedullary nails for proximal third fractures.[27] Recommendations included using a lateral starting point placed just anterior to the articular margin and an insertion angle that is parallel to the anterior cortex of the tibia. A cadaver study on starting portals made on the lateral tibial plateau in the lateral third, middle third, and medial third to evaluate the effectiveness of correcting valgus malalignment typical in proximal third fractures demonstrated that using the most lateral starting portal allowed for correction of up to 20° of valgus.[28] However, varus malalignment can occur when the nail starting point is made too far laterally; therefore, the optimal nail starting point is in the middle of the lateral tibial plateau for proximal fractures.

A concern about possible damage to intra-articular structures when a lateral approach is used led the same authors to investigate the effect of a medial parapatellar approach for proximal fractures located at different levels.[29] Fresh frozen cadavers were used, and osteotomies were created between 2 cm and 9 cm below the tibial tubercle, followed by fixation with a 9-mm intramedullary nail. Coronal and sagittal plane alignment as well as coronal and sagittal plane displacement of the distal fragment were recorded. The authors found that fractures located 8 cm below the tibial tuberosity could be nailed using a medial parapatellar approach without malalignment or displacement, whereas the same technique applied in more proximal fractures resulted in valgus and apex anterior malalignment.

Distal third tibial fractures also can be difficult to treat. The use of intramedullary nails can result in fracture malalignment, and ORIF can lead to infections, wound complications, and hardware irritation. A prospective randomized trial compared intramedullary nails with plate fixation for distal third fractures.[30] One hundred four extra-articular distal tibial fractures located between 4 cm and 11 cm proximal to the tibial plafond were randomized to either nailing or plate fixation. There was a similar rate of infection and secondary procedures for the two procedures, and there was a nonstatistically significant higher rate of malalignment when using an intramedullary nail. A trend toward a higher rate of nonunion was observed in fractures treated with distal fibula fixation. Another prospective randomized trial compared nails with percutaneously placed plates for the fixation of extra-articular distal fractures located at least 3 cm from the tibial plafond. Surgical and imaging times, time to fracture union, complications, and functional outcomes were assessed.[31] The intramedullary nailing group had a statistically significant decrease in surgical and imaging times. There was no difference in the time to union, and the 1-year rate of union was 100%. Better American Orthopaedic Foot and Ankle Society (AOFAS) scores were found for the nailing group, but this difference was not statistically significant.

Plate fixation using minimally invasive percutaneous techniques has been developed in an attempt to decrease the complications of infection, soft-tissue issues, and nonunion associated with standard open plating approaches.[32] Two recent studies reported the results and outcomes of minimally invasive plate osteosynthesis of distal tibial fractures. A retrospective analysis of 21 patients with distal tibial fractures treated with minimally invasive plate osteosynthesis and locked plates reported on the union rate, deformity, limb-length discrepancy, ankle range of motion, return to preinjury activity level, and infection and complication rates.[33] Twenty of 21 fractures were united by 24 weeks, 4 patients experienced healing with a deformity of less than 7°, no limb-length discrepancies greater than 1.1 cm were noted, and a late infection developed in 3 patients. The authors thought the high rate of union and the low complication rate with this technique indicated that it is a safe and effective treatment method. Locking plate implants with hybrid screw constructs were applied using minimally invasive approaches to 38 distal tibial fractures with minimal or no intra-articular extension.[34] Acceptable length and alignment were restored in all but one case, and union was achieved in all cases at an average of 21 weeks. Secondary procedures were required in 3 of the 38 patients to achieve union. The functional outcomes scores for the ankle were mostly good to excellent. The authors concluded that this technique was effective for low metaphyseal fractures of the distal tibia.

Open Fractures

Open fractures are classified using the Gustilo and Anderson classification[10,11] (**Table 2**) and require prompt antibiotic administration, tetanus prophylaxis, surgical irrigation and débridement, and fracture stabilization. First- or second-generation cephalosporins are recommended for type I and II open fractures to cover gram-positive bacteria. For type III open fractures, the addition of an aminoglycoside is recommended for coverage of gram-negative bacteria. Soil- or farm-related injuries require the addition of penicillin to combat anaerobic bacteria. The optimal duration of antibiotic therapy is unknown but is typically continued for 24 to 72 hours postoperatively.

There is considerable debate about the effect of time to débridement on the infection rate, and the 6-hour rule has limited evidence-based support. A recent study examined the factors associated with a delay from emergency department presentation to surgical irrigation and débridement.[35] More than 6,000 patients with blunt trauma and open tibial fractures comprised the cohort that was obtained from the National Trauma Data Bank. The median time to irrigation and débridement was 4.9 hours. Fifty-eight percent of the patients underwent irrigation and débridement within 6 hours of emergency department presentation, whereas 42% had a delay greater than 6 hours. Irrigation and débridement within 24 hours was performed for 76% of the patients, whereas 24% had a delay of 24 hours or more. Multiple variables were analyzed, including age, sex, the Injury Severity Score (ISS), and the time of admission (separated into 2 am to 6 pm and 6 pm to 2 am) to determine which factors were associated with a delay. Increasing patient age, the presence of a closed head injury or a thoracic injury, and admission after 6 pm were statistically associated with a delay greater than 6 hours. Other factors statistically associated with a delay greater than 6 hours were admission to a service other than orthopaedic surgery and presentation to a level I trauma center. Both of these factors may be associated with a more severely injured patient, which was also shown to be associated with a delay.

Urgent surgical débridement continues to be part of the recommended treatment of open tibial fractures and was the focus of a recent report that attempted to identify modifiable predictors of poor outcomes after open tibial fractures.[36] This prospective observational study of consecutive open tibial fractures assessed demographics, the mechanism of injury, time to antibiotics, time to débridement, ISS, fracture type and grade, and local contamination to determine their effect on length of stay, infection, secondary procedures, and union at 6 and 12 months. The authors found that controlling for timely débridement left only patient factors and injury severity as predictors of poor outcome. Only an ISS greater than 15 was statistically significantly associated with increased time to fracture union.

Tibial Malunion

Acceptable alignment for a healed tibial shaft fracture is defined as less than 5° of varus or valgus angulation, less than 10° of sagittal plane angulation, more than 50% cortical apposition, less than 1 cm of shortening, and less than 10° to 15° of rotational malalignment. The definition of malalignment is fractures that fall outside these parameters. The rate of malalignment is variable and has been reported to be as high as 84%.[37] Proximal third fractures have been the most challenging to achieve anatomic alignment after intramedullary nailing and tend to have a typical deformity consisting of valgus, apex anterior, and posterior translation of the distal fragment. A better understanding of nail insertion techniques[20-22] and the use of reduction aids[23,24] have reduced the malunion rate.

The long-term results of tibial malunion include knee and ankle osteoarthritis because malalignment/malunion alters the mechanics of the knee and ankle joint. Radiographic evidence of osteoarthritis does not always correlate with clinical symptoms. A study performed on joint malalignment and clinical outcomes following tibial shaft fractures demonstrated that greater degrees of distal tibial malunions that resulted in ankle malalignment had statistically significant poorer clinical results compared with more proximal malunions.[38] Alignment should be evaluated using full-length standing radiographs from the hip to the ankle of bilateral lower extremities. In addition, CT is valuable to assess rotational alignment and deformity. The treatment of a symptomatic malunion is achieved with a corrective osteotomy.

Tibial Nonunions

It is generally accepted that tibial shaft fractures unite between 16 and 19 weeks.[13,15,39] Open fractures have a longer average time to union, which can be 1 year or longer.[40] Because of a lack of agreement among surgeons as to which fractures are healed, the Radiographic Union Scale in Tibial Fractures (RUST) was developed. This method has been used to assess healing in fractures treated with intramedullary nails. The scoring system is based on AP and lateral radiographs of the tibia, and 1 to 3 points are allocated based on the presence or the absence of fracture callus as well as visible or invisible fracture lines[41] (Table 3). The RUST method has shown excellent interobserver reliability, and investigation is under way to demonstrate its validity.[41]

The definition of nonunion is less clear. Historically, nonunion of the tibia was defined as a fracture that has not healed after 9 months. Another common definition is a fracture that will not heal without surgical intervention. At any time, a lack of evidence of healing and/or the absence of progression of radiologic union combined with persistent pain and motion at the fracture site are signs of nonunion.

As with all fractures, tibial nonunions are classified as aseptic or infected, hypertrophic, oligotrophic, or atrophic, and the treatment differs based on the diagnosis. Dynamization, or the removal of screws from the intramedullary nail to allow motion at the fracture site, has not consistently led to fracture healing.[39] Exchange nailing has been studied for the treatment of aseptic nonunions. This treatment involves removing the intramedullary nail, reaming the canal, and placing a larger diameter nail. One study followed 547 tibial shaft fractures treated with intramedullary nails; 33 went on to develop aseptic nonunions and were treated with exchange nailing. At an average of 15 to 16 weeks, 29 of the 33 patients (87.9%) experienced healing and the 4 remaining patients required a second exchange nailing procedure to achieve union.[40] The use of circular external fixation such as the Ilizarov or Taylor spatial frame and bone transport is another treatment option typically reserved for bone defects greater than 4 cm.

As an alternative to or in conjunction with surgery for nonunion, extracorporeal shock wave therapy (ESWT) has recently been described. This treatment involves regional or general anesthesia and fluoroscopy to identify the proximal and distal extents of the nonunion site. A specialized device is used to focus the ESWT at the nonunion, and a voltage of 26 to 28 kV is used to administer a median of 4,000 pulses. A retrospective analysis of 192 consecutive nonunions treated with ESWT alone (8 patients), ESWT and immobilization (174 patients), or ESWT and external fixation (10

patients) was performed to assess fracture healing and factors associated with success or failure of the ESWT technique.[42] Of the 172 patients with complete treatment and follow-up records, 138 (80.2%) demonstrated healing at an average of 4.8 ± 4.0 months. The authors found that the number of orthopaedic operations, shock wave treatments, and pulses delivered were significantly associated with complete healing. This technique shows promise and requires further investigation.

Table 3

Radiographic Union Scale in Tibial Fractures (RUST) Classification

[a]Score per Cortex	Radiographic Citeria Callus Fracture Line
1	Absent visible
2	Present visible
3	Present invisible

[a]The individual cortical scores (anterior, posterior, medial, lateral) are added to provide a RUST value for a set of radiographs of 4 (definitely not healed) to 12 (definitely healed).
(Reproduced with permission from Kooistra BW, Dijkman BG, Busse JW, et al: The radiographic union scale in tibial fractures: Reliability and validity. *J Orthop Trauma* 2010;24 [suppl] 1:S81–S86.)

Summary

Tibial shaft fractures are common. These fractures are classified descriptively by the AO/OTA classification system. Compartment syndrome is most often found in fractures of the tibial diaphysis; therefore, a careful physical examination should be performed, and close monitoring is recommended. The goal of treatment is near anatomic restoration of length, alignment, and rotation. Functional bracing is an effective nonsurgical treatment method involving casting followed by early functional bracing with weight bearing. Although select fractures can be treated closed, tibial shaft fractures are most often treated surgically with intramedullary nailing, ORIF with plate application, or less often with external fixation. Open fractures are a separate case and demand the prompt administration of intravenous antibiotics and surgical irrigation and débridement. Healing time varies but typically occurs in 16 to 19 weeks. Malunions do occur and can be treated with a corrective osteotomy. Nonunions require a thorough workup to determine the etiology and further surgical intervention to achieve union.

Key Study Points

- Intramedullary nailing with a statically locked nail is the preferred treatment for most tibial shaft fractures, and fracture union typically occurs between 16 and 19 weeks.

- For tibial shaft fractures, acceptable alignment is less than 5° of varus or valgus angulation, less than 10° of sagittal plane angulation, more than 50% cortical apposition, less than 1 cm of shortening, and less than 10° of rotational malalignment.

- Compartment syndrome is one of the most common complications of tibial fractures. Preoperative diastolic blood pressure should be used to calculate delta P with a threshold of less than 30 mm Hg for fasciotomy.

Annotated References

1. Praemer A, Furner S, Rice DP: *Musculoskeletal Conditions in the United States.* Rosemont, IL, American Academy of Orthopaedic Surgeons, 1999.

2. Bucholz RW: *Rockwood and Green's Fractures in Adults.* New York, NY, Lippincott Williams & Wilkins, 2009, pp 2084-2085.

3. McQueen MM, Gaston P, Court-Brown CM: Acute compartment syndrome: Who is at risk? *J Bone Joint Surg Br* 2000;82(2):200-203.

4. Whitesides TE, Heckman MM: Acute compartment syndrome: Update on diagnosis and treatment. *J Am Acad Orthop Surg* 1996;4(4):209-218.

5. Kakar S, Firoozabadi R, McKean J, Tornetta P III: Diastolic blood pressure in patients with tibia fractures under anaesthesia: Implications for the diagnosis of compartment syndrome. *J Orthop Trauma* 2007;21(2):99-103.

6. Schmidt AH: The impact of compartment syndrome on hospital length of stay and charges among adult patients admitted with a fracture of the tibia. *J Orthop Trauma* 2011;25(6):355-357.

   This retrospective review of uncomplicated tibial shaft fractures compared the hospital length of stay and associated costs for patients with and without acute compartment syndrome.

7. Wind TC, Saunders SM, Barfield WR, Mooney JF III, Hartsock LA: Compartment syndrome after low-energy tibia fractures sustained during athletic competition. *J Orthop Trauma* 2012;26(1):33-36.

   In this retrospective review, the rate of acute compartment syndrome was reported for 626 consecutive tibial fractures, with a subgroup analysis for fractures sustained during soccer or football participation.

8. Tinetti ME, Speechley M, Ginter SF: Risk factors for falls among elderly persons living in the community. *Engl J Med* 1988;319(26):1701-1707.

9. Tscherne H, Oestern HJ: A new classification of soft-tissue damage in open and closed fractures (author's transl). *Unfallheilkunde* 1982;85(3):111-115.

10. Gustilo RB, Anderson JT: Prevention of infection in the treatment of one thousand and twenty-five open fractures of long bones: Retrospective and prospective analyses. *J Bone Joint Surg Am* 1976;58(4):453-458.

11. Gustilo RB, Mendoza RM, Williams DN: Problems in the management of type III (severe) open fractures: A new classification of type III open fractures. *J Trauma* 1984;24(8):742-746.

12. Lindsey RW, Blair SR: Closed tibial-shaft fractures: Which ones benefit from surgical treatment? *J Am Acad Orthop Surg* 1996;4(1):35-43.

13. Sarmiento A, Sharpe FE, Ebramzadeh E, Normand P, Shankwiler J: Factors influencing the outcome of closed tibial fractures treated with functional bracing. *Clin Orthop Relat Res* 1995;315:8-24.

14. Littenberg B, Weinstein LP, McCarren M, et al: Closed fractures of the tibial shaft: A meta-analysis of three methods of treatment. *J Bone Joint Surg Am* 1998;80(2):174-183.

15. Hooper GJ, Keddell RG, Penny ID: Conservative management or closed nailing for tibial shaft fractures: A randomised prospective trial. *J Bone Joint Surg Br* 1991;73(1):83-85.

16. Antich-Adrover P, Martí-Garin D, Murias-Alvarez J, Puente-Alonso C: External fixation and secondary intramedullary nailing of open tibial fractures: A randomised, prospective trial. *J Bone Joint Surg Br* 1997;79(3):433-437.

17. Bhandari M, Zlowodzki M, Tornetta P III, Schmidt A, Templeman DC: Intramedullary nailing following external fixation in femoral and tibial shaft fractures. *J Orthop Trauma* 2005;19(2):140-144.

18. Bhandari M, Guyatt G, Tornetta P III, et al: Randomized trial of reamed and unreamed intramedullary nailing of tibial shaft fractures. *J Bone Joint Surg Am* 2008;90(12):2567-2578.

19. Gaebler C, McQueen MM, Vécsei V, Court-Brown CM: Reamed versus minimally reamed nailing: A prospectively randomised study of 100 patients with closed fractures of the tibia. *Injury* 2011;42(suppl 4):S17-S21.

   The authors present the results of a randomized trial comparing standard reaming to minimal reaming for closed tibial shaft fractures.

20. Tornetta P III, Collins E: Semiextended position of intramedullary nailing of the proximal tibia. *Clin Orthop Relat Res* 1996;328:185-189.

21. Eastman JG, Tseng SS, Lee MA, Yoo BJ: The retropatellar portal as an alternative site for tibial nail insertion: A cadaveric study. *J Orthop Trauma* 2010;24(11): 659-664.

    Using a cadaver study, the authors described the surgical technique for the retropatellar portal for tibial nail insertion.

22. Eastman J, Tseng S, Lo E, Li CS, Yoo B, Lee M: Retropatellar technique for intramedullary nailing of proximal tibia fractures: A cadaveric assessment. *J Orthop Trauma* 2010;24(11):672-676.

    In a follow-up study to the authors' publication on the retropatellar portal for tibial nail insertion, this cadaver study describes the use of the retropatellar technique in proximal third fractures.

23. Ricci WM, O'Boyle M, Borrelli J, Bellabarba C, Sanders R: Fractures of the proximal third of the tibial shaft treated with intramedullary nails and blocking screws. *J Orthop Trauma* 2001;15(4):264-270.

24. Krettek C, Stephan C, Schandelmaier P, Richter M, Pape HC, Miclau T: The use of Poller screws as blocking screws in stabilising tibial fractures treated with small diameter intramedullary nails. *J Bone Joint Surg Br* 1999;81(6):963-968.

25. Rüedi T, Webb JK, Allgöwer M: Experience with the dynamic compression plate (DCP) in 418 recent fractures of the tibial shaft. *Injury* 1976;7(4):252-257.

26. Hoenig M, Gao F, Kinder J, Zhang LQ, Collinge C, Merk BR: Extra-articular distal tibia fractures: A mechanical evaluation of 4 different treatment methods. *J Orthop Trauma* 2010;24(1):30-35.

    Surgical techniques of standard plate fixation, locking plate fixation, intramedullary nailing, and angular stable intramedullary nailing are compared for extraarticular distal tibial fractures.

27. Liporace FA, Stadler CM, Yoon RS: Problems, tricks, and pearls in intramedullary nailing of proximal third tibial fractures. *J Orthop Trauma* 2013;27(1):56-6.

    The authors report on surgical techniques and modifications for intramedullary nailing of proximal third fractures and include supporting literature for each topic. Level of evidence: V.

28. Weninger P, Tschabitscher M, Traxler H, Pfafl V, Hertz H: Intramedullary nailing of proximal tibia fractures: An anatomical study comparing three lateral starting points for nail insertion. *Injury* 2010;41(2):220-225.

    This cadaver study compared lateral, middle, and medial starting portals on the lateral tibial plateau for intramedullary nailing and the potential to correct coronal plane malalignment.

29. Weninger P, Tschabitscher M, Traxler H, Pfafl V, Hertz H: Influence of medial parapatellar nail insertion on alignment in proximal tibia fractures—special consideration of the fracture level. *J Trauma* 2010;68(4): 975-979.

    The results of this study showed that a medial parapatellar approach for nail entry can be performed without misalignment or fragment dislocation in patients with fractures of the proximal tibia that are located 8 cm or more below the tibial tuberosity.

30. Vallier HA, Cureton BA, Patterson BM: Randomized, prospective comparison of plate versus intramedullary nail fixation for distal tibia shaft fractures. *J Orthop Trauma* 2011;25(12):736-741.

    The authors reported results and complications in this prospective randomized trial of locked plating compared with intramedullary nailing for metaphyseal fractures of the distal tibia.

31. Guo JJ, Tang N, Yang HL, Tang TS: A prospective, randomised trial comparing closed intramedullary nailing with percutaneous plating in the treatment of distal metaphyseal fractures of the tibia. *J Bone Joint Surg Br* 2010;92(7):984-988.

    In this prospective randomized trial comparing intramedullary nailing with percutaneous plating for distal tibial fractures, the authors report on surgical and imaging times, time to union, complications, and functional outcomes.

32. Collinge CA, Sanders RW: Percutaneous plating in the lower extremity. *J Am Acad Orthop Surg* 2000;8(4): 211-216.

33. Ronga M, Longo UG, Maffulli N: Minimally invasive locked plating of distal tibia fractures is safe and effective. *Clin Orthop Relat Res* 2010;468(4):975-982.

    The authors assessed factors such as bone union rate, deformity, leg-length discrepancy, infection, and return to preinjury activities in individuals who underwent minimally invasive osteosynthesis of closed distal tibial fractures with a locking plate. Results showed that the locking plate is an acceptable device for the treatment of distal tibial fractures. Level of evidence: IV.

34. Collinge C, Protzman R: Outcomes of minimally invasive plate osteosynthesis for metaphyseal distal tibia fractures. *J Orthop Trauma* 2010;24(1):24-29.

    The authors report their results and complications using minimally invasive plate osteosynthesis with locked plating and hybrid constructs for metaphyseal distal tibial fractures.

35. Namdari S, Baldwin KD, Matuszewski P, Esterhai JL, Mehta S: Delay in surgical débridement of open tibia fractures: An analysis of national practice trends. *J Orthop Trauma* 2011;25(3):140-144.

    This study describes the national practice trends in time to débridement for open tibial fractures and the factors associated with delays greater than 6 hours and greater than 24 hours.

4: Lower Extremity

36. Enninghorst N, McDougall D, Hunt JJ, Balogh ZJ: Open tibia fractures: Timely debridement leaves injury severity as the only determinant of poor outcome. *J Trauma* 2011;70(2):352-357.

This prospective observational study of open tibial fractures assessed demographics, mechanism of injury, time to antibiotics, time to débridement, ISS, fracture type and grade, and local contamination to determine their effect on length of stay, infection, secondary procedures, and union.

37. Cannada LK, Anglen JO, Archdeacon MT, Herscovici D Jr, Ostrum RF: Avoiding complications in the care of fractures of the tibia. *Instr Course Lect* 2009;58:27-36.

38. Puno RM, Vaughan JJ, Stetten ML, Johnson JR: Long-term effects of tibial angular malunion on the knee and ankle joints. *J Orthop Trauma* 1991;5(3):247-254.

39. Court-Brown CM, Christie J, McQueen MM: Closed intramedullary tibial nailing: Its use in closed and type I open fractures. *J Bone Joint Surg Br* 1990;72(4): 605-611.

40. Court-Brown CM, Keating JF, Christie J, McQueen MM: Exchange intramedullary nailing: Its use in aseptic tibial nonunion. *J Bone Joint Surg Br* 1995;77(3): 407-411.

41. Kooistra BW, Dijkman BG, Busse JW, Sprague S, Schemitsch EH, Bhandari M: The radiographic union scale in tibial fractures: Reliability and validity. *J Orthop Trauma* 2010;24(suppl 1):S81-S86.

The authors found that the RUST method is associated with increased interrater reliability compared with conventional radiographic measures such as surgeons' general impression or number of cortices bridged by callus.

42. Elster EA, Stojadinovic A, Forsberg J, Shawen S, Andersen RC, Schaden W: Extracorporeal shock wave therapy for nonunion of the tibia. *J Orthop Trauma* 2010;24(3):133-141.

In this retrospective review, the authors report on ESWT for tibial nonunions, the effect on fracture healing, and factors associated with success or failure with this technique.

Chapter 43

Ankle Fractures

Kenneth A. Egol, MD   Jodi Siegel, MD   Paul Tornetta III, MD

Fractures of the Tibial Plafond

Mechanism of Injury

Generally, there are two different mechanisms of injury that produce pilon fractures. The low-energy, sports-related, rotational injury is the less common mechanism. Impaction fractures associated with high-energy axial loading are more common and are the result of motor vehicle accidents or a fall from a height. The common characteristic of pilon fractures is forced dorsiflexion of the talus, with the wider, anterior part driven into the tibial plafond. First, the medial malleolus is split off. Second, the anterior articular surface is disrupted. Third, the distal end of the fibula is fractured. Fourth, the tibial metaphysis fractures transversely above the anterior lip.

History and Physical Examination

A pilon fracture should be considered in the differential diagnosis whenever a patient reports pain and swelling about the ankle following major or minor trauma. Decision making regarding the treatment of periarticular fractures about the tibial plafond is dependent on the mechanism of injury, clinical stability, radiographic findings, and associated soft-tissue injuries. Initial evaluation of the distal tibia following trauma includes palpation to elicit tenderness over a potential fracture or site of ligamentous disruption. Careful neurovascular examination of the extremity should follow documentation of the skin condition and presence of swelling. Because many of these injuries are high energy, compartment syndrome should be ruled out. If pulses are not palpable, a reduction should be attempted. If pulses do not return, Doppler studies and/or ankle brachial index testing should be performed. If the clinical signs of an impending compartment syndrome (pain out of pro-

portion, pallor, pain on passive stretch of the toes, or impaired neurologic status) are present, compartment pressures can be measured. Pressures should also be measured in the unconscious patient with a tense, swollen foot. Any open wound should be evaluated for the possibility of an open joint injury. When there is a high degree of suspicion for an open joint wound, it should be explored in the operating room. Because of the high-energy forces responsible for most pilon fractures, other fractures associated with vertical compression must be ruled out, including calcaneal fractures, tibial plateau fractures, pelvic fractures, and vertebral fractures.

Imaging

Following the clinical examination, radiographic evaluation should be performed. An ankle trauma series includes AP, lateral, and mortise views. Plain films will elicit specific fracture patterns and direct the treating physician toward a certain clinical pathway. CT scans, with or without two- and three-dimensional reconstruction, aid in the identification of impacted articular segments (Figure 1). These studies are excellent adjuncts in the preoperative planning of lag screw placement when percutaneous fixation is to be undertaken.

Dr. Egol or an immediate family member has received royalties from Exactech and has received research or institutional support from Stryker, Synthes, and Orthopaedic Research Education Foundation. Dr. Tornetta or an immediate family member has received royalties from Smith & Nephew. Neither Dr. Siegel nor any immediate family member has received anything of value from or has stock or stock options held in a commercial company or institution related directly or indirectly to the subject of this chapter.

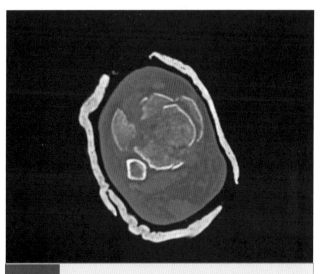

Figure 1   An axial CT scan cut demonstrating a type C pilon fracture.

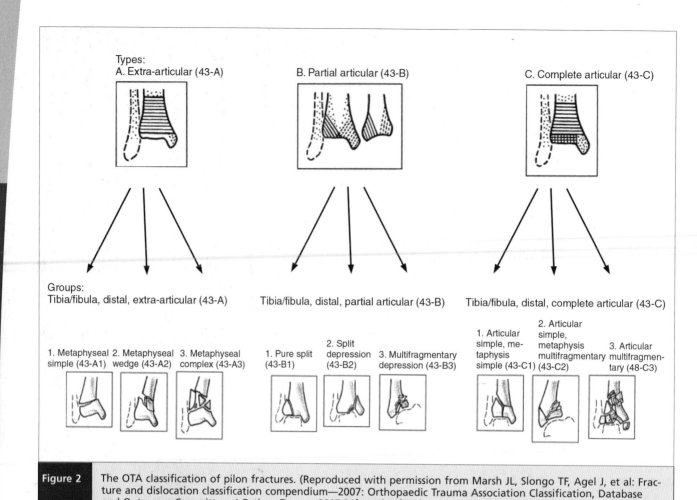

Figure 2 The OTA classification of pilon fractures. (Reproduced with permission from Marsh JL, Slongo TF, Agel J, et al: Fracture and dislocation classification compendium—2007: Orthopaedic Trauma Association Classification, Database and Outcomes Committee. *J Orthop Trauma* 2007;21[suppl 10]:S1.)

Classification

The Orthopaedic Trauma Association (OTA) classification divides pilon fractures into three main categories (**Figure 2**). Type A fractures are extra-articular and are subdivided into simple, wedge, and complex. Type B fractures are partially articular and are subdivided into B1, pure split; B2, split-depression; and B3, multifragmentary depression. Type C fractures are complete articular fractures and are also subdivided into: C1, articular and metaphyseal simple; C2, articular simple and metaphyseal multifragmentary; and C3, articular multifragmentary.[1]

Anatomic Considerations

Lower energy torsional fractures may be reduced and splinted, whereas higher energy impaction fractures may require reduction under anesthesia. All limbs are strictly elevated until definitive fixation is chosen to allow for soft-tissue swelling resolution. The decision regarding timing for open reduction and internal fixation (ORIF) is based on the overall health of the patient and the status of the soft-tissue envelope about the distal tibia. For pilon fractures with an associated fibula fracture, the fibula can be plated through a lateral approach, and a bridging external fixator can be placed across the ankle

joint on the night of admission. It should be noted that controversy exists regarding the need to plate the fibula when an external fixator is used. Patients with higher energy fractures who have undergone temporary spanning external fixations may be discharged to home and followed in the outpatient clinic until soft-tissue concerns, such as swelling and blistering, have resolved. Waiting 7 to 14 days before definitive surgery is attempted has become the standard of care. The exact nature of the fracture should be understood before surgical intervention is attempted. Preoperative planning is essential for any complex injury because it forces the surgeon to understand the "personality" of the fracture and mentally prepare a strategy for surgery. When definitive fixation is performed, all aspects of fracture reduction and fixation should be planned to avoid technical pitfalls, and the surgeon must make sure that all of the needed equipment is available. The general principles for the open treatment of these fractures, which were developed in 1969, are in current use: restoration of tibial length, reconstruction of the articular surface, bone void filling of the metaphyseal defect, and provision of a neutralization device (plate or fixator) to stabilize the tibial shaft. The advent of locked plates altered the traditional approach.

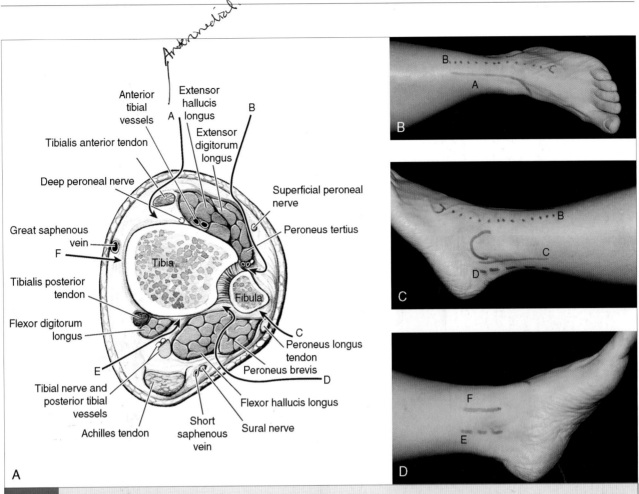

Anteromedial (handwritten annotation)

Figure 3 A, Cross-sectional anatomy demonstrating the various intervals for approaches to the distal tibia. B through D, Anterior, lateral, and medial views, respectively, of the ankle. Line A represents the anteromedial approach. Line B represents the anterolateral approach. Line C represents the direct lateral approach. Line D represents the posterolateral approach. Line E represents the posteromedial approach. Line F represents the medial approach. (Reproduced from Crist BD, Khazzam M, Murtha YM, Della Rocca GJ: Pilon fractures: Advances in surgical management. *J Am Acad Orthop Surg* 2011;19[10]:612-622.)

Open Approaches

Anteromedial

The various intervals for approaches to the distal tibia and the ankle are shown in Figure 3. The anteromedial approach to the distal tibia begins just lateral to the tibial crest and distally curves posteromedially at the level of the joint. The incision is carried down to the extensor retinaculum as one thick flap. Care is taken to avoid entering the sheath of the tibialis anterior and creating subcutaneous flaps. This traditional approach allows for most fracture patterns. The downside is the lack of soft-tissue coverage on the anteromedial surface of the tibia, which can be problematic in cases of wound compromise.

Anterolateral

The anterolateral approach has recently become popular. This approach is centered over the ankle between the tibia and the fibula. The incision is carried down and exploits the interval between the peroneous tertius and the extensor digitorum communis. The superficial peroneal nerve must be identified and protected. Next,

the extensor retinaculum is incised down to the capsule.[2,3] The advantage of this approach is the presence of a more robust soft-tissue envelope around the bone. Injuries with the major fracture line laterally are amenable to this fixation approach.

Posterolateral

This approach is based on the interval between the peroneals and the flexor hallucis longus. The sural nerve must be protected superficially. After the flexor hallucis longus is elevated off the fibula, the posterior compartment musculature is elevated off the posterior tibia. It is often difficult to visualize articular impaction via this approach. Large fragments can be compressed, lagged, or buttressed directly.[4-6] This approach is well suited for fractures with the major displacement involving the posterior tibia. Sometimes this approach is used in concert with anterior approaches in staged fixation scenarios.

Management

Nonsurgical care is reserved for nondisplaced fractures or for those who are too ill or high risk to undergo

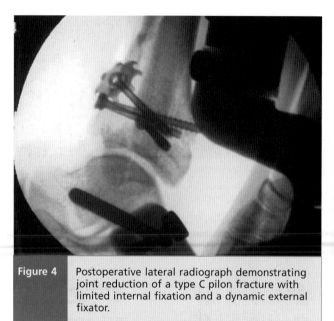

Figure 4 Postoperative lateral radiograph demonstrating joint reduction of a type C pilon fracture with limited internal fixation and a dynamic external fixator.

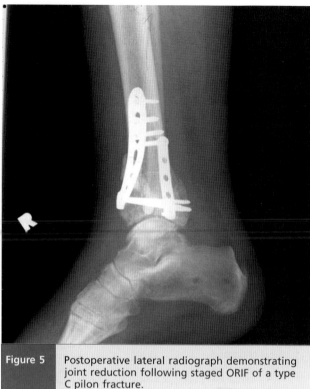

Figure 5 Postoperative lateral radiograph demonstrating joint reduction following staged ORIF of a type C pilon fracture.

surgical intervention. In these cases, complete ankle immobilization should be maintained in a cast or a cast brace for a minimum of 8 to 12 weeks. For those patients in whom surgical treatment is selected, several options exist. Definitive external fixation with or without limited internal fixation theoretically diminishes the amount of surgical soft-tissue injury, which decreases the risk of postoperative soft-tissue complications. Some reports have found that general health status is diminished, and patients are limited in their recreational activities following a pilon fracture. Definitive external fixation frames may be joint spanning, with or without articulation at the ankle, or nonspanning frames. If a nonspanning frame is chosen, tensioned, thin wires must be used to gain purchase in comminuted metaphyseal bone. Joint reduction is performed percutaneously or through very small incisions, and well-placed lag screws are used to stabilize the major fragments. The use of external fixation results in radiographic signs of arthritic change, yet very few patients who have had external fixation undergo secondary procedures. Patients tend to improve clinically, even after 2 years following their injuries when treated with these devices[7] (Figure 4).

ORIF is a popular method of treatment of these injuries. The recommendations for the timing of definitive ORIF has changed over the years, but the surgical principles remain the same. If fibular fixation is chosen, two incisions may be needed. In this case, the fibula is usually approached posterolaterally and the tibia anteromedially. If the fibula is to be stabilized early as part of a temporizing procedure, care should be taken to allow for a future anteromedial incision. This is accomplished by drawing out both incisions at the time of initial surgery. Recently, the dogma of a 7-cm skin bridge between incisions has been called into question.[8] Both bones may be addressed if an anterolateral approach is chosen. Indirect reduction techniques have the advan-

tage of minimal soft-tissue stripping and fragment devitalization. A femoral distractor with threaded pins is placed into the calcaneus or the talus and the tibial shaft to help provide the indirect reduction; however, ligamentotaxis will not work on centrally depressed articular fragments. For badly comminuted fractures, if an external fixation has been used as a temporizing measure, it is now used intraoperatively for assistance with reduction. Manipulation and reduction of comminuted fragments is performed using small forceps or a dental pick. Reduction of the joint is accomplished under direct vision. Small incisions can be used over the fracture lines. The anterolateral fragment will be left in its anatomic position by virtue of its attachment to the fibula (already reduced and plated) through the syndesmotic ligaments. If the articular surface is severely comminuted, the dome of the talus can be used as a template. Provisional reduction is confirmed on image intensification before definitive fixation. With the joint reconstructed, the articular surface is fixed to the metaphysis. This is accomplished by using well-contoured, low-profile plates (Figure 5). Some type of bone void filer is then placed in the metaphyseal defect. Wound closure is performed in two layers. The skin is then closed with atraumatic soft-tissue handling.

The key to the closure, regardless of the suture technique chosen, is that it is tension free. Negative pressure wound therapy has recently been shown to be helpful in managing damaged soft tissues about the distal tibia and fibula by minimizing postoperative hematoma drainage.[9]

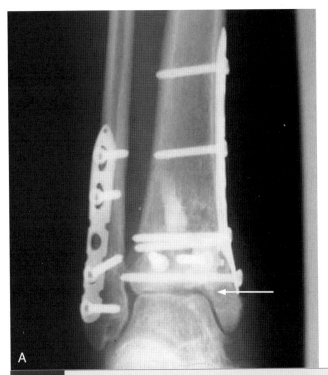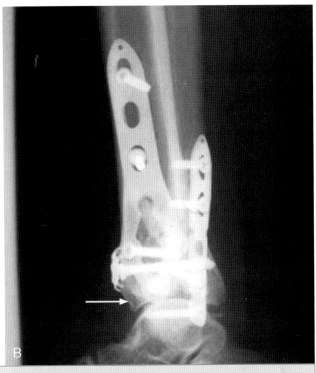

Figure 6	A and B, Mortise views 2 years following ORIF for a type C pilon fracture. Note the joint space narrowing (arrows) that is present.

Results

Outcomes

Outcomes following pilon fractures demonstrate a wide multifactorial range. In general, patients with pilon fracture report poorer function than the general population, limitations in ankle range of motion, and some baseline chronic pain. Poor patient outcomes can lead to significant financial burden on patients, especially if they are unable to return to work.[10]

Early studies reported excellent outcomes following early ORIF. Because these results could not be duplicated and were associated with high rates of complications, surgeons sought alternate methods of treatment. Over the past 30 years, the pendulum has swung from ORIF to hybrid external fixation to joint-spanning external fixation with limited internal fixation to staged ORIF back to ORIF with limited approaches. Poorer outcomes have previously been related to higher energy injuries, lower socioeconomic status, and external fixation as definitive treatment.[11]

In several recent retrospective studies comparing two cohorts of patients, one treated with staged ORIF and the other with joint spanning external fixation with limited internal fixation, the authors found no significant functional differences at 1 year between groups, although the external fixation group did have more arthritic change on radiographs at 1 year.[12-14] A long-term outcomes study also demonstrated a lack of correlation between radiographic and functional outcomes in a series of patients with pilon fractures who were treated with external fixation at 80 months after surgery.[15]

These authors found that patient symptoms stabilized and did not progress, and there were few secondary procedures in the 32 patients studied.

Despite trends toward staged ORIF, a recent study described success in the management of these injuries using immediate ORIF by specialized surgeons.[16] These authors reported acceptable complication rates consistent with those seen using staged protocols. It should be noted that these specialized surgeons are very experienced and thought that acute management of these injuries was safe.

Complications

Early and late complications occur following the treatment of pilon fractures. Wound breakdown and infection are the most common complications seen early after surgical fixation. Rates have been reported as high as 31% using modern techniques. Several strategies have been used to help reduce this complication rate, including staged internal fixation protocols, definitive external fixation, alternate approaches, and minimally invasive approaches. As a result, the rate of superficial infection has decreased to zero to 3%.[17,18] However, in other series, deep infection rates and osteomyelitis have been reported as high as 25%.[14,19,20] Longer term complications include malunion, nonunion, posttraumatic arthritis, and complex regional pain syndrome. Malunion is reported to occur in 2% to 42% of patients[12,14,18,21-25] and nonunion in 2% to 27%.[14,21,23-26] Complex regional pain syndrome is thought to be caused by prolonged immobilization and is reported to

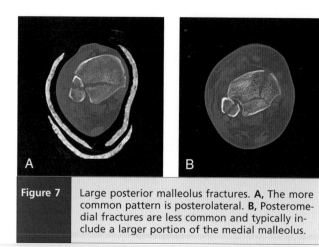

Figure 7 Large posterior malleolus fractures. **A,** The more common pattern is posterolateral. **B,** Posteromedial fractures are less common and typically include a larger portion of the medial malleolus.

occur in 2% to 4% of cases.[25,26] Radiographic evidence of arthritic change is present in up to 81% of patients 1 year after a pilon fracture[12,16] (**Figure 6**).

Rotational Ankle Fractures

Rotational ankle fractures are among the most common fractures treated by orthopaedic surgeons. Patients typically describe a twisting injury and report pain isolated to the ankle. Medical comorbidities affect outcomes and are important to document and discuss with the patient. Significant swelling or compromised soft-tissue envelopes will delay surgical treatment of unstable, displaced fractures.

Imaging

Plain radiographs, including AP, mortise, and lateral views, provide adequate radiographic evaluation for the treatment of most ankle fractures. Full-length views of the tibia are necessary to identify an associated proximal fibula fracture when ankle films indicate a widened mortise without fracture or an isolated medial malleolus fracture. In addition, when the physical examination findings are indicative of bony injury but no ankle fracture is found, other less common injuries, such as a lateral process of the talus fracture, should be considered. High-quality images allow inspection of the medial, lateral, and posterior malleoli for any bony injury. Medial clear space widening, tibiofibular overlap, and tibiofibular clear space alignment provide clues to the integrity of the deltoid ligament and the syndesmosis. External rotation stress radiographs performed in the AP or the ankle mortise plane provide additional information regarding stability. Recently, the relationship of the distal tibiofibular syndesmosis has been more accurately described with substantial variation in the anatomic normal appearance[27] and with significant sex differences in tibiofibular overlap and the anterior tibiofibular interval.[28] CT scans are helpful in cases with posterior malleolar fractures that appear large enough to require reduction and fixation. These frac-

tures can be in different planes, and the CT scan will accurately demonstrate the size of the fragment and the plane of the injury, be it posterolateral (most common) or more posteromedial (**Figure 7**).

Classification

The Danis-Weber, AO, and OTA classification systems all describe the level of the fibula fracture in relationship to the syndesmosis. Weber type A, B, and C fractures are below, at, or above the level of the joint, respectively. Although reliable and reproducible, this identifying characteristic of the fracture does not indicate ankle stability and has little value beyond identifying likely syndesmotic disruption. The Lauge-Hansen classification system (**Figure 8**) is a mechanism-based system derived from cadaver studies to improve the understanding of fracture patterns. The first element in the classification is the position of the foot at the time of the injury and the second element is the direction of the deforming force. Although interobserver and intraobserver reliability has been questioned, this system is often referenced and will aid in determining treatment plans. In addition, fractures may present with dislocation or subluxation or in a reduced position. In this situation, fractures may be stable or unstable to stress examination. The position and the stability of the fracture at presentation also guides management and should be part of any classification.

Management

Ankle fractures can be treated successfully both with and without surgery. The goal of either treatment method is to hold the ankle mortise reduced until fracture union, with equal outcomes regardless of the method used if the mortise is maintained. Indications for surgical management differ based on the location of the bony injury.

Lateral Malleolus Fractures

Oblique distal fibular fractures, Lauge-Hansen supination external rotation (SER) type 2, are associated with external rotation stress negative radiographs and can be treated nonsurgically with immediate weight bearing. Stress-positive ankle fractures may be treated either surgically or nonsurgically. A randomized trial reported equivalent functional outcomes at 1 year; however, there was a 10% loss of reduction in the nonsurgical arm.[29] A second series used a more individualized approach of ORIF for patients with greater instability, and closed treatment for those with less instability; there was no loss of reduction.[30] Isolated lateral malleolus ankle fractures that cannot be maintained with a reduced mortise in a cast have failed nonsurgical management and are indicated for surgery.

Posterolateral antiglide and lateral plating techniques are both used successfully for SER pattern ankle fractures. Although both plating techniques have benefits and risks, no agreement regarding optimal plate position exists.[31]

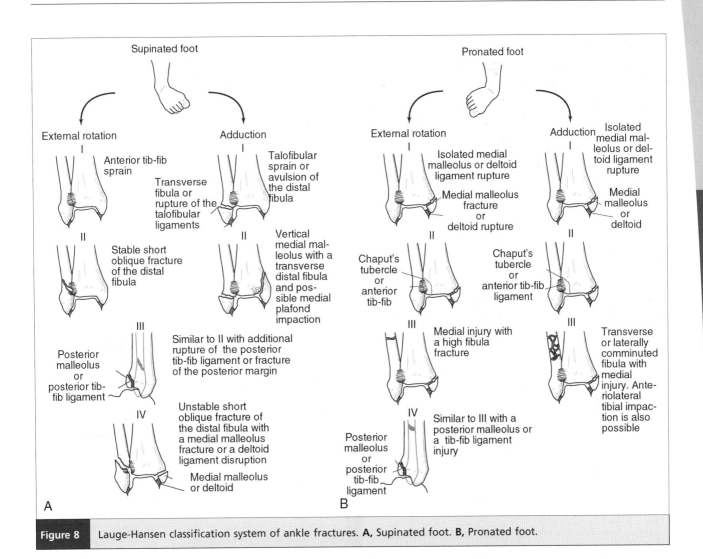

Supinated foot

External rotation — Adduction

External rotation

I
Anterior tib-fib sprain

II
Stable short oblique fracture of the distal fibula

III
Posterior malleolus or posterior tib-fib ligament

Adduction

I
Talofibular sprain or avulsion of the distal fibula

II
Vertical medial malleolus with a transverse distal fibula and possible medial plafond impaction

Transverse fibula or rupture of the talofibular ligaments

Similar to II with additional rupture of the posterior tib-fib ligament or fracture of the posterior margin

IV
Unstable short oblique fracture of the distal fibula with a medial malleolus fracture or a deltoid ligament disruption

Medial malleolus or deltoid

A

Pronated foot

External rotation — Adduction

External rotation

I
Isolated medial malleolus or deltoid ligament rupture

Medial malleolus fracture or deltoid rupture

II
Chaput's tubercle or anterior tib-fib

III
Medial injury with a high fibula fracture

IV
Similar to III with a posterior malleolus or a tib-fib ligament injury

Posterior malleolus or posterior tib-fib ligament

Adduction

I
Isolated medial malleolus or deltoid ligament rupture

Medial malleolus or deltoid

II
Chaput's tubercle or anterior tib-fib ligament

III
Transverse or laterally comminuted fibula with medial injury. Anteriolateral tibial impaction is also possible

B

Figure 8 Lauge-Hansen classification system of ankle fractures. **A,** Supinated foot. **B,** Pronated foot.

Medial Malleolus Fractures

Several types of medial malleolus fractures exist. The difference between anterior collicular fractures and supracollicular fractures is important to recognize because each provides different levels of stability to the ankle based on the attachments and the competence of the deltoid ligament.[32] Fixation of an anterior collicular fracture, with the superficial deltoid ligament attachment, will impart no additional stability to the ankle; therefore, the likely benefit of this procedure would be reduced incidence of painful nonunion. Stabilizing larger supracollicular fractures restores medial stability and also realigns the articular surface at the corner of the joint. Fixation with bicortical, fully threaded screws placed by a lag technique are biomechanically stronger and exhibit less screw loosening than partially threaded cancellous lag screws.[33] Isolated medial malleolus fractures, unless large, vertical, or associated with an articular component, can be successfully treated nonsurgically.[34] Supination adduction or vertical medial malleolar fractures behave differently and should be reduced and stabilized. These fractures have an articular component with a 42% incidence of joint impaction.[35]

Posterior Malleolus Fractures

The posterior malleolus contributes to syndesmotic stability based on the attachment site of the posterior inferior tibiofibular and inferior transverse tibiofibular ligaments.[36] Also, it carries a large articular segment, which when fractured can alter the contact pressures of the tibiotalar joint and the stability of the talus in the ankle mortise. Most posterior malleolar fractures are treated without reduction and fixation because they are small and assumed not to contribute significantly to tibiotalar stability or future posttraumatic arthritis.[37] The authors of a 2010 study favor fixation of the posterior malleolus to restore syndesmotic stability, although this method has not received wide acceptance.[38] Large fragments, classically defined as compromising greater than 25% to 30% of the articular surface, but more recently described to include a segment of the medial malleolus,[39] comprise a significant portion of the joint. A survey of surgeon practice patterns in the treatment of posterior malleolar fractures indicated that stability and large fragment size are frequently the indications for open treatment,[40] and open reduction through a posterolateral approach to the distal tibia is being more commonly used and leads to excellent access,

4: Lower Extremity

control, and results.[41] Less commonly, when the fracture pattern includes a posteromedial fragment, a posteromedial approach is needed.[42]

Syndesmosis

Instability of the distal tibiofibular syndesmosis is important to recognize and treat accurately in an attempt to avoid long-term arthrosis. Accurate diagnosis of instability, the degree of relevant instability, and evaluation of the reduction continue to be controversial. Although high fibula fractures or cases without fibula fracture that demonstrate clear syndesmotic widening are diagnostic, preoperative plain radiographs have limited use in determining syndesmotic instability in low (Weber B) fibula fractures. In addition, ankle fractures that include a posterior malleolus fragment must be carefully evaluated because this is a sign of potential instability as a result of the attachments of syndesmotic ligaments.[36] Multiple clinical tests exist to evaluate the syndesmosis, including the Cotton test, the hook test, the squeeze test, the gravity stress test, and the external rotation stress test; the interpretation of these tests is very subjective. The rate of syndesmotic instability has been reported from 11% to 40% depending on the definition used. Interestingly, even in stress positive SER type 4 injuries, the rate is unchanged.[30] An attempt to standardize the intraoperative external rotation stress test using a modified F-tool to apply 7.5-Nm torque has been described.[43] The authors of another study then compared the hook test and the external rotation stress test while using the modified F-tool device as the standard.[44] Although interobserver reliability and specificity were excellent, the sensitivity was insufficient in adequately detecting intraoperative syndesmotic instability after fixation of SER ankle fractures.

A randomized trial was performed to evaluate whether stabilization of an unstable syndesmosis is necessary in SER ankle fractures.[45] Although the study was terminated early because of a low incidence of syndesmotic injuries in the study population, leading to questions about generalizability and opening the study to type II error, the authors' conclusion that relevant syndesmotic injuries are rare introduces the concept of a spectrum of instability.[30,46]

Traditionally, position screws across the distal tibiofibular articulation are used to stabilize the syndesmosis. Recently, suture button fixation has been introduced based on the theory of preserving the micromotion of the joint to improve functional outcomes. Cadaver studies report adequate stability while allowing physiologic movement.[47] The longest clinical follow-up reported is an average of 20 months in 24 patients; radiographic reductions were maintained and the average American Orthopaedic Foot and Ankle Society (AOFAS) score was 94.[48] The definitive answer remains unknown because larger studies with long-term outcomes are still needed, but adoption should be slow because the standard methods have given excellent results.

Accurate reduction of the syndesmosis is universally agreed to be important. Given that many surgeons choose to repair the syndesmosis if there is any question of instability because cases of untreated instability have worse long-term results[49] and malreductions as small as 1.5 mm[50] also have poor results, the challenge lies in determining when an accurate reduction has been performed. A recent cadaver study supports the difficulties of intraoperative fluoroscopic detection of rotational malreductions.[51] The authors of a 2012 study reviewed 251 consecutive cases of patients with an unstable syndesmosis treated with stabilization that was deemed reduced under fluoroscopic guidance in the three standard views.[52] A three-dimensional scan was obtained of the injured ankle, and if an accurate reduction was not found, a re-reduction was performed. The authors reported no specific method of evaluation of the fluoroscopic images. The most common malreductions identified were anterior displacement of the fibula on the tibia (54%) and internal rotation of the distal fibula (24%). The importance of the lateral radiograph, with its more pronounced displacement of the fibula in relationship to the tibia with syndesmotic instability, has been previously reported[53] but seems often overlooked (**Figure 9**). Similarly, the authors of a 2012 study evaluated 68 of 107 patients with syndesmotic injury at least 2 years postinjury with radiographs and a CT scan.[27] All of the plain radiographs revealed anatomic reduction of the syndesmosis although no criteria were given; based on one reviewer's assessment, the axial CT scans showed 27 of 68 malreductions (39.7%), with the most common deformity fibular translation in the anterior-posterior plane (64%). Fewer malreductions occurred with open than percutaneous reduction, although there was no comparison of the types of injury patterns between those two groups demonstrating that they were the same.

Special Considerations
Ankle Fractures in Patients With Diabetes
Patients with diabetes who sustain an ankle fracture are a challenge to treat to union and have a well-established high risk for complications.[54-56] Nonsurgical management in a well-molded cast is not risk free because the associated diabetic neuropathy can result in a patient's inability to feel a developing pressure ulcer. In addition, diabetes increases the risk for superficial and deep infection.[54,55] A recent study compared early outcomes of 105 surgically treated ankle fractures in patients with complicated (peripheral neuropathy, nephropathy, and/or peripheral artery disease) and uncomplicated diabetes.[56] Thirty-six of the 105 patients (34.2%) had a complication; one half of the patients with complicated diabetes (23/46, 50%) had a complication compared with 13 patients (22.8%) with uncomplicated diabetes. Open fractures were associated with a higher rate of overall complications, total infections, superficial infections, and amputation. Supplemental fixation, including fibular screw fixation into the tibia, was associated with significantly fewer complications than other techniques.

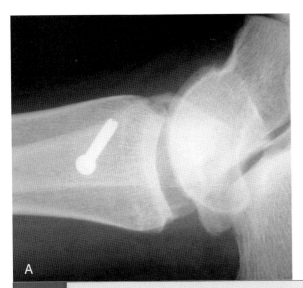
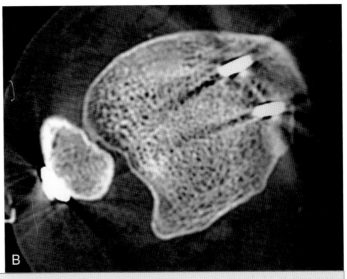

| Figure 9 | Malreduction of the distal tibiofibular syndesmosis as evident on both a lateral radiograph (**A**) and an axial CT scan (**B**). |

Ankle Fractures in Elderly Patients

Ankle fractures in the elderly are the third most common fracture in this population, after hip fractures and distal radius fractures. Previous studies have indicated that this group of patients has better outcomes when treated surgically;[57] most of these studies have not examined octogenerians. A retrospective review of 92 patients older than 80 years at the time of surgical treatment of closed or type 1 open ankle fractures was performed to evaluate postoperative mobility and complication rates.[58] Seventy-six patients (82.6%) lived independently, and 66 patients (71.7%) ambulated without an assistive device. Six patients (7%) with superficial wound infection or breakdown healed without further surgical intervention; 4 cases (4.6%) of deep infection required additional surgical treatment. By 3 to 6 months, 86% of the patients (75 of 87) had returned to preinjury mobility. The 30-day mortality was 5.4%, with death caused by cerebrovascular accident, myocardial infarction, and sepsis as a result of pneumonia.[27,28] Radiographic union occurred in 84 of 87 patients, with 1 asymptomatic medial malleolus nonunion and 2 fixation failures that required prolonged cast treatment.

Results

Outcomes

Functional and radiographic evaluation of the treatment methods of ankle fractures has been extensively researched over the past several decades. Longer term follow-up is helpful because the prevention of osteoarthritis and the restoration of patient function are ultimate goals. A recent minimum 17-year follow-up study including 148 of 276 patients with surgically and nonsurgically managed SER types 2-4 ankle fractures reported that 93% of the patients had a good Olerud score (median Olerud score 95).[59] Radiographic arthri-

tis was good or excellent in 79%, and medial clear space widening was 1 mm or less in 92%. Of the SER type 2 fractures, 23 were treated surgically and had outcomes equal to those of the 53 nonsurgically treated patients. Stress radiographs were not done at this time. Seven surgically treated patients with SER type 4 fractures did as well as the 61 patients with nonsurgically treated fractures except for range of motion; the medial injury in this group was unknown.

A similar study was done on 68 of 98 patients with pronation external rotation (PER) type 3-4 fractures sustained between 1985 and 1990 with minimum 19-year follow-up.[60] The authors reported statistically similar outcomes between the surgically and nonsurgically treated groups. Overall, the median Olerud score was 98, with 90% of the patients scoring good or excellent results. The Cedell score, a radiographic classification, showed 45 of 59 patients maintained good or excellent scores after 22 years.

Functional outcomes after malreduction of an unstable syndesmosis are known to be worse than when an accurate reduction is performed. CT scans have been used to confirm misalignment and reported worse Short Musculoskeletal Function Assessment general health questionnaire scores in that group.[27] In a prospective series of 347 patients requiring malleolar fixation, worse AOFAS function scores and worse pain scores were reported in those requiring syndesmotic fixation.[61]

The distal tibiofibular syndesmosis is a dynamic articulation; during dorsiflexion of the ankle, the distal fibula externally rotates, and the mortise widens to accommodate the wider anterior trapezoidal-shaped talus. The placement of screws across this articulation provides stability to allow an injury to heal. Because no consensus exists as to whether to remove these screws, two recent studies evaluated outcomes in association with syndesmotic screw removal. One study examined 25 patients stabilized with a locked transsyndesmotic screw construct.[62] Two weeks after screw removal, improvement in both average range of motion and functional outcomes scores was noted. The second study retrospectively evaluated outcomes on 76 patients with syndesmotic fixation.[63] Functional outcome scores for those with intact screws were less than for those with removed or compromised screws; the medial clear space and tibiofibular overlap were similar in both groups. A complication rate of 22.4% from routine screw removal at 6 to 8 weeks after fixation was reported in a retrospective study of 76 patients.[64] Recurrent syndesmotic instability was associated with the time of removal.

Chronic syndesmotic instability with evidence of radiographic arthrosis is associated with pain and dysfunction. Salvage of the ankle joint with fusion of the distal tibiofibular articulation yielded improvements in pain, function, and patient satisfaction at 2 years in a cohort of 10 patients with a previous rotational ankle fracture.[65]

Complications

The care of patients with ankle fractures is generally considered to be low risk with good outcomes expected. The discussion of possible complications is minimal until they appear. Cigarette smoking has been shown previously to affect wound and bony healing in other areas. A 2011 study investigated the effect of smoking on postoperative complications in ankle fracture patients; higher complication rates were reported in the smoking group, including 4.9% deep and 14.8% superficial infections.[55]

A thromboembolic event after a musculoskeletal injury is not uncommon and can lead to death. Prophylaxis against these events is often discussed and remains controversial with regard to ambulatory patients with surgically treated ankle fractures. The American College of Chest Physician guidelines have been extrapolated from the recommendations for arthroplasty or hip fracture patients.[66] A retrospective study on a large cohort of patients who underwent surgery for an ankle fracture reported data that supports the American College of Chest Physician statement that prophylaxis is not recommended.[67]

Summary

Fractures involving the tibial plafond denote some impaction injury to the tibial articular surface. Because these injuries usually are the result of high-energy mechanisms, compromise of the thin, soft-tissue envelope can lead to complications if certain principles of treatment are not respected. Displaced fractures should be reduced and stabilized to allow for early ankle range of motion. Two schools of thought guide treatment: either early spanning external fixation, followed by definitive internal fixation after the soft-tissue concerns have resolved, or articulated external fixation with limited joint reduction and percutaneous fixation. Radio-

graphic results in general do not predict functional outcomes, but complications will universally lead to poor outcomes.

Rotational ankle fractures are common. The management of the associated subtle nuances can affect functional outcomes. Careful evaluation of overall ankle stability and the syndesmosis is important. Avoiding complications, performing accurate reductions including the syndesmosis, and providing attentive follow-up care is necessary to improve long-term outcomes.

Key Study Points

- The issues related to the timing of surgery of pilon fractures must be understood. In general, if ORIF is to be undertaken, surgeons should wait 10 to 14 days from injury to allow soft-tissue resolution.

- The advantages and the limitations of the anterolateral and anteromedial approach to the distal tibia must be understood. There may be fewer soft-tissue complications with the anteromedial approach. With the use of locked plating, the medial buttress is less important.

- Evaluation of the distal tibiofibular syndesmosis is important and requires careful attention.

- Stress examination of Weber B SER ankle fractures presenting with an intact mortise is needed to determine deltoid ligament competence.

- Patients with diabetes who have ankle fractures require frequent follow-up care and supplemental fixation to reduce the risk of complications.

Annotated References

1. Marsh JL, Slongo TF, Agel J, et al: Fracture and dislocation classification compendium—2007: Orthopaedic Trauma Association classification, database and outcomes committee. *J Orthop Trauma* 2007;21(10, suppl):S1-S133.

2. Hak DJ: Anterolateral approach for tibial pilon fractures. *Orthopedics* 2012;35(2):131-133.

   The anterolateral approach for the treatment of tibial pilon fractures is advantageous because of improved soft-tissue coverage and the potential for fewer wound-healing complications.

3. Grose A, Gardner MJ, Hettrich C, et al: Open reduction and internal fixation of tibial pilon fractures using a lateral approach. *J Orthop Trauma* 2007;21(8):530-537.

4. Amorosa LF, Brown GD, Greisberg J: A surgical approach to posterior pilon fractures. *J Orthop Trauma* 2010;24(3):188-193.

This report describes the posterolateral approach to the tibia and the fibula. The authors also report on its use in successfully treating 15 patients with posterior fractures. Level of evidence: IV.

5. Sirkin M, Sanders R: The treatment of pilon fractures. *Orthop Clin North Am* 2001;32(1):91-102.

6. Ketz J, Sanders R: Staged posterior tibial plating for the treatment of Orthopaedic Trauma Association 43C2 and 43C3 tibial pilon fractures. *J Orthop Trauma* 2012; 26(6):341-347.

   This review of 19 patients who sustained a type B or C fracture looked at the ability of a separate staged posterior incision to enhance reduction of the posterior malleolar fragment. Ten patients with a separate posterolateral approach following an anteromedial approach were compared with a group of nine patients who underwent the anteromedial approach only. Postoperative CT showed improved articular reduction in the two-incision group. No differences, however, were seen in functional outcomes at 1 year. Level of evidence: IV.

7. Marsh JL: External fixation is the treatment of choice for fractures of the tibial plafond. *J Orthop Trauma* 1999;13(8):583-585.

8. Howard JL, Agel J, Barei DP, Benirschke SK, Nork SE: A prospective study evaluating incision placement and wound healing for tibial plafond fractures. *J Orthop Trauma* 2008;22(5):299-306.

9. Stannard JP, Robinson JT, Anderson ER, McGwin G Jr, Volgas DA, Alonso JE: Negative pressure wound therapy to treat hematomas and surgical incisions following high-energy trauma. *J Trauma* 2006;60(6):1301-1306.

10. Volgas D, DeVries JG, Stannard JP: Short-term financial outcomes of pilon fractures. *J Foot Ankle Surg* 2010; 49(1):47-51.

    This retrospective review of 25 patients who sustained pilon fractures examined financial outcomes and return to work 1 year following injury. Most patients belonged to a low socioeconomic class (salary < $40,000). Only 30% of the patients returned to work. All of the white-collar workers and 14% of the blue-collar workers returned to their preinjury employment. Sixty-five percent of the patients reported that the injury caused them financial stress. More than one half of the patients needed to apply for financial assistance. Level of evidence: IV.

11. Pollak AN, McCarthy ML, Bess RS, Agel J, Swiontkowski MF: Outcomes after treatment of high-energy tibial plafond fractures. *J Bone Joint Surg Am* 2003; 85(10):1893-1900.

12. Davidovitch RI, Elkhechen RJ, Romo S, Walsh M, Egol KA: Open reduction with internal fixation versus limited internal fixation and external fixation for high grade pilon fractures (OTA type 43C). *Foot Ankle Int* 2011;32(10):955-961.

    This single surgeon, retrospective review compared 20 patients with 21 high-grade pilon fractures treated with dynamic external fixation and limited internal fixation to a similar group of 26 patients with 26 high-grade pilon fractures. At a minimum of 1 year, no differences were seen between treatment types with regard to ankle range of motion, ultimate healing, and functional outcomes based on AOFAS and Short Musculoskeletal Function Assessment scores. However, patients who were treated with external fixation underwent more procedures and took longer to heal. Level of evidence: IV.

13. Wang C, Li Y, Huang L, Wang M: Comparison of two-staged ORIF and limited internal fixation with external fixator for closed tibial plafond fractures. *Arch Orthop Trauma Surg* 2010;130(10):1289-1297.

    Fifty-six patients who sustained a type B or C pilon fracture were treated over a 3-year period. All of the patients were initially placed in calcaneal pin traction. At a mean of 13 days, patients were randomly allocated to definitive fixation with either ORIF or closed reduction, application of a dynamic external fixator, and limited internal fixation. No differences in demographics and injury patterns existed between the groups. There were no differences in range of motion, complications, radiographs, or functional outcomes between groups based on Mazur scores. Level of evidence: IV.

14. Bacon S, Smith WR, Morgan SJ, et al: A retrospective analysis of comminuted intra-articular fractures of the tibial plafond: Open reduction and internal fixation versus external Ilizarov fixation. *Injury* 2008;39(2): 196-202.

15. Marsh JL, Weigel DP, Dirschl DR: Tibial plafond fractures: How do these ankles function over time? *J Bone Joint Surg Am* 2003;85(2):287-295.

16. White TO, Guy P, Cooke CJ, et al: The results of early primary open reduction and internal fixation for treatment of OTA 43.C-type tibial pilon fractures: A cohort study. *J Orthop Trauma* 2010;24(12):757-763.

    The authors of this study retrospectively reviewed 93 of 95 patients who sustained a high-grade pilon fracture and were treated with definitive ORIF within 48 hours of injury. Only six patients (6%) had wound dehiscence or deep infection, and four of these were open fracture cases. The radiographic and functional results were similar to the reported series. These authors suggest that, in the face of low complications, early surgery may decrease healthcare costs. Level of evidence: IV.

17. Patterson MJ, Cole JD: Two-staged delayed open reduction and internal fixation of severe pilon fractures. *J Orthop Trauma* 1999;13(2):85-91.

18. Helfet DL, Koval K, Pappas J, Sanders RW, DiPasquale T: Intraarticular "pilon" fracture of the tibia. *Clin Orthop Relat Res* 1994;298:221-228.

19. Blauth M, Bastian L, Krettek C, Knop C, Evans S: Surgical options for the treatment of severe tibial pilon fractures: A study of three techniques. *J Orthop Trauma* 2001;15(3):153-160.

4: Lower Extremity

20. Boraiah S, Kemp TJ, Erwteman A, Lucas PA, Asprinio DE: Outcome following open reduction and internal fixation of open pilon fractures. *J Bone Joint Surg Am* 2010;92(2):346-352.

Fifty-nine patients who sustained an open pilon fracture were followed for a minimum of 1 year and 38 for a minimum of 2 years. All were treated with a standard protocol. Most of the injuries were Gustillo type 3. The overall infection rate was 8%. The average Mazur foot and ankle scores were poor. There was only one amputation, which occurred because of failed soft-tissue reconstruction. Level of evidence: IV.

21. Kellam JF, Waddell JP: Fractures of the distal tibial metaphysis with intra-articular extension—the distal tibial explosion fracture. *J Trauma* 1979;19(8):593-601.

22. McCann PA, Jackson M, Mitchell ST, Atkins RM: Complications of definitive open reduction and internal fixation of pilon fractures of the distal tibia. *Int Orthop* 2011;35(3):413-418.

The authors report on a series of 49 pilon fractures in 48 patients treated by ORIF with limited soft-tissue stripping. The authors report a 2% incidence of infection, which is attributed to meticulous soft-tissue handling and a direct surgical approach to the fracture. However, 20 patients had secondary low-energy mechanisms that may represent a distinct injury from higher grade pilons. Level of evidence: IV.

23. McFerran MA, Smith SW, Boulas HJ, Schwartz HS: Complications encountered in the treatment of pilon fractures. *J Orthop Trauma* 1992;6(2):195-200.

24. Teeny SM, Wiss DA: Open reduction and internal fixation of tibial plafond fractures: Variables contributing to poor results and complications. *Clin Orthop Relat Res* 1993;292:108-117.

25. Ovadia DN, Beals RK: Fractures of the tibial plafond. *J Bone Joint Surg Am* 1986;68(4):543-551.

26. Etter C, Ganz R: Long-term results of tibial plafond fractures treated with open reduction and internal fixation. *Arch Orthop Trauma Surg* 1991;110(6):277-283.

27. Sagi HC, Shah AR, Sanders RW: The functional consequence of syndesmotic joint malreduction at a minimum 2-year follow-up. *J Orthop Trauma* 2012;26(7):439-443.

The authors of this study evaluated 68 patients with unstable syndesmotic injuries reduced and stabilized at a minimum of 2 years with clinical, radiographic, and CT scans. Malreduced injuries had worse SFMA and Olerud/Molander outcomes. The authors recommended direct, open reduction of the syndesmosis. There was no distinction in low versus high fibula fractures and no indication of whether the group with open treatment was the same as those with percutaneous management. Level of evidence: II.

28. Dikos GD, Heisler J, Choplin RH, Weber TG: Normal tibiofibular relationships at the syndesmosis on axial CT imaging. *J Orthop Trauma* 2012;26(7):433-438.

Thirty healthy volunteers received bilateral ankle CT scans to establish normal distal tibiofibular relationships. Significant sex differences were identified; however, using the contralateral ankle for comparison is reliable.

29. Sanders DW, Tieszer C, Corbett B; Canadian Orthopedic Trauma Society: Operative versus nonoperative treatment of unstable lateral malleolar fractures: A randomized multicenter trial. *J Orthop Trauma* 2012;26(3):129-134.

The authors studied 81 patients with isolated fibula fractures and showed similar functional outcomes with less risk of displacement and less delayed union or nonunion with surgical management compared with nonsurgical treatment. Level of evidence: I.

30. Tornetta P III, Axelrad W, Sibai T, Creevy W: Treatment of the stress positive ligamentous SE4 ankle fracture: Incidence of syndesmotic injury and clinical decision making. *J Orthop Trauma* 2012;26(11):659-661.

The authors report their outcomes with 114 patients with stress position ligamentous SER type 4 ankle fractures treated by shared decision making after informed consent of the advantages and the disadvantages of surgical and nonsurgical management. Almost one half of the patients (54 of 114) opted for closed management; 46% of the surgical patients (27 of 60) had an associated syndesmotic injury. All of the fractures united without medial clear space widening. Level of evidence: III.

31. Lamontagne J, Blachut PA, Broekhuyse HM, O'Brien PJ, Meek RN: Surgical treatment of a displaced lateral malleolus fracture: The antiglide technique versus lateral plate fixation. *J Orthop Trauma* 2002;16(7):498-502.

32. Tornetta P III: Competence of the deltoid ligament in bimalleolar ankle fractures after medial malleolar fixation. *J Bone Joint Surg Am* 2000;82(6):843-848.

33. Ricci WM, Tornetta P, Borrelli J Jr: Lag screw fixation of medial malleolar fractures: A biomechanical, radiographic, and clinical comparison of unicortical partially threaded lag screws and bicortical fully threaded lag screws. *J Orthop Trauma* 2012;26(10):602-606.

This cadaver and clinical study reported that two 3.5-mm fully threaded screws placed by a lag technique to stabilize medial malleolus fractures generated three times the insertion torque and had less radiographic screw loosening compared with partially threaded cancellous lag screws.

34. Herscovici D Jr, Scaduto JM, Infante A: Conservative treatment of isolated fractures of the medial malleolus. *J Bone Joint Surg Br* 2007;89-B(1):89-93.

35. McConnell T, Tornetta P III: Marginal plafond impaction in association with supination-adduction ankle fractures: A report of eight cases. *J Orthop Trauma* 2001;15(6):447-449.

36. Gardner MJ, Brodsky A, Briggs SM, Nielson JH, Lorich DG: Fixation of posterior malleolar fractures provides greater syndesmotic stability. *Clin Orthop Relat Res* 2006;447:165-171.

37. Donken CC, Goorden AJ, Verhofstad MH, Edwards MJ, van Laarhoven CJ: The outcome at 20 years of conservatively treated 'isolated' posterior malleolar fractures of the ankle: A case series. *J Bone Joint Surg Br* 2011;93-B(12):1621-1625.

    Nineteen patients with isolated posterior malleolus fractures treated closed were evaluated at 2-year follow-up; 74% had good or excellent Olerud scores. The median size of the fragment as a proportion of the tibial plafond on the lateral radiograph was 12% (range, 3% to 47%). Level of evidence: IV.

38. Miller AN, Carroll EA, Parker RJ, Helfet DL, Lorich DG: Posterior malleolar stabilization of syndesmotic injuries is equivalent to screw fixation. *Clin Orthop Relat Res* 2010;468(4):1129-1135.

    The authors prospectively treated 31 patients with ankle fractures that included a syndesmotic injury to evaluate methods of syndesmotic stabilization. The outcomes of posterior malleolus fracture stabilization were equal to locked transsyndesmotic screw fixation. Level of evidence: II.

39. Haraguchi N, Haruyama H, Toga H, Kato F: Pathoanatomy of posterior malleolar fractures of the ankle. *J Bone Joint Surg Am* 2006;88(5):1085-1092.

40. Gardner MJ, Streubel PN, McCormick JJ, Klein SE, Johnson JE, Ricci WM: Surgeon practices regarding operative treatment of posterior malleolus fractures. *Foot Ankle Int* 2011;32(4):385-393.

    Web-based questionnaires completed by 20% of the members of the OTA and the AOFAS revealed that significant variation exists regarding the treatment of posterior malleolar fractures, including factors other than fragment size, notably stability, cited as most impacting surgical decision making.

41. Tornetta P III, Ricci W, Nork S, Collinge C, Steen B: The posterolateral approach to the tibia for displaced posterior malleolar injuries. *J Orthop Trauma* 2011;25(2):123-126.

    The authors describe their technique for direct reduction and stabilization of large posterior malleolus fractures using prone positioning and the flexor hallucis longus–peroneal interval. Accurate reductions within 1 mm were achieved on all 72 patients evaluated.

42. Bois AJ, Dust W: Posterior fracture dislocation of the ankle: Technique and clinical experience using a posteromedial surgical approach. *J Orthop Trauma* 2008;22(9):629-636.

43. Jenkinson RJ, Sanders DW, Macleod MD, Domonkos A, Lydestadt J: Intraoperative diagnosis of syndesmosis injuries in external rotation ankle fractures. *J Orthop Trauma* 2005;19(9):604-609.

44. Pakarinen H, Flinkkilä T, Ohtonen P, et al: Intraoperative assessment of the stability of the distal tibiofibular joint in supination-external rotation injuries of the ankle: Sensitivity, specificity, and reliability of two clinical tests. *J Bone Joint Surg Am* 2011;93(22):2057-2061.

    The authors of this study evaluated the hook test and external rotation stress test in SER ankle fractures after internal fixation of the fracture. Interobserver reliability was excellent for both tests, but the sensitivity was insufficient to detect instability. Level of evidence: I.

45. Pakarinen HJ, Flinkkilä TE, Ohtonen PP, et al: Syndesmotic fixation in supination-external rotation ankle fractures: A prospective randomized study. *Foot Ankle Int* 2011;32(12):1103-1109.

    The authors performed a prospective comparative study of 140 patients with SER type 4 ankle fractures with positive stress tests after bony fixation randomized to syndesmotic fixation with 3.5-mm screw or no fixation. Twenty-four patients (17%) were stress positive; Olerud and visual analog scale pain scores did not differ between the groups at 1 year. Level of evidence: II.

46. Hoshino CM, Nomoto EK, Norheim EP, Harris TG: Correlation of weightbearing radiographs and stability of stress positive ankle fractures. *Foot Ankle Int* 2012;33(2):92-98.

    Thirty-eight patients with stress positive ankle fractures were treated in a short leg walking cast, reevaluated 7 days later with weight-bearing radiographs, and then treated definitively based on the standing films. Three patients converted to surgical management because of medial clear space widening. The average AOFAS score was 98 at final follow-up. Level of evidence: IV.

47. Klitzman R, Zhao H, Zhang LQ, Strohmeyer G, Vora A: Suture-button versus screw fixation of the syndesmosis: A biomechanical analysis. *Foot Ankle Int* 2010;31(1):69-75.

    Using cadavers, the authors evaluated the biomechanical properties of the intact syndesmosis, suture button stabilized syndesmosis, and tricortical transsyndemotic screw stabilization. After submaximal load cycling, the suture button fixation maintained reduction while allowing physiologic fibular movement as compared to screw fixation.

48. Degroot H, Al-Omari AA, El Ghazaly SA: Outcomes of suture button repair of the distal tibiofibular syndesmosis. *Foot Ankle Int* 2011;32(3):250-256.

    The authors of this study present a case series with an average 20-month follow-up and evaluate suture button repair of unstable syndesmotic injuries, reporting an average AOFAS score of 94 and no loss of reduction. The authors note unexpected local irritation requiring hardware removal and osteolysis of the bone around the suture button construct. Level of evidence: IV.

49. Leeds HC, Ehrlich MG: Instability of the distal tibiofibular syndesmosis after bimalleolar and trimalleolar ankle fractures. *J Bone Joint Surg Am* 1984;66(4):490-503.

4: Lower Extremity

50. Wikerøy AK, Høiness PR, Andreassen GS, Hellund JC, Madsen JE: No difference in functional and radiographic results 8.4 years after quadricortical compared with tricortical syndesmosis fixation in ankle fractures. *J Orthop Trauma* 2010;24(1):17-23.

The authors provide mean 8.4-year follow-up of a randomized controlled trial of comparing types of syndesmotic screw fixation. Similar outcomes between groups are reported with the presence of a posterior fracture fragment indicative of a poorer outcomes. Level of evidence: II.

51. Marmor M, Hansen E, Han HK, Buckley J, Matityahu A: Limitations of standard fluoroscopy in detecting rotational malreduction of the syndesmosis in an ankle fracture model. *Foot Ankle Int* 2011;32(6):616-622.

The authors fluoroscopically evaluated syndesmotic malreductions in cadavers and reported radiographic indices, including tibiofibular clear space, tibiofibular overlap, and posterior fibular subluxation, could not detect external rotation malreductions of up to 30°.

52. Franke J, von Recum J, Suda AJ, Grützner PA, Wendl K: Intraoperative three-dimensional imaging in the treatment of acute unstable syndesmotic injuries. *J Bone Joint Surg Am* 2012;94(15):1386-1390.

The authors of this study evaluated three-dimensional imaging compared with standard fluoroscopy in detecting syndesmotic malreduction. The authors found that conventional images cannot reliably evaluate correct positioning of the distal fibula into the incisura. The authors recommend intraoperative or postoperative three-dimensional imaging. Level of evidence: III.

53. Xenos JS, Hopkinson WJ, Mulligan ME, Olson EJ, Popovic NA: The tibiofibular syndesmosis: Evaluation of the ligamentous structures, methods of fixation, and radiographic assessment. *J Bone Joint Surg Am* 1995; 77(6):847-856.

54. SooHoo NF, Krenek L, Eagan MJ, Gurbani B, Ko CY, Zingmond DS: Complication rates following open reduction and internal fixation of ankle fractures. *J Bone Joint Surg Am* 2009;91(5):1042-1049.

55. Nåsell H, Ottosson C, Törnqvist H, Lindé J, Ponzer S: The impact of smoking on complications after operatively treated ankle fractures—a follow-up study of 906 patients. *J Orthop Trauma* 2011;25(12):748-755.

A cohort study of 906 patients with ankle fracture comparing postoperative complications in smokers versus nonsmokers is presented. Smokers were more likely to develop any complication (30.1% versus 20.3%, P = 0.005) and deep infection (4.9% vs 0.8%, P < 0.001) than nonsmokers.

56. Wukich DK, Joseph A, Ryan M, Ramirez C, Irrgang JJ: Outcomes of ankle fractures in patients with uncomplicated versus complicated diabetes. *Foot Ankle Int* 2011; 32(2):120-130.

A retrospective review of 105 patients with diabetes and ankle fractures comparing complications in those with complicated versus uncomplicated diabetes is presented. Complicated diabetes carried a 3.8 times increased risk of complication and a five times higher likelihood of needing additional procedures.

57. Ali MS, McLaren CA, Rouholamin E, O'Connor BT: Ankle fractures in the elderly: Nonoperative or operative treatment. *J Orthop Trauma* 1987;1(4):275-280.

58. Shivarathre DG, Chandran P, Platt SR: Operative fixation of unstable ankle fractures in patients aged over 80 years. *Foot Ankle Int* 2011;32(6):599-602.

A retrospective review of 92 patients older than 80 years with closed or type 1 open unstable ankle fractures revealed surgical management yielded a return to preinjury mobility status in 86% and a 30-day mortality of 5.4%.

59. Donken CC, Verhofstad MH, Edwards MJ, van Laarhoven CJ: Twenty-one-year follow-up of supination-external rotation type II-IV (OTA type B) ankle fractures: A retrospective cohort study. *J Orthop Trauma* 2012;26(8):e108-e114.

A retrospective, cohort study with 21-year follow-up of 148 of 276 patients treated both surgically and nonsurgically who had SER ankle fractures revealed good or excellent Olerud scores in 92%. No outcome differences were reported between the treatment methods or between the type of fractures. Level of evidence: IV.

60. Donken CC, Verhofstad MH, Edwards MJ, van Laarhoven CJ: Twenty-two-year follow-up of pronation external rotation type III-IV (OTA type C) ankle fractures: A retrospective cohort study. *J Orthop Trauma* 2012; 26(8):e115-e122.

Median 22-year follow-up is reported in this retrospective cohort study of PER ankle fractures treated both surgically and nonsurgically. Good or excellent Olerud scores were reported in 90%, with no differences based on treatment method. Level of evidence: III.

61. Egol KA, Pahk B, Walsh M, Tejwani NC, Davidovitch RI, Koval KJ: Outcome after unstable ankle fracture: Effect of syndesmotic stabilization. *J Orthop Trauma* 2010;24(1):7-11.

Outcomes were evaluated in 347 patients with ankle fractures with syndesmotic disruption (N = 79, 23%) compared with those with an intact syndesmosis (N = 268, 77%). At 12 months, the outcomes were worse in the group that required both malleolar fixation and syndesmotic fixation. Level of evidence: III.

62. Miller AN, Paul O, Boraiah S, Parker RJ, Helfet DL, Lorich DG: Functional outcomes after syndesmotic screw fixation and removal. *J Orthop Trauma* 2010; 24(1):12-16.

Functional outcomes were evaluated before and after syndesmotic screw removal in 25 patients with unstable ankle fractures that included MRI-diagnosed syndesmotic injury. Range of motion and outcome scores were improved, and no radiographic loss of reduction was reported after hardware removal. Level of evidence: IV.

63. Manjoo A, Sanders DW, Tieszer C, MacLeod MD: Functional and radiographic results of patients with

syndesmotic screw fixation: Implications for screw re-moval. *J Orthop Trauma* 2010;24(1):2-6.

Ankle fracture treatment, including syndesmotic screw fixation, in 106 patients was retrospectively reviewed to compare the outcomes regarding intact screws with loose, fractured, or removed screws. Intact screws are associated with a worse outcome; there is no difference between loose, fractured, or removed screws. Level of evidence: IV.

64. Schepers T, Van Lieshout EM, de Vries MR, Van der Elst M: Complications of syndesmotic screw removal. *Foot Ankle Int* 2011;32(11):1040-1044.

Complications of syndesmotic screw removal were ret-rospectively evaluated in 76 patients. Infection occurred in 9.2%. Recurrent syndesmotic instability was reported in 6.6%. Screws were removed by protocol at 6 to 8 weeks; the authors recommended delaying removal until at least 8 to 12 weeks. Level of evidence: IV.

65. Olson KM, Dairyko GH Jr, Toolan BC: Salvage of chronic instability of the syndesmosis with distal tibio-fibular arthrodesis: Functional and radiographic results. *J Bone Joint Surg Am* 2011;93(1):66-72.

Ten patients with chronic syndesmotic instability who underwent fusion were reviewed after 2 years. All pa-tients reported satisfaction with the procedure and a willingness to undergo it again because it improved pain, activity, and maximum walking distance. Level of evidence: IV.

66. Geerts WH, Pineo GF, Heit JA, et al: Prevention of ve-nous thromboembolism: The seventh ACCP conference on antithrombotic and thrombolytic theray. *Chest* 2004;126(3, suppl):338S-400S.

67. Pelet S, Roger ME, Belzile EL, Bouchard M: The inci-dence of thromboembolic events in surgically treated ankle fracture. *J Bone Joint Surg Am* 2012;94(6):502-506.

A retrospective study of 2,478 patients evaluated throm-boembolic events and risk factors in ambulatory ankle fracture patients and revealed that clinically detectable events after surgery are uncommon. These events do not appear to be influenced by the use of prophylaxis. In a subgroup with at least one risk factor, the event rate also was not influenced by the use of thromboprophylaxis. Level of evidence: III.

4: Lower Extremity

Chapter 44

Foot Trauma

David B. Karges, DO

4: Lower Extremity

Introduction

The foot is a dynamic structure. Gait begins as the hindfoot receives load following heel strike. The gastrocnemius-soleus and tibialis posterior muscles contract to invert the heel-locking midtarsal joints, creating a rigid lever with which to promote locomotion. As the body axis advances forward over the midfoot, momentum is generated with the power of toe-off, propelling the forefoot and the body forward. When this single-stance gait cycle ends, the midtarsus unlocks and the ipsilateral foot swings forward, allowing the contralateral foot to perform its cycle.

Injury severity associated with foot trauma depends on the energy associated with the injury mechanism; the severity of chondral, bone, and soft-tissue damage; and their eventual influence on lower extremity function. The practical application of all posttraumatic foot reconstruction, acute and delayed, is to protect joint motion and increase stability necessary for normal gait. These goals are achieved through advances in fracture fixation and surgical soft-tissue management and improved techniques in anatomic reduction of hindfoot and midfoot trauma, which play key roles in the return to preinjury status.

Talar Fractures

Fractures and dislocations of the talus present a surgical challenge to orthopaedic surgeons because of the nature of the displacement patterns and the fact that bone is partially concealed by adjacent osseous articulations. Depending on the clinical practice, these injuries may be seen infrequently. Open reduction and internal fixation (ORIF) is generally mandatory for displaced fractures to restore talar anatomy precisely and allow early motion. The outcomes of talar fractures correlate with injury severity.[1,2] Outcome variables include ankle and subtalar joint stiffness, posttraumatic arthrosis, and osteonecrosis of the talus.

Neither Dr. Karges nor any immediate family member has received anything of value from or has stock or stock options held in a commercial company or institution related directly or indirectly to the subject of this chapter.

Anatomy

The talus receives its blood supply from each of the three main vessels perfusing the foot and the ankle: the posterior tibial, dorsalis pedis, and peroneal arteries.[3,4] Disruption of talar circulation correlates with fracture displacement, fracture-dislocation, and open injuries, leading to increased risks for osteonecrosis. A 2011 latex injection cadaver study evaluated talar vascularity using gadolinium-enhanced MRI followed by gross dissection. The results showed that the peroneal artery contributed 17% of talar perfusion, the anterior tibial artery contributed 36%, and the posterior tibial artery contributed 47%.[5] The study demonstrated substantial vascular contribution to the posterior talus, which helps explain why talar neck fractures may not result in osteonecrosis (Figures 1 and 2).

Knowledge of talar blood supply is of substantial value when planning surgical approaches for fracture

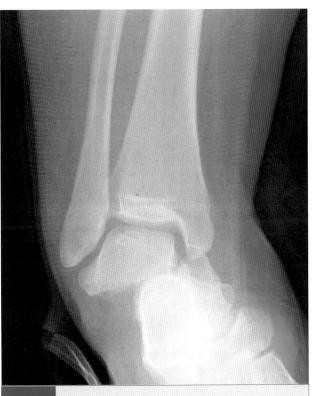

Figure 1   Radiograph showing a displaced Hawkins type II talar neck fracture.

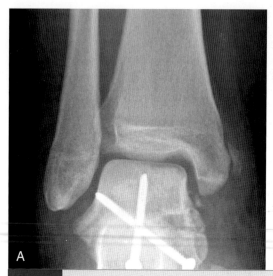
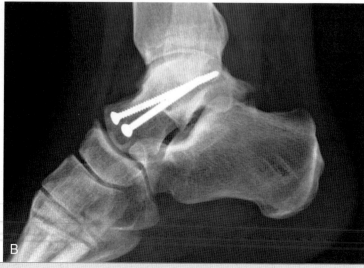

Figure 2 **A,** AP view obtained 6 weeks postoperatively shows talar dome Hawkins sign. **B,** Lateral view obtained at 2 years postoperatively shows limited ankle and subtalar arthrosis.

reconstruction. An anteromedial and anterolateral (dual-incision) approach is a well-regarded technique for repairing displaced fractures of the talar head, neck, and body.[6] Upon initial impression of this dual-incision approach, surgeons may perceive disregard for the biology of the bone and its extraosseous blood supply, but neither plantar nor direct dorsal circulation to the talus is violated. If a reconstruction requires fixation of a talar dome fracture, a medial malleolar osteotomy must be planned to gain exposure and preserve circulation from the talar dome's artery of the tarsal canal.[7]

Imaging

Three-view ankle radiographs provide routine evaluation of a talar fracture. A Canale view (foot internally rotated 15° with the x-ray beam tilted 15° cephalad) is recommended with minimally displaced fractures to assess talar neck alignment.[8] Because of the high-energy nature of a talar fracture, a three-view series of the foot should be a standard addition to this imaging protocol. Posteromedial fractures of the talus are reliably identified by implementing a 30° external rotation view.

CT is valuable to determine nondisplacement of the talar neck when deciding on nonsurgical management or when planning the reconstruction of talar body fractures. CT has been reported as the most precise method with which to measure postoperative malunion and rotational deformity of the talar neck.[9]

Immediate Management of Talus Fractures

All open fractures of the talus are an emergency. One study surveying the opinion of orthopaedic trauma experts on closed, displaced fractures of the talar neck concluded that the fracture is safely managed in an early but not emergent manner following adequate closed reduction with splinting.[10] It is important to differentiate compromised extraosseous blood flow of the talar body from neurovascular injury, soft-tissue injury,

or a severe pressure phenomenon to the skin envelope of the hindfoot attributable to a talar fracture as an orthopaedic emergency.

No consensus exists regarding the most appropriate treatment of the extruded talus. This is an uncommon injury with a potentially ominous prognosis. A report evaluating sterile reimplantation of an extruded talus injury identified definitive external fixation as an effective immediate option to treat the dislocated talus.[11]

Fractures of the Talar Neck

Fractures of the talar neck are defined as fractures anterior to the lateral process of the talus. A previous study of vertical fractures of the talar neck characterized an injury of extraosseous perfusion to the bone by classifying three types of talar neck fractures.[12]

A type I fracture is nondisplaced, with disruption of blood flow limited to the anterolateral region of the bone. A nondisplaced fracture of the talar neck is best determined by a CT scan. A type II fracture is associated with posterior subluxation of the body, with possible dislocation of the subtalar joint. In a type III injury, the transverse fracture of the talar neck is associated with dislocation of the talar body. A talar neck fracture-dislocation of the body with an associated talonavicular dislocation is classified as a type IV injury.

A type I fracture can be managed nonsurgically with cast immobilization and nonweight-bearing activity, but surgical treatment controls late displacement of the fracture and allows patients early range of motion. If treated surgically, a type I fracture conveniently allows posterior to anterior percutaneous screw fixation.[13] ORIF using the dual anteromedial and anterolateral approach and countersunk interfragmentary screw fixation and mini-fragment periarticular talar neck plating is the recommended fixation for displaced talar neck injuries.[14,15]

Fractures of the Talar Body

Talar body fractures are defined as fractures extending posterior to the lateral process. Reconstruction of the talar body fracture is best performed using the dual anteromedial and anterolateral approach, with the addition of a medial malleolar osteotomy.[16] Fracture patterns of the body of the talus occur in both the coronal and sagittal planes. Countersunk small and minifragment cortical screws and headless screws are effective forms of fixation.

Lateral Process and Posterior Talar Body Fractures

Isolated lateral process fragments with extension into the subtalar joint are best repaired with interfragmentary bicortical mini-screw fixation. Comminuted lateral process fractures should be additionally buttressed laterally by mini-screw and plate fixation to resist displacement.

Small extra-articular posteromedial talar ligamentous avulsion fractures, which precipitate secondary to a violent dislocation of the flexor hallucis longus tendon, are routinely managed nonsurgically with nonweight-bearing activity and cast immobilization for 4 weeks, followed by protected weight bearing and active range of motion for 3 weeks. Larger, intra-articular posterior talar body fractures, which may involve up to one third of the body, are wisely treated surgically in a prone position. Initially, a temporary medial external fixator that is placed to distract the ankle and the subtalar joint is followed by medial or lateral approaches, reduction, interfragmentary posterior-to-anterior minifragment screw fixation, and mini-buttress plating.

Postoperative Care

Patients treated nonsurgically for type I talar neck fractures are immobilized in a short-leg, non–weight-bearing cast for 8 weeks. Nonsurgical management of isolated talar process fractures requires similar cast immobilization for 4 to 6 weeks with subsequent application of a removable fracture boot and gradual progressive weight bearing in the boot until full weight bearing is tolerated.

Postoperative care should dictate 8 weeks of protected non–weight-bearing activity in a removable fracture boot to allow early motion. The Hawkins sign can be visualized with an AP radiograph of the ankle at 6 to 8 weeks postinjury. This sign is identified when an early subchondral radiolucent transverse line to the body of the talus is detected. Its presence indicates bone resorption, which is a biologic process requiring vascularity and documented to have a radiographic accuracy as a predictor of osteonecrosis of 75%.[1] The lack of a Hawkins sign does not confirm osteonecrosis. Patients surgically treated for fractures of the talar neck should begin progressive weight bearing at 8 weeks. There are no data to support extended periods of non–weight-bearing activity in patients with partial osteonecrosis of the talar dome. The effect of weight bearing on the progression of osteonecrosis is unknown. It is recommended that patients with fractures of the dome and body of the talus avoid weight-bearing activity for up to 12 weeks.

Outcomes

Data evaluating the surgical timing of talar fractures maintain that there is no association between surgical delay and osteonecrosis, provided an early reduction of the talar fracture is achieved.[12] Risk factors leading to poorer functional outcomes include comminution, higher Hawkins classification, open fracture, and associated ipsilateral lower extremity injuries.[2]

Osteonecrosis of the talus, posttraumatic arthrosis, joint stiffness, and varus malalignment of the hindfoot secondary to fractures of the talus negatively influence outcomes. Studies evaluating talar neck fractures maintain an overall 50% incidence of osteonecrosis, with evidence of collapse of the talar dome in approximately 30% of the cases.[17] Posttraumatic arthrosis associated with talar neck fractures is more common and predominates in the subtalar joint. Ankle arthrosis is seen in combination with subtalar joint degeneration but has not been found to be an isolated complication associated with these injuries. Reports of talar body fractures show that the incidence of osteonecrosis increases with the severity of the injury, with most patients displaying radiographic osteonecrosis and posttraumatic arthrosis.

Calcaneal Fractures

The calcaneus is the largest bone in the foot and commonly is fractured as a result of direct axial loading and shear mechanisms, such as when the talus comes into contact with the calcaneus after a height-related fall, or when there is a high-energy intrusion to the floor panel of a car. During the initial clinical evaluation of calcaneal fractures, the axial skeleton must be inspected, particularly the low thoracic and high lumbar spine for associated compression fractures. The internal design of the os calcis features powerful superomedial cortical thickness (3 to 5 mm) in the region of the sustentaculum, superolaterally in the anterior process of the calcaneus and anterolaterally in the posterior facet and the posteroinferior tuberosity, reflecting the bone's key weight-bearing components. These regions of calcaneal bone play a significant role when reconstructing fractures of the os calcis.

Management

Nonsurgical treatment of os calcis fractures is suitable for simple fractures with displacement of the posterior facet less than 2 mm; contraindications include a neuropathic foot and ankle, severe peripheral vascular disease, a history of hindfoot infection, and, possibly, tobacco smoking. The benefits of nonsurgical care for patients at least 50 years of age have been documented.[18,19] A 2010 study compared outcomes of surgically treated patients older than 50 years with a cohort of surgical patients younger than 50 years. Contrary to

4: Lower Extremity

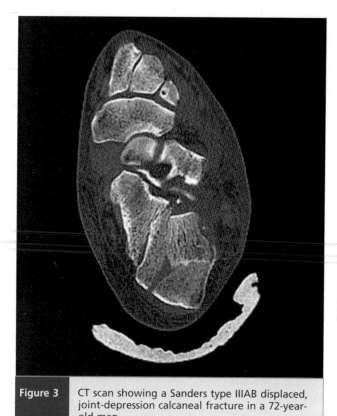

Figure 3   CT scan showing a Sanders type IIIAB displaced, joint-depression calcaneal fracture in a 72-year-old man.

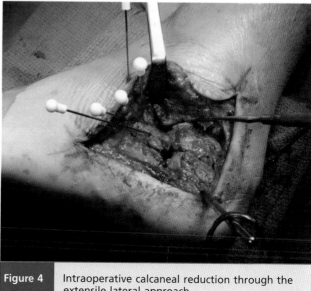

Figure 4   Intraoperative calcaneal reduction through the extensile lateral approach.

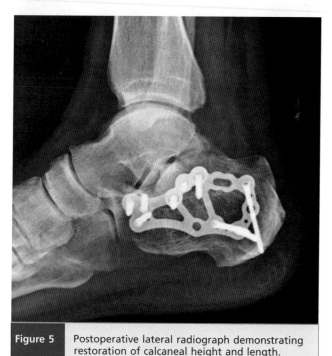

Figure 5   Postoperative lateral radiograph demonstrating restoration of calcaneal height and length.

studies analyzed the biomechanical performance of locking versus nonlocking calcaneal plates in osteoporotic bone models. No significant difference was revealed between the two plating systems.[21,22]

Nonsurgical treatment of an acute os calcis fracture initially involves the application of a compressive bulky Jones dressing with a posterior splint for approximately 2 weeks. Afterward, the patient's treatment should include elevation, a removable splint, and absolute non–weight-bearing activity with daily active ankle and subtalar motion for 8 to 12 weeks. Reported long-term follow-up of nonsurgically treated calcaneal fractures at 20 years revealed 53% of the patients had fair to poor results.[23] A randomized trial comparing the outcomes of surgical and nonsurgical articular fractures of the calcaneus reported that subtablar fusions developed in 17% of the nonsurgically treated patients, compared with 3% of surgically treated patients.[24]

Displaced intra-articular fractures of the calcaneus are clear indications for surgical treatment. A recent meta-analysis synthesizing data of six randomized and four controlled clinical trials evaluating ORIF versus nonsurgical treatment in 891 patients identified better anatomic and functional outcomes with the surgical groups. However, complications were significantly more common in the surgical groups. Meticulous soft-tissue management is critical, with 25% complication rates reported when the extensile exposure is used.[25]

The tongue-type calcaneal pattern maintains a connection between the tuberosity and, possibly, the entire posterior facet, yet an extra-articular pattern may present with the tuberosity segment, extending posterosuperiorly just behind the posterior articular facet. These tongue patterns of the calcaneus are commonly amenable to indirect reduction and percutaneous fixation, yet even open reductions of a tongue-type calcaneal fracture can prove challenging to anatomically reduce in

older studies, the functional outcomes of those older than 50 years were significantly better than for the younger group. The authors concluded that chronologic age does not appear to be a contraindication for surgery[20] (Figures 3, 4, and 5). In addition, two 2011

select cases. A 2012 study identified a helpful intraoperative open technique to convert a challenging tongue-type fracture into a joint-depression pattern by way of an oblique osteotomy through the posterosuperior tongue fragment, which allows removal of the posterior facet segment.[26] The most posterior tongue component may be rotated out of the way, allowing an anatomic repositioning of the posterior facet fragment and subsequent reduction of the osteotomized tongue fragments.[26] Percutaneous reduction and screw fixation of Sanders types IIB, IIC, and III intra-articular fractures of the os calcis have resulted in nonsignificant trends toward fewer wound complications and the ability to maintain overall fracture reduction without plate fixation.[27,28] A 2011 randomized study compared ORIF without grafting in 45 cases to percutaneous reduction with calcium sulfate grafting in 45 cases using both 6.5-mm and 3.5-mm screw fixation. Sanders types IIB, IIC, and III fractures were inclusion criteria. The percutaneous group had less blood loss, and at 24 months, the patients displayed better ankle and subtalar motion and improved outcome scoring (American Orthopaedic Foot and Ankle Society [AOFAS] score and Maryland Foot Score). There was no difference in wound infection, Bohler angle, or calcaneal length and width between treatment groups.[29] However, the authors did not discuss assessing articular reduction and presence of arthrosis.

Indirect percutaneous reduction and fixation of calcaneal fractures must be performed selectively and with extreme caution. The ability to directly visualize, reduce, and fix calcaneal fractures through an open approach leads to a more accurate reduction and, possibly, improved control of patient outcomes.

Midfoot Fractures

Midfoot fractures and dislocations are historically uncommon, with little outcome reported in the orthopaedic literature. The most frequently injured tarsal bone is the navicular; however, isolated fractures and dislocations of the midfoot are the exception rather than the rule. To avoid overlooking foot injuries, a three-view series of foot radiographs is required for diagnosis. Clinical evaluation, however, will play a large role in diagnosing subtle injuries. A CT scan is a valuable tool with which to identify ligamentous injury in an isolated, injured foot with midfoot swelling, plantar ecchymosis, and pain but no obvious sign of fracture.

Fractures of the Tarsal Navicular

The navicular articulates with all four tarsal bones, including the talus and the calcaneus. Because of its extensive chondral articulations, extraosseous perfusion is limited to the medial, plantar, and dorsal surfaces, which are compromised with any fracture to the bone.

Body fractures are commonly the result of increased energy and were further subclassified into three types.[30] A type I fracture is transverse in the coronal plane. A

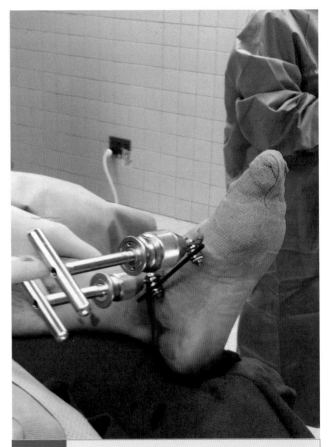

Figure 6 | A temporary medial column spanning external fixator is shown.

displaced dorsal fragment may create pressure compromise to the skin envelope if not reduced promptly. A simple type I fracture does not present with medial column shortening and is managed with a limited medial incision to achieve fracture reduction while percutaneously fixed with dorsal-to-plantar interfragmentary screw fixation.

A type II body fracture is comminuted plantar-medial, extending dorsally-laterally. The dorsal-medial segment displaces medially at the time of injury, shortening the inside column of the midfoot. The type III fracture is commonly mutifragmentary with central comminution of the body, which shortens the medial column of the midfoot. This injury is associated with cuboid fractures, which shorten the lateral column of the midfoot as well. Loss of midfoot alignment in type II and III navicular body fractures is associated with intense swelling, which precludes safe, immediate ORIF. A medial external fixator spanning the neck of the talus and the base of the first metatarsal will maintain column length until soft tissues allow an index procedure (Figure 6). Plain radiographs provide an understanding of the fracture type, but a CT scan after external fixation is recommended for surgical planning (Figure 7). Reconstruction of the navicular by open reduction and mini-fragment plate-screw or medial bridge-plate fixation is recommended[31] (Figure 8).

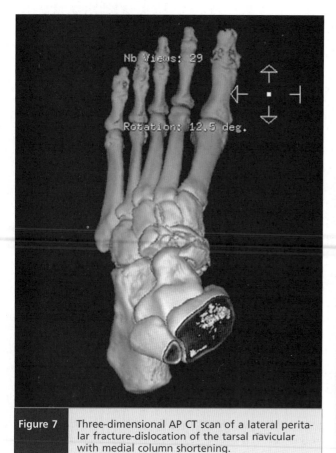

Figure 7 Three-dimensional AP CT scan of a lateral peritalar fracture-dislocation of the tarsal navicular with medial column shortening.

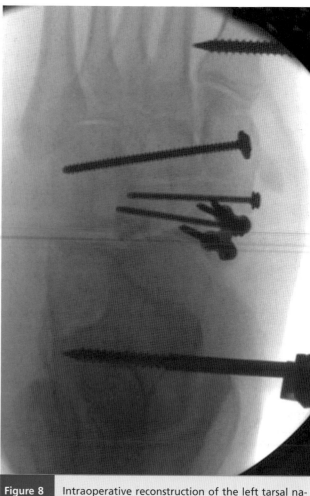

Figure 8 Intraoperative reconstruction of the left tarsal navicular is shown.

Postoperatively, the patient does not bear weight for 10 to 12 weeks. The medial column of the midfoot is supported long-term with a full-length orthotic and rocker-bottom sole modification of the shoe. Secondary talonavicular and naviculocuneiform arthrosis is best managed by medial column midfoot arthrodesis.

In a recent study evaluating mini-plate fixation of 24 navicular body fractures with only 9 patients sustaining isolated navicular fractures, all of the fractures healed with no deep infection. No patient underwent a secondary midfoot fusion.[32]

Fractures of the Cuboid

The cuboid is the only lateral column bone of the midfoot and a stabilizer to the lateral longitudinal arch of the foot. The bone articulates with the calcaneus, the navicular, the lateral cuneiform, and the lateral two metatarsals. Fracture mechanisms are associated with direct lateral forefoot forces and indirect abduction forces received from the medial column.[33] Injury to the cuboid is routinely diagnosed with radiographs of the foot. The oblique image best depicts the lateral column length of the bone. If surgery is planned, a CT scan may be indicated to determine the fracture pattern, comminution, and implant selection.

Displaced fractures with articular impaction are strong indications for surgery. These injuries present with severe soft-tissue swelling, which warrants a staged approach with early spanning external fixation of the calcaneus to the base of the fifth metatarsal. This approach preserves alignment and lateral column length while tissue swelling resolves.[34] ORIF is considered the standard of care for displaced fractures; however, the spanning external fixator or the transarticular spanning internal fixator also are treatment options.[35] The bridging internal fixator should be removed after healing.

Postoperative complications associated with the management of cuboid fractures include sural neuritis, delay in soft-tissue incision healing, painful hardware, arthrosis, nonunion, and loss of lateral column length. It is important to manage these complications. Sural neuritis commonly resolves without treatment but can be treated medically with agents that suppress somatic nerve pain and the application of adhesive patches that transdermally emanate local anesthetic. In a recalcitrant case, a supramalleolar sural neurectomy may be recommended. Delay in soft-tissue healing commonly requires only local wound care, but outpatient use of a negative pressure wound dressing can exacerbate the

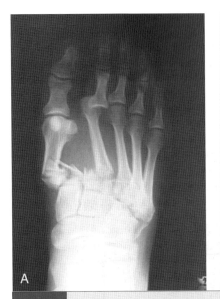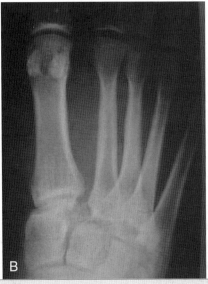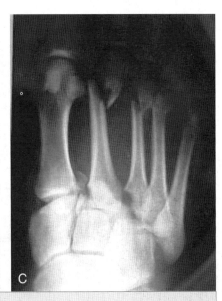

Figure 9 Radiographs showing the classification of TMT injuries. **A,** Divergent pattern. **B,** Isolated pattern. **C,** Homolateral pattern.

problem. Nonunion is best managed by bone graft and revision fixation. Arthrosis of the fourth and fifth tarsometatarsal (TMT) joints presents a difficult problem. All attempts must be made to avoid TMT fusion. Severe lateral midfoot pain is often the result of secondary arthrosis to both the medial and lateral columns of the midfoot; clinicians must look for a short lateral column. If such a column is present, counseling regarding a medial column fusion and a cuboid osteotomy with lengthening of the lateral column is needed because this procedure can substantially improve patient symptoms.

TMT Fracture-Dislocations

Adult TMT injuries were rarely reported in the early literature, with a reported incidence of 1 per 55,000 yearly.[36] Anecdotal views among contemporary level I orthopaedic trauma and academic foot and ankle services providers, however, indicate underrepresentation of the incidence of this injury. There is a spectrum of TMT bone, ligamentous, and combined-injury patterns ranging from intermetatarsal sprain to pure ligamentous dislocation to irreducible fracture-dislocation of the TMT joints with tendon interposition. Subluxated and dislocated TMT injuries, whether partial or complete, are indications for surgical management. The transverse arch of the midfoot is an inherently stable construct, but when disrupted, the flat vertical joints of the metatarsal base will assume a displaced, subluxed position, and, if left malreduced, subside, with motion poorly tolerated by the patient.

Anatomy

The intermetatarsal ligaments are divided into dorsal, plantar, and interosseous fibers, of which the intermetatarsal interosseous ligaments are the most powerful stabilizers for the second through fifth TMT joints.[37] There is no intermetatarsal ligament between the first and second metatarsal bases. Plantar ligaments are stronger than dorsal ligaments, which likely contribute to the common dorsal direction of dislocation.[38] The intimate bony interposition of the medial and middle intercuneiforms and their ligamentous attachments, the TMT capsules, the dorsal and plantar intrinsic muscles, the distal transverse ligaments, the plantar fascia, and the peroneal tendons, are secondary stabilizers of the TMT joints.

Mechanism of Injury

There are two types of injury mechanisms: direct and indirect. The direct mechanism is commonly a crush injury associated with a high-energy blunt force to the dorsum of the midfoot. Indirect injury is most commonly attributable to hindfoot axial loading of a plantar flexed foot or a fixed hindfoot with abduction force to the forefoot.

Classification

More than one classification system exists. The initial classification was first documented in 1909, and divergent, isolated, and homolateral patterns were identified[39] (**Figure 9**). Currently, a columnar classification identifies three mechanical columns of the foot.[40-42] The medial column consists of the first TMT joint and the medial naviculocuneiform joints. The middle column is composed of the second and third TMT joints, the middle and lateral cuneiforms, and the navicular. The lateral column is defined by the fourth and fifth TMT articulations and the cuboid. These classifications describe injury patterns but provide little to no information regarding management or prognosis.

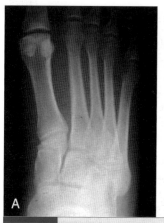
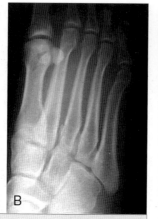

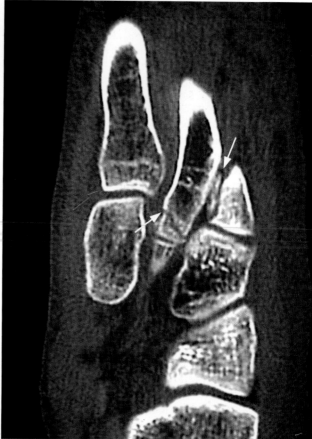

Figure 10   **A,** AP radiograph of the right TMT joints without obvious displacement. **B,** Oblique radiograph of a subtle second TMT subluxation and medial avulsion of the third metatarsal base.

Diagnosis

Acutely, patients with a high-energy TMT injury will present with intense circumferential midfoot swelling and deformity. Radiographically, laterally displaced fracture-dislocations of the second through fifth TMT joints are common presentations. A first TMT joint injury may show either medial or lateral displacement. An intercuneiform injury is best defined by a gap between the medial and middle cuneiforms. With severe pain and foot swelling, a concurrent foot compartment syndrome diagnosis can be determined by loss of plantar sensation and increased pain with the passive dorsiflexion of digits. An assessment of compartment pressures is warranted if the diagnosis is uncertain or if a patient cannot assist in the examination.

The diagnosis of a low-energy indirect TMT injury is far less straightforward. Immediate swelling may be mild; however, diagnosis of the injury is associated with a patient being unable to bear weight, with a display of plantar ecchymosis. Radiographic diagnosis requires AP, lateral, and 30° oblique views of the foot. The AP view evaluates the first and second TMT joints, and an oblique view assesses the lateral three TMT articulations. The first metatarsal should be centrally aligned with no lateralization. The medial cortex of the second metatarsal base should be anatomic with the medial cortex of the middle cuneiform. On the oblique view, the medial cortex of the fourth metatarsal base should be aligned precisely with the medial border of the cuboid. On the lateral view, the dorsal surface of the second metatarsal should align anatomically with the dorsal surface of tarsal bones. Overlap of the metatarsals makes it a challenge to decipher any plantar injury with radiography.

Subtle ligamentous injuries may spontaneously reduce and conceal a true medial column dislocation; consequently, the radiographic evaluation should include comparative weight-bearing AP views of both feet. A CT scan evaluation of the TMT joints can easily identify ligamentous plantar bony avulsions to further

Figure 11   CT scan confirmation of first TMT lateral subluxation (red arrow) and plantar ligamentous avulsions (white arrows) of the second and third TMT joints.

increase the accuracy of the diagnosis[43] (Figures 10 and 11).

Treatment

The goal of management is anatomic restoration of TMT arc geometry and a painless, functional foot. A poorer prognosis is associated with delay in treatment or a concomitant compensation claim.[44] Surgical management includes open anatomic reduction and rigid set screw fixation to the first through third TMT joints; pin fixation is applied to the fourth and fifth TMT joints following reduction.[44] With anatomic reduction, good and excellent results occur in 50% to 95% of cases.[45,46]

After undergoing anatomic reduction of the transverse arch of the foot, patients may develop symptomatic arthrosis and instability attributable to medial column creep of scar and capsular tissue, particularly in the pure ligamentous injury pattern; this condition warrants further surgery.[47] A randomized prospective study comparing the outcomes of acute reconstruction to primary medial column fusions of TMT injuries reported better AOFAS midfoot scoring with primary arthrodesis and advocated medial column fusion, particularly in cases of pure ligamentous TMT injuries.[48] A 2012 retrospective comparative study evaluated the outcomes of 25 Lisfranc fracture-dislocations (12 ligamentous, 13 combined) treated with primary medial column arthrodesis.[49] Patients were followed an average of 42 months, with a reported 85% return to their preinjury state and 84% clinical satisfaction. There was no statistical difference in Medical Outcomes Study 36-Item Short Form results between the injury groups. The authors concluded primary medial column TMT fusions were an indication for both pure ligamentous and combined ligamentous and osseous-type Lisfranc injuries.[50]

Cast application is deferred until immediate postoperative swelling of soft tissues is resolved. The well-padded, short-leg cast is maintained for 4 to 6 weeks; then the lateral column pins are removed. A non–weight-bearing removable fracture boot and compression stocking are then applied. Weight bearing is initiated progressively after 10 to 12 weeks, and boot weaning is supervised by physical therapy. The patient is then fitted with a full-length semirigid orthotic and rocker-bottom sole modification. There is no consensus regarding the timing of screw removal; however, with repetitive loading, fatigue failure of hardware generally will ensue, and removal is recommended at approximately 1 year. However, to the benefit of patients and surgeons, screws that fail because of fatigue are found to break distal to subchondral joint lines and are free of chondral impingement when removed.

Forefoot Fractures

The forefoot's function is to provide a platform during stance and a lever for push-off during gait. The first metatarsal and the first metatarsophalangeal joint accept up to one third of body weight, whereas the second through fifth metatarsals bear the remaining two thirds of weight equally. Injuries to the forefoot are attributable to both direct and indirect trauma.[51] Although direct forefoot trauma associated with industrial injuries has diminished thanks to the use of protective work boots, indirect high-energy forefoot injuries associated with vehicular trauma have increased.

Treatment

Metatarsal fractures associated with multiple fractures of the lower extremities, open-foot fractures, and metatarsal fractures with gross displacement warrant surgical management. Displaced first and second metatarsal fractures with proximal articular extension must be evaluated for TMT instability and are best managed with ORIF. First metatarsal fractures have a lower threshold for surgical management because of the potential for displacement. Fractures of the fifth metatarsal middiaphysis are safely treated with closed reduction and cast immobilization similar to the treatment for central metatarsal fractures, which can splint one another by way of the transverse metatarsal ligaments, holding length, and alignment.[52]

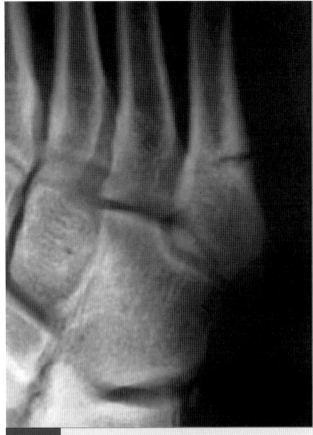

Figure 12 Oblique radiograph of an acute metaphyseal-diaphyseal proximal fifth metatarsal fracture.

Fractures of the metatarsal neck are commonly multiple fractures with plantar, lateral, and proximal displacement. Multiple neck fractures will displace and align in concert as a result of intermetatarsal ligament attachment. These injuries are routinely managed as central shaft fractures with a short-leg cast and non–weight-bearing activity for displacements up to 4 mm and angulation limited to 10°.[53] Larger displacements warrant open reduction and dorsal mini T-plate fixation of the most medial fracture. Additional lateral neck fractures will indirectly align in good position and heal, provided surgical dissection is isolated to the dorsal approach.

Proximal Fifth Metatarsal Fractures

The fifth metatarsal is reported to comprise 25% of all metatarsal fractures, whereas up to 90% of these fractures involve the metaphyseal tuberosity.[54] The proximal fifth metatarsal is anatomically divided into three zones. A tuberosity fracture occurs only in metaphyseal bone and is classified as a zone I injury. The fracture is managed symptomatically with an immediate postoperative shoe or cast boot and progressive weight bearing until it is healed.[54]

Fractures isolated to the proximal metaphyseal-diaphyseal junction of the fifth metatarsal are known as Jones fractures and occur in zone II (Figure 12). This fracture should not be confused with a diaphyseal

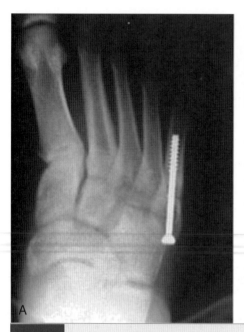
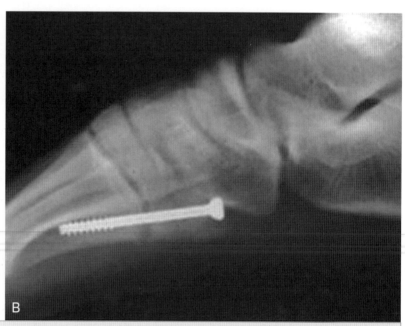

Figure 13 **A** and **B**, Radiographs showing reamed intramedullary fixation with a 4.0-mm compression screw.

stress fracture of the fifth metatarsal. The natural history of nonsurgical treatment has shown an increased risk of delayed healing and nonunion attributable to a watershed of arterial perfusion at this location. Early management of acute fractures entails short-leg non–weight-bearing cast immobilization for 6 weeks. Surgical management is considered for athletes or patients seeking early mobilization. Reamed surgical intramedullary screw treatment is usually reserved for patients in whom nonsurgical care has failed (**Figure 13**). A zone III fracture is located in the distal dimetaphyseal region and is commonly a stress fracture. Patients present with a history of lateral foot pain and radiographs demonstrating a lateral diaphyseal cortical gap and little or no callus. The treatment depends on the severity of symptoms. Patients are counseled to consider cast immobilization and 6 weeks of non–weight-bearing activity versus intramedullary screw fixation and possible local bone grafting of the fracture.

Summary

Interest in the management of and advances in technology for foot and ankle trauma has increased during the past 10 years, possibly in response to a heightened interest in developing surgical skill sets required to treat the high-energy injury sustained by the foot and the ankle during vehicular trauma in the current era of the airbag-equipped vehicle. Despite advances in restoring foot biomechanics and specific joint function in foot and ankle trauma, areas of controversy remain. Examples are the acceptable displacement of articular fractures of the calcaneus when treated by percutaneous and mini-open technique when compared with the extensile, direct open approach to the os calcis fracture;

or when midfoot and forefoot injuries associated with the ipsilateral proximal foot and extremity trauma are left undermanaged or untreated, possibly to become the chief cause of chronic pain and long-termdisability.

It is imperative that sound principles and techniques in foot and ankle trauma management are applied to predictably achieve the most acceptable long-term functional outcomes.

Key Study Points

- The outcome of surgical treatment of the calcaneus is difficult to characterize and is influenced by multiple variables, including patient selection, complex pathoanatomy, and fixation strategies.

- Acute isolated and combined fractures of the tarsal navicular and the cuboid are best treated with immediate spanning and medial and/or lateral column external fixtion, CT imaging of the midfoot, and index surgery after soft-tissue swelling has resolved.

- Diagnosis of the low-energy, indirect TMT injury is often difficult because of an inability to see noticeable TMT displacement on radiographs.

Annotated References

1. Lindvall E, Haidukewych G, DiPasquale T, Herscovici D Jr, Sanders R: Open reduction and stable fixation of isolated, displaced talar neck and body fractures. *J*

Bone Joint Surg Am* 2004;86(10):2229-2234.

2. Sanders DW, Busam M, Hattwick E, Edwards JR, McAndrew MP, Johnson KD: Functional outcomes following displaced talar neck fractures. *J Orthop Trauma* 2004;18(5):265-270.

3. Haliburton RA, Sullivan CR, Kelly PJ, Peterson LF: The extra-osseous and intra-osseous blood supply of the talus. *J Bone Joint Surg Am* 1958;40(5):1115-1120.

4. Mulfinger GL, Trueta J: The blood supply of the talus. *J Bone Joint Surg Br* 1970;52-B(1):160-167.

5. Miller AN, Prasarn ML, Dyke JP, Helfet DL, Lorich DG: Quantitative assessment of the vascularity of the talus with gadolinium-enhanced magnetic resonance imaging. *J Bone Joint Surg Am* 2011;93(12):1116-1121.

   This latex injection cadaver study delineated talar vascularity using gadolinium-enhanced MRI imaging followed by gross dissection. The results showed that the peroneal artery contributed 17% of talar perfusion, the anterior tibial artery contributed 36%, and the posterior tibial artery contributed 47%. This study demonstrates vascular contribution to the posterior talus, which helps explain why talar neck fractures may not result in osteonecrosis. Level of evidence: III.

6. Mayo KA: Fractures of the talus: Principles of management and techniques of treatment. *Tech Orthop* 1987; 2(3):42-54.

7. Vallier HA, Nork SE, Benirschke SK, Sangeorzan BJ: Surgical treatment of talar body fractures. *J Bone Joint Surg Am* 2003;85(9):1716-1724.

8. Canale ST, Kelly FB Jr: Fractures of the neck of the talus: Long-term evaluation of seventy-one cases. *J Bone Joint Surg Am* 1978;60(2):143-156.

9. Rammelt S: Secondary correction of talar fractures: Asking for trouble? *Foot Ankle Int* 2012;33(4):359-362.

   This retrospective series of 22 secondary anatomic reconstructions of talar malunions and nonunions reported on preoperative evaluation using CT and MRI scans was used to assess deformity, displacement, and osteonecrosis. Following anatomic reduction, fixation, and autogenous bone grafting, solid union was achieved in all 22 cases. There were no signs of new osteonecrosis, and the mean AOFAS score increased from 36.8 to 87.5 following correction. Three patients underwent salvage fusion at a minimum of 18 months because of posttraumatic arthritis. Level of evidence: III.

10. Patel R, Van Bergeyk A, Pinney S: Are displaced talar neck fractures surgical emergencies? A survey of orthopaedic trauma experts. *Foot Ankle Int* 2005;26(5): 378-381.

11. Smith CS, Nork SE, Sangeorzan BJ: The extruded talus: Results of reimplantation. *J Bone Joint Surg Am* 2006; 88(11):2418-2424.

12. Hawkins LG: Fractures of the neck of the talus. *J Bone Joint Surg Am* 1970;52(5):991-1002.

13. Ebraheim NA, Mekhail AO, Salpietro BJ, Mermer MJ, Jackson WT: Talar neck fractures: Anatomic considerations for posterior screw application. *Foot Ankle Int* 1996;17(9):541-547.

14. Fleuriau Chateau PB, Brokaw DS, Jelen BA, Scheid DK, Weber TG: Plate fixation of talar neck fractures: Preliminary review of a new technique in twenty-three patients. *J Orthop Trauma* 2002;16(4):213-219.

15. Attiah M, Sanders DW, Valdivia G, et al: Comminuted talar neck fractures: A mechanical comparison of fixation techniques. *J Orthop Trauma* 2007;21(1):47-51.

16. Ziran BH, Abidi NA, Scheel MJ: Medial malleolar osteotomy for exposure of complex talar body fractures. *J Orthop Trauma* 2001;15(7):513-518.

17. Vallier HA, Nork SE, Barei DP, Benirschke SK, Sangeorzan BJ: Talar neck fractures: Results and outcomes. *J Bone Joint Surg Am* 2004;86(8):1616-1624.

18. Buckley R, Tough S, McCormack R, et al: Operative compared with nonoperative treatment of displaced intra-articular calcaneal fractures: A prospective, randomized, controlled multicenter trial. *J Bone Joint Surg Am* 2002;84-A(10):1733-1744.

19. Tofescu TV, Buckley R: Age, gender, work capability, and worker's compensation in patients with displaced intraarticular calcaneal fractures. *J Orthop Trauma* 2001;15(4):275-279.

20. Gaskill T, Schweitzer K, Nunley J: Comparison of surgical outcomes of intra-articular calcaneal fractures by age. *J Bone Joint Surg Am* 2010;92(18):2884-2889.

   This retrospective study compared outcomes of surgically treated patients older than 50 years with a cohort of surgical patients younger than 50 years. Functional outcomes of those older than 50 years were significantly better than those in the younger group. The authors concluded that chronologic age does not appear to be a contraindication for surgery. Level of evidence: III.

21. Illert T, Rammelt S, Drewes T, Grass R, Zwipp H: Stability of locking and non-locking plates in an osteoporotic calcaneal fracture model. *Foot Ankle Int* 2011;32(3): 307-313.

   This cadaver study of 16 fresh-frozen bone mineral density–matched calcaneal Sanders type IIB fractures compared locking calcaneal plates to nonlocking plates in osteoporotic bone. The specimens were subject to cyclic loading, and displacement of the posterior facet was measured with an optical tracking system. No significant differences were observed between the nonlocking and locking plates with respect to cycles to failure or displacement of the posterior facet.

22. Blake MH, Owen JR, Sanford TS, Wayne JS, Adelaar RS: Biomechanical evaluation of a locking and non-

locking reconstruction plate in an osteoporotic calcaneal fracture model. *Foot Ankle Int* 2011;32(4): 432-436.

This biomechanical performance study evaluated 10 matched pairs of osteoporotic cadaveric Sanders type IIB calcaneus fractures fixed with locking and nonlocking calcaneal reconstruction plates. The specimens were axially loaded for 1,000 cycles through the talus, followed by load to failure. Comparisons were made between locking and nonlocking constructs on displacements during cyclic loading and construct stiffness. There were no significant differences detected in fracture displacements during cyclic loading or stiffness between locking and nonlocking calcaneal constructs.

23. Allmacher DH, Galles KS, Marsh JL: Intra-articular calcaneal fractures treated nonoperatively and followed sequentially for 2 decades. *J Orthop Trauma* 2006;20(7): 464-469.

24. Csizy M, Buckley R, Tough S, et al: Displaced intra-articular calcaneal fractures: Variables predicting late subtalar fusion. *J Orthop Trauma* 2003;17(2):106-112.

25. Jiang N, Lin QR, Diao XC, Wu L, Yu B: Surgical versus nonsurgical treatment of displaced intra-articular calcaneal fracture: A meta-analysis of current evidence base. *Int Orthop* 2012;36(8):1615-1622.

This meta-analysis, which synthesized data from six randomized and four controlled clinical trials evaluating ORIF versus nonsurgical treatment of 891 patients, reported better anatomic and functional outcomes with the surgical groups. However, complications were significantly more common in the surgical groups, confirming the risks associated with surgical care. Meticulous soft-tissue management is imperative, with 25% of the complication rates reported when using the extensile exposure. Level of evidence: II.

26. Sanders R: Turning tongues into joint depressions: A new calcaneal osteotomy. *J Orthop Trauma* 2012;26(3): 193-196.

A calcaneal osteotomy performed to convert a challenging tongue-type fracture into a joint-depression pattern by way of an oblique osteotomy through the posterosuperior tongue fragment is described. This process allows removal of the posterior facet segment of the tongue component. Subsequently, the most posterior tongue component is rotated out of the way, allowing anatomic repositioning of the posterior facet fragment and subsequent reduction of the osteotomized posterior tongue fragment. Level of evidence: III.

27. Carr JB: Surgical treatment of intra-articular calcaneal fractures: A review of small incision approaches. *J Orthop Trauma* 2005;19(2):109-117.

28. Smerek JP, Kadakia A, Belkoff SM, Knight TA, Myerson MS, Jeng CL: Percutaneous screw configuration versus perimeter plating of calcaneus fractures: A cadaver study. *Foot Ankle Int* 2008;29(9):931-935.

29. Chen L, Zhang G, Hong J, Lu X, Yuan W: Comparison of percutaneous screw fixation and calcium sulfate cement grafting versus open treatment of displaced intraarticular calcaneal fractures. *Foot Ankle Int* 2011; 32(10):979-985.

This randomized study compares ORIF without grafting (n = 45) and percutaneous reduction with calcium sulfate grafting (n = 45) using both 6.5-mm and 3.5-mm screw fixation. Sanders type IIB, IIC, and III fractures were inclusion criteria. The results demonstrated the percutaneous group had less blood loss, and at 24 months, the patients displayed better ankle and subtalar motion and improved outcome scoring (AOFAS score and Maryland Foot Score). There was no difference in wound infection, Bohler angle, or calcaneal length and width between the treatment groups. Level of evidence: II.

30. Sangeorzan BJ, Benirschke SK, Mosca V, Mayo KA, Hansen ST Jr: Displaced intra-articular fractures of the tarsal navicular. *J Bone Joint Surg Am* 1989;71(10): 1504-1510.

31. Schildhauer TA, Nork SE, Sangeorzan BJ: Temporary bridge plating of the medial column in severe midfoot injuries. *J Orthop Trauma* 2003;17(7):513-520.

32. Evans J, Beingessner DM, Agel J, Benirschke SK: Minifragment plate fixation of high-energy navicular body fractures. *Foot Ankle Int* 2011;32(5):S485-S492.

This retrospective study evaluated mini-plate fixation of 24 navicular body fractures with 8 type II and 16 type III fractures. Associated ipsilateral midfoot and hindfoot injuries were common, with only 9 patients sustaining isolated navicular fractures. All of the fractures healed with no deep infection. No patient underwent a secondary midfoot fusion. Level of evidence: IV.

33. Jahn H, Freund KG: Isolated fractures of the cuboid bone: Two case reports with review of the literature. *J Foot Surg* 1989;28(6):512-515.

34. Sangeorzan BJ, Swiontkowski MF: Displaced fractures of the cuboid. *J Bone Joint Surg Br* 1990;72-B(3): 376-378.

35. Weber M, Locher S: Reconstruction of the cuboid in compression fractures: Short to midterm results in 12 patients. *Foot Ankle Int* 2002;23(11):1008-1013.

36. English TA: Dislocations of the metatarsal bone and adjacent toe. *J Bone Joint Surg Br* 1964;46-B:700-704.

37. de Palma L, Santucci A, Sabetta SP, Rapali S: Anatomy of the Lisfranc joint complex. *Foot Ankle Int* 1997; 18(6):356-364.

38. Kadel N, Boenisch M, Teitz C, Trepman E: Stability of Lisfranc joints in ballet pointe position. *Foot Ankle Int* 2005;26(5):394-400.

39. Quenu E, Kuss G: Etude sur luxations du metatarse du diastasis entre 1er et 2e metatarsien. *Rev Chir* 1909;39: 281-336.

40. Hardcastle PH, Reschauer R, Kutscha-Lissberg E,

Schoffmann W: Injuries to the tarsometatarsal joint: Incidence, classification and treatment. *J Bone Joint Surg Br* 1982;64-B(3):349-356.

41. Myerson MS, Fisher RT, Burgess AR, Kenzora JE: Fracture dislocations of the tarsometatarsal joints: End results correlated with pathology and treatment. *Foot Ankle* 1986;6(5):225-242.

42. Chiodo CP, Myerson MS: Developments and advances in the diagnosis and treatment of injuries to the tarsometatarsal joint. *Orthop Clin North Am* 2001;32(1):11-20.

43. Rosenbaum A, Dellenbaugh S, Dipreta J, Uhl R: Subtle injuries to the lisfranc joint. *Orthopedics* 2011;34(11):882-887.

   This updated review of the literature on TMT injuries discusses the diagnostic and radiographic findings that can increase the accuracy of TMT injury diagnoses. Level of evidence: IV.

44. Calder JD, Whitehouse SL, Saxby TS: Results of isolated Lisfranc injuries and the effect of compensation claims. *J Bone Joint Surg Br* 2004;86-B(4):527-530.

45. Arntz CT, Hansen ST Jr: Dislocations and fracture dislocations of the tarsometatarsal joints. *Orthop Clin North Am* 1987;18(1):105-114.

46. Arntz CT, Veith RG, Hansen ST Jr: Fractures and fracture-dislocations of the tarsometatarsal joint. *J Bone Joint Surg Am* 1988;70(2):173-181.

47. Lee CA, Birkedal JP, Dickerson EA, Vieta PA Jr, Webb LX, Teasdall RD: Stabilization of Lisfranc joint injuries: A biomechanical study. *Foot Ankle Int* 2004;25(5):365-370.

48. Kuo RS, Tejwani NC, Digiovanni CW, et al: Outcome after open reduction and internal fixation of Lisfranc joint injuries. *J Bone Joint Surg Am* 2000;82(11):1609-1618.

49. Ly TV, Coetzee JC: Treatment of primarily ligamentous Lisfranc joint injuries: Primary arthrodesis compared with open reduction and internal fixation: A prospective, randomized study. *J Bone Joint Surg Am* 2006;88(3):514-520.

50. Reinhardt KR, Oh LS, Schottel P, Roberts MM, Levine D: Treatment of Lisfranc fracture-dislocations with primary partial arthrodesis. *Foot Ankle Int* 2012;33(1):50-56.

   This retrospective comparative study evaluated the outcomes of 25 Lisfranc fracture-dislocations (12 ligamentous, 13 combined) treated with primary medial column arthrodesis. Patients were followed for an average of 42 months, with a reported 85% return to their preinjury state and 84% clinical satisfaction. There was no statistical difference in outcome per Medical Outcomes Study 36-Item Short Form results between the injury groups. The authors concluded that primary medial column TMT fusion was an indication for both pure ligamentous and combined ligamentous and osseous-type Lisfranc injuries. Level of evidence: III.

51. Reinherz RP, Sink CA, Westerfield M: Management of trauma to the fifth metatarsal bone. *J Foot Surg* 1989;28(4):301-307.

52. Shereff MJ: Complex fractures of the metatarsals. *Orthopedics* 1990;13(8):875-882.

53. Johnson V: *Foot Science*. Philadelphia, PA, WB Saunders, 1976, pp 257-265.

54. Egol K, Walsh M, Rosenblatt K, Capla E, Koval KJ: Avulsion fractures of the fifth metatarsal base: A prospective outcome study. *Foot Ankle Int* 2007;28(5):581-583.

Chapter 45

Foot and Ankle Reconstruction

Eric Giza, MD   Michael Sirkin, MD   Brad Yoo, MD

4: Lower Extremity

Introduction

Pathology of the foot and ankle can arise from myriad sources, creating symptoms ranging from minor functional impairment to severe incapacitation. Each condition requires an individualized treatment approach, with the goal of reconstructive efforts to maximize functional recovery and rectifying deformity while minimizing irreversible changes to the patient's structural anatomy. In this chapter, both traumatic and acquired pathologies will be discussed, with an emphasis on current data useful in clarifying the disease process as well as optimal treatment modalities.

Arthritis

Arthritis is the end result following an insult to the articular cartilage. The initial damage is commonly traumatic but may also result from autoimmune disorders, intra-articular sepsis, blood dyscrasias, or unknown causes yet to be discovered by modern medicine. As the condition progresses, synovitis and subchondral bone wear creates a painful condition that restricts the joint's typical mobility. Distortion of the normal anatomy may occur, often resulting in malalignment that only predisposes the appendage to further deformity.

Syndesmosis

A growing body of literature documents the incidence of syndesmotic malreductions following traumatic dislocations. Anatomic reduction can be obtained either

Dr. Giza or an immediate family member serves as a paid consultant to or is an employee of Arthrex and Zimmer and has received research or institutional support from Arthrex. Dr. Sirkin or an immediate family member has received royalties from Biomet; is a member of a speakers' bureau or has made paid presentations on behalf of Biomet; serves as a paid consultant to or is an employee of Biomet; and serves as a board member, owner, officer, or committee member of the Orthopaedic Trauma Association. Dr. Yoo or an immediate family member has received research or institutional support from Synthes.

through direct articular visualization or by re-creating the radiographic appearance of the syndesmosis, using the contralateral limb as a template. Intraoperative or postoperative CT may clarify the position of the fibula within the syndesmosis, although it is unclear what degree of malreduction is an indication for reoperation.[1-3] A patient with a grossly malreduced syndesmosis, especially associated with clinical symptoms of pain and dorsiflexion restriction, is a candidate for revision surgery. As the malreduction becomes chronic, the concern is the syndesmosis will not be readily reduced anatomically because of changes in the bony architecture and scarring. In these instances, an arthrodesis may be more appropriate. This particular dilemma has been recently addressed.[4] The authors of a 2011 study concluded that delayed reduction and syndesmotic arthrodesis resulted in improved outcome scores, primarily from improving pain symptoms.[4] During the 2-year follow up period, there was no progression of radiographic arthritic appearance, theoretically because of the corrections in ankle alignment. The effect of the arthrodesis on ankle range of motion could not be assessed.[4]

Tibiotalar Joint

The long-term effects of ankle fractures may have been previously underestimated. Up to 80% of patients evaluated for ankle arthritis will relate a history of trauma.[5] Clinical symptoms can remain latent for up to 20 years.[5] Cartilage injuries at the time of injury are suggested as the cause, with a fivefold increased risk of posttraumatic arthritis. Cartilage lesions over the anterior and lateral talus, as well as the medial malleolus, have the poorest prognosis.[6] Progression to posttraumatic arthritis is more predictable for pilon injuries. The dramatic axial load results in increased chondrocyte apoptosis, lower proteoglycan synthesis, and higher water content in the area of direct impact.[7,8]

When nonsurgical treatments of arthritis have been exhausted to no avail, surgical intervention is based on the severity of symptoms. Anterior osteophyte formation at the level of the tibiotalar joint is common, resulting in impingement during dorsiflexion. If impingement symptoms are present without arthritic pain, resection of the talar osteophyte can improve symptoms. Caution should be implemented with resection of the tibial ostophyte because anterior tibiotalar subluxation may result. Early tibiotalar arthritis associated

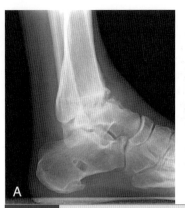
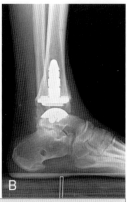

Figure 1   A, Preoperative lateral radiograph demonstrating ankle arthritis and anterior/distal tibial bone loss. B, Radiograph obtained 6 months after surgery demonstrating a stable implant with restoration of limb length.

with excessive talar tilt or medial clear space widening caused by a malreduced fibula may undergo a lengthening osteotomy of fibula to decrease the medial clear space and neutralize the pathologic talar tilt.[9] Distal tibia coronal plane malalignment predisposes the ankle joint to asymmetric load. A supramalleolar osteotomy to correct coronal plane malalignment improves the loading environment of the tibiotalar joint.[10,11] Excessive correction of the varus deformity can result in subfibular impingement, especially in patients with preexisting heel valgus. For this reason, it is recommended that supramalleolar osteotomies be performed in isolation for patients with varus or neutral heel alignment. Patients with preoperative heel valgus should undergo both a medial opening wedge osteotomy as well as a medial sliding calcaneal osteotomy.[10]

Although tibiotalar arthrodesis is considered the gold standard for end-stage arthritis, the procedure has a complication rate between 26% and 49%.[5,12,13] With either open or arthroscopic techniques, potential short-term complications include nonunion (10% of cases), malalignment, and infection.[14] Adjacent joint arthritis has also been described in up to 60% of arthrodeses.[5,12] Gait disturbances and leg-length inequality are typical. These complications, combined with the effect of arthrodesis on physiologic motion, results in decreased Medical Outcomes Study Short Form-36 (SF-36) scores for physical function, emotional disturbances, and bodily pain.[5,12] For these reasons, during preoperative counseling, patients should be informed of the near-inevitable appearance of symptomatic adjacent joint arthritis and the expectation of progressive pain and functional limitations over time.[5]

Total ankle arthroplasty is an attractive option to mitigate the functional limitations associated with both end-stage ankle arthritis and ankle arthrodesis (Figure 1). Proper candidate selection is crucial to minimize postoperative complications and maximize patient satisfaction following the procedure. When examined 2 years postoperatively, the outcomes of total ankle re-

placement and ankle arthrodesis, with regard to both pain relief and function, were comparable.[13] This was especially true for total ankle arthroplasties selected for older and less active patients, despite a higher incidence of complications in the arthroplasty group.[13] The rate of subtalar fusion following ankle arthroplasty was lower than in the arthrodesis group.[15] Although comparable outcomes between the two treatment groups exist, the rates for reoperation were higher for ankle arthroplasty at both 1 and 5 years.[15]

In 2009, the results of a large multicenter trial comparing ankle fusion to total ankle replacement were published, and the positive outcome of this study has increased the popularity of total ankle replacement as a viable treatment option for ankle arthritis.[16] Another report found that the probability of implant survival was 96% at 5 years and 90% at 10 years.[17]

One advantage of total ankle replacement is the ability to maintain ankle range of motion, thus reducing stress on the subtalar and tarsal joints and decreasing the future likelihood of talonavicular or subtalar osteoarthritis. Short-term follow-up has demonstrated improvements in gait for patients with a total ankle arthroplasty compared with those with ankle fusion.[18] The changes in gait mechanics in 51 ankle replacement patients were compared from before surgery to 1 and 2 years after surgery, and improvements in pain and gait were found for up to 2 years following implantation.[19] As more data for total ankle arthroplasty become available, an improved understanding of the time needed for patient recovery has developed.[20]

As the numbers of total ankle arthroplasties increase, there has also been an evolution of surgical techniques and technical pearls. Traditionally, patients with a varus or valgus deformity greater than 10° or patients with medial or lateral ligament instability were not considered as candidates for total ankle arthroplasty. The advent of modern arthroplasty techniques has led to a systematic approach of deformity correction, either in a staged fashion or at the time of implantation. Ligament balancing about the ankle for optimal placement of the ankle can be challenging. The selective release of components of the deltoid ligament complex may provide a means for achieving optimal ligament balancing in total ankle arthroplasty.[21]

The varus arthritic ankle can be corrected and balanced in a systematic fashion intraoperatively with deltoid release, lateral allograft reconstruction, calcaneus/tibial osteotomy, or subtalar arthrodesis.[22] Axial correction can also be attained with osteotomies at the same time of ankle replacement as long as great care is taken to ensure soft-tissue viability.[23]

Subtalar Joint

The subtalar articulation involves interfaces at the talocalcaneal, talonavicular, and calcaneocuboid joints. Each interface can be involved individually or in combination. Displaced intra-articular fractures of the calcaneus can result in solitary involvement of the talocalcaneal articulation. An isolated arthrodesis of the talocalcaneal articulation, sparing the talonavicular and calcaneocuboid joints, will maintain more physiologic motion than fusion of all three articulations, otherwise referred to as a triple arthrodesis. Regardless of the procedure performed, improved functional outcomes and fewer wound complications were associated with subtalar fusion after initial open reduction and internal fixation (ORIF) of displaced calcaneal fractures compared with arthrodesis secondary to malunion following initial nonsurgical treatment.[24]

In severe cases of diabetic Charcot arthropathy or pantalar arthritis, an arthrodesis of both the subtalar and tibiotalar articulations may be required. Implant fixation in this setting of deformity and poor bone quality can be especially challenging.[25,26] Locking screw fixation, an inverted proximal humeral locking plate, and blade fixation have been described. Retrograde intramedullary hindfoot nails, because of their central placement within the tibial axis, have also been proven to be effective and durable in pantalar arthrodesis.[27]

Midfoot

The midfoot comprises the naviculocuneiform, intercuneiform, and tarsometatarsal articulations. These rela-

Video 45.1: Midfoot Anatomy, Pathology and Physical Examination. Matthias Vanhees, MD; Sakia Van Bouwel, MD; Francis van Glabbeek, PhD; Geoffroy S. Vandeputte, MD (15.30 min).

tionships can be subclassified into essential and nonessential articulations. Essential articulations are those that are critical to the normal motion of the foot, such as the fourth and fifth metatarsal cuboid joints. All attempts should be made to preserve motion at these sites. Arthodesis at this site may relieve symptoms of arthritis but creates a rigid foot on which ambulation is uncomfortable. Solutions in this case include tissue arthroplasty or joint arthroplasty.[28,29] The remainder of the midfoot can be classified as nonessential, being primarily rigid and nonmobile. These articulations include the first, second, and third tarsometatarsal articulations, the intercuneiform joints, and the naviculocuneiform joints. Arthrodesis at these sites will have significantly less effect on motion.

Instability at the midfoot caused by ligamentous or osseous disruption can lead to weight-bearing pain and deformity at the midfoot. Lisfranc injuries can occur in either instance, with a loss of normal relationship between the medial cuneiform and the base of the second metatarsal. Instability at the first tarsometatarsal joint, intercuneiform, and naviculocuneiforms may occur. Typically, the diagnosis is readily performed by the

combination of patient interrogation, physical examination, and conventional radiographs. The pain experienced at the time of injury is severe and is accompanied by severe soft-tissue swelling. Because of the osteology of the midfoot, instability may be occult, with static plain radiographs appearing normal. In these instances, stress radiographs, weight-bearing radiographs, or MRI may be useful in determining the presence of instability.[30,31] The reconstructive efforts of a chronic Lisfranc injury are controversial. Nonsurgical management of chronically displaced medial column midfoot injuries is associated with poor pain scores and functional disability. Indeed, stable anatomic reduction of the Lisfranc complex leads to the best long-term outcomes.[32] All attempts should be made to restore this architecture. Surgical treatment can include ORIF of the displaced articulations or fusion of the tarsometatarsal articulations of the medial column. Fusions may best be reserved for purely ligamentous patterns because it is this subset of patients that appear to function better following fusion than ORIF.[33]

Charcot arthropathy most commonly affects the midfoot. This neuropathic condition, along with the presence of concomitant long-standing diabetes, is a particularly difficult condition to treat. Initial management is nonsurgical, with shoe wear modification and bracing. As the disease process progresses, deformity and skin ulceration can occur, forcing the need for a reconstructive procedure. Realignment fusions require judicious soft-tissue handling as well as atypical implant placement, such as locking screw fixation for poor bone quality. Long retrograde intramedullary screw fixation has also been described to address poor insertional screw torques with diabetic osteoporotic bone.[34]

Major and Minor Acquired Deformities

Acquired deformities of the foot may be broadly classified as major or minor types. Major deformities describe structural pathologies that are painful, preclude a normal gait pattern, or predispose the patient to arthritic changes. Major deformities may be congenital, posttraumatic, or neuropathic in origin. Minor acquired deformities refer to pathology of the foot and ankle that may be initially addressed with either nonsurgical management or simple, noncomplex surgical procedures. Although considered minor, the significance of these pathologic processes should not be underestimated because permanent deformity and disability may result if the condition is left untreated. In other words, minor acquired deformities may lead to major acquired deformities. As a result, in this section, both types of deformity will be discussed simultaneously.

Hallux Valgus

Hallux valgus describes the lateral deviation of the proximal phalanx, and metatarsus varus describes medial deviation of the first metatarsal. The etiology is multifactorial with the incidence being 10 times higher

Table 1

Parameters for Radiographic Assessment of Hallux Rigidus

Radiographs	Normal	Mild	Moderate	Severe
Hallux valgus angle	< 15°	< 30°	> 30° < 40°	> 40°
1-2 Intermetatarsal angle	< 9°	< 15°	> 15°< 20°	> 20°
Lateral sesamoid subluxation	0 to 25%	<50%	50% to 75%	> 75%

in women. Other factors include family history of bunion, inappropriate shoe wear, congenital deformity, flexible pes planus, neuromuscular disorders, trauma, and inflammatory arthropathy.

To understand the bunion deformity and potential surgical correction, one must understand the delicate balance of the anatomy of the first metatarsophalangeal (MTP) joint. The medial capsule is a short, strong structure that creates static deviation of the joint and is aided dynamically by the abductor hallucis. The sesamoids glide under the metatarsal head and are held in place by the crista ridge on the plantar surface of the metatarsal. The adductor hallucis pulls on the lateral capsule and the sesamoid complex. The medial ligaments and capsule can fail because of medial deviation of the metatarsal or from the aforementioned causes. After the medial capsule begins to attenuate and the hallux assumes a more pronated position, the thinner dorsal capsule moves more medial and has a diminished capacity to resist adductor pull. After the crista erodes, the sesamoids can dislocate laterally.[35]

If the deformity is passively correctable, it will likely be amenable to standard treatment; however, a fixed hallux valgus with crepitus or dorsal osteophytes indicates a combined hallux valgus/hallux rigidus. The relationship of any lesser toe deformities must be considered because second MTP plantar callosities and hammer toes often are secondary to progressive bunion deformities and the relative shortening/varus of the first metatarsal.

Weight-bearing three-view radiographs of the bilateral feet should be obtained to properly assess the hallux (Table 1). The most common finding is an incongruent joint in which the proximal phalanx assumes a more lateral position relative to the articular surface of the first metatarsal head. A line connecting the centers of the first metatarsal head and the proximal articular surface of the first metatarsal to define its longitudinal axis yields the best intraobserver and interobserver reliability for the measurement of hallux valgus and intermetatarsal angles.[36]

The initial treatment of all bunion deformities consists of shoe wear modifications. The current position of the American Orthopaedic Foot and Ankle Society asserts that cosmesis is not a valid surgical indication. If the patient is pain free and able to function with no complaints, surgical correction is not indicated.

Many different types of surgical correction have been described, with success rates in the range of 75% to 95%.[37] Regardless of the variation of technique, the

Table 2

Surgical Treatment Guidelines for Hallux Rigidus

Bunion Deformity	Suggested Correction
IM angle < 15° + HV angle < 30°	Distal MT osteotomy with STC Distal STC with proximal MT osteotomy
IM angle > 15° + HV angle < 40°	Distal STC with proximal MT osteotomy Distal STC with first TMT arthrodesis Distal STC with cuneiform osteotomy
IM angle > 20° + HV angle > 40°	Distal STC with proximal MT osteotomy Distal STC with first TMT arthrodesis Distal STC with cuneiform osteotomy First MTP arthrodesis

HV = hallux valgus; MT = metatarsal; STC = soft-tissue correction; TMT = tarsometatarsal.

principles of repair must include medial soft-tissue tightening, removal of the medial prominence, lateral soft-tissue release, correction of the intermetatarsal angle (most often via a distal or proximal metatarsal osteotomy) and relocation of the sesamoids under the metatarsal head. Incomplete reduction of the sesamoids has been recognized as a risk factor for recurrence of a bunion postoperatively.[36]

The general guidelines for correction depend on the amount of deformity, and the choice of osteotomy can vary on surgeon preference (Table 2).

The standard surgical approach involves a medial first MTP joint incision, proximal incision of the metatarsal or first tarsometatarsal (TMT) joint, and an incision in the 1-2 webspace for a lateral release. One study demonstrated that percutaneous techniques were unreliable and not recommended for hallux valgus greater than 30°.[38] Another study showed that outcome scores were significantly higher for patients younger than 60 years.[39] The use of a proximal opening wedge on the first metatarsal (Figure 2) can decrease the intermetatarsal angle.[40] The use of local anesthesia can substantially improve postoperative pain control and patient recovery.[41]

Postoperatively, most patients are permitted to bear weight through the hindfoot; it is placed in a soft elastic wrap that is changed weekly or biweekly for 6 weeks.[42]

Deltoid Ligament Insufficiency

The deltoid ligament complex is an extremely important component of stability of the ankle joint. Careful reconstruction of the original geometry of the ligaments is necessary after injury or during total ankle replacement.[43] Traditionally, deltoid ligament repair was not performed for ankle fracture-dislocations, unless there was an associated medial malleolus fracture. Deltoid insufficiency can lead to medial instability with increased contact pressure on the medial joint, with subsequent development of ankle arthritis with a valgus hindfoot deformity. Thus, selective repair in the setting of deltoid rupture has been suggested.[44]

Although most cases of chronic ankle instability are caused by lateral ligament instability, deltoid instability and chronic changes can be associated with lateral instability.[45]

Although rare, subtle clinical deltoid instability can occur after trauma or secondary to chronic attenuation from a tibial valgus deformity. Patients will report medial giving way or rolling out of the ankle. Increased hindfoot valgus without a visible pes planus or medial foot collapse will be evident when the patient is observed from behind (**Figure 3, A**). In the absence ankle arthritis or excessive talar tilt on standing AP ankle radiographs, ankle arthroscopy can be helpful in the diagnosis. If there is sufficient tissue for repair with minimal valgus tilt, then a primary repair can be performed with reliable excellent outcome[46] (**Figure 3, B**).

Deltoid instability in the setting of severe ankle arthritis has few surgical treatment options other than fusion. The advent of reliable total ankle arthroplasty has allowed deltoid allograft reconstruction to provide successful maintenance of ankle alignment.[47,48]

Cavus Foot Deformity

The term cavus foot is used to describe a spectrum of foot shapes that have a high arch in common. The arch may be high because of a high pitch angle of the hindfoot, excessive plantar flexion of the forefoot, or excessive bend in the midfoot.[49] The components of cavus are increased pitch and varus of the hindfoot, plantar flexion of the midfoot, and varus and adduction of the forefoot.[49]

Approximately one fifth to one quarter of the population has a cavovarus foot, which has traditionally been associated with neuromuscular conditions and severe deformity. The four main causes of adult cavovarus foot deformity can be grouped into neurologic, traumatic, residual clubfoot, and idiopathic etiologies.[22] In general, there are imbalances between the intrinsic

4: Lower Extremity

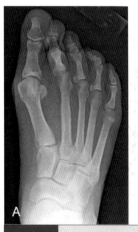
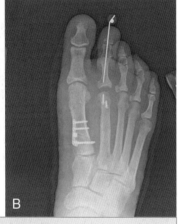

Figure 2 Preoperative (**A**) and postoperative (**B**) radiographs in a moderate bunion corrected with an opening wedge proximal metatarsal osteotomy. A second metatarsal osteotomy and proximal interphalangeal arthroplasty were performed in the same setting for a second metatarsophalangeal metatarsalgia and hammertoe.

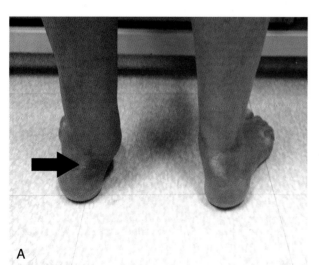
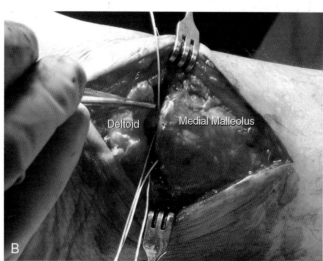

Figure 3 **A,** Hindfoot valgus associated with deltoid insufficiency (arrow). **B,** Intraoperative photograph demonstrating the repair of the attenuated but intact deltoid to the medial malleolus.

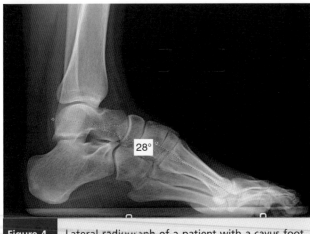

Figure 4 Lateral radiograph of a patient with a cavus foot. Note the positive lateral talo-first metatarsal angle.

and extrinsic muscles of the foot, between the tibialis anterior and peroneus longus muscles, and between the peroneus brevis and tibialis posterior muscles. In the cavovarus foot, the intrinsic muscles are generally weaker than the extrinsics, the tibialis anterior is weaker than the peroneus longus, and the peroneus brevis is weaker than the tibialis posterior.

Over the past few years, there has been increased interest in the diagnosis and the treatment of the subtle cavovarus foot, a less severe form of the cavovarus foot.[50] The subtle cavovarus foot typically presents with lateral symptoms commonly seen in patients with ankle or hindfoot instability, peroneal tendon injury, lateral column pain (pain along the anterior process of the calcaneus, the cuboid, ans the fourth and fifth metatarsals), and even stress fractures of the fourth and fifth rays.[50]

Standing three-view radiographs will often demonstrate overlapping of the base of the second through fifth metatarsals on the AP view as well an increase in the medial cuneiform height on the lateral view. The talo-first metatarsal angle will often be positive, indicating a plantar flexion through the midfoot (**Figure 4**).

Depending on the severity and the flexibility of the deformity, a combination of surgical treatments is needed to achieve the goals of creating a neutral, plantigrade hindfoot, a decrease in arch height, and a correction of forefoot adductus. Soft-tissue and contracture release procedures will include gastrocnemius-soleus complex lengthening, plantar fascia release, flexor digitorum longus/flexor hallucis longus lengthening or transfer, posterior/medial ankle capsule release, talonavicular joint release, and lateral ligament stabilization. Osteotomies can include a lateralizing calcaneal osteotomy, dorsiflexion osteotomy of the first ray, distal metatarsal osteotomies of the lesser metatarsals, dorsiflexion osteotomies of the midfoot through the naviculocunieform joints, and cuboid and lateral column shortening for forefoot varus. Tendon transfers may also be included, which can consist of peroneus longus to brevis transfer, extensor hallucis longus trans-

fer with interphalangeal joint fusion of the hallux, and posterior tibial tendon transfer.[50,51]

A commonly recognized cause of cavus foot is Charcot-Marie-Tooth (CMT) disease, which can range from subtle to a severe fixed ankle varus with arthritis. The disorder is a phenotypic manifestation of a complex genetic disorder, with variable underlying causative genetic abnormalities resulting in greatly variable clinical severity. Type 1 is a condition in which the myelin surrounding the nerve is abnormal; however, in type 2 the axonal function is abnormal. Approximately two thirds of patients who have CMT disease have type 1, and one third have type 2.[52]

The tibial nerve innervated intrinsic musculature often fails first, which can lead to hammertoes/claw toes. Further deinnervation of the peroneus brevis and tibialis anterior can lead to overpull from the peroneus longus. One study of 41 feet with an average follow-up of 26 years found that correction of the cavus deformity was well maintained, although most patients had some recurrence of hindfoot varus as seen on radiographic examination.[53]

Calcaneal Malunion

Fractures of the calcaneus are accompanied by a predictable deformity that has been previously discussed. If left to heal in this pathologic position, a calcaneal malunion creates several secondary problems. First, expulsion of the lateral wall results in impingement of the peroneal tendons in the subfibular space. Chronic irritation may result in degenerative changes or scarring of the tendons within their sheaths. Debulking of the lateral wall can improve symptoms, along with specific treatment to the peroneal tendons themselves. This complication may be avoided by performing fracture reduction surgery, during which time the lateral wall expulsion is reduced and the medial to lateral dimensions of the burst calcaneus is restored.

Cutaneous nerve entrapment, commonly the posterior tibial nerve, can be observed following a malunited fracture.[54] Patients report pain in the medial heel and paresthesias in the distribution of the posterior tibial nerve. If nonsurgical supportive measures fail, then surgical decompression may provide relief.

Varus malpositioning of the tuberosity will affect the normal talocalcaneal mechanics. Patients will report deformity, with prominence of the fibula distally. Patient shoe wear is asymetrically worn on the lateral border. If nonsurgical management with lateral shoe wedges is unsuccessful, a correctional osteotomy may be required.

Tendinopathies

Posterior tibial tendon dysfunction has been well documented as a distinct disease process. In addition to the common etiologies, the posterior tibial tendon is particularly susceptible to attrition because of a regressing blood supply. This watershed area is located 2 to 3 cm proximal to the medial malleolus and invariably is the location where ruptures occur.[55] Four stages of poste-

Table 3

Clinical Grading System for Adult Acquired Flatfoot Deformity

Stage	Posterior Tibial Tendonopathy	Planovalgus Foot Description
1	Peritendinitis and/or tendon degeneration	Minimal/no deformity
2a	Tendon elongation	Minimal/no deformity
2b	Tendon elongation	Correctable deformity
3	Tendon elongation	Fixed planovalgus deformity
4	Tendon elongation	Valgus tilt of the talus within the ankle mortise with degenerative changes

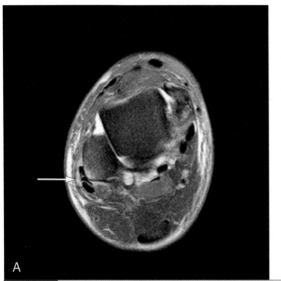 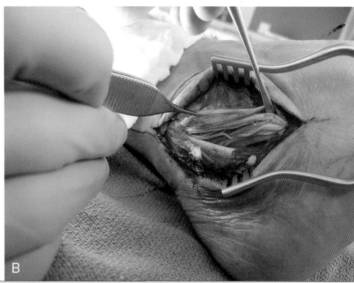

Figure 5 **A,** Axial MRI demonstrating a peroneal tendon dislocation (arrow) and superior peroneal retinaculum tear. **B,** Intraoperative photograph demonstrating a split tear of the peroneus brevis tendon (held in forceps).

rior tibial tendon dysfunction have been described[56,57] (Table 3). An additional classification system has recently been described, which breaks down the deformity into rearfoot, ankle, and midfoot (RAM classification), thus providing a more systematic algorithm for flatfoot treatment.[58]

As mentioned previously, initial management is nonsurgical, with strengthening exercises and bracing. Type 1 conditions may be treated with tenosynovectomy and tendon repair for intrasubstance or longitudinal tears. Type 2 pathology may be treated with either a flexor digitorum longus or split tibialis anterior transfer to the medial column. Flexible deformities associated with more than 15° of resting forefoot supination should also undergo a medializing calcaneal osteotomy and possibly a lateral column lengthening procedure.[55]

Type III and IV conditions are usually treated with corrective osteotomies or a triple arthrodesis. However, some studies have demonstrated that the long-term follow-up of patients after a triple arthrodesis has shown that many develop adjacent joint arthritis at the ankle or the midfoot. Therefore, a double or modified double arthrodesis in selected patients can correct rigid deformity and provide acceptable outcomes.[59]

Peroneal tendinopathy occurs distal to the tip of the fibula. Overuse and traumatic etiologies are most common, for instance, following a subtalar dislocation. Intrasubtance tears and frank rupture involve the peroneus brevis typically because of its proximity to the distal fibula at its inflection point (**Figure 5**). Acute traumatic injuries are often associated with an avulsion of the superior peroneal retinaculum from the lateral border of the fibula, which can be detected radiographically. Intrasubstance degeneration is to be débrided, and the remainder of the tendon can be tubularized if 50% or less of the tendon is involved. Tenodesis is indicated for tears involving more than 50%.[60] Chronic subluxation of the peroneal tendons may be associated with a shallow fibular groove, which should be deepened to provide more reliable stability to tendon excursion.

Achilles tendinopathy is another frequent source of problems for patients, with various afflictions occurring at the site of tendon insertion into the calcaneus.

Patients should be cautioned that preexisting tendinitis of the tendoachilles can predispose patients to frank rupture. In the absence of tendon incompetence, nonsurgical modalities are taken first. Stretching exercises and modalities are the mainstays of initial treatment. More recalcitrant cases may require débridement, resection of a cranial calcaneal prominence or a Haglund deformity, or gastrocnemius release. Currently, there is no consensus on the definite treatment algorithm for Achilles tendon ruptures. Surgical intervention naturally has a higher incidence of surgical complications, such as wound edge necrosis or suppuration. Nonsurgical management has a higher rate of tendon rerupture. Patients followed prospectively for either surgically or nonsurgically treated tendon ruptures demonstrated comparable functional results.[61]

Isolated gastrocnemius tightness can be determined by the Silverskiold maneuver, whereby the degree of dorsiflexion is compared with the knee flexed compared with the knee fully extended. A patient bearing weight on a contracted plantar flexed ankle is susceptible to a host of secondary conditions, such as plantar fasciitis, flatfoot deformity, hallux valgus, or plantar ulcerations.[62] In the absence of spasticity, the best solution is prevention. Non–weight-bearing patients should wear a splint in neutral ankle positioning, and passive stretching exercises are strongly encouraged. Dorsiflexion exercises should be performed with full knee extension to affect the gastrocnemius. If nonsurgical measures fail, patients are candidates for an isolated gastrocnemius release or an Achilles tendon lengthening.

Neuropathy

Nerve-related pain stems from a multitude of causes. Intrinsic damage to the intraneural architecture during crushing or tearing of the foot can result in persistent neuropathic pain. Extrinsic causes are also common as a result of trauma-related scar formation or other space-occupying lesions. Particularly with tarsal tunnel syndrome, the physical findings are variable, resulting in misdiagnosis of the condition. Classically, the patient is unable to abduct the small toe, which is consistent with dysfunction of the lateral plantar nerve. Passive maximal ankle dorsiflexion, heel eversion, and toe dorsiflexion with reproduction of local tenderness posterior to the medial malleolus will help confirm the diagnosis.[63] Common etiologies include talocalcaneal coalition, ganglia, and anomalous muscular anatomy. Decompression, including release of the laciniate ligament, should be performed if the surgical indications are met.

Osteochondral Injury of the Talus

Talar articular injury is the major cause of advanced joint disease in the ankle.[64] Both acute injuries and chronic lateral ligament insufficiency can lead to talar osteochondral lesions. In the setting of an ankle fracture, up to 69% of ankles can have chondral defects or cartilage injury. Cartilage injury was found in 69% of

228 fractures at the time of arthroscopy and fracture fixation.[65]

Routine radiographs fail to identify approximately 50% of the lesions identified with other modalities. MRI possesses increased sensitivity for diagnosis and the identification of lesions in preparation for possible surgical intervention.[66] Nonsurgical treatment is guided by the potential for a lesion to heal and patient preferences. Minor, stable injuries can be treated nonsurgically with immobilization and protected weight bearing for 6 weeks. The initial surgical treatment of most lesions involves arthroscopy with curettage and/or microfracture. Microfracture involves placing small holes in the bone underneath the damaged cartilage to stimulate a healing response. Arthroscopy is indicated for unstable lesions and those in whom nonsurgical treatment has failed with stable lesions. Best results are seen in

Video 45.2: 21 Point Arthroscopic Examination of the Ankle. Mark James Albritton, MD; Richard D. Ferkel, MD (7:48 min).

patients with small lesions (less than 1.29 cm²) and stable surrounding cartilage.[67]

After microfracture, pain improvement is seen in 85% of people.[68] Although the goals of drilling and microfracture are to stimulate healing and restoration of hyaline cartilage, defects usually heal with fibrocartilage. Patients with continued pain and swelling after 6 months of healing and physical therapy should be evaluated with a repeat MRI and considered candidates for other procedures, such as allograft or autograph, osteochondral plugs, or autologous chondrocyte implantation.[69-71] Matrix-based chondrocyte implantation obviates the need for a medial malleolar osteotomy and has results similar to autologous chondrocyte implantation.[72]

Postoperative Thromboprophylaxis

In 2012, the American College of Chest Physicians Evidence-Based Clinical Practice Guidelines (9th edition) was issued.[73] Based on their recommendations, no prophylaxis other than pharmacologic thromboprophylaxis was recommended for patients with isolated lower leg injuries requiring immobilization. For all patients undergoing major or minor orthopaedic surgery, there are no recommendations supporting the use of Doppler ultrasound screening for deep vein thrombosis before discharge.

Summary

Foot and ankle reconstruction can return patients to high levels of function but frequently involves corrective surgical techniques. Recent advancements in ankle arthroplasty and arthroscopy have had a distinct effect on the treatment of these conditions. Conditions that historically were associated with poor outcomes, such as talar osteochondral defects, can now be successfully ameliorated with newer innovations, such as chondrocyte transplantation techniques. Regardless of the treatment technique, a strong knowledge of normal form and function is critical.

Key Study Points

- Articulations of the lower leg and ankle each possess their own unique osteology as well as surgical and nonsurgical options when afflicted with cartilage wear. A primary objective in treating these patients is restoration of a mechanical weight-bearing alignment prior to arthrodesis or arthroplasty.

- Tendinopathies are typically the result of vascular insufficiency to the tendon substance or abrasion from an external source. The initial treatment is supportive first, with excision of diseased tendon or the external aggravating cause if nonsurgical treatment fails.

Annotated References

1. Leeds HC, Ehrlich MG: Instability of the distal tibiofibular syndesmosis after bimalleolar and trimalleolar ankle fractures. *J Bone Joint Surg Am* 1984;66(4): 490-503.

2. Richter M, Geerling J, Zech S, Goesling T, Krettek C: Intraoperative three-dimensional imaging with a motorized mobile C-arm (SIREMOBIL ISO-C-3D) in foot and ankle trauma care: A preliminary report. *J Orthop Trauma* 2005;19(4):259-266.

3. Gardner MJ, Demetrakopoulos D, Briggs SM, Helfet DL, Lorich DG: Malreduction of the tibiofibular syndesmosis in ankle fractures. *Foot Ankle Int* 2006; 27(10):788-792.

4. Olson KM, Dairyko GH Jr, Toolan BC: Salvage of chronic instability of the syndesmosis with distal tibiofibular arthrodesis: Functional and radiographic results. *J Bone Joint Surg Am* 2011;93(1):66-72.

   Salvage of chronic syndesmotic instabity can be achieved by distal tibiofibular arthrodesis. Reconstruction of an incongruous or arthritic ankle joint can delay the need for ankle fusion. Level of evidence: IV.

5. Coester LM, Saltzman CL, Leupold J, Pontarelli W: Long-term results following ankle arthrodesis for post-traumatic arthritis. *J Bone Joint Surg Am* 2001;83(2): 219-228.

6. Stufkens SA, Knupp M, Horisberger M, Lampert C, Hintermann B: Cartilage lesions and the development of osteoarthritis after internal fixation of ankle fractures: A prospective study. *J Bone Joint Surg Am* 2010;92(2): 279-286.

   Cartilage damage that occurs as a result of ankle fractures is associated with clinical outcomes. Specifically, lesions on the anterior and lateral aspects of the talus and on the medial malleolus correlate with an unfavorable outcome. Level of evidence: III.

7. Borrelli J Jr, Tinsley K, Ricci WM, Burns M, Karl IE, Hotchkiss R: Induction of chondrocyte apoptosis following impact load. *J Orthop Trauma* 2003;17(9): 635-641.

8. Borrelli J Jr, Torzilli PA, Grigiene R, Helfet DL: Effect of impact load on articular cartilage: Development of an intra-articular fracture model. *J Orthop Trauma* 1997; 11(5):319-326.

9. Weber BG, Simpson LA: Corrective lengthening osteotomy of the fibula. *Clin Orthop Relat Res* 1985;199: 61-67.

10. Lee W-C, Moon JS, Lee K, Byun WJ, Lee SH: Indications for supramalleolar osteotomy in patients with ankle osteoarthritis and varus deformity. *J Bone Joint Surg Am* 2011;93(13):1243-1248.

    Patients with ankle arthritis may have relief from a supramalleolar osteotomy but only when associated with minimal talar tilt greater than or equal to 5° and neutral or varus heel alignment. Level of evidence: IV.

11. Lee W-C, Moon J-S, Lee HS, Lee K: Alignment of ankle and hindfoot in early stage ankle osteoarthritis. *Foot Ankle Int* 2011;32(7):693-699.

    In early stages of ankle arthritis, the alignment of the tibial plafond and the hindfoot are variable. Level of evidence: III.

12. Fuchs S, Sandmann C, Skwara A, Chylarecki C: Quality of life 20 years after arthrodesis of the ankle: A study of adjacent joints. *J Bone Joint Surg Br* 2003;85-B(7): 994-998.

13. Krause FG, Windolf M, Bora B, Penner MJ, Wing KJ, Younger AS: Impact of complications in total ankle replacement and ankle arthrodesis analyzed with a validated outcome measurement. *J Bone Joint Surg Am* 2011;93(9):830-839.

    When comparing total ankle replacement and ankle fusion, both groups have significant improvement in their American Orthopaedic Society (AOS) scores, with no difference between groups. There are more complications associated with replacement than arthrodesis (54% versus 26%). A complication in either group has a negative effect on the AOS score. Level of evidence: III.

14. Zwipp H, Rammelt S, Endres T, Heineck J: High union rates and function scores at midterm followup with ankle arthrodesis using a four screw technique. *Clin Orthop Relat Res* 2010;468(4):958-968.

    The authors found that a four-screw technique for ankle arthrodesis provided high union rates, good pain relief, and favorable functional midterm results. Level of evidence: IV.

15. SooHoo NF, Zingmond DS, Ko CY: Comparison of reoperation rates following ankle arthrodesis and total ankle arthroplasty. *J Bone Joint Surg Am* 2007;89(10):2143-2149.

16. Saltzman CL, Mann RA, Ahrens JE, et al: Prospective controlled trial of STAR total ankle replacement versus ankle fusion: Initial results. *Foot Ankle Int* 2009;30(7):579-596.

17. Mann JA, Mann RA, Horton E: STAR™ ankle: Long-term results. *Foot Ankle Int* 2011;32(5):S473-S484.

    The medium- to long-term follow up of 84 STAR ankle replacements is discussed. Ninety-one percent survived at average follow-up of 9.1 years, 96% at 5 years, and 90% at 10. Average improvement of American Orthopaedic Foot and Ankle Society score was 39 points, with a mean of 82 with significant improvement in pain and function subscores. Ninety-two percent were satisfied with the outcome. Level of evidence: IV.

18. Hahn ME, Wright ES, Segal AD, Orendurff MS, Ledoux WR, Sangeorzan BJ: Comparative gait analysis of ankle arthrodesis and arthroplasty: Initial findings of a prospective study. *Foot Ankle Int* 2012;33(4):282-289.

    A comparison of ankle arthroplasty and fusion showed improved gait function and decreased pain in both groups 12 months after surgery. Level of evidence: II.

19. Queen RM, De Biassio JC, Butler RJ, DeOrio JK, Easley ME, Nunley JA: J. Leonard Goldner Award 2011: Changes in pain, function, and gait mechanics two years following total ankle arthroplasty performed with two modern fixed-bearing prostheses. *Foot Ankle Int* 2012;33(7):535-542.

    A 2-year follow-up study of 51 patients who received a total ankle replacement is presented. All observed changes improved or maintained functioning in patients with the greatest improvement in the first year. Level of evidence: IV.

20. Pagenstert G, Horisberger M, Leumann AG, Wiewiorski M, Hintermann B, Valderrabano V: Distinctive pain course during first year after total ankle arthroplasty: A prospective, observational study. *Foot Ankle Int* 2011;32(2):113-119.

    The authors studied the pain course of 28 patients undergoing ankle arthroplasty over a 1-year period. At 6 weeks, all measured variables had improved; however, at 3 months, there was deterioration of these same variables. These variables then improved asymptomatically at the 6-, 9-, and 12-month assessments. This pain course should influence patient education. Level of evidence: II.

21. Merian M, Glisson RR, Nunley JA: J. Leonard Goldner Award 2010: Ligament balancing for total ankle arthroplasty. An in vitro evaluation of the elongation of the hind- and midfoot ligaments. *Foot Ankle Int* 2011;32(5):S457-S472.

    Components of the deltoid ligament elongate largest at the ankle joint with hindfoot movement, except inversion. Optimal ligament balancing may require selective deltoid release when ankle arthroplasty is performed.

22. Ryssman DB, Myerson MS: Total ankle arthroplasty: Management of varus deformity at the ankle. *Foot Ankle Int* 2012;33(4):347-354.

    By balancing the varus ankle during surgery, ankle arthroplasty becomes a more durable, viable option. Level of evidence: IV.

23. DeOrio JK: Peritalar symposium: Total ankle replacements with malaligned ankles. Osteotomies performed simultaneously with TAA. *Foot Ankle Int* 2012;33(4):344-346.

    Osteotomies can be performed at the time of total ankle replacement to correct malalignment. Level of evidence: IV.

24. Radnay CS, Clare MP, Sanders RW: Subtalar fusion after displaced intra-articular calcaneal fractures: Does initial operative treatment matter? *J Bone Joint Surg Am* 2009;91(3):541-546.

25. Ahmad J, Pour AE, Raikin SM: The modified use of a proximal humeral locking plate for tibiotalocalcaneal arthrodesis. *Foot Ankle Int* 2007;28(9):977-983.

26. Chodos MD, Parks BG, Schon LC, Guyton GP, Campbell JT: Blade plate compared with locking plate for tibiotalocalcaneal arthrodesis: A cadaver study. *Foot Ankle Int* 2008;29(2):219-224.

27. Boer R, Mader K, Pennig D, Verheyen CC: Tibiotalocalcaneal arthrodesis using a reamed retrograde locking nail. *Clin Orthop Relat Res* 2007;463:151-156.

28. Berlet GC, Hodges Davis W, Anderson RB: Tendon arthroplasty for basal fourth and fifth metatarsal arthritis. *Foot Ankle Int* 2002;23(5):440-446.

29. Shawen SB, Anderson RB, Cohen BE, Hammit MD, Davis WH: Spherical ceramic interpositional arthroplasty for basal fourth and fifth metatarsal arthritis. *Foot Ankle Int* 2007;28(8):896-901.

30. Coss HS, Manos RE, Buoncristiani A, Mills WJ: Abduction stress and AP weightbearing radiography of purely ligamentous injury in the tarsometatarsal joint. *Foot Ankle Int* 1998;19(8):537-541.

31. Raikin SM, Elias I, Dheer S, Besser MP, Morrison WB, Zoga AC: Prediction of midfoot instability in the subtle Lisfranc injury: Comparison of magnetic resonance imaging with intraoperative findings. *J Bone Joint Surg Am* 2009;91(4):892-899.

32. Kuo RS, Tejwani NC, Digiovanni CW, et al: Outcome after open reduction and internal fixation of Lisfranc joint injuries. *J Bone Joint Surg Am* 2000;82(11):1609-1618.

33. Ly TV, Coetzee JC: Treatment of primarily ligamentous Lisfranc joint injuries: Primary arthrodesis compared with open reduction and internal fixation. A prospective, randomized study. *J Bone Joint Surg Am* 2006;88(3):514-520.

34. Sammarco VJ, Sammarco GJ, Henning C, Chaim S: Surgical repair of acute and chronic tibialis anterior tendon ruptures. *J Bone Joint Surg Am* 2009;91(2):325-332.

35. Perera AM, Mason L, Stephens MM: The pathogenesis of hallux valgus. *J Bone Joint Surg Am* 2011;93(17):1650-1661.

    A more scientific approach to the treatment of hallux valgus will be possible when pathogenetic factors are more clearly identified. Level of evidence: V.

36. Okuda R, Kinoshita M, Yasuda T, Jotoku T, Kitano N, Shima H: Postoperative incomplete reduction of the sesamoids as a risk factor for recurrence of hallux valgus. *J Bone Joint Surg Am* 2009;91(7):1637-1645.

37. Easley ME, Trnka H-J: Current concepts review: Hallux valgus part 1. Pathomechanics, clinical assessment, and nonoperative management. *Foot Ankle Int* 2007;28(5):654-659.

38. Huang P-J, Lin Y-C, Fu Y-C, Yang Y-H, Cheng Y-M: Radiographic evaluation of minimally invasive distal metatarsal osteotomy for hallux valgus. *Foot Ankle Int* 2011;32(5):S503-S507.

    In a retrospective review, 125 hallux valgus deformities treated with minimally invasive distal metatarsal osteotomy were studied. If the hallux valgus angle was greater than 30°, poor radiographic results occurred in 64% of the patients. When the hallux valgus angle was less than 30°, only 6.7% of the patients had a poor radiographic result. Patients with moderate to severe deformity should be treated by more traditional methods. Level of evidence: IV.

39. Trnka HJ, Hofstaetter SG, Hofstaetter JG, Gruber F, Adams SB Jr, Easley ME: Intermediate-term results of the Ludloff osteotomy in one hundred and eleven feet. *J Bone Joint Surg Am* 2008;90(3):531-539.

40. Shurnas PS, Watson TS, Crislip TW: Proximal first metatarsal opening wedge osteotomy with a low profile plate. *Foot Ankle Int* 2009;30(9):865-872.

41. Kim BS, Shim DS, Lee JW, Han SH, Ko YK, Park EH: Comparison of multi-drug injection versus placebo after hallux valgus surgery. *Foot Ankle Int* 2011;32(9):856-860.

    The use of multidrug injection is effective in reducing pain after hallux valgus surgery. The technique is safe and effective. Level of evidence: I.

42. Pentikäinen IT, Ojala R, Ohtonen P, Piippo J, Leppilahti JI: Radiographic analysis of the impact of internal fixation and dressing choice of distal chevron osteotomy: Randomized control trial. *Foot Ankle Int* 2012;33(5):420-423.

    A prospective randomized trial compared fixation/no fixation and dressing choice when a distal chevron osteotomy was performed. There was a statistical difference in shift of the osteomy in the fixation group when compared to the no fixation group, but the clinical significance did not affect outcome. There was no difference in choice of dressing type. When the preoperative hallux valgus angle was greater than 30°, the correction was worse. Level of evidence: I.

43. Leardini A, O'Connor JJ, Catani F, Giannini S: The role of the passive structures in the mobility and stability of the human ankle joint: A literature review. *Foot Ankle Int* 2000;21(7):602-615.

44. Bluman EM: Deltoid ligament injuries in ankle fractures: Should I leave it or fix it? *Foot Ankle Int* 2012;33(3):236-238.

    The treatment of deltoid ligament injuries is discussed. Level of evidence: V.

45. Crim JR, Beals TC, Nickisch F, Schannen A, Saltzman CL: Deltoid ligament abnormalities in chronic lateral ankle instability. *Foot Ankle Int* 2011;32(9):873-878.

    Deltoid ligament injuries are common in 72% of patients with chronic lateral ankle instability and no pain medially. Twenty-three percent had superficial injury, 6% had deep infection, and 43% had both injuries. Level of evidence: IV.

46. Hintermann B, Valderrabano V, Boss A, Trouillier HH, Dick W: Medial ankle instability: An exploratory, prospective study of fifty-two cases. *Am J Sports Med* 2004;32(1):183-190.

47. Jeng CL, Bluman EM, Myerson MS: Minimally invasive deltoid ligament reconstruction for stage IV flatfoot deformity. *Foot Ankle Int* 2011;32(1):21-30.

    A new technique to perform minimally invasive deltoid ligament reconstruction for stage IV flatfoot deformity was described. This should be performed only in patients with less than 10° of valgus tibiotalar tilt on preoperative standing ankle radiographs. Level of evidence: IV.

48. Haddad SL, Dedhia S, Ren Y, Rotstein J, Zhang L-Q: Deltoid ligament reconstruction: A novel technique with biomechanical analysis. *Foot Ankle Int* 2010;31(7):639-651.

    This article describes a utilitarian reconstruction of the deltoid ligament under low torque that was able to restore eversion and rotation stability to the talus. Biome-

4: Lower Extremity

chanical analysis was performed of the construct. Level of evidence: IV.

49. Aminian A, Sangeorzan BJ: The anatomy of cavus foot deformity. *Foot Ankle Clin* 2008;13(2):191-198, v.

50. Maskill MP, Maskill JD, Pomeroy GC: Surgical management and treatment algorithm for the subtle cavovarus foot. *Foot Ankle Int* 2010;31(12):1057-1063.

    A successful treatment algorithm is presented for the surgical management of the subtle cavus foot. Procedures performed included a combination of the following: lateral displacement calcaneus osteotomy, peroneus longus to peroneus brevis transfer, dorsiflexion first metatarsal osteotomy, and Achilles tendon lengthening. Symptomatic relief, long-standing correction, and patient satisfaction were obtained. Level of evidence: III.

51. Kroon M, Faber FW, van der Linden M: Joint preservation surgery for correction of flexible pes cavovarus in adults. *Foot Ankle Int* 2010;31(1):24-29.

    When performing joint-preserving correction of flexible pes cavovarus feet, patient satisfaction is generally good. The procedures performed included soft-tissue releases, tendon transfers and lengthenings, and osteotomies of either the first metatarsal or the calcaneus. Radiographic alignment of the foot was not significantly acssociated with patient-based outcomes. Level of evidence: IV.

52. Beals TC, Nickisch F: Charcot-Marie-Tooth disease and the cavovarus foot. *Foot Ankle Clin* 2008;13(2):259-274, vi-vii.

53. Ward CM, Dolan LA, Bennett DL, Morcuende JA, Cooper RR: Long-term results of reconstruction for treatment of a flexible cavovarus foot in Charcot-Marie-Tooth disease. *J Bone Joint Surg Am* 2008;90(12):2631-2642.

54. Myerson M, Quill GE Jr: Late complications of fractures of the calcaneus. *J Bone Joint Surg Am* 1993; 75(3):331-341.

55. Parsons S, Naim S, Richards PJ, McBride D: Correction and prevention of deformity in type II tibialis posterior dysfunction. *Clin Orthop Relat Res* 2010;468(4):1025-1032.

    This study describes a method of reconstruction in Johnson and Strom type II tibialis posterior dysfunction (TPD) using a split tibialis anterior musculotendinous graft (the Cobb method). The study prospectively followed 32 patients with an average follow-up of 5.1 years. All of the osteotomies healed, and 29 of the 32 patients could perform a single heel rise test at 12 months. The mean postoperative American Orthopaedic Foot and Ankle Society hindfoot score was 89. Level of evidence: IV.

56. Johnson KA, Strom DE: Tibialis posterior tendon dysfunction. *Clin Orthop Relat Res* 1989;239:196-206.

57. Myerson MS: Adult acquired flatfoot deformity: Treatment of dysfunction of the posterior tibial tendon. *Instr Course Lect* 1997;46:393-405.

58. Raikin SM, Winters BS, Daniel JN: The RAM classification: A novel, systematic approach to the adult-acquired flatfoot. *Foot Ankle Clin* 2012;17(2):169-181.

    A systematic approach to adult acquired flatfoot is presented. The deformity is classified into rearfoot, ankle, and midfoot. Level of evidence: V.

59. Gentchos CE, Anderson JG, Bohay DR: Management of the rigid arthritic flatfoot in the adults: Alternatives to triple arthrodesis. *Foot Ankle Clin* 2012;17(2):323-335.

    The management of the rigid arthritic flatfoot in adults is presented. The focus is on avoiding arthrodesis with thoughtful patient evaluation and examination, the use of joint preparation, careful positioning with rigid fixation, and the use of adjunctive procedures to achieve a plantigrade foot. Level of evidence: V.

60. Heckman DS, Reddy S, Pedowitz D, Wapner KL, Parekh SG: Operative treatment for peroneal tendon disorders. *J Bone Joint Surg Am* 2008;90(2):404-418.

61. Twaddle BC, Poon P: Early motion for Achilles tendon ruptures: Is surgery important? A randomized, prospective study. *Am J Sports Med* 2007;35(12):2033-2038.

62. DiGiovanni CW, Kuo R, Tejwani N, et al: Isolated gastrocnemius tightness. *J Bone Joint Surg Am* 2002;84(6): 962-970.

63. Kinoshita M, Okuda R, Morikawa J, Jotoku T, Abe M: The dorsiflexion-eversion test for diagnosis of tarsal tunnel syndrome. *J Bone Joint Surg Am* 2001;83(12): 1835-1839.

64. Athanasiou KA, Niederauer GG, Schenck RC Jr: Biomechanical topography of human ankle cartilage. *Ann Biomed Eng* 1995;23(5):697-704.

65. Loren GJ, Ferkel RD: Arthroscopic assessment of occult intra-articular injury in acute ankle fractures. *Arthroscopy* 2002;18(4):412-421.

66. Loomer R, Fisher C, Lloyd-Smith R, Sisler J, Cooney T: Osteochondral lesions of the talus. *Am J Sports Med* 1993;21(1):13-19.

67. Choi WJ, Kim BS, Lee JW: Osteochondral lesion of the talus: Could age be an indication for arthroscopic treatment? *Am J Sports Med* 2012;40(2):419-424.

    Older patients are less likely to have a history of trauma and a longer duration of symptoms, smaller osteochondral defects, and more associated intra-articular lesions. Increased age was not an independent risk factor for poor clinical outcome after arthroscopic treatment of an osteochondral lesion of the talus. Level of evidence: IV.

68. Schuman L, Struijs PA, van Dijk CN: Arthroscopic treatment for osteochondral defects of the talus: Results at follow-up at 2 to 11 years. *J Bone Joint Surg Br* 2002;84-B(3):364-368.

69. Mandelbaum BR, Gerhardt MB, Peterson L: Autologous chondrocyte implantation of the talus. *Arthroscopy* 2003;19(suppl 1):129-137.

70. Nam EK, Ferkel RD, Applegate GR: Autologous chondrocyte implantation of the ankle: A 2- to 5-year follow-up. *Am J Sports Med* 2009;37(2):274-284.

71. Giannini S, Battaglia M, Buda R, Cavallo M, Ruffilli A, Vannini F: Surgical treatment of osteochondral lesions of the talus by open-field autologous chondrocyte implantation: A 10-year follow-up clinical and magnetic resonance imaging T2-mapping evaluation. *Am J Sports Med* 2009;37(suppl 1):112S-118S.

72. Giza E, Sullivan M, Ocel D, et al: Matrix-induced autologous chondrocyte implantation of talus articular defects. *Foot Ankle Int* 2010;31(9):747-753.

The purpose of this study was to assess the results of matrix-induced autologous chondrocyte implantation (MACI) for the treatment of osteochondral defects of the talar dome using a technique that does not require an osteotomy of the tibia or the fibula. A prospective investigation of MACI was performed on 10 patients with full thickness lesions of the talus. At both 1 and 2 years postoperatively, the results of the SF-36 evaluation demonstrated a significant improvement in the Physical Functioning ($P = 0.002$) and Bodily Pain ($P < 0.001$)

components. Subjectively, all 10 patients believed this procedure helped them. Level of evidence: IV.

73. Guyatt GH, Akl EA, Crowther M, Gutterman DD, Schuünemann HJ; American College of Chest Physicians Antithrombotic Therapy and Prevention of Thrombosis Panel: Executive summary: Antithrombotic Therapy and Prevention of Thrombosis, 9th ed: American College of Chest Physicians Evidence-Based Clinical Practice Guidelines. *Chest* 2012;141(2, suppl):7S-47S.

A summary of the recommendations is presented.

Video References

45.1: Vanhees M, Van Bouwel S, van Glabbeek F, Vandeputte GS: Video. *Midfoot Anatomy, Pathology and Physical Examination.* Available at http://orthoportal.aaos.org/emedia/singleVideoPlayer.aspx?resource=EMEDIA_OSVL_13_01. Accessed January 15, 2014.

45.2: Albritton MJ, Ferkel RD: Video. *21 Point Arthroscopic Examination of the Ankle.* Available at http://orthoportal.aaos.org/emedia/singleVideoPlayer.aspx?resource=EMEDIA_OSVL_06_01. Accessed January 15, 2014.

4: Lower Extremity

Chapter 46

Lower Extremity Amputations

Daniel R. Dziadosz, MD   Karl A. Bergmann, MD

4: Lower Extremity

Background

Amputation is the most ancient surgical procedure. The earliest amputations were performed on patients who were not anesthetized; among those who survived, the result was a stump that often could not accommodate a prosthesis.[1] In the United States, approximately 185,000 amputations are performed on an annual basis, and, as of 2005, an estimated 1.6 million people are living with the loss of a limb.[2] The etiology of these amputations includes trauma, infection, neoplastic disease, congenital deformity, and systemic disease. Regardless of the need for amputation, the goal is the same: to create an end-bearing limb/stump that can accommodate a prosthesis and allow for locomotion.

Historically, it was believed that those undergoing a traumatic amputation adapted quickly to the loss of the limb and returned to their activities of daily living (ADLs) with ease. This, however, has not been the case.[3] The postoperative course often is complicated by infection, pain, and anatomic problems related to the stump.[4]

The financial burden following lower extremity amputation is also considerable. The costs related to an amputation (initial hospitalization, rehospitalizations, inpatient/outpatient rehabilitation, and the purchase and maintenance of prosthetic devices) create a financial burden that can exceed the costs associated with limb salvage.[5] The decision to perform amputation should be made with extreme care by a surgeon who is comfortable with performing the amputation and with postoperative rehabilitation and prosthetic design.

Preoperative Assessment and Initial Management

The assessment of all trauma patients begins in the field by emergency medical personnel; at this point, resuscitation also begins. After a patient reaches the hospital, resuscitation continues and decisions are made regarding extremity injuries. An orthopaedic consultation and evaluation that includes a thorough history and examination of the extremity is initiated; however, if the patient is unconscious on arrival to the hospital, the history must be obtained from the emergency medical services personnel, family, and/or friends.

The history is a vital component of the evaluation because preinjury health, comorbidities, and functional limitations can guide decisions. Many factors must be considered before deciding on amputation or limb salvage. Several points were highlighted through the Lower Extremity Assessment Project (LEAP), and the findings of this multicenter trial were reviewed.[6] This study provides a wide variety of preinjury, injury, treatment, and outcome variables with which to evaluate lower extremity injuries (**Table 1**).

The physical examination must include documentation of any soft-tissue wounds and nerve function, as well as the vascular status of the extremity. The use of ankle-brachial indices is an objective measure that can help determine the presence of an arterial injury.[7] Radiographic imaging of the affected extremity should include the joint above and below the injury. After this assessment is complete and a patient has been medically optimized, he or she may be taken to the operating room.

When amputations are performed on a delayed basis, screening tests for nutritional status and immunocompetency can be performed. In a retrospective review of a series of patients who had undergone amputation, patients who had a serum albumin level higher than 3.5 g/dL and a total lymphocyte count of at least 1,500 mm³ demonstrated improved healing compared with those who did not meet these preoperative levels.[8] This finding confirms that, if time allows, nutritional and immune status can be optimized. If time does not allow, however, an amputation level that is out of the zone of injury and allows for a nontraumatized margin of tissue may have an improved opportunity to heal.

Performing amputations on a delayed basis also allows more time for preoperative counseling. Members of the treatment team can evaluate patients and lay the

Dr. Dziadosz or an immediate family member is a member of a speakers' bureau or has made paid presentations on behalf of Synthes and AO North America. Neither Dr. Bergmann nor any immediate family member has received anything of value from or has stock or stock options held in a commercial company or institution related directly or indirectly to the subject of this chapter.

Table 1

Lower Extremity Assessment Project Study Review

1. Two years after injury, there was no significant difference in the Sickness Impact Profile (SIP) between those undergoing primary amputation and reconstruction.
   Self-efficacy and social support are highlypredictive of outcome in those undergoing reconstruction.

2. Patients treated with above-knee amputations showed no significant difference in their SIP scores compared with those treated with below-knee amputations.
   Patients undergoing below-knee amputations had the fastest walking speeds.
   There was no link between outcomes and the technological sophistication of the prosthetic device.

3. The Lower Extremity Assessment Project (LEAP) study did not support any of the lower extremity injury severity indices for determining those who require amputation and those who can undergo salvage.

4. Absent plantar sensation at the time of presentation is not an indication for amputation, a predictor of functional outcome, or a predictor of eventual plantar sensation.

5. The timing of wound débridement (< 6 hours versus 6-24 hours), the timing of soft-tissue coverage (more or less than 3 days), and the timing of bone grafting (more or less than 3 months) had no influence on infection rates, union rates, or functional outcomes.

6. Current smokers were
   37% less likely to achieve union.
   2.2 times more likely to develop infection.
   3.7 times more likely to develop osteomyelitis.

7. Past smokers were
   At no higher risk for infection than nonsmokers.
   2.8 times more likely to develop osteomyelitis.

8. Primary amputation
   5.4% revision amputation rate
   24.8% 3-month complication rate (one third wound infections)

9. Limb salvage
   3.9% require late amputation
   37.7% 6-month complication rate (one quarter wound infection; 23.7% nonunion; 7.7% osteomyelitis)

10. Factors influencing patient satisfaction
    Return to work
    Depression
    Physical functioning of the SIP
    Self-selected walking speed
    Pain intensity

11. Rate of psychologic distress
    48% tested positive after 3 months
    42% tested positive at 2 years
    20% had severe phobic anxiety/depression

12. Knee dislocation + vascular injury
    4 of 18 knees required amputation
    Prolonged warm ischemia time → Highest association with amputation

13. Factors favoring return to work
    Younger age
    Caucasian race
    Higher education level
    Nonsmoking
    Self-efficiency
    Preinjury job tenure
    Absence of litigation

14. At 7 years, more than 50% reported severe disability based on SIP scores.

15. Patient characteristics associated with prolonged disability
    Increasing age
    Female sex
    Nonwhite race
    Lower education level
    Poverty
    Smoking
    Litigation

16. Chronic pain (7 years) predictors
    23% pain-free (42% general population)
    High-school-level education
    Less than college education
    Low self-efficacy
    High ethyl alcohol consumption

(Adapted with permission from Higgins TF, Klatt JB, Beals TC: Lower Extremity Assessment Project (LEAP)—the best available evidence on limb-threatening lower extremity trauma. *Orthop Clin North Am* 2010;41(2):233-239.)

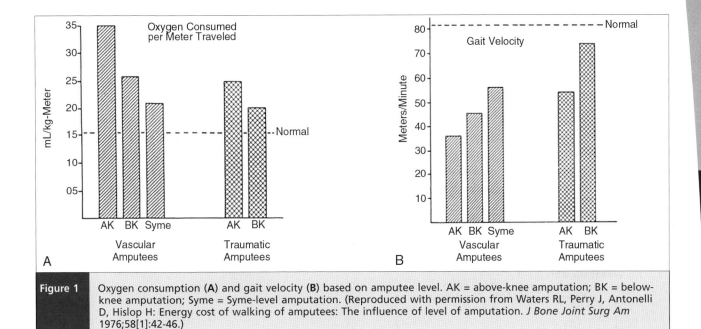

Figure 1 Oxygen consumption (**A**) and gait velocity (**B**) based on amputee level. AK = above-knee amputation; BK = below-knee amputation; Syme = Syme-level amputation. (Reproduced with permission from Waters RL, Perry J, Antonelli D, Hislop H: Energy cost of walking of amputees: The influence of level of amputation. *J Bone Joint Surg Am* 1976;58[1]:42-46.)

groundwork for the postoperative treatment course. Initiating psychologic evaluation and treatment early helps patients navigate the stages of grief[9] that often occur after amputation. A preoperative pain management evaluation and the initiation of psychologic treatment before surgical intervention can help patients address postoperative pain. If time permits, a preoperative evaluation by the prosthetic team can educate patients about the postoperative stages of prosthetic design, fitting, and function. When educating and treating patients in advance, the transition to dealing with limb loss is eased for patients.

Whether surgery is delayed or acute, a detailed informed consent must be obtained and documentation of all aspects of the surgery must be reviewed. From intraoperative assessment of the limb at risk to the potential for amputation, all aspects must be discussed with the patient, and informed consent must be obtained with a witness present.

Surgical Considerations

The extremity can be assessed completely in the operating room. The degree of contamination, the amount of bone injury or loss, and the condition of large motor nerves are assessed. A thorough débridement of all devitalized muscle, skin, and bone without articular cartilage is performed. At this point, the decision to perform an immediate or a delayed amputation can be made.

The decision to perform an immediate amputation is a difficult one; however, there are a few absolute indications: (1) blunt or contaminated traumatic amputation, (2) a mangled extremity in a critically injured patient in shock, and (3) a crushed extremity with arterial injury and a warm ischemia time of longer than 6 hours.

Other relative indications for acute amputation include severe bone/soft-tissue loss, an anatomic transection of the major motor nerves, an open tibial fracture with serious associated polytrauma or a severe ipsilateral foot injury, and/or a prolonged predicted course to obtain soft-tissue coverage.[2,10]

If amputation is imminent, a staged approach should be undertaken. For severely contaminated wounds, multiple surgical débridements are often required to decrease the bacterial burden and risk for infection. Antibiotic-impregnated polymethyl methacrylate can be placed in wounds to help decrease the bacterial load. The use of negative-pressure wound therapy (NPWT) on open wounds also reduces the rate of deep infection[11] and can decrease the risk for wound dehiscence when used on closed incisions.[12] In wounds with minimal contamination but a high degree of contused tissue, staged débridements can help eliminate progressively dying tissue. The removal of dead tissue is imperative because it can become a nidus for infection.

Amputation Level

Determining the appropriate level of amputation requires an understanding of the tradeoffs between increased function with a more distal level of amputation and a decreased complication rate with amputation at a more proximal level.[1] The patient's long-term function is influenced by residual limb length, which affects rehabilitation and dictates the ability for independent ambulation. Both gait velocity and energy expenditure are significantly improved in below-knee amputations[13] (**Figure 1**). Walking speeds were 21% slower and induced aerobic demands 49% higher for the amputees. Across specified paced speeds, aerobic demands were 55% to 83% higher for the amputees than for the able-

Table 2

Lower Extremity Amputation Types

Amputation	Eponym	Type	Advantages	Common Complications
Midfoot	Transmetatarsal/Lisfranc	Transosseous/disarticulation	Cosmesis	Limited propulsion strength; cumbersome prosthesis
Hindfoot	Boyd/Chopart	Disarticulation		Late ankle equinus
Ankle	Syme	Disarticulation	End-bearing, beneficial in children	Shoe-fitting; bulky prosthesis
Transtibial		Transosseous	Prosthetic use	Wound complications; ulceration from prosthesis
Knee disarticulation		Disarticulation	End-bearing	Loss of quadriceps lever arm
Transfemoral		Transosseous		Loss of quadriceps lever arm; increased energy demands for ambulation
Hip disarticulation		Disarticulation		Few functional prosthetic users; sitting imbalance

bodied subjects. This suggests that the higher metabolic costs for the amputees resulted from greater demands for maintaining balance and posture and for performing the walking movement.[14]

Differentiation among etiologies revealed that subjects with a vascular amputation had a lower VO_2 (peak) of 29.1%, compared with that of able-bodied control patients ($P < 0.001$), whereas the aerobic capacity of those who underwent traumatic amputation did not differ from able-bodied control patients ($P = 0.127$). After correcting for etiology, no association between the level of amputation and $Vo(2)(peak)$ was found ($P = 0.534$).

Although residual limb length is of paramount importance, it should not compromise the soft-tissue envelope, which acts as an interface/cushion during the loading process. An optimal soft-tissue envelope functions to distribute the load to the underlying bone and dissipate the pressures and forces applied during weight bearing.[15]

There are two general types of lower extremity amputations: disarticulation and transosseous. In general, when the amputation occurs through a joint, there is direct load transfer from the extremity to the prosthesis, which allows force to be dissipated over a larger surface area and through metaphyseal bone. With a well-constructed soft-tissue envelope to cushion the residual osseous platform, the direct-transfer prosthetic sock need only suspend the prosthesis. In a transosseous amputation at the transtibial or transfemoral level, the bone end is small and less resilient, which concentrates the same force seen in a disarticulation over a much smaller area. When constructing the prosthesis, the end of the bone must be "unweighted" by dissipating the load over the entire surface of the residual limb. This indirect load transfer requires a durable and mobile soft-tissue envelope that can tolerate the shearing

forces associated with weight bearing.[16]

There are several classic types of lower extremity amputations (**Table 2**). Amputations through the midfoot are described, but there is a limited role for their use, considering the inability to preserve a powerful lever arm for ambulation. To maintain this lever arm, preserving the metatarsal heads allows those who undergo amputation to take advantage of the ankle's contribution to walking. This type of amputation involves several soft-tissue requirements to maintain a functional residual limb. A high degree of equinus occurs with midfoot amputations, and Achilles tendon lengthening should be performed at the time of definitive surgery.

Tendon balancing plays a critical role in maintaining a balanced residual limb. There is a high incidence of varus deformity, and transfer of the tibialis anterior tendon to a more lateral position on the midfoot eliminates this tendency. Considering that amputation proximal to the metatarsal heads compromises the normal propulsive function of the foot and ankle, surgery should not strive to preserve residual foot length to maintain function but instead aim to achieve good distal tissue coverage and healing, particularly considering that the hip joint(s), not the ankle, become the primary source of power for walking.[17]

Hindfoot amputations such as the Syme amputation provide an end-bearing stump, which has its advantages. The Syme amputation also is a viable option for young children. Because it is not a transosseous amputation, there is no risk of overgrowth, and, with preservation of the physis, there are minimal issues regarding leg length and the need for stump revision. If the amputation occurs before a child learns to walk, he or she will adapt quite easily.[18] Considering that the soft-tissue flap consists of the glabrous skin of the hindfoot, patients can walk without a prosthesis. This can eliminate the fiscal burden of prosthetic construction and care, as well as the social stigma of using a prosthesis. The technical difficulty with this amputation relates to the posterior skin flap. Great care must be taken to preserve the posterior tibial artery when excising the tarsal bones because flap viability is based on its patency.

Transtibial amputations are the most common amputation performed for trauma patients and have been associated with the best functional outcomes. These patients have a high rate of prosthetic use and often exhibit minimal disability when in isolation.[19] The goal of this amputation type is to create the longest viable residual limb with a soft-tissue envelope that provides enough area to distribute the forces of weight bearing and can withstand the shear forces of a prosthesis. The optimal length of the residual tibia should be 12 cm to 15 cm, although walking propulsion from the retained quadriceps can be accomplished if the residual tibia retains the tibial tubercle and patellar tendon attachment.[20] The importance of maintaining maximal length of the residual limb is paramount, and several procedures will aid in this task. One such procedure that has been described to help maintain limb length when the zone of injury involves the proximal part of the tibia, or in cases of massive tibial bone/soft-tissue loss, is the osteocutaneous pedicle flap. This is a hindfoot rotational flap that is a functional alternative and does not require a microvascular free tissue transfer.[21]

Knee disarticulations provide an end-bearing residual limb on a much broader area of metaphyseal bone and preserves the quadriceps musculature. A meta-analysis of 27 studies revealed that patients with a knee disarticulation have a better physical quality of life (QOL) than those with a transfemoral amputation; this supports the surgical strategy of maintaining maximum length when possible.[22] Results from another study showed worse Sickness Impact Profile scores in patients undergoing through-knee amputation compared with above-knee and below-knee amputations.[23] Reasons for this finding include an insufficient soft-tissue envelope and the lack of skilled prosthetists to create the appropriate prosthesis for this particular amputation.

Loss of the knee joint in transfemoral amputations results in a less efficient gait with higher energy expenditure.[13] Great care must be taken with the myodesis; the femoral shaft axis can be maintained as nearly "normal" by preserving the adductor magnus and performing myodesis of the muscle to the residual femur. These steps allow a patient to be fitted with a prosthesis and provide the best opportunity for independent ambulation.

Another reconstructive option for patients whose knee joint has been sacrificed is rotationplasty. This procedure involves the rotation of the distal tibia 180° externally so that the ankle joint becomes a functional knee joint. Ankle plantar flexion becomes knee extension, and ankle dorsiflexion becomes knee flexion.[24] This reconstruction technique often is reserved for children undergoing oncologic resection. One study looked at QOL measures in patients undergoing a Van Ness rotationplasty; the authors found that patients' physical functioning was poorer than that of healthy peers but better compared with chronically ill patients. Levels of psychosocial functioning, general QOL, and social support were highly comparable with those of healthy peers. One third to one half of patients reported negative effects of the surgery on initiating social and/or intimate contacts, body image, and sexuality. With respect to physical functioning, two thirds of patients engaged actively in sports. Patients reported wearing the prosthesis continuously and were, in general, satisfied with its fit.[25]

Postoperative Management

The postoperative management of amputations requires a multidisciplinary approach. From the treating surgeons and prosthetists to behavioral therapists, all are charged with optimizing outcomes. Often, general principles are overlooked. Anticoagulation, for example, can be forgotten. The potential for pulmonary embolism (PE) in a patient who has lost an extremity must be addressed. The authors of a 2011 study[26] showed that the cumulative incidence of PE is significantly higher (5.7%) with trauma-associated amputation than with extremity long-bone fracture without amputation (1.9%), and they recommended aggressive prophylaxis, deep vein thrombosis screening with ultrasonography, and the potential use of inferior vena cava filters in this population.[26,27]

Dressings

After surgical closure, there are many options for postoperative dressings. Most wounds are covered with nonadhesive gauze, then dry gauze, and ultimately a compressive elastic wrap; the goal is to isolate wounds from the outside environment and limit postoperative swelling.

For transtibial amputation, soft dressings have several advantages, such as low cost, ease of application, and wound accessibility. The disadvantages of elastic dressing include (1) high local pressures that impair skin survival or healing; (2) limited durability with motion; (3) increased risk of knee flexion contracture; (4) limited mobilization/prolonged bed rest, which increases the length of hospital days and admissions; and (5) risk for pulmonary complications, strokes, and pneumonia. Despite these drawbacks, management with soft dressings is still believed to be among the least expensive and least time-consuming options.[28]

An alternative and often more effective postoperative dressing involves a rigid support that incorporates the knee. This type of dressing typically consists of an inner, soft gauze layer for wound protection, a postoperative residual limb sock for compression, a variable amount of soft cast padding (felt or polyurethane for bony prominences), and a foam end-pad. After these layers are in place, the final step is to apply a plaster cast that is molded to fit the residual limb. This dressing can be changed anywhere between 5 and 21 days (there is no consensus in the literature).

The advantage of a thigh-level rigid dressing is that it helps to prevent knee flexion contractures and protects the residual limb. The disadvantages include difficult wound access; delayed weight bearing and physical therapy for the knee; and the complexity of application, for which a surgeon or skilled prosthetist is required (which will increase cost). Some studies claim that rigid plaster dressings reduce edema, pain, and healing times, but there are no level I data to support this claim.[28] Although some sort of revision surgery was required for only 6% of thigh-level rigid cast procedures (versus a 22% surgery rate for the soft gauze dressing group), this was not statistically significant.[29]

Rigid thigh-level dressings can also incorporate an immediate postoperative prosthesis (IPOP). These are similar to rigid dressings; however, there is the addition of a connector, a pylon, and a foot at the time of surgery. This configuration allows for immediate weight bearing when the cast is dry (approximately 12 hours). The advantage of the IPOP is that it has been shown to produce a significantly lower number of limb complications, few surgical revisions, and a shorter time to a custom prosthetic fitting.[28] There is also a documented emotional benefit associated with the IPOP because patients are less troubled postoperatively regarding their self-image because a foot is present.[30] IPOP disadvantages include decreased visualization of the wound, tissue necrosis resulting from improper wrapping of the gauze layer, mechanical trauma to the residual limb tissue, and the requirement of a skilled prosthesis team.[28] An IPOP variation involves using a shorter rigid dressing, attaching a polyvinyl chloride pipe to the end, and then attaching a prosthetic foot. This variation results in an intermediate prosthesis that molds the residual limb, is quick to fabricate (usually 2 hours), and allows patients to move about more easily.[31]

Prefabricated pneumatic prostheses are similar to other IPOP methods but use air bladders that line the socket or an "airbag" system to surround the residual limb. The pneumatic portion is placed over a layer of gauze dressing and is inflated to 20 to 40 mm Hg to externally compress the limb. Options include above- and below-knee lengths. These pneumatic layers are covered with a plastic prosthetic unit. These prostheses tend to maintain the advantages of a rigid dressing: the ability to splint the knee, protect the end of the limb, and allow earlier weight bearing but are lighter, create better control of limb compression, allow easy removal for wound care, and serve as intermediate prostheses during limb maturity.[28] Because these are prefabricated systems, the need for a highly trained prosthetic staff is eliminated. These systems are associated with fewer postoperative complications than soft dressings only (16% and 65%, respectively).[32]

Pain Control

Pain control is essential to help patients physically and emotionally. Using a standard pain scale helps to monitor the effectiveness of pain interventions, with most

hospitals using the Visual Analog Scale. Pain after an amputation is usually thought of as either phantom limb pain (PLP) or residual limb pain (RLP). PLP is the sensation of pain in an amputated extremity, whereas RLP pain occurs in the unamputated residual limb. PLP is thought to develop when there is a long-lasting noxious stimulus to the limb (chronic preamputation pain). This leads to the development of a cortical pain memory, which has enhanced excitability. When the amputation occurs, this leads to a reorganization in the somatosensory area of the cortex associated with the amputated limb. Postoperative inputs from the limb, such as a neuroma, and changes in the dorsal root ganglion contribute to the abnormal sensation and pain.[33] Pain also may develop in other areas. One study showed that between 46% and 90% of patients who undergo amputation continue to have pain at 1 year.[34] Of those, 69% reported PLP, and 42% reported RLP.[34] A more recent retrospective review analyzed potential triggers for PLP. These triggers included psychologic, emotional, and autonomic triggers; behavioral triggers that involved forgetting the limb's absence and trying to use the phantom; weather-induced PLP; and sensations referred from other parts of the body[27].

This review also showed that those who underwent traumatic amputation were more likely to report emotional triggers. Managing spontaneously triggered phantom phenomena requires residual limb and neuroma management, restoration of central pain networks, limb movement, and effective coping with amputation-related memories.[27]

Pain management methods include local, regional, and oral analgesia. Local/regional analgesia requires the placement of a catheter within the nerve sheath during surgery or performing a block in a more proximal area (sciatic or epidural). Surgical techniques involving burying of the cut nerve ends within the muscle also can help to decrease painful neuromas. Most studies that evaluate regional pain control involve epidural use. A randomized prospective study showed that preoperative epidural analgesia 24 hours before amputation was less effective in decreasing PLP than a perineural catheter.[35] Local or regional analgesia has not been shown to be effective in preventing PLP.[36] Another study found that RLP was reduced by both morphine and lidocaine, whereas PLP was reduced by morphine only.[37] This alludes to the fact that PLP has a more centralized basis. Neither intervention completely resolved PLP; therefore, the authors concluded that a multifaceted approach is best.[5,37]

Pain treatment has included pharmacologic agents such as gabapentin (antiseizure), amitriptyline (a tricyclic antidepressant), selective serotonin reuptake inhibitors, NSAIDs, N-methyl-D-aspartate receptor agonists, and long-acting narcotics. Other interventions have included scar desensitization, biofeedback, relaxation, transcutaneous electrical stimulation, and mirror therapy. Mirror therapy involves placing a mirror between the legs to make it look as if there are two limbs when viewed off center. According to a 2010 study, this therapy may lead to a decrease in PLP.[38] An earlier study

Table 3

Amputation and the Five Stages of Grief

1. **Denial and Isolation**: "This is impossible. It's not really happening! I feel nothing at all."

2. **Anger**: "Why is this happening to me? I'm enraged! God is unjust."

3. **Bargaining**: "If I promise to do such and such, maybe I'll get my old life back."

4. **Depression**: "I feel hopeless. Everything is beyond my control. Why bother trying? I give up."

5. **Acceptance**: "I don't like it, but the amputation is a reality. I'll find ways to make the best of it and go on."

(Adapted with permission from Military In-step: Dealing with Grief and Depression. Manassas, VA, Amputee Coalition, 2008.)

found that use of a mirror does not necessarily reduce PLP, but it may halt cortical reorganization.[10]

Preamputation pain and immediate postoperative pain are predictors of chronic pain intensity. At-risk patients should be identified and placed in an early and intensive pain intervention program.[39] Investigators have found that acute pain intensity was the best predictor of chronic pain at 6 months and at 1 year. Preamputation pain was found to be the best predictor of chronic PLP at 2 years. A multimodal intervention was thought to be more appropriate than any single modality because PLP has been attributed to psychosocial factors.

Psychosocial Management

Amputations result in a variety of limitations that have emotional consequences. The authors of a 2012 study reported a high prevalence (43%) of mental disorders related to the number of morbid conditions and dependency among those who have had lower-limb amputations, and, as a result, a psychological and social assessment of this population is recommended to ease their adaptation and social reintegration.[40]

Patients who undergo amputation must adapt to physical changes and limitations, and psychologic changes. Depression, anxiety, altered body perception, decreased social function, and an altered sense of self-worth can all occur during the postoperative period. The stages of grief experienced after amputation are presented in **Table 3**.

Depression has been reported among those with recent amputations as a reason for decreased prosthesis use and lower levels of mobility. Older studies have yielded mixed results; some cite no increase in levels of depression,[41] and others report that those who undergo amputation are vulnerable to developing depression.[42] According to more recent studies, depression among those who undergo amputation is common but tends to resolve between 2 and 10 years after the event.[43]

According to one study,[43] anxiety can peak at 1 year after amputation, but it will gradually decline to levels consistent with the uninjured population. Both body image anxiety and body image distortion occur; however, body image anxiety is associated with higher levels of depression, poorer perceived QOL, lower levels of self-esteem, and higher levels of anxiety. Amputees will also experience self-stigmatization. They must endure an overt difference in appearance; they are physically limited compared with their own standards and the standards of those who are uninjured, and uninjured people tend to overemphasize their disability.[44]

Several physical (amputation) and social factors are associated with the degree of psychologic adjustment.[44] Amputation-related factors include the amputation cause, the amputation level, the elapsed postoperative time, the presence of PLP and residual limb pain, and the prosthesis.

Most patients will experience an initial period of denial after traumatic amputation, whereas those who are chronically infirmed (with vascular-related amputations) experience anger. Overall, the cause of amputation has little effect on psychiatric symptoms, anxiety, depression, or social discomfort. Studies evaluating QOL have shown that the level of the amputation predicts success. Those who undergo transfemoral amputations have more difficulty with ADLs than those with transtibial amputations and have lower QOL scores.[45] Elapsed postsurgical time is associated with more favorable outcomes that are associated, in part, with adjustment and acceptance of a changed body image.[43] Pain negatively influences a patient's ability to adjust. Regardless of the pain type, its presence will negatively affect psychosocial adaptation. The prosthesis type has also been proven to influence a patient's ability to adjust. It has been shown that more functional prostheses allowed for better psychosocial adjustment.[46]

Social factors that influence psychological adjustment include sex, age, marital and social support, and personality and coping skills. Demographic factors such as gender and age do not influence psychological adjustment, but marital status and available social support, college-level education, and income level do. According to one study, college-level education was associated with a better physical functioning outcome.[47] Income level also affects activity level. People with lower income levels were more likely to be restricted in their activities.[43] Personality and coping skills have been shown to influence adjustment to life after amputation. People who are extroverts and risk takers before an amputation tend to have better levels of social integration after recovery.[48] Coping skills also play a role in social integration and rehabilitation. Another study found that people who can find something positive about their experience have better self-ratings of health and physical capabilities, better adjustment to limitations, and less athletic restriction.[49] Support groups that recognize these factors, strengthen positive skills, and redirect the negative will better socialize, reintegrate, and rehabilitate this population.

Table 4

Prosthesis Components

Components	Transtibial	Transfemoral
Suspension	Total contact socket	Quadrilateral socket
	Patellar tendon bearing (PTB)	Cad cam socket
	Patellar tendon supporting	Suction contour socket
	PTB with supracondylar cuff	
	PTB with sleeve suspension	
Liners	Soft PTB sockets	Soft socket
	Hard sockets	Hard sockets
	Pylete	Pylete
	Thermoplastic elastomer (TEM)	TEM
Knee	N/A	Constant friction knee
		Variable friction knee
		Polycentric
		Fluid control (hydraulic)
Foot	Solid ankle, cushion heel (SACH) foot	SACH foot
	Single-axis foot	Single axis foot
	Multiaxis foot	Multiaxis foot
	Energy storing	Energy storing

(Reproduced with permission from Pasquina PF, Cooper RA: *Care of the Combat Amputee*. Falls Church, VA, Washington, DC, United States Department of the Army, Office of the Surgeon General Borden Institute, 2009.)

Therapy

The goal of physical therapy is to maximize functionality for people who undergo amputation. Depending on the reason for the amputation, vascular or traumatic, therapy that entails working on range of motion and strengthening of the extremity can begin after surgery. In a traumatic amputation scenario, there is no preamputation therapy. Each level of amputation has a distinct potential for contractures. A transtibial amputation usually results in a knee flexion contracture, and a transfemoral amputation can result in a hip flexion contracture. Some studies have looked at preventive strategies such as prone lying, side lying, and aggressive pain control. These strategies, along with prosthetic gait training, resulted in higher rates of successful prosthetic use.[50] With the use of different postamputation dressings (for example, elastic with a knee immobilizer, rigid dressing, or IPOP, the risk for each contraction type may be alleviated, but a patient will also need to undergo therapy to increase strength and conditioning of the limb and the overall body.

Prosthesis

Once a patient can start wearing a prosthesis, he or she will progress from an intermediate to a permanent prosthesis. Lower-extremity prostheses contain the socket, the suspension, the pylon, and the foot. Those who undergo a transfemoral amputation will have an articulation to compensate for the loss of the knee. The design of the prosthesis depends on the patient's functional level. The Centers for Medicare and Medicaid Services requires a determination of the patient's functional level, often referred to as the K level, before prosthesis design. These levels include the following: (1) K1 level: unlimited household ambulatory (may do transfers or ambulate on level surfaces); (2) K2 level: limited community ambulatory (may have potential to ambulate with the ability to traverse low-level environmental barriers such as curbs, stairs, and uneven surfaces); (3) K3 level: community ambulator (can ambulate with variable cadence and traverse most environmental barriers; and (4) K4 level: exceeds basic ambulation (high stresses will be placed on the prosthesis because the patient is a child, an active adult, or an athlete. A list of prosthesis components is presented in **Table 4**.

Follow-up Care

People who undergo amputation require long-term follow-up care to ensure that they are functioning at the highest possible level. Continuous monitoring allows minor issues such as prosthesis fit and gait pattern to be evaluated, and changes can be addressed before they escalate into bigger issues that affect function.

Because of gait alteration and body realignment after amputation, the kinematic and loading characteristics of the native joints change. This change, in addition to residual limb maturation, necessitates long-term monitoring by the orthopaedic surgeon. Routine follow-up by the prosthetist also is required to monitor the condition of the prosthesis and its components.[52] Both are forms of preventive maintenance that can optimize patient outcome and function.

If the amputation was needed because of a medical condition, follow up with the appropriate specialist (an endocrinologist for diabetes mellitus or a vascular surgeon for vascular disease) also is required. Complications have been reported to be as high as 21% within the first 18 months after surgery.[52] As people age after an amputation, there is a decrease in independent walking. One third of young adults who underwent successful lower-extremity amputation and rehabilitation were noted to have limitations in mobility after an extended follow-up of about 30 years.[53] With the increase in prosthesis technology and improvements in medicine, it is imperative that these patients be followed so that they can continue to maintain the best possible functionality.

Heterotopic Bone Formation

Heterotopic ossification (HO) refers to the formation of mature lamellar bone in nonosseous tissue. In the setting of high-energy wartime extremity wounds, HO is expected to affect as many as 64% of patients, tends to form on residual limbs of those who undergo amputation, and remains a significant source of disability. Although the inciting events and the definitive cell(s) of origin remain elusive, animal models and human histology samples suggest that HO formation follows a predictable sequence of events, culminating in endochondral ossification. The authors of a 2011 study showed that the number of connective tissue progenitor cells was increased in traumatized tissue. Furthermore, wounds in which HO eventually forms have a higher percentage of connective tissue progenitor cells committed to osteogenic differentiation than do wounds in which HO does not form.[54] In a 2012 study of 36 penetrating extremity war wounds in 24 patients, the observed rate of HO in the study population was 38%. Of the 36 wounds, 13 (36%) demonstrated HO at a minimum follow-up of 2 months. An elevated injury severity score was associated with the development of HO ($P = 0.006$). Wound characteristics that correlated with the development of HO included impaired healing ($P = 0.005$) and bacterial colonization ($P = 0.001$). Both serum (interleukin [IL]-6, IL-10, and monocyte chemotactic protein-1) and wound effluent (IL-10) were characteristics that demonstrated favorable diagnostic performance in the detection of ectopic bone formation.[55]

Primary prophylaxis is not medically or logistically practical in most cases because patients have generally sustained massive wounds and are undergoing serial débridements during an intercontinental aeromedical evacuation. Surgical excision of symptomatic lesions is warranted only after an appropriate trial of nonsurgical measures and is associated with low recurrence rates in appropriately selected patients. Future research regarding prognostication and definition as the early molecular biology of ectopic bone may permit individualized prophylaxis and the development of novel targeted therapies.[56]

Another potential treatment can be related to retinoic acid receptor-γ (RAR-γ) agonist. HO was prevented in mice receiving a nuclear RAR-γ agonist.[57] Side effects were minimal, and there was no significant rebound effect. To uncover the mechanisms of these responses, mouse mesenchymal stem cells were treated with an RAR-γ agonist and transplanted into nude mice. Whereas control cells formed ectopic bone masses, cells that had been pretreated with the RAR-γ agonist did not, suggesting that they had lost their skeletogenic potential. The cells became unresponsive to recombinant bone morphogenetic protein-2 treatment in vitro and showed decreases in phosphorylation of SMAD1, SMAD5, and SMAD8 and overall levels of SMAD proteins. In addition, an RAR-γ agonist blocked HO in transgenic mice expressing activin receptor-like kinase-2 (ALK2) Q207D, a constitutively active form of the receptor that is related to ALK2 R206H found in individuals with fibrodysplasia ossificans progressiva. The data indicate that RAR-γ agonists are potent inhibitors of HO in mouse models and may also be effective against injury-induced and congenital HO in humans.[57]

Summary

Traumatic amputations are a procedure with which the practicing orthopaedic surgeon should be familiar. Several factors must be taken into consideration before and after the procedure. From the level of amputation and the effort to conserve as much length as possible to help with long-term energy expenditure to the management of complications such as heterotopic bone formation and psychological acceptance, all factors must be optimized to create the best possible outcome. The overall treatment of patients requiring an amputation requires a multidisciplinary approach with the involvement of pain management specialists, psychologists, and skilled prosthetists. Patients will require counseling from all the specialists involved to prepare them for short- and long-term outcomes. Traumatic amputations are an unfortunate circumstance, but careful planning and a cohesive treatment team can lead to a positive outcome.

Key Study Points

- The level of ampuation is critical in determing the energy expenditure and the cadence of ambulation. However, as per the LEAP studies, patients with a through-the-knee amputation did worse than those with below-knee and above-knee amputations.

- Current smokers were less likely to achieve fracture union than nonsmokers. Those who quit smoking were at no greater risk of infection overall but were at 2.8 times greater risk for developing osteomyelitis.

- When all factors are included, the lifetime healthcare cost for patients who had undergone amputation was three times higher than for those treated with reconstruction.

Annotated References

1. Campbell WC, Canale ST, Beaty JH: *Campbell's Operative Orthopaedics*. Philadelphia, PA, Mosby/Elsevier, 2008.

2. Ziegler-Graham K, MacKenzie EJ, Ephraim PL, Travison TG, Brookmeyer R: Estimating the prevalence of limb loss in the United States: 2005 to 2050. *Arch Phys Med Rehabil* 2008;89(3):422-429.

3. Tintle SM, Keeling JJ, Shawen SB, Forsberg JA, Potter BK: Traumatic and trauma-related amputations: Part I. General principles and lower-extremity amputations. *J Bone Joint Surg Am* 2010;92(17):2852-2868.

   This is a current concepts review of the general principles of lower extremity amputations. Level of evidence: III.

4. Harris AM, Althausen PL, Kellam J, Bosse MJ, Castillo R; Lower Extremity Assessment Project (LEAP) Study Group: Complications following limb-threatening lower extremity trauma. *J Orthop Trauma* 2009;23(1):1-6.

5. MacKenzie EJ, Jones AS, Bosse MJ, et al: Health-care costs associated with amputation or reconstruction of a limb-threatening injury. *J Bone Joint Surg Am* 2007; 89(8):1685-1692.

6. Higgins TF, Klatt JB, Beals TC: Lower Extremity Assessment Project (LEAP)—the best available evidence on limb-threatening lower extremity trauma. *Orthop Clin North Am* 2010;41(2):233-239.

   This is a review of all publications derived from LEAP. Level of evidence: II.

7. Mills WJ, Barei DP, McNair P: The value of the ankle-brachial index for diagnosing arterial injury after knee dislocation: A prospective study. *J Trauma* 2004;56(6): 1261-1265.

8. Dickhaut SC, DeLee JC, Page CP: Nutritional status: importance in predicting wound-healing after amputation. *J Bone Joint Surg Am* 1984;66(1):71-75.

9. Kübler-Ross E, Wessler S, Avioli LV: On death and dying. *JAMA* 1972;221(2):174-179.

10. Brodie EE, Whyte A, Niven CA: Analgesia through the looking-glass? A randomized controlled trial investigating the effect of viewing a "virtual" limb upon phantom limb pain, sensation and movement. *Eur J Pain* 2007; 11(4):428-436.

11. Blum ML, Esser M, Richardson M, Paul E, Rosenfeldt FL: Negative pressure wound therapy reduces deep infection rate in open tibial fractures. *J Orthop Trauma* 2012;26(9):499-505.

    In this retrospective cohort study, data were collected from medical records and radiographs at two level I trauma centers. Data included patients who sustained open tibial fractures and underwent delayed soft-tissue coverage. The main outcome measure was the deep infection rate. A total of 229 open tibial fractures in 220 patients met the inclusion criteria and received either NPWT (72%) or conventional dressings (28%). There was a decreased rate of deep infection in the NPWT group compared with the conventional dressing group (8.4% versus 20.6%; *P* = 0.01). Level of evidence: III.

12. Stannard JP, Volgas DA, McGwin G III, et al: Incisional negative pressure wound therapy after high-risk lower extremity fractures. *J Orthop Trauma* 2012;26(1): 37-42.

    This prospective randomized multicenter clinical trial investigated NPWT to prevent wound dehiscence and infection after high-risk lower extremity trauma in four level I trauma centers. Among subjects, 122 were randomized to Group A (controls) and 141 to Group B (NPWT). There were a total of 23 infections in Group A and 14 in Group B, which represented a significant difference in favor of NPWT (*P* = 0.049). The relative risk for developing an infection was 1.9 times higher in the control patients than in patients treated with NPWT. Level of evidence: I.

13. Waters RL, Perry J, Antonelli D, Hislop H: Energy cost of walking of amputees: The influence of level of amputation. *J Bone Joint Surg Am* 1976;58(1):42-46.

14. Hoffman MD, Sheldahl LM, Buley KJ, Sandford PR: Physiological comparison of walking among bilateral above-knee amputee and able-bodied subjects, and a model to account for the differences in metabolic cost. *Arch Phys Med Rehabil* 1997;78(4):385-392.

15. Pinzur MS: *Skeletal Trauma*. Philadelphia, PA, Saunders, 2009, p 2863.

16. Pinzur MS, Beck J, Himes R, Callaci J: Distal tibiofibular bone-bridging in transtibial amputation. *J Bone Joint Surg Am* 2008;90(12):2682-2687.

17. Dillon MP, Barker TM: Preservation of residual foot length in partial foot amputation: A biomechanical analysis. *Foot Ankle Int* 2006;27(2):110-116.

18. Kirkup J: *A History of Limb Amputation.* London, United Kingdom, Springer, 2007.

19. Dougherty PJ: Transtibial amputees from the Vietnam War: Twenty-eight-year follow-up. *J Bone Joint Surg Am* 2001;83(3):383-389.

20. Browner BD: *Skeletal Trauma Basic Science, Management, and Reconstruction.* Philadelphia, PA, Saunders/ Elsevier, 2009.

21. Vallier HA, Fitzgerald SJ, Beddow ME, Sontich JK, Patterson BM: Osteocutaneous pedicle flap transfer for salvage of transtibial amputation after severe lower-extremity injury. *J Bone Joint Surg Am* 2012;94(5): 447-454.

    In this retrospective review, 14 patients underwent osteocutaneous pedicle flap transfer for salvage of transtibial amputation. Level of evidence: IV.

22. Penn-Barwell JG: Outcomes in lower limb amputation following trauma: A systematic review and meta-analysis. *Injury* 2011;42(12):1474-1479.

    This meta-analysis of 27 studies, including 3,105 patients (1,855 with below-knee amputations, 104 with a total knee arthroplasty [TKA], 888 with above-knee amputation [AKA], and 258 with bilateral amputations), shows progressively and significantly worsening outcomes as unilateral amputation height becomes more proximal. Patients who underwent TKA wore their prosthesis less and had significantly more pain than those who underwent AKA. Level of evidence: II.

23. MacKenzie EJ, Bosse MJ, Castillo RC, et al: Functional outcomes following trauma-related lower-extremity amputation. *J Bone Joint Surg Am* 2004;86(8):1636-1645.

24. Campbell WC, Canale ST, Beaty JH: *Campbell's Operative Orthopaedics.* Philadelphia, PA, Elsevier/Mosby, 2013.

25. Veenstra KM, Sprangers MA, van der Eyken JW, Taminiau AH: Quality of life in survivors with a Van Ness-Borggreve rotationplasty after bone tumour resection. *J Surg Oncol* 2000;73(4):192-197.

26. Gillern SM, Sheppard FR, Evans KN, et al: Incidence of pulmonary embolus in combat casualties with extremity amputations and fractures. *J Trauma* 2011;71(3): 607-613.

    The incidence of PE is significantly higher (15.7%) with trauma-associated amputation than with extremity long-bone fracture without amputation. The cumulative incidence of PE was 5.7%. Bilateral amputations, multiple long-bone fractures, and pelvic fractures are independent risk factors for the development of PE. The use of aggressive prophylaxis, deep vein thrombosis screening with ultrasonography, and prophylactic inferior vena cava filters should be considered in this population. Level of evidence: IV.

27. Giummarra MJ, Georgiou-Karistianis N, Nicholls ME, Gibson SJ, Chou M, Bradshaw JL: The menacing phantom: What pulls the trigger? *Eur J Pain* 2011;15(7): e1-e8.

    The triggers of phantom phenomena are reviewed in a heterogeneous sample of 264 adult patients with upper and lower limb amputations who have phantom sensations. Participants completed a structured questionnaire to determine the prevalence and nature of the triggers of phantom phenomena. The four categories of triggers identified include psychologic, emotional, or autonomic triggers; behavioral triggers ("forgetting" the limb's absence and attempting to use the phantom); weather-induced triggers; and triggers referred from parts of the body. Level of evidence: III.

28. Smith DG, McFarland LV, Sangeorzan BJ, Reiber GE, Czerniecki JM: Postoperative dressing and management strategies for transtibial amputations: A critical review. *J Rehabil Res Dev* 2003;40(3):213-224.

29. Mooney V, Harvey JP Jr, McBride E, Snelson R: Comparison of postoperative stump management: Plaster vs. soft dressings. *J Bone Joint Surg Am* 1971;53(2):241-249.

30. Kihn RB, Golbranson FL, Hutchinson RH, Moore WS, Premer RF: The immediate postoperative prosthesis in lower extremity amputations: An evaluation. *Arch Surg* 1970;101(1):40-44.

31. Wu Y, Brncick MD, Krick HJ, Putnam TD, Stratigos JS: Scotchcast P.V.C. interim prosthesis for below-knee amputees. *Bull Prosthet Res* 1981;10(36):40-45.

32. Schon LC, Short KW, Soupiou O, Noll K, Rheinstein J: Benefits of early prosthetic management of transtibial amputees: A prospective clinical study of a prefabricated prosthesis. *Foot Ankle Int* 2002;23(6):509-514.

33. Nikolajsen L, Ilkjaer S, Jensen TS: Relationship between mechanical sensitivity and postamputation pain: A prospective study. *Eur J Pain* 2000;4(4):327-334.

34. Gallagher P, Allen D, Maclachlan M: Phantom limb pain and residual limb pain following lower limb amputation: A descriptive analysis. *Disabil Rehabil* 2001; 23(12):522-530.

35. Lambert Aw, Dashfield Ak, Cosgrove C, Wilkins Dc, Walker Aj, Ashley S: Randomized prospective study comparing preoperative epidural and intraoperative perineural analgesia for the prevention of postoperative stump and phantom limb pain following major amputation. *Reg Anesth Pain Med* 2001;26(4):316-321.

36. Nikolajsen L, Finnerup NB, Kramp S, Vimtrup AS, Keller J, Jensen TS: A randomized study of the effects of gabapentin on postamputation pain. *Anesthesiology* 2006;105(5):1008-1015.

4: Lower Extremity

37. Wu CL, Tella P, Staats PS, et al: Analgesic effects of intravenous lidocaine and morphine on postamputation pain: A randomized double-blind, active placebo-controlled, crossover trial. *Anesthesiology* 2002;96(4): 841-848.

38. Hanling SR, Wallace SC, Hollenbeck KJ, Belnap BD, Tulis MR: Preamputation mirror therapy may prevent development of phantom limb pain: A case series. *Anesth Analg* 2010;110(2):611-614.

    This case series reported on four patients who performed daily mirror therapy for 2 weeks before undergoing elective limb amputation. One patient experienced no PLP. Two patients experienced rare episodes of mild PLP without effect on their participation in physical therapy or their QOL. One patient reported daily, brief episodes of moderate PLP without effect on his participation in physical therapy or his stated QOL. Level of evidence: IV.

39. Osborne TL, Jensen MP, Ehde DM, Hanley MA, Kraft G: Psychosocial factors associated with pain intensity, pain-related interference, and psychological functioning in persons with multiple sclerosis and pain. *Pain* 2007;127(1-2):52-62.

40. Nunes MA, de Barros N Jr, Miranda F Jr, Baptista-Silva JC: Common mental disorders in patients undergoing lower limb amputation: A population-based sample. *World J Surg* 2012;36(5):1011-1015.

    This cross-sectional study assessed the association of sociodemographic and clinical variables in relation to psychiatric disorders evaluated through the Self Reporting Questionnaire for patients undergoing lower limb amputation. Among the 138 patients interviewed, a prevalence of 43% was observed for patients with mental disorders. Level of evidence: III.

41. Fisher K, Hanspal RS: Phantom pain, anxiety, depression, and their relation in consecutive patients with amputated limbs: Case reports. *BMJ* 1998;316(7135):903-904.

42. Williams RM, Ehde DM, Smith DG, Czerniecki JM, Hoffman AJ, Robinson LR: A two-year longitudinal study of social support following amputation. *Disabil Rehabil* 2004;26(14-15):862-874.

43. Horgan O, MacLachlan M: Psychosocial adjustment to lower-limb amputation: A review. *Disabil Rehabil* 2004; 26(14-15):837-850.

44. Social DS: *Handbook of Rehabilitation Psychology.* Washington, DC, American Psychological Association, 2000, p 565.

45. Hagberg K, Brånemark R: Consequences of non-vascular trans-femoral amputation: A survey of quality of life, prosthetic use and problems. *Prosthet Orthot Int* 2001;25(3):186-194.

46. Murray CD, Fox J: Body image and prosthesis satisfaction in the lower limb amputee. *Disabil Rehabil* 2002; 24(17):925-931.

47. Pezzin LE, Dillingham TR, Mackenzie EJ, Ephraim P, Rossbach P: Use and satisfaction with prosthetic limb devices and related services. *Arch Phys Med Rehabil* 2004;85(5):723-729.

48. Gerhards F, Florin I, Knapp T: The impact of medical, reeducational, and psychological variables on rehabilitation outcome in amputees. *Int J Rehabil Res* 1984;7(4): 379-388.

49. Gallagher P, MacLachlan M: Psychological adjustment and coping in adults with prosthetic limbs. *Behav Med* 1999;25(3):117-124.

50. Munin MC, Espejo-De Guzman MC, Boninger ML, Fitzgerald SG, Penrod LE, Singh J: Predictive factors for successful early prosthetic ambulation among lower-limb amputees. *J Rehabil Res Dev* 2001;38(4):379-384.

51. Gailey R, Allen K, Castles J, Kucharik J, Roeder M: Review of secondary physical conditions associated with lower-limb amputation and long-term prosthesis use. *J Rehabil Res Dev* 2008;45(1):15-29.

52. Skoutas D, Papanas N, Georgiadis GS, et al: Risk factors for ipsilateral reamputation in patients with diabetic foot lesions. *Int J Low Extrem Wounds* 2009;8(2): 69-74.

53. Burger H, Marincek C, Isakov E: Mobility of persons after traumatic lower limb amputation. *Disabil Rehabil* 1997;19(7):272-277.

54. Davis TA, O'Brien FP, Anam K, Grijalva S, Potter BK, Elster EA: Heterotopic ossification in complex orthopaedic combat wounds: Quantification and characterization of osteogenic precursor cell activity in traumatized muscle. *J Bone Joint Surg Am* 2011;93(12):1122-1131.

    Muscle biopsies were obtained from military service members who had sustained high-energy wartime injuries and from patients undergoing harvest of a hamstring tendon autograft. Plastic-adherent cells were isolated in single-cell suspension and plated to assess the prevalence of colony-forming cells. Phenotypic characteristics were assessed with flow cytometry. Individual colony-forming units were counted after an incubation period of 7 to 10 days, and replicate cultures were incubated in lineage-specific induction media. Immunohistochemical staining was performed to determine the percentage of colonies that had differentiated along an osteogenic lineage. Quantitative real-time reverse-transcription polymerase chain reaction was used to identify changes in osteogenic gene expression. Level of evidence: III.

55. Evans KN, Forsberg JA, Potter BK, et al: Inflammatory cytokine and chemokine expression is associated with heterotopic ossification in high-energy penetrating war injuries. *J Orthop Trauma* 2012;26(11):e204-e213.

    Patients with high-energy penetrating extremity wounds were prospectively enrolled in this study. Surgical débridement along with the use of a pulse lavage and vacuum-assisted closure device was performed every 48-72 hours until definitive wound closure. Wound bed tissue biopsy, wound effluent, and serum were collected before each débridement. Effluent and serum were analyzed for 22 relevant cytokines and chemokines. Tissue was analyzed quantitatively for bacterial colonization. Correlations between specific wound and patient characteristics were also analyzed. The primary clinical outcome measure was the formation of HO as confirmed with radiographs at a minimum of 2 months of follow-up. Level of evidence: II.

56. Forsberg JA, Potter BK: Heterotopic ossification in wartime wounds. *J Surg Orthop Adv* 2010;19(1):54-61.

The authors present a general review of wartime HO. There was a 64% HO incidence among those sustaining lower extremity amputation attributable to combat-related activity. Level of evidence: IV.

57. Shimono K, Tung WE, Macolino C, et al: Potent inhibition of heterotopic ossification by nuclear retinoic acid receptor-γ agonists. *Nat Med* 2011;17(4):454-460.

HO was essentially prevented in mice receiving a nuclear RAR-γ agonist. Side effects were minimal, and there was no significant rebound effect.

4: Lower Extremity

Section 5

Spine

SECTION EDITOR:

Mitchel B. Harris, MD

Chapter 47

Cervical Spine Trauma

Rowan Schouten, MBChB, FRACS   Charles G. Fisher, MD, MHSc, FRCSC

Introduction

The use of a systematic, evidence-based medicine approach is necessary to achieve an optimal outcome after a cervical spine injury. A failure to recognize or appropriately manage a cervical injury can have catastrophic consequences. Many practice guidelines and clinical decisions are based on low-level evidence because level I studies are difficult to perform and often are ethically inappropriate.

Initial Treatment and Evaluation

According to the Advanced Trauma Life Support protocol, the potentially injured cervical spine requires protection during initial assessment and resuscitation. Immobilization using a cervical orthosis supplemented with lateral supports (with or without forehead tape) is recommended. For a child, an occipital recess or mattress under the torso is required to accommodate a head that is disproportionately larger than the body. For a patient known to have an ankylosed cervical spine, immobilization must take into account any preexisting and often kyphotic deformity. A comprehensive neurologic examination that includes the lower sacral segments is critical for a patient with cervical trauma. A complete assessment often is not possible if the patient is multitraumatized, intoxicated, or unresponsive. The importance of a thorough secondary evaluation that includes imaging of the entire spine was highlighted in a recent retrospective review of 468 patients with a cervical injury, which found associated extraspinal injury in 267 (57%) and noncontiguous spine injury in 89 (19%).[1]

The National Emergency X-Radiography Utilization Study criteria and the Canadian C-Spine rule are highly sensitive decision-making tools that can be used to clinically exclude significant cervical injury in an alert, stable patient with trauma, allowing rationalization of C-spine imaging without jeopardizing patient outcomes.[2,3] In a patient requiring radiologic evaluation, CT has been shown to be more sensitive, efficient, and cost-effective than plain radiography, and in major trauma centers it is now considered the primary screening modality.[4] CT is particularly effective for identifying trauma in the upper cervical and cervicothoracic regions. MRI should be used if ligamentous, disk, or neural element pathology is suspected. In the presence of neurologic deficits, the ability of MRI to illustrate causes of extrinsic cord compression (for example, disk disruption, hematoma) assists surgical planning, while intrinsic cord signal changes are useful for spinal cord injury (SCI) prognostication.[5,6]

Isolated injuries to the diskoligamentous structures alone can create an unstable injury pattern. If spontaneous reduction and/or the placement of cervical collars leads to bony realignment, an isolated unstable injury may be undetectable on CT. This possibility is responsible for the controversy as to whether CT is sufficient for ruling out a clinically significant cervical injury in a patient who cannot be examined or whether both CT and MRI are necessary for definitive clearance. A recent meta-analysis pooled data on 1,550 patients with negative cervical CT after blunt trauma.[7] MRI revealed a clinically significant injury that altered treatment in 96 patients (6%) and 12 (1%) needed surgical stabilization. Counterarguments include the low incidence of clinically significant injuries missed on CT, the risk of prolonged collar use before MRI, the logistics of transporting an obtunded patient to and from the MRI scanner, and the cost incurred.

Because the integrity of diskoligamentous structures after a cervical injury influences treatment decisions, surgeons need to be aware that signal change on MRI may not be clinically relevant. A comparison of preoperative MRI findings with intraoperative inspection in patients with subaxial cervical trauma found that MRI had high sensitivity but only moderate specificity in detecting an injury of the posterior ligamentous complex.[8]

Dynamic radiography, including flexion-extension views and stretch tests, has a limited role in detecting occult injury of the cervical spine and should be avoided if the patient is obtunded. In a patient who is

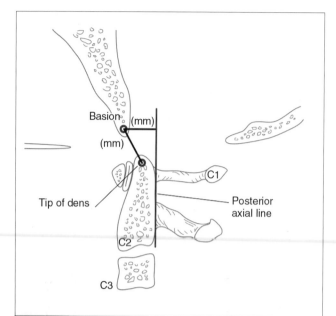

Figure 1 Schematic drawing showing the Harris rule of 12 mm. A basion-dens interval or basion–posterior axial interval greater than 12 mm is highly suggestive of occipitocervical dissociation. (Adapted with permission from Bono CM, Vaccaro AR, Fehlings M, et al: Measurement techniques for upper cervical spine injuries: Consensus statement of the Spine Trauma Study Group. *Spine (Phila Pa 1976)* 2007;32[5]:593-600.)

Occipitocervical Dissociation

Considerable force is required to destabilize the occipitoatlantoaxial articulation. Severe neurologic morbidity and mortality are common with occipitocervical dissociation. Increasing numbers of patients are surviving this highly unstable, potentially devastating injury because of improved prehospitalization management, and a good outcome is possible with early diagnosis and appropriate treatment.[11] Reliable radiographic diagnostic parameters include the basion-dens interval and basion–posterior axial interval, which are best measured on a midsagittal CT reconstruction.[11-13] According to the Harris rule, occipitocervical dissociation is strongly suggested if either of these intervals is larger than 12 mm (Figure 1). MRI of the stabilizing capsuloligamentous structures can reveal an occult injury and guide treatment decisions.

After occipitocervical dissociation is recognized, great caution must be taken to maintain alignment until surgical fixation. Prompt provisional stabilization, using a halo vest or tongs to help control head position, should be followed by immediate surgery. If static imaging shows preserved alignment but the MRI findings are abnormal, provocative traction has been recommended to identify occult instability.[11] If traction creates a distraction of the occipitoatlantal joint greater than 2 mm, internal fixation is recommended. High rates of clinical success have been reported after posterior occipitocervical fixation and fusion using modern segmental instrumentation, in which contoured rods are used to connect midline occipital plates or screws with suboccipital polyaxial screws to achieve fixation from C0 to C2 or lower.[11]

neurologically intact but has persistent neck pain after trauma and a normal initial CT, delayed flexion-extension radiographs can be a valid alternative to MRI.[4] If the radiographic findings are both adequate and negative, a cervical collar can be safely removed.

Occipital Condyle Fracture

An occipital condyle fracture is often difficult to detect on plain radiographs but increasingly is recognized with CT trauma screening. Occipital condyle fractures are rarely an isolated injury, given their typically high-energy mechanism; a noncontiguous spine fracture or an extraspinal injury was reported in 30% or 85% of patients, respectively.[1] Lower cranial nerve palsy, often involving the hypoglossal nerve, can also coexist.

The stability of the occipitocervical junction and any associated cervical injuries are the primary factors dictating the treatment and the ultimate functional outcome.[9] Classification systems are available but offer limited additional clinical value.[10] If the integrity of the occipitocervical junction remains preserved (that is, no malalignment on reformatted CT images or ligamentous disruption on MRI), treatment with a cervical orthosis is appropriate, even for bilateral fractures.[10] If the occipital fracture represents part of a destabilizing injury to the occipitocervical articulation, internal fixation is necessary.

Odontoid Fracture

Fracture of the odontoid has a bimodal age distribution and is commonly described using the anatomically based Anderson-D'Alonzo classification[14] (Figure 2). Most surgeons agree that an Anderson-D'Alonzo type I or III fracture is effectively managed with external immobilization. The rates of mortality and complications are high when a halo orthosis is used in patients 65 years or older. Collar immobilization is recommended for a type III odontoid fracture in these patients and has favorable union rates.[15] Because bony avulsion of the alar ligament can exist with occipitocervical dissociation, careful assessment is required before an isolated type I odontoid fracture is diagnosed.

Fracture through the base of the odontoid (an Anderson-D'Alonzo type II fracture), where blood supply and trabecular bone are limited, has diminished healing potential. The treatment options include external immobilization or surgical stabilization through an anterior or posterior approach. The management of this injury remains controversial, particularly in the elderly. The only relevant evidence is of low or very low quality.[15,16] The threat of selection bias has thwarted attempts to compare the outcomes of patients who were nonrandomly selected for nonsurgical or surgical treatment. Many published studies have focused on radiologic outcomes, such as osseous union, despite uncertainty as to the incidence of neurologic sequelae and secondary pain in patients with a stable fibrous union. Recent systematic reviews have combined the best available evidence with expert opinion to provide evidence-based recommendations on optimal clinical care.[15,16]

The need for surgery is generally undisputed for patients with a neurologic deficit and often is considered appropriate for patients with risk factors for nonunion, such as advanced age, posterior fracture displacement greater than 5 mm, fracture comminution, or tobacco use.[15] Nonsurgical treatment often is effective but may be poorly tolerated, particularly by patients older than 65 years. A trend toward surgical management of these injuries has been reported, in part as a result of advances in internal fixation techniques.[17] Contemporary fixation options include arthrodesis with the use of a single anterior odontoid screw or a rigid posterior construct (C1-C2 transarticular or segmental). Only low-quality evidence is available to help determine the optimal surgical strategy.[16] Anterior screw fixation is suitable for an acute, reducible simple fracture (with little or no comminution) that is obliquely oriented from anterosuperior to posteroinferior so that screw insertion can create perpendicular compression. The patient must have good bone quality as well as neck geometry conducive to achieving the necessary drill-screw trajectory and intraoperative imaging.[16] An anterior odontoid screw is presumed to preserve C1-C2 motion, but in some studies, particularly those of elderly patients, a posterior approach led to superior union rates.[15,16] Anterior and posterior approaches lead to equivalent overall rates of complications, but the complication profiles differ. Anterior surgery can be complicated by screw misplacement, dislodgement with loss of reduction, swallowing difficulty, or aspiration pneumonia. Posterior surgery is more likely to lead to blood loss, C2 nerve root injury, vertebral artery injury, or postoperative pain. Patient characteristics and preferences as well as surgeon expertise and resources have pivotal roles in the choice of treatment.[16]

As the population ages, increasing numbers of patients older than 65 years sustain an odontoid fracture, often as the result of a low-energy fall.[17] The 1-year mortality rate after a type II odontoid fracture is 31% in patients older than 65 years, regardless of the treatment method.[15,18] Patients and their families should be informed of the high morbidity and mortality rates after an odontoid fracture. Factors such as patient preference, life expectancy, preinjury functional status, and surgical suitability often determine the ideal treatment modality. Increasingly, surgical treatment of type II odontoid fracture is recommended for patients older than 65 years.[15] Although anterior screw fixation has been successfully used for these patients, many surgeons prefer a posterior surgical technique because of higher fusion rates and lower surgical morbidity.[15,19] If

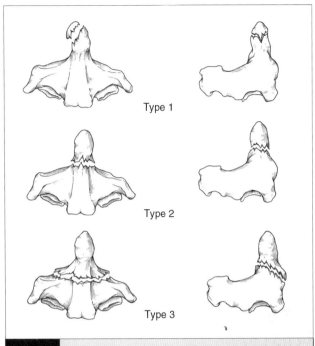

Figure 2 Schematic drawing showing the Anderson-D'Alonzo classification of odontoid fractures. Type I is an avulsion of the tip of the odontoid process, type II is a fracture through the base of the odontoid, and type III is a fracture extending into the vertebral body and C1-C2 articulation. (Reproduced from Hsu WK, Anderson PA: Odontoid fractures: Update on management. *J Am Acad Orthop Surg* 2010;18:383-394.)

nonsurgical treatment is chosen, a hard collar is preferable to a halo vest because the complication rates are lower with the hard collar and the fusion rates are comparable.[15]

C2 Traumatic Spondylolisthesis (Hangman's Fracture)

Traumatic spondylolisthesis of the axis results from bilateral C2 pars interarticularis fractures and, depending on the trauma mechanism, varying degrees of disruption of the anterior and/or posterior longitudinal ligaments and the C2-C3 disk. The amount of resulting translation, angulation, and facet joint dislocation between the second and third cervical vertebrae is the basis of the popular Levine-Edwards modification of the original Effendi classification.[20] This system highlights the unique qualities of fractures with severe angulation of C2 on C3 but little or no translation (a Levine-Edwards type IIA injury). Because the mechanism of this specific injury pattern involves flexion-distraction, traction can be harmful.

Displacement of these injuries typically results in spinal canal expansion, and therefore most hangman's fractures are neurologically benign. One exception is a neural arch fracture that extends into the posterior portion of the vertebral body. Subluxation of this atypical

5: Spine

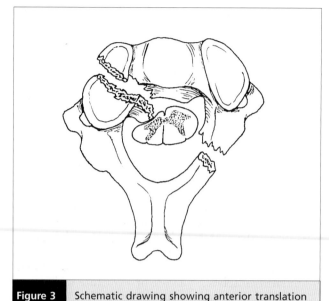

Figure 3 Schematic drawing showing anterior translation in an atypical hangman's fracture, which creates spinal cord compression against the posterior C2 vertebral body component that remains fixed to the posterior elements. (Reproduced with permission from Starr JK, Eismont FJ: Atypical hangman's fractures. *Spine (Phila Pa 1976)* 1993;18[14]:1954-1957.)

Table 1

The Subaxial Cervical Spine Injury Classification and Severity Scale

Injury Characteristic	Score
Morphology	
No abnormality	0
Compression	1
Burst	+ 1 = 2
Distraction (facet joint perch, hyperextension)	3
Rotation-translation (facet joint dislocation, unstable teardrop fracture, advanced-stage flexion compression injury)	4
Diskoligamentous complex	
Intact	0
Indeterminate (isolated interspinous widening, MRI spine change only)	1
Disrupted (widening of disk space, facet joint perch, dislocation)	2
Neurologic status	
Intact	0
Root injury	1
Complete spinal cord injury	2
Incomplete spinal cord injury	3
Continuous spinal cord compression in setting of neurologic deficit (neuromodifier)	+ 1

Nonsurgical treatment is recommended if the total score is lower than 4; surgical treatment is recommended if the total score is higher than 4. A score of 4 is considered equivocal.
(Reproduced with permission from Vaccaro AR, Hulbert RJ, Patel AA, et al: The Subaxial Cervical Spine Injury Classification system: A novel approach to recognize the importance of morphology, neurology, and integrity of the disco-ligamentous complex. *Spine (Phila Pa 1976)* 2007;32[21]:2365-2374.)

fracture has the potential to create canal compromise and lead to neurologic sequelae[21] (**Figure 3**).

The literature on the optimal treatment strategy and surgical indications for hangman's fractures is weak; consequently, the treatment varies widely.[22] For Levine-Edwards type I injuries and many type II injuries, external immobilization with or without prior traction reduction has been reported as reliable.[23] Surgical stabilization is considered if there is significant C2-C3 disk disruption, severe angulation, and fracture with C2-C3 facet dislocation (a Levine-Edwards type III injury). Anterior or posterior surgical strategies can be effective. Anterior procedures include C2-C3 diskectomy, plating, and fusion. Posterior procedures typically involve C1-C3 fixation and fusion or, in an effort to preserve motion, direct pars articularis osteosynthesis using lag screws alone (for minimal C2-C3 disk injury) or connected to C3 segmental fixation.

Subaxial Cervical Injury

In 2007, the Spine Trauma Study Group introduced the Subaxial Cervical Spine Injury Classification (SLIC), a simple but comprehensive system to stratify subaxial spine injuries.[24] The SLIC focuses on three integral variables: injury morphology, integrity of the diskoligamentous complex, and neurologic status (**Table 1**). A severity-related score is assigned to each variable, and the total score is used to guide treatment. The simplicity of the SLIC system, coupled with its clinical relevance, reliability, and ability to direct treatment in a manner that is highly correlated with spine surgeon preferences, has led to its widespread adoption.[24,25]

An evidence-based algorithm based on the SLIC system is useful for selecting the surgical approach (anterior, posterior, or circumferential) to use for common subaxial injury patterns.[26] The algorithm recommends treatment of a burst-type compression injury with neurologic deficits using anterior vertebrectomy, fusion, and plating.[26] Distraction injuries secondary to hyperflexion, which range from unilateral facet joint subluxation to bilateral perched facet joints without dislocation or fracture, can be treated with anterior or posterior fixation, but anterior diskectomy and fusion are recommended if there is a traumatic disk herniation. A hyperextension injury causes primarily anterior diskoligamentous disruption, and anterior stabilization therefore is preferred. If this injury occurs in an ankylosed spine, a biomechanically superior multilevel posterior construct may be required.[26] Surgical treatment generally is required for an injury that results in translation (such as a bilateral facet dislocation) or rotation (such as a displaced unilateral facet joint fracture or dislocation) relative to an adjacent vertebra.

Cervical Dislocation

The well-established treatment goals for a cervical unilateral or bilateral facet joint dislocation are to achieve a timely controlled realignment, decompression, and appropriate surgical stabilization leading to an optimal neurologic outcome. No universally accepted algorithm exists, however, and there is considerable variation in the use of prereduction MRI, a preference for closed or open reduction, and the surgical approach.[27,28] Factors pertinent to these decisions include the patient's level of consciousness, the patient's neurologic status, and local access to MRI and an operating room.

Each treatment choice has benefits and drawbacks. By restoring spine alignment, closed reduction allows rapid decompression of the spinal cord and has the potential to limit neurologic impairment. However, a traumatic disk herniation could further displace into the canal during the reduction maneuver and cause neurologic consequences. If prereduction MRI identifies a traumatic disk herniation, many surgeons prefer to perform an open anterior diskectomy before a reduction to mitigate the risk of further displacement. The drawback of obtaining prereduction MRI includes the time required, the risk of transporting the patient to and from the scanner, and the need to accurately interpret the findings. Worldwide experience has shown that closed reduction using sequential traction is effective and safe in an alert and cooperative patient who can communicate any change in neurologic status during the maneuver.[28]

The neurologic status of the patient is often considered critical. Prereduction MRI may be preferred for a cooperative patient who has escaped neurologic injury. In contrast, many surgeons believe that an examinable patient with profound neurologic impairment is more likely to benefit from a prompt indirect decompression through closed reduction than from a procedure that was delayed to obtain baseline MRI. Considerable controversy exists between these two philosophies for a patient with an incomplete neurologic deficit. A further option, if an operating room is immediately available, is to proceed directly to open anterior diskectomy and reduction of facet joint dislocations.

Although the need for surgical stabilization after reduction is widely accepted, there is little agreement on the optimal surgical approach.[29] A posterior approach may be required after unsuccessful open anterior reduction or as a supplement to anterior fixation if bilateral facet joint fractures or a superior end plate fracture is present.[30] The final choice of approach often is influenced by the surgeon's training and experience as well as unique patient factors and preferences, which often are based on the adverse event profile of each procedure. Compared with an anterior approach, a posterior approach carries a greater risk of surgical site infection and segmental kyphosis as well as more severe postoperative pain. The risks of anterior surgery include voice and swallowing dysfunction as well as complications associated with inferior biomechanical properties.

Combined anterior-posterior stabilization generally is recommended for a teardrop fracture, which is characterized by a significant vertebral body fracture that includes a triangular fragment from the anteroinferior corner, retrodisplacement of the posterior vertebral body cortex, and tensile failure of the posterior elements.[26]

Unilateral Facet Joint Injury

The wide variety of unilateral facet joint injuries includes fractures, subluxations, and dislocations as well as fractures that involve the ipsilateral lamina and pedicle and lead to separation (or "floating") of the lateral mass from the vertebral body. Surgical stabilization generally is recommended for subluxation or dislocation. In contrast, a neurologically intact nondisplaced or minimally displaced fracture or a fracture with a stable or improving radicular neurologic deficit can be treated with an external orthosis for 6 to 8 weeks. Close follow-up is necessary to detect a delayed subluxation or new-onset or progressive neurologic symptoms. A unilateral facet joint fracture with a height of more than 1 cm or 40% of the intact lateral mass has been associated with an increased risk of failure of nonsurgical treatment.[31] The largest reported study of unilateral facet joint fractures, subluxations, and dislocations included 90 patients.[32] This study concluded that surgery should be strongly considered for all facet joint injuries because patients treated nonsurgically were found to have worse pain and disability at long-term follow-up (more than 18 months) than those treated surgically, even though patients treated nonsurgically almost exclusively had so-called benign nondisplaced superior facet joint fractures.

Vertebral Artery Injury

Cervical trauma can cause a vertebral artery injury ranging from an intimal flap to a complete occlusion. Modern CT angiography and magnetic resonance angiography are noninvasive and capable of accurately identifying clinically relevant injuries.[33-35] A recent prospective study found a particularly high incidence of vertebral artery injury associated with facet joint subluxation-dislocation (31%), upper cervical injury (24%), and fracture extending into the transverse foramen (20%).[33] The consequences of these lesions vary greatly, and many patients remain asymptomatic. In contrast, patients with insufficient collateral blood supply may have a spectrum of neurologic symptoms ranging from headaches, dizziness, vertigo, and visual disturbances to catastrophic posterior circulation stroke and death.

The prevention of delayed vertebrobasilar ischemia is the rationale for screening patients at risk and treating those in whom a vertebral artery injury is identified. No randomized comparative studies are available

5: Spine

to guide clinical decision making.[34,35] Consequently, much debate remains about which, if any, patients without symptoms should be screened and whether observation, anticoagulation therapy, or endovascular treatment is advisable if a vertebral artery injury is identified. The adverse effects of systemic anticoagulation therapy and, in particular, the risk of hemorrhage from coexisting injuries, such as a traumatized spinal cord or intracranial hemorrhage, is included in the decision-to-treat process. When anticoagulation is selected, variation exists in the choice of therapeutic agent (antiplatelet agents, heparin, or warfarin) and the duration of treatment (1 to 6 months).[33-35] At the very least, the existence of a vertebral artery injury can be factored into the surgical tactics to ensure protection of the opposite, intact vertebral artery.

Cervical Spinal Cord Injury

Because of the devastating ramifications of cervical SCI, strategies aimed at achieving an optimal neurologic outcome continue to be the focus of extensive research into both the surgical and medical aspects of care.

Surgical Treatment

The potential neurologic benefits and the feasibility of early decompression after a traumatic cervical SCI remains a subject of research. A survey of 971 spine surgeons worldwide revealed that more than 80% favored decompression within 24 hours after a cervical SCI and even earlier intervention (within 12 hours) for an incomplete SCI (except for central cord syndrome).[36] Emergency reduction of bilateral facet joint dislocations is a widespread practice, and it may be even more critical after low-velocity trauma, such as a sports injury.[37] Until recently, the belief that early decompression improves neurologic outcome was based on biologic rationale, animal studies, evidence from low-quality clinical studies, and anecdotal reports. Affirmation from high-quality human studies was lacking until the 2012 publication of the Surgical Timing in Acute Spinal Cord Injury Study, a prospective North American multicenter nonrandomized study of 313 patients with an acute cervical SCI and spinal cord compression.[38] At 6-month follow-up, improvement of two or more grades on the American Spinal Injury Association Impairment Scale (AIS) was documented in more patients who underwent decompression within 24 hours than in patients who had later decompression (19.8% and 8.8% of patients, respectively). Even after controlling for baseline differences in the patient groups, the odds of a minimum two-grade AIS improvement remained 2.8 times higher in the patients who received early decompression.

Central Cord Syndrome

An exception to the emerging consensus on the role of early surgical decompression involves central cord injuries in patients who have background cervical stenosis, do not have evidence of acute fracture or instability, and have static or improving neurology. The most common incomplete SCI pattern, central cord syndrome occurs mainly in elderly patients after traumatic hyperextension of a stenotic, spondylitic cervical spine. Central cord syndrome involves incomplete tetraplegia characterized by disproportionate impairment in the upper extremities compared with the lower limbs, with variable degrees of sensory and sacral root involvement that cause bladder, bowel, and sexual dysfunction.

Despite the reputation of central cord syndrome for significant spontaneous neurologic recovery, persistent motor deficits, dysesthetic pain, bowel and bladder dysfunction, and loss of hand dexterity can be disabling. Lower initial AIS motor scores are associated with inferior ultimate functional outcomes.[6,39] It is unclear whether surgical decompression of background stenosis within 24 hours improves the neurologic prognosis of patients with acute central cord syndrome or whether surgery should be reserved for patients whose neurologic recovery reaches a plateau. This debate is reflected in the significant variability in current practice.[22,36] The Spine Trauma Study Group recently combined the available low-quality studies with analysis of a prospective observational cohort study and consensus expert opinion to conclude that surgical decompression within 24 hours is "a reasonable and safe option" for patients with a significant neurologic deficit (AIS type C). Initial observation was recommended for patients with less severe initial neurologic involvement (AIS type D).[40]

Medical Treatment

After the initial mechanical insult to the spinal cord, a sequence of secondary pathophysiologic processes is initiated that leads to further neurologic damage.[41] Sparing neurologic tissue by attenuating these events and promoting subsequent axonal regeneration or remyelination is the goal of neuroprotective and neuroregenerative therapies. These interventions are administered systemically or less commonly applied directly to the injured spinal cord or overlying dura.[42] Earlier strategies involved methylprednisolone, but more current interventions include anti-Nogo antibodies, minocycline, riluzole, magnesium, human embryonic stem cell–derived oligodendrocyte progenitors, and systemic hypothermia. Many of these recent therapies have bridged the translational gap, and human studies have begun.[43] Clinical efficacy has yet to be determined.

The neuroprotective effect of methylprednisolone was assessed in human studies conducted during the 1980s and 1990s, collectively known as the National Acute Spinal Cord Injury Study (NASCIS).[44] Although the use of methylprednisolone initially was heralded as a standard of care, independent scrutiny of the original study results found serious associated complications and only modest clinical benefits.[45] Methylprednisolone use subsequently was abandoned or relegated to treatment-option status in many practice guidelines.

Nonetheless, the possibility of any mitigation of neurologic loss as well as medicolegal concerns have contributed to the enduring use of methylprednisolone; 62% of patients received methylprednisolone in the recent multicenter Surgical Timing in Acute Spinal Cord Injury Study.[38]

Like the injured brain, the traumatized spinal cord is vulnerable to ischemic damage from hypoperfusion. Uncontrolled studies found that prevention and aggressive treatment of hypotension following SCI is associated with a favorable neurologic outcome.[46,47] The ideal mean arterial pressure and duration of hemodynamic support are yet to be defined, but the belief that optimization of spinal cord perfusion improves neurologic outcomes has gained widespread support.

The Ankylosed Cervical Spine

Ankylosing spinal disorders, such as ankylosing spondylitis, diffuse idiopathic skeletal hyperostosis, and end-stage degenerative spondylosis, often create an osteoporotic cervical spine with altered biomechanical properties that render it prone to fracture. A high index of suspicion is necessary when a patient with an ankylosed cervical spine has neck pain after an injury. Recent studies have reiterated that even a minor or supposedly trivial event, such as a ground-level fall, is capable of producing an unstable fracture with potentially devastating repercussions.[48-51] Particularly vulnerable are the lower cervical levels (C5-C7), in which hyperextension-type injury patterns predominate, and associated SCI is common.[49,50] Secondary neurologic deterioration can result from a delay in presentation or diagnosis, improper immobilization that fails to respect their preexisting alignment, or the formation of an epidural hematoma. CT or MRI is mandatory because the injury often is unrecognized on plain radiographs.[48] Noncontiguous fractures are also frequent (8%).[48] Caution is required when alignment alone is used to gauge fracture stability because the altered spinal biomechanics mean that even a minimally displaced fracture may be unstable.

The currently available low-quality studies reported high complication rates associated with the treatment of these injuries, which typically occur in patients who are of advanced age and have multiple comorbidities.[49] Definitive treatment using a rigid cervical orthosis typically is reserved for a nondisplaced fracture in a neurologically intact patient or a patient considered to be a high-risk surgical candidate. In these patients, a halo vest often is poorly tolerated.[51] Close monitoring is required.

Surgical stabilization has the advantage of restoring immediate stability, protecting neurologic status, and avoiding excessive mobility restrictions, but surgical complications are common. It is possible to acutely correct severe kyphotic deformities through the cervical fracture site, but, in general, stabilization that restores preinjury alignment is preferred. Posterior instrumentation extending at least three levels above and below the fracture is favored to offset the long lever arms and osteoporosis typical of a fused spine.[50] Aberrant anatomy can make implant placement difficult, and the use of intraoperative navigation can be advantageous. An anterior approach rarely is used in isolation but is considered if supplemental fixation is necessary or ventral pathology requires decompression.

Summary

Evidence-based treatment of cervical trauma is essential to optimize the outcome of these potentially devastating injuries. High-quality evidence to guide treatment is lacking for many injury scenarios; consequently, variability currently exists among treating surgeons. Research continues, with a particular spotlight on the management of fractures typical in an aging population and strategies to maximize neurologic function after SCI.

Key Study Points

- The treatment of cervical trauma often is based on low-level evidence, and the result can be variability in treatment preferences, particularly for bilateral facet joint dislocation and odontoid fracture in elderly patients.

- Clinical evidence increasingly suggests that early decompression after a traumatic cervical SCI may lead to an optimal neurologic outcome, but the effectiveness of medical therapies is unproved.

- A high index of suspicion is necessary for a patient with an ankylosed cervical spine because minor trauma has the potential to cause an unstable fracture that can have devastating consequences if left untreated.

Annotated References

1. Miller CP, Brubacher JW, Biswas D, Lawrence BD, Whang PG, Grauer JN: The incidence of noncontiguous spinal fractures and other traumatic injuries associated with cervical spine fractures: A 10-year experience at an academic medical center. *Spine (Phila Pa 1976)* 2011; 36(19):1532-1540.

   A retrospective chart review of 468 patients with a cervical fracture or a dislocation documented the incidence of associated extraspinal injuries (57%) and noncontiguous spine injuries (19%). Level of evidence: IV.

2. Hoffman JR, Mower WR, Wolfson AB, Todd KH, Zucker MI; National Emergency X-Radiography Utilization Study Group: Validity of a set of clinical criteria to rule out injury to the cervical spine in patients with blunt trauma. *N Engl J Med* 2000;343(2):94-99.

5: Spine

3. Stiell IG, Wells GA, Vandemheen KL, et al: The Canadian C-spine rule for radiography in alert and stable trauma patients. *JAMA* 2001;286(15):1841-1848.

4. Como JJ, Diaz JJ, Dunham CM, et al: Practice management guidelines for identification of cervical spine injuries following trauma: Update from the Eastern Association for the Surgery of Trauma practice management guidelines committee. *J Trauma* 2009;67(3):651-659.

5. Bozzo A, Marcoux J, Radhakrishna M, Pelletier J, Goulet B: The role of magnetic resonance imaging in the management of acute spinal cord injury. *J Neurotrauma* 2011;28(8):1401-1411.

   A literature review on the usefulness of MRI in patients with acute SCI found that MRI was able to predict neurologic outcomes, exclude injury in a patient who is obtunded, and identify vertebral artery injuries.

6. Hohl JB, Lee JY, Horton JA, Rihn JA: A novel classification system for traumatic central cord syndrome: The central cord injury scale (CCIS). *Spine (Phila Pa 1976)* 2010;35(7):E238-E243.

   In a retrospective review of 37 patients with central cord syndrome, initial AIS motor score and signal change on MRI were combined to create a classification system predictive of 1-year functional outcomes. Level of evidence: IV.

7. Schoenfeld AJ, Bono CM, McGuire KJ, Warholic N, Harris MB: Computed tomography alone versus computed tomography and magnetic resonance imaging in the identification of occult injuries to the cervical spine: A meta-analysis. *J Trauma* 2010;68(1):109-114.

   A meta-analysis of level III studies of 1,550 patients with cervical trauma and negative cervical CT found that 96 patients (6%) had a clinically relevant injury that was identified on subsequent MRI, and 12 patients (1%) required surgical stabilization.

8. Rihn JA, Yang N, Fisher C, et al: Using magnetic resonance imaging to accurately assess injury to the posterior ligamentous complex of the spine: A prospective comparison of the surgeon and radiologist. *J Neurosurg Spine* 2010;12(4):391-396.

   Preoperative MRI of the posterior ligamentous complex was compared with intraoperative assessment in 47 patients with cervical trauma. A high rate of false-positive MRI findings was noted. Level of evidence: I.

9. Malham GM, Ackland HM, Jones R, Williamson OD, Varma DK: Occipital condyle fractures: Incidence and clinical follow-up at a level 1 trauma centre. *Emerg Radiol* 2009;16(4):291-297.

10. Maserati MB, Stephens B, Zohny Z, et al: Occipital condyle fractures: Clinical decision rule and surgical management. *J Neurosurg Spine* 2009;11(4):388-395.

11. Bellabarba C, Mirza SK, West GA, et al: Diagnosis and treatment of craniocervical dislocation in a series of 17 consecutive survivors during an 8-year period. *J Neurosurg Spine* 2006;4(6):429-440.

12. Bono CM, Vaccaro AR, Fehlings M, et al: Measurement techniques for upper cervical spine injuries: Consensus statement of the Spine Trauma Study Group. *Spine (Phila Pa 1976)* 2007;32(5):593-600.

13. Horn EM, Feiz-Erfan I, Lekovic GP, Dickman CA, Sonntag VK, Theodore N: Survivors of occipitoatlantal dislocation injuries: Imaging and clinical correlates. *J Neurosurg Spine* 2007;6(2):113-120.

14. Anderson LD, D'Alonzo RT: Fractures of the odontoid process of the axis. *J Bone Joint Surg Am* 1974;56(8):1663-1674.

15. Harrop JS, Hart R, Anderson PA: Optimal treatment for odontoid fractures in the elderly. *Spine (Phila Pa 1976)* 2010;35(21, suppl):S219-S227.

    A systematic review of the available low- and very low–quality studies and expert opinion were used to answer focused questions on the optimal treatment strategies for type II and III odontoid fractures in patients older than 65 years.

16. Patel AA, Lindsey R, Bessey JT, Chapman J, Rampersaud R; Spine Trauma Study Group: Surgical treatment of unstable type II odontoid fractures in skeletally mature individuals. *Spine (Phila Pa 1976)* 2010;35(21, suppl):S209-S218.

    Based on a systematic literature review and consensus expert opinion, the optimal surgical choices for unstable type II odontoid fractures in skeletally mature patients were reviewed. Ideal indications and techniques for anterior or posterior fixation were included.

17. Smith HE, Kerr SM, Fehlings MG, et al: Trends in epidemiology and management of type II odontoid fractures: 20-year experience at a model system spine injury tertiary referral center. *J Spinal Disord Tech* 2010;23(8):501-505.

    A retrospective review of all neurologically intact type II odontoid fractures at a single center between 1985 and 2006 found a higher incidence over time as well as a higher rate of surgical management. Level of evidence: IV.

18. Schoenfeld AJ, Bono CM, Reichmann WM, et al: Type II odontoid fractures of the cervical spine: Do treatment type and medical comorbidities affect mortality in elderly patients? *Spine (Phila Pa 1976)* 2011;36(11):879-885.

    Retrospective analysis found a 21% mortality rate at 3 months and a 31% rate at 12 months in 156 patients age 65 years or older with a type II odontoid fracture. The patients were further stratified by age, comorbidities, and treatment modality. Level of evidence: IV.

19. Dailey AT, Hart D, Finn MA, Schmidt MH, Apfelbaum RI: Anterior fixation of odontoid fractures in an elderly population. *J Neurosurg Spine* 2010;12(1):1-8.

    A retrospective review of 57 patients (mean age, 81.2 years) with type II or III odontoid fracture treated with anterior screw fixation found an 81% rate of radiologic stability at a mean 14-month follow-up. Perioperative complications included dysphagia (35%), pneumonia (19%), and myocardial infarction (5%). Level of evidence: IV.

20. Levine AM, Edwards CC: The management of traumatic spondylolisthesis of the axis. *J Bone Joint Surg Am* 1985;67(2):217-226.

21. Starr JK, Eismont FJ: Atypical hangman's fractures. *Spine (Phila Pa 1976)* 1993;18(14):1954-1957.

22. Lenehan B, Dvorak MF, Madrazo I, Yukawa Y, Fisher CG: Diversity and commonalities in the care of spine trauma internationally. *Spine (Phila Pa 1976)* 2010; 35(21, suppl):S174-S179.

    Significant regional differences were identified when 77 spine surgeons worldwide were surveyed as to preferred methods of managing common spine injuries. Level of evidence: V.

23. Li XF, Dai LY, Lu H, Chen XD: A systematic review of the management of hangman's fractures. *Eur Spine J* 2006;15(3):257-269.

24. Vaccaro AR, Hulbert RJ, Patel AA, et al: The subaxial cervical spine injury classification system: A novel approach to recognize the importance of morphology, neurology, and integrity of the disco-ligamentous complex. *Spine (Phila Pa 1976)* 2007;32(21):2365-2374.

25. Patel AA, Hurlbert RJ, Bono CM, Bessey JT, Yang N, Vaccaro AR: Classification and surgical decision making in acute subaxial cervical spine trauma. *Spine (Phila Pa 1976)* 2010;35(21, suppl):S228-S234.

    A Spine Trauma Study Group review of available subaxial cervical spine injury classification systems concluded with a strong recommendation for adopting the SLIC system. Clinical examples were presented.

26. Dvorak MF, Fisher CG, Fehlings MG, et al: The surgical approach to subaxial cervical spine injuries: An evidence-based algorithm based on the SLIC classification system. *Spine (Phila Pa 1976)* 2007;32(23):2620-2629.

27. Arnold PM, Brodke DS, Rampersaud YR, et al: Differences between neurosurgeons and orthopedic surgeons in classifying cervical dislocation injuries and making assessment and treatment decisions: A multicenter reliability study. *Am J Orthop (Belle Mead NJ)* 2009; 38(10):E156-E161.

28. Grauer JN, Vaccaro AR, Lee JY, et al: The timing and influence of MRI on the management of patients with cervical facet dislocations remains highly variable: A survey of members of the Spine Trauma Study Group. *J Spinal Disord Tech* 2009;22(2):96-99.

29. Nassr A, Lee JY, Dvorak MF, et al: Variations in surgical treatment of cervical facet dislocations. *Spine (Phila Pa 1976)* 2008;33(7):E188-E193.

30. Johnson MG, Fisher CG, Boyd M, Pitzen T, Oxland TR, Dvorak MF: The radiographic failure of single seg-

ment anterior cervical plate fixation in traumatic cervical flexion distraction injuries. *Spine (Phila Pa 1976)* 2004;29(24):2815-2820.

31. Spector LR, Kim DH, Affonso J, Albert TJ, Hilibrand AS, Vaccaro AR: Use of computed tomography to predict failure of nonoperative treatment of unilateral facet fractures of the cervical spine. *Spine (Phila Pa 1976)* 2006;31(24):2827-2835.

32. Dvorak MF, Fisher CG, Aarabi B, et al: Clinical outcomes of 90 isolated unilateral facet fractures, subluxations, and dislocations treated surgically and nonoperatively. *Spine (Phila Pa 1976)* 2007;32(26):3007-3013.

33. Mueller CA, Peters I, Podlogar M, et al: Vertebral artery injuries following cervical spine trauma: A prospective observational study. *Eur Spine J* 2011;20(12):2202-2209.

    In a prospective observational study of 69 cervical spine injuries suspicious for vertebral artery injury because of facet joint subluxation or dislocation or extension into the transverse foramen, vertebral artery injury was identified in 19 (27.5%) and treated using a standardized clinical protocol. Level of evidence: III.

34. Fassett DR, Dailey AT, Vaccaro AR: Vertebral artery injuries associated with cervical spine injuries: A review of the literature. *J Spinal Disord Tech* 2008;21(4): 252-258.

35. Desouza RM, Crocker MJ, Haliasos N, Rennie A, Saxena A: Blunt traumatic vertebral artery injury: A clinical review. *Eur Spine J* 2011;20(9):1405-1416.

    The literature on traumatic vertebral artery injury was comprehensively reviewed with attention to current controversies.

36. Fehlings MG, Rabin D, Sears W, Cadotte DW, Aarabi B: Current practice in the timing of surgical intervention in spinal cord injury. *Spine (Phila Pa 1976)* 2010;35(21, suppl):S166-S173.

    A systematic literature review of preclinical and clinical data focused on early surgical decompression for SCI. The responses of 971 surgeons worldwide to questions about their current practices indicated that most preferred to decompress an acute spine injury within 24 hours.

37. Newton D, England M, Doll H, Gardner BP: The case for early treatment of dislocations of the cervical spine with cord involvement sustained playing rugby. *J Bone Joint Surg Br* 2011;93(12):1646-1652.

    The neurologic outcomes of 57 patients with acute SCI after low-velocity trauma (rugby injury) were compared with the time to achieve a closed reduction. Of the 34 patients who were completely paralyzed on admission, 5 of the 8 whose injury was reduced within 4 hours of injury made a full recovery, but none of the 24 patients who received a later reduction recovered fully.

38. Fehlings MG, Vaccaro A, Wilson JR, et al: Early versus delayed decompression for traumatic cervical spinal

5: Spine

cord injury: Results of the Surgical Timing in Acute Spinal Cord Injury Study (STASCIS). *PLoS One* 2012;7(2): e32037.

A multicenter (United States and Canada) prospective cohort study of 313 adult patients with a cervical SCI at 6-month follow-up found improvement of at least two AIS grades in 19.8% of patients who received decompression within 24 hours compared with 8.8% of patients who received later decompression.

39. Dvorak MF, Fisher CG, Hoekema J, et al: Factors predicting motor recovery and functional outcome after traumatic central cord syndrome: A long-term follow-up. *Spine (Phila Pa 1976)* 2005;30(20):2303-2311.

40. Lenehan B, Fisher CG, Vaccaro A, Fehlings M, Aarabi B, Dvorak MF: The urgency of surgical decompression in acute central cord injuries with spondylosis and without instability. *Spine (Phila Pa 1976)* 2010; 35(21, suppl):S180-S186.

The findings of a systematic literature review, data from an observational cohort of patients, and expert opinion were combined to conclude that early surgical decompression is safe and reasonable in the presence of a profound neurologic deficit (AIS type C). Initial observation can be justified for those with less neurologic impairment (AIS type D).

41. Gupta R, Bathen ME, Smith JS, Levi AD, Bhatia NN, Steward O: Advances in the management of spinal cord injury. *J Am Acad Orthop Surg* 2010;18(4):210-222.

A comprehensive review of SCI pathophysiology describes surgical strategies as well as pharmacologic and cellular transportation therapies aimed at maximizing neurologic outcomes.

42. Kwon BK, Okon EB, Plunet W, et al: A systematic review of directly applied biologic therapies for acute spinal cord injury. *J Neurotrauma* 2011;28(8):1589-1610.

Traumatic SCI therapies applied directly to the spinal cord or overlying dura were described. An outline of preclinical animal model data and the challenges of translating these interventions into human studies was included.

43. Kwon BK, Sekhon LH, Fehlings MG: Emerging repair, regeneration, and translational research advances for spinal cord injury. *Spine (Phila Pa 1976)* 2010;35(21, suppl):S263-S270.

The pathophysiologic processes initiated by spinal cord trauma were described, with an overview of novel therapies for SCI scheduled for or currently undergoing human studies.

44. Bracken MB, Shepard MJ, Collins WF, et al: A randomized, controlled trial of methylprednisolone or naloxone in the treatment of acute spinal-cord injury: Results of the Second National Acute Spinal Cord Injury Study. *N Engl J Med* 1990;322(20):1405-1411.

45. Coleman WP, Benzel D, Cahill DW, et al: A critical appraisal of the reporting of the National Acute Spinal Cord Injury Studies (II and III) of methylprednisolone in acute spinal cord injury. *J Spinal Disord* 2000;13(3): 185-199.

46. Levi L, Wolf A, Belzberg H: Hemodynamic parameters in patients with acute cervical cord trauma: Description, intervention, and prediction of outcome. *Neurosurgery* 1993;33(6):1007-1017.

47. Vale FL, Burns J, Jackson AB, Hadley MN: Combined medical and surgical treatment after acute spinal cord injury: Results of a prospective pilot study to assess the merits of aggressive medical resuscitation and blood pressure management. *J Neurosurg* 1997;87(2): 239-246.

48. Anwar F, Al-Khayer A, Joseph G, Fraser MH, Jigajinni MV, Allan DB: Delayed presentation and diagnosis of cervical spine injuries in long-standing ankylosing spondylitis. *Eur Spine J* 2011;20(3):403-407.

A retrospective review of 32 cervical fractures in patients with ankylosing spondylitis found delayed identification in 27 (84%). Three of 15 patients who initially were neurologically intact had neurologic deterioration before admission. Initial plain radiographs were nondiagnostic in 19 (59%) of patients.

49. Schoenfeld AJ, Harris MB, McGuire KJ, Warholic N, Wood KB, Bono CM: Mortality in elderly patients with hyperostotic disease of the cervical spine after fracture:An age- and sex-matched study. *Spine J* 2011;11(4): 257-264.

A review of 43 patients with cervical fracture in a hyperostotic spine found that those with ankylosing spondylitis had an increased risk of mortality compared with age- and sex-matched control subjects or patients with diffuse idiopathic skeletal hyperostosis. Level of evidence: IV.

50. Caron T, Bransford R, Nguyen Q, Agel J, Chapman J, Bellabarba C: Spine fractures in patients with ankylosing spinal disorders. *Spine (Phila Pa 1976)* 2010;35(11): E458-E464.

A retrospective analysis of 122 spine fractures in patients with an ankylosing spine disorder described an increased incidence over time, fracture characteristics, rates of SCI, delayed diagnosis, surgical intervention, and complications. Level of evidence: IV.

51. Whang PG, Goldberg G, Lawrence JP, et al: The management of spinal injuries in patients with ankylosing spondylitis or diffuse idiopathic skeletal hyperostosis: A comparison of treatment methods and clinical outcomes. *J Spinal Disord Tech* 2009;22(2):77-85.

Chapter 48
Thoracolumbar Trauma

Christopher Chambliss Harrod, MD   Jeffrey A. Rihn, MD   Alexander R. Vaccaro, MD, PhD

Introduction

Thoracolumbar fractures are estimated to affect more than 700,000 individuals worldwide each year.[1] These fractures range from low-energy osteoporotic compression fractures to high-energy fracture-dislocations. Approximately 15,000 surgical thoracolumbar fractures occur in the United States annually, and approximately one third of these injuries cause significant neurologic damage.[2]

Anatomically, the thoracolumbar spine consists of the upper thoracic region, the thoracolumbar junction, and the lower lumbar region (T1-T9, T10-L2, and L3-L5, respectively). Sixteen percent of thoracolumbar fractures are in the upper thoracic spine, 52% are in the thoracolumbar junction, and 32% are in the lower lumbar spine.[2] Controversy remains as to the comparative benefits of surgical and nonsurgical management, the timing of surgical intervention, the optimal surgical approach and construct length, complication management, the management of osteoporotic vertebral compression fracture, and the use of evolving surgical techniques such as minimally invasive surgery, cement augmentation, and bone morphogenetic proteins.

Anatomy

Normal thoracic kyphosis is produced and maintained at T1-T10 by wedge-shaped vertebral bodies that have a greater posterior height than anterior height. Because of its articulations with the rib cage and the sternum, the thoracic spine is significantly stiffer than the subjacent lumbar spine, and there is a hypermobile transition zone at the thoracolumbar junction (T10-L2). Sternal fractures are often associated with high-energy thoracolumbar fractures and result in a loss of the anterior-most flexion restraint. This transitional region is characterized by the loss of costal articulations, the transition from a relatively small thoracic spinal canal diameter to a larger lumbar spinal canal, and a change in facet joint orientation from coronal to sagittal. Because the ideal center of the head, arm, and trunk weight is located anterior to T10, the thoracolumbar junction is exposed to a flexion moment. Positive sagittal balance after a thoracolumbar fracture has been associated with a poor outcome, and, therefore, the goal of treatment is to maintain sagittal balance and an upright posture.

Dr. Rihn or an immediate family member has received research or institutional support from DePuy and serves as a board member, owner, officer, or committee member of the North American Spine Society. Dr. Vaccaro or an immediate family member has received royalties from Aesculap/B. Braun; DePuy, Globus Medical, Medtronic Sofamor Danek, Stout Medical, Progressive Spinal Technology, and Applied Spinal Intellectual Properties; has stock or stock options held in Globus Medical, Progressive Spinal Technologies, Advanced Spinal Intellectual Properties, Computational Biodynamics, Stout Medical, Paradigm Spine, K2M, Replication Medica, Spinology, Spine Medica, Orthovita, Vertiflex, Small Bone Technologies, NeuCore, Crosscurrent, Syndicom, In Vivo, Flagship Surgical, Location Based Intelligence, Gamma Spine, and Spinicity; has received research or institutional support from AO North America and Cerapeutics; has received nonincome support (such as equipment or services), commercially derived honoraria, or other non–research-related funding (such as paid travel) from Neuvasive; and serves as a board member, owner, officer, or committee member of the CSRS and AO North America. Neither Dr. Harrod nor any immediate family member has received anything of value from or has stock or stock options held in a commercial company or institution related directly or indirectly to the subject of this chapter.

Epidemiology

Six percent of all bony fractures involve the spine, and 90% of all spine fractures (including osteoporotic vertebral fractures) involve the thoracolumbar spine (compared with the occipital, cervical, or sacral regions).[3,4] Most fractures occur in the T10-L2 transitional area, and as many as 40% of such injuries result in a spinal cord injury.[5] Thoracolumbar burst fractures are most common in boys and men in the second or third decade of life, although they are bimodally distributed as high-energy fractures among young patients and as osteoporotic fractures in patients older than 70 years.

6. Smith AB, Dillon WP, Lau BC, et al: Radiation dose reduction strategy for CT protocols: Successful implementation in neuroradiology section. *Radiology* 2008; 247(2):499-506.

7. Rihn JA, Fisher C, Harrop J, Morrison W, Yang N, Vaccaro AR: Assessment of the posterior ligamentous complex following acute cervical spine trauma. *J Bone Joint Surg Am* 2010;92(3):583-589.

   MRI was sensitive for evaluating injury to the PLC after acute cervical trauma but had a relatively low positive predictive value and specificity. Injury to the PCL may be overread on MRI. Level of evidence: II.

8. Haba H, Taneichi H, Kotani Y, et al: Diagnostic accuracy of magnetic resonance imaging for detecting posterior ligamentous complex injury associated with thoracic and lumbar fractures. *J Neurosurg* 2003; 99(suppl 1):20-26.

9. Bernstein M: Easily missed thoracolumbar spine fractures. *Eur J Radiol* 2010;74(1):6-15.

   The most commonly missed thoracolumbar fractures were described.

10. Harrop JS, Vaccaro AR, Hurlbert RJ, et al: Intrarater and interrater reliability and validity in the assessment of the mechanism of injury and integrity of the posterior ligamentous complex: A novel injury severity scoring system for thoracolumbar injuries. Invited submission from the Joint Section Meeting on Disorders of the Spine and Peripheral Nerves, March 2005. *J Neurosurg Spine* 2006;4(2):118-122.

11. Han S, Wan S, Ning L, Tong Y, Zhang J, Fan S: Percutaneous vertebroplasty versus balloon kyphoplasty for treatment of osteoporotic vertebral compression fracture: A meta-analysis of randomised and non-randomised controlled trials. *Int Orthop* 2011;35(9): 1349-1358.

   A meta-analysis compared vertebroplasty and kyphoplasty for a compression fracture. Level of evidence: II.

12. Wood KB, Harrod CC, Mehbod AA, Buttermann GR: Operative versus nonoperative treatment of thoracolumbar burst fractures without neurological deficit: 15- to 20-year follow-up. *Spine J* 2012;12(9, suppl): 523.

   Long-term follow-up of prospective randomized control trial comparing surgical versus nonsurgical management of neurologically intact thoracolumbar burst fractures demonstrates superior long-term clinical outcomes in nonsurgically managed patients. Level of evidence: II.

13. Lakshmanan P, Jones A, Mehta J, Ahuja S, Davies PR, Howes JP: Recurrence of kyphosis and its functional implications after surgical stabilization of dorsolumbar unstable burst fractures. *Spine J* 2009;9(12):1003-1009.

14. Koller H, Acosta F, Hempfing A, et al: Long-term investigation of nonsurgical treatment for thoracolumbar and lumbar burst fractures: An outcome analysis in

15. Bailey CS, Dvorak MF, Thomas KC, et al: Comparison of thoracolumbosacral orthosis and no orthosis for the treatment of thoracolumbar burst fractures: Interim analysis of a multicenter randomized clinical equivalence trial. *J Neurosurg Spine* 2009;11(3):295-303.

16. Gnanenthiran SR, Adie S, Harris IA: Nonoperative versus operative treatment for thoracolumbar burst fractures without neurologic deficit: a meta-analysis. *Clin Orthop Relat Res* 2012;470(2):567-577.

   Surgical management of thoracolumbar burst fractures without neurologic deficit may improve residual kyphosis but does not appear to improve pain or function at an average of 4 years after injury and is associated with higher complication rates and costs. Level of evidence: II.

17. Tisot RA, Avanzi O: Laminar fractures as a severity marker in burst fractures of the thoracolumbar spine. *J Orthop Surg (Hong Kong)* 2009;17(3):261-264.

18. Kong W, Sun Y, Hu J, Xu J: Modified posterior decompression for the management of thoracolumbar burst fractures with canal encroachment. *J Spinal Disord Tech* 2010;23(5):302-309.

   Clinical and radiographic results were presented for posterior reduction and instrumentation of burst fractures for a transpedicular decompression using a surgical instrument developed by the authors. Level of evidence: IV.

19. Prabhakar MM, Rao BS, Patel L: Thoracolumbar burst fracture with complete paraplegia: Rationale for second-stage anterior decompression and fusion regarding functional outcome. *J Orthop Traumatol* 2009; 10(2):83-90.

20. Dai LY, Jiang LS, Jiang SD: Conservative treatment of thoracolumbar burst fractures: A long-term follow-up results with special reference to the load sharing classification. *Spine (Phila Pa 1976)* 2008;33(23):2536-2544.

21. McCormack T, Karaikovic E, Gaines RW: The load sharing classification of spine fractures. *Spine (Phila Pa 1976)* 1994;19(15):1741-1744.

22. Dai LY, Jiang LS, Jiang SD: Posterior short-segment fixation with or without fusion for thoracolumbar burst fractures: A five to seven-year prospective randomized study. *J Bone Joint Surg Am* 2009;91(5):1033-1041.

23. Yang H, Shi JH, Ebraheim M, et al: Outcome of thoracolumbar burst fractures treated with indirect reduction and fixation without fusion. *Eur Spine J* 2011;20(3): 380-386.

   A retrospective review of thoracolumbar burst fractures treated with indirect reduction without fusion found that 54 of 62 patients had an excellent or good result; neurologic status was improved or normal in 61 of 64 patients.

5: Spine

24. Palmisani M, Gasbarrini A, Brodano GB, et al: Minimally invasive percutaneous fixation in the treatment of thoracic and lumbar spine fractures. *Eur Spine J* 2009; 18(suppl 1):71-74.

25. Marco RA, Kushwaha VP: Thoracolumbar burst fractures treated with posterior decompression and pedicle screw instrumentation supplemented with balloon-assisted vertebroplasty and calcium phosphate reconstruction. *J Bone Joint Surg Am* 2009;91(1):20-28.

26. Liao JC, Fan KF, Keorochana G, Chen WJ, Chen LH: Transpedicular grafting after short-segment pedicle instrumentation for thoracolumbar burst fracture: Calcium sulfate cement versus autogenous iliac bone graft. *Spine (Phila Pa 1976)* 2010;35(15):1482-1488.

   A retrospective clinical and radiographic study compared transpedicular cancellous bone and transpedicular calcium sulfate for anterior augmentation of thoracolumbar burst fractures. Both grafting materials can be effective.

27. Sasani M, Özer AF: Single-stage posterior corpectomy and expandable cage placement for treatment of thoracic or lumbar burst fractures. *Spine (Phila Pa 1976)* 2009;34(1):E33-E40.

28. Dai LY, Ding WG, Wang XY, Jiang LS, Jiang SD, Xu HZ: Assessment of ligamentous injury in patients with thoracolumbar burst fractures using MRI. *J Trauma* 2009;66(6):1610-1615.

29. Kallemeier PM, Beaubien BP, Buttermann GR, Polga DJ, Wood KB: In vitro analysis of anterior and posterior fixation in an experimental unstable burst fracture model. *J Spinal Disord Tech* 2008;21(3):216-224.

30. Yadla S, Lebude B, Tender GC, et al: Traumatic spondyloptosis of the thoracolumbar spine. *J Neurosurg Spine* 2008;9(2):145-151.

31. Kerwin AJ, Frykberg ER, Schinco MA, et al: The effect of early surgical treatment of traumatic spine injuries on patient mortality. *J Trauma* 2007;63(6):1308-1313.

32. Cengiz SL, Kalkan E, Bayir A, Ilik K, Basefer A: Timing of thoracolomber spine stabilization in trauma patients; impact on neurological outcome and clinical course: A real prospective (rct) randomized controlled study. *Arch Orthop Trauma Surg* 2008;128(9):959-966.

33. Pakzad H, Roffey DM, Knight H, Dagenais S, Yelle JD, Wai EK: Delay in operative stabilization of spine fractures in multitrauma patients without neurologic injuries: Effects on outcomes. *Can J Surg* 2011;54(4): 270-276.

   A prospective study of 83 consecutive patients with spine fracture without neurologic injury found that a delay of more than 72 hours had a negative effect on complication rates. Level of evidence: III.

34. Reinhold M, Knop C, Beisse R, et al: Operative treatment of 733 patients with acute thoracolumbar spinal injuries: Comprehensive results from the second, prospective, Internet-based multicenter study of the Spine Study Group of the German Association of Trauma Surgery. *Eur Spine J* 2010;19(10):1657-1676.

   The results of a survey of German spine trauma surgeons described injury patterns, surgical patterns, and outcomes at 2-year follow-up. Level of evidence: IV.

5: Spine

Chapter 49
Cervical Disk Disease

Justin W. Miller, MD   Rick C. Sasso, MD

Introduction

The somewhat vague term, cervical disk disease, most often is used to describe degenerative pathology involving the cervical disk itself as well as associated clinical symptoms. So-called cervical disk disease encompasses a broad clinical spectrum in which the symptoms range from minimal axial neck pain to symptoms characteristic of myelopathy. Between these two extremes, patients may have a combination of symptoms, depending on severity of the disease, including debilitating axial pain, loss of motion, radiculopathy, numbness, tingling, gait imbalance, and fine motor dysfunction. For the purpose of treatment decision making, three overlapping clinical categories can be used: axial neck pain, radiculopathy, and cervical spondylotic myelopathy.

Axial Neck Pain

Etiology

Axial neck pain is one of the most common initial symptoms related to the cervical spine. This condition often is self-limiting, and in almost all patients, it can be resolved with minimal intervention. Some patients will have persistent pain, however, and further evaluation and treatment will be required. Axial or referred pain can occur in the paraspinal musculature, the occipital or periorbital region, or the trapezial or interscapular areas. The presence of several potential pain generators in the neck region complicates the ability to provide an accurate and prompt diagnosis. The often vague and subjective nature of symptoms, the lack of physical examination findings, and the paucity of specific tests to diagnose the anatomic source of the axial

pain mean that the evaluation can be difficult. Axial pain related to degenerative disease can stem from the disk, the facet joint, the atlantoaxial joint, and/or neurologic compression. Although radicular pain typically radiates into the arm, the most severe pain usually is proximal, and neck pain may be a significant component of radicular symptoms.

The cervical disk is composed of the outer anulus fibrosus and the nucleus pulposus, both of which undergo degeneration with aging. Within the intervertebral disk, metabolic changes, annular tearing, herniation of disk material, dehydration of the nucleus, and loss of disk height can occur. One theory locates the origin of pain in the disk itself, as a result of vascular or neurologic ingrowth into the anulus.[1] Other causes of axial pain probably are directly related to disk degeneration.

Facet joint pain results from spondylotic changes, the action of inflammatory mediators, and increased stress, which presumably occur with progressive degeneration of the intervertebral disk. As the anterior column of the cervical spine becomes less able to support the physiologic load, the posterior structures and facet joints undergo increased stress. With time, the joint can become hypertrophic, arthritic, and painful (Figure 1).

Arthritic changes involving the atlantoaxial joint are known to be a cause of axial pain[2] (Figure 2). Discomfort primarily occurs with rotation to the affected side, involves the occipitocervical region, and often radiates into the occiput. The diagnosis is easily missed because the focus may be on the subaxial spine.

Evaluation

A valid and reliable test to identify symptomatic degenerative disks remains elusive. Diskography is unreliable and inconsistent. Imaging, including MRI, has a significant false-positive rate because most of the degenerative changes shown on imaging studies are not the source of pain.[3] Conversely, facet joint injections are valuable for elucidating pain and can be guided by clinically distinct pain distributions.[4,5] These injections are both diagnostic and therapeutic.

Treatment

The key issue in treatment decision making is identifying the true pain generator. This task is difficult if the patient has axial pain only. Treatment should begin with nonsurgical intervention. Anti-inflammatory

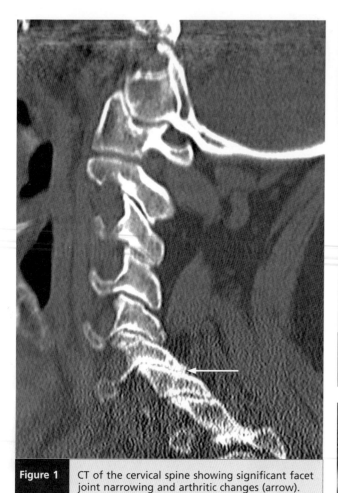

Figure 1 · CT of the cervical spine showing significant facet joint narrowing and arthritic changes (arrow).

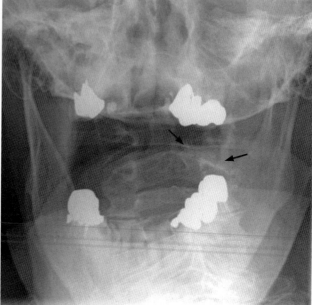

Figure 2 · Open-mouth odontoid radiograph showing bilateral C1-C2 joints with unilateral arthritic changes (arrows).

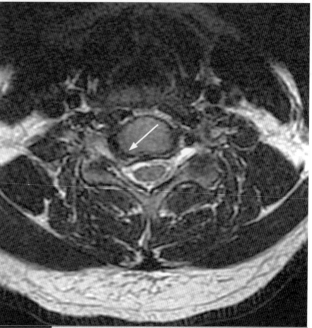

Figure 3 · Axial T2-weighted MRI of the cervical spine showing a soft disk herniation causing significant neurologic impingement (arrow).

medication, activity modification, and a short course of immobilization are of potential benefit. Moderate-quality evidence supports the use of physical therapy for chronic cervical pain.[6] Injection of local anesthetic with or without a steroid can provide benefit after a pathologic diagnosis is made. Surgical fusion is the last recourse for treating axial neck pain. Although there is controversy and a lack of level I evidence, the surgical treatment of axial neck pain has provided clinical benefit.[7,8]

Radiculopathy

Etiology

Radiculopathy is caused by nerve root pathology with etiologies including mechanical compression, ischemia, and inflammation. The signs and symptoms of radiculopathy include pain in a dermatomal pattern, myotomal weakness, hyporeflexia, and paresthesias. The factors determining the response of the nerve are not entirely understood. However, it is well known that relieving the nerve from any offensive lesion often alleviates the radiculopathy. The nerve rarely sustains permanent damage.

Mechanical compression can occur directly in the presence of a soft or hard disk herniation, osteophyte, or facet capsule infolding, or it can occur indirectly through foraminal narrowing or instability (Figures 3 and 4). Ischemic changes can result from direct compression and possibly from inflammation of the root. Inflammation occurs as a result of exposure to disk material, joint irritation, or mechanical instability.

Evaluation

Detection of radicular pathology often is fairly straightforward and is based on a complete history, a detailed neurologic examination, and correlation with imaging and diagnostic studies. The history and physical examination are crucial. Classic dermatome distributions and provocative testing of muscles and reflexes involving the upper extremities are shown in **Figures 5** and **6**.

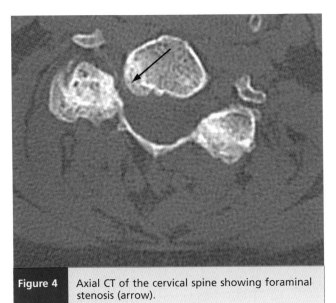

| Figure 4 | Axial CT of the cervical spine showing foraminal stenosis (arrow). |

The Spurling maneuver, in which the patient extends the neck and rotates the head toward the side of typical pain, can help differentiate a true cervical root etiology from other potential sources of pain. In a positive Spurling sign, the maneuver re-creates or enhances the patient's typical pain. During the examination, the clinician must keep in mind the need to rule out other sources of upper extremity pain, such as the shoulder or a peripheral nerve.

The use of imaging studies (plain radiographs, MRI, and CT myelogram) and diagnostic selective nerve root injections should be primarily confirmatory in nature. Imaging studies may reveal the pathology, though the results can be equivocal or show multiple abnormalities. Selective nerve root injections can be used to precisely identify the symptomatic area if the imaging findings are equivocal.[9] The placement of the selective nerve root injection is guided by the history and examination findings. Electromyography and nerve conduction testing can be used to identify nonradicular pathology, such as peripheral neuropathy.

Treatment

Treatment should begin with nonsurgical measures because most cervical radicular pain will improve over time. During the acute phase, the patient can be given steroids, NSAIDs, and a short course of narcotic medication.[10] Typically, narcotic medications have a limited ability to control nerve-related pain and should be used sparingly. The key is to break the cycle of acute pain so

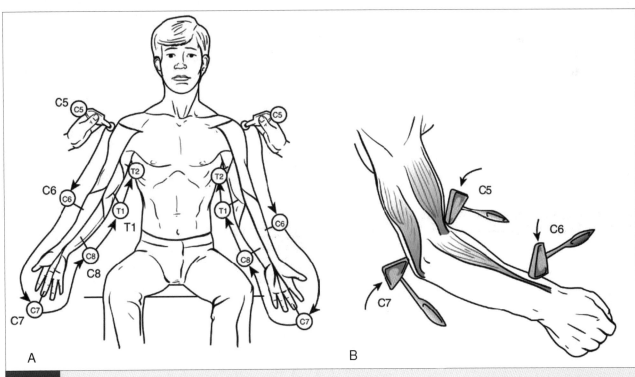

| Figure 5 | Schematic drawings showing the upper extremity dermatome distribution (**A**) and reflex examination (**B**). (Reproduced from Grauer NJ, Beiner JM, Albert TJ: Cervical disk disease, in Vaccaro AR, ed: *Orthopaedic Knowledge Update*, ed 8. Rosemont, IL, American Academy of Orthopaedic Surgeons, 2005, pp 527-534.) |

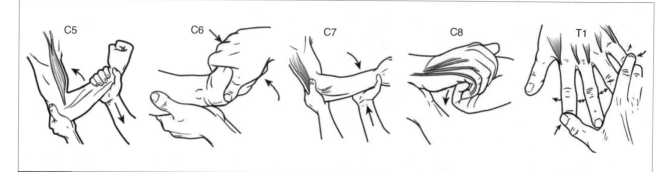

Figure 6 Schematic drawing showing the upper extremity motor examination. (Reproduced from Grauer NJ, Beiner JM, Albert TJ: Cervical disk disease, in Vaccaro AR, ed: *Orthopaedic Knowledge Update*, ed 8. Rosemont, IL, American Academy of Orthopaedic Surgeons, 2005, pp 527-534.)

that the patient can tolerate gradual healing of the radiculopathy, with resolution of paresthesias or weakness over a period of months. To avoid exacerbating the discomfort, a structured physical therapy program is delayed until the pain has been alleviated.

Steroids should be used sparingly, if at all, because of the potential adverse effects.[11] Although the use of oral steroids can quickly and dramatically diminish radicular pain, no good data have shown their long-term effectiveness for treating radicular symptoms. If the patient's symptoms are not relieved by oral medical therapy, a selective nerve root injection may be beneficial. The therapeutic benefit of selective nerve root injection is a topic of controversy, but it certainly has diagnostic value.[9] A patient who continues to have incapacitating nerve root pain, has undergone at least 6 weeks of nonsurgical treatment, or has a progressive neurologic deficit may be a candidate for surgical treatment.[12]

Several surgical options are available for treating radicular pathology. The goal is to remove the agent causing the radiculopathy. Standard anterior procedures include anterior cervical diskectomy and fusion (ACDF) and anterior cervical disk arthroplasty (ACDA).

ACDA is a relatively new surgical option for symptomatic cervical disk disease after unsuccessful nonsurgical treatment. Although long-term data are lacking, the early results are promising compared with those of ACDF. A 4-year follow-up study of ACDA using the Bryan Cervical Disc implant (Medtronic Sofamor Danek) found outcomes significantly superior to those of ACDF.[13] The measures included the Neck Disability Index, the Medical Outcomes Survey 36-Item Short Form physical component, scales for neck and arm pain, and overall success. The potential for long-term complications after ACDA, as related to durability and wear, requires further study.

Posterior pathology can be treated through laminoforaminotomy, which has been well described elsewhere.[14,15]

Cervical Spondylotic Myelopathy

Etiology

The all-encompassing term, myelopathy, is used to describe spinal cord dysfunction with its associated signs and symptoms. Myelopathy in cervical degenerative disease is believed to directly result from static or dynamic spinal cord compression. Spondylotic changes include loss of disk height, disk bulging or herniation, osteophyte development, pathology of the posterior longitudinal ligament, buckling of the ligamentum flavum, instability, and loss of lordosis. All of these anatomic and physiologic conditions can lead to compression of the spinal cord (**Figure 7**). Congenital narrowing of the spinal canal can predispose the spinal cord to compression. It is not entirely clear how compression of the spinal cord leads to clinical dysfunction. Theories include ischemia, inflammation, edema, gliosis, and demyelination.[16,17] It is most likely a combination of these factors that result in cervical spondylotic myelopathy.

Evaluation

The signs and symptoms of clinically diagnosed cervical spondylotic myelopathy depend on the severity of the disease, chronicity, levels of involvement, and factors that are not fully understood.[18] A thorough history and physical examination are crucial but may not be as straightforward as with radicular pathology.

Patients typically describe difficulty in hand and other fine motor functions, including writing and gait, as well as diffuse weakness or numbness. If the condition is severe, the patient may have disturbance in bowel and bladder function. Examination findings may include both upper and lower motor neuron abnormalities. Long tract signs include hyperreflexia, clonus, the Babinski sign, the Hoffman sign, the Lhermitte sign, and an inverted radial reflex. With concomitant nerve root compression, concurrent lower motor neuron findings may be seen in the upper extremities. These classic findings are completely absent in approximately one fifth of patients with cervical spondylotic myelopathy, however.

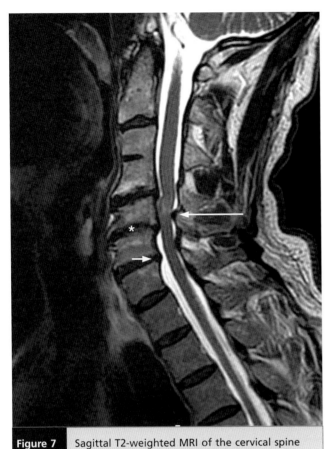

Figure 7 Sagittal T2-weighted MRI of the cervical spine showing spondylotic changes, including disk height collapse (*), disk bulging (small arrow), and buckling of the ligamentum flavum (large arrow), with intrinsic cord changes just anterior.

Plain radiographs, CT myelogram, and MRI are useful for diagnosing and evaluating pathology associated with cervical spondylotic myelopathy. Plain radiographs are used to assess gross spondylotic changes and overall alignment of the cervical spine. CT myelograms are superior for assessing bony pathology, such as osteophytes or ossification of the posterior longitudinal ligament, as well as indirect compression of the neurologic structures. MRI is superior for evaluating the neurologic structures (the spinal cord and nerve roots) and soft-tissue structures, such as the disk, ligamentum flavum, and posterior longitudinal ligament. MRI can be used to detect the extent and cause of compression as well as intrinsic changes within the spinal cord (Figure 7). Changes in signal intensity on T2-weighted (hyperintense) or T1-weighted (hypointense) sequences are believed to indicate cord pathology. There is no consensus on the meaning of these changes; however, theories include ischemia, inflammation, edema, gliosis, and demyelination.[16,17]

Electrodiagnostic studies are used to diagnose spinal cord dysfunction. Motor-evoked and sensory-evoked potentials can show abnormalities in central conduction patterns. Patients with subclinical cervical spondylotic myelopathy (with subtle or no physical signs) may have electrophysiologic changes. Motor-evoked potentials have proved to be more sensitive than sensory-evoked potentials.[19,20]

Treatment

The natural history of cervical spondylotic myelopathy is not well understood, although the disease appears to progress slowly over time with variable periods of quiescence and gradual stepwise decline.[21] Rapid neurologic decline is the exception and requires that the patient be treated with surgical decompression. There is much debate as to the best treatment of patients with subclinical myelopathy.

Nonsurgical treatment of cervical spondylotic myelopathy is limited to activity modification, anti-inflammatory medications, and an orthosis. These modalities do not affect the overall condition and may be detrimental to a patient's condition by masking further decline and leading to a delay in surgical treatment.[22]

Surgical treatment entails decompression of the neurologic elements. There is debate as to whether an anterior (ACDF, ACDA, corpectomy), a posterior (laminectomy, fusion laminoplasty), or a combined procedure is most efficacious for treating cervical spondylotic pathology.

An anterior procedure can directly treat anterior pathology and improve lordosis, with fusion of the involved levels providing stability to the spine and spinal cord. Stability is believed to provide an optimal environment for recovery of the neurologic elements; however, this belief may be unfounded. One indication for ACDA may be single-level myelopathy with cord compression caused by a large retrodiscal fragment. The choice of multilevel ACDF or corpectomy should be based on the location of the pathology as well as the patient's healing potential because multilevel ACDF requires fusion of more surfaces than corpectomy.

A posterior procedure can be used to treat posterior pathology directly. Lordosis can be partially corrected with fusion. Both fusion and laminoplasty decrease motion and thereby improve stability. A posterior cervical fusion clearly provides stability, and overall motion is decreased with laminoplasty, which is meant to indirectly decompress the spinal cord and preserve motion. Laminoplasty should be avoided if the cervical spine is kyphotic because the spinal cord will not drift posterior, and progression of the deformity and myelopathy will be allowed to continue. Lordosis or neutral alignment is a necessary prerequisite for a laminoplasty. A posterior laminectomy and decompression should routinely be accompanied by instrumentation and fusion to prevent postlaminectomy kyphosis.

Recent research found that surgical decompression led to significant improvement in the outcomes of patients with mild to severe cervical spondylotic myelopathy, with the greatest improvement in those who had severe myelopathy.[23] This research justifies a strong recommendation for surgical intervention to treat mild or moderate myelopathy and a definite recommendation to treat severe myelopathy.

5: Spine

Surgical Complications

Surgical treatment of cervical degenerative disk disease can lead to complications, the most common of which is dysphagia. Although dysphagia is more prevalent after an anterior procedure, it also can occur with a posterior procedure.[24] The reported incidence of dysphagia is as high as 50% during the first month after anterior surgery, typically with significant improvement over time.[25] The etiology of dysphagia is not entirely clear, but identifiable risk factors include extended length of surgery, wound retraction, a multilevel procedure, and high endotracheal cuff pressure. The assessment of patients with dysphagia is difficult because diagnostic criteria and measurement tools are poorly defined.[26,27] Patients undergoing surgery for cervical degenerative disk disease should be counseled to expect dysphagia, with gradual improvement over time.

Other complications include wound infection, nerve root palsy, epidural hematoma, retropharyngeal hematoma, cerebrospinal fluid leakage, blindness, instrumentation or graft failure, pseudarthrosis, instability, vascular injury, and neurologic injury. Medical comorbidities or cardiopulmonary complications can result from any surgical procedure. Most of these complications are rare, and often they are self-limiting and resolve with time.

Summary

Degenerative changes of the cervical spine present in many ways and vary from axial neck pain to severe myelopathy. Most symptoms related to cervical disk disease are self-limiting and benign; however, indicated surgical treatments result in high success rates. The key to a positive outcome is prompt diagnosis of the problem, development of a treatment plan, and sound execution. Fortunately, with adherence to these principles, complications rarely occur.

Key Study Points

- Atlantoaxial arthritis is an easily missed cause of axial neck pain.

- Arthroplasty using the Bryan Cervical Disc had significantly better outcomes than anterior cervical diskectomy and fusion.

- Cervical spondylotic myelopathy is a clinical diagnosis with a constellation of signs and symptoms, and surgical treatment often is required to halt its progression.

Annotated References

1. Brisby H: Pathology and possible mechanisms of nervous system response to disc degeneration. *J Bone Joint Surg Am* 2006;88(suppl 2):68-71.

2. Ghanayem AJ, Leventhal M, Bohlman HH: Osteoarthrosis of the atlanto-axial joints: Long-term follow-up after treatment with arthrodesis. *J Bone Joint Surg Am* 1996;78(9):1300-1307.

3. Boden SD, McCowin PR, Davis DO, Dina TS, Mark AS, Wiesel S: Abnormal magnetic-resonance scans of the cervical spine in asymptomatic subjects: A prospective investigation. *J Bone Joint Surg Am* 1990;72(8): 1178-1184.

4. Dwyer A, Aprill C, Bogduk N: Cervical zygapophyseal joint pain patterns: I. A study in normal volunteers. *Spine (Phila Pa 1976)* 1990;15(6):453-457.

5. Aprill C, Dwyer A, Bogduk N: Cervical zygapophyseal joint pain patterns: II. A clinical evaluation. *Spine (Phila Pa 1976)* 1990;15(6):458-461.

6. Kay TM, Gross A, Goldsmith CH, et al: Exercises for mechanical neck disorders. *Cochrane Database Syst Rev* 2012;8:CD004250.

    A literature review of randomized controlled studies of therapeutic exercise for adult neck pain found moderate evidence of symptom improvement with combined therapies specific to the cervicoscapular region, including stretching and strengthening. Nonspecific upper extremity therapy provided no benefit for neck pain.

7. Palit M, Schofferman J, Goldthwaite N, et al: Anterior discectomy and fusion for the management of neck pain. *Spine (Phila Pa 1976)* 1999;24(21):2224-2228.

8. Garvey TA, Transfeldt EE, Malcolm JR, Kos P: Outcome of anterior cervical discectomy and fusion as perceived by patients treated for dominant axial-mechanical cervical spine pain. *Spine (Phila Pa 1976)* 2002;27(17):1887-1895.

9. Sasso RC, Macadaeg K, Nordmann D, Smith M: Selective nerve root injections can predict surgical outcome for lumbar and cervical radiculopathy: Comparison to magnetic resonance imaging. *J Spinal Disord Tech* 2005;18(6):471-478.

10. Levine MJ, Albert TJ, Smith MD: Cervical radiculopathy: Diagnosis and nonoperative management. *J Am Acad Orthop Surg* 1996;4(6):305-316.

11. Young IA, Hyman GS, Packia-Raj LN, Cole AJ: The use of lumbar epidural/transforaminal steroids for managing spinal disease. *J Am Acad Orthop Surg* 2007;15(4): 228-238.

12. Albert TJ, Murrell SE: Surgical management of cervical radiculopathy. *J Am Acad Orthop Surg* 1999;7(6): 368-376.

13. Sasso RC, Anderson PA, Riew KD, Heller JG: Results of cervical arthroplasty compared with anterior discectomy and fusion: Four-year clinical outcomes in a prospective, randomized controlled trial. *J Bone Joint Surg Am* 2011;93(18):1684-1692.

A multicenter prospective randomized study compared the Bryan artificial disk with fusion for treatment of cervical spondylosis. Early and midterm (48-month) results revealed significantly superior results after arthroplasty. Level of evidence: I.

14. Murrey DB: Degenerative disease of the cervical spine, in Fischgrund JS, ed: *Orthopaedic Knowledge Update*, ed 9. Rosemont, IL, American Academy of Orthopaedic Surgeons, 2008, pp 541-549.

15. Rhee JM, Riew KD: Cervical degenerative disease, in Flynn JM, ed: *Orthopaedic Knowledge Update*, ed 10. Rosemont, IL, American Academy of Orthopaedic Surgeons, 2011, pp 611-622.

Cervical degenerative disease results in axial neck pain, radiculopathy, and myelopathy. The treatment of such disease involves nonsurgical and surgical means depending on the severity and symptoms. There are a multitude of successful surgical options according to the type of pathology, including decompression, fusion, laminoplasty, and arthroplasty.

16. Mehalic TF, Pezzuti RT, Applebaum BI: Magnetic resonance imaging and cervical spondylotic myelopathy. *Neurosurgery* 1990;26(2):217-227.

17. Nurick S: The pathogenesis of the spinal cord disorder associated with cervical spondylosis. *Brain* 1972;95(1): 87-100.

18. Rhee JM, Heflin JA, Hamasaki T, Freedman B: Prevalence of physical signs in cervical myelopathy: A prospective, controlled study. *Spine (Phila Pa 1976)* 2009; 34(9):890-895.

19. Chistyakov AV, Soustiel JF, Hafner H, Kaplan B, Feinsod M: The value of motor and somatosensory evoked potentials in evaluation of cervical myelopathy in the presence of peripheral neuropathy. *Spine (Phila Pa 1976)* 2004;29(12):E239-E247.

20. Simó M, Szirmai I, Arányi Z: Superior sensitivity of motor over somatosensory evoked potentials in the diagnosis of cervical spondylotic myelopathy. *Eur J Neurol* 2004;11(9):621-626.

21. Lees F, Turner JW: Natural history and prognosis of cervical spondylosis. *Br Med J* 1963;2(5373):1607-1610.

22. Sampath P, Bendebba M, Davis JD, Ducker TB: Outcome of patients treated for cervical myelopathy: A prospective, multicenter study with independent clinical review. *Spine (Phila Pa 1976)* 2000;25(6):670-676.

23. Fehlings MG, Kopjar B, Arnold PM, et al: AOSpine North America Cervical Spondylotic Study: 2-year surgical outcomes of a prospective multicenter study in 280 patients. *Neurosurgery* 2010;67(2):543.

A prospective study followed 278 patients with mild, moderate, or severe cervical spondylotic myelopathy for 1 year after surgical decompression. Outcome measures included the modified Japanese Orthopaedic Association score, the Nurick Scale, the Neck Disability Index, and Medical Outcomes Study 36-Item Short Form (version 2). On all measures, there was a statistically significant improvement from baseline, and with the exception of the modified Japanese Orthopaedic Association score, the measures showed that improvement was not dependent on the preoperative severity of myelopathy. Level of evidence: II.

24. Fehlings MG, Smith JS, Kopjar B, et al: Perioperative and delayed complications associated with the surgical treatment of cervical spondylotic myelopathy based on 302 patients from the AOSpine North America Cervical Spondylotic Myelopathy Study. *J Neurosurg Spine* 2012;16(5):425-432.

An analysis of outcomes data for 302 patients included adverse events, complications within 30 days of the procedure, and complications 31 days to 2 years after the procedure. Early complications were more likely among patients who were older or had a combined anterior-posterior procedure, a longer surgical time, and greater blood loss compared with other patients. Surgical treatment of cervical spondylotic myelopathy had a low rate of neurologic complications and minimal risk of long-term morbidity.

25. Bazaz R, Lee MJ, Yoo JU: Incidence of dysphagia after anterior cervical spine surgery: A prospective study. *Spine (Phila Pa 1976)* 2002;27(22):2453-2458.

26. Riley LH III, Vaccaro AR, Dettori JR, Hashimoto R: Postoperative dysphagia in anterior cervical spine surgery. *Spine (Phila Pa 1976)* 2010;35(9, suppl):S76-S85.

A systematic review of dysphagia after cervical spine surgery found 17 appropriate articles from 1990 to 2008. The reported rates of dysphagia varied significantly but were found to decline, with a plateau at 1 year of 13% to 21%. Associated risk factors included multilevel surgery and female sex.

27. Lee MJ, Bazaz R, Furey CG, Yoo J: Risk factors for dysphagia after anterior cervical spine surgery: A two-year prospective cohort study. *Spine J* 2007;7(2):141-147.

Chapter 50

Lumbar Stenosis and Degenerative Spondylolisthesis

Adam Pearson, MD, MS   William A. Abdu, MD, MS

Introduction

Lumbar stenosis and degenerative spondylolisthesis are common degenerative conditions that are affecting increasing numbers of patients as the population ages. These two conditions lead to narrowing of the spinal canal and can cause low back pain, neurogenic claudication, and radiculopathy. Degenerative spondylolisthesis sometimes is considered a subdiagnosis of lumbar stenosis, but the two conditions affect different patient populations, require different treatments, and have different surgical outcomes.[1] The Spine Patient Outcomes Research Trial (SPORT) compared surgical and nonsurgical outcomes for patients with lumbar stenosis or degenerative spondylolisthesis, and the findings have implications for clinical practice.[2-5]

Lumbar Stenosis

Epidemiology

Lumbar stenosis is a disease of aging that rarely affects patients younger than 50 years. A cross-sectional Japanese study found that no patients younger than 40 years had symptomatic lumbar stenosis, but approximately 10% of patients older than 60 years met the radiographic and clinical diagnostic criteria.[6] Lumbar stenosis often is asymptomatic, however. More than 75% of patients (mean age, 66 years) had at least one area of moderate or severe stenosis on MRI.[6] Lumbar stenosis was found to affect more men than women younger than 70 years, but there was no sex-based difference in patients older than 70 years. These findings are similar to those of the SPORT, in which the average patient age was 65 years and approximately 60% of the patients were men.[5]

Neither of the following authors nor any immediate family member has received anything of value from or has stock or stock options held in a commercial company or institution related directly or indirectly to the subject of this chapter: Dr. Pearson and Dr. Abdu.

Pathophysiology

The most common cause of spinal stenosis is osteoarthritic change affecting the intervertebral disk and facet joints. Less common etiologies include idiopathic congenital stenosis, achondroplasia, osteopetrosis, acromegaly, Paget disease, fluorosis, and ankylosing spondylitis. Postoperative changes, tumor, trauma, and infection can lead to compression of the neural structures and cause symptoms of stenosis. Typically, a loss of disk hydration and height leads to increased loading and hypertrophy of the facet joints. The ligamentum flavum and the facet capsule also become hypertrophic and can become redundant with loss of disk height. This combination of factors can lead to central, lateral recess, or foraminal stenosis (**Figure 1**).

Central stenosis typically is caused by a combination of central disk bulging, facet hypertrophy, and ligamen-

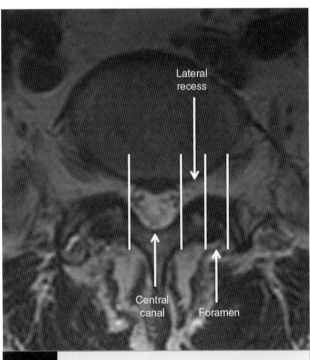

Figure 1   MRI showing the central canal, the lateral recess, and the foramen, all of which can be affected by spinal stenosis.

5: Spine

tum flavum and capsular hypertrophy. These factors cause a decrease in the cross-sectional area of the spinal canal and circumferential compression of the thecal sac. Central stenosis generally is believed to cause claudication. Lateral recess stenosis results in compression of the traversing nerve root from the point at which it leaves the dural tube until it enters the foramen, and typically is caused by compression of the nerve root between a bulging posterolateral disk and a hypertrophic superior articulating process. For example, the traversing L5 nerve root can be compressed between the superior articulating process of L5 and a posterolateral disk bulge at L4-5. Foraminal stenosis often is caused by a decrease in the cranial-caudal dimension of the foramen resulting from disk height loss and a decrease in the anterior-posterior dimension resulting from facet hypertrophy. Foraminal disk material can contribute to foraminal stenosis. In general, lateral recess and foraminal stenosis give rise to radicular symptoms. Extension of the motion segment decreases the cross-sectional area of the central canal, the lateral recess, and the foramen, giving rise to symptoms when the patient stands or walks. The symptoms improve with lumbar flexion or sitting.

On a microscopic level, compression of the thecal sac and nerve roots restricts blood flow through capillaries and causes venous congestion.[7] As the pressure increases above 50 mm Hg, electrophysiologic changes in nerve function can be measured.[8] It is believed that decreased perfusion and oxygenation cause neural dysfunction, giving rise to pain and sometimes to motor or sensory deficits. Efforts to define a cross-sectional area threshold at which stenosis becomes symptomatic have revealed that no threshold exists, and the extent of cross-sectional narrowing is not always correlated with symptoms.[9] The segmental nature of the spinal vasculature may allow perfusion to be maintained in single-level stenosis; multilevel stenosis would be more likely to give rise to symptoms. The effects of single-level and multilevel stenosis were compared in the SPORT. In the absence of spondylolisthesis, no differences were found between patients with single-level or multilevel stenosis in baseline symptoms or improvement after surgical or nonsurgical treatment.[10] However, patients who had degenerative spondylolisthesis and single-level disease had greater improvement after surgery compared with those who had multilevel disease. Thus, the clinical effect of single-level stenosis compared with multilevel stenosis remains somewhat obscure.

Clinical Presentation

Patients with lumbar stenosis typically have neurogenic claudication or radicular symptoms. Neurogenic claudication is classically described as lower extremity pain, heaviness, numbness, and subjective weakness brought on by standing and walking and improved with flexion or sitting down. Both lower extremities often are affected, and the pain usually does not occur in a dermatomal fashion. The pain typically radiates distally from the buttocks and frequently extends below the knees,

although some patients report claudication primarily in the back and the buttocks. Unlike claudication, radiculopathic pain or numbness is in a dermatomal pattern and may be associated with weakness in a myotomal distribution, in which the muscles are innervated by a specific nerve root. Patients with stenosis frequently have low back pain as well as claudication with standing and walking or have mechanical symptoms. In the SPORT, patients with stenosis tended to have slightly more severe leg pain than back pain, and 80% reported neurogenic claudication.[5] The finding that almost 80% also had pain in a dermatomal fashion indicates that most patients have a mixture of claudication and radicular symptoms.

Physical examination findings are not consistent in patients with lumbar stenosis. These patients often have normal neurologic examination results. In some patients, symptoms can be re-created with prolonged extension. In the SPORT, 55% of the patients with stenosis had one or more findings on neurologic examination: 28% had a motor deficit, 28% had a sensory deficit, and 27% had asymmetric depressed reflexes.[5] Approximately 20% had a positive straight leg raise. Given the lack of sensitivity and specificity of these findings in patients with stenosis, the physical examination is particularly important for ruling out other causes of a patient's symptoms. Pulse palpation is important to rule out vascular claudication, which can have similar symptoms. Examination of the hip can rule out hip arthritis as a cause of buttock and groin pain. Tests for upper motor neuron dysfunction, such as hyperreflexia, clonus, and the Babinski sign, should be used because myelopathy is common in patients older than 60 years. Diminished sensation in a stocking distribution should alert the clinician to the possibility of a peripheral neuropathy. Because of the high prevalence of radiographic stenosis in individuals older than 60 years, the diagnosis of lumbar stenosis must be made clinically, and a thorough history and physical examination are essential.

Diagnostic Studies

MRI without contrast is the gold standard for the radiographic diagnosis of lumbar stenosis (Figure 2). T2-weighted studies provide the highest imaging resolution of the contributing neural elements and soft tissues, including the disk, the ligamentum flavum, the capsule, and any facet cysts. Attempts to define radiographic criteria for diagnosis based on measurements of the central canal, the lateral recess, and the foramen have not been successful because of the high prevalence of radiographic stenosis in asymptomatic individuals.[9] The extent of stenosis varies with body position, and this fact has prompted investigators to evaluate the use of upright and axially loaded MRI.[11,12] Decreases in the cross-sectional area of the spinal canal have been reported with both techniques, but it is unclear whether these findings have the potential to alter surgical treatment and, ultimately, outcomes. Supine MRI remains the standard imaging modality.

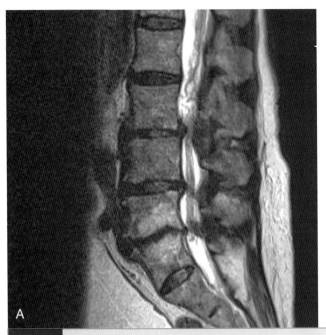
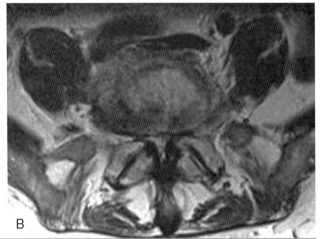

Figure 2 **A,** Sagittal T2-weighted MRI showing multilevel lumbar stenosis. **B,** Axial T2-weighted MRI showing central and lateral recess stenosis.

CT with and without myelography is the second-line imaging modality, typically used if a patient has a pacemaker or another contraindication to MRI. CT without myelography provides low-resolution imaging of neural and soft-tissue structures and allows the evaluation of bony compression from osteophytes or foraminal narrowing. The addition of myelography is essential for evaluating neural structures. Weight-bearing plain radiographs, including flexion-extension views, are most useful for defining dynamic features of the spine, including spondylolisthesis and scoliosis that can contribute to stenosis and affect surgical treatment. Most surgeons consider standing radiographs to be essential for the preoperative workup.

The use of electrodiagnostic studies for lumbar stenosis is controversial and not well established because of the lack of a consistent relationship between clinical and electrodiagnostic findings.[13] If peripheral neuropathy is expected, electrodiagnostic studies can be useful for establishing the diagnosis. The evaluation of electromyographic changes after a patient walks on a treadmill was proposed as an electrodiagnostic test for lumbar stenosis, but differences in findings for patients with lumbar stenosis, patients with peripheral neuropathy, and healthy control subjects were not sufficiently consistent to establish the test as clinically useful.[14]

Nonsurgical Treatment

Before surgical treatment of lumbar stenosis is considered, most experts recommend at least 6 to 12 weeks of nonsurgical treatment. Nonsurgical treatments include medications, physical therapy, bracing, and injections. In general, the evidence to support any of these treatment modalities is of low or very low quality, and none

have been shown to alter the natural history of lumbar stenosis.[15] The medication options include NSAIDs, acetaminophen, gabapentin, calcitonin, and prostaglandins. Physical therapy can be based on modality or exercise, but the greatest support is for symptom-guided exercises.[16] The use of a lumbosacral corset modestly improved walking distance while the corset was being worn.[17] Although epidural steroid injections are widely used, there is only very low-quality evidence to suggest any short-term benefit and no evidence to suggest long-term benefit.[15]

Because of the lack of evidence supporting any specific nonsurgical treatment modality, the SPORT defined nonsurgical treatment as usual care and suggested that it include, at a minimum, education, NSAIDs, and physical therapy. Of the SPORT patients with lumbar stenosis, 44% were treated with physical therapy, 49% with NSAIDs, 37% with opioids, and 45% with an injection. Over 4 years, the patients who were exclusively treated nonsurgically had improvement of approximately 12 points on the Medical Outcomes Study 36-Item Short Form (SF-36) bodily pain and physical function components and improvement of approximately 9 points on the Oswestry Disability Index (ODI). Most of the improvement occurred within the first year. "Substantial clinical benefit" on the ODI is approximately 18 points, and therefore the improvement with nonsurgical treatment was modest at best.

Surgical Treatment

Surgical treatment is indicated after bothersome symptoms have persisted at least 6 to 12 weeks and nonsurgical treatment options have been exhausted. The standard surgical treatment of lumbar stenosis is an open

5: Spine

Table 1

Surgical Treatments for Lumbar Stenosis and Degenerative Spondylolisthesis

Surgical Procedure	Lumbar Stenosis	Degenerative Spondylolisthesis
Decompression	Yes	Yes
Interbody fusion	No	No
Instrumentation	No	Controversial
Posterolateral fusion	No	Yes

central laminectomy followed by medial facetectomies and foraminotomies, as needed (**Table 1**). This procedure involves a midline approach with elevation of the paraspinal muscles off the spinous processes and laminae. To avoid instability, care must be taken not to disrupt the pars interarticularis or remove more than 50% of each facet joint. Most experts agree that arthrodesis is not needed after decompression for lumbar stenosis in the absence of evidence of instability, and a small randomized controlled study found no differences in the outcomes of patients who underwent decompression with or without fusion.[18]

The most common complication associated with laminectomy is a dural tear, which occurred in 9% of the patients with lumbar stenosis in the SPORT.[4] This complication typically is treated with direct suture repair, if possible, with or without a hydrogel or fibrin sealant or a collagen matrix scaffold. A dural tear not amenable to suture repair can be treated using a sealant and a collagen scaffold, although inability to obtain a watertight closure may necessitate an extended period of bed rest. In the SPORT, patients with lumbar stenosis who underwent a durotomy had a longer surgical time, a longer inpatient stay, and greater blood loss but no significant differences in long-term clinical outcomes compared with those who did not have a durotomy.[19] Less common surgical complications include nerve root injury (none were reported), epidural hematoma (1%), wound infection (2%), and iatrogenic instability (not reported). Medical complications are more common in elderly patients with stenosis; the rate of complications probably is twice as high in patients who undergo spine surgery after age 65 years than in patients younger than 65 years.[20]

Less invasive techniques for direct decompression have been developed. The use of an operating microscope and tubular retractors allows bilateral decompression from a unilateral approach. Although the risk of infection and the amount of blood loss probably are reduced with this technique, the risk of complications, such as dural tears, probably is increased, especially early in the surgeon's learning curve.[21] No large-scale level I study has compared tubular decompression with open laminectomy, although one small study suggested that patients treated with tubular decompression have similar neurologic outcomes and less back pain.[22]

In another attempt to minimize surgical morbidity, interspinous spacers have been developed to indirectly decompress the neural elements. These devices are placed between the spinous processes and result in flexion of the motion segment, with the goal of enlarging the spinal canal and the foramina. Most surgeons believe that the use of an interspinous spacer is indicated in patients whose symptoms are resolved with flexion and whose comorbidities put them at high risk of a perioperative medical complication. The use of an interspinous spacer is contraindicated in patients with spondylolisthesis that is more severe than grade I, significant scoliosis, or osteoporosis (which puts the patient at risk of spinous process fracture). Initial industry-sponsored studies comparing interspinous devices to nonsurgical treatment found a clear benefit for the devices. No study has compared the use of an interspinous device to open laminectomy, however.[23] Concern about high reoperation rates and the recurrence of symptoms has tempered enthusiasm for this technique.[24] The use of interspinous spacers represents a less invasive treatment option for elderly patients with stenosis and who have medical comorbidities, although the results may be less predictable or durable than that of a traditional decompression.

Surgical Versus Nonsurgical Outcomes

Both the Maine Lumbar Spine Study and a relatively small Finnish randomized controlled study comparing surgical and nonsurgical outcomes in patients with lumbar stenosis reported a clear benefit to surgery during the first 2 years after surgery.[25-27] The magnitude of the benefit of surgery decreased over time but remained significant on some outcome measures at 6 to 10 years.

The SPORT was undertaken as a large-scale effort to compare surgical and nonsurgical outcomes for patients with lumbar stenosis or degenerative spondylolisthesis in the United States. The study was designed with both randomized and observational cohorts; patients who declined randomization were followed as part of the observational group. All patients with lumbar stenosis had claudication or radicular symptoms of at least 3 months' duration and had radiographic evidence of stenosis consistent with their symptoms. Patients with degenerative spondylolisthesis were studied separately. Somewhat unexpectedly, there was a large rate of crossover, with approximately 40% of the patients assigned to nonsurgical treatment undergoing surgery and 40% of the patients assigned to surgical treatment never undergoing surgery. The intention-to-treat analysis was uninformative because the treatment received by patients in the two groups became almost identical. The researchers elected to report the results as an observational study with an as-treated analysis. After controlling for the important baseline differences between patients in the two treatment groups, the researchers found that those in the surgery group improved significantly more than those in the nonsurgical group on all major outcome measures over the first 4 years.[4] At 4-year follow-up, patients in the surgery group had improved more than 18 points on the ODI compared with 9 points for those treated nonsurgically. Similar differences were found on the SF-36 bodily pain and physical function components. The SPORT represents level II evidence, but evaluation in the context of earlier studies indicates that there is strong evidence that surgical treatment of lumbar stenosis leads to better short-term and long-term outcomes than nonsurgical treatment.[28]

The SPORT confirmed what most spine care providers believed was true: surgery leads to a better outcome than nonsurgical treatment. The SPORT also provided a large database of prospectively collected comparative data that could be analyzed to answer many additional questions. Surgeons had long believed that patients with pain predominantly in the back had less improvement after surgery than those with pain predominantly in the leg; this belief was confirmed for patients with lumbar stenosis or degenerative spondylolisthesis.[29] A second hypothesis based on anecdotal data was that patients with lumbar stenosis who had a long duration of symptoms improved less than those who had a shorter duration of symptoms; SPORT confirmed this hypothesis for both surgical and nonsurgical treatment.[30] However, the treatment effect of surgery (the difference between surgical and nonsurgical outcomes) was not affected by the duration of symptoms. Therefore, patients should have greater improvement with surgery than with nonsurgical treatment, regardless of symptom duration. In an attempt to determine independent treatment-effect predictors in lumbar stenosis, more than 50 variables were analyzed using the SPORT data. Smokers were found to be the only subgroup of patients that did not have greater improvement with surgery than with nonsurgical treatment. This finding echoes that of a Swedish Spine Registry study whereby surgical outcomes were worse in patients who were smokers than in those who were nonsmokers.[31,32] A greater treatment effect also was seen for patients whose baseline ODI score was below the top quartile or who had neuroforaminal stenosis, predominant leg pain, a neurologic deficit, or a job not requiring lifting.

Degenerative Spondylolisthesis

Epidemiology

Because lumbar stenosis and degenerative spondylolisthesis have a similar clinical presentation and both conditions involve compression of the lumbar nerve roots,

patients with either condition traditionally have been studied together. The demographic characteristics of the two patient populations are substantially different, however, as are the approaches to treatment and the outcomes. In the SPORT, the cohort of patients with degenerative spondylolisthesis included a much higher proportion of women (69% versus 39% of the patients in the lumbar stenosis cohort) and patients with single-level stenosis (65% versus 39% of the patients in the lumbar stenosis cohort). However, there were no differences in baseline SF-36, ODI, or leg or back pain scores between patients in the two diagnostic cohorts.[1] Degenerative spondylolisthesis is known to be far more common in women than in men; the Copenhagen Osteoarthritis Study reported an incidence of 8.4% in women and 2.7% in men.[33] This longitudinal study found that risk factors for degenerative spondylolisthesis in women were obesity, greater-than-normal lumbar lordosis, and advancing age. In men, only advancing age was associated with degenerative spondylolisthesis. It has been suggested that greater ligamentous laxity and estrogen exposure create a predisposition to degenerative spondylolisthesis in women. This hypothesis has not been proved, and one study found that degenerative spondylolisthesis was more common in women who had undergone oophorectomy.[34] The same study also reported an increased risk of degenerative spondylolisthesis in patients with diabetes.

Pathophysiology

The caudal tilt of the L4-L5 interspace and the relative stiffness of the L5-S1 interspace mean that degenerative spondylolisthesis affects L4-L5 in most patients. In the SPORT, 90% of the patients with degenerative spondylolisthesis had a listhesis at L4-L5, and only 10% had a listhesis at L3-L4.[2] A variety of morphologic factors are associated with degenerative spondylolisthesis, including an L4-L5 interspace above the intercrestal line, relatively slender L5 transverse processes, greater-than-normal sacral inclination and lumbar lordosis, and hemisacralization of L5.[34,35] Sagittal orientation of the L4-L5 facet joint also has been implicated as creating a predisposition to degenerative spondylolisthesis, although it remains unclear whether this orientation is the etiology of the slip or part of the degenerative process.[36,37] These factors cause increased shear stress at the L4-L5 interspace or decreased resistance to these forces, leading to anterolisthesis accompanying the degenerative cascade. The facet joints hypertrophy as they are exposed to increasing loads with disk degeneration, according to the Wolff law. The combination of anterolisthesis of L4, facet hypertrophy, L4-5 disk bulge, and ligamentum flavum and capsular hypertrophy contributes to central and lateral recess stenosis, which frequently is severe. The traversing L5 nerve root typically is compressed in the lateral recess between the superior articular process of L5 and the L4-5 disk, and radicular symptoms typically occur in an L5 distribution. Foraminal stenosis also can develop at L4-L5, resulting in compression of the L4 root. Foraminal

5: Spine

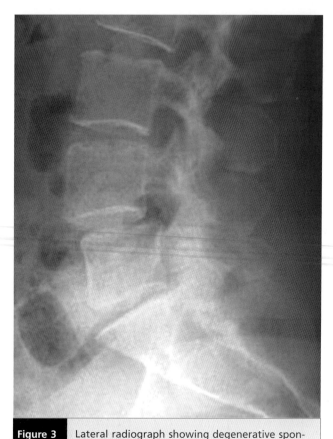

Figure 3 | Lateral radiograph showing degenerative spondylolisthesis at L4-L5.

In the SPORT, 85% of the patients with degenerative spondylolisthesis reported claudication, and 78% also had pain in a dermatomal distribution.[2] Approximately one half of the patients had a detectable neurologic deficit, including asymmetric reflex depression in 15%, sensory deficit in 28%, and motor weakness in 25%. Straight leg raise caused radicular pain in only 15% of the patients with degenerative spondylolisthesis. As with lumbar stenosis, physical examination findings are neither sensitive nor specific for the diagnosis of degenerative spondylolisthesis. The physical examination is most important for ruling out other possible diagnoses, including vascular claudication, hip or knee arthritis, myelopathy, peripheral neuropathy, and a systemic neurologic disorder.

Diagnostic Studies

The same diagnostic imaging techniques are used for degenerative spondylolisthesis and lumbar stenosis. Plain radiographs and MRI are the first-line modalities. Weight-bearing radiographs are essential for making the diagnosis because a subtle listhesis may be reduced if the patient is supine during MRI (Figure 3). Most patients with degenerative spondylolisthesis have a grade I listhesis (less than 25%), and listhesis beyond grade II does not occur. In the SPORT, 86% of the patients had grade I listhesis, with the remaining 14% having progressed to grade II.[38] Flexion-extension radiographs show the extent of mobility at the level of the listhesis, and some experts have suggested that the presence of hypermobility indicates the need for an instrumented fusion.[39,40] The effect of hypermobility (defined as more than 4 mm of translation or 10° of rotation on flexion-extension radiographs) was examined in the SPORT and was found to have no effect on surgical outcomes. Nonsurgical outcomes were actually better in patients with hypermobility.[38]

MRI findings in patients with degenerative spondylolisthesis typically include marked facet degeneration and hypertrophy, loss of disk height with a broad-based disk bulge, severe central and lateral recess stenosis, foraminal stenosis of variable severity, and fluid in the facet joints (**Figure 4**). The amount of fluid in the facet joint on the MRI was found to be correlated with the amount of increase in listhesis between the supine MRI and standing plain radiographs.[41] The presence of facet joint effusion was not associated with a poorer outcome in patients with degenerative spondylolisthesis who were treated with decompression alone, and therefore it is not helpful in determining the need for a fusion.[42]

Nonsurgical Treatment

The nonsurgical treatments for lumbar stenosis also are used for patients with degenerative spondylolisthesis, and include medication, physical therapy, and epidural steroid injections. There is very little evidence to support the use of any of these modalities in lumbar stenosis, and no studies have evaluated nonsurgical treatment exclusively in patients with degenerative

stenosis is less common than severe central and lateral recess stenosis, however. The pathophysiology of nerve root compression leading to claudication and radicular symptoms is similar to that of lumbar stenosis.

Clinical Presentation

Like patients with lumbar stenosis, those with degenerative spondylolisthesis typically have neurogenic claudication or radicular symptoms. Anecdotal reports suggest that patients with degenerative spondylolisthesis may be more likely to have severe back pain than those with lumbar stenosis because of the instability associated with the listhesis. However, the SPORT found no significant between-group differences in back pain scores.[1] Similarly, 26% of the patients with degenerative spondylolisthesis or lumbar stenosis reported that their back pain was more severe than their leg pain.[29] Radicular symptoms are common in patients with degenerative spondylolisthesis, usually with L5 radiculopathy. Pain classically occurs in the buttocks, the posterolateral thigh, the lateral leg, and the dorsum of the foot, with extensor hallucis longus weakness and numbness on the dorsum of the foot. L4 radiculopathy is less common and most often occurs in patients with L4-L5 foraminal stenosis. The symptoms are pain in the buttocks, the anterolateral thigh, and the anteromedial leg; tibialis anterior weakness; numbness in the medial leg and ankle; and decreased patellar tendon reflex.

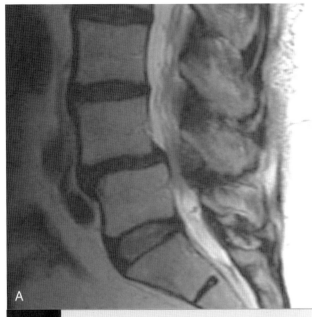

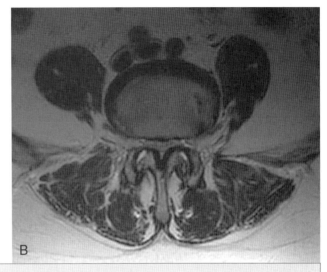

Figure 4 **A,** Sagittal T2-weighted MRI showing degenerative spondylolisthesis at L4-L5. **B,** Axial T2-weighted MRI showing fluid in degenerative facet joints as well as central and lateral recess stenosis.

spondylolisthesis. In the SPORT, which defined nonsurgical treatment as usual care, at 4-year follow-up the patients who received nonsurgical treatment had improved 16 points on the SF-36 bodily pain component, 8 points on the SF-36 physical function component, and 9 points on the ODI. As with the patients in the lumbar stenosis group, the improvements were modest.

Surgical Treatment

Surgery is considered for patients who have had claudication or radicular symptoms at least 6 to 12 weeks despite adequate nonsurgical treatment and whose imaging studies show degenerative spondylolisthesis with stenosis. A seminal prospective study comparing decompression with and without uninstrumented fusion in 50 patients with degenerative spondylolisthesis found that the addition of fusion led to significantly better clinical outcomes at 3-year follow-up.[43] Decompression with fusion has more recently been considered the standard treatment of degenerative spondylolisthesis (Table 1). Some experts have questioned the need for fusion in all patients, but there is no strong clinical evidence to show that certain subgroups of patients with degenerative spondylolisthesis do not benefit from fusion in addition to decompression. An observational study using modern patient-reported outcome measures found better outcomes when patients were treated using decompression with fusion rather than decompression alone.[44] Some researchers have suggested that facet-sparing or minimally invasive decompression may yield results comparable to those of traditional laminectomy and fusion, but no high-quality study has validated this hypothesis. Unless new data emerge to show that fusion does not lead to improved outcomes in some subgroups of patients with degenerative spon-

dylolisthesis, decompression with fusion will remain the standard of care.

More controversial than the need for fusion in patients with degenerative spondylolisthesis is the choice of a fusion technique to achieve the best results. The fusion techniques for treating degenerative spondylolisthesis include uninstrumented posterolateral fusion, instrumented posterolateral fusion, posterior lumbar interbody fusion, transforaminal lumbar interbody fusion, extreme lateral interbody fusion, and 360° fusion. No level I data have shown the superiority of any one of these fusion techniques for treating degenerative spondylolisthesis. The only truly randomized study comparing instrumented and uninstrumented fusion found a higher fusion rate when instrumentation was used, but fusion with instrumentation did not lead to better clinical outcomes at 2-year follow-up.[45] There was no correlation between fusion status and clinical outcome. A longer term follow-up of the patients who were treated without instrumentation found relatively poor outcomes in patients with a pseudarthrosis. Some researchers believe this finding provides support for the use of instrumentation to promote fusion and prevent the poor outcomes associated with pseudarthrosis.[46] This argument falls short, however, because the study did not include patients treated with instrumentation to compare the long-term outcomes of the two techniques, and no long-term studies have compared uninstrumented and instrumented fusion. Although the use of instrumentation leads to a higher fusion rate, it also may be associated with a higher rate of adjacent-level degeneration. A Finnish study comparing 5-year outcomes of patients with degenerative spondylolisthesis who were treated with or without instrumentation found that instrumentation led to slightly better clinical outcomes but a much higher rate of reoperation (28% and 14%, respectively).[47] It remains unclear whether the possible benefits of a solid fusion outweigh the adverse effects of instrumentation. A long-term comparison study is needed to answer this question.

Although determining the most effective arthrodesis technique was not a primary objective of the SPORT, a post-hoc subgroup analysis compared the 4-year outcomes of patients treated with uninstrumented posterolateral fusion, instrumented posterolateral fusion, or 360° fusion.[48] There was a trend toward better clinical outcomes in the patients treated without instrumentation rather than with instrumentation during the first 3 months and toward better outcomes in the patients treated with 360° fusion at 2-year follow-up, but at 3- to 4-year follow-up, there were no significant between-group differences. As in earlier studies, the patients in the instrumentation and 360° groups had higher fusion rates than those in the uninstrumented group. Fusion status was not associated with clinical outcome, however. This study was not randomized or powered to detect differences among the different techniques, but it is the largest comparative study on the topic and the only one using modern outcome measures. Most fusions for degenerative spondylolisthesis currently involve instrumentation (73% in the SPORT), despite a lack of clinical evidence showing whether the additional cost and the risk of complications associated with pedicle screw instrumentation leads to a measurable clinical benefit.

Interspinous devices were developed to treat lumbar stenosis, but some experts advocate their use for degenerative spondylolisthesis. High failure rates have been reported for these devices; a study of 12 patients treated for degenerative spondylolisthesis with an interspinous device found a 2-year reoperation rate of 58%.[49] Another investigation found that patients with degenerative spondylolisthesis had a 52% rate of spinous process fracture after the placement of an interspinous device, compared with 0% among patients without a listhesis.[50] Degenerative spondylolisthesis probably should be considered a relative contraindication to the use of an interspinous device.

Surgical Versus Nonsurgical Treatment

Many relatively early studies that compared the surgical and nonsurgical outcomes of patients with lumbar stenosis included patients with degenerative spondylolisthesis, although these patients often undergo different surgical treatments and have different outcomes. The SPORT was the first study to compare outcomes in a cohort exclusively composed of patients with degenerative spondylolisthesis.[2] As in the lumbar stenosis SPORT, the approximately 40% crossover rates from surgical to nonsurgical treatment and vice versa precluded any conclusions from the intention-to-treat analysis. In the adjusted as-treated analysis, patients who underwent surgery were found to have improved substantially more than those treated nonsurgically.[3] At 4-year follow-up, the patients who were surgically treated had a 23-point improvement on the ODI, compared with a 9-point improvement for those treated nonsurgically. The SPORT showed that patients with degenerative spondylolisthesis improved significantly more after surgery than patients with lumbar stenosis; the difference was approximately 5 points on the ODI at 2-year follow-up. Patients in the two diagnostic cohorts had similar outcomes after nonsurgical treatment.[1] The cause of these differences is not clear and could be related to the characteristics of the two patient populations, the underlying pathology, the number of levels involved, or the type of surgery performed.

Summary

Patients with lumbar stenosis and those with degenerative spondylolisthesis have similar symptoms, including neurogenic claudication, radiculopathy, and low back pain. Both conditions become more prevalent with advancing age. Degenerative spondylolisthesis is much more common in women than in men. The standard diagnostic workup includes plain radiographs and MRI. The nonsurgical treatment options include medications, physical therapy, and epidural steroid injections. These modalities should be attempted before surgery is considered. The surgery for lumbar stenosis in the absence of listhesis is decompression without fusion. Degenerative spondylolisthesis is best treated with decompression and fusion. The most effective fusion technique for degenerative spondylolisthesis remains controversial because no level I evidence has established the superiority of any technique. For patients who have had symptoms at least 12 weeks, have not had improvement with nonsurgical treatment, and have MRI findings showing stenosis with or without listhesis, surgery leads to a better outcome than nonsurgical treatment.

Key Study Points

- Surgery for lumbar stenosis or degenerative spondylolisthesis leads to a better outcome than nonsurgical treatment.

- It remains unclear whether the use of pedicle screw instrumentation for posterolateral fusion leads to a better clinical outcome in patients with degenerative spondylolisthesis.

- The use of an interspinous device is associated with a high failure rate in patients with degenerative spondylolisthesis.

Annotated References

1. Pearson A, Blood E, Lurie J, et al: Degenerative spondylolisthesis versus spinal stenosis: Does a slip matter?

Comparison of baseline characteristics and outcomes (SPORT). *Spine (Phila Pa 1976)* 2010;35(3):298-305.

Baseline characteristics and surgical and nonsurgical outcomes were compared in patients in the lumbar stenosis and degenerative spondylolisthesis SPORT cohorts. The degenerative spondylolisthesis cohort included more women, and patients had better surgical outcomes and similar nonsurgical outcomes compared with patients in the lumbar stenosis cohort. Level of evidence: II.

2. Weinstein JN, Lurie JD, Tosteson TD, et al: Surgical versus nonsurgical treatment for lumbar degenerative spondylolisthesis. *N Engl J Med* 2007;356(22):2257-2270.

3. Weinstein JN, Lurie JD, Tosteson TD, et al: Surgical compared with nonoperative treatment for lumbar degenerative spondylolisthesis: Four-year results in the Spine Patient Outcomes Research Trial (SPORT) randomized and observational cohorts. *J Bone Joint Surg Am* 2009;91(6):1295-1304.

4. Weinstein JN, Tosteson TD, Lurie JD, et al: Surgical versus nonoperative treatment for lumbar spinal stenosis four-year results of the Spine Patient Outcomes Research Trial. *Spine (Phila Pa 1976)* 2010;35(14):1329-1338.

The 4-year outcomes data for patients with lumbar stenosis from SPORT showed that patients who underwent surgery continued to have better outcomes than those who had nonsurgical treatment. There were minimal changes in outcomes from 2- to 4-year follow-up.

5. Weinstein JN, Tosteson TD, Lurie JD, et al: Surgical versus nonsurgical therapy for lumbar spinal stenosis. *N Engl J Med* 2008;358(8):794-810.

6. Ishimoto Y, Yoshimura N, Muraki S, et al: Prevalence of symptomatic lumbar spinal stenosis and its association with physical performance in a population-based cohort in Japan: The Wakayama Spine Study. *Osteoarthritis Cartilage* 2012;20(10):1103-1108.

This cross-sectional study evaluated the prevalence of lumbar stenosis using clinical and radiographic criteria. Approximately 10% of the population older than 60 years had symptomatic lumbar stenosis, and more than 75% had stenosis on MRI. Level of evidence: III.

7. Rydevik B, Brown MD, Lundborg G: Pathoanatomy and pathophysiology of nerve root compression. *Spine (Phila Pa 1976)* 1984;9(1):7-15.

8. Rydevik BL, Pedowitz RA, Hargens AR, Swenson MR, Myers RR, Garfin SR: Effects of acute, graded compression on spinal nerve root function and structure: An experimental study of the pig cauda equina. *Spine (Phila Pa 1976)* 1991;16(5):487-493.

9. Steurer J, Roner S, Gnannt R, Hodler J; LumbSten Research Collaboration: Quantitative radiologic criteria for the diagnosis of lumbar spinal stenosis: A systematic literature review. *BMC Musculoskelet Disord* 2011; 12:175.

A systematic review of radiographic criteria for the diagnosis of lumbar stenosis found that canal diameter or cross-sectional area could not be reliably used to diagnose lumbar stenosis. Level of evidence: III.

10. Park DK, An HS, Lurie JD, et al: Does multilevel lumbar stenosis lead to poorer outcomes? A subanalysis of the Spine Patient Outcomes Research Trial (SPORT) lumbar stenosis study. *Spine (Phila Pa 1976)* 2010; 35(4):439-446.

A SPORT subgroup analysis found no differences in baseline symptoms or outcomes between patients with lumbar stenosis who had single-level or multilevel stenosis, although patients with degenerative spondylolisthesis who had multilevel stenosis had worse surgical outcomes than those with single-level disease. Level of evidence: II.

11. Alyas F, Connell D, Saifuddin A: Upright positional MRI of the lumbar spine. *Clin Radiol* 2008;63(9):1035-1048.

12. Kinder A, Filho FP, Ribeiro E, et al: Magnetic resonance imaging of the lumbar spine with axial loading: A review of 120 cases. *Eur J Radiol* 2012;81(4):e561-e564.

The addition of an axial load of 50% of body weight to MRI resulted in a decrease in the cross-sectional area of the canal of at least 15 mm^2 in 82 (68%) of 120 patients. Level of evidence: IV.

13. Haig AJ, Tong HC, Yamakawa KS, et al: Spinal stenosis, back pain, or no symptoms at all? A masked study comparing radiologic and electrodiagnostic diagnoses to the clinical impression. *Arch Phys Med Rehabil* 2006; 87(7):897-903.

14. Adamova B, Vohanka S, Dusek L: Dynamic electrophysiological examination in patients with lumbar spinal stenosis: Is it useful in clinical practice? *Eur Spine J* 2005;14(3):269-276.

15. Ammendolia C, Stuber K, de Bruin LK, et al: Nonoperative treatment of lumbar spinal stenosis with neurogenic claudication: A systematic review. *Spine (Phila Pa 1976)* 2012;37(10):E609-E616.

A systematic review of nonsurgical treatment modalities for lumbar stenosis found only very low or low-quality evidence to support the use of medication, physical therapy, bracing, or injections. Level of evidence: II.

16. Albert HB, Manniche C: The efficacy of systematic active conservative treatment for patients with severe sciatica: A single-blind, randomized, clinical, controlled trial. *Spine (Phila Pa 1976)* 2012;37(7):531-542.

A randomized controlled study compared symptom-guided exercise with sham exercise consisting of low-level cardiovascular exercises for patients with sciatica. A modest benefit was found for the symptom-guided exercises. Level of evidence: I.

17. Prateepavanich P, Thanapipatsiri S, Santisatisakul P, Somshevita P, Charoensak T: The effectiveness of lumbosacral corset in symptomatic degenerative lumbar spinal stenosis. *J Med Assoc Thai* 2001;84(4):572-576.

5: Spine

18. Grob D, Humke T, Dvorak J: Degenerative lumbar spinal stenosis: Decompression with and without arthrodesis. *J Bone Joint Surg Am* 1995;77(7):1036-1041.

19. Desai A, Ball PA, Bekelis K, et al: SPORT: Does incidental durotomy affect long-term outcomes in cases of spinal stenosis? *Neurosurgery* 2011;69(1):38-44.

    A SPORT subgroup analysis found that the 9% of patients with lumbar stenosis who had a durotomy had greater inpatient length of stay, surgical time, and blood loss but no differences in long-term clinical outcomes compared with those without durotomy. Level of evidence: II.

20. Glassman SD, Carreon L, Dimar JR: Outcome of lumbar arthrodesis in patients sixty-five years of age or older: Surgical technique. *J Bone Joint Surg Am* 2010; 92(suppl 1, pt 1):77-84.

    This cohort study demonstrated similar patient-reported outcomes for patients older and younger than 65 years undergoing lumbar fusion. Although the complication rate was higher for the older patients, the 2-year outcomes were similar. Level of evidence: II.

21. Asgarzadie F, Khoo LT: Minimally invasive operative management for lumbar spinal stenosis: Overview of early and long-term outcomes. *Orthop Clin North Am* 2007;38(3):387-399.

22. Yagi M, Okada E, Ninomiya K, Kihara M: Postoperative outcome after modified unilateral-approach microendoscopic midline decompression for degenerative spinal stenosis. *J Neurosurg Spine* 2009;10(4):293-299.

23. Zucherman JF, Hsu KY, Hartjen CA, et al: A prospective randomized multi-center study for the treatment of lumbar spinal stenosis with the X STOP interspinous implant: 1-year results. *Eur Spine J* 2004;13(1):22-31.

24. Tuschel A, Chavanne A, Eder C, Meissl M, Becker P, Ogon M: Implant survival analysis and failure modes of the X STOP interspinous distraction device. *Spine (Phila Pa 1976)* 2013;38:1826-1831.

    A case study of 46 patients with lumbar stenosis who were treated using an interspinous device found a reoperation rate of 30% at a mean follow-up of 40 months, with most revision surgeries performed during the first year. Level of evidence: IV.

25. Atlas SJ, Keller RB, Wu YA, Deyo RA, Singer DE: Long-term outcomes of surgical and nonsurgical management of lumbar spinal stenosis: 8 to 10 year results from the maine lumbar spine study. *Spine (Phila Pa 1976)* 2005; 30(8):936-943.

26. Malmivaara A, Slätis P, Heliövaara M, et al: Surgical or nonoperative treatment for lumbar spinal stenosis? A randomized controlled trial. *Spine (Phila Pa 1976)* 2007;32(1):1-8.

27. Slätis P, Malmivaara A, Heliövaara M, et al: Long-term results of surgery for lumbar spinal stenosis: A randomised controlled trial. *Eur Spine J* 2011;20(7):1174-1181.

    A randomized controlled study evaluated almost 100 patients treated with either surgery or nonsurgical care over 6 years. Those treated surgically improved significantly more on all outcome measures at 2-year follow-up, but the benefit decreased over time. Level of evidence: I.

28. Kovacs FM, Urrútia G, Alarcón JD: Surgery versus conservative treatment for symptomatic lumbar spinal stenosis: A systematic review of randomized controlled trials. *Spine (Phila Pa 1976)* 2011;36(20):E1335-E1351.

    A systematic review of surgical and nonsurgical treatment of lumbar stenosis found a clear benefit to surgery. Level of evidence: II.

29. Pearson A, Blood E, Lurie J, et al: Predominant leg pain is associated with better surgical outcomes in degenerative spondylolisthesis and spinal stenosis: Results from the Spine Patient Outcomes Research Trial (SPORT). *Spine (Phila Pa 1976)* 2011;36(3):219-229.

    A SPORT subgroup analysis found that patients with lumbar stenosis or degenerative spondylolisthesis who had predominant back pain improved less with surgery than those who had predominant leg pain. There was less consistent difference in nonsurgical outcomes. Level of evidence: II.

30. Radcliff KE, Rihn J, Hilibrand A, et al: Does the duration of symptoms in patients with spinal stenosis and degenerative spondylolisthesis affect outcomes? Analysis of the Spine Outcomes Research Trial. *Spine (Phila Pa 1976)* 2011;36(25):2197-2210.

    A SPORT analysis compared surgical and nonsurgical outcomes in patients with lumbar stenosis or degenerative spondylolisthesis who were stratified by the duration of symptoms. Patients with lumbar stenosis who had symptoms for less than 12 months had greater improvement after surgical or nonsurgical treatment than patients with degenerative spondylolisthesis. Level of evidence: II.

31. Pearson A, Lurie J, Tosteson T, Zhao W, Abdu W, Weinstein JN: Who should have surgery for spinal stenosis? Treatment effect predictors in SPORT. *Spine (Phila Pa 1976)* 2012;37(21):1791-1802.

    SPORT data were analyzed to determine treatment effect predictors. A baseline ODI score below the top quartile, nonsmoking, neuroforaminal stenosis, predominant leg pain, no lifting at work, and a neurologic deficit predicted greater treatment effect. Level of evidence: II.

32. Sandén B, Försth P, Michaëlsson K: Smokers show less improvement than nonsmokers two years after surgery for lumbar spinal stenosis: A study of 4555 patients from the Swedish spine register. *Spine (Phila Pa 1976)* 2011;36(13):1059-1064.

    A review of the Swedish Spine Registry found that patients who were smokers improved significantly less with decompressive surgery than those who were nonsmokers. Level of evidence: II.

33. Jacobsen S, Sonne-Holm S, Rovsing H, Monrad H, Gebuhr P: Degenerative lumbar spondylolisthesis: An epidemiological perspective. The Copenhagen Osteoarthritis Study. *Spine (Phila Pa 1976)* 2007;32(1):120-125.

34. Frymoyer JW: Degenerative spondylolisthesis: Diagnosis and treatment. *J Am Acad Orthop Surg* 1994;2(1): 9-15.

35. Hosoe H, Ohmori K: Degenerative lumbosacral spondylolisthesis: Possible factors which predispose the fifth lumbar vertebra to slip. *J Bone Joint Surg Br* 2008; 90(3):356-359.

36. Boden SD, Riew KD, Yamaguchi K, Branch TP, Schellinger D, Wiesel SW: Orientation of the lumbar facet joints: Association with degenerative disc disease. *J Bone Joint Surg Am* 1996;78(3):403-411.

37. Love TW, Fagan AB, Fraser RD: Degenerative spondylolisthesis: Developmental or acquired? *J Bone Joint Surg Br* 1999;81(4):670-674.

38. Pearson AM, Lurie JD, Blood EA, et al: Spine patient outcomes research trial: Radiographic predictors of clinical outcomes after operative or nonoperative treatment of degenerative spondylolisthesis. *Spine (Phila Pa 1976)* 2008;33(25):2759-2766.

39. Yone K, Sakou T: Usefulness of Posner's definition of spinal instability for selection of surgical treatment for lumbar spinal stenosis. *J Spinal Disord* 1999;12(1): 40-44.

40. Yone K, Sakou T, Kawauchi Y, Yamaguchi M, Yanase M: Indication of fusion for lumbar spinal stenosis in elderly patients and its significance. *Spine (Phila Pa 1976)* 1996;21(2):242-248.

41. Lattig F, Fekete TF, Grob D, Kleinstück FS, Jeszenszky D, Mannion AF: Lumbar facet joint effusion in MRI: A sign of instability in degenerative spondylolisthesis? *Eur Spine J* 2012;21(2):276-281.

    A radiographic study showed that the amount of fluid seen in the facet joints on supine MRI was correlated with the magnitude of increase in listhesis observed when the MRI and standing lateral radiographs were compared. Level of evidence: III.

42. Lattig F, Fülöp Fekete T, Kleinstück FS, Porchet F, Jeszenszky D, Mannion AF: Lumbar facet joint effusion on MRI as a sign of unstable degenerative spondylolisthesis: Should it influence the treatment decision? *J Spinal Disord Tech* 2012. Epub ahead of print.

    Outcomes of patients with degenerative spondylolisthesis who were treated with decompression alone or decompression and fusion were compared. No relationship between the presence of facet joint effusion and outcomes was found in either patient group. Level of evidence: II.

43. Herkowitz HN, Kurz LT: Degenerative lumbar spondylolisthesis with spinal stenosis: A prospective study comparing decompression with decompression and intertransverse process arthrodesis. *J Bone Joint Surg Am* 1991;73(6):802-808.

44. Kleinstueck FS, Fekete TF, Mannion AF, et al: To fuse or not to fuse in lumbar degenerative spondylolisthesis: Do baseline symptoms help provide the answer? *Eur Spine J* 2012;21(2):268-275.

    An observational study of 213 patients with degenerative spondylolisthesis reported better outcomes in patients treated with decompression and fusion than in those treated with decompression alone. Level of evidence: II.

45. Fischgrund JS, Mackay M, Herkowitz HN, Brower R, Montgomery DM, Kurz LT: 1997 Volvo Award winner in clinical studies: Degenerative lumbar spondylolisthesis with spinal stenosis. A prospective, randomized study comparing decompressive laminectomy and arthrodesis with and without spinal instrumentation. *Spine (Phila Pa 1976)* 1997;22(24):2807-2812.

46. Kornblum MB, Fischgrund JS, Herkowitz HN, Abraham DA, Berkower DL, Ditkoff JS: Degenerative lumbar spondylolisthesis with spinal stenosis: A prospective long-term study comparing fusion and pseudarthrosis. *Spine (Phila Pa 1976)* 2004;29(7):726-734.

47. Bjarke Christensen F, Stender Hansen E, Laursen M, Thomsen K, Bünger CE: Long-term functional outcome of pedicle screw instrumentation as a support for posterolateral spinal fusion: Randomized clinical study with a 5-year follow-up. *Spine (Phila Pa 1976)* 2002; 27(12):1269-1277.

48. Abdu WA, Lurie JD, Spratt KF, et al: Degenerative spondylolisthesis: Does fusion method influence outcome? Four-year results of the Spine Patient Outcomes Research Trial. *Spine (Phila Pa 1976)* 2009;34(21): 2351-2360.

    A subgroup analysis of the SPORT patients with degenerative spondylolisthesis who were treated surgically found similar outcomes in those treated with uninstrumented fusion, instrumented fusion, or 360° fusion at 4-year follow-up. Level of evidence: II.

49. Verhoof OJ, Bron JL, Wapstra FH, van Royen BJ: High failure rate of the interspinous distraction device (X-Stop) for the treatment of lumbar spinal stenosis caused by degenerative spondylolisthesis. *Eur Spine J* 2008;17(2):188-192.

50. Kim DH, Shanti N, Tantorski ME, et al: Association between degenerative spondylolisthesis and spinous process fracture after interspinous process spacer surgery. *Spine J* 2012;12(6):466-472.

    A cohort study of patients treated using an interspinous device found a 52% rate of spinous process fracture in patients with a spondylolisthesis compared with 0% in patients without a slip. Level of evidence: II.

5: Spine

Chapter 51

Lumbar and Thoracic Disk Herniations

John S. Clapp, MD   Rachel M. Deering, MPH   Christopher M. Bono, MD

Lumbar Disk Herniations

Epidemiology and Demographics

Symptomatic lumbar disk herniation is common and has a lifetime prevalence of approximately 2%.[1] Lumbar disk herniation occurs across a wide age range but is most common during the fourth to sixth decades of life. The cause can be a specific trauma, although most herniations are not attributable to an identifiable event. Herniation of the nucleus pulposus occurs through a disruption of the outer anulus fibrosus of the disk and resulting intrusion into the spinal canal. Symptomatic herniation typically is part of a degenerative cascade in which the patient has prodromal pain in the back or buttock that progresses to the lower extremities in a dermatomal pattern. Nerve dysfunction and symptoms can be the result of mechanical insult to the nerve, leading to ischemia, or a chemical irritation from the inflammatory cascade in response to exposure to disk material.

Most lumbar disk herniations are asymptomatic. The prevalence of asymptomatic herniations increases with age as part of the natural degenerative progression of the aging spine. However, an MRI study of patients without back or leg pain found that 36% of those older than 60 years had a herniated disk, compared with 43% of those younger than 60 years.[2] These data highlight the importance of correlating a patient's history

Dr. Bono or an immediate family member has received nonincome support (such as equipment or services), commercially derived honoraria, or other non–research-related funding (such as paid travel) from the Harvard Clinical Research Institute and Intrinsic Therapeutics and serves as a board member, owner, officer, or committee member of the American Academy of Orthopaedic Surgeons, the International Society for the Advancement of Spinal Surgery, and the North American Spine Society. Neither of the following authors nor any immediate family member has received anything of value from or has stock or stock options held in a commercial company or institution related directly or indirectly to the subject of this chapter: Dr. Clapp and Dr. Deering.

and physical examination with findings from imaging studies.

Classification

The goal of a classification system should be to provide the practitioner with a consistent and reproducible means of identifying and describing a condition and provide guidance in treatment decisions. Lumbar disk herniations often are classified and discussed using descriptive terminology based on the anatomic location of the herniation and its morphologic characteristics.

A lumbar disk herniation can be central, posterolateral (also called subarticular or lateral recess), foraminal, or extraforaminal (**Figure 1**). The location can be important for correlating symptoms and examination findings with a particular radicular pattern. Central disk herniation causes more low back pain than posterolateral disk herniation.[3] Recognizing the exact location of the disk material is critical for determining a surgical approach. Ideally, the patient's symptoms, clinical examination, and imaging findings all corroborate

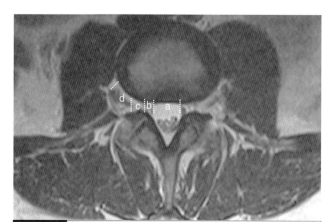

Figure 1   Axial MRI showing the description of lumbar disk herniation based on its location in the transverse plane. The central zone (a) is delineated between the borders of the cauda equina sac. The posterolateral zone (b) is between the lateral border of the cauda equina and the foramen. The foraminal zone (c) and the extraforaminal zone (d) are relatively uncommon locations for lumbar disk herniation.

5: Spine

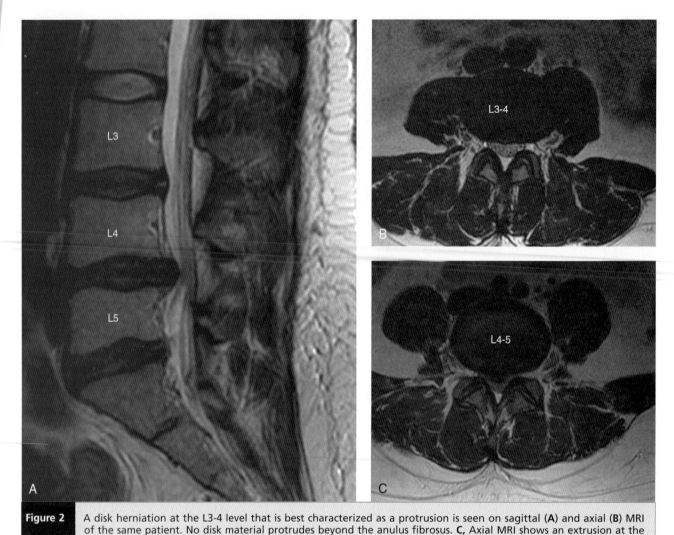

Figure 2 A disk herniation at the L3-4 level that is best characterized as a protrusion is seen on sagittal (**A**) and axial (**B**) MRI of the same patient. No disk material protrudes beyond the anulus fibrosus. **C,** Axial MRI shows an extrusion at the L4-5 level, with abundant disk material protruding beyond the anulus fibrosus and clearly compressing the cauda equina. A disk sequestration (not shown) is not connected to the parent disk and usually lies directly posterior to the vertebral body.

the diagnosis of radiculopathy of a single nerve root.

A lumbar disk herniation also can be described based on its morphology at the time of diagnosis. The traditional classifications are disk bulge, protrusion, extrusion, and sequestration (**Figure 2**). Further distinction can be made based on containment of disk fragments and the amount of protrusion.[4] Disk material that remains beneath the posterior longitudinal ligament is considered contained, and material extending through or around the ligament is considered uncontained. Uncontained material is more likely to be resorbed over time without surgery.

Herniation size and shape on MRI were found to be more predictive of outcome than clinical parameters, such as workers' compensation status, age, and sex.[5] Nonsurgical treatment is relatively unlikely to be successful in patients with a primarily central disk herniation in a spinal canal with a relatively small cross-sectional area; these patients are more likely to require surgery than other patients with a herniation.[6] In a prospective observational study of 187 consecutive pa-

tients undergoing diskectomy, intraoperative findings were found to be more predictive of outcome than demographic, socioeconomic, or other clinical variables at a minimum 2-year follow-up.[7] Patients with a larger, extruded disk herniation tended to have relatively good results after surgery, particularly if the remaining annular defect was small. A disk fragment with a large annular defect was associated with a 21% rate of symptomatic recurrence.

Clinical Evaluation and Diagnosis

Patients with symptomatic lumbar disk herniation typically have leg pain in a dermatomal distribution, with or without back pain. Some patients have a sudden onset of leg pain and little or no back pain, but others experience a prodrome of acute back pain, with subsequent onset of leg symptoms. The acute back pain is believed to stem from tearing of the outer annular disk fibers, which are innervated by nociceptive sinuvertebral nerve fibers.

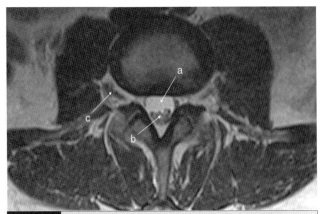

Figure 3 Axial MRI offers a so-called myelography effect in which the cerebrospinal fluid (a) is bright on T2-weighted studies, allowing clear visualization of the nerve rootlets within the thecal sac (b). The dorsal root ganglion of the exiting nerve root is readily seen (c), with surrounding perineural fat.

A thorough history is an important part of diagnosis and management. Some patients describe an onset of symptoms after a traumatic event, such as a fall, or an incident of heavy lifting, bending, or twisting. Pain is the most common symptom, but a patient also may have numbness or weakness. The level of the herniation should be correlated with the distribution of radicular pain. Typically, an upper herniation (at L1-2 or L2-3) causes proximal lower extremity symptoms, and a lower herniation (at L3-4, L4-5, or L5-S1) causes pain that extends below the knee and into the foot. The history should target red flag issues such as unexplained weight loss, fevers, chills, history of cancer, significant trauma, progressive weakness, and bowel or bladder incontinence or dysfunction. The presence of one or more of these indicates a need for early advanced imaging.

It is important to consider other possible causes of leg and back pain during a workup for suspected disk herniation. The differential diagnoses that should be considered are vascular (peripheral vascular disease, claudication, aneurysm, or thromboembolic disease), peripheral nerve-related (nerve tumor or peripheral compression such as tarsal tunnel syndrome, meralgia paresthetica, or diabetic neuropathy), and musculoskeletal (hip or knee joint pathology, muscle sprain or strain, piriformis syndrome, obturator internus syndrome, pudendal nerve entrapment, or sacroiliac joint pain).

Several well-described maneuvers are useful in the diagnosis of symptomatic lumbar disk herniation. The straight leg raise test is used to evaluate the lower nerve roots (at L3-S1); a positive test produces leg pain below the knee with 30° to 70° of hip flexion when the patient is supine. The femoral stretch test is intended to reproduce pain from upper lumbar herniation (at L1-2 or L2-3) and is performed by flexing the knee and extending the hip with the patient prone or in the lateral decubitus position. A Cochrane review found that the straight leg raise has reported sensitivity of approximately 90% but specificity ranging from 10% to 100%.[8] The contralateral or crossed straight leg raise had 90% specificity. Specificity was increased by performing the maneuver bilaterally. The reliability of the straight leg raise test recently was called into question by a study of patients with known MRI disk herniation and a radiculopathy. Sensitivity of 36% and specificity of 74% were found, and the positive and negative predictive values were 0.69 and 0.52, respectively.[9] The slump test is a variation of the straight leg raise that adds cervical and thoracic flexion with dorsiflexion of the ipsilateral foot. The additional flexion is intended to cause proximal migration of the spinal cord as well as tension on the more caudal roots. This maneuver was found to be more sensitive but less specific than the straight leg raise in patients with a known disk herniation.[10] The use of the slump test was promoted as a means of adding sensitivity when a patient has a negative straight leg raise test.

In the absence of a red flag, imaging is not necessary before treatment is initiated based on a presumptive diagnosis of a lumbar disk herniation. Symptoms often quickly improve, sometimes within a few days of onset, thus obviating the usefulness of advanced imaging modalities. For patients with refractory or worsening symptoms, plain radiographs may be helpful. Although the images do not allow characterization of a disk herniation, they do allow assessment of alignment and degree of spondylosis. Plain radiographs also are helpful in surgical planning to ensure the accurate numbering of vertebral levels and detect an anomaly such as spina bifida occulta.

MRI is the primary imaging modality for lumbar disk herniation. Sagittal and axial studies clearly show the size and the location of the herniations. T2-weighted studies provide a so-called myelography effect, in which the cerebrospinal fluid is bright in relation to the nerve roots and disk material (**Figure 3**). It is common to obtain a gadolinium contrast–enhanced MRI if the patient has had earlier spine surgery. The contrast-enhanced MRI preferentially enhances vascular tissue, such as epidural scarring, which can be useful in distinguishing it from recurrent disk herniation material. However, MRI without contrast enhancement usually is sufficient before surgery. If a patient has a contraindication to MRI, a CT myelogram can be obtained.

Natural History

Much of the knowledge of the natural history of lumbar disk herniation is derived from the nonsurgical treatment arm of studies that compared surgical and nonsurgical treatments (**Table 1**). The success rates of nonsurgical treatments ranged from 51% to 90%, but few of the controlled studies used the same nonsurgical modalities.[11-15] Another confounding factor is the high crossover rates between patients assigned to surgical or nonsurgical treatment. Few, if any, data reflect the natural history of lumbar disk herniation in the absence of treatment.

Table 1

Large Prospective Studies Documenting the Nonsurgical Treatment (Natural History) of Lumbar Disk Herniation

Study (Year)	Study Type	Summary of Results
Weber[11] (1983)	Prospective randomized controlled (nonsurgical cohort)	89% good or fair outcome (4-year follow-up)
Saal and Saal[12] (1989)	Retrospective cohort	92% return to work; 90% good or excellent outcome
Atlas et al[13] (2005)	Prospective case control	61% improvement in predominant symptom; 56% satisfaction rate (10-year follow-up)
Weinstein et al[14] (2008)	Prospective case control (nonsurgical cohort)	51% major improvement (4-year follow-up)
Peul et al[15] (2008)	Prospective randomized controlled (nonsurgical cohort)	56% success, defined as ability to avoid surgery (2-year follow-up)

A frequently cited retrospective study of the nonsurgical management of lumbar disk herniation reported outcomes for patients with a primary symptom of leg pain, a positive straight leg raise test, lumbar disk pathology on imaging, and a positive electromyogram. After treatment with back school and a rehabilitation program, 90% of patients had a good or excellent outcome, and 92% returned to work.[12] Critics of this study point out that 10% of the patients dropped out of the study to undergo surgery, and the 58 patients in the study cohort were enrolled from 347 patients identified as candidates. Many of the patients in this study were referred for a second opinion regarding surgery, and this step may have acted to select those who were reluctant to proceed with surgery. A follow-up study by the same researchers found a greater than 50% decrease in disk herniation size on imaging in 11 of the 58 patients.[16]

In another frequently cited study, 49 patients with lumbar disk herniation were randomly assigned to nonsurgical treatment consisting of a week of full-time bed rest followed by a second week of partial rest and inpatient back school. A good or fair result was reported in 89%.[11] The crossover rate was high, however (17 patients left the nonsurgical group to have surgery), and patients with relatively severe symptoms were excluded. Nonsurgically treated patients in the Spine Patient Outcomes Research Trial (SPORT) had a 51% rate of major improvement in symptoms at 4-year follow-up.[14]

Nonsurgical Treatment

A prospective cohort study compared outcomes after nonsurgical treatment in patients who were older or younger than 60 years. The outcome measures included the Oswestry Disability Index (ODI), back pain, and leg pain. Patients in the two age groups had similar improvement in back-related disability and pain over a 6-month follow-up period.[17] These data suggest that age does not preclude a favorable outcome after nonsurgical treatment of lumbar disk herniation.

Epidural steroid injections are commonly used as a nonsurgical treatment of patients with lumbar disk herniation. The goal is to provide pain relief and possibly avoid the need for surgery. SPORT data on 154 patients treated with an epidural steroid injection for lumbar disk herniation within the first 3 months of the study were compared with data on 453 patients who did not receive an injection.[18] None of the patients had received an earlier injection. There were no differences between patients in the two groups at 4-year follow-up, as measured on the bodily pain component of the Medical Outcomes Study 36-Item Short Form or the ODI. In addition, no between-group differences were found on secondary outcome measures at any follow-up point. Patients assigned to surgery had a higher crossover rate than those who received an epidural steroid injection. However, the baseline preference among patients who chose an injection was significantly in favor of avoiding surgery, and this factor may have confounded the results. No between-group differences were found in surgical complications or the rate of revision surgery based on whether patients had received an epidural steroid injection.

It is recommended that an epidural steroid injection be used if a patient's condition does not respond to initial nonsurgical measures. Rarely, an injection may be indicated earlier in the course of a rehabilitation regimen if the patient's pain is too intense to allow participation.

Surgical Versus Nonsurgical Treatment

Several studies have compared surgical and nonsurgical treatment of lumbar disk herniation, but most studies in which randomization was attempted were affected by a high crossover rate.[14,19,20] Both a high crossover rate and the use of an intent-to-treat analysis can dilute the effect of surgery. It becomes more difficult to accurately interpret the effects of nonsurgical treatment if many of the patients actually underwent surgery.

The prospective nonrandomized Maine Lumbar Spine Study followed 400 patients who received nonsurgical or surgical treatment of lumbar disk herniation. The outcome measures included patient-reported symptoms, work status, and functional status. At 1-year follow-up, patients who chose surgery had a significant reduction in their primary symptom, and at 10-year follow-up they had a satisfaction rate higher than that of the patients who were nonsurgically treated (71% versus 56%), with more complete relief of leg pain and improved function. There was no between-group statistical difference in work or disability status or in the severity of the primary symptom at 10-year follow-up.[13]

Surgical Outcomes and Influential Covariables

Time to Surgery

Urgent decompressive surgery for lumbar disk herniation is primarily indicated in or for patients with cauda equina syndrome characterized by saddle anesthesia, bowel and/or bladder dysfunction, and lower extremity pain and weakness. A progressive neurologic deficit, such as a new-onset foot drop, can be a relative indication for early surgery. In most other patients, surgery can be considered elective and performed in a delayed fashion. Nonetheless, timing is important in surgical decision making. A criterion threshold beyond which the results of elective diskectomy may be less favorable compared with earlier surgery has been suggested. Recent analysis of SPORT data on patients in the randomized and observational groups found that patients with symptoms of more than 6 months' duration before treatment had worse outcomes than other patients at all points up to 4-year follow-up.[21] Patients treated after 6 months did have improvement, but in both the surgical and nonsurgical groups the improvement was less than in patients treated before 6 months.

Level of Herniation

The SPORT data were analyzed to determine the role of herniation level in outcomes. A comparison of surgical and nonsurgical treatment of upper lumbar herniations (defined as L2-3 and L3-4) found more benefit from surgical treatment.[22] This finding was related to relatively unsuccessful nonsurgical treatment at the upper lumbar levels.

Surgical Techniques

The term minimally invasive diskectomy has been used to describe surgery with the use of a small incision, tubular retractors, microscopes, and even endoscopic techniques. Research has not yet shown a benefit to long-term outcomes of these techniques compared with open surgery. Proponents believe that avoidance of extensive muscle damage and other soft-tissue injury reduces the amount of postoperative back pain. As a result, patients are believed to recover more quickly and possibly have an improved clinical outcome.

A prospective randomized study compared patients who underwent a first surgical procedure for radiculopathy using a 3-cm or a 7-cm fascial incision.[23] No difference in outcomes was found in terms of length of hospital stay, use of pain medication, or back or leg pain. In another prospective randomized study, 112 patients were assigned to microendoscopic or open diskectomy after 6 weeks of unsuccessful nonsurgical therapy.[24] The outcome measures were ODI score, length of hospital stay, surgical time, amount of blood loss, and complication rates. Patients in the minimally invasive surgery group had longer surgical procedures with less blood loss and a shorter hospital stay than those in the open surgery group, but between-group ODI scores and complication rates were similar. The two techniques were found to be equally effective.

Tubular system diskectomy was compared with open microdiskectomy in a prospective randomized study.[25] Importantly, patient and observer blinding was done after a same-size incision was made, and the procedure continued as an open or a tubular diskectomy intended to spare the multifidus muscle. Patients in the tubular diskectomy group had more low back pain during the year after surgery, as measured on the visual analog scale (VAS). Creatine phosphokinase levels measured the day before and the day after surgery showed no significant between-group difference. There was no significant difference in measurements of the cross-sectional area of the multifidus muscle.

A prospective comparison of outcomes after minimally invasive diskectomy was based on medical center level of experience with the procedure.[26] One hundred patients were randomly assigned to one of two centers. The outcome measures included duration of surgery, hospital length of stay, VAS leg and back pain scores, ODI scores, complications, and return to work. The clinical results and complication rates were similar for patients treated at the two centers, but patients treated at the center with the higher level of experience had a shorter surgical time and more rapid recovery.

A diskectomy may involve the removal of only the extruded fragment or a more aggressive débridement of a large amount of tissue from within the disk space in an attempt to limit recurrent herniation. Reported rates of recurrence range from 5% to 18%, depending on the definition of the term. Subtotal diskectomy, an aggressive method of removing disk material to reduce the amount of herniation, was prospectively studied in 30 patients.[27] The 9% rate of recurrent herniation in the patients treated with subtotal diskectomy was lower than that of historical control subjects (18%), but the patients had a longer time to return to work and were less satisfied at 2-year follow-up.

Intraoperative Topical Steroids

Many surgeons apply topical steroids intraoperatively in an attempt to reduce inflammation and irritation of the nerve after removal of the herniated disk. The underlying belief is that inflammation is associated with a lowering of the threshold for nociceptive sense organs, and the inflammatory process is partly responsible for postoperative pain. In a prospective randomized study of patients undergoing lumbar diskectomy, 61 patients were randomly assigned to receive 80 mg of methylprednisolone or saline topically over the decompressed nerve root.[28] The VAS was used to assess pain outcomes. At 2-week follow-up, patients who had received the steroid had significant relief of back pain, but there was no between-group difference in leg pain at 2-week or 1-year follow-up.

Topical steroids sometimes are used in the diskectomy wound in conjunction with bupivacaine or a local anesthetic. In a prospective study of 151 patients with L4-5 and L5-S1 disk herniations, patients received methylprednisolone and bupivacaine, bupivacaine and saline, or saline only.[29] No difference was found among patients in the three groups in the intensity of back or leg pain 24, 36, 72, and 96 hours after surgery, as recorded using the VAS. In another prospective study, 84 patients were randomly assigned to receive topical methylprednisolone or saline at the end of a microdiskectomy.[30] No between-group differences were found in length of stay, postoperative use of pain medication, functional status, or return to work. At best, the results of using steroids after diskectomy are mixed, and long-term benefit has not been found.

Thoracic Disk Herniation

Epidemiology and Demographics

Symptomatic thoracic disk herniation is uncommon and has been reported to occur in one individual per one million population. MRI of individuals without symptoms found a 40% prevalence, however.[31] Most symptomatic herniations appear in the fourth to sixth decades of life, with the peak incidence in the fifth decade.

Clinical Evaluation and Diagnosis

The clinical appearance of thoracic disk herniation varies widely and can be similar to that of other disorders. Often symptoms do not follow a characteristic pattern. The findings on examination depend on the location and the size of the herniation as well as the general health of the patient. The anatomic features of the thoracic region also have a role. Because the thoracic spinal canal has relatively little space available for the neural elements, herniation is less well tolerated than in the lumbar region. The tenuous blood supply to the spinal cord in the middle thoracic segments creates a greater susceptibility to compression than is found in the cauda equina in the lumbar spine.

The initial symptoms range from axial pain and discomfort to radiculopathy or myelopathy. Radicular pain follows the distribution of the involved thoracic nerve root; patients usually describe a bandlike pain around the chest wall. The diagnosis may be delayed if initially there is a less obviously spine-related symptom, such as centralized sternal or chest pain, abdominal pain, bowel or bladder dysfunction, or groin pain. The physical examination should include a complete neurologic examination to specifically assess for long tract signs, such as Babinski reflex, clonus, ataxia, and lower extremity hyperreflexia. The patient should be observed walking to assess for wide-based gait. The upper extremities also should be examined to rule out concomitant cervical spinal cord compression or stenosis.

The differential diagnoses include transverse myelitis, multiple sclerosis, trauma (rib fracture or vertebral compression fracture), cardiac pathology (angina, ischemia, or myocardial infarction), abdominal visceral pathology (cholecystitis or pleuritic syndromes), paraspinal muscle strain or sprain, herpes zoster, kidney stones, and scapulothoracic bursitis.

The evaluation of a patient with suspected symptomatic thoracic disk herniation should include standing plain radiographs to rule out deformity, spine imbalance, tumor, and fracture. MRI and CT also should be performed (Figure 4). CT myelography is a reasonable alternative to MRI in patients with a contraindication. The anatomic and examination findings must be correlated. CT can help determine whether the disk material appears calcified. If surgery is planned, the presence of disk calcification or dural adhesions can affect decision making as to the approach.

Incidental MRI findings can make diagnosis even more difficult in the thoracic spine than in the lumbar spine. Disk herniation was found in 33% of individuals without symptoms, disk bulging in 53%, cord deformation in 29%, annular tear in 58%, and end plate irregularity in 38%.[31] These figures suggest the need for caution when interpreting MRI results. Imaging should be used as a tool for confirmation and diagnosis in conjunction with a thorough physical examination and a carefully obtained history.

Nonsurgical Versus Surgical Treatment

An incidentally found thoracic disk herniation should be observed. The natural history in a patient without symptoms is favorable. In one study, all 20 patients (with 48 herniations) remained asymptomatic during the follow-up period.[32] Symptomatic thoracic disk herniation also can have a favorable natural history. A study of 55 individuals with symptoms over a 3-year period found that 73% were adequately treated without surgery and did not require surgical intervention, and 77% returned to their previous level of activity.[33]

The indications for surgical treatment remain unclear. Surgery for patients with myelopathy from a thoracic disk herniation is the least debated, despite the lack of direct comparison studies of surgical and nonsurgical treatment for these patients. Patients with radiculopathy from a thoracic disk herniation may be candidates for surgery after unsuccessful nonsurgical treatment, including physical therapy, activity modification, NSAIDs, analgesics, and possibly injections. Activity modification can include the avoidance of rotational stresses that can exacerbate symptoms. Surgery for the treatment of axial pain related to a thoracic disk herniation is controversial. Surgical intervention is not believed to have high value for patients with isolated

5: Spine

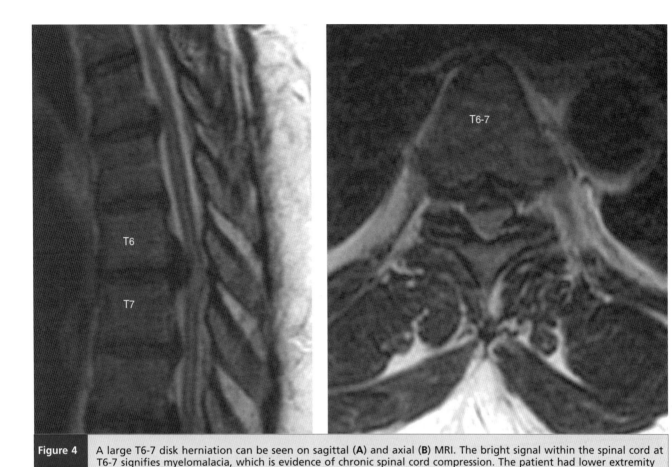

Figure 4 A large T6-7 disk herniation can be seen on sagittal (**A**) and axial (**B**) MRI. The bright signal within the spinal cord at T6-7 signifies myelomalacia, which is evidence of chronic spinal cord compression. The patient had lower extremity hyperreflexia and difficulty with balance when walking. Incidentally found disk degeneration and protrusion at other levels made diagnosis of the symptomatic level challenging.

axial pain in the absence of neurologic signs or symptoms.

Surgical Techniques

The surgical options for the removal of a thoracic disk herniation include anterior transthoracic (standard or video-assisted) diskectomy, posterior transpedicular diskectomy, costotransversectomy, and lateral extracavitary techniques. In addition, minimally invasive and pedicle-sparing posterior techniques have been described. Imaging studies should be reviewed to determine whether the disk material is central, paracentral, or lateral. The cranial-caudal level of the disk also affects the decision because access to a high thoracic herniation is difficult through a thoracotomy. The factors that should be considered when planning a thoracic diskectomy include the central, paracentral, or lateral location of the disk within the canal; the region within the thoracic spine (because access to the upper and lower ends of the thoracic spine can be difficult from an anterior approach); the surgeon's experience with the approach; and patient comorbidities such as previous thoracic surgery or large body habitus.

In general, thoracic disk herniations are more central than lumbar herniations. The most important distinction between surgery for thoracic and lumbar disk her-

niations is that surgery in the thoracic spine is at the spinal cord level. Manipulation and retraction of the spinal cord should be minimized or altogether avoided. Standard laminectomy through a posterior approach is no longer recommended because of the high reported rate of neurologic complications from manipulation of the spinal cord.[34] Central and large herniations may be better suited for anterior excision in an effort to prevent or avoid neural element retraction. As in an anterior cervical diskectomy and fusion, anterior excision allows the surgeon direct access to the disk material while avoiding manipulation of the neural elements. Morbidity can be associated with the transthoracic approach. Posterolateral approaches have been developed that can allow posterior access to the disk with minimal retraction of the cord (Figure 5). CT can be helpful in decision making by identifying any disk calcification, which can increase the likelihood of adhesions, dural tearing, or neural injury.

It is important to have a reliable and reproducible method of confirming the spine level during surgical excision. Preoperative MRI or CT can be used to count vertebrae cranially from the lumbar spine. However, the recommended method is to use the ribs as a reference. Starting from the cervical or lumbar spine, axial images should be carefully examined to confirm the

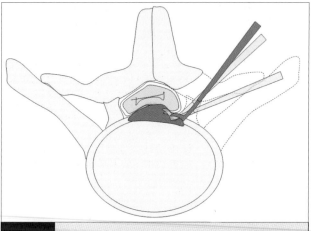

Figure 5 Schematic drawing showing a posterolateral approach for removing thoracic disk herniation. The pedicle, the hemilamina, and the rib head have been removed on one side (dotted lines). Downward curettes are used to carefully push herniated disk material into the disk space for ultimate removal.

presence of the first or last rib and its relation to the level of pathology. It is important to determine the number of thoracic and lumbar vertebrae present on imaging studies. The rib heads at T1, T11, and T12 articulate with the corresponding vertebral body; the rib heads at T2 through T10 span a disk space and articulate with both the corresponding and next most cranial vertebral bodies. Some surgeons recommend preoperative placement of a marker, such as polymethyl methacrylate or a fiduciary screw, that can be easily identified at the time of surgery.[35,36]

Although each decision is made on a per-patient basis, most researchers agree that the anterolateral approach is safer and more suited for large, central, and calcified disks than posterior or posterolateral approaches.[37] From the more direct anterior approach, there is less potential for cord injury and intraoperative dural tearing.

The role of fusion remains controversial. Fusion can be considered if an extensive decompression is necessary (as with the removal of most of a vertebral body) and iatrogenic destabilization is anticipated. Iatrogenic destabilization is believed to occur if an entire facet joint has been removed. Some surgeons believe that a full laminectomy at the apex of the kyphosis, even with preservation of the facet joints, can create a disposition to kyphotic deformity. An underlying deformity such as kyphosis or scoliosis also may be an indication for fusion after thoracic diskectomy.

Surgical Outcomes

A 10-year prospective study followed 167 patients with single-level thoracic disk herniation causing myelopathy or radiculopathy, all of whom were treated with a thoracoscopic anterior approach.[38] Seventy-nine percent of the patients had a excellent or good outcome on the VAS pain scale, and 80% reported an excellent or

good outcome for motor function. The overall complication rate was 15.6%. Other case studies found similar postoperative neurologic recovery and pain improvement after other surgical techniques were used.[38-46] One study compared minimally invasive posterolateral extracavitary diskectomy with a standard open anterolateral diskectomy. The two procedures led to similar clinical and radiographic outcomes at 1-year follow-up, but patients who underwent the minimally invasive procedure had better VAS scores and less narcotic usage immediately after surgery.[40] It is critically important for the surgeon to choose the approach based on an understanding of disk location, herniation size, the presence of calcification, and the surgeon's personal experience.

Summary

Most thoracic and lumbar disk herniations can be treated nonsurgically. Surgery is reserved for patients who have a progressive neurologic deficit, cauda equina syndrome (with lumbar herniation), or myelopathy (with thoracic herniation), as well as patients who have undergone unsuccessful nonsurgical treatment. High-level comparison studies found that surgery was more effective than nonsurgical treatment of lumbar disk herniation in the early to intermediate period. Open or minimally invasive laminotomy and diskectomy is ideal for almost all lumbar herniations. The choice of procedure is more difficult for thoracic disk herniations. There are more options, and they are associated with varying morbidities and risks. In appropriately selected patients, surgery for lumbar or thoracic disk herniation can lead to significant functional improvement.

Key Study Points

- Patients with larger, extruded disk herniations tend to have relatively good results after surgery, particularly if the remaining annular defect was small, which is associated with a low rate of recurrence.

- Recent analysis of prospective data suggest that patients with symptoms from a lumbar disc herniation of more than 6 months' duration before treatment have worse outcomes than patients treated before 6 months.

- For symptomatic thoracic disc herniations, the anterolateral approach is safer and more suited for large, central, and calcified disks than posterior or posterolateral approaches.

Annotated References

1. Deyo RA, Loeser JD, Bigos SJ: Herniated lumbar intervertebral disk. *Ann Intern Med* 1990;112(8):598-603.

2. Boden SD, Davis DO, Dina TS, Patronas NJ, Wiesel SW: Abnormal magnetic-resonance scans of the lumbar spine in asymptomatic subjects: A prospective investigation. *J Bone Joint Surg Am* 1990;72(3):403-408.

3. Pearson AM, Blood EA, Frymoyer JW, et al: SPORT lumbar intervertebral disk herniation and back pain: Does treatment, location, or morphology matter? *Spine (Phila Pa 1976)* 2008;33(4):428-435.

4. Spengler DM, Ouellette EA, Battié M, Zeh J: Elective discectomy for herniation of a lumbar disc: Additional experience with an objective method. *J Bone Joint Surg Am* 1990;72(2):230-237.

5. Knop-Jergas BM, Zucherman JF, Hsu KY, DeLong B: Anatomic position of a herniated nucleus pulposus predicts the outcome of lumbar discectomy. *J Spinal Disord* 1996;9(3):246-250.

6. Carlisle E, Luna M, Tsou PM, Wang JC: Percent spinal canal compromise on MRI utilized for predicting the need for surgical treatment in single-level lumbar intervertebral disc herniation. *Spine J* 2005;5(6):608-614.

7. Carragee EJ, Han MY, Suen PW, Kim D: Clinical outcomes after lumbar discectomy for sciatica: The effects of fragment type and anular competence. *J Bone Joint Surg Am* 2003;85(1):102-108.

8. van der Windt DA, Simons E, Riphagen II, et al: Physical examination for lumbar radiculopathy due to disc herniation in patients with low-back pain. *Cochrane Database Syst Rev* 2010;2:CD007431.

   A large meta-analysis studied the reliability of physical examination tests for lumbar disk herniation by determining their diagnostic performance.

9. Capra F, Vanti C, Donati R, Tombetti S, O'Reilly C, Pillastrini P: Validity of the straight-leg raise test for patients with sciatic pain with or without lumbar pain using magnetic resonance imaging results as a reference standard. *J Manipulative Physiol Ther* 2011;34(4):231-238.

   A retrospective study determined the validity of the straight leg raise for the diagnosis of lumbar disk herniation by comparing the test results to MRI findings.

10. Majlesi J, Togay H, Unalan H, Toprak S: The sensitivity and specificity of the slump and the straight leg raising tests in patients with lumbar disc herniation. *J Clin Rheumatol* 2008;14(2):87-91.

11. Weber H: Lumbar disc herniation: A controlled, prospective study with ten years of observation. *Spine (Phila Pa 1976)* 1983;8(2):131-140.

12. Saal JA, Saal JS: Nonoperative treatment of herniated lumbar intervertebral disc with radiculopathy: An outcome study. *Spine (Phila Pa 1976)* 1989;14(4):431-437.

13. Atlas SJ, Keller RB, Wu YA, Deyo RA, Singer DE: Long-term outcomes of surgical and nonsurgical management of sciatica secondary to a lumbar disc herniation: 10 year results from the Maine Lumbar Spine Study. *Spine (Phila Pa 1976)* 2005;30(8):927-935.

14. Weinstein JN, Lurie JD, Tosteson TD, et al: Surgical versus nonoperative treatment for lumbar disc herniation: Four-year results for the Spine Patient Outcomes Research Trial (SPORT). *Spine (Phila Pa 1976)* 2008;33(25):2789-2800.

15. Peul WC, van den Hout WB, Brand R, Thomeer RT, Koes BW; Leiden-The Hague Spine Intervention Prognostic Study Group: Prolonged conservative care versus early surgery in patients with sciatica caused by lumbar disc herniation: Two year results of a randomised controlled trial. *BMJ* 2008;336(7657):1355-1358.

16. Saal JA, Saal JS, Herzog RJ: The natural history of lumbar intervertebral disc extrusions treated nonoperatively. *Spine (Phila Pa 1976)* 1990;15(7):683-686.

17. Suri P, Hunter DJ, Jouve C, et al: Nonsurgical treatment of lumbar disk herniation: Are outcomes different in older adults? *J Am Geriatr Soc* 2011;59(3):423-429.

    A prospective longitudinal comparative cohort study determined whether adults age 60 years or older experienced less improvement in disability and pain with nonsurgical treatment of lumbar disk herniation than younger adults.

18. Radcliff K, Hilibrand A, Lurie JD, et al: The impact of epidural steroid injections on the outcomes of patients treated for lumbar disc herniation: A subgroup analysis of the SPORT trial. *J Bone Joint Surg Am* 2012;94(15):1353-1358.

    SPORT data were analyzed to determine the efficacy of epidural steroid injections for improving patient outcomes and whether this nonsurgical treatment lowered the rate of crossover to surgical treatment.

19. Buttermann GR: Treatment of lumbar disc herniation: Epidural steroid injection compared with discectomy: A prospective, randomized study. *J Bone Joint Surg Am* 2004;86(4):670-679.

20. Weinstein JN, Tosteson TD, Lurie JD, et al: Surgical vs nonoperative treatment for lumbar disk herniation: The Spine Patient Outcomes Research Trial (SPORT). A randomized trial. *JAMA* 2006;296(20):2441-2450.

21. Rihn JA, Hilibrand AS, Radcliff K, et al: Duration of symptoms resulting from lumbar disc herniation: Effect on treatment outcomes. Analysis of the Spine Patient Outcomes Research Trial (SPORT). *J Bone Joint Surg Am* 2011;93(20):1906-1914.

    An as-treated analysis of SPORT patients was performed to determine whether duration of symptoms

5: Spine

affects the outcome of surgical or nonsurgical treatment of lumbar disk herniation.

22. Lurie JD, Faucett SC, Hanscom B, et al: Lumbar discectomy outcomes vary by herniation level in the Spine Patient Outcomes Research Trial. *J Bone Joint Surg Am* 2008;90(9):1811-1819.

23. Henriksen L, Schmidt K, Eskesen V, Jantzen E: A controlled study of microsurgical versus standard lumbar discectomy. *Br J Neurosurg* 1996;10(3):289-293.

24. Garg B, Nagraja UB, Jayaswal A: Microendoscopic versus open discectomy for lumbar disc herniation: A prospective randomised study. *J Orthop Surg (Hong Kong)* 2011;19(1):30-34.

    A prospective randomized controlled study compared the outcomes of microendoscopic and open diskectomy for lumbar disk herniations.

25. Arts M, Brand R, van der Kallen B, Lycklama à Nijeholt G, Peul W: Does minimally invasive lumbar disc surgery result in less muscle injury than conventional surgery? A randomized controlled trial. *Eur Spine J* 2011;20(1):51-57.

    Analysis of data from a Netherlands-conducted randomized study determined the effectiveness of minimally invasive lumbar disk surgery for reducing muscle injury. Creatine phosphokinase in serum and the cross-sectional area of the multifidus muscle on MRI were used as indicators of muscle injury.

26. Franke J, Greiner-Perth R, Boehm H, et al: Comparison of a minimally invasive procedure versus standard microscopic discotomy: A prospective randomised controlled clinical trial. *Eur Spine J* 2009;18(7):992-1000.

27. Carragee EJ, Spinnickie AO, Alamin TF, Paragioudakis S: A prospective controlled study of limited versus subtotal posterior discectomy: Short-term outcomes in patients with herniated lumbar intervertebral discs and large posterior anular defect. *Spine (Phila Pa 1976)* 2006;31(6):653-657.

28. Debi R, Halperin N, Mirovsky Y: Local application of steroids following lumbar discectomy. *J Spinal Disord Tech* 2002;15(4):273-276.

29. Lotfinia I, Khallaghi E, Meshkini A, Shakeri M, Shima M, Safaeian A: Interaoperative use of epidural methylprednisolone or bupivacaine for postsurgical lumbar discectomy pain relief: A randomized, placebo-controlled trial. *Ann Saudi Med* 2007;27(4):279-283.

30. Lavyne MH, Bilsky MH: Epidural steroids, postoperative morbidity, and recovery in patients undergoing microsurgical lumbar discectomy. *J Neurosurg* 1992;77(1):90-95.

31. Wood KB, Garvey TA, Gundry C, Heithoff KB: Magnetic resonance imaging of the thoracic spine: Evaluation of asymptomatic individuals. *J Bone Joint Surg Am* 1995;77(11):1631-1638.

32. Wood KB, Schellhas KP, Garvey TA, Aeppli D: Thoracic discography in healthy individuals: A controlled prospective study of magnetic resonance imaging and discography in asymptomatic and symptomatic individuals. *Spine (Phila Pa 1976)* 1999;24(15):1548-1555.

33. Brown CW, Deffer PA Jr, Akmakjian J, Donaldson DH, Brugman JL: The natural history of thoracic disc herniation. *Spine (Phila Pa 1976)* 1992;17(6, suppl): S97-S102.

34. Love JG, Kiefer EJ: Root pain and paraplegia due to protrusions of thoracic intervertebral disks. *J Neurosurg* 1950;7(1):62-69, illust.

35. Binning MJ, Schmidt MH: Percutaneous placement of radiopaque markers at the pedicle of interest for preoperative localization of thoracic spine level. *Spine (Phila Pa 1976)* 2010;35(19):1821-1825.

    A small retrospective review found that the preoperative placement of radiopaque markers at the thoracic spine level of interest is safe and effective for avoiding wrong-level surgery if standard localization techniques are difficult to implement.

36. Upadhyaya CD, Wu JC, Chin CT, Balamurali G, Mummaneni PV: Avoidance of wrong-level thoracic spine surgery: Intraoperative localization with preoperative percutaneous fiducial screw placement. *J Neurosurg Spine* 2012;16(3):280-284.

    The placement of preoperatively placed percutaneous fiducial screws for intraoperative localization at the level of intended surgery was determined to be safe and accurate.

37. Bohlman HH, Zdeblick TA: Anterior excision of herniated thoracic discs. *J Bone Joint Surg Am* 1988;70(7):1038-1047.

38. Quint U, Bordon G, Preissl I, Sanner C, Rosenthal D: Thoracoscopic treatment for single level symptomatic thoracic disc herniation: A prospective followed cohort study in a group of 167 consecutive cases. *Eur Spine J* 2012;21(4):637-645.

    A prospective study found that thoracoscopic microdiskectomy for single-level symptomatic disk herniation was highly effective, reliable, and safe, with a low complication rate.

39. Hott JS, Feiz-Erfan I, Kenny K, Dickman CA: Surgical management of giant herniated thoracic discs: Analysis of 20 cases. *J Neurosurg Spine* 2005;3(3):191-197.

40. Khoo LT, Smith ZA, Asgarzadie F, et al: Minimally invasive extracavitary approach for thoracic discectomy and interbody fusion: 1-year clinical and radiographic outcomes in 13 patients compared with a cohort of traditional anterior transthoracic approaches. *J Neurosurg Spine* 2011;14(2):250-260.

    A minimally invasive lateral extracavitary tubular approach was described for diskectomy and fusion to treat thoracic disk herniation.

5: Spine

41. Levi N, Gjerris F, Dons K: Thoracic disc herniation: Unilateral transpedicular approach in 35 consecutive patients. *J Neurosurg Sci* 1999;43(1):37-43.

42. Malawski S, Lukawski S: Results of surgical treatment for the intervertebral disc protrusion within thoracic spine. *Chir Narzadow Ruchu Ortop Pol* 1998;63(6): 585-590.

43. Mulier S, Debois V: Thoracic disc herniations: Transthoracic, lateral, or posterolateral approach? A review. *Surg Neurol* 1998;49(6):599-608.

44. Ohnishi K, Miyamoto K, Kanamori Y, Kodama H, Hosoe H, Shimizu K: Anterior decompression and fusion for multiple thoracic disc herniation. *J Bone Joint Surg Br* 2005;87(3):356-360.

45. Sheikh H, Samartzis D, Perez-Cruet MJ: Techniques for the operative management of thoracic disc herniation: Minimally invasive thoracic microdiscectomy. *Orthop Clin North Am* 2007;38(3):351-361, abstract vi.

46. Simpson JM, Silveri CP, Simeone FA, Balderston RA, An HS: Thoracic disc herniation: Re-evaluation of the posterior approach using a modified costotransversectomy. *Spine (Phila Pa 1976)* 1993;18(13):1872-1877.

5: Spine

Chapter 52

Disk Degeneration and Pain in the Lumbar Spine

Eugene J. Carragee, MD   Michael P. Stauff, MD

Introduction

Lumbar disk degeneration and the associated syndromes are a significant socioeconomic burden in modern society. The direct and indirect costs are estimated to be $100 to $200 billion per year in the United States.[1] A large portion of the cost is attributable to lost wages and productivity because of pain, disability, and psychological illness resulting from lumbar disk degeneration. Research has established that lumbar disk degeneration is common, and most individuals with lumbar disk degeneration are asymptomatic. The degenerative changes commonly seen on MRI are unlikely to be the sole primary pathology causing low back pain.[2,3]

In the absence of serious pathology, such as a tumor, infection, spinal instability, or deformity, it is difficult to attribute all or even most of a patient's isolated axial low back pain to common degenerative changes in a lumbar disk. The diagnostic difficulty is multifactorial but most likely is related to the large number of conditions directly or indirectly leading to perceived back pain. Consequently, surgical treatment of axial low back pain and lumbar disk degeneration has had unpredictable and often disappointing levels of success.

In its more advanced stages, lumbar disk degeneration can lead to disk height narrowing, disk protrusion, disk herniation, secondary instability, and spinal stenosis. In these situations, the patient may report radiculopathy or neurogenic claudication, which are associated with nerve root compression and neurologic

Dr. Carragee or an immediate family member has stock or stock options held in Simpirica and Intrinsic Orthopaedics; has received research or institutional support from Kaiser (National Institutes of Health grant), the AO Foundation, and the Orthopaedic Research and Education Foundation; and serves as a board member, owner, officer, or committee member of the North American Spine Society. Neither Dr. Stauff nor any immediate family member has received anything of value from or has stock or stock options held in a commercial company or institution related directly or indirectly to the subject of this chapter.

impairment. These clinical syndromes are more readily identifiable and treatable. This chapter reviews the risk factors for lumbar disk degeneration, the diagnostic and treatment modalities for suspected primary discogenic low back pain, the negative effect of psychosocial comorbidities on the results of treatment, and new directions in diagnosis and treatment.

Risk Factors

The likelihood of having lumbar disk degeneration increases with age. Historically, clinicians attributed lumbar disk degeneration to normal aging, and back pain syndromes to humoral imbalances or rheumatic disease. During the mid to late 20th century, common back pain syndromes were associated with mechanical events acting on a degenerative spine. More recent work has found strong evidence for a genetic predisposition to lumbar disk degeneration. The Finnish Twin Spine Study investigated monozygotic twins who were discordant for multiple environmental exposures, including physical loading, driving or other whole-body vibration, and smoking.[4] The results confirmed a strong genetic basis for the development of lumbar disk degeneration. This work led to other clinical and population-based studies, which also found a genetic link. A genetic predisposition to lumbar disk degeneration was supported by the results of a recent study of the Utah Population Database.[5] The Genealogical Index of Familiality was used to identify excess relatedness in 1,264 patients ($P < 0.001$) in whom lumbar disk herniation or lumbar disk degeneration was diagnosed (using the *International Classification of Diseases*, Ninth Revision). Data analysis revealed a significant relative risk among first- and third-degree relatives for the development of symptomatic lumbar disk disease.[5] Furthermore, several gene loci have been implicated in the development of disk degeneration (Table 1).

In the mid-20th century, many experts believed that repetitive minor trauma from physical loading or other occupational exposure was a significant risk factor for symptomatic lumbar disk degeneration. These theories implicated abnormal mechanical stress as a cause of radial fissures, disk bulges, disk herniations, and vertebral end plate injury. Experimental induction of disk

Table 1

Factors Associated With Lumbar Disk Degeneration

A disintegrin and metalloproteinase domain (ADAM) metallopeptidase with thrombospondin, type 1 motif, 7 (ADAMTS7)

ADAM metallopeptidase with thrombospondin, type 1 motif, 12 (ADAMTS12)

Aggrecan (AGC)

B cell CLL/lymphoma 2 (BCL-2)

Cartilage intermediate layer protein (CILP)

Collagen, type 1, alpha 1 (COL1A1)

Collagen, type 2, alpha 1(9) (COL2A1[9])

Collagen, type 9, alpha 1 (COL9A1)

Collagen, type 11, alpha 2 (COL11A2)

Cyclo-oxygenase 2 (COX2)

Estrogen receptor (ER)

Hyaluronan and proteoglycan link protein 1 (HAPLN1)

Interleukin 1α (IL-1α)

Interleukin 1β (IL-1β)

Interleukin 6 (IL-6)

Interleukin 10 (IL-10)

Matrilin 3 (MATN3)

Matrix metalloproteinase 3 (MMP-3)

Matrix metalloproteinase 9 (MMP-9)

Thrombospondin, type 1, domain containing 2 (THSD2)

Tumor necrosis factor–receptor superfamily member 6 (FAS)

Tumor necrosis factor–receptor superfamily member 6 ligand (FAS-L)

Vitamin D receptor (VDR)

degeneration by scalpel-induced annular injury appeared to support the theory that trauma was a significant risk factor for lumbar disk degeneration.[6] During the past 20 years, in the wake of an established link between genetics and lumbar disk degeneration, epidemiologic studies have suggested that minor trauma is only a modest risk factor for the development or the acceleration of lumbar disk degeneration or serious low back pain. Monozygotic twins who were discordant for exposure to minor trauma were found to have no significant difference in lumbar disk degeneration.[7] Moreover, changes seen on MRI were found not to be associated with a first episode of serious low back pain.[8] Monozygotic twins who were discordant for exposure to minor trauma were found to have no significant difference in lumbar disk degeneration.[7]

Other possible risk factors for lumbar disk degeneration include occupational vibration from operating a vehicle, smoking, and anthropometric factors. The Twin Spine Study, based on the Finnish Twin Cohort, provided the best data on the effects of occupational vibration from driving.[4] Forty-five pairs of matched monozygotic twins discordant for occupational driving exposure had no significant differences in lumbar disk degeneration. A similar design was used to show that smoking was a small but significant risk factor for lumbar disk degeneration.[4] A more recent study of female twin pairs in the United Kingdom found no association between smoking and lumbar disk degeneration, but these twin pairs did not have a high rate of discordance for smoking exposure.[9] Anthropometric factors may be more important than occupational vibration and smoking. In multiple well-designed studies, relatively high weight, height, and body mass index were found to have a significant effect on the development of lumbar disk degeneration.[4,9,10]

The current literature underscores that lumbar disk degeneration is an oligogenic, multifactorial condition. A genetic predisposition can create a significant risk of developing lumbar disk degeneration and its associated disorders. A host of environmental exposures may accelerate the degenerative process, but usually they are not a major factor in degenerative conditions of the spine.

Diagnosis

In some patients, the association of degenerative changes and a pain syndrome is clear, as in unstable degenerative spondylolisthesis or collapsing sagittal imbalance with degenerative scoliosis. However, it is very difficult for a spine provider to care for a patient with chronic low back pain and common lumbar degenerative changes on MRI but no instability, deformity, or root irritation. Although the lumbar disk may be the source of pain, many other conditions can cause back pain unrelated to the disk. The current diagnostic armamentarium lacks the accuracy to determine whether a patient's disabling low back pain emanates from an isolated disk or another source.

The initial evaluation of a patient with chronic low back pain begins with a history and a physical examination to rule out serious disease, such as tumor, infection, or referred visceral pain. Dynamic radiographs and MRI are vital for ruling out serious disease and can be expected to show common degenerative findings.

Magnetic Resonance Imaging

The signs of lumbar disk degeneration on MRI may include decreased disk hydration, disk height collapse, Schmorl nodes, disk prolapse, disk bulges, annular tears, high intensity zones, vertebral syndesmophytes, and Modic changes (Figure 1). Multiple studies have found that these signs are present in most individuals, regardless of whether they are symptomatic, and in almost all who are older than 60 years.[2] Follow-up studies have found no association between MRI findings for a patient without symptoms and the patient's future development of low back pain or neurologic symptoms.[3]

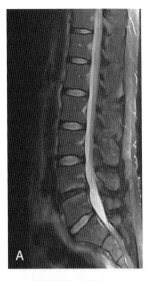
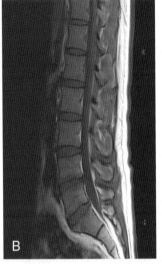
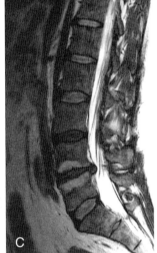
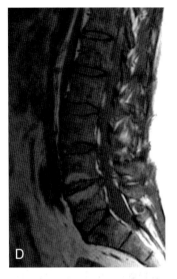

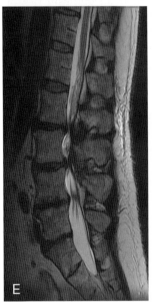
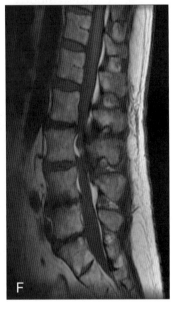
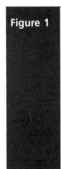

Figure 1 Sagittal MRI of the lumbar spine showing Modic changes. Type I Modic end plate changes can be seen at L4-L5 with hyperintense end plate signal on a T2-weighted sequence (**A**) and hypointense end plate signal on a T1-weighted sequence (**B**). Type 2 Modic end plate changes can be seen at L4-L5 with end plate enhancement on both T2- (**C**) and T1-weighted (**D**) sequences. Type 3 Modic end plate changes at L4-L5 appear with hypointense signal on both T2- (**E**) and T1-weighted (**F**) sequences.

Multiple recent studies have attempted to correlate specific MRI findings with chronic low back pain. One recent study found a high prevalence of Modic changes in patients with chronic low back pain.[11] Other studies found that end plate lesions, such as Schmorl nodes, erosions, fractures, and calcifications, may indicate more severe disk degeneration.[12] Most spine specialists recommend against the routine use of MRI for patients with chronic low back pain except to rule out serious underlying disease.

Diskography

Diskography is a testing modality that combines imaging findings from radiographs or CT with a subjective pain response from the patient. The test involves introducing a contrast medium into a clinically suspicious disk while recording the pressure and the patient's pain response. The test is positive if the pain response is concordant, meaning that it reproduces the patient's typical low back pain. Control levels above and/or below the suspected level also may be tested. Although there is a less than 1% possibility that the test will lead to diskitis, there is a risk that the test will cause or accelerate disk degeneration.[13]

The use of diskography has been controversial because some studies found a high rate of false-positive results and poor specificity.[14-16] The rate of false-positive results was 50% in patients who underwent posterior iliac crest bone harvest, 40% in patients with chronic cervical spine pain, and 83% in patients with a somatization disorder.[14,15]

In another study, a gold standard evaluation of diskography was performed using outcomes after fusion and demonstrated a positive predictive value of 43% for a positive single-level, low-pressure test in patients with no psychosocial comorbidity.[16] Patients with isthmic spondylolisthesis formed the control group for surgical morbidity. Studies have consistently found that

5: Spine

psychosocial factors adversely affect the validity of diskography results.[17,18]

Investigators have attempted to increase the accuracy of diskography by injecting local anesthetic into the disk to monitor recovery from concordant pain. A comparison of the results of standard provocative diskography with those of functional anesthetic diskography found that the test results differed in 46% of patients.[19] The anesthetic test frequently was negative when standard provocative diskography was positive in patients with abnormal psychometric testing or a compensation claim.

Two studies found better outcomes after fusion in patients who were selected by using a disk injection with a local anesthetic rather than provocative diskography.[20,21] A 3-year follow-up study of patients with normal psychometric testing and no compensation claim who had undergone anterior lumbar interbody fusion for discogenic low back pain found that those who had a positive "diskoblock" (relief of back pain with injection of local anesthetic into a suspected disk) had significantly better results than those who had a positive result after provocative diskography without a control level.[20] A randomized prospective study of 41 patients who had a positive result after standard diskography as well as relief of concordant pain after diskoblock found significantly better 2-year results in those who underwent surgical treatment of discogenic low back pain than in those who were treated nonsurgically.[21] These data suggest that an anesthetic disk injection is more useful than provocative diskography for selecting patients with single-level disk degeneration who will benefit from fusion (in the presence of normal psychometric testing and no compensation claim). The use of an anesthetic disk injection for diagnosing discogenic low back pain needs to be investigated further before it can be recommended as a routine diagnostic test.

The diagnosis of discogenic low back pain using diskography is difficult. Diskography may be particularly misleading in patients with other chronic pain issues, psychological distress, or a compensation claim. Despite extensive research, consistent results will continue to be elusive after surgical or nonsurgical treatment until there is a reliable method for distinguishing a discogenic pain syndrome from a generalized pain syndrome complicated by psychosocial issues.

Treatment

Nonsurgical Treatment

The nonsurgical treatment of low back pain in patients with disk degeneration is similar to the treatment of nonspecific low back pain and can include reassurance and support, nonnarcotic medications, narcotic pain medications (rarely), physical therapy, chiropractic manipulation, and massage therapy. Often the patient or a primary care provider initiates the use of one or more of these treatments simultaneously.

Medications can be useful for relieving low back pain. NSAIDs typically are used first. A Cochrane review of 65 studies found that NSAIDs were superior to placebo for treating low back pain, but the effect size was small and there was a statistically significant risk of adverse effects.[22] A similar review found some benefit to the use of muscle relaxants but noted that they should be used with caution because of central nervous system effects.[23] The use of herbal medicines may be beneficial, but high-quality evidence is lacking. Narcotic pain medication is an option but should be avoided for first-line or chronic treatment of nonspecific low back pain because of concern for dependence, abuse, and altered sensorium.

For decades, physical therapy has been a mainstay treatment for low back pain. The therapy can be supervised, self-directed, high intensity, low intensity, extension based (McKenzie method), or flexion based (Williams method). Most variations have some benefit, but no single technique or protocol has demonstrated superiority. Some clinicians stipulate that patients with low back pain should be stratified and placed into a program that best treats their symptoms.[24] Proponents note that the properly applied McKenzie method includes an assessment and classification, the results of which allow the patient to be treated with a matched exercise-based intervention.[25] The McKenzie method was found to provide greater benefit than nonspecific low back pain protocols and equal or marginally better outcomes than other therapies.[25]

Proponents of chiropractic care for low back pain state that spine manipulation and mobilization can be as effective as physical therapy or NSAIDs.[26] However, most studies have not found chiropractic care to be more beneficial than other nonsurgical treatments, especially in patients with chronic pain. Most studies of chiropractic manipulation, like those of other nonsurgical treatment modalities, have lacked adequate patient subgrouping.

Choosing the best nonsurgical treatment for a patient is difficult because the literature directly comparing most treatments is mixed. A recent randomized controlled study compared the efficacy of home-based exercise, supervised exercise, and chiropractic care.[27] Benefit was found with all treatment modalities, but some superiority was found with supervised exercises. A recent systematic review found that methodologic limitations precluded any firm conclusions as to the superiority of particular methods.[28]

A large body of evidence has established the importance of behavioral health in patients with low back pain. Many spine care providers have suggested that by treating a patient's psychosocial well-being using antidepressant medications and cognitive therapy, they may be able to improve the results of nonsurgical treatment of low back pain. A randomized controlled study that compared minimal care with a 6-week course of exercise and cognitive behavioral therapy found no significant differences in outcomes between groups.[29] A back school is one means of structuring a multifaceted approach to low back pain, including cognitive behavioral therapy and exercise. A back school requires significant resources, however, and strong evidence is lacking regarding the efficacy of this type of treatment.

When initiating nonsurgical treatment for a patient with nonspecific low back pain, the provider should attempt to individualize the treatment to the patient's specific symptoms and expectations, while being cognizant of costs. Many of the available treatment modalities can lead to symptom improvement, and the patient can choose the modalities that best suit his or her needs. For most patients, a trial use of an NSAID combined with some form of therapeutic exercise will provide some relief. In a patient who has significant psychosocial comorbidities, the addition of cognitive behavioral therapy may be beneficial.

Percutaneous Treatments

After unsuccessful nonsurgical treatment, percutaneous treatments have been considered for patients who have back pain and only common degenerative changes in the spine. Unfortunately, no percutaneous treatment for discogenic low back pain is clearly more effective than general supportive care. Analysis of the results of the percutaneous treatment options for presumed discogenic low back pain has been marred by the lack of ability to diagnose discogenic low back pain with confidence.

Intradiskal electrothermal therapy for discogenic pain was investigated in two well-designed studies and was found to have minimal or no significant benefit.[30,31] Some investigators have promoted the use of epidural steroid injections for the treatment of discogenic low back pain, but there is a dearth of evidence for efficacy in patients without radicular pain. Similarly, the use of radiofrequency neurotomies of the ramus communicans or intradiskal corticosteroid injections to treat low back pain in patients with degenerative MRI findings is not supported by strong evidence.

Fusion

Fusion remains a controversial treatment for patients with discogenic low back pain. It seems reasonable to assume that if a disk is identified as the pain generator, removal of the disk accompanied by fusion should result in significant symptom reduction. The current body of literature contains only limited support for this treatment, at least partly because of the difficulty of consistently ascribing low back symptoms to a degenerative lumbar disk.

Five randomized, placebo-controlled studies have compared lumbar fusion with nonsurgical treatment of discogenic low back pain.[21,29-32] A 2001 study from the Swedish Lumbar Spine Study Group found significantly better results in patients with discogenic low back pain who received fusion rather than typical nonsurgical treatment.[32] Three later randomized controlled studies found no significant difference after surgical or nonsurgical treatment of patients with discogenic low back pain.[33-35] The most important differences between two of the studies and the original 2001 study were a more

rigorously scripted nonsurgical treatment protocol and a shorter follow-up period (1 year versus 2 years).[33,34] One of these studies had a significantly smaller sample size (64 patients versus 294 patients) and probably was underpowered for finding a small effect size.[33] A third study, conducted in Great Britain at the behest of the National Health Service, had a rigorous nonsurgical treatment control arm, a large sample size (349 patients), and a 2-year follow-up period.[35] A small but statistically significant improvement in Oswestry Disability Index scores was found in patients who underwent fusion rather than nonsurgical treatment. The improvement was not clinically significant, however, and no difference was found in any other outcome measure. Most recently, discogenic low back pain was diagnosed using a refined diskography technique with bupivacaine and the careful selection of patients (to exclude those with psychological distress or a compensation claim).[21] This small, randomized, placebo-controlled study found statistically and clinically significant improvement in patients who were surgically treated compared with those who were minimally treated.

These five randomized controlled studies should be evaluated in light of several considerations: the techniques used for fusion were not uniform, the methods used for diagnosing discogenic low back pain were heterogeneous, the burden of psychosocial comorbidity was highly variable, and the nonsurgical treatment protocols were poorly defined or heterogeneous. The evidence supporting fusion for treating discogenic low back pain leaves spine care providers with more questions than answers. Overall, these studies show that fusion has better results than no treatment, but the results may be similar to those of an intense, structured nonsurgical protocol. Methodologic concerns have caused many to question the conclusions of these studies. One central issue is the lack of diagnostic accuracy when a disk is labeled as the pain generator in chronic low back pain. A large study similar to the Swedish Lumbar Spine study would be ideal if it used a refined means of diagnosing discogenic low back pain.[32] There may be a decreasing likelihood that a study of this scale will be conducted, given the current level of interest and resources dedicated to elucidating the use of motion-sparing technology for treating discogenic low back pain. Until a large, rigorously designed study is conducted, the routine use of fusion cannot be recommended for treating discogenic low back pain, especially in patients who have psychological distress, compensation litigation, additional distant or widespread pain, or substance dependence.

Disk Arthroplasty

Lumbar total disk arthroplasty has been used in Europe for treating discogenic low back pain since the 1980s but has gained traction in the United States only in the past 10 years. Two total disk prostheses have been approved by the FDA: the CHARITÉ Artificial Disk and the ProDisc-L Total Disk Replacement (both manufactured by DePuy Synthes). Lumbar disk arthroplasty of-

5: Spine

fers the advantage of sparing motion at the involved level, theoretically mitigating issues related to adjacent segment deterioration after arthrodesis.[36,37] The approved indication for lumbar total disk replacement is one- or two-level discogenic low back pain without evidence of instability.

The most robust research on lumbar disk arthroplasty comes from the FDA Investigational Device Exemption (IDE) noninferiority studies for the CHARITÉ and ProDisc-L prostheses, which were conducted to achieve FDA approval in the United States.[38-41] In the original FDA IDE study of the CHARITÉ device, noninferiority was established in a comparison at 2-year follow-up of one-level total disk arthroplasty with stand-alone anterior lumbar interbody fusion using threaded cages and iliac crest autograft.[38] Noninferiority also was reported at 5-year follow-up.[39] A similar FDA IDE study of the ProDisc-L showed noninferiority in a comparison of one-level 360° fusion to one-level total disk arthroplasty.[40] A second FDA IDE study of the ProDisc-L found noninferiority by comparing the results of two-level circumferential fusion to two-level arthroplasty.[41] These studies in essence proved that lumbar disk arthroplasty is equivalent to fusion, which is the current gold standard surgical treatment for discogenic low back pain.

The parameters of the control group were a fundamental difficulty in the FDA IDE studies of the CHARITÉ and ProDisc-L prostheses. Research has not unequivocally shown that fusion is preferable to nonsurgical treatment of discogenic low back pain. Furthermore, stand-alone anterior lumbar interbody fusion, the technique used for patients in the control group arm of the CHARITÉ study, is known to lead to poor fusion rates.[42] The circumferential technique used in the ProDisc-L studies has a higher fusion rate, but a comparison of patients who had two separate surgical exposures to patients who had one surgical exposure may create bias against those with two exposures, especially in the early follow-up period. The harvest of iliac crest autograft for all fusions may have further confounded the results by adding a significant source of early postoperative pain for patients in the control groups.[38-41]

At best, there is some evidence that disk arthroplasty is equivalent to fusion for treating discogenic low back pain, although long-term data are minimal. One recent study compared the results of single-level arthroplasty with structured exercise and behavioral therapy for treating chronic low back pain.[43] The patients who underwent arthroplasty had significantly better Oswestry Disability Index scores at 2-year follow-up than those who received therapy, but the differences did not meet the standard of minimally important clinical difference.[42] Although no prospective long-term results are available for disk arthroplasty, a retrospective review found spontaneous ankylosis in 60% of patients after having a CHARITÉ disk arthroplasty and an 11% reoperation rate.[43] These results are particularly troubling because of the theoretic advantage of maintained motion with disk arthroplasty. Currently, the treatment of discogenic low back pain involves a spectrum of care that generally begins with supportive care and NSAIDs. Eventually, patients with chronic symptoms may consider surgical treatment in the form of fusion or disk arthroplasty. Unfortunately, most current studies have found minimal benefit to surgical treatments of discogenic low back pain. Improving the ability to accurately diagnose discogenic low back pain may ultimately improve treatment results.

The Effect of Psychosocial Comorbidity

Clinicians have long observed the influence of psychosocial factors on patients with chronic low back pain. Spine surgeons were found to detect psychological distress during a clinical encounter with a sensitivity of only 19.6%, whereas nonsurgical spine specialists had a sensitivity of 41.7%.[44] Based on these findings, the routine use of a psychological questionnaire was recommended as part of the diagnostic workup for a patient with chronic low back pain. In 100 patients at risk for serious low back pain, psychosocial factors were found to be more predictive of serious low back pain illness than morphologic characteristics on MRI or diskography.[17] A cross-sectional examination of 149 US military veterans evaluated in a Veterans Health Administration spine clinic found severe psychological stress in 43%, and the rate was 59.1% for veterans who had been exposed to combat.[45]

The importance of identifying psychosocial factors during the diagnostic workup of a patient with a lumbar spine condition has been underscored in studies that found a link between the results of treatment and the presence of psychosocial comorbidities. In a study of patients selected for lumbar fusion on the basis of a highly specific provocative diskography procedure (one positive level, a negative control level, and a low pressure injection), those with a psychological concern (defined as a score lower than 40 on the mental component scale of the Medical Outcomes Study 36-Item Short Form [SF-36]) were unimproved based on the primary outcome (the mean score on the SF-36 physical component scale).[18] Similarly, outcomes after lumbar fusion were poorer in patients with a score lower than 40 on the mental component scale of the SF-36.[46] Most patients did not report substantial clinical improvement on the Oswestry Disability Index.

Preoperative depression was found to be an independent predictor of functional outcome after revision lumbar surgery for adjacent segment deterioration, pseudarthrosis, or recurrent spinal stenosis.[47] A prospective study of patients who underwent surgery for spinal stenosis found that preoperative and 3-month postoperative depression scores predicted self-reported outcomes at 1-year follow-up.[48]

Although it is clear that psychosocial factors play a role in chronic low back pain, providers have not universally considered psychosocial comorbidity in determining the appropriate treatment for a patient. A recent systematic review suggested that patients with certain personality disorders, neuroticism, or a relatively high score on a depression scale should preferentially be treated nonsurgically. This recommendation was rated as weak, however, because only one relevant study met the inclusion criteria.[49] Future outcomes research into surgical and nonsurgical treatment of discogenic low back pain should include a thorough comparison of patients with or without a significant psychosocial comorbidity.

Future Directions

An increased understanding of the biochemical milieu and biologic mechanisms of intervertebral disk degeneration has resulted in a push to use relatively new methods of diagnosing and treating discogenic low back pain. The discovery of biochemical mediators having a high concentration in disks has spawned efforts to use a biochemical marker to accurately identify a painful lumbar disk.[50] The numerous candidates include matrix metalloproteinases, nitric oxide, prostaglandin E_2, interleukin-6, interferon-γ, interleukin-1, tumor necrosis factor–α, and others. A recent investigation systematically analyzed diskographic lavage fluid from patients with presumed discogenic low back pain and patients with scoliosis without back pain.[51] Of the analyzed biochemical markers, interferon-γ was found to have a significantly higher concentration in patients with discogenic back pain.[51] These preliminary results raise the prospect of improving the current diagnostic armamentarium for discogenic low back pain.

Multiple biologic treatment modalities including molecular therapy, gene therapy, and stem cell therapy are being developed for discogenic low back pain. Molecular therapy is the introduction of exogenous biologics into the disk to slow the degenerative process or to tip the anabolic-catabolic balance toward anabolism, thereby reversing degeneration. The different molecules can be categorized as anticatabolics, such as tissue inhibitors of metalloproteinase; mitogens, such as insulin-like growth factor–1; platelet-derived growth factor; chondrogenic morphogens, such as transforming growth factor–β and bone morphogenetic proteins; and intracellular regulators, such as LIM mineralization protein–1 and sex-determining region-Y box 9 (Sox9).[52] Multiple in vitro and in vivo animal studies have shown the beneficial effects of different molecular therapies, but enthusiasm has waned because of the ephemeral nature of the compounds in vivo.[53-55]

Using mesenchymal stem cells or gene therapy, researchers have attempted to sustain adequate levels of molecular anabolites in the disk for continued disk regeneration. Stem cells have been found to survive and incorporate themselves into the host tissue, where they can help synthesize and maintain healthy extracellular matrix and act as a means of implanting exogenous genes into the disk.[56] Gene therapy using viruses as vectors also holds promise for treating lumbar disk degeneration. Gene therapy is a means of inserting an exogenous DNA sequence into a target cell to allow the production or overexpression of specific molecules that

aid in maintaining disk integrity. Recently, researchers have successfully treated rabbit degenerative disks with gene therapy using adeno-associated virus serotype 2 as a vector for genes encoding TIMP metallopeptidase inhibitor 1 or bone morphogenetic protein 2.[57] These results are encouraging, but application of the gene therapy model has yet to be tested in humans.

Summary

Lumbar disk degeneration is a complex condition. The diagnosis, natural history, and treatment options are well established for progressive disk degeneration causing neurogenic claudication or radiculopathy. In contrast, the diagnosis and treatment of disk degeneration leading to chronic low back pain are enigmatic. Research during the past 20 years has advanced the understanding of the pathophysiology of disk degeneration and the interplay between genetic and environmental risk factors leading to disk degeneration. Despite these gains in knowledge, more accurate ways are needed to identify the pain generator in a patient with disk degeneration and chronic low back pain. An accurate diagnosis may lead to better results from common treatments such as exercise therapy, cognitive behavioral therapy, fusion, and disk arthroplasty. Successful diagnosis and treatment must account for the psychosocial comorbidities intimately associated with chronic discogenic low back pain.

Key Study Points

- Lumbar disk degeneration is an oligogenic condition that may be influenced by multiple environmental factors.

- The mixed results of nonsurgical and surgical treatments for discogenic low back pain are directly linked to the inability to accurately ascribe low back pain to an intervertebral disk or other structure.

- Pain syndromes associated with lumbar disk degeneration can be affected by psychosocial comorbidities.

Annotated References

1. Katz JN: Lumbar disc disorders and low-back pain: Socioeconomic factors and consequences. *J Bone Joint Surg Am* 2006;88(suppl 2):21-24.

2. Boden SD, Davis DO, Dina TS, Patronas NJ, Wiesel SW: Abnormal magnetic-resonance scans of the lumbar spine in asymptomatic subjects: A prospective investigation. *J Bone Joint Surg Am* 1990;72(3):403-408.

5: Spine

ferential fusion for the treatment of 1-level degenerative disc disease. *Spine (Phila Pa 1976)* 2007;32(11):1155-1163.

41. Delamarter R, Zigler JE, Balderston RA, Cammisa FP, Goldstein JA, Spivak JM: Prospective, randomized, multicenter Food and Drug Administration investigational device exemption study of the ProDisc-L total disc replacement compared with circumferential arthrodesis for the treatment of two-level lumbar degenerative disc disease: Results at twenty-four months. *J Bone Joint Surg Am* 2011;93(8):705-715.

    The 2-year results of a level I FDA IDE noninferiority study showed that two-level lumbar disk arthroplasty with the ProDisc-L device was equivalent to circumferential fusion in the treatment of degenerative disk disease.

42. Hellum C, Johnsen LG, Storheim K, et al: Surgery with disc prosthesis versus rehabilitation in patients with low back pain and degenerative disc: Two year follow-up of randomised study. *BMJ* 2011;342:d2786-d2796.

    A prospective randomized controlled study at five Norwegian hospitals found significantly better results if patients were treated with a disk prosthesis, but the difference between the groups did not exceed the minimum clinically important difference.

43. Putzier M, Funk JF, Schneider SV, et al: Charité total disc replacement—clinical and radiographical results after an average follow-up of 17 years. *Eur Spine J* 2006;15(2):183-195.

44. Daubs MD, Patel AA, Willick SE, et al: Clinical impression versus standardized questionnaire: The spinal surgeon's ability to assess psychological distress. *J Bone Joint Surg Am* 2010;92(18):2878-2883.

    A prospective comparative study found that a standardized questionnaire had more sensitivity than clinical impression in detecting psychological distress of patients with spine symptoms. Level of evidence: III.

45. Patton CM, Hung M, Lawrence BD, et al: Psychological distress in a Department of Veterans Affairs spine patient population. *Spine J* 2012;12(9):798-803.

    A cross-sectional examination of 149 patients with spine symptoms at a Veterans Health Administration hospital revealed that 80% had some psychological distress, and 43% had severe psychological stress (twice as high as the rate in a civilian practice).

46. Carreon LY, Glassman SD, Howard JH: Fusion and nonsurgical treatment for symptomatic lumbar degenerative disease: A systematic review of Oswestry Disability Index and MOS Short Form-36 outcomes. *Spine J* 2008;8(5):747-755.

47. Adogwa O, Parker SL, Shau DN, et al: Preoperative Zung Depression Scale predicts outcome after revision lumbar surgery for adjacent segment disease, recurrent stenosis, and pseudarthrosis. *Spine J* 2012;12(3):179-185.

    A retrospective cohort study of 150 patients found that a higher preoperative Zung Depression Score is an inde-pendent predictor of a poor 2-year outcome after revision lumbar surgery.

48. Sinikallio S, Aalto T, Airaksinen O, Herno A, Kröger H, Viinamäki H: Depressive burden in the preoperative and early recovery phase predicts poorer surgery outcome among lumbar spinal stenosis patients: A one-year prospective follow-up study. *Spine (Phila Pa 1976)* 2009;34(23):2573-2578.

49. Daubs MD, Norvell DC, McGuire R, et al: Fusion versus nonoperative care for chronic low back pain: Do psychological factors affect outcomes? *Spine (Phila Pa 1976)* 2011;36(21, suppl):S96-S109.

    A systematic review of randomized controlled studies found a tendency to better outcomes after treatment for chronic low back pain if patients are stratified for psychological disorders.

50. Kang JD, Georgescu HI, McIntyre-Larkin L, Stefanovic-Racic M, Donaldson WF III, Evans CH: Herniated lumbar intervertebral discs spontaneously produce matrix metalloproteinases, nitric oxide, interleukin-6, and prostaglandin E2. *Spine (Phila Pa 1976)* 1996;21(3):271-277.

51. Cuellar JM, Golish SR, Reuter MW, et al: Cytokine evaluation in individuals with low back pain using discographic lavage. *Spine J* 2010;10(3):212-218.

    A cohort study found modestly increased interferon-γ in disk lavage samples from patients with positive provocative diskography and degenerative findings on MRI.

52. Yoon ST: Molecular therapy of the intervertebral disc. *Spine J* 2005;5(6, suppl):280S-286S.

53. Thompson JP, Oegema TR Jr, Bradford DS: Stimulation of mature canine intervertebral disc by growth factors. *Spine (Phila Pa 1976)* 1991;16(3):253-260.

54. Walsh AJ, Bradford DS, Lotz JC: In vivo growth factor treatment of degenerated intervertebral discs. *Spine (Phila Pa 1976)* 2004;29(2):156-163.

55. Gruber HE, Norton HJ, Hanley EN Jr: Anti-apoptotic effects of IGF-1 and PDGF on human intervertebral disc cells in vitro. *Spine (Phila Pa 1976)* 2000;25(17):2153-2157.

56. Sobajima S, Vadala G, Shimer A, Kim JS, Gilbertson LG, Kang JD: Feasibility of a stem cell therapy for intervertebral disc degeneration. *Spine J* 2008;8(6):888-896.

57. Leckie SK, Bechara BP, Hartman RA, et al: Injection of AAV2-BMP2 and AAV2-TIMP1 into the nucleus pulposus slows the course of intervertebral disc degeneration in an in vivo rabbit model. *Spine J* 2012;12(1):7-20.

    A prospective randomized controlled study with rabbits showed that gene therapy can slow the course of disk degeneration based on MRI, histologic, and biochemical analysis.

Chapter 53

Spine Infections

Andrew J. Schoenfeld, MD

Introduction

The continuum of spine infections extends from superficial postoperative surgical site infection (SSI) to spontaneous epidural abscess and destructive granulomatous osteomyelitis. These conditions represent 2% to 7% of all skeletal infections and are a complication in 0.3% to 20% of all spine surgeries.[1-4] Infections were among the first disorders of the spine to be recognized as necessitating surgical intervention, and spine arthrodesis initially was developed as a treatment of tuberculous spondylitis and osteomyelitis.[5,6] The incidence of spine infections has increased along with the number of spine surgical procedures and the number of individuals who are of advanced age or immunocompromised.[1,3,6-8]

Postoperative infection can have a deleterious effect on outcome and has been shown to increase the rate of perioperative morbidity.[3,9-12] Depending on the virulence of the infectious organism and the extent of the process, postoperative infection may lead to neurologic compromise and mortality. Epidural abscess carries similar risks, and pyogenic or granulomatous osteomyelitis can lead to spinal instability or deformity. During the later years of the 20th century, granulomatous infection of the spine caused by tuberculosis or a fungus was found only in the economically developing world, but these conditions now are also occurring in highly developed countries.[13-15]

Postoperative Surgical Site Infections

Epidemiology

Postoperative SSI is reported to occur after 0.3% to 20% of all spine surgeries.[3,4] This wide variation represents the heterogeneity of spine surgical procedures as well as the disparate indications for surgery. Study findings have been heavily influenced by sample size, population characteristics, institution of origin, type of surgery, surgical approach, and the use of instrumentation. In studies of more than 1,000 patients, however, an infection rate of approximately 3% has consistently been reported.[10,16] A prospective review of more than 100,000 spine procedures found that infection occurred after posterolateral spinal arthrodesis in 3% of patients.[4] Diskectomy was associated with a 1% risk of infection. Of all adult procedures, surgery for osteomyelitis or diskitis carried the greatest risk of SSI (5%). In revision procedures, the risk of infection increased by 65%. The incidence of infection was significantly lower when a minimally invasive technique was used.[4]

Risk Factors

Numerous studies have examined the risk factors for SSI, but many of the findings cannot readily be generalized. Several recent studies may be more translatable to the treatment of typical patients undergoing spine surgery, however. Diabetes, obesity, and increased surgical time were found to be significant risk factors for SSI after adult spine surgery.[3,10,11] The effect of obesity on infection risk may be related to a patient's nutritional status, a relatively large surgical dead space after intervention, longer surgical time related to the duration of the approach, an enhanced environment for microbial colonization because of the poor blood supply of adipose tissue, or a combination of these factors.[10] An examination of the influence of perioperative hyperglycemia on the development of SSI found that a preoperative blood glucose level in excess of 125 mg/dL elevated the risk of infection by a factor of 5.[11] The risk of SSI was greater after an instrumented procedure than after a comparable noninstrumented procedure.[4,12]

Clinical Presentation

The symptoms of SSI can depend on individual patient factors, the type of surgical intervention, the depth and degree of infection, and the time since surgery. The classic findings of fever, malaise, greater than expected pain at the surgical site, peri-incisional erythema, induration, and purulent drainage may not be present in every instance. The surgeon must maintain a high level of vigilance during the postoperative period. Fever, incisional erythema, or persistent drainage raises suspicion for SSI, and seropurulent drainage, frank pus, wound dehiscence, increasing pain at the surgical site, or a new-onset neurologic deficit are even more concerning. The initial examination findings may be misleading; for example, a small amount of superficial serosanguineous drainage may be communicating with gross infection below the fascia, and a benign-appearing wound may mask a smoldering deep infection with no evidence of

5: Spine

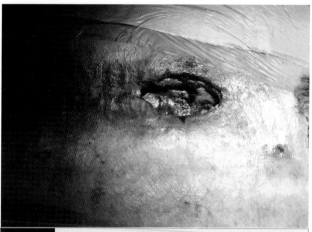

Figure 1 Clinical photograph showing wound breakdown in an 80-year-old man. The patient had dehiscence at the inferior margin of the wound. The wound had polymicrobial colonization. The patient was treated with irrigation and débridement with negative pressure wound therapy and long-term antibiotic therapy.

drainage because of the watertight closure of the fascial layer.

Laboratory Studies and Imaging

The diagnosis of SSI is readily apparent if the patient has a wound dehiscence or purulent drainage from the surgical site (**Figure 1**). Nonetheless, laboratory and radiographic assessments should be completed (**Figure 2**). A patient who may have an SSI should receive prompt measurement of body temperature, white blood cell (WBC) count with differential, erythrocyte sedimentation rate (ESR), C-reactive protein (CRP) levels, and blood cultures.[12,17] If the diagnosis of SSI remains indeterminate, serial laboratory studies can establish trends.[17] During treatment of SSI, serial laboratory studies can gauge the response to antibiotic therapy or surgical débridement and may indicate a need to change the drug regimen or perform additional surgery.

The WBC count, ESR, and CRP levels are nonspecific and may be elevated during the immediate postoperative period, even in the absence of infection. Postoperative CRP levels peak 3 days after spine surgery, trend downward beginning on day 5, and return to near normal 10 to 14 days after surgery.[17] The ESR may require as long as 40 days to reach normative values. An elevated CRP level 2 weeks after surgery or a trend of increasing CRP levels may indicate a deep, inconspicuous SSI.[17]

CT and MRI are useful for evaluating paraspinal soft tissues and identifying abnormal fluid collections within the spinal canal, the intervertebral disk, or adjacent structures. When evaluating enhanced imaging studies, the surgeon must keep in mind that many postoperative changes can mimic an early infectious process, and image resolution may be limited at the surgical site, particularly in the presence of instrumentation. The use of a contrast medium can enhance the specificity of CT or MRI to some extent. A fluid collection on MRI that is enhanced after gadolinium administration is pathognomonic for infection.

Treatment

The initial treatment of most SSIs is prompt irrigation and débridement.[8,12,18-21] There is anecdotal evidence that superficial infections can be managed with antibiotic therapy alone, but there is no consistent description of the clinical entity or reliable high-quality supporting evidence. Inappropriate treatment of an SSI can have substantial long-term consequences, and only intraoperative examination can truly ascertain the depth of an infectious process.[9,16] If a presumptive superficial infection is treated with antibiotics alone, the patient should be monitored closely, and serial laboratory studies should be obtained to ensure adequate resolution.[17]

Surgical irrigation and débridement offer the opportunity to remove necrotic tissue and hematoma, decompress pockets of seromatous or purulent material, and obtain intraoperative cultures. Depending on the indication for the index procedure, most surgeons advocate retaining well-seated instrumentation and any viable, adherent bone graft to avoid precipitating instability or compromising the capacity to obtain solid arthrodesis.[9,18-20,22] This practice is safe and effective.[9,19,20,22] Early removal of instrumentation (without replacement) has been found to lead to loss of lordosis, disk space collapse, and pseudarthrosis.[21]

Many surgeons close the surgical site over drains after a single irrigation and débridement procedure for SSI. Until the results of intraoperative cultures are available, surgery is followed by the administration of vancomycin or another broad-spectrum intravenous antibiotic that is effective against resistant organisms. If the infection is severe or the patient is septic, some physicians place a negative pressure wound therapy device and return to the operating room at a later date for further débridement and an attempt at closure.[18,22] A 97% success rate (defined as resolution of infection and retention of hardware) was reported in 73 patients treated with negative pressure wound therapy for spine SSI.[22]

Appropriate antibiotics, as determined by culture results, typically are administered for 6 to 8 weeks. If the organism is resistant or instrumentation is present, oral antibiotics may be continued for an additional 4 to 6 weeks, for a total of 12 weeks of antibiotic therapy. During the 24- to 48-hour period after surgical débridement and initial antibiotic administration, a substantial decrease in CRP levels and body temperature should occur. Laboratory values that remain high or decrease initially only to spike again are indicative of a need for further débridement and/or a change in the antibiotic regimen.[12,17,18]

A recently formulated scoring system, the Postoperative Infection Treatment Score for the Spine, is in-

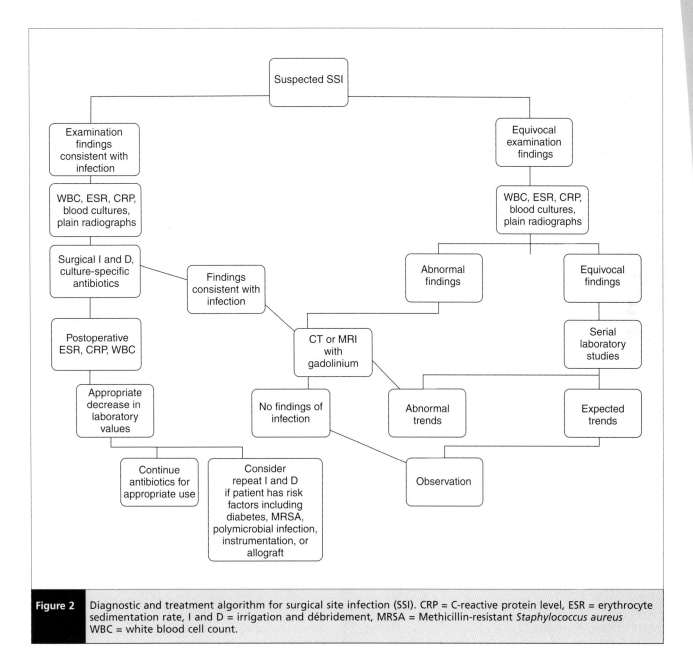

Figure 2 Diagnostic and treatment algorithm for surgical site infection (SSI). CRP = C-reactive protein level, ESR = erythrocyte sedimentation rate, I and D = irrigation and débridement, MRSA = Methicillin-resistant *Staphylococcus aureus* WBC = white blood cell count.

tended to determine whether multiple irrigation and débridement procedures are needed.[18] This system uses surgical location, patient comorbidities, the infectious organism, and the presence of instrumentation to determine a numeric score. A patient with a score of 21 or higher is believed to be at high risk for multiple procedures. The most influential factors in the scoring system include the presence of diabetes, methicillin-resistant *Staphylococcus aureus* (MRSA), polymicrobial infection, instrumentation, and allograft.[18]

Outcomes

The effect of an SSI on final outcome depends on the indication for the index procedure, the patient's age, the presence of comorbidities, and organism virulence. A young, healthy patient with an SSI after diskectomy is likely to recover without adverse effects, but a pa-

tient of advanced age with multiple comorbidities who has MRSA after a multilevel arthrodesis may have serious long-term consequences. The evidence with respect to the long-term effects of SSI is controversial, and several factors probably contribute to the quality of the outcome.

Some studies support the belief that an appropriately treated SSI does not negatively affect results.[19,20] A retrospective study of 32 patients found no significant difference in the Medical Outcomes Study 36-Item Short Form (SF-36) physical function, bodily pain, and general health domains between patients who had SSI after instrumented posterior arthrodesis and those who did not.[20] Early and aggressive surgical treatment was believed to facilitate resolution of the SSI and allow the instrumentation to be retained. Multiple débridement was believed to increase the risk of pseudarthrosis.

Another retrospective study had similar findings, but the researchers cautiously pointed out that, although there were no significant differences in outcome metrics between those who developed SSI after instrumented arthrodesis and those who did not, the patients with SSI were more likely to be dissatisfied with their results at final follow-up.[19]

A comparison of outcomes in 30 patients who had an SSI after instrumented arthrodesis and a propensity-matched cohort of control subjects found no significant differences in SF-36 or Oswestry Disability Index scores.[9] However, the patients with SSI had significantly higher back pain scores 2 years after surgery and were less likely to reach a minimum clinically important difference on the Oswestry Disability Index. These results point to the potential for SSI to have a deleterious effect on outcome, even if managed appropriately. Increased back pain in patients with SSI could be attributable to direct sequelae of the infection and surgical débridement, including devitalization of muscle, denervation, atrophy, and biomechanical dysfunction.[9]

Epidural Abscess

Epidemiology and Pathophysiology

Epidural abscess is reported to represent only 7% of all spine infections.[23] Primary epidural abscess occurs as a result of hematogenous seeding of bacteria, and secondary abscess results from direct inoculation of the epidural space during surgery or a less invasive spinal procedure, such as an epidural steroid injection.[24] In most instances, hematogenous seeding takes place within the disk space, and an epidural abscess develops as the infection progresses. As the abscess increases in size, it can exert a mass effect on the neural elements, leading to radicular-type symptoms or paresis.[23-25] Direct pressure from the abscess as well as the associated inflammation and immunologic response can precipitate infarction in the microcirculation, resulting in vascular insult to the spinal cord or nerve roots. Deficits resulting from such a vascular event have an extremely poor prognosis for recovery.

Although there is no good supporting evidence, it is widely believed that the rising incidence of epidural abscess is a consequence of an increasing prevalence of highly virulent organisms as well as increasing numbers in the population of individuals who are of advanced age, immunocompromised, or intravenous drug abusers.[1,7,8,15,23-26] Studies cited an epidural abscess incidence rate of 0.2 to 3.0 per 10,000 hospital admissions.[23,24] An epidemiologic study documented an incidence of epidural abscess of 0.88 per 100,000 person years from 1990 to 2000 in Olmstead County, Minnesota.[27] S aureus remains the most common causative organism. The prevalence of MRSA-associated epidural abscess has increased dramatically during the past 20 years.[1,23,24,26] Coagulase-negative staphylococci, streptococci, and Escherichia coli are less common pathogens.[24] Pseudomonas aeruginosa is a characteristic organism in patients who are intravenous drug abusers.[1,15]

Risk Factors and Clinical Presentation

The risk factors for epidural abscess are well described and include patient age, immunocompromise (as in HIV or posttransplant immunosuppression), diabetes, cancer, chronic inflammatory disease, endocarditis, end-stage renal disease, chronic hepatitis or cirrhosis, an indwelling vascular catheter, or intravenous drug use.[1,8,15,23,24,26,27] The patient's symptoms can range from moderate back or neck pain to severe sepsis or paralysis. Pain is the most common initial symptom. Approximately one half of patients have fever, and one third have neurologic involvement.[23,26,28] Only 1 of 55 patients (2%) with epidural abscess had the classic triad of axial pain, fever, and neural compromise at the time of presentation in a prospective clinical study.[28] Patients with a ventral abscess are most likely to have systemic symptoms, and those with a dorsal abscess frequently have neural impairment.[23]

Laboratory Studies and Imaging

A patient who may have an epidural abscess should be clinically evaluated with a comprehensive physical examination and assessment of body temperature, WBC count with differential, ESR, CRP level, and blood cultures.[1,7,15,23,24,26,28] Plain radiographs yield little information unless the infectious process has advanced to cause osseous destruction. MRI is the preferred imaging modality for the diagnosis of epidural abscess because it has high sensitivity for the condition and increased specificity when gadolinium contrast is used.[25] A ring-enhancing fluid collection within the spinal canal on postgadolinium images is indicative of epidural abscess (Figure 3).

Insidious onset and an inconsistent clinical picture often lead to the delayed diagnosis of epidural abscess. A recently devised clinical decision guideline was intended to aid in the diagnosis of epidural abscess.[28] The guideline recommends that neurologically stable patients with fever, any risk factor for epidural abscess, a neurologic deficit, or radicular pain receive ESR and CRP level testing. If the ESR or CRP level is elevated, the patient should immediately undergo MRI. ESR was found to be highly sensitive and moderately specific for epidural abscess in patients with at least one risk factor. The adjunct use of CRP levels did not increase the algorithm's specificity. The assessment guideline was claimed to have 100% sensitivity and 67% specificity for epidural abscess.[28]

Treatment and Outcomes

Many patients with an epidural abscess require surgical decompression and evacuation of the abscess material, at a minimum.[23,24,26] There is insufficient high-quality evidence to support a specific approach to treatment. Relatively few studies have measured outcomes or compared treatment results. Patients with paresis or neurologic deficit typically are treated with a decompressive procedure that spans the abscess, as determined by MRI. The abscess location (dorsal or ventral) and the region of spine involvement often dictates the surgical approach. If the abscess involves the cervical spine, spine reconstruction (arthrodesis with instrumentation) usually is required in conjunction with the decompression.[23] Based on the extent of infection and patient comorbidities, an arthrodesis may be delayed. In the thoracic or lumbar region, the decision to perform an arthrodesis in conjunction with the decompression is based on the abscess location and the extent of instability incurred during the procedure. After surgery, patients are generally treated with culture-specific intravenous antibiotics for 8 weeks or for a longer period if ESR and CRP levels remain elevated.[23-26]

Some experts believe that some epidural abscesses without neural involvement, particularly in the low lumbar region, may be amenable to stand-alone antibiotic treatment.[23,25] There is limited evidence to support this contention, however. Although no study has conclusively shown that surgical intervention significantly alters outcomes compared with antibiotic administration alone, it is important to recognize that the literature almost exclusively consists of retrospective studies, and a strong selection bias probably influenced the findings.[23]

Neurologic status at the time of surgery consistently has been identified as the most important predictor of final outcome.[23,24,26] The mortality rate after epidural abscess may be as high as 20%, and it does not appear to be influenced by surgery.[23] A prospective study of 36 patients found that 25 (70%) achieved complete recovery after treatment, with no residual deficits.[24] At final follow-up, 9 patients (26%) had residual paraparesis or complete tetraplegia. A retrospective analysis documented 25% improvement in neurologic status after surgical intervention, but the plurality (45%) of patients had no functional change from the preoperative level.[23] Advanced age, diabetes, chronic heart failure, and chronic liver failure have been identified as prognostic indicators of a poor outcome in patients with epidural abscess.[8,23-26]

Spondylodiskitis (Pyogenic Diskitis and Vertebral Osteomyelitis)

Epidemiology
The clinical entity spondylodiskitis encompasses both pyogenic diskitis and vertebral osteomyelitis. Spondylodiskitis is the most common spontaneous spinal infection; it represents approximately 5% of all skeletal infections.[6] In some recent studies, MRSA was identified as the causative organism in as many as 80% of the patients, but methicillin-susceptible *S aureus* remains the most commonly encountered pathogen.[6,7,14,25] During the past decade, an increase in the percentage of cases caused by a coagulase-negative staphylococcus has also been reported.[7] *P aeruginosa* remains a characteristic organism in intravenous drug users.[1,7]

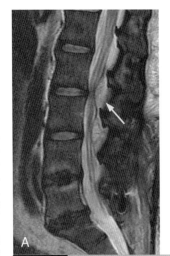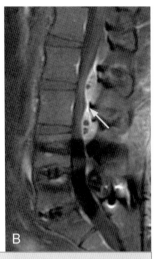

Figure 3 **A,** T2-weighted MRI showing a dorsal epidural abscess at L2-L4 (arrow) in a 33-year-old man who had severe back pain, sensory abnormalities, and lower extremity weakness. **B,** MRI with gadolinium contrast showing the characteristic ring-enhancing pattern (arrow). The patient underwent emergency irrigation and débridement.

The lumbar spine is the most common site of infection and is involved in almost 50% of incidences. The thoracic spine is the site of disease in 30%.[7] In the cervical spine, C5-6 and C6-7 are the most frequent sites of spondylodiskitis.[2,6]

Pathophysiology
The exact pathophysiology of spondylodiskitis remains unknown. The condition appears to exist on a continuum, with pyogenic diskitis being an early manifestation and vertebral osteomyelitis representing a more advanced stage. Hematogenous bacteria may become trapped in the tortuous end plate arterioles adjacent to the disk space, or seeding may occur as a result of stasis in the Batson plexus. The poor vascular supply to the disk space allows bacteria to proliferate in a nutrient-rich and relatively immunoprivileged environment. Pyogenic enzymes destroy the disk and end plate cartilage.[14] In more advanced disease, bone destruction can lead to pathologic fracture or spinal instability. Phlegmon within the spinal canal can cause nerve root irritation, compression, or spinal cord compromise. In the most severe instances, abscesses spread along tissue planes to involve adjacent soft tissues.

Risk Factors and Clinical Presentation
Advanced age, diabetes, chronic renal failure, chronic liver disease, obesity, alcohol abuse, and intravenous drug abuse are important risk factors for the development of spondylodiskitis.[1,6-8,14] Intravenous drug use was proposed as the most significant risk factor for spine osteomyelitis,[6] and spondylodiskitis was found to be the most common type of spine infection among such drug abusers.[1]

5: Spine

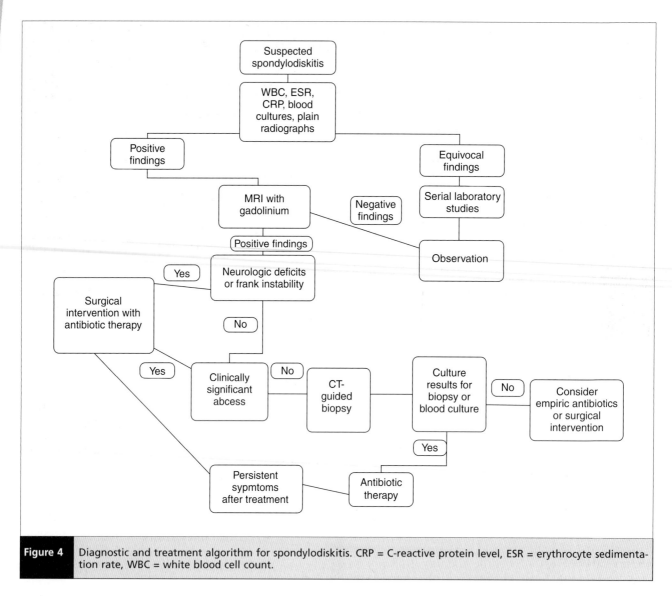

Figure 4   Diagnostic and treatment algorithm for spondylodiskitis. CRP = C-reactive protein level, ESR = erythrocyte sedimentation rate, WBC = white blood cell count.

Pain in the affected spinal region is the most consistent clinical manifestation of pyogenic diskitis or vertebral osteomyelitis and occurs in almost 90% of patients.[7] Other symptoms, including fever, malaise, and radiculitis, are documented in fewer than 50% of patients. A more subtle examination finding, such as diminished deep tendon reflexes or motor strength impairment, occurred in 70% or 60% of individuals with vertebral osteomyelitis, respectively.[7] The symptoms and physical examination findings are varied, individualized, and highly influenced by the location and extent of the infectious process. Neurologic compromise is uncommon in true spondylodiskitis. Spinal cord involvement is more likely in cervical or thoracic infection than in lumbar infection.[2,6,7] Paralysis reportedly occurs in only 1% of patients with vertebral osteomyelitis.[7]

Laboratory Studies and Imaging
The diagnostic studies for spondylodiskitis are similar to those for other spine infections and include blood cultures, plain radiographs, WBC count, ESR, and CRP

levels (**Figure 4**). Total lymphocyte count and albumin levels should be ascertained to evaluate a patient's nutritional status, especially if surgery is being considered. Blood cultures are positive in as many as 85% of patients with vertebral osteomyelitis, but, depending on the responsible organism, inflammatory markers are not always elevated.[7] CT can be useful in providing guidance for biopsy and showing the extent of osseous destruction in the vertebral bodies (**Figure 5, A**). MRI with gadolinium contrast is useful for identifying areas of abscess formation, evaluating the condition of the spinal cord and nerve roots, and determining whether the infection has spread to adjacent soft tissues such as the psoas musculature or the mediastinal region. Within the past two decades, the use of bone scanning to identify spine infection has largely been supplanted by a reliance on MRI (**Figure 5, B**).

Treatment
The mainstay treatment of spondylodiskitis is long-term antibiotic therapy guided by culture results.[6,7]

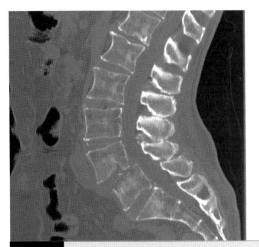
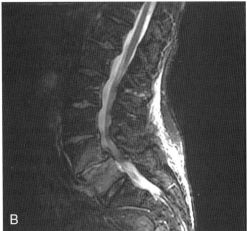
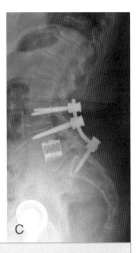

Figure 5 **A,** Sagittal CT reconstruction showing osteomyelitis in a 74-year-old woman with a 6-week history of diskitis at L4-5. The patient had incapacitating back pain but was neurologically intact. The diskitis had progressed to osteomyelitis despite adequate intravenous antibiotic therapy. **B,** Short-tau inversion recovery MRI revealed diffuse osteomyelitis involving the L4 vertebral body and most of L5. **C,** Lateral radiograph after a staged anterior-posterior procedure that included partial corpectomies of L4 and L5, with anterior reconstruction using a titanium interbody cage and posterior instrumented fusion from L3 to the sacrum.

Bracing may be used as an adjunct to reduce pain by providing external support.[6] There is no good evidence to support the contention that bracing can prevent disk or vertebral body collapse and deformity in spondylodiskitis. In the absence of neurologic findings, spinal instability, or a clinically significant abscess, patients are treated with an appropriate intravenous antibiotic regimen, usually for 8 to 12 weeks[6,7] (**Figure 4**). Predictors of successful treatment with antibiotics alone include patient age younger than 60 years, immunocompetence, infection with methicillin-susceptible *S aureus*, and a significant reduction in inflammatory markers with antibiotic administration (**Table 1**).

CT-guided biopsy of the involved vertebrae often is sufficient for obtaining a culture capable of informing treatment. In the absence of culture growth from CT-guided biopsy, blood culture results can be used. Many physicians prefer an open biopsy for identifying the infectious pathogen in the absence of positive blood cultures or tissue cultures obtained by needle biopsy. The risks of surgery may outweigh the potential benefit of obtaining a precise diagnosis, however, if the patient can be treated using a broad-spectrum combination therapy that covers resistant organisms. There is no high-quality evidence that surgical intervention for the sole purpose of obtaining tissue for diagnosis has a positive influence on patient outcomes. The absolute indications for surgical intervention include a progressive neurologic deficit and frank instability that jeopardizes the neural structures[6,7] (**Table 1**). Relative indications include the failure of an appropriate course of antibiotic therapy to relieve persistent symptoms or the presence of a clinically significant spondylodiskitis-associated abscess. The choice of surgical approach and extent of intervention are greatly influenced by the location and the extent of the infectious process.[2,7] In the cervical spine, instrumented arthrodesis almost always

Table 1

Indications for Treating Spondylodiskitis With Antibiotic Therapy Alone or With Surgery

Predictors of Successful Treatment With Antibiotic Therapy Alone

Age younger than 60 years

Substantial reduction in ESR after initiation of antibiotics

Immunocompetence

Infection with methicillin-susceptible *S aureus*

Indications for Surgery

Absolute Indications:

Progressive neurologic deficit

Spinal instability that puts neurologic structures at risk

Relative Indications:

Persistent symptoms after an appropriate course of antibiotic therapy

Clinically significant abscess (large abscess in the psoas musculature, mediastinum, or perirectal region) in the absence of an absolute indication

Inability to identify the infectious organism using blood culture or percutaneous needle biopsy, if surgery is deemed to be in the best interest of the patient

is required after radical débridement.[2] In the thoracic and lumbar regions, an extensive anterior-posterior procedure may be necessary, consisting of débridement followed by reconstruction using posterior instrumentation and anterior strut grafting with autogenous bone and/or interbody cages[6,29] (**Figure 5, C**).

Documented mortality rates after surgery are 5% to

20%, and complications occur in as many as 50% of patients.[2,6,14,29] The infectious process recurs in approximately 4% of patients, with the risk of recurrence heavily influenced by the quality of the débridement.[6,29] Placement of instrumentation during the index débridement does not appear to play a substantial role in recurrence risk, particularly if titanium products were used.[6] SSI is reported to occur in 6% of patients and can be treated like other postoperative infections.[6]

Recently, some surgeons have promoted single-stage reconstruction after débridement for spondylodiskitis to diminish surgical time, blood loss, and the consequent risk of morbidity.[6,29] Patients who undergo single-stage surgery may have a faster rehabilitation and a shorter hospital stay, with an associated impact on healthcare costs. The safety and the efficacy of a single-stage posterior interbody method have been documented in the treatment of spondylodiskitis.[29] Use of the posterior approach may lower the risk of perioperative complications and enhance postoperative stabilization.[29] The evidence is insufficient, however, and does not allow a recommendation to be made on the optimal surgical approach for treating spondylodiskitis.

Granulomatous and Tuberculous Spondylitis

Epidemiology and Pathophysiology

Granulomatous and tuberculous spondylitis are rarely encountered in economically developed countries.[15,30] Granulomatous, or nonpyogenic, infections are caused by fungi, atypical bacteria, and spirochetes such as *Aspergillus, Cryptococcus, Coccidioides, Actinomyces,* and *Treponema pallidum.* Tuberculous spondylitis results from infection with *Mycobacterium tuberculosis* and is more common than the other granulomatous infections.

Only 1% of all patients with tuberculosis develop osseous disease, but 50% of patients with skeletal tuberculosis have spine involvement.[13,14,30] Prolonged infection can lead to kyphotic deformity, spinal instability, and spinal cord compression.[5,13,30] Neural impairment occurs in 10% to 50% of patients because of prolonged spinal cord compression, pathologic fracture, spine subluxation, or vascular infarction from an infectious thrombus.[13,30]

Clinical Presentation, Laboratory Studies, and Imaging

Patients with a granulomatous infection are maintained to have long-standing back pain and deformity as well as systemic fever, weight loss, night sweats, and lymphadenopathy. It is unclear how many patients with nonpyogenic spine infections have such textbook manifestations of the disease. Any individual with a suspected granulomatous spondylitis should be evaluated with a chest radiograph, plain radiographs of the spine, sputum cultures, blood cultures, and a purified tuberculin protein-derivative test. Although WBC count, ESR, and CRP levels generally are ordered as part of the standard battery of tests, they are not always elevated in patients with long-standing granulomatous spondylitis. Patients who are immunocompromised also may not have a positive purified tuberculin protein-derivative test.

CT and MRI with gadolinium contrast are effective for identifying areas of osseous destruction, locating intraosseous abscesses, and evaluating the status of the spine elements. A CT-guided or open tissue biopsy with culture on appropriate media and evaluation using special stains (such as acid fast for mycobacteria) is the only means of obtaining a definitive diagnosis. Sometimes identification of the pathogen can be elusive, and empiric treatment becomes necessary.

Treatment

In patients with stable spine involvement and no evidence of neurologic compromise, the treatment is an extended course of antibiotics, even if future surgical intervention is expected.[30] Initial treatment with an appropriate course of antibiotics can diminish the risk of perioperative complications and increase the likelihood that the infectious process will be eradicated after surgery.

Urgent indications for surgical intervention include a progressive neurologic deficit or spinal instability.[5,13,30] Otherwise, elective intervention is considered if the patient has severe and unremitting pain, kyphotic deformity, and granulomatous spondylitis after unsuccessful antibiotic treatment of appropriate duration. The goals of surgery are to eliminate the infection through débridement, decompress the neural elements, and correct any existing deformity.[5,13] Extensive anterior-posterior constructs traditionally have been used.[5,6] An anterior approach is used to débride involved bone and evacuate any abscess. The quality of débridement is the most important factor in ensuring disease remission.[5,13] Reconstruction is achieved with an anterior strut graft and instrumentation, followed by the application of a posterior spanning construct.

Some surgeons recently have used a less invasive approach for treating tuberculous conditions in the spine. In a two-stage technique, the spine initially is stabilized using stand-alone posterior instrumentation, and anterior débridement and strut grafting with autogenous rib is done an average 9 weeks after the index procedure.[5] The initial posterior fixation is believed to provide immediate stability, enhance pain reduction, and allow rehabilitation. A stand-alone anterior procedure also was described for the treatment of tuberculous spine infection in 42 patients.[13] An extensive anterior débridement was followed by anterior reconstruction using rib grafts and instrumentation. All patients reportedly had a successful arthrodesis, no implant failures occurred, and all had some neurologic recovery.

Summary

Spinal infections represent 2% to 7% of all skeletal infections and can complicate up to 20% of all spine surgeries. As the number of spine surgical procedures has increased, along with concomitant elevation in the elderly population and the number of immunocompromised individuals, so too has the incidence of infectious processes involving the spine. All spinal infections may have a deleterious effect on patient quality of life and may even threaten neurologic function and survival. Regardless of the type of infection or causative organism, all are associated with elevated healthcare costs and periods of disability (be they acute or chronic). Orthopaedic surgeons should maintain high levels of suspicion for infectious processes involving the spine and initiate prompt and appropriate treatment to mitigate the potential for long-term functional compromise, neurologic impairment, and mortality.

Key Study Points

- All spinal infections are associated with elevated healthcare costs and periods of patient disability, and many carry the risk of permanent neurologic sequelae and/or mortality.

- Surgeons should maintain a high level of suspicion for infectious processes involving the spine and should initiate prompt and appropriate treatment to mitigate the potential for long-term functional compromise.

- The use of diagnostic and treatment algorithms in the care of a patient with suspected postoperative infection, epidural abscess, or spondylodiskitis may enhance detection and improve results.

Annotated References

1. Chuo CY, Fu YC, Lu YM, et al: Spinal infection in intravenous drug abusers. *J Spinal Disord Tech* 2007; 20(4):324-328.

2. Shousha M, Boehm H: Surgical treatment of cervical spondylodiscitis: A review of 30 consecutive patients. *Spine (Phila Pa 1976)* 2012;37(1):E30-E36.

   A large study of outcomes in cervical osteomyelitis found associated epidural abscess in 24 of 30 patients (80%). A 10% mortality rate and approximately 20% complication rate were reported. Five patients (42%) of the 12 with neurologic deficit did not improve neurologically after surgery. Level of evidence: IV.

3. Pull ter Gunne AF, Cohen DB: Incidence, prevalence, and analysis of risk factors for surgical site infection following adult spinal surgery. *Spine (Phila Pa 1976)* 2009; 34(13):1422-1428.

4. Smith JS, Shaffrey CI, Sansur CA, et al: Rates of infection after spine surgery based on 108,419 procedures: A report from the Scoliosis Research Society Morbidity and Mortality Committee. *Spine (Phila Pa 1976)* 2011; 36(7):556-563.

   A large study of the Scoliosis Research Society database found a 1.2% incidence of deep infection after adult spine surgery. The rate of infection after posterolateral fusion was 3%. Surgery for an infectious process carried a 5.1% risk. Level of evidence: II.

5. Hirakawa A, Miyamoto K, Masuda T, et al: Surgical outcome of 2-stage (posterior and anterior) surgical treatment using spinal instrumentation for tuberculous spondylitis. *J Spinal Disord Tech* 2010;23(2):133-138.

   A prospective study of 10 patients found that all responded well to staged anterior débridement and grafting and posterior instrumentation for tuberculous spondylitis and achieved successful arthrodesis. Pain was diminished, and neurologic status improved in all patients. Level of evidence: III.

6. Rayes M, Colen CB, Bahgat DA, et al: Safety of instrumentation in patients with spinal infection. *J Neurosurg Spine* 2010;12(6):647-659.

   A retrospective review of 47 patients who received spinal instrumentation as treatment of an infectious process found complications in 25% and recurrent infection in 4%. The authors maintained that spinal instrumentation after thorough surgical débridement is safe and does not carry an increased risk of infection recurrence. Level of evidence: IV.

7. Bhavan KP, Marschall J, Olsen MA, Fraser VJ, Wright NM, Warren DK: The epidemiology of hematogenous vertebral osteomyelitis: A cohort study in a tertiary care hospital. *BMC Infect Dis* 2010;10:158.

   One of the largest studies of patients with vertebral osteomyelitis at a US center found a 4% in-hospital mortality rate. The lumbar spine was most frequently involved. Chronic renal failure and diabetes were the most common medical comorbidities. Level of evidence: IV.

8. Urrutia J, Bono CM, Mery P, Rojas C, Gana N, Campos M: Chronic liver failure and concomitant distant infections are associated with high rates of neurological involvement in pyogenic spinal infections. *Spine (Phila Pa 1976)* 2009;34(7):E240-E244.

9. Petilon JM, Glassman SD, Dimar JR II, Carreon LY: Clinical outcomes after lumbar fusion complicated by deep wound infection: A case-control study. *Spine (Phila Pa 1976)* 2012;37(16):1370-1374.

   A case control study found that patients with postoperative infection had greater back pain and a decreased probability of reaching a minimal clinically important difference on the Oswestry Disability Index compared with patients without infection. Level of evidence: III.

10. Koutsoumbelis S, Hughes AP, Girardi FP, et al: Risk factors for postoperative infection following posterior lumbar instrumented arthrodesis. *J Bone Joint Surg Am* 2011;93(17):1627-1633.

5: Spine

In consecutive patients undergoing spinal fusion during a period of 6 years, a 2.6% infection rate was reported. Obesity and obstructive pulmonary disease were the strongest predictors of infection risk. Osteoporosis and diabetes also increased the risk of postoperative infection. Level of evidence: II.

11. Olsen MA, Nepple JJ, Riew KD, et al: Risk factors for surgical site infection following orthopaedic spinal operations. *J Bone Joint Surg Am* 2008;90(1):62-69.

12. Collins I, Wilson-MacDonald J, Chami G, et al: The diagnosis and management of infection following instrumented spinal fusion. *Eur Spine J* 2008;17(3):445-450.

13. Li M, Du J, Meng H, Wang Z, Luo Z: One-stage surgical management for thoracic tuberculosis by anterior debridement, decompression and autogenous rib grafts, and instrumentation. *Spine J* 2011;11(8):726-733.

    A retrospective study promoted less invasive anterior-only radical débridement and instrumented fusion for tuberculous spondylitis involving only the anterior column and no more than two disk spaces. Level of evidence: IV.

14. Kim CJ, Song KH, Jeon JH, et al: A comparative study of pyogenic and tuberculous spondylodiscitis. *Spine (Phila Pa 1976)* 2010;35(21):E1096-E1100.

    A retrospective study compared the clinical and radiographic differences between patients with tuberculous and pyogenic spondylodiskitis. Pyogenic spondylodiskitis carried a 5% perioperative mortality rate. Chronic renal disease, cirrhosis, and earlier spine procedures were significantly associated with a risk of spondylodiskitis. Level of evidence: III.

15. Bono CM: Spectrum of spine infections in patients with HIV: A case report and review of the literature. *Clin Orthop Relat Res* 2006;444:83-91.

16. Abdul-Jabbar A, Takemoto S, Weber MH, et al: Surgical site infection in spinal surgery: Description of surgical and patient-based risk factors for postoperative infection using administrative claims data. *Spine (Phila Pa 1976)* 2012;37(15):1340-1345.

    A retrospective review of a dataset at a tertiary medical center revealed an infection rate of 3% over 5 years. Surgery for tumors, surgery involving the sacrum or pelvis, and a history of coagulopathy or heart disease increased the risk of infection. Level of evidence: II.

17. Kang BU, Lee SH, Ahn Y, Choi WC, Choi YG: Surgical site infection in spinal surgery: Detection and management based on serial C-reactive protein measurements. *J Neurosurg Spine* 2010;13(2):158-164.

    A prospective study found that CRP levels reach their maximum 3 days after surgery and decline thereafter. Abnormal responses, such as a second rise after day 5 or a steady rise, may be indicative of infection. Level of evidence: II.

18. Dipaola CP, Saravanja DD, Boriani L, et al: Postoperative infection treatment score for the spine (PITSS): Construction and validation of a predictive model to define need for single versus multiple irrigation and debridement for spinal surgical site infection. *Spine J* 2012;12(3):218-230.

    A prognostic system with good internal and external validity was presented to determine the need for multiple irrigation and débridement procedures in spine infection. Level of evidence: II.

19. Falavigna A, Righesso O, Traynelis VC, Teles AR, da Silva PG: Effect of deep wound infection following lumbar arthrodesis for degenerative disc disease on long-term outcome: A prospective study. Clinical article. *J Neurosurg Spine* 2011;15(4):399-403.

    A prospective matched-cohort study found no significant difference in outcome measures between patients who had infection after lumbar arthrodesis and those without infectious complications. However, patients with postoperative infection had significantly lower satisfaction scores. Level of evidence: II.

20. Mok JM, Guillaume TJ, Talu U, et al: Clinical outcome of deep wound infection after instrumented posterior spinal fusion: A matched cohort analysis. *Spine (Phila Pa 1976)* 2009;34(6):578-583.

21. Kim JI, Suh KT, Kim SJ, Lee JS: Implant removal for the management of infection after instrumented spinal fusion. *J Spinal Disord Tech* 2010;23(4):258-265.

    A retrospective review of 21 patients who underwent implant removal and wide débridement for postoperative spinal infection found that patients without solid fusion at the time of débridement had greater disk height loss and loss of lordosis, which did not affect outcome. Level of evidence: IV.

22. Ploumis A, Mehbod AA, Dressel TD, Dykes DC, Transfeldt EE, Lonstein JE: Therapy of spinal wound infections using vacuum-assisted wound closure: Risk factors leading to resistance to treatment. *J Spinal Disord Tech* 2008;21(5):320-323.

23. Karikari IO, Powers CJ, Reynolds RM, Mehta AI, Isaacs RE: Management of a spontaneous spinal epidural abscess: A single-center 10-year experience. *Neurosurgery* 2009;65(5):919-924.

24. Zimmerer SM, Conen A, Müller AA, et al: Spinal epidural abscess: Aetiology, predisponent factors and clinical outcomes in a 4-year prospective study. *Eur Spine J* 2011;20(12):2228-2234.

    In a prospective study of 36 patients with epidural abscess, 34 (94%) were treated surgically; 77% had complete neurologic recovery, and 25% had partial recovery with persistent paresis. Level of evidence: II.

25. Uchida K, Nakajima H, Yayama T, et al: Epidural abscess associated with pyogenic spondylodiscitis of the lumbar spine; evaluation of a new MRI staging classification and imaging findings as indicators of surgical management: A retrospective study of 37 patients. *Arch Orthop Trauma Surg* 2010;130(1):111-118.

    A scale was proposed for grading epidural abscess based

on MRI appearance. Stage I and II lesions, as determined by certain physiologic criteria, are amenable to nonsurgical treatment. Stage IV and V abscesses require surgery. Level of evidence: IV.

26. Chen SH, Chang WN, Lu CH, et al: The clinical characteristics, therapeutic outcome, and prognostic factors of non-tuberculous bacterial spinal epidural abscess in adults: A hospital-based study. *Acta Neurol Taiwan* 2011;20(2):107-113.

    A retrospective study compared outcomes and prognostic factors for patients with epidural abscess treated surgically or nonsurgically. Although indications were different, no significant difference was encountered based on treatment. Advanced age and diabetes were predictors of poor outcome. Level of evidence: III.

27. Ptaszynski AE, Hooten WM, Huntoon MA: The incidence of spontaneous epidural abscess in Olmsted County from 1990 through 2000: A rare cause of spinal pain. *Pain Med* 2007;8(4):338-343.

28. Davis DP, Salazar A, Chan TC, Vilke GM: Prospective evaluation of a clinical decision guideline to diagnose spinal epidural abscess in patients who present to the emergency department with spine pain. *J Neurosurg Spine* 2011;14(6):765-770.

    A prospective analysis defined historical risk factors for epidural abscess. In the presence of these risk factors, elevated ESR was 100% sensitive and 67% specific for epidural abscess. The addition of CRP level did not increase specificity. Level of evidence: II.

29. Hempelmann RG, Mater E, Schön R: Septic hematogenous lumbar spondylodiscitis in elderly patients with multiple risk factors: Efficacy of posterior stabilization and interbody fusion with iliac crest bone graft. *Eur Spine J* 2010;19(10):1720-1727.

    A stepwise approach to surgical treatment was studied in 18 patients with vertebral osteomyelitis. The mortality rate approached 20%, and 50% of the patients had a complication. Level of evidence: IV.

30. Dunn R, Zondagh I, Candy S: Spinal tuberculosis: Magnetic resonance imaging and neurological impairment. *Spine (Phila Pa 1976)* 2011;36(6):469-473.

    A retrospective review of outcomes of 82 patients with surgically managed spine tuberculosis over a 4-year period found substantial neurologic recovery is presented. Preoperative MRI findings were not always indicative of outcome. Level of evidence: IV.

5: Spine

Chapter 54

Adult Lumbar and Thoracolumbar Deformity

Kirkham B. Wood, MD

Introduction

Adult scoliosis and kyphosis are deformities of the spine that are diagnosed after skeletal maturity, which occurs at age 18 years or later according to the Scoliosis Research Society.[1] The two basic types are idiopathic scoliosis, which was present during the growing years but not diagnosed or symptomatic until skeletal maturity, and degenerative scoliosis, which occurs relatively late in life as the disks and other spine elements age. Kyphotic conditions of the adult spine can occur in many different settings. The most commonly treated conditions are Scheuermann kyphosis, which also occurs in adolescents; senile kyphosis, which typically results from the collapse of aging disk space and vertebral body fracture; and kyphosis from a posttraumatic condition. Any curvature in the coronal plane with a Cobb measurement exceeding 10° can be considered scoliosis. In the sagittal plane, the normal angulations of the thoracic and lumbar spines are variable across the population and thus are more difficult to describe as pathologic. However, the typical range of thoracic kyphosis in the adult spine is 20° to 50°, as measured from T2 to T12.

Idiopathic Scoliosis

Natural History

The principal clinical appearance of adult scoliosis is progressive deformity and mechanical pain, with or without lower extremity radicular or stenotic symptoms. Although pain is unusual in an adolescent with scoliosis, frequently it is the primary reason an adult decides to seek treatment.[2] An adult may be somewhat concerned about the cosmesis of the deformity, such as a rib hump, shoulder imbalance, waist asymmetry, or

Dr. Wood or an immediate family member has stock or stock options held in TranS1 and has received nonincome support (such as equipment or services), commercially derived honoraria, or other non–research-related funding (such as paid travel) from Globus Medical, the Orthopaedic Research and Education Foundation, and Synthes.

loss of height. Another concern of adults with scoliosis is the possible progression of the curvature. Although an adult is not at the same risk of progression as an adolescent, a curve greater than 50° or 60° or with significant apical rotation has an increased risk of progression, as does the lumbar aspect of a double major curve.[3] A small increase in curvature has been reported during pregnancy.[3,4] The average progression is 0.5° and 1° per year, but in some circumstances, it can be as much as 2°. As the spine ages and the disk spaces between the vertebrae collapse, the measured curvatures will increase. In adolescents with scoliosis, follow-up examinations usually are scheduled every 4 to 6 months, but in adults, radiographic evaluation to assess progression is needed only every 2 to 3 years.

Rotatory subluxation can occur in the mechanical portion of the lumbar spine (L2-L5) as the spine ages. This translation can lead to neural compression if it advances, and radiculopathy or claudication can develop. This phenomenon is much more common in patients with late-onset degenerative scoliosis. A patient with idiopathic adult scoliosis may report leg symptoms, but mechanical axial pain is more common even in patients with dramatic curvatures and degenerative subluxations. Disk space narrowing at L5-S1 can lead to foraminal stenosis.

When evaluating a patient with adult scoliosis, it is important to remember that there are many sources of mechanical back, hip, or extremity pain other than a spine deformity. Pathologies of the retroperitoneal space, abnormalities of the descending aorta, and pancreatic and splenic conditions can mimic the vague pain of the low back that occurs with scoliosis. Lumbar radiculopathy from a degenerative condition or herniated disk must be assessed separately from the curvature itself.

The pain from thoracolumbar scoliosis or midlumbar to low lumbar scoliosis emanates from arthritic facet capsules, degenerative disks, or muscle tension from the deformity, especially if the deformity is in the setting of sagittal plane imbalance. Spine fatigue pain from such a deformity often can be diagnosed by providing upright correction, thereby relieving the tension in the muscles and allowing the patient to experience relief of discomfort. Thoracic curves are somewhat more variable and typically less painful than lumbar curves in an adult. A relatively large thoracic curve can lead to similar muscle tension pain, however, especially when combined with increased thoracic kyphosis and facet arthrosis as well as shoulder girdle irritation on the convex side of the curve.

The physical examination of an adult with scoliosis is similar to that of an adolescent and focuses on the patient's overall upright appearance, the location of the curve, the nature and timing of pain, and any neurologic sequelae. Shoulder balance is noted, and a plumb line is dropped from the C7 level to measure coronal and sagittal plane balance. The overall shift of the trunk and any asymmetry of the waist are noted, although most adult patients bring these features to the examiner's attention. The flexibility of the spine can be assessed through forward flexion and extension maneuvers, with particular attention to pain as well as the degree of flexibility. Especially in a patient who is bent forward into imbalance in the sagittal plane, flexibility of the spine can be assessed when the patient attempts to lie flat on the examining table. A patient who can comfortably lie flat with the head down and the legs extended may not have the need for surgery suggested by examination in the standing position. A rigid lumbar curvature bent into kyphosis will prevent the patient from placing the head and shoulders down or extending the legs fully onto the table. The examiner must take into account the contribution of any fixed flexion contractures of the hips to the overall sagittal plane imbalance, along with the degenerative flattened lumbar spine. The patient's attempt to lie supine on the examining table allows the examiner to gauge ability and ease of lying flat and fully extending the lower limbs at the hips.

The radiographic evaluation includes full-length PA and lateral radiographs of the spine. Both the cervical spine and the femoral heads should be visible. The patient should stand unassisted with the hips and knees extended and the fingers resting bilaterally on the clavicles. From these radiographs, Cobb angle measurements can be made, pelvic parameters such as pelvic incidence can be measured, and global spine alignments such as C7 sagittal balance can be assessed. Significant information also can be obtained from dynamic bending or flexion-extension radiographs to assess instability, fusion status, or the rigidity and correctability of the curves.

CT provides valuable information on bony anatomy, spinal canal dimensions, and the integrity of any earlier fusion masses. Myelography can be useful when combined with CT to understand the spinal canal's patency. In a patient with no instrumentation, MRI allows visualization of the soft tissues, the physiology of the intervertebral disks, and the contents of the neural canal.

A thorough neurologic examination is necessary to detect radiculopathy caused by arthritic compression or myelopathy from a remote region, such as the cervical spine. Attention should be paid to the patient's gait; motor and sensory testing; and any upper motor neuron signs, such as the Babinski sign or clonus. MRI or CT myelography of the thoracic or cervical spine may be warranted.

Nonsurgical Treatment

Physical therapy, the judicious use of NSAIDs, changes in lifestyle, weight reduction, and exercise may provide pain relief and improve function in a patient with adult idiopathic scoliosis. The most lasting effects seem to be associated with patient-driven active physical exercise programs aimed at both anaerobic and aerobic conditioning and emphasizing abdominal strength and lumbar flexibility. Patients with thoracolumbar or lumbar deformity tend to have better results than those with a primarily thoracic curve.

Bracing generally is not indicated for adult deformity because the curves do not progress as they do in an adolescent, and prolonged use of a brace can lead to muscular deconditioning, dependence on the device, and worsened pain and disability. Rare exceptions occur, however, especially for patients of advanced age for whom major surgery is not considered safe.

Surgical Treatment

The principal reasons for considering surgery to treat adult idiopathic scoliosis are to relieve pain and halt any identified progression of the curvature. Rarely, neurologic symptoms are a reason for surgery. Patients who elect surgery, compared with those who elect nonsurgical treatment, tend to be older; have more comorbidities; have worse health-related quality-of-life scores; and have worse sagittal, coronal, and spinopelvic alignment.[5] A thorough course of nonsurgical treatment first should be tried. In patients with symptomatic thoracolumbar scoliosis, nonsurgical treatment, unlike surgery, did not improve quality-of-life scores, and the cost of the treatment frequently was substantial.[6,7] As with other types of fusions for spine pathologies, the success rate is good but not perfect, and it is important to carefully study the nature, location, and temperament of the pain. Surgical success comes from a combination of stabilization of the spine, treatment of arthritic facet joints and degenerative disks, and lessening of the spine muscle fatigue that comes from being out of balance in the coronal or the sagittal plane. Sagittal alignment correction is the most important parameter related to success.[8] Cobb angle correction is of less importance than it is in adolescents. Many patients undergoing such surgery have a coexisting medical condition that can lead to an adverse outcome if inadequately recognized and treated.[9,10]

Pulmonary morbidity in the form of atelectasis, effusions, or infiltrates is a common postoperative finding. Patients most at risk are those who are older than 70 years, have a history of smoking, have chronic obstructive pulmonary disease, or are scheduled for an extended anterior-posterior approach. These patients should be evaluated for pulmonary morbidity before surgery. Patients should be encouraged to avoid all tobacco products for at least 2 months before surgery. An exercise tolerance test should be considered; a patient who cannot exercise his or her heart to a rate of 100 beats per minute for 2 minutes is at increased risk of pulmonary complications.[10] Pneumonia is the second most common postoperative infection, after urinary tract infection, and rates as high as 4% have been reported.[10]

A patient with a history of coronary artery disease should be evaluated using a cardiac stress test. A patient with ischemic heart disease, cerebrovascular disease, insulin-dependent diabetes, a history of smoking, chronic renal failure, or hypertension should be considered for perioperative treatment with a β-blockade.[11] This treatment was found to reduce the risk of cardiac events during the first 30 days after surgery and the mortality rate of patients undergoing major vascular surgery. Patients with diabetes should make sure their blood glucose is well controlled before and after surgery.

Protocols designed to lower the incidence of adverse events and improve surgical outcomes have been developed for patients with adult spine deformity and who are at high risk. These protocols include specific preoperative evaluations and testing; a recommended intraoperative course for blood loss and replacement, fluid balances, and other factors; and the length of time in the postoperative intensive care and surgical recovery units. Early results have shown a definite decrease in the length of stay and complications, with improved outcomes.[12]

The successful components of surgery for adult spine deformity include a thorough arthrodesis rigidly immobilized with adequate segmental fixation. Scoliotic curves in an adult with arthritic changes and osteopenic bone can be much stiffer than those in a younger patient. In an adolescent, Cobb angle curve correction is of primary concern, but the most important aspect of treating an adult is to achieve a well-aligned, well-balanced spine in both the coronal and sagittal planes.[13] Absolute curve correction is of much less concern. The best results appear when the sagittal vertical axis is within 50 mm of the lumbosacral disk space and the pelvic tilt is less than 25°.

Most idiopathic curves, especially those smaller than 70° or 80°, can be treated through a posterior approach.[14] Most thoracic, thoracolumbar, double-major, and flexible lumbar curves are included in this group. Fusion and instrumentation in an adult is not dramatically different from the same procedure in an adolescent, and it should extend from end vertebral body to end vertebral body for each structural or painful curve.

Anterior fusion is indicated for an adult with idiopathic scoliosis in the presence of some types of flexible thoracolumbar curves, especially if the patient is relatively young; has regional kyphotic malalignment within the lumbar spine; has poor bone quality; or requires fusion extending to the sacrum. A younger adult who has a primary lumbar curve with a flexible compensatory curve can be treated with an anterior instrumented fusion alone, if desired.

Fusion to the sacrum is indicated if the patient has a fixed lumbosacral curvature with related spine-pelvis obliquity, needs some form of release and fusion of the lowermost segments to achieve spine balance (as in a rigid fractional lumbosacral curve below the primary lumbar curve that cannot correct with side bending), or

has painful degenerative segments below a primary curve. In these patients, some form of structural anterior support is needed (Figure 1). A patient with severe coronal decompensation may be a candidate for vertebral column resection and both anterior and posterior fusion and instrumentation.[15]

Anterior approaches, especially the lateral thoracolumbar approach for a large fusion from T10 to the sacrum, are associated with an increased risk of complications. Untoward events include a sympathectomy effect in the ipsilateral leg; denervation of the abdominal wall musculature, leading to an uncomfortable and unsightly hernia; and deep vein thrombosis caused by mobilization of the pelvic vessels. During the past several years, the use of bone graft extenders, including allograft and bone morphogenetic protein, has been introduced in an attempt to achieve successful fusion through a posterior-only approach. Anterior surgery increasingly is done through a miniopen retroperitoneal approach to achieve vital structural support at L4-L5 and L5-S1 for long fusions to the sacrum. With the use of bone graft extenders, many types of fusion for deformity that formerly required two approaches can now be safely and successfully done from a posterior approach alone, as long as there is rigid and capable segmental fixation.[16,17]

Following anterior diskectomies, interbody fusion can be done with rib autograft (with a thoracolumbar approach), femoral rings, or synthetic (polyether-ether-ketone) cages filled with autograft or a synthetic fusion extender. The number of anterior levels treated and fused is correlated with the likelihood of achieving curve correction. For biomechanical purposes, anterior interbody support improves the chances of a successful fusion at the lumbosacral junction by lessening strain on the posterior instrumentation. The two most important levels to support and fuse are the lowest: L4-L5 and L5-S1.

The basic rule for posterior instrumentation is to extend the instrumentation from the proximal neutral vertebra, which tends to be the most centered vertebra on a thoracic or chest radiograph, to the neutral distal vertebrae. Whether distal vertebrae are included depends on a careful review of the radiography, MRI, and diskography. Fusion of the adult scoliotic spine extending into the lower lumbar spine can end at L4 or L5 if the distal disk segments are without deformity, the patient is otherwise in good sagittal and coronal balance, and there appears to be little or no disk degeneration.

Pedicle screws have replaced hooks as the anchor of choice for most surgeons, although many continue to use hooks at the upper end of the construct in the thoracic spine, where the pedicles may be small and the use of a hook may lessen the risk of a junctional kyphosis. Sublaminar wires or cable systems can be used in a patient with osteopenic bone or relatively small pedicles. Sacral screws should be bicortical to increase the likelihood of successful fusion at the lumbosacral junction. Iliac fixation also increases the likelihood of success and especially should be considered in the presence of osteoporosis because a long construct extending

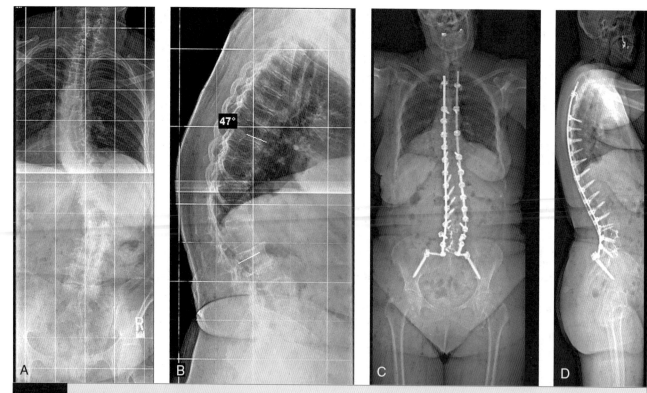

Figure 1 Full-spine radiographs showing painful scoliosis in a 74-year-old woman. **A**, AP radiograph showing that the lower curve is structural and measures 38°; the upper thoracic curve, also painful, measures 29°. **B**, Weight-bearing lateral radiograph showing 47° of thoracolumbar kyphosis and moderately severe anterior sagittal imbalance. **C**, Postoperative PA radiographs with segmental fixation from T3 to bilateral iliac screws. **D**, Postoperative lateral radiograph showing excellent sagittal alignment. Anterior structural interbody support can be seen at L4-5 and L5-S1.

to the sacrum-pelvis places significant strain on the distal fixation points, and the sacrum may fracture in osteoporotic bone with sacral screws alone (Figure 2). It is important to remember that the iliac screw heads can be prominent, especially in a thin patient, and should be buried well within the posterior iliac spine, preferably at the level of the sacrum itself.

The gold standard bone-grafting material remains posterior iliac crest bone, although many surgeons have complemented iliac crest bone with a bone graft extender such as cancellous allograft, synthetic allograft, or bone morphogenetic protein.[18] The use of bone morphogenetic protein remains off-label because it has been approved by the FDA only for placement in an interbody cage anteriorly in the lower lumbar spine. In addition, some concern has been expressed as to potential carcinogenicity. Some researchers have reported that the rate of major complications is no different from that of other fusion materials.[16,19] A thoracoplasty can be performed to correct a cosmetically unacceptable rib hump, material from which can serve as a source of additional autograft bone. It should be remembered that a violation of the chest wall, as with thoracoplasty, has a detrimental effect on pulmonary function for as long as 2 years after surgery.

The 10% to 50% complication rate associated with the surgical treatment of adult scoliosis is much higher than the rate for surgical treatment of adolescent scoliosis.[10] Infection (4% to 7%), neurologic complications (1% to 7%), pulmonary complications (13% to 64%), pseudarthrosis (5% to 20%), and a reoperation rate as high as 44% have been reported.[20-23] Proximal or distal junctional kyphosis is a complication associated with the overcorrection of sagittal curves, low bone mineral density, long posterior fusion to the sacrum, inappropriate spine alignment, a substantial sagittal vertical axis change, or combined anterior-posterior surgery.[21,24-27]

Despite the high overall rate of complications, the clinical success rate of instrumented fusion for adult spine deformity can be quite good when it is used for well-selected patients.[28,29] Patients older than 65 years tend to have greater disability, poorer health status, and more severe back and leg pain than younger patients. However, their improvement in outcome scores often is much greater than that of younger patients, however, despite an elevated risk of major postoperative complications, especially in men and with an increasing number of fusion levels.[30]

Degenerative Scoliosis

Degenerative (or de novo) scoliosis appears with advancing age, as the previously straight lumbar spine ages and collapses into a curve in the coronal plane. Degenerative scoliosis typically is associated with disk

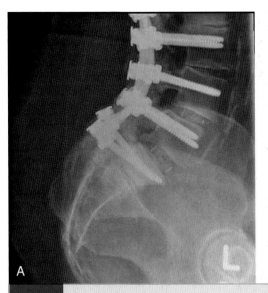
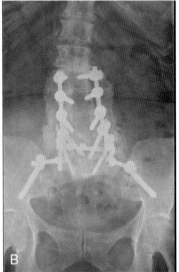
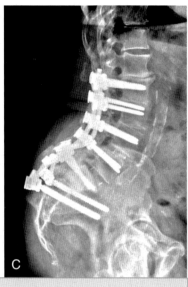

Figure 2 **A,** Lateral radiograph showing a horizontal fracture through the upper sacrum just below the sacral pedicle screws after fusion from the sacrum to the thoracolumbar junction in a 66-year-old woman. AP (**B**) and lateral (**C**) radiographs showing reinstrumentation and fixation to the ilium with posterior sacral bone grafting.

space narrowing, loss of lumbar lordosis, and spinal stenosis. The principal symptoms of a patient with degenerative scoliosis are leg pain, in the form of neurogenic claudication or radiculopathy, and back pain. These symptoms result from disk degeneration, facet arthritis, and degenerative laxity. Cobb angle measurements in degenerative scoliosis typically are lower than in idiopathic scoliosis, and the typical curve patterns and rotational abnormalities of idiopathic curves are lacking. Degenerative scoliosis may be more likely to progress than idiopathic scoliosis, especially in the presence of more than one segment of rotatory subluxation, increased distance of the apical vertebrae from the midsagittal line, and a lack of bridging osteophytes.[31,32] The most common curve types are on the left side from T12 to L3 and/or on the right side from L3 to the sacrum (Figure 3). Subluxation secondary to disk degeneration especially occurs at L3-L4 and L4-L5.

A formal exercise program, injections, and physical therapy will help some patients. Instrumentation and fusion are indicated in patients who have more severe back pain and spine deformity with rotatory subluxations within the areas that require decompression. Decompression with both anterior and posterior fusion can be considered if there is substantial loss of lordosis, sagittal plane imbalance, and a need for fusion to the sacrum. The reconstruction of the anterior disk space with femoral ring allograft or polyether ether ketone cages can not only improve lordosis but also indirectly decompress the spinal canal at the central and foraminal levels. The distal instrumented vertebrae typically is L5, unless the lumbosacral level is symptomatically degenerated. The choice of the cephalad instrumented vertebrae depends on the neutral vertebra superiorly as well as the sagittal profile, with care to include any abnormal thoracolumbar kyphosis. Transition zones or areas of subluxation should be included in the instrumentation and fusion.

Postoperative sagittal decompensation can occur in a patient with degenerative scoliosis as well as a patient with idiopathic deformity. A patient with significant preoperative sagittal imbalance or a high pelvic incidence is most at risk for postoperative malalignment.[33]

Sagittal Plane Disorders

In the sagittal plane of the normal spine, balanced curves of cervical and lumbar lordosis and thoracic kyphosis align and complement one another, so that a plumb line from the base of the cervical spine (C7) falls into the disk space at the lumbosacral junction (L5-S1). This measurement is called the sagittal balance. In a positive sagittal balance, the plumb line drops anterior to the lumbosacral disk; in a substantial positive sagittal imbalance, with clinical implications of pain and disability, the C7 plumb line falls more than 5 cm anteriorly. In a negative sagittal balance, the plumb line falls posteriorly. Even mildly positive sagittal balance is detrimental, and the severity of symptoms increases in a linear fashion with greater anterior sagittal imbalance.[34]

Flatback Deformity

Flatback deformity is the loss of normal sagittal plane alignment, resulting in a fixed anterior displacement of C7 relative to the sacrum. No specific measurement or angle defines flatback deformity. The syndrome principally is represented by clinical symptoms of low back pain and fatigue from overexertion of the erector spinae musculature as it attempts to overcome a fixed and flexed spine while in the upright position. Typically, the patient has few or no symptoms and has a normal ap-

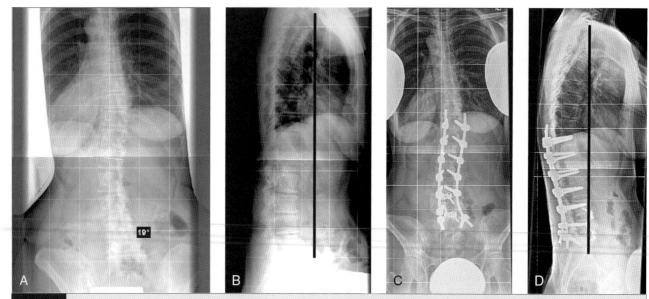

Figure 3 Full-spine radiographs showing degenerative scoliosis in a 57-year-old woman. **A,** AP radiograph showing minimal 19° rotation. **B,** Lateral radiograph showing loss of lumbar lordosis, disk space collapse throughout the lumbar spine, and mild anterior sagittal plane imbalance. Postoperative AP (**C**) and lateral (**D**) radiographs showing anterior structural supporting fusions at L4-L5 and L5-S1 and an instrumented posterior fusion from T12 to S1. Lumbar lordosis has been restored and the sagittal imbalance corrected.

pearance when supine or seated. A pitched-forward, flexed posture becomes apparent when standing or walking. The patient is unable to sit or stand for an extended period of time (**Figure 4**).

Flatback deformity is most commonly associated with a loss of normal lumbar lordosis but can be described as any anterior displacement of the C7 plumb line that forces the patient to flex the hips and bend the knees to stay as upright as possible and keep the head over the pelvis. This position eventually causes quadriceps fatigue. Flatback deformity was first identified when it occurred with the use of Harrington rod distraction instrumentation in the lower lumbar spine for the treatment of scoliosis. Many other clinical situations can lead to a flatback syndrome, including inadequate restoration of lumbar lordosis after fusion for lumbar degeneration; the breakdown of spine segments above a previously fused lumbar spine; and idiopathic conditions such as diffuse idiopathic skeletal hyperostosis, ankylosing spondylitis, tumor, trauma, and infection. Flatback deformity also is called fixed sagittal imbalance or sagittal imbalance syndrome.

Nonsurgical Treatment

Most flatback conditions are truly fixed, and the sagittal plane deformity can be corrected only by surgery. In a patient with relatively little malpositioning, extension strengthening and conditioning sometimes can improve the length of time an upright position can be maintained. The use of NSAIDs sometimes lessens the discomfort. Brace wear is contraindicated because it can decondition the musculature.

Surgical Treatment

A patient with a fixed flatback deformity is surgically treated to relieve pain or correct pseudarthrosis. An unfused, flexible spine that has degenerated and fallen into a flatback deformity can be treated with a solid fusion and properly contoured spine instrumentation. A more severe or less flexible deformity with anteriorly narrow or ossified disk spaces requires anterior release, either transforaminally or directly from an anterior approach, to release the contracted disk spaces and regain height and proper lordosis at the affected levels. If an unsuccessful posterior fusion has led to a flatback deformity, an anterior fusion is advisable to increase the fusion area and improve the likelihood of obtaining a solid arthrodesis.

In a previously fused spine, the surgical options include a Smith-Petersen osteotomy, a pedicle subtraction osteotomy, and a vertebral column resection for the most severe deformities, especially if complicated by a scoliotic deformity.[35,36] A Smith-Petersen osteotomy involves resection of a wedge from the posterior column which, when closed through a hyperextension maneuver, achieves correction through a mobile or ossified disk space as in ankylosing spondylitis. Thus, the posterior column is shortened while the anterior column hinges open on the posterior aspect of the vertebral column. A Smith-Petersen osteotomy most often is performed when the needed correction is modest and the segments being treated do not extend to the sacrum. A general rule is that approximately 1° of correction is obtained for each millimeter of resected posterior column. A typical Smith-Petersen osteotomy can be expected to achieve a 10° to 15° correction.

A pedicle subtraction osteotomy is a resection of a wedge that involves both the anterior and posterior columns and is based at the anterior vertebral body wall and ligament. The posterior column is shortened, but the anterior column is not opened. Because it involves a larger wedge of resection than a Smith-Petersen osteotomy, a typical pedicle subtraction osteotomy can be expected to achieve a 30° to 35° correction in the lumbar spine, and thus it is preferable if a larger correction is required. The blood loss can be more significant than with a Smith-Petersen osteotomy because part of the vertebral body is removed and the epidural veins are exposed. Nonetheless, the overall morbidity, blood loss, and surgical time are less than when a combined anterior-posterior approach is used.[37] The preferred location for a pedicle subtraction osteotomy is the midlumbar spine for two principal reasons: the amount of correction required to restore the position of C7 over the sacrum is greater the more caudad the procedure is, and resecting a vertebral body in the region of the cauda equina rather than the spinal cord or the conus level reduces the risk of serious neurologic injury.

A vertebral column resection involves the removal and the morcellization of one or more vertebral bodies combined with resection of the posterior elements. Vertebral column resection is powerful for obtaining correction in both the coronal and sagittal planes, and it is indicated for the most severe sagittal plane deformities or coronal scoliosis conditions, such as a rigid, fixed curve of more than 120°. Spinal cord monitoring is strongly recommended during the procedure, which probably should be performed only by a surgeon with a substantial history of surgically treating complex spine deformities.

The complication rate after the treatment of fixed sagittal plane deformities is similar to that of adult scoliosis and ranges from 25% to 40%.[38] Durotomy, infection, new neurologic deficits, implant failure, and hematoma can occur. The procedure most associated with a complication is a pedicle subtraction osteotomy.[38]

Kyphosis

In the sagittal plane, there is a wide range of normal values for lumbar lordosis and thoracic kyphosis. Lumbar lordosis ranges from 40° to 70°, and thoracic kyphosis as measured from T2 to T12 ranges from 20° to 50°.[39,40] Thoracic kyphosis of more than 50° tends to be considered abnormal, although there is little correlation between any measurement and the patient's symptoms.

As an adult ages and the disks degenerate between the vertebrae, the average kyphosis slowly increases over time, whereas the lumbar lordosis tends to decrease. The anterior column of the thoracic spine resists compressive forces, and the posterior column (the facets and the ligaments) resists tensile forces. An alteration in either column can lead to an increase in the kyphosis and potentially to pain and deformity.

Scheuermann kyphosis is a disorder of the thoracic spine that occurs in many adolescents, often without

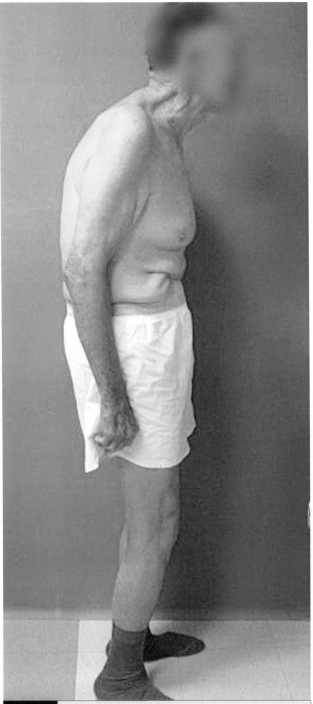

Figure 4 Clinical photograph showing the characteristic flexion of the hips and knees and forward posture in a patient with a flatback deformity.

pain, but also can occur later in life. Pain and deformity prompt most adults with Scheuermann kyphosis to seek treatment. This long-radius kyphotic deformity is a uniform curvature over many segments of the spine that can be flexible or quite rigid. The diagnosis is made when three consecutive vertebrae of the midthoracic spine can be measured to subtend an angle of more than 5°.

5: Spine

In senile kyphosis, the loss of disk space and anterior vertebral body fractures secondary to osteoporosis combine with the loss of posterior muscle and ligamentous tone to produce a long, sweeping painful kyphotic deformity. Posttraumatic kyphosis is difficult to define in terms of a Cobb angle measurement but tends to be a short-radius kyphotic deformity (an acute angular kyphosis over a few vertebral segments) that can be flexible or, if the trauma was in the distant past, quite rigid. The most common scenarios leading to the development of a painful kyphosis are a neglected or inadequately treated flexion-distraction fracture of the thoracolumbar junction, with attendant damage to the ligamentous structures, or a severe burst fracture at the same location. In the thoracic spine, posttraumatic kyphosis can lead to a progressive, painful deformity and occasionally to neurologic changes. In the normally lordotic lumbar spine, a kyphotic angulation can lead to pain and neurologic changes as well as a stooped forward posture. The pain can arise not only from the fracture itself but also from damaged disks adjacent to a fractured vertebra and from altered facet joint motion in adjacent segments as the spine attempts to compensate for the kyphosis with local hyperextension above and below a fracture.

Nonsurgical Treatment

In some patients, extension strengthening and conditioning exercises aimed at the posterior musculature can reduce the fatigue and aching back pain of a kyphotic deformity, especially during prolonged upright posture. NSAIDs should be used judiciously. Bracing is relatively contraindicated in an adult patient to avoid muscle deconditioning.

Surgical Treatment

The general goals of surgical treatment of a kyphotic deformity are to realign the spine as closely as possible to the normal sagittal contour and stabilize the painful arthritic segments. Both goals are designed to relieve posture-related aching back pain caused by stretching of the posterior musculature. Posterior fusion and instrumentation are designed to restore the integrity of posterior column while maintaining the anterior load-bearing capacity of the vertebral column.

The traditional surgical treatment of Scheuermann kyphosis depends on whether the kyphosis is rigid or flexible as well as the severity of the Cobb angle. Most flexible curves smaller than 80° to 90° can be successfully treated from a posterior approach alone using pedicle screw instrumentation and aggressive facetectomies. The goal is to correct the curvature to the higher range of normal kyphosis, without overcorrection. If preoperative hyperextension lateral radiographs obtained with the patient supine over a bolster placed at the kyphotic apex do not suggest flexibility, a first-stage anterior release of the contracted anterior column structures, including the anterior longitudinal ligament and the intervertebral disks, can aid in the final correction (**Figure 5**). Nonstructural bone graft can effect a

fusion anteriorly, and the posterior instrumentation can correct the deformity. The posterior-only Ponte osteotomy technique can achieve correction through multilevel interlaminar closing-wedge osteotomies and compression forces from segmental fixation to shorten the posterior column.

In general, the overall correction should not exceed 50% of the preoperative Cobb sagittal measurement or greatly exceed the preoperative flexibility shown on hyperextension radiographs. The reason for this rule is the risk of developing junctional kyphosis at the superior or the inferior end of the posterior construct. Even with aggressive anterior releases, too much posterior correction can lead to symptomatic junctional angulations. The risk of distal junctional abnormalities is lessened if the construct includes not only the entire Cobb angle measurement of the kyphotic deformity but also the first lordotic segment of the lumbar spine. To reduce the risk of a late junctional deformity, it has been suggested that the inferior aspect of the instrumentation should extend down to the vertebral body bisected by a vertical line drawn superiorly from the posterosuperior sacral corner; according to the the sagittal stable vertebra concept.[41] In addition to junctional kyphosis, the principal complications of surgically treating Scheuermann kyphosis are neurologic injury, infection, and instrumentation failure.[42]

Senile osteoporotic kyphotic deformities tend to be somewhat more flexible than Scheuermann kyphosis, but the attempt to correct a rigid deformity must be judicious because of soft bone. Because of general health and comorbidity concerns, the surgical treatment often is with a posterior instrumented construct with multiple fixation points.

Surgical intervention for posttraumatic kyphosis is considered if the kyphotic deformity is progressive over time, the patient has significant local pain, or there is evidence of a new or progressive neurologic deficit. Decision making is individualized. Posterior stabilization alone often is insufficient because of long-standing anterior bony bridging from the fracture. In addition, there may be significant tension as the instrumentation and bone graft attempt to overcome the anterior column's rigidity; therefore, an initial anterior release is often necessary. Anterior-alone surgeries also tend to be ineffective because of arthrosis and contracture of the facet joints posteriorly. The successful treatments usually involve an anterior release and corpectomy followed by posterior instrumentation or pedicle subtraction osteotomy from the posterior approach. Severe kyphotic angulations may require an extensive vertebral decancellation corpectomy.[43]

Revision Surgery

Adults treated for spine deformity are much more likely to need revision surgery than adolescents because of the risk of pseudarthrosis, poor bone quality, instrumentation dissociation, neurologic complications, postoperative malalignment or sagittal plane imbalance, adjacent segment degeneration or deformity, infection, and instru-

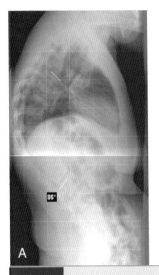
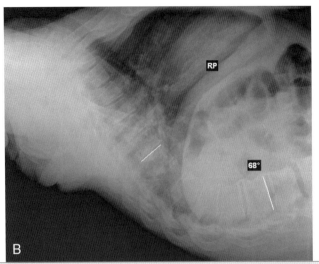
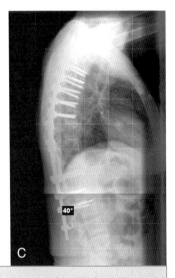

Figure 5   **A,** Weight-bearing lateral radiograph showing rigid and painful Scheuermann kyphosis measuring 86° in a 47-year-old man. **B,** Hyperextension lateral radiograph obtained with the patient supine over a bolster shows little correction. **C,** Correction to a more normal 40° was obtained after anterior transthoracic releases of the disk spaces (arrow) and posterior instrumentation and fusion.

mentation complications. The risk of nonunion is particularly high because so many fusions in adults extend down to the sacrum and the pelvis, where the failure rate is the highest. Reoperation rates after an index spine fusion for idiopathic scoliosis range from 3% to 13%.[44,45]

The most important symptoms after surgery for spine deformity are pain, disability, or progressive or new deformity. The challenges are to understand the patient's deformity before the index surgery, appreciate the current situation, and develop the optimal treatment approach. The patient's sagittal plane balance is most closely aligned with symptoms, and most revision procedures are performed to correct malalignment in this plane. The goal is to do whatever is necessary to bring the C7 plumb line into line with the lumbosacral disk space and restore the appropriate anterior column load bearing. Assessment radiography should be done with the patient upright and standing unassisted, with the fingers to the clavicles. The hips and knees must be as extended, as possible.

Adequate neural decompression must be performed (if needed), the internal fixation must be made secure, and appropriate autologous or synthetic bone graft must be obtained and used. With an already-fused spine, posterior osteotomies such as the pedicle subtraction osteotomy can be used, particularly in a spine with a circumferential fusion. For a spine with open disk spaces anteriorly, one or more Smith-Petersen osteotomies may be adequate, especially if there is no need for dramatic angular correction.

Many patients already have a solid posterior fusion and instrumentation in place. If the instrumentation involves the mid or low lumbar spine and is to be extended further (as to the sacrum), often it can be left in place, and pedicle screws or hooks can be positioned around it and connected to the sacrum and the ilium. If an osteotomy is needed, however, some or all of the in-

strumentation should be removed.

For a severe, rigid coronal deformity, it may be necessary to perform an apical vertebral body resection with rigid segmental posterior fixation.[35,46] If the risks of an anterior approach are increased by earlier anterior surgery or medical comorbidities, a posteriorly based eggshell or decancellation osteotomy (in which the bone of an apical vertebra is removed through a transpedicular approach, and the vertebra is converted into a controlled compression fracture) often can effect a reasonable correction in both the coronal and the sagittal planes.

The complication rate of revision surgery for adult deformity ranges from 30% to 40%.[47] The risk of complications is related to age older than 60 years, medical comorbidities, obesity, and the use of a pedicle subtraction osteotomy.

Summary

Adult spinal deformity is a collection of complex diagnoses that involve not only scoliosis but also kyphosis, degenerative scoliosis, and flatback deformities, otherwise known as sagittal plane deformities. Pain is the principal issue that drives consideration for surgical treatment, although many nonsurgical trials, including medication, physical therapy, weight loss, and changes in lifestyle, are always encouraged first. When surgery is undertaken, it must be counseled that it can be significantly more complex than that for the adolescent. The exposure takes longer, the curves are stiffer, the instrumentation is often times more robust, the bleeding is greater, the patients are sicker, and the complication rate is much more. Yet, despite these obstacles, the satisfaction rate when patients complete function and outcome scores can be quite strong, especially in the elderly.

5: Spine

Key Study Points

- Adult scoliosis can be associated with severe disability. Nonsurgical treatment is initially recommended, but in most patients the long-term outcome appears to be most favorable with surgical stabilization. The risk of surgical complications remains relatively high.

- Deformities in the sagittal plane (flatback deformity, loss of lordosis, posttraumatic kyphosis) are among the most debilitating. Osteotomies often are required to realign the spine. Pedicle subtraction osteotomies are the most effective, although the blood loss can be significant.

- Hyperkyphosis of the thoracic spine can cause disabling pain and be cosmetically unappealing. Surgical correction is achieved with a combination of careful cantilever bending techniques and small osteotomies to return the spine to a more normal contour. The choice of distal levels is important to minimize the risk of junctional kyphosis.

Annotated References

1. Carl AC: *Spinal Deformities: The Comprehensive Text.* Thieme, New York, NY, 2003, pp 809-818.

2. Bess S, Boachie-Adjei O, Burton D, et al: Pain and disability determine treatment modality for older patients with adult scoliosis, while deformity guides treatment for younger patients. *Spine (Phila Pa 1976)* 2009; 34(20):2186-2190.

3. Weinstein SL, Ponseti IV: Curve progression in idiopathic scoliosis. *J Bone Joint Surg Am* 1983;65(4): 447-455.

4. Bradford DS, Tay BK, Hu SS: Adult scoliosis: Surgical indications, operative management, complications, and outcomes. *Spine (Phila Pa 1976)* 1999;24(24):2617-2629.

5. Terran J, Schwab F, Shaffrey CI, et al: The Schwab-SRS Adult Spinal Deformity Classification: Assessment and clinical correlations based on a prospective operative and nonoperative cohort. *Neurosurgery* 2013;73(4): 559-568.

   Prospectively collected data on 757 patients with adult spine deformity revealed that patients treated surgically were older and had more comorbidities, greater disability, and worse spinopelvic alignment than other patients.

6. Bridwell KH, Glassman S, Horton W, et al: Does treatment (nonoperative and operative) improve the two-year quality of life in patients with adult symptomatic lumbar scoliosis: A prospective multicenter evidence-based medicine study. *Spine (Phila Pa 1976)* 2009; 34(20):2171-2178.

7. Glassman SD, Carreon LY, Shaffrey CI, et al: The costs and benefits of nonoperative management for adult scoliosis. *Spine (Phila Pa 1976)* 2010;35(5):578-582.

   Sixty-eight adult scoliosis patients who received nonsurgical treatment modalities over a 2-year period were compared with 55 similar patients who received no real treatment. Health-related quality-of-life scores were no different, but the mean cost over the period was more than $10,000 for those receiving treatment. Level of evidence: II.

8. Blondel B, Schwab F, Ungar B, et al: Impact of magnitude and percentage of global sagittal plane correction on health-related quality of life at 2-years follow-up. *Neurosurgery* 2012;71(2):341-348.

   The best quality-of-life outcomes in surgically treated patients with adult spine deformity were in those whose preoperative sagittal balance was corrected by at least 66% or 120 mm.

9. Fu KM, Smith JS, Polly DW Jr, et al: Correlation of higher preoperative American Society of Anesthesiology grade and increased morbidity and mortality rates in patients undergoing spine surgery. *J Neurosurg Spine* 2011;14(4):470-474.

   In a retrospective review of the Scoliosis Research Society's morbidity and mortality database, the complication rates related to American Society of Anesthesiology grades 1 through 5 were 5.4%, 9.0%, 14.4%, 20.3%, and 50.0%, respectively.

10. Baron EM, Albert TJ: Medical complications of surgical treatment of adult spinal deformity and how to avoid them. *Spine (Phila Pa 1976)* 2006;31(suppl 19):S106-S118.

11. Hu SS, Berven SH: Preparing the adult deformity patient for spinal surgery. *Spine (Phila Pa 1976)* 2006; 31(suppl 19):S126-S131.

12. Halpin RJ, Sugrue PA, Gould RW, et al: Standardizing care for high-risk patients in spine surgery: The Northwestern high-risk spine protocol. *Spine (Phila Pa 1976)* 2010;35(25):2232-2238.

    Standardizing preoperative risk assessment using a multidisciplinary team of hospitalists, critical care physicians, anesthesiologists, and spine surgeons led to improved outcomes and less morbidity.

13. Lafage V, Bharucha NJ, Schwab F, et al: Multicenter validation of a formula predicting postoperative spinopelvic alignment. *J Neurosurg Spine* 2012;16(1):15-21.

    A review of a multicenter retrospective study of pedicle subtraction osteotomies found that a formula of sagittal vertical axis of less than 50 mm and pelvic tilt of less than 25° was strongly predictive of a good outcome.

14. Good CR, Lenke LG, Bridwell KH, et al: Can posterior-only surgery provide similar radiographic and clinical results as combined anterior (thoracotomy/thoracoabdominal)/posterior approaches for adult scoliosis? *Spine (Phila Pa 1976)* 2010;35(2):210-218.

    A comparison of 24 patients treated with anterior-posterior fusion and 24 patients treated with posterior-only techniques involving osteotomies, pedicle screws, transforaminal lumbar interbody fusions, and bone morphogenetic protein found similar outcomes, but those treated with combined surgery had statistically longer surgical times and length of stay and were at greater risk for pseudarthrosis.

15. Bradford DS, Tribus CB: Vertebral column resection for the treatment of rigid coronal decompensation. *Spine (Phila Pa 1976)* 1997;22(14):1590-1599.

16. Williams BJ, Smith JS, Fu KM, et al: Does bone morphogenetic protein increase the incidence of perioperative complications in spinal fusion? A comparison of 55,862 cases of spinal fusion with and without bone morphogenetic protein. *Spine (Phila Pa 1976)* 2011; 36(20):1685-1691.

    A review of 55,862 spine fusions from a multi-institutional, multisurgeon database revealed that the use of bone morphogenetic protein with anterior cervical fusions was associated with higher rates of overall complications and wound infections than other fusions. There were no other significant differences between fusions with or without bone morphogenetic protein with regard to overall complications, wound infections, or hematomas or seromas.

17. Bess S, Line BG, Boachie-Adjei O, et al: Does recombinant human bone morphogenetic protein-2 (BMP) use in adult spinal deformity (ASD) increase complications and are complications dose related? A prospective, multicenter study of 257 consecutive patients. *Neurosurgery* 2012;71(2):E556-E557.

    In a prospective multicenter study of 257 patients treated for adult spine deformity, 155 were treated with bone morphogenetic protein-2 without an increase in major, wound, or neurologic complications or a return to the operating room.

18. Maeda T, Buchowski JM, Kim YJ, Mishiro T, Bridwell KH: Long adult spinal deformity fusion to the sacrum using rhBMP-2 versus autogenous iliac crest bone graft. *Spine (Phila Pa 1976)* 2009;34(20):2205-2212.

19. Lubelski D, Abdullah KG, Steinmetz MP, et al: Adverse events with the use of rhBMP-2 in thoracolumbar and lumbar spine fusions: A nine year institutional analysis. *J Spinal Disord Tech* 2013. Epub ahead of print.

    A retrospective chart review of 547 patient charts revealed an incidence of radiculitis, pseudarthrosis, and reoperation that was similar to historical controls.

20. Charosky S, Guigui P, Blamoutier A, Roussouly P, Chopin D; Study Group on Scoliosis: Complications and risk factors of primary adult scoliosis surgery: A multicenter study of 306 patients. *Spine (Phila Pa 1976)* 2012;37(8):693-700.

    A retrospective multicenter study of 306 adults older than 50 years with scoliosis treated surgically. Three fourths were treated with a posterior-only approach. The complication rate was 39% (175 complications in 119 patients). The rate of neurologic complications was 7%.

21. O'Shaughnessy BA, Bridwell KH, Lenke LG, et al: Does a long-fusion "T3-sacrum" portend a worse outcome than a short-fusion "T10-sacrum" in primary surgery for adult scoliosis? *Spine (Phila Pa 1976)* 2012;37(10): 884-890.

    In a group of 58 patients with adult scoliosis, those who received instrumentation to the upper thoracic spine had more perioperative complications, pseudarthrosis, and revision surgery than those who received instrumentation to the thoracolumbar junction. Those with thoracolumbar junction fusion had more proximal junctional kyphosis. Functional outcomes were similar.

22. Sansur CA, Smith JS, Coe JD, et al: Scoliosis research society morbidity and mortality of adult scoliosis surgery. *Spine (Phila Pa 1976)* 2011;36(9):E593-E597.

    A review of adult idiopathic and degenerative scoliosis from the Scoliosis Research Society's morbidity and mortality database from 2004 to 2007 revealed a complication rate of 11%. Most common were dural tearing, superficial infection, deep wound infection, implant complication, acute neurologic deficit, delayed neurologic deficit, hematoma, pulmonary embolism, and deep vein thrombosis.

23. Pull ter Gunne AF, van Laarhoven CJ, Cohen DB: Incidence of surgical site infection following adult spinal deformity surgery: An analysis of patient risk. *Eur Spine J* 2010;19(6):982-988.

    Obesity and an earlier surgical site infection were most strongly associated with a risk of surgical site infection.

24. Lowe TG, Kasten MD: An analysis of sagittal curves and balance after Cotrel-Dubousset instrumentation for kyphosis secondary to Scheuermann's disease: A review of 32 patients. *Spine (Phila Pa 1976)* 1994;19(15): 1680-1685.

25. Yagi M, Akilah KB, Boachie-Adjei O: Incidence, risk factors and classification of proximal junctional kyphosis: Surgical outcomes review of adult idiopathic scoliosis. *Spine (Phila Pa 1976)* 2011;36(1):E60-E68.

    In a review of 157 consecutive patients with adult scoliosis treated with long instrumented spine fusion, 32 patients (20%) had proximal junctional kyphosis, most of which was classified as ligamentous and mild. Outcome and disability scores did not reveal significant differences based on whether patients had proximal junctional kyphosis.

26. Yagi M, King AB, Boachie-Adjei O: Incidence, risk factors, and natural course of proximal junctional kyphosis: Surgical outcomes review of adult idiopathic scoliosis. Minimum 5 years of follow-up. *Spine (Phila Pa 1976)* 2012;37(17):1479-1489.

    At an average follow-up of more than 7 years, proximal junctional kyphosis had occurred in 17 of 76 patients. Seventy-six percent were identified within the first 3 months, and they tended to continuously progress to follow-up. The risk factors were preexisting low bone mineral density, posterior spine fusion, fusion to the sacrum, and greater change in the sagittal vertical axis.

5: Spine

27. Kim HJ, Yagi M, Nyugen J, Cunningham ME, Boachie-Adjei O: Combined anterior-posterior surgery is the most important risk factor for developing proximal junctional kyphosis in idiopathic scoliosis. *Clin Orthop Relat Res* 2012;470(6):1633-1639.

In a review of 249 patients, risk factors for proximal junctional kyphosis were a T1 to T3 upper instrumented level, combined anterior-posterior surgery, and an increased sagittal sacral vertical line correction.

28. Zimmerman RM, Mohamed AS, Skolasky RL, Robinson MD, Kebaish KM: Functional outcomes and complications after primary spinal surgery for scoliosis in adults aged forty years or older: A prospective study with minimum two-year follow-up. *Spine (Phila Pa 1976)* 2010;35(20):1861-1866.

In a prospective study of 35 patients older than 40 years, 26% had a major complication and 31% a minor one. Despite the complications, there were significant improvements in postoperative disability and outcome scores. Patients whose fusions ended at L4 or L5 had greater improvement in some of component scores than those whose fusions involved the sacrum.

29. Smith JS, Shaffrey CI, Glassman SD, et al: Risk-benefit assessment of surgery for adult scoliosis: An analysis based on patient age. *Spine (Phila Pa 1976)* 2011;36(10):817-824.

A retrospective review of 206 patients in prospective studies from multiple spine centers found a complication rate of 17% for those age 25 to 44 years, 48% for those age 45 to 64 years, and 71% for those age 65 to 85 years. At baseline, the older patients had greater disability, poorer health status, and more severe back and leg pain. At follow-up, however, improvement on the Oswestry Disability Index was greatest for these patients, and there were trends to greater improvement in back pain and outcomes scores.

30. Cloyd JM, Acosta FL Jr, Cloyd C, Ames CP: Effects of age on perioperative complications of extensive multilevel thoracolumbar spinal fusion surgery. *J Neurosurg Spine* 2010;12(4):402-408.

In a retrospective review of 124 patients who underwent surgery from 2000 to 2007, the risk factors for complications were increasing age, increasing numbers of fusion levels, and male sex.

31. Seo JY, Ha KY, Hwang TH, Kim KW, Kim YH: Risk of progression of degenerative lumbar scoliosis. *J Neurosurg Spine* 2011;15(5):558-566.

In 27 patients followed for a mean of 10 years, the sum of the segmental wedge angles above L3 and the initial disk index at the apical vertebra were correlated with the last Cobb angle measurement. The final Oswestry Disability Index score was correlated with the last coronal measurement but not with age, sex, direction of the scoliosis, or listhesis.

32. Chin KR, Furey C, Bohlman HH: Risk of progression in de novo low-magnitude degenerative lumbar curves: Natural history and literature review. *Am J Orthop (Belle Mead NJ)* 2009;38(8):404-409.

33. Cho KJ, Suk SI, Park SR, et al: Risk factors of sagittal decompensation after long posterior instrumentation and fusion for degenerative lumbar scoliosis. *Spine (Phila Pa 1976)* 2010;35(17):1595-1601.

Postoperative sagittal decompensation was found in 19 of 45 patients. Preoperative sagittal imbalance and a high pelvic incidence were risk factors, but hypolordosis was not.

34. Glassman SD, Bridwell K, Dimar JR, Horton W, Berven S, Schwab F: The impact of positive sagittal balance in adult spinal deformity. *Spine (Phila Pa 1976)* 2005;30(18):2024-2029.

35. Zhou C, Liu L, Song Y, et al: Anterior and posterior vertebral column resection for severe and rigid idiopathic scoliosis. *Eur Spine J* 2011;20(10):1728-1734.

A combined anterior posterior approach for treating severe scoliosis of more than 90° with flexibility of less than 20% was found to be effective.

36. Bridwell KH: Decision making regarding Smith-Petersen vs. pedicle subtraction osteotomy vs. vertebral column resection for spinal deformity. *Spine (Phila Pa 1976)* 2006;31(suppl 19):S171-S178.

37. Burkett B, Ricart-Hoffiz PA, Schwab F, et al: Comparative analysis of surgical approaches and osteotomies for the correction of sagittal plane spinal deformity in adults. *Spine (Phila Pa 1976)* 2013;38(2):188-194.

The radiographic correction of severe sagittal plane deformity in adults was similar in combined anterior-posterior and posterior-only approaches, but morbidity was significantly higher in combined surgery.

38. Smith JS, Sansur CA, Donaldson WF III, et al: Short-term morbidity and mortality associated with correction of thoracolumbar fixed sagittal plane deformity: A report from the Scoliosis Research Society Morbidity and Mortality Committee. *Spine (Phila Pa 1976)* 2011;36(12):958-964.

A retrospective review of the Scoliosis Research Society's morbidity and mortality database revealed 578 incidences of fixed sagittal imbalance treated surgically. There were 170 complications in 132 patients, the most common of which were durotomy, wound infection, new neurologic deficit, and implant failure.

39. Macagno AE, O'Brien MF: Thoracic and thoracolumbar kyphosis in adults. *Spine (Phila Pa 1976)* 2006;31(suppl 19):S161-S170.

40. Bernhardt M, Bridwell KH: Segmental analysis of the sagittal plane alignment of the normal thoracic and lumbar spines and thoracolumbar junction. *Spine (Phila Pa 1976)* 1989;14(7):717-721.

41. Cho KJ, Lenke LG, Bridwell KH, Kamiya M, Sides B: Selection of the optimal distal fusion level in posterior instrumentation and fusion for thoracic hyperkyphosis: The sagittal stable vertebra concept. *Spine (Phila Pa 1976)* 2009;34(8):765-770.

42. Coe JD, Smith JS, Berven S, et al: Complications of spinal fusion for scheuermann kyphosis: A report of the scoliosis research society morbidity and mortality committee. *Spine (Phila Pa 1976)* 2010;35(1):99-103.

    A retrospective review of a prospectively collected, multicentered database revealed a complication rate of 14%, the most common being wound infection. The mortality rate was 0.6%. Level of evidence: IV.

43. Chen Z, Zeng Y, Li W, Guo Z, Qi Q, Sun C: Apical segmental resection osteotomy with dual axial rotation corrective technique for severe focal kyphosis of the thoracolumbar spine. *J Neurosurg Spine* 2011;14(1):106-113.

    Anterior and posterior approaches to the spine through one incision for the correction of severe kyphotic angulations were described.

44. Luhmann SJ, Lenke LG, Bridwell KH, Schootman M: Revision surgery after primary spine fusion for idiopathic scoliosis. *Spine (Phila Pa 1976)* 2009;34(20):2191-2197.

45. Pichelmann MA, Lenke LG, Bridwell KH, Good CR, O'Leary PT, Sides BA: Revision rates following primary adult spinal deformity surgery: Six hundred forty-three consecutive patients followed-up to twenty-two years postoperative. *Spine (Phila Pa 1976)* 2010;35(2):219-226.

    A retrospective review of patients treated from 1985 to 2008 found a 9.0% rate of revision surgery and a 2.3% rate of more than one revision. The most common reasons for revision surgery were pseudarthrosis (41%), curve progression (20%), infection (15%), and painful implant (7%).

46. Wang Y, Lenke LG: Vertebral column decancellation for the management of sharp angular spinal deformity. *Eur Spine J* 2011;20(10):1703-1710.

    Management and surgical techniques for vertebral decancellation for severe angular deformity were described.

47. Cho SK, Bridwell KH, Lenke LG, et al: Major complications in revision adult deformity surgery: Risk factors and clinical outcomes with 2- to 7-year follow-up. *Spine (Phila Pa 1976)* 2012;37(6):489-500.

    In this retrospective study of 166 patients, 34% had a major complication in the perioperative period or at 3.5-year follow-up. Risk factors for perioperative complications included age older than 60 years, medical comorbidities, obesity, and a pedicle subtraction osteotomy. Risk factors for late complications were a three-column osteotomy and progressive loss of sagittal correction.

5: Spine

Chapter 55

Spine Tumors

Marco Ferrone, MD   Joe Schwab, MD, MS

Introduction

Primary tumors of the spine are rare, and they are encountered far less often than metastatic disease to the spine. A primary spine tumor can be benign or malignant. The initial symptom or constellation of symptoms often is nonspecific, but advanced imaging may lead to a diagnosis that can be confirmed with a tissue biopsy. The spine is the most common site of osseous metastases.

Clinical Evaluation

History and Physical Examination

A thorough history and physical examination are useful for determining the diagnosis. A patient's age and sex can be important factors in the differential diagnosis. Patients younger than 30 years usually have a benign condition, with the exception of Ewing sarcoma and osteosarcoma. Patients older than 30 years are more likely to have a malignant disease, such as multiple myeloma or metastasis, although benign conditions, such as an enostosis (a bone island) or a hemangioma, also are common. The factors that aggravate or alleviate a patient's symptoms can help differentiate mechanical instability from the pain of periosteal swelling. These factors may be pathognomonic, as in pain relief with the use of NSAIDs in a patient with osteoid osteoma. A patient's medical comorbidities, health maintenance screening, and past treatments can help guide the differential diagnosis. A history of radiation exposure can be helpful for establishing a diagnosis of radiation-

---

Dr. Schwab or an immediate family member is a member of a speakers' bureau or has made paid presentations on behalf of Synthes and Stryker Spine; serves as a paid consultant to or is an employee of Biom'up; has received nonincome support (such as equipment or services), commercially derived honoraria, or other non–research-related funding (such as paid travel) from Globus Medical and Stryker; and serves as a board member, owner, officer, or committee member of Biom'up. Neither Dr. Ferrone nor any immediate family member has received anything of value from or has stock or stock options held in a commercial company or institution related directly or indirectly to the subject of this chapter.

associated malignancy. A detailed neurologic examination and subsequent serial examinations always are important for detecting disease progression.

Laboratory Data

The basic laboratory tests for a patient with a new spine lesion include the complete blood cell count; the erythrocyte sedimentation rate; a liver function test; serum and urine immunoelectrophoresis; and calcium, phosphorous, alkaline phosphatase, blood urea nitrogen, creatinine, and glucose measurements. If metastatic disease is strongly suspected, C-reactive protein level and tumor marker assays (such as the α-fetoprotein–carcinoembryonic antigen–prostate-specific antigen panel) should be added. These laboratory tests are not diagnostic by themselves, but they can direct the differential diagnosis and are an important part of understanding the host environment of the lesion.

Imaging

Orthogonal standing plain radiographs always should be obtained, even if axial radiographs are available, because instability may be more apparent with standing rather than supine positioning. MRI with and without gadolinium contrast can delineate soft-tissue components. Contrast-enhanced MRI can be useful for biopsy targeting of the tissue with the greatest diagnostic potential. Dedicated CT with coronal and sagittal reformatting often provides more information about bony architecture than MRI. If malignancy or metastasis is suspected, CT of the chest, abdomen, and pelvis with contrast is necessary for staging or finding the primary source of the metastasis. A bone scan is useful for identifying other sites of bony disease, particularly if biopsy of a spine lesion is being considered. The bone scan may identify lesions in an extremity, where biopsy would be safer than in the spine. If the serum or urine immunoelectrophoresis is positive, a skeletal survey is useful to assess the extent of bony involvement from multiple myeloma. Bone scan results often are normal in patients with multiple myeloma. Recently developed MRI sequences can screen the entire spine to look for sites of metastasis. These sequences often include only sagittal studies, and axial MRI may be necessary after the disease burden has been defined.

5: Spine

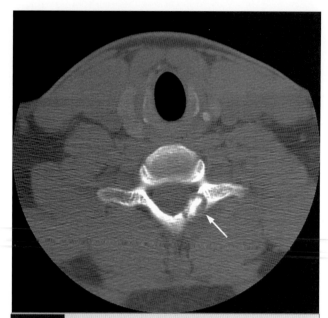

Figure 1   Axial CT showing an osteoid osteoma in the posterior elements of C7 (arrow). An osteoid osteoma is bone forming and usually smaller than 1.5 cm.

Location-Related Spine Tumor Characteristics

A bone tumor in a vertebral body most often is benign but is more likely to be malignant than a tumor found in the posterior elements. The malignant diagnoses include chordoma, osteosarcoma, and multiple myeloma–plasmacytoma. Almost all spine metastases occur in the vertebral body. The benign pathologies include hemangioma, giant cell tumor, and eosinic granuloma.

Most posterior element lesions are benign; only 35% are malignant.[1] The malignant diagnoses include Ewing sarcoma and chondrosarcoma, and the benign diagnoses include aneurysmal bone cyst, osteoid osteoma, osteoblastoma, and osteochondroma.

Benign Bone Tumors of the Spine

A patient with a benign tumor of the spine may have pain, deformity, neurologic dysfunction, or no symptoms. Some lesions are found incidentally on imaging studies. The treatment ranges from observation to excision, depending on the symptoms and the histology.

The optimal surgical management of a benign bone tumor of the spine is less clear than that of a malignant bone tumor, in which en bloc resection often is the treatment of choice. Benign bone tumors have a very low to nonexistent risk of metastasis, and the focus is on local control of the tumor. After a benign bone tumor is diagnosed, the first question is whether any treatment is warranted. Most benign tumors are indolent and can simply be observed. However, a locally aggressive benign tumor, such as an osteoblastoma, an aneurysmal bone cyst, or a giant cell tumor, may require treatment to prevent local progression. An osteoid osteoma is not locally aggressive, in that it is not associated with a breach in the cortex, but it can be active and cause pain. It is important to understand the natural history of such a tumor before deciding on a treatment. Many nonsurgical treatments can be used in conjunction with surgery or alone.

Classification

The Enneking classification of benign bone tumors continues to be relevant.[2] The three categories are based on tumor aggressiveness. Stage 1 tumors are indolent and generally do not require treatment but may require observation. The stage 1 tumors include enostosis, enchondroma, hemangioma, and monostotic fibrous dysplasia. Stage 2 tumors are active and may cause symptoms but generally are contained within the bone. Osteoid osteoma is a stage 2 tumor. Stage 3 tumors are considered aggressive and are defined by their ability to break through the cortex of bone. Osteoblastoma, aneurysmal bone cysts, and giant cell tumors most often are stage 2 or 3, depending on whether there is an associated soft-tissue mass.

Enostosis

An enostosis, or a bone island, is a benign, asymptomatic lesion that is incidentally found in a patient of any age. The condition represents a developmental anomaly rather than a neoplasm and consists of compact bone in the spongiosa. Plain radiographs and CT show an osteoblastic lesion with a brush border, and MRI shows signal dropout, with hypointense imaging on T1- and T2-weighted studies. Enostosis must be distinguished from an osteoblastic metastasis. No intervention is required.

Osteoid Osteoma

Osteoid osteoma tends to occur during the second or third decade of life, with an almost 3:1 ratio of men to women. Osteoid osteoma represents 11% of all benign bone tumors. Ten percent of osteoid osteomas occur in the spine, and 90% of these are in the posterior elements (Figure 1). These tumors are most common in the thoracic and lumbar regions and less common in the cervical and sacral regions. Night pain is common, and NSAIDs offer pain relief. The pain often is described as constant and progressive, but it can have radicular features.

Osteoid osteoma is the most common cause of painful scoliosis.[3] Plain radiographs and CT may show a nidus of less than 1.5 cm; a dense center of osteoblastic bone is surrounded by a less dense matrix and rimmed by reactive sclerotic bone. The lesion is seen as intensely hot on bone scan. On MRI, the T1-weighted signal is low and the T2-weighted signal is high, with uptake seen on gadolinium-enhanced studies. Histologic findings are a nidus of woven bone with a surrounding fibrovascular matrix. The treatment options include symptom management with NSAIDs, which

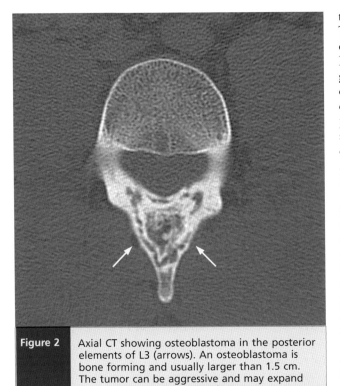

Figure 2 Axial CT showing osteoblastoma in the posterior elements of L3 (arrows). An osteoblastoma is bone forming and usually larger than 1.5 cm. The tumor can be aggressive and may expand into or destroy surrounding bone.

have been shown to successfully eliminate pain after 30 to 40 months (pain control), but associated scoliosis is not treated.[4] Radiofrequency ablation is safe and effective when used outside the spine, and it is safe in the spine if cortical bone is separating the lesion from neural elements.[5] Nonetheless, the risk of neurologic injury remains a concern. Surgical excision has had great success; local control was reported in 76 of 81 patients (94%), and the associated scoliosis rarely required treatment.[6]

Osteoblastoma

Osteoblastoma tends to occur during the second or third decade of life, with an almost 2:1 ratio of men to women. This condition represents only approximately 1% of benign bone tumors. Thirty percent to 40% of osteoblastomas are in the spine, and more than 95% of these are in the posterior elements (**Figure 2**). Tumors occur in the lumbar spine slightly more often than in the cervical or thoracic spine.[7] Osteoblastoma and osteoid osteoma share histologic features, although osteoblastoma is a larger tumor and tends to expand. Most patients have dull pain that may be progressive and often occurs at night or at rest. Radicular and even myelopathic features can occur. On bone scan, the most sensitive study, there is intense radiotracer uptake. Osteoblastoma may be associated with painful scoliosis. Plain radiographs may show a destructive expansile lesion with a narrow to broad zone of transition. On CT the lesion may be lytic, and irregularly mottled radiopacities may be seen. The MRI findings are similar to those for osteoid osteoma in that the signal is likely to be low with T1 weighting, intermediate to high with T2 weighting, and enhanced with gadolinium. A zone of increased T2 signal often appears around the tumor. It is crucial to distinguish these tumors from a low-grade malignant tumor, such as low-grade osteosarcoma, which has similar radiographic and histologic characteristics. Malignant transformation has been reported but has been disputed as an initial misdiagnosis.[8,9] When the histologic diagnosis is confirmed, surgical planning can ensue. Angioembolization has been recommended as a means of reducing intraoperative blood loss.

Osteoblastomas typically are active or aggressive (Enneking stage 2 or 3).[2] Stage 2 lesions can be managed effectively with piecemeal or intralesional resection. No local recurrences were found in the 10 patients with an Enneking stage 2 lesion treated with intralesional curettage alone, but 5 of 22 patients with an Enneking stage 3 lesion had a recurrence after treatment with intralesional curettage alone.[7] In contrast, no local recurrences occurred in five patients with Enneking stage 3 lesions who were treated with intralesional resection and postoperative radiation. Similarly, no local recurrences occurred in 10 patients treated with en bloc resection with negative margins. Two of three patients had a recurrence after en bloc excision with positive margins.[7] These data suggest that a stage 2 lesion should be treated with a piecemeal intralesional resection alone to achieve local control without the additional morbidity risk of en bloc resection or radiation. The recommendations are less clear with regard to stage 3 lesions. The question is whether a local recurrence can be managed well with further surgery. The answer depends on the size and the location of the recurrence as well as patient factors. The risks of en bloc resection and/or radiation must be balanced with the risks of recurrence for a patient with a stage 3 lesion. The type of surgery must be chosen on an individual patient basis.

Giant Cell Tumor

Giant cell tumor tends to occur after closure of the physes in patients age 20 to 40 years; it is slightly more common among women than men and is most common in patients of Asian descent. Giant cell tumor occurs in the spine, most often in a vertebral body, in 5% to 10% of patients.[10] Extraosseous extension is common. The sacrum is the most common site of disease in the spine; disease occurs more often in the thoracic or lumbar spine than in the cervical spine.

Histologically, giant cell tumors are composed of three cell populations: giant cell tumor stromal cells, mononuclear histiocytic cells, and the characteristic multinucleated giant cells. Most patients have pain, and some have neurologic compromise.[10] Most bone scans show increased uptake at the site of the lesion, although a negative bone scan is possible. The tumor is radiolucent, and the cortex may be expanded or destroyed. The features seen on CT are similar to those on radiographs, but CT may also show the extraosseous soft-tissue component of the tumor, cystic areas of hemorrhage, or an associated aneurysmal bone cyst. MRI findings may be heterogeneous with T1 and T2 weighting. Like osteoblastoma, giant cell tumor usually is seen at Enneking stage 2 or 3.[2] A recent large study reported excellent local control of Enneking stage 2 tumors and relatively poor local control of stage 3 tumors with piecemeal resection.[10] En bloc resection led to good local control of stage 3 lesions. These results mirror those reported for osteoblastoma.[7]

A promising systemic adjuvant therapy for giant cell tumors is available. Denosumab is a monoclonal antibody targeting the receptor activator for nuclear factor κ B ligand (RANKL) expressed by the giant cells in giant cell tumors.[11] A study of 35 giant cell tumors in an extremity found that 86% had responded at 25-week follow-up. Denosumab is being used before surgery in an ongoing study, and the results of this study may affect how patients with giant cell tumor in the spine are treated. One important drawback to using denosumab is that tumors seem to recur when the antibody is discontinued. The long-term adverse effects of denosumab are unknown, but at least one incidence of osteonecrosis of the jaw has been reported, and there are likely to be other complications with long-term use.[12] For this reason, denosumab may be best used as a neoadjuvant or an adjuvant treatment in conjunction with surgery.

Aneurysmal Bone Cyst

Aneurysmal bone cysts constitute 1.4% to 2.3% of all primary bone tumors, and 3% to 20% of them involve the spine.[13] These tumors usually appear during the second decade of life but can occur at any age. The ratio of women to men is 1.04:1. Aneurysmal bone cysts of the spine most often occur in the posterior elements of the thoracic region, followed by the lumbar, cervical, and sacral regions. This vascular tumor is composed of spindle-lined cysts and osteoid. Approximately one third of all aneurysmal bone cysts are found in conjunction with another tumor, most commonly a giant cell tumor. Other associated lesions are osteoblastoma, chondroblastoma, angioma, nonossifying fibroma, chondromyxoid fibroma, fibrous dysplasia, osteosarcoma, and metastatic carcinoma.[14]

The initial symptoms vary with the tumor's position and size. Pain is the most common symptom, but neurologic symptoms related to spinal cord or nerve root compression occur in more than one third of patients.[15] Plain radiography often reveals an aneurysmal or ballooned thin cortex with a lytic core. CT and MRI reveal characteristic but not pathognomonic fluid-fluid levels. Contrast is used to highlight the septations and any solid component. The treatment can include embolization, sclerotherapy, surgery, and possibly radiation.

The treatment goals center on decompression of the neural structures and stabilization of weakened areas of the spine. Three large studies reported a local recurrence rate of 5%, 10%, or 14%, respectively.[13,15,16] Most recurrences occurred during the first year, but some were as late as 8 years after surgery. Arterial em-

bolization has been used as a stand-alone treatment of aneurysmal bone cyst, but no large study has evaluated this treatment in the spine.[17] Radiotherapy used in conjunction with surgery or as a stand-alone treatment has local control rates comparable to those of surgery alone.[13,18] However, the long-term risk of a radiation-associated sarcoma must be considered when radiation is used to treat a benign tumor in a relatively young person.[15] Excellent local control rates were reported in a clinical study of sclerotherapy compared with surgery alone to treat aneurysmal bone cysts in the pelvis or an extremity.[19] It is unclear whether sclerotherapy is safe to use in the mobile spine.[20]

Eosinophilic Granuloma

Eosinophilic granuloma represents the benign end of the disease spectrum of Langerhans cell histiocytosis. The estimated annual incidence of this tumor in the United States is 0.05 to 0.5 per 100,000 population.[21] The disease occurs during the first two decades of life; 80% of patients are younger than 10 years, and slightly more boys than girls are affected. The disease is rare among people of African descent. The spine is involved in 8% to 25% of incidences.[22] Cervical spine involvement is most common, followed by thoracic and lumbar spine involvement.

The characteristic appearance of vertebra plana with preserved disk spaces is the result of sparing of the posterior elements. Histologically, the tumor appears as sheets of Langerhans cells with a variable presence of lymphocytes, polymorphonuclear cells, and eosinophils. The initial symptom often is focal or radicular pain, sometimes with fever, an elevated erythrocyte sedimentation rate, leukocytosis, or normochromic anemia. Neurologic compromise is rare. The characteristic vertebra plana with preserved disk spaces can be seen on plain radiographs in 40% of patients. CT often shows a lytic area and is useful for biopsy guidance. On MRI the lesion is dark with T1 weighting and bright with T2 weighting.[22]

The treatment of eosinophilic granuloma usually is nonsurgical. Bracing or casting is used if the patient's condition is stable and there is no neurologic impairment.[22] Steroid injection at the time of biopsy has had good results.[23] The patient should be followed until skeletal maturity. Outcomes generally are excellent, with restoration of vertebral body height by the time the patient reaches skeletal maturity.[22]

Osteochondroma

Osteochondroma is the most common benign bone tumor, but only 1% to 4% of incidences are in the spine.[24] Most tumors are solitary, unless they are associated with multiple hereditary exostosis and the exostosin 1, 2, or 3 gene mutation. Most patients are in the first or second decade of life. The ratio of boys to girls is 1.5:1. The tumor most commonly occurs in the posterior elements and in the cervical spine region, followed by the thoracic and lumbar regions. Pain is the most common symptom.

Unlike osteochondroma in the extremities, a tumor in the spine often cannot be diagnosed on plain radiographs because of the complex overlapping osseous structure of the spine. CT is the imaging modality of choice because it reveals the diagnostic features of continuous cortical integrity and a communicating shared medullary canal. MRI can show the cartilage cap that normally thins with age. A cap thicker than 1 cm may be associated with malignant degeneration. Histologically, osteochondromas mimic the physis.

The lesion can be observed if it was found incidentally. If symptoms develop or there is concern about spinal cord compromise, en bloc resection should be done, with care to avoid violating the cartilaginous cap or its overlying pseudocapsule.

Hemangioma

Hemangioma of bone most often occurs in the spine. The tumor often is solitary and is found in the lower thoracic or upper lumbar vertebral bodies, usually during the fifth decade of life. Slightly more women than men are affected. Many tumors are asymptomatic and found incidentally, but some lead to pain or, uncommonly, neurologic compromise or pathologic fracture. The histologic characteristics include endothelial-lined vessels with prominent trabeculae and interspersed fat. Radiographs often show sclerotic or ivory vertebrae with characteristic coarse, thickened trabeculae that create an appearance described as corduroy or honeycomb. CT shows the coarse, thickened trabeculae in a polka dot pattern. On MRI hemangioma has a component of hyperintensity because of its fat content on T1-weighted studies, and the vascular content is reflected in the high signal on T2-weighted studies and with contrast enhancement. Usually it is not necessary to obtain contrast studies to identify hemangioma. The presence of fat within the lesion on MRI, coupled with plain radiographs and CT, is sufficient for diagnosis.

Primary Malignant Tumors of the Spine

Three surgeons laid the foundation for surgical treatment of primary malignant tumors of the spine. Surgical techniques for primary malignant spine tumors had lagged behind those for extremity sarcomas because of the rarity of spine tumors. In addition, few surgeons had sufficient expertise with the anatomy of the axial skeleton to attempt en bloc resection of tumors. The way in which primary malignant spine tumors were treated changed in the early 1970s, when the oncologic principles developed for extremity sarcomas were applied.[25,26] En bloc removal of tumors in the thoracic spine was first described from a posterior-only approach, by using a Gigli saw to cut the spine above and below the tumor.[27] The bony cut was stopped before the saw reached the spinal canal, and the remaining bone was cut using instruments directed anteriorly away from the canal. The technique was modified and improved by using a threaded fiber wire saw, which is better suited for use around the spinal cord.[28]

Staging and Classification

Tumor staging is an important aspect of all surgical decision making. A staging system should provide insight into the likelihood of local or distant recurrence, the appropriate resection plan, and guidelines for using adjuvant treatments.[29] The Enneking extremity tumor system was first adapted for the spine by Campanacci.[29,30] During the 1990s, a spine tumor classification system was developed around each of the Enneking criteria by Weinstein, Boriani, and Biagini to provide a common language for researchers as well as clinicians.[31] The system provides insight into the local aggressiveness of tumors by identifying tumors that have progressed outside the bony cortex. Most importantly, the classification of a tumor suggests whether it is suitable for en bloc resection. Oncologically appropriate margins can be determined by following the classification guidelines.[31]

The Weinstein-Boriani-Biagini system is based on an axial view of the vertebrae divided into 12 zones. Zone 1 begins at the lateral half of the spinous process, and subsequent zones proceed in a counterclockwise fashion to zone 12 at the opposite half of the spinous process. Zones 3 through 10 encompass the posterior elements, and zones 4 through 9 include the vertebral body and pedicles. According to the Weinstein-Boriani-Biagini system, four types of resection can be performed in the thoracic and lumbar spine.[32] The type of resection is dictated by the location of the tumor.

A posterior-only approach is reserved for a tumor that is restricted to the posterior elements. In this situation, the laminae above and below the tumor must be removed to allow access to the spinal canal. The pedicles of the involved level are transected and the tumor is removed.

Tumors involving the vertebral body are removed in a staged fashion with a posterior approach first, followed by an anterior approach. When a tumor involves the vertebral body, close attention must be paid to zones 4 and 9 because they represent each of the two pedicles. At least one of the pedicles must be free of tumor for an oncologically sound margin to be obtained.[31] The importance of surgical margins is well known in extremity sarcoma and has been confirmed in malignant spine tumors.[33]

A tumor involving half of the vertebral body may be amenable to hemivertebrectomy via a sagittal cut through the vertebral body. If the tumor is located eccentrically within the vertebral body, a posterior-only, sagittal resection of the vertebral body can be considered. This type of resection is commonly associated with a Pancoast tumor.[34] Another approach to vertebral body tumors involves a posterior-only approach.[35] This method involves removing the posterior elements at the level of the tumor, followed by bluntly developing an anterior plane between the vertebrae and the vessels. After this plane is developed, threaded wire saws are passed anterior to the vertebral body but posterior to the vessels. The spine is transected above and below the level of the tumor by sawing from anterior to posterior

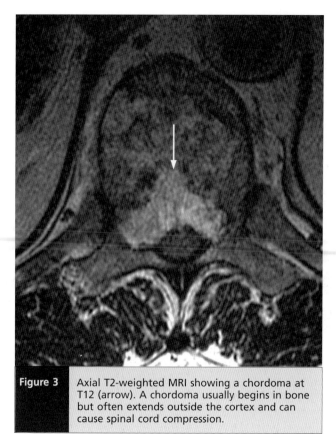

Figure 3 Axial T2-weighted MRI showing a chordoma at T12 (arrow). A chordoma usually begins in bone but often extends outside the cortex and can cause spinal cord compression.

while taking care to protect the spinal cord. This approach is attractive because it spares the patient a second stage, with the trade-off of additional technical challenges.

Surgical Margins

En bloc resection means that the tumor is removed in one piece, but it does not imply that negative margins are achieved. The status of the margins is determined after histologic review by a pathologist. Margins are classically described as wide, marginal, or intralesional. A wide margin is outside the reactive zone of the tumor, a marginal resection is within the reactive zone, and an intralesional margin is microscopically positive. From a practical perspective, it is useful to know whether the margin was positive or negative. Defining the tumor's reactive zone can be difficult because the concept is somewhat subjective. If the tumor is removed in multiple pieces rather than en bloc, it is important to note whether a gross total resection is achieved or gross residual disease remains.

The standard of care for a malignant bone tumor in an extremity or the spine is to attempt a wide resection. In practice, en bloc resection of a solitary bony tumor in the spine should be considered whenever possible. The morbidity associated with en bloc resection and the goals of the patient also must be considered.[36,37] Some malignant bone tumors respond more favorably than others to adjuvant therapies, such as radiation or chemotherapy. It is imperative that the surgeon has a

thorough understanding of the pathophysiology of the tumor and the possible usefulness of adjuvant therapies.

Chondrosarcoma

Chondrosarcoma is a malignant cartilaginous tumor whose propensity to metastasize is correlated with its grade. This tumor is characterized by a lobular pattern of growth with areas of irregular calcification throughout the lesion. Chemotherapy has not been effective and is not generally used except in experimental protocols. En bloc resection with negative margins is an effective means of control. A local recurrence rate of 8% was found when negative margins were obtained, compared with a 100% local failure rate after piecemeal removal of the tumor.[38] Radiation therapy is controversial, but the results were promising when dosages higher than 70 Gy were used in small studies.[39,40] No local recurrences were found in eight patients after en bloc resection combined with high-dosage radiation, although negative margins were obtained in only four of the patients.[40] Local control was maintained in 8 of 13 patients after intralesional resection combined with high-dosage radiation.

Chordoma

Chordomas are believed to originate in notochord cells and have a high local recurrence rate as well as a tendency to late metastasis. Chordoma in the mobile spine often appears as a soft-tissue mass with spinal cord compression (Figure 3). Chemotherapy has not been effective, although there have been modestly promising results with the use of targeted therapies.[41] Radiation therapy has been used as an adjuvant to surgery.[42] Radiation alone has been used to manage chordoma but is considered experimental.[43] Wide en bloc resection remains the standard of care for the management of sacral chordoma as well as chordoma of the mobile spine.[44,45]

Ewing Sarcoma

Ewing sarcoma is a malignancy characterized by small, round blue cells. This tumor commonly is treated with systemic chemotherapy and radiation or with surgery. Despite improvements in the ability to treat Ewing sarcoma in an extremity, a tumor in the mobile spine or sacrum has a poor prognosis, regardless of whether surgery is used. Five-year disease-free survival rates of 37% to 49% were reported in several studies.[46-48] Many patients in these studies were not treated surgically. En bloc resection led to positive results in a small number of patients, but no statistical comparison could be made.[48]

Osteosarcoma

Osteosarcoma is a malignant bone-forming tumor. The use of chemotherapy with wide resection for extremity osteosarcoma led to improvement in overall 5-year survival rates from approximately 20% in 1970 to 75% currently.[49,50] Chemotherapy combined with wide resection has been the standard of care for more than 20 years for the management of osteosarcoma in the extremities. Despite improvements in surgical technique and the increased use of en bloc resection for osteosarcoma in the spine, survival rates remain low compared with those of lesions in an extremity. Two recent studies of modern chemotherapy used with advanced surgical resection techniques found mortality rates of 71% and 73%.[51,52] In both studies, there was a trend toward an improved overall survival rate when en bloc resection was used.

Metastases to the Spine

The spine is the most common site of osseous metastasis and the third most common site of all metastases, after the lungs and the liver. At autopsy, as many as 90% of patients with cancer have evidence of spine involvement. Common primary carcinomas that metastasize to the spine include breast, lung, prostate, and kidney carcinomas. The posterior two thirds of the vertebral body most often is affected, but the intervertebral disk is spared. Lesions may be lytic, blastic, or mixed. The thoracic spine is the most common site of metastasis, followed by the lumbar and cervical spines, in a 4:2:1 ratio. Plain radiographs often fail to detect spine involvement until 30% to 50% destruction has occurred. MRI should be considered for all patients after unsuccessful nonsurgical management of localized back pain of at least 6 weeks' duration. This is particularly true for patients with a history of cancer or a so-called red flag symptom, such as night pain, unexplained weight loss, fever, or neurologic deficit.

The orthopaedic surgeon may be responsible for identifying an unknown primary cancer in a patient with metastatic lesions in the spine. Plain radiography and axial MRI of the entire spine are necessary because noncontiguous metastases are common. A bone scan is useful for assessing the burden of disease in carcinoma. It may also identify a site that is more amenable to biopsy than the spine. A skeletal survey is the better option when myeloma is suspected, which would be strongly considered if a serum protein electrophoresis is consistent with myeloma. CT of the chest, abdomen, and pelvis is an important component of the workup of a patient with an unknown primary cancer. A large renal mass or lung mass may help determine the site of the primary cancer. Laboratory studies are an important part of the initial workup and include the aforementioned serum protein electrophoresis. It is important to check calcium levels because hypercalcemia can be associated with rapid bone destruction seen in some aggressive cancers, and it is important to treat hypercalcemia promptly, starting with fluid resuscitation. Other important laboratory studies include serum hemoglobin, which may be low in patients with a gastrointestinal primary cancer. Liver function tests should be performed when liver involvement is suspected. Thyroid function tests may help identify a primary cancer of the thyroid gland. Tissue biopsy should be considered; however, the optimum site for biopsy may not become apparent until all imaging studies are completed.

Surgical Decision Making

The treatment of metastatic disease to the spine by definition almost always is palliative, and its goals must reflect this truth. Palliative care is centered on preventing and relieving suffering. These goals must be realistically communicated to the patient and the family, with consideration of the patient's expectations as well as those of the treating team. Treatment can take different forms and is best considered by a team that includes a spine surgeon, a radiation oncologist, a medical oncologist, an interventional radiologist, and a palliative pain specialist. The factors to be weighed include the patient's tumor type, disease burden, number and location of involved spine levels, neurologic status, ambulatory status, and overall health. Surgery with radiation is superior to radiation alone for some patients with spinal cord compression.[53]

One of the main considerations in deciding whether to surgically intervene is the likelihood that the patient will outlive the procedure's recovery period. This factor is easy to articulate but difficult to predict. Several scoring systems can be used in deciding on surgical intervention. A recent retrospective study compared seven prognostic scoring systems by analyzing records from 254 patients with proven spine metastases from a variety of primary cancers (not including multiple myeloma).[54] Sixty-two of the patients had been treated surgically, and 192 had been treated nonsurgically. Each system was designed to guide treatment by predicting patient survival. The factors weighed include functional scores (Karnofsky and/or Eastern Cooperative Oncology Group); the number and sites of metastases, including the viscera; the primary site of the cancer; and the presence of neurologic signs or symptoms. Only the Bauer and the modified Bauer scores achieved significance in all prediction groups; the other systems failed to significantly differentiate a good prognosis from a moderate prognosis.

The simplicity of the modified Bauer score adds to its versatility. The modified Bauer score omits pathologic fracture but otherwise is identical to the original Bauer score. Four factors are scored by assigning one point for each positive answer: absence of visceral metastasis, a solitary skeletal metastasis, primary tumor is breast, or kidney, or lymphoma, and primary cancer not lung cancer. Life expectancy is predicted as follows: a score of 0 or 1, 4.8 months; 2, 18.2 months, and 3 or 4, 28.4 months.[54]

Spine surgeons often are asked to determine whether a lesion has rendered the spine unstable. A recent classification from the Spine Oncology Study Group is useful for making this determination.[55] The Spine Instability Neoplastic Score is based six categories: location, pain relief with recumbency, type of bony lesion (lytic or blastic), spine alignment based on radiographs, extent of vertebral body collapse, and involvement of the posterolateral spine elements (**Table 1**). This system

Table 1

The Spine Instability Neoplastic Score

Criterion	Score
Location	
Junctional (occiput-C2, C7-T2, L5-S1)	3
Mobile spine (C3-C6, L2-L4)	2
Semirigid spine (T3-T10)	1
Rigid spine (S2-S5)	0
Pain relief with recumbency	
Yes	3
Occasional, but not mechanical	1
No	0
Bone lesion	
Lytic	2
Mixed (lytic and blastic)	1
Blastic	0
Radiographic spine alignment	
Subluxation or translation	4
De novo deformity (kyphosis or scoliosis)	2
Normal alignment	0
Vertebral body collapse	
More than 50%	3
Less than 50%	2
No collapse, with more than 50% of body involved	1
None	0
Posterolateral involvement of the spine elements[a]	3
Bilateral	1
Unilateral	0
None	

Spine stability prediction	Total score (0 to 18)
Stable	0 to 6
Indeterminate (possibly unstable)	7 to 12
Unstable	13 to 18

[a] Implies a fracture or replacement of the facet, the pedicle, or the costovertebral joint with tumor.
(Adapted with permission from Fourney DR, Frangou EM, Ryken TC, et al: Spinal Instability Neoplastic Score: An analysis of reliability and validity from the Spine Oncology Study Group. *J Clin Oncol* 2011;29[22]:3072-3077.)

was reported to have excellent interobserver and intraobserver reliability, 95.7% sensitivity, and 79.5% specificity for predicting lesion stability.[56]

The risk of complications after surgery for spine metastasis most be considered. One study reviewed various factors, including the Charlson index, as a means of predicting complications after surgical procedures for spinal metastases. The Charlson index assigns values to known medical comorbidities. A complication rate of 34% was reported, and the Charlson index was found to be the most robust predictor of postoperative complications in the first 30 days after the surgery.[57,58] Higher complication rates were found in prospective rather than retrospective studies, and the rates were found to be related to surgical approach.[59] A prospective study of 128 consecutive patients found major complication rates of 18.7% after posterior surgery, 50.0% after anterior surgery, and 29.8% after a combined approach was used for thoracic or lumbar surgery.[59]

The effect of surgical treatment of metastatic disease on a patient's quality of life is of primary concern because a cure is rarely, if ever, obtained. A recent large multicenter prospective study found improved quality of life after surgery in patients who were carefully selected.[60] The use of a minimally invasive technique offers the theoretic benefit of a relatively short hospital stay and decreased postoperative morbidity. Although such techniques hold promise, the level of evidence supporting their use is low.[61,62]

Cement augmentation of pathologic vertebral compression fractures recently was evaluated through the Cancer Patient Fracture Evaluation study.[63] Kyphoplasty was compared with nonaugmentation-based treatment. The primary outcome measure was back-specific functional status, as measured on the Roland-Morris Disability Questionnaire at 1-month follow-up. The scores of patients who received kyphoplasty improved from 17.6 to 9.1, compared with a decrease from 18.2 to 18.0 in the scores of patients who received the usual treatment. Kyphoplasty was favored as a safe and effective treatment.[63]

Radiation for Spine Tumors

Conventional external beam radiation remains the standard of care for painful vertebral metastasis. Most centers use dosages of 30 to 40 Gy delivered in 5 to 10 fractions. Conventional radiotherapy was found to relieve pain in 50% to 70% of patients; 60% to 80% of patients remained ambulatory, and 20% to 60% regained ambulation.[64] The field of radiation oncology has changed dramatically during the past several decades with the development of high-precision radiation delivery. Most radiation therapy is delivered with photons, although some centers use carbon ion radiation. The physical properties of the proton or the carbon ion allow precise delivery of radiation. Photon radiation can be delivered even more precisely by stabilizing the patient in a custom-molded brace, using real-time CT so that the position of the tumor is known rather than assumed, using a table that can be adjusted with six degrees of freedom to allow for precise patient positioning, using radiation beam filters designed to shield normal structures, and altering the beams themselves (as in intensity-modulated radiation therapy). The goal of these measures is to reliably protect the normal structures around the tumor, thus allowing higher radiation dosages to be delivered directly to the tumor and increasing the efficacy of the therapy. In this way, tumors that were once radiation resistant have become radiation sensitive. No cell is completely radiation resistant; the dosage-limiting factor is not the amount of radiation that can be delivered but the ability to protect normal structures from off-target effects of radiation.

These changes in radiation oncology will affect the care of patients with spine tumors. In patients with metastasis, limited surgery is being combined with postoperative radiation therapy.[65] Surgery is used to separate the tumor from the spinal cord, thus allowing radiation to be delivered more safely. Significant debulking of the tumor is not attempted, in favor of using radiation for local control. Conventional radiation therapy remains the standard of care and is highly effective for palliating pain. The indications for high-precision radiation therapy are evolving. In patients who have recurrence after radiation therapy or surgery, a radiation-resistant tumor, or oligometastatic disease, high-precision radiation therapy may have an important role.[66,67]

Summary

General principles and recent advances in the management of primary spinal tumors were reviewed in this chapter. Over the past several decades, surgical techniques have evolved and en bloc resection is being used more frequently. However, the field continues to change as advances in radiation therapy and chemotherapy are ongoing; therefore, it is important to remain vigilant regarding the treatment of these tumors.

Key Study Points

- Radiation therapy continues to evolve and will likely play a larger role in the management of spinal tumors.

- En bloc resection should be performed selectively, particularly when the tumor is metastatic.

- Adjuvant therapies such as RANKL inhibitors are changing the field, and the surgeon must remain up to date on these modalities to provide the best patient care.

Annotated References

1. Weinstein JN, McLain RF: Primary tumors of the spine. *Spine (Phila Pa 1976)* 1987;12(9):843-851.

2. Enneking WF, Spanier SS, Goodman MA: A system for the surgical staging of musculoskeletal sarcoma: 1980. *Clin Orthop Relat Res* 2003;415:4-18.

3. Ransford AO, Pozo JL, Hutton PA, Kirwan EO: The behaviour pattern of the scoliosis associated with osteoid osteoma or osteoblastoma of the spine. *J Bone Joint Surg Br* 1984;66(1):16-20.

4. Frassica FJ, Waltrip RL, Sponseller PD, Ma LD, McCarthy EF Jr: Clinicopathologic features and treatment of osteoid osteoma and osteoblastoma in children and adolescents. *Orthop Clin North Am* 1996;27(3):559-574.

5. Hadjipavlou AG, Tzermiadianos MN, Kakavelakis KN, Lander P: Percutaneous core excision and radiofrequency thermo-coagulation for the ablation of osteoid osteoma of the spine. *Eur Spine J* 2009;18(3):345-351.

6. Gasbarrini A, Cappuccio M, Bandiera S, Amendola L, van Urk P, Boriani S: Osteoid osteoma of the mobile spine: Surgical outcomes in 81 patients. *Spine (Phila Pa 1976)* 2011;36(24):2089-2093.

   A large study of patients with osteoid osteoma found conventional open surgery to be successful and described the use of minimally invasive surgical techniques.

7. Boriani S, Amendola L, Bandiera S, et al: Staging and treatment of osteoblastoma in the mobile spine: A review of 51 cases. *Eur Spine J* 2012;21(10):2003-2010.

   Adequate local control was achieved with intralesional techniques for Enneking stage 2 tumors. Stage 3 tumors required more aggressive en bloc treatment or adjuvant radiation to achieve local control.

8. Merryweather R, Middlemiss JH, Sanerkin NG: Malignant transformation of osteoblastoma. *J Bone Joint Surg Br* 1980;62(3):381-384.

9. Mayer L: Malignant degeneration of so-called benign osteoblastoma. *Bull Hosp Joint Dis* 1967;28(1):4-13.

10. Boriani S, Bandiera S, Casadei R, et al: Giant cell tumor of the mobile spine: A review of 49 cases. *Spine (Phila Pa 1976)* 2012;37(1):E37-E45.

    Adequate local control of Enneking stage 2 tumors was achieved using intralesional techniques. Stage 3 tumors required more aggressive treatment. The risks of en bloc resection should be carefully compared with the benefit of local control.

11. Thomas D, Henshaw R, Skubitz K, et al: Denosumab in patients with giant-cell tumour of bone: An open-label, phase 2 study. *Lancet Oncol* 2010;11(3):275-280.

    This study demonstrated the effect of denosumab, a monoclonal antibody against RANKL, in giant cell tumors. The authors reported objective radiographic responses as well as histologic changes that result in a decrease in the number of giant cells in patients treated with this new therapy.

12. Neuprez A, Coste S, Rompen E, Crielaard JM, Reginster JY: Osteonecrosis of the jaw in a male osteoporotic patient treated with denosumab. *Osteoporos Int* 2013, July 9 [Epub ahead of print].

    The authors report a rare case of osteonecrosis of the jaw in a male patient after treatment with denosumab.

13. Boriani S, De Iure F, Campanacci L, et al: Aneurysmal bone cyst of the mobile spine: Report on 41 cases. *Spine (Phila Pa 1976)* 2001;26(1):27-35.

14. Bonakdarpour A, Levy WM, Aegerter E: Primary and secondary aneurysmal bone cyst: A radiological study of 75 cases. *Radiology* 1978;126(1):75-83.

5: Spine

validity from the spine oncology study group. *J Clin Oncol* 2011;29(22):3072-3077.

The Spine Instability Neoplastic Score was found to have almost perfect interobserver and intraobserver reliability in determining three clinically relevant categories of stability.

57. Arrigo RT, Kalanithi P, Cheng I, et al: Charlson score is a robust predictor of 30-day complications following spinal metastasis surgery. *Spine (Phila Pa 1976)* 2011; 36(19):E1274-E1280.

The Charlson index was retrospectively applied to 200 patient records to determine whether it predicted 30 complications. Patients with a score of 2 or higher were five times more likely to have a complication compared with patients with a lower score.

58. Charlson ME, Pompei P, Ales KL, MacKenzie CR: A new method of classifying prognostic comorbidity in longitudinal studies: Development and validation. *J Chronic Dis* 1987;40(5):373-383.

59. Campbell PG, Malone J, Yadla S, et al: Early complications related to approach in thoracic and lumbar spine surgery: A single center prospective study. *World Neurosurg* 2010;73(4):395-401.

This study demonstrated higher complication rates associated with anterior/posterior approaches than posterior-only approaches to the spine. The authors took great care to document their complications and reported rates well over 50%.

60. Ibrahim A, Crockard A, Antonietti P, et al: Does spinal surgery improve the quality of life for those with extradural (spinal) osseous metastases? An international multicenter prospective observational study of 223 patients: Invited submission from the Joint Section Meeting on Disorders of the Spine and Peripheral Nerves, March 2007. *J Neurosurg Spine* 2008;8(3):271-278.

61. Zairi F, Arikat A, Allaoui M, Marinho P, Assaker R: Minimally invasive decompression and stabilization for the management of thoracolumbar spine metastasis. *J Neurosurg Spine* 2012;17(1):19-23.

In 10 patients, the spinal canal was decompressed using a tubular retractor system and percutaneous fixation. The compression was caused by metastasis.

62. Schwab JH, Gasbarrini A, Cappuccio M, et al: Minimally invasive posterior stabilization improved ambulation and pain scores in patients with plasmacytomas and/or metastases of the spine. *Int J Surg Oncol* 2011; 2011:239230.

Clinical outcomes were reported for patients with metastatic spine disease treated with minimally invasive stabilization. Patients had improved pain and function after surgery compared with their preoperative status. Level of evidence: IV.

63. Berenson J, Pflugmacher R, Jarzem P, et al: Balloon kyphoplasty versus non-surgical fracture management for treatment of painful vertebral body compression fractures in patients with cancer: A multicentre, randomised controlled trial. *Lancet Oncol* 2011;12(3):225-235.

The effect of kyphoplasty on function was measured with the Roland-Morris scoring system 1 month after treatment. Kyphoplasty was found to have superior results compared with usual care. Level of evidence: I.

64. Gerszten PC, Mendel E, Yamada Y: Radiotherapy and radiosurgery for metastatic spine disease: What are the options, indications, and outcomes? *Spine (Phila Pa 1976)* 2009;34(22, suppl):S78-S92.

65. Laufer I, Iorgulescu JB, Chapman T, et al: Local disease control for spinal metastases following "separation surgery" and adjuvant hypofractionated or high-dose single-fraction stereotactic radiosurgery: Outcome analysis in 186 patients. *J Neurosurg Spine* 2013;18(3): 207-214.

A retrospective study reviewed the use of a combination of less aggressive surgery and high-dosage hypofractionated radiation.

66. Rades D, Schild SE, Abrahm JL: Treatment of painful bone metastases. *Nat Rev Clin Oncol* 2010;7(4): 220-229.

A review from the perspective of a radiation oncologist on the management of metastatic bone disease is presented.

67. Rades D, Abrahm JL: The role of radiotherapy for metastatic epidural spinal cord compression. *Nat Rev Clin Oncol* 2010;7(10):590-598.

A review from the perspective of a radiation oncologist on the topic of epidural spinal cord compression. The authors provide insight into this disease process from a nonsurgical point of view.

5: Spine

Chapter 56

Vertebral Compression Fractures

Ejovi Ughwanogho, MD   Xiaobang Hu, MD, PhD   Isador H. Lieberman, MD, MBA, FRCSC

Introduction

Vertebral compression fractures are a common cause of morbidity and are the most common fragility fractures in postmenopausal women. Men older than 65 years are also at increased risk of vertebral compression fracture but their risk is less than that of women of the same age. The estimated annual incidence is 500,000 in the United States.[1] The incidence probably is underestimated, however, because most patients with this fracture pattern do not have clinical symptoms. One estimate was that 30% of vertebral compression fractures in women receive clinical attention. Most diagnosed fractures are found incidentally.[2] Vertebral compression fractures most often occur in women who are postmenopausal. Primary osteoporosis is the most likely etiology. The natural history of isolated vertebral compression fractures generally is benign, and most patients attain relief of symptoms as the fracture heals.

Dr. Hu or an immediate family member has received nonincome support (such as equipment or services), commercially derived honoraria, or other non–research-related funding (such as paid travel) from MAZOR Surgical Technologies. Dr. Lieberman or an immediate family member has received royalties from AxioMed, MAZOR Surgical Technologies, Stryker, and Merlot Orthopedix; is a member of a speakers' bureau or has made paid presentations on behalf of Synthes and Orthofix; serves as a paid consultant to or is an employee of AxioMed, MAZOR Surgical Technologise, Merlot Orthopedix, Trans 1, Zyga, and Crosstrees; has stock or stock options held in AxioMed, MAZOR Surgical Technologies, Merlot Orthopedix, CrossTrees, Zyga, and Pearldiver; has received nonincome support (such as equipment or services), commercially derived honoraria, or other non–research-related funding (such as paid travel) from AxioMed, MAZOR Surgical Technologies, and Merlot Orthopedix; and serves as a board member, owner, officer, or committee member of the American Academy of Orthopaedic Surgeons, the Scoliosis Research Society, the Spine Arthroplasty Society, and the North American Spine Society. Neither Dr. Ugwanogho nor any immediate family member has received anything of value from or has stock or stock options held in a commercial company or institution related directly or indirectly to the subject of this chapter.

A patient with a symptomatic vertebral compression fracture may have disabling back pain, loss of mobility, and ultimately impaired function and quality of life. In the long term, the fracture increases the risk of additional vertebral compression fractures; the highest risk is within the first year after the initial injury.[3]

Kyphosis or a scoliotic deformity can result from multiple untreated vertebral compression fractures. Progressive deformity caused by multiple fractures can lead to diminished lung volume and compromised pulmonary function. Restrictive lung disease, as shown by a reduction of forced vital capacity, occurs with multiple vertebral fractures.[4] Patients with untreated vertebral compression fractures have an increased mortality risk.[5] The economic impact of these fractures in the United States in 2005 was estimated at $1 billion.[1]

Pathogenesis

Vertebral compression fractures usually occur in patients with primary osteoporosis. Primary osteoporosis is caused by uncoupling of the osteoclast-osteoblast function, as naturally occurs with aging, and leads to an increase in osteoclast-mediated bone resorption. In osteoporosis, there is a quantitative reduction of vertebral cancellous trabeculae and a qualitative disruption of vertebral microarchitecture. Osteoclast-osteoblast uncoupling is accelerated by estrogen deficiency, which naturally occurs after menopause. Consequently, primary osteoporosis is most prevalent in women who are postmenopausal.[6] Although osteoporosis is much less prevalent in men than in women, it does occur in men older than 80 years with decreasing levels of testosterone, which has an effect on bone metabolism mediated through aromatization to estradiol.[7]

The normal vertebral body consists of a cancellous core enclosed within a compacted cancellous bone outer shell. The cancellous core consists of vertical trabecular columns with horizontal struts supporting the vertebral end plates. In contrast, the osteoporotic vertebra has diminished trabecular thickness and quantity within the cancellous core. The thickness of the compacted cancellous shell significantly diminishes with osteoporosis. This quantitative and qualitative alteration of the vertebra ultimately reduces its mechanical strength and the threshold for failure of each vertebra.

Spondylosis, as often seen in the elderly, also renders the vertebra susceptible to compression fracture. The

5: Spine

nondegenerated disk is viscoelastic and normalizes forces across the adjacent vertebra by dissipating axial forces through the anulus fibrosus. With disk degeneration and loss of viscoelasticity, the vertebral end plates are eccentrically loaded, and the periphery is subjected to higher loads that can directly and indirectly increase the risk of fracture. Preferential loading of the periphery of the end plate accelerates bone resorption in the center of the spondylotic vertebra, in accordance with the Wolff law. The loss of lordosis or outright kyphosis caused by global spondylosis, especially in the lumbar spine, results in increased loading of the anterior column.

Tumors can cause vertebral compression fractures, although this cause is unusual. A lytic primary tumor or a metastatic tumor activates osteoclasts, leading to bone resorption and an increased risk of fracture. In addition, radiotherapy and antineoplastic agents diminish bone strength and further increase the risk of fracture. Several primary and metastatic tumors commonly involve the spine. Multiple myeloma, the most prevalent primary lytic tumor, has an annual incidence of 20,000 in the United States.[8,9] Most patients have vertebral body lesions at the time multiple myeloma is diagnosed, and a compression fracture often is the initial symptom. The spine is the most common site of skeletal metastasis from tumors, including those of the breast, lung, and prostate.[10]

Secondary, drug-induced osteoporosis or osteopenia can be the cause of a vertebral compression fracture. The long-term use of glucocorticoids, chemotherapy, gonadotrophin-releasing hormone antagonist, and aromatase inhibitors accelerates bone loss.[11] In the elderly, the presence of one or more of these risk factors significantly increases the risk of an insufficiency fracture.

Clinical Evaluation

Patients with a vertebral compression fracture may have acute pain after a low-energy traumatic events such as a fall from a standing position. The patient often reports poorly localized back pain adjacent to the site of injury. The fracture may appear as intractable back pain without an identifiable antecedent traumatic event. Fracture in this setting can be secondary to extensive subfailure loading of the osteoporotic vertebral body, leading to a slow, progressive collapse.

A primary goal of the clinical evaluation of patients with a vertebral compression fracture is to assess for symptoms and signs of tumor or infection. A systemic symptom such as unexplained weight loss, fever, or dyspnea may suggest a pathologic fracture. A comprehensive physical examination should include abdominal, musculoskeletal, chest, and neurologic examinations. Neurologic deficits are uncommon in fractures resulting from primary osteoporosis.

Laboratory studies, including a complete blood cell count, erythrocyte sedimentation rate, C-reactive protein level, and serum electrophoresis, should be obtained if indicated. Additional blood tests, such as serum calcium, phosphate, vitamin D, parathyroid hormone, and creatinine, may be useful to assess for other types of metabolic bone disease. These values usually are within normal limits in a patient with primary osteoporosis.

Vertebral compression fractures often are seen incidentally on imaging studies obtained for another indication. Plain radiographs of the spine should be obtained for a patient with a suspected vertebral fracture. Vertebral compression fractures are characterized by a loss of anterior vertebral body height, typically less than 50% of total anterior height (Figure 1, A). The radiographs should be scrutinized to determine the extent of anterior height collapse; global and focal sagittal alignment; and involvement of the posterior cortex or posterior elements, including the pedicles, facets, and laminae. Lytic lesions at the involved or adjacent vertebra may indicate the presence of a tumor. Radiographic findings that suggest an unstable pattern include a fracture of the posterior elements or the spinous processes, with significant local segmental kyphosis. Often, multiple fractures of indeterminate age are identified on radiographs (Figure 1, B).

Vertebral body height collapse may not be clearly identifiable on plain radiographs, and advanced imaging may be needed to identify a subtle compression fracture.[12] Increased signal intensity within the vertebral body on T2-weighted MRI may indicate a vertebral fracture. This finding is verified by increased signal intensity on the T2-weighted short tau inversion recovery (STIR) sequence, which suggests edema and fracture acuity (Figure 2). In addition, MRI is useful for differentiating tumor from infection. MRI findings suggestive of infection include increased signal intensity within the disk and a peripherally enhancing epidural collection. The avascular nature of the disk precludes tumor involvement. However, findings of bone loss or osteolysis in the posterior elements, paravertebral soft tissue, or multiple vertebral bodies may suggest tumor involvement (Figure 3). MRI also shows extrinsic compression of the neurologic elements in the spinal canal or the foramen.

Nonsurgical Treatment

The initial treatment of a vertebral compression fracture involves pain control, early mobilization, and rehabilitation. Analgesic agents such as NSAIDs and acetaminophen can be used for pain management during the acute phase, despite inconclusive evidence of their efficacy.[13] These medications should be used judiciously because of their adverse effects, particularly in patients of advanced age. The use of narcotic pain medications should be minimized because of their sedating effects and addictive properties. Patients with a compression fracture should be mobilized early to minimize complications associated with prolonged immobilization, such as further bone loss, general deconditioning, the development of pressure sores, and pulmonary compromise. Rehabilitation should emphasize strengthening of the

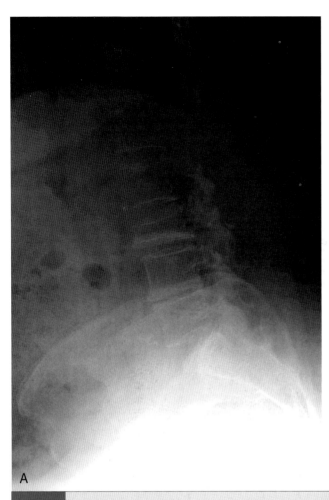
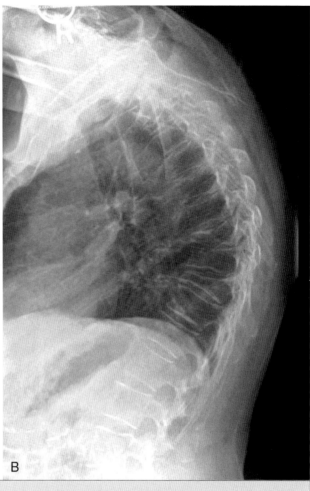

Figure 1   **A,** Lateral radiograph showing a compression fracture at L3 in a 70-year-old woman. There is an approximate 40% loss of L3 anterior height. Note the integrity of the posterior cortex and the posterior elements. **B,** Lateral radiograph showing multiple compression fractures and thoracic hyperkyphosis in a 56-year-old woman.

core muscles, especially the extensor muscles, to improve dynamic stabilization of the spine.[14,15]

The use of bracing to manage a vertebral compression fracture remains controversial. The brace unloads the compromised anterior column by placing a lordotic moment on the spine and theoretically minimizes gross spine motion at the injured segment. A custom-molded thoracolumbosacral orthosis or a Jewett hyperextension-type orthosis frequently is used in managing an acute fracture, but patient compliance is unpredictable and generally poor, even with the use of a modern low-profile brace. A brace often is ineffective in a patient who is obese, and it can be difficult for a patient with functional limitations to put on or remove. The evidence is insufficient to show the efficacy of brace treatment in patients with an osteoporotic vertebral compression fracture. However, a prospective randomized controlled study found increased core muscle strength, pain reduction, and improved posture in patients treated with bracing of an osteoporotic vertebral compression fracture.[13,16]

Prevention and treatment of osteoporosis are primary goals in the medical management of patients in

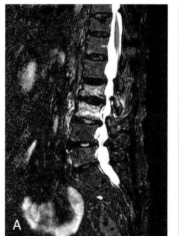
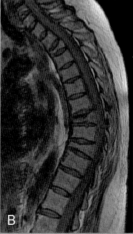

Figure 2   **A,** Sagittal STIR MRI showing edema within the L2-L3 vertebral body and an absence of disk space involvement in an 85-year-old woman with back pain. **B,** Sagittal T2-weighted MRI showing a lack of edema in a caudal fracture in the patient shown in Figure 1, B, which suggests that the fracture was chronic.

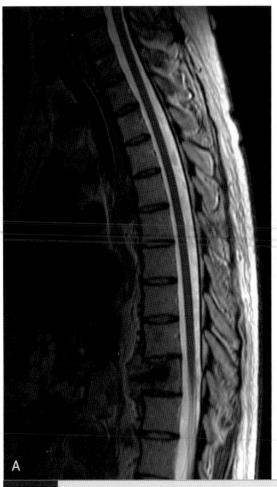
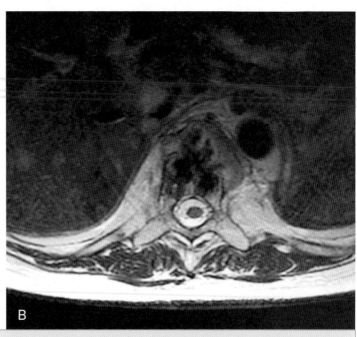

Figure 3   Sagittal (**A**) and axial (**B**) T2-weighted MRI showing a lesion at T10 with a retroperitoneal mass suggestive of a tumor in a 33-year-old man with persistent back pain.

whom a vertebral compression fracture has been diagnosed. The presence of a such a fragility fracture without a history of high-energy trauma is diagnostic of osteoporosis and significantly increases the risk of additional fragility fracture.[17] Consequently, the prompt treatment of osteoporosis is paramount in these patients.

Surgical Treatment

Most patients with an osteoporotic vertebral compression fracture are asymptomatic and initially have few or no functional limitations. However, a substantial number of patients with vertebral compression fractures have persistent symptoms despite appropriate medical management. These patients are candidates for percutaneous vertebral augmentation.[18] Vertebral augmentation involves fluoroscopically guided percutaneous infusion of polymethyl methacrylate cement into the collapsed cancellous cavity of the affected vertebrae. The technique was first described in 1987 for the treatment of vertebral hemangioma.[19] Traditional vertebroplasty with cement interdigitation within the cancel-

lous bone stabilizes the fracture, minimally restores vertebral height, and ultimately relieves pain. In 1998, kyphoplasty was introduced as an extension of the vertebroplasty technique[20,21] (**Figure 4**). Kyphoplasty involves inflating a balloon within the collapsed vertebra before the infusion of cement. Cancellous impaction by the balloon before cement infusion creates a cavity and theoretically allows lower filling pressures than vertebroplasty, thus reducing the risk of a cement leak. The use of the balloon in an acute or central fracture configuration may allow a close-to-normal vertebral height to be restored, especially in an acute fracture.[22,23]

The natural history of isolated vertebral compression fractures generally is benign, and most patients gain relief of symptoms as the fracture heals. However, patients may benefit from vertebral augmentation if nonsurgical treatment of approximately 6 weeks' duration does not lead to symptom relief. Patients of advanced age who cannot tolerate prolonged nonsurgical treatment and patients who are immobile because of pain from the fracture may benefit from earlier treatment. Before augmentation, the fracture acuity and configuration should be confirmed by MRI of the index vertebra showing increased signal intensity on T2-

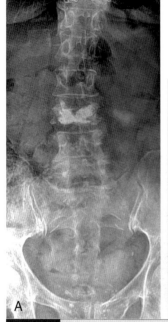
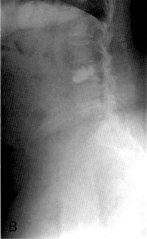

Figure 4   AP (**A**) and lateral (**B**) radiographs after kypho-plasty at L3 in the patient shown in Figure 1, **A**.

weighted and T2-weighted STIR studies. On examination, the pain should be localized to the fractured vertebra by tenderness to palpation over the spinous process. Vertebral augmentation allows normalization of spine alignment and force transmission through the spine by virtue of passive correction resulting from surgical positioning or direct correction resulting from the use of an inflatable balloon. The risk of progressive deformity and its adverse sequelae is thus reduced.[24,25]

The efficacy of vertebral augmentation has been well documented but was challenged in 2009 in two highly publicized studies.[26-29] A prospective randomized controlled study of 131 patients found no significant differences in pain scores between patients treated with vertebroplasty and those treated with a sham procedure, immediately after surgery and at all points up to 6-month follow-up.[28] A prospective randomized controlled study of 78 patients also found no beneficial effects of vertebroplasty over placebo treatment at 1-week and 1-, 3- and 6-month follow-up.[29] Postpublication scrutiny revealed limitations in both studies that tempered the validity of their conclusions.[30]

In contrast, several recent studies reaffirmed the efficacy of vertebral augmentation. Patients with an acute (of less than 6 weeks' duration), intractable, MRI-diagnosed vertebral compression fracture had a 5.7-point reduction in pain on the visual analog scale (VAS) after treatment with vertebroplasty, compared with a 3.7-point reduction for similar patients who were treated nonsurgically.[31] This study is more generalizable and consistent with current surgical and medical care practice patterns than the two 2009 studies. Nonsurgical treatment consisted of as-needed oral analgesia, as directed by an internist. Patients in both treatment

arms received bisphosphonates and calcium supplementation. A prospective randomized study in 308 patients found greater improvement on the VAS, the Medical Outcomes Study 36-Item Short Form physical component, and narcotic use after kyphoplasty compared with nonsurgical care.[32]

Two additional recent prospective randomized controlled studies that compared vertebral augmentation with the usual nonsurgical treatment also supported the efficacy of augmentation. Significant pain resolution was found at 12-month follow-up in patients who received vertebral augmentation or nonsurgical treatment, but those who underwent vertebral augmentation had more rapid pain resolution.[33] A study of 105 patients compared the efficacy of vertebroplasty and optimal nonsurgical treatment for acute vertebral compression fractures at several points up to 36 months. Over a 24-month period, patients treated with vertebral augmentation had greater improvement in VAS and quality-of-life scores than those who received optimal nonsurgical treatment. In the patients treated with vertebral augmentation, vertebral height was maintained over 36 months without an increase in the risk of adjacent segment fracture.[17]

Vertebral augmentation also is useful for treating osteolytic vertebral collapse caused by tumor.[34,35] These fractures are unlikely to heal spontaneously, and the patient often is too frail to undergo a major open reconstructive spine procedure. As with all bony tumors, a definitive diagnosis must be obtained before treatment is initiated. The diagnosis must differentiate among a primary bone tumor (which may require a curative treatment strategy), multiple myeloma, and a metastatic lesion, which should be treated palliatively. A solitary lesion without evidence of a primary tumor must be biopsied to obtain a diagnosis. A percutaneous transpedicular approach can be used for the biopsy. The presence of multiple spine lesions with or without a known primary origin suggests multiple myeloma or metastasis. Vertebral augmentation in the setting of metastatic or osteolytic involvement may be contraindicated if there is a tumor in the epidural space or extensive destruction of the posterior vertebral body wall. The appropriate treatment may be vertebral augmentation, chemotherapy and radiotherapy, or open surgical decompression and reconstruction, depending on the individual patient. Vertebral augmentation in a patient with primary or secondary osteoporosis should be avoided if the patient also has osteomyelitis, gross instability, cord compression, or neurologic deficit. Such a patient should be treated using the most appropriate and least invasive surgical procedure. Augmentation should be used judiciously if the patient has a posterior wall defect or an upper thoracic spine lesion.[36,37]

The role of vertebral augmentation in the treatment of vertebral compression fractures continues to be defined. In September 2010 the AAOS published clinical practice guidelines related to the treatment of osteoporotic vertebral compression fractures. This was based on the guideline committee's review of the available evidence up to 2009.[39] There have been several high-

5: Spine

quality articles since the guidelines were approved, and both vertebroplasty and kyphoplasty are commonly used by many practitioners. Despite studies questioning its use, the preponderance of evidence seems to confirm the efficacy of vertebroplasty and kyphoplasty. [38] Open surgical intervention is rarely indicated in patients with isolated vertebral compression fractures. In some patients, however, a progressive disabling deformity or neurologic compromise may necessitate surgical stabilization with multilevel instrumentation, and selective augmentation may enhance pedicle screw fixation. Pretreatment of these patients with an anabolic agent, such as teriparatide, may increase bone mass before surgery to facilitate a robust and predictable fusion.

Summary

Vertebral compression fractures are common and disabling. The diagnosis can be verified with an appropriate clinical examination and MRI. Pharmacologic treatment of osteoporosis is critical to prevent the sequelae of osteoporotic vertebral fractures. In patients who cannot tolerate prolonged nonsurgical treatment or have under-

Key Study Points

- Vertebral compression fractures are a common but often silent consequence of osteoporosis. Occasionally, the fracture results from a neoplasm, an infection, or trauma.

- A comprehensive history and physical examination with radiographic studies and appropriate blood work are important when evaluating a patient with a vertebral compression fracture.

- Pharmacologic treatment of osteoporosis is critical to preventing the sequelae of osteoporotic fractures. Vertebral augmentation can reduce pain and improve function in a patient for whom prolonged nonsurgical treatment is not appropriate.

gone unsuccessful nonsurgical treatment, vertebral augmentation can reduce pain and improve function.

Annotated References

1. Burge R, Dawson-Hughes B, Solomon DH, Wong JB, King A, Tosteson A: Incidence and economic burden of osteoporosis-related fractures in the United States, 2005-2025. *J Bone Miner Res* 2007;22(3):465-475.

2. Cooper C, O'Neill T, Silman A; European Vertebral Osteoporosis Study Group: The epidemiology of vertebral fractures. *Bone* 1993;14(suppl 1):S89-S97.

3. Lindsay R, Silverman SL, Cooper C, et al: Risk of new

vertebral fracture in the year following a fracture. *JAMA* 2001;285(3):320-323.

4. Schlaich C, Minne HW, Bruckner T, et al: Reduced pulmonary function in patients with spinal osteoporotic fractures. *Osteoporos Int* 1998;8(3):261-267.

5. Edidin AA, Ong KL, Lau E, Kurtz SM: Mortality risk for operated and nonoperated vertebral fracture patients in the medicare population. *J Bone Miner Res* 2011;26(7):1617-1626.

   Mortality was higher in patients age 65 years or older with a vertebral compression fracture who did not undergo surgical treatment compared with those who underwent vertebral augmentation. The study included 858,978 patients treated from 2005 to 2008.

6. McDonnell P, McHugh PE, O'Mahoney D: Vertebral osteoporosis and trabecular bone quality. *Ann Biomed Eng* 2007;35(2):170-189.

7. Greendale GA, Edelstein S, Barrett-Connor E: Endogenous sex steroids and bone mineral density in older women and men: The Rancho Bernardo Study. *J Bone Miner Res* 1997;12(11):1833-1843.

8. Durie BG, Kyle RA, Belch A, et al: Myeloma management guidelines: A consensus report from the Scientific Advisors of the International Myeloma Foundation. *Hematol J* 2003;4(6):379-398.

9. Jemal A, Siegel R, Ward E, Murray T, Xu J, Thun MJ: Cancer statistics, 2007. *CA Cancer J Clin* 2007;57(1):43-66.

10. Aghayev K, Papanastassiou ID, Vrionis F: Role of vertebral augmentation procedures in the management of vertebral compression fractures in cancer patients. *Curr Opin Support Palliat Care* 2011;5(3):222-226.

    The differences between osteoporotic and tumor-related vertebral compression fractures was discussed, with implications for treatment. The prospective randomized Cancer Fracture Evaluation study showed the efficacy and safety of vertebral augmentation in the management of tumor-related vertebral compression fractures.

11. Orcel P, Funck-Brentano T: Medical management following an osteoporotic fracture. *Orthop Traumatol Surg Res* 2011;97(8):860-869.

    This review article states that the medical management for patients with osteoporotic fractures is often insufficient. The authors suggest that orthopaedic and trauma surgeons must emphasize to these patients there need to consult with their general practitioner or rheumatologist to decide on the diagnosis and treatment of their osteoporosis.

12. Mao H, Zou J, Geng D, et al: Osteoporotic vertebral fractures without compression: Key factors of diagnosis and initial outcome of treatment with cement augmentation. *Neuroradiology* 2012;54(10):1137-1143.

    A retrospective study of 45 patients who underwent vertebral augmentation for a vertebral compression fracture showed the role of MRI in identifying fracture acuity. Bony edema on STIR or TI-weighted studies were found to be specific for acute fracture.

13. Esses SI, McGuire R, Jenkins J, et al: The treatment of symptomatic osteoporotic spinal compression fractures. *J Am Acad Orthop Surg* 2011;19(3):176-182.

    The American Academy of Orthopaedic Surgeons provided recommendations on the management of vertebral compression fractures based on the best available evidence.

14. Sinaki M, Brey RH, Hughes CA, Larson DR, Kaufman KR: Balance disorder and increased risk of falls in osteoporosis and kyphosis: Significance of kyphotic posture and muscle strength. *Osteoporos Int* 2005;16(8): 1004-1010.

15. Sinaki M, Itoi E, Wahner HW, et al: Stronger back muscles reduce the incidence of vertebral fractures: A prospective 10 year follow-up of postmenopausal women. *Bone* 2002;30(6):836-841.

16. Pfeifer M, Begerow B, Minne HW: Effects of a new spinal orthosis on posture, trunk strength, and quality of life in women with postmenopausal osteoporosis: A randomized trial. *Am J Phys Med Rehabil* 2004;83(3): 177-186.

17. Farrokhi MR, Alibai E, Maghami Z: Randomized controlled trial of percutaneous vertebroplasty versus optimal medical management for the relief of pain and disability in acute osteoporotic vertebral compression fractures. *J Neurosurg Spine* 2011;14(5):561-569.

    A prospective randomized controlled study compared vertebroplasty and optimal medical treatment for acute painful vertebral compression fractures in 82 patients. Those who underwent vertebroplasty had better early and long-term improvement on VAS and quality-of-life scores, with less risk of adjacent segment fracture.

18. Muijs SP, van Erkel AR, Dijkstra PD: Treatment of painful osteoporotic vertebral compression fractures: A brief review of the evidence for percutaneous vertebroplasty. *J Bone Joint Surg Br* 2011;93(9):1149-1153.

    This brief review discusses the history of percutaneous vertebroplasty as well as two 2009 studies.

19. Galibert P, Deramond H, Rosat P, Le Gars D: Preliminary note on the treatment of vertebral angioma by percutaneous acrylic vertebroplasty. *Neurochirurgie* 1987; 33(2):166-168.

20. Garfin SR, Yuan HA, Reiley MA: New technologies in spine: Kyphoplasty and vertebroplasty for the treatment of painful osteoporotic compression fractures. *Spine (Phila Pa 1976)* 2001;26(14):1511-1515.

21. Lieberman IH, Dudeney S, Reinhardt MK, Bell G: Initial outcome and efficacy of "kyphoplasty" in the treatment of painful osteoporotic vertebral compression fractures. *Spine (Phila Pa 1976)* 2001;26(14):1631-1638.

22. Kim KH, Kuh SU, Chin DK, et al: Kyphoplasty versus vertebroplasty: Restoration of vertebral body height and correction of kyphotic deformity with special attention to the shape of the fractured vertebrae. *J Spinal Disord Tech* 2012;25(6):338-344.

    A retrospective study compared height restoration, sagittal alignment, and cement extravasation in 103 patients undergoing kyphoplasty or vertebroplasty. Kyphoplasty was superior in all three outcomes.

23. Ma XL, Xing D, Ma JX, Xu WG, Wang J, Chen Y: Balloon kyphoplasty versus percutaneous vertebroplasty in treating osteoporotic vertebral compression fracture: Grading the evidence through a systematic review and meta-analysis. *Eur Spine J* 2012;21(9):1844-1859.

    A meta-analysis compared the efficacy and the safety of vertebroplasty and balloon kyphoplasty. Twelve studies involving 1,081 patients met the inclusion criteria. Both procedures were found to effectively treat vertebral fractures, but kyphoplasty may better restore vertebral height and sagittal alignment.

24. Kayanja MM, Togawa D, Lieberman IH: Biomechanical changes after the augmentation of experimental osteoporotic vertebral compression fractures in the cadaveric thoracic spine. *Spine J* 2005;5(1):55-63.

25. Kayanja MM, Evans K, Milks R, Lieberman IH: Adjacent level load transfer following vertebral augmentation in the cadaveric spine. *Spine (Phila Pa 1976)* 2006; 31(21):E790-E797.

26. Gill JB, Kuper M, Chin PC, Zhang Y, Schutt R Jr: Comparing pain reduction following kyphoplasty and vertebroplasty for osteoporotic vertebral compression fractures. *Pain Physician* 2007;10(4):583-590.

27. Taylor RS, Fritzell P, Taylor RJ: Balloon kyphoplasty in the management of vertebral compression fractures: An updated systematic review and meta-analysis. *Eur Spine J* 2007;16(8):1085-1100.

28. Kallmes DF, Comstock BA, Heagerty PJ, et al: A randomized trial of vertebroplasty for osteoporotic spinal fractures. *N Engl J Med* 2009;361(6):569-579.

29. Buchbinder R, Osborne RH, Ebeling PR, et al: A randomized trial of vertebroplasty for painful osteoporotic vertebral fractures. *N Engl J Med* 2009;361(6):557-568.

30. Bono CM, Heggeness M, Mick C, Resnick D, Watters WC III: North American Spine Society: Newly released vertebroplasty randomized controlled trials: A tale of two trials. *Spine J* 2010;10(3):238-240.

    This commentary questions the conclusions of two highly publicized randomized controlled studies, namely, that vertebral augmentation did not provide significantly more relief of symptoms than placebo.

31. Klazen CA, Lohle PN, de Vries J, et al: Vertebroplasty versus conservative treatment in acute osteoporotic vertebral compression fractures (Vertos II): An open-label randomised trial. *Lancet* 2010;376(9746):1085-1092.

5: Spine

This prospective randomized controlled study involved 202 patients randomly assigned to vertebroplasty or nonsurgical treatment. Vertebroplasty had greater efficacy for the treatment of acute vertebral compression fractures. Patients undergoing vertebroplasty had significantly better pain relief at 1-month and 1-year follow-up.

32. Wardlaw D, Cummings SR, Van Meirhaeghe J, et al: Efficacy and safety of balloon kyphoplasty compared with non-surgical care for vertebral compression fracture (FREE): A randomised controlled trial. *Lancet* 2009; 373(9668):1016-1024.

33. Blasco J, Martinez-Ferrer A, Macho J, et al: Effect of vertebroplasty on pain relief, quality of life, and the incidence of new vertebral fractures: A 12-month randomized follow-up, controlled trial. *J Bone Miner Res* 2012;27(5):1159-1166.

A prospective randomized study compared vertebroplasty and nonsurgical treatment in 125 patients, using the VAS at 12-month follow-up as a primary outcome measure. Both arms showed significant improvement in VAS scores at all time points. Significant improvement in the Qualeffo total score was seen in the vertebroplasty group throughout the study but was not seen in the conservative treatment arm until the 6-month follow-up.

34. Hussein MA, Vrionis FD, Allison R, et al: The role of vertebral augmentation in multiple myeloma: International Myeloma Working Group Consensus Statement. *Leukemia* 2008;22(8):1479-1484.

35. Köse KC, Cebesoy O, Akan B, Altinel L, Dinçer D, Yazar T: Functional results of vertebral augmentation techniques in pathological vertebral fractures of myelomatous patients. *J Natl Med Assoc* 2006;98(10):1654-1658.

36. Eleraky M, Papanastassiou I, Setzer M, Baaj AA, Tran ND, Vrionis FD: Balloon kyphoplasty in the treatment of metastatic tumors of the upper thoracic spine. *J Neurosurg Spine* 2011;14(3):372-376.

Fourteen patients with metastatic lesions to the upper thoracic spine were treated with kyphoplasty. All patients had significant improvement in VAS and Oswestry Disability Index scores at final follow-up, without neurologic or pulmonary complications. Cement extravasation was seen in 3 of 30 treated vertebral bodies (10%).

37. Masala S, Anselmetti GC, Muto M, Mammucari M, Volpi T, Simonetti G: Percutaneous vertebroplasty relieves pain in metastatic cervical fractures. *Clin Orthop Relat Res* 2011;469(3):715-722.

A retrospective case study evaluated clinical outcomes in 62 patients undergoing vertebroplasty for a metastatic cervical spine fracture. Most of the patients had immediate and significant pain relief after vertebroplasty. Two patients had asymptomatic cement leakage.

38. Goz V, Koehler SM, Egorova NN, et al: Kyphoplasty and vertebroplasty: Trends in use in ambulatory and inpatient settings. *Spine J* 2011;11(8):737-744.

Kyphoplasty and vertebroplasty procedures were identified from California, New York, and Florida inpatient and ambulatory discharge databases. The authors found a continued increase in vertebral augmentation procedures from 2004 to 2008. Kyphoplasty substantially outpaces the use of vertebroplasty.

39. American Academy of Orthopaedic Surgeons: Clinical Practice Guideline on Treatment of Symptomatic Osteoporotic Compression Fractures. Rosemont, IL, American Academy of Orthopaedic Surgeons, September 2010. http://www.aaos.org/research/guidelines/SCFguideline.asp.

Section 6

Pediatrics

SECTION EDITOR:
Todd A. Milbrandt, MD

Shoulder, Upper Arm, and Elbow Trauma: Pediatrics

Derek M. Kelly, MD   Joshua Meier, MD

Introduction

An understanding of the immature skeleton and fracture patterns unique to the growing skeleton is necessary in discussing pediatric fractures. In the upper extremity, experience is helpful in evaluating the normal proximal and distal humeral growth centers. The proximal humeral physis has a classic tent-shaped appearance and is responsible for 80% of the growth of the humerus. An AP radiograph of the shoulder often shows the anterior and posterior portions of the physis superimposed, which can be mistaken for a fracture. The distal humerus has multiple secondary ossification centers, and these have an ordered appearance. The mnemonic CRITOE can be used to remember the order of ossification: capitellum, radial head, internal (medial) epicondyle, trochlea, olecranon, and external (lateral) epicondyle. A contralateral radiograph of the uninjured elbow can be used for comparison if uncertainty exists.

The Salter-Harris classification is the most commonly used system for classifying pediatric physeal fractures.[1] This system is used for any fracture that involves the physis. Salter-Harris type I fractures are those that go directly through the physis and do not have a metaphyseal fragment. Salter-Harris type II fractures involve the physis and the adjacent metaphysis. Salter-Harris type III fractures consist of a fracture through the physis and the epiphysis, and type IV fractures extend through both the metaphysis and the epiphysis. Salter-Harris type V fractures have been described as a crushed epiphysis and are not commonly encountered.

Dr. Kelly or an immediate family member serves as a board member, owner, officer, or committee member of the Pediatric Orthopaedic Society of North America. Neither Dr. Meier nor any immediate family member has received anything of value from or has stock or stock options held in a commercial company or institution related directly or indirectly to the subject of this chapter.

Sternoclavicular Joint and Proximal Humeral Injuries

The medial clavicular ossification center does not appear until late adolescence, and the physis does not close until the middle of the third decade of life. For this reason, sternoclavicular injuries in children and adolescents often are physeal fractures, not true joint dislocations. Injury to the medial clavicle and the sternoclavicular joint often occurs from a direct blow or a force applied laterally to the acromion. A sternoclavicular injury is suggested by pain at that location and a history consistent with an appropriate mechanism of injury. Axial imaging often is required to further characterize the extent of the injury and the direction of displacement because clinical examinations and plain radiography often are inadequate (Figure 1).

Anterior displacement of a medial clavicular fracture often can be treated nonsurgically with excellent remodeling potential. Posterior displacement of a medial physeal injury or a true posterior sternoclavicular dislocation carries a much greater risk of serious complications because these injuries can compress the trachea,

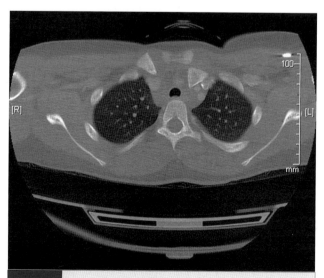

Figure 1 CT scan showing the typical appearance of a medial clavicular fracture with posterior displacement.

the esophagus, and the great vessels. Patients should be carefully questioned and examined for signs and symptoms of compression, including dysphagia, dyspnea, and asymmetric pulses and blood pressures. Posteriorly displaced injuries typically are treated with open reduction and internal fixation if stable closed reduction is unsuccessful. There is little role for nonsurgical treatment in these injuries.[2] Stable fixation often can be obtained with a large, nonabsorbable, figure-of-8 suture between the stable bony clavicle and the sternum. Smooth pin fixation is not recommended because of the proximity of vital structures and the risk of implant migration. Because of the possibility of damage to major vessels, a vascular surgeon should be immediately available to assist when these procedures are performed.

Fractures of the Clavicle

Diaphyseal clavicular fractures are common in children and occur in all age groups, including newborns. Clavicular fractures in infants can occur with obstetric injury from shoulder dystocia or nonaccidental trauma. Patients often present with pseudoparalysis of the affected limb. In a newborn with a clavicular fracture, brachial plexus injury, although rare, should be suspected and ruled out with a careful follow-up examination. Clavicular fractures in newborns can be stabilized with immobilization with a simple sling or cloth bandage. Rapid union and complete remodeling can be expected.

The management of diaphyseal and distal clavicular fractures in children and adolescents remains largely nonsurgical despite increased support for the surgical treatment of many of these injuries in adults.[3] Indications for the surgical management of clavicular fractures in children include open injuries, impending open injuries, neurovascular compromise, and some fractures with severe shortening or angulation. A comparison of surgical and nonsurgical treatment of displaced clavicular fractures in adolescents reported uniform union rates but a more rapid return to activities in the surgically treated group, and higher rates of symptomatic malunion in the nonsurgically treated group.[4] Many fixation methods have been proposed, including plate fixation and intramedullary pinning. With all methods, implant prominence and irritation are concerns and can often necessitate implant removal.[5] Despite the increasing role of surgery in treating displaced clavicular fractures in adolescents and children, nonsurgical treatment is generally appropriate because most of these injuries have minimal displacement, shortening, or angulation, and rapid union is expected in almost all patients.

Fractures of the Proximal Humerus

The proximal humeral physis contributes 80% of the overall adult length of the humerus. Excellent growth and remodeling potential along with close proximity to the highly mobile shoulder joint allows for nonsurgical management of almost all proximal humeral physeal injuries. The proximal humeral physis typically fractures in a Salter-Harris type II pattern. The Neer and

Horowitz system is used to classify the degree of displacement of the fragments.[6] Type I injuries have less than 5 mm of displacement, type II fractures are displaced between 5 mm and less than one third of the humeral shaft diameter, type III fractures are displaced from one third to two thirds of the diameter of the shaft, and type IV injuries are displaced more than two thirds of the width of the diaphysis.

Nondisplaced fractures can be treated nonsurgically with simple sling immobilization in most pediatric patients. The initial treatment of displaced proximal humeral fractures includes closed reduction and immobilization with a sling, a hanging arm cast, or a coaptation splint, followed by early graduated range of motion. Surgical treatment is indicated for open injuries and those with neurovascular compromise, as well as for irreducible or unstable injuries after attempted closed reduction (particularly in older children with less remodeling potential). Soft-tissue entrapment of the periosteum or the biceps tendon may prevent closed reduction and may require exploration and removal of the entrapped tissue, followed by internal fixation with pins or elastic intramedullary nails.[7,8] Intramedullary nails are introduced distally, driven across the reduced fracture, and left under the skin for later surgical removal. Percutaneous pins can remain outside the skin for nonsurgical removal, but the rate of skin irritation and local infection is much greater.

Complications are rare in proximal humeral fractures. Growth disturbance is uncommon. Symptomatic malunion is rare when care is taken to obtain and maintain a successful closed reduction or intervene with surgical reduction when required. Neurovascular compromise has been reported in fewer than 1% of patients and occurs most commonly with medial displacement of the humeral shaft.[9]

Elbow Injuries

Elbow injuries are common in children. The initial evaluation should always include a careful neurovascular examination, with close attention paid to the presence of a radial artery pulse and motor function of the anterior interosseous, posterior interosseous, and ulnar nerves. This examination can be challenging in a child with a painful elbow injury, but knowledge of neurovascular injuries before treatment is of paramount importance.

At a minimum, the radiographic evaluation should include AP and lateral radiographs. An internal oblique radiograph can be helpful if a minimally displaced lateral condylar fracture is suspected. A true lateral radiograph of the pediatric elbow should show the hourglass appearance of the coronoid and olecranon fossae. Obliquely obtained lateral radiographs can be difficult to interpret. The anterior humeral line (a line drawn down the anterior shaft of the humerus) should always bisect the capitellum (Figure 2, A). The anterior humeral line commonly passes through the anterior third of the capitellum in children younger than 4 years.[10] If

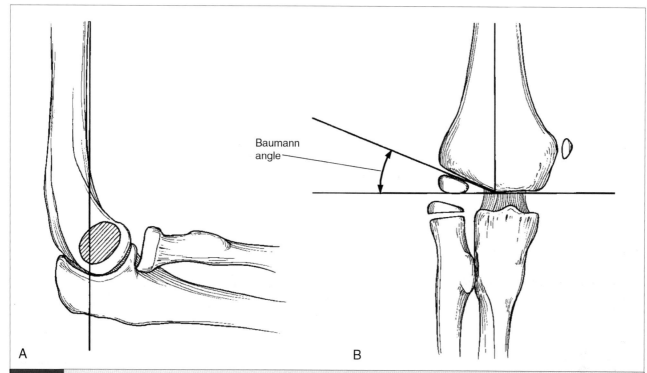

| Figure 2 | Illustrations of anatomic relationships in the elbow. **A,** A line drawn along the anterior humeral cortex normally bisects the capitellum. If the center of the capitellum is posterior to this line, an extension-type supracondylar fracture is likely; if it is anterior, a flexion-type supracondylar or transphyseal fracture is likely. **B,** The Baumann angle (shown as measured on an AP view) is formed by the intersection of the capitellar physis and a line perpendicular to the humeral axis. (Reproduced from Skaggs DL: Elbow fracture in children: Diagnosis and management. *J Am Acad Orthop Surg* 1997;5:303-312.) |

this line does not touch the capitellum, substantial deformity exists. Coronal alignment can be assessed on the AP radiograph. The Baumann angle is formed by a line drawn through the long axis of the humerus and a line drawn along the flat metaphyseal region adjacent to the capitellar physis (**Figure 2, B**). The normal Baumann angle is approximately 72° in children (range, 64° to 81°). The radiocapitellar line (a line drawn along the shaft of the radius) should intersect the capitellum on all radiographic views.

Supracondylar Humeral Fractures

Supracondylar humeral fractures are among the most common injuries in children. Most are caused by a fall with the elbow extended, causing a hyperextension force through the distal humerus. These fractures by definition do not involve the physis.

Classification

The Gartland classification describes extension-type fractures and consists of three types[11] (**Figure 3**). Type I Gartland injuries are nondisplaced or minimally displaced. Often a posterior and/or anterior fat pad sign, which is caused by the fracture hematoma displacing the fat pads of the olecranon fossa, is the only evidence of this injury in an immature elbow (**Figure 4**). Displacement of the posterior fat pad is highly suggestive

of an occult fracture.[12] Type II Gartland fractures are incomplete, with angulation of the distal segment and one intact cortex (typically the posterior cortex), with

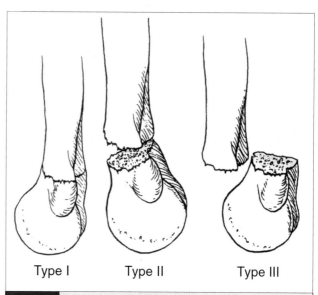

| Figure 3 | Illustration of the Gartland classification system for supracondylar humeral fractures. (See text for a description of each type of fracture.) |

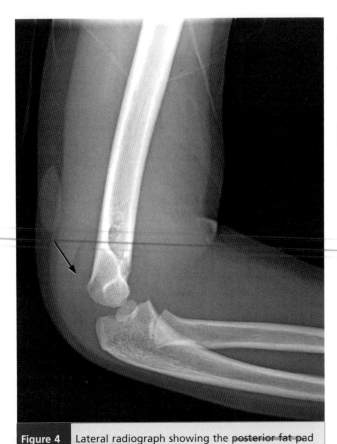

Figure 4 Lateral radiograph showing the posterior fat pad sign (arrow), which indicates hemarthrosis and often is associated with an occult supracondylar humeral fracture.

fracture of the opposite cortex. There also may be angulation in the coronal plane. Attention must be paid to medial column disruption, which can lead to varus alignment. A type III Gartland fracture is completely displaced. A modification of the Gartland classification has described a type IV fracture with multidirectional instability.[13]

Radiographic Evaluation

Proper AP and lateral radiographs, with the addition of oblique views in selected cases, are essential for evaluating supracondylar humeral fractures. Oblique radiographs can isolate the lateral and medial columns. Occasionally, comparison views of the contralateral elbow can be helpful if uncertainty exists.

Treatment

Type I fractures can be adequately treated in a long-arm cast for 3 to 4 weeks. The key principles include extending the cast proximally to the axilla and having a good supracondylar mold. Some type I fractures (such as those with a clear transverse fracture line) require close follow-up because displacement in the cast can occur.

Treatment options for types II and III fractures include closed reduction, traction, and open reduction.

Currently, closed reduction and stabilization with percutaneous pins is the most common treatment. Pin stabilization allows the elbow to be immobilized in slight extension rather than hyperflexion. Type II fractures

Video 57.1: Percutaneous Pinning of Supracondylar Humerus Fractures. John D. Koerner, MD; Sanjeev Sabharwal, MD (11.26 min)

with minimal posterior angulation can be initially treated in a long arm cast after gentle closed reduction but should be closely followed to ensure that alignment is maintained. In type II injuries, closed reduction and percutaneous pinning have had good results and a low complication rate.[14,15]

Some controversy exists in the treatment of type II fractures with mild posterior angulation, although most authors agree that closed reduction and percutaneous pinning is the treatment of choice.[16] Angulation or displacement in the coronal plane on the AP radiograph should be an indication for closed reduction and percutaneous pinning; however, mild translation and rotation can be accepted. Although the potential for fracture remodeling is high in children, hyperextension of the distal humerus shows little capacity for improvement, even with continued growth. Increased angulation and soft-tissue shadows (indicating a larger arm) may be predictors of the failure of closed treatment.[17,18]

Type III supracondylar humeral fractures can be treated with closed or open reduction and pinning. A consistent reduction technique that reproducibly first corrects the coronal plane followed by the sagittal plane, combined with modern pinning techniques, leads to good results and minimal complications.[19,20] The procedure can be performed using a full sterile setup or a semisterile technique. Postoperatively, the arm is placed in a bivalved cast or a long arm splint. Care must be taken to leave the elbow semiextended because increased elbow flexion leads to increased forearm compartment pressures.[21,22] Open reduction is occasionally required, most often because of muscle interposition. A milking maneuver can aid in removing the interposed muscle and soft tissues. Open approaches can be anterior or lateral. The anterior approach can be made through the elbow flexion crease and can directly expose the neurovascular structures and minimize scarring.[23,24] The anterior approach typically is used for open fractures because most are extension-type injuries with the open wound positioned in the antecubital fossa (**Figure 5**).

The lateral approach for supracondylar humeral fractures is the same as that used for lateral condylar fractures and often is more familiar to surgeons. A recent report showed that a posterior percutaneous approach with a mosquito forceps was a safe and effective alternative method to true open reduction.[25]

Historically, a cross-pinning technique was used with good results and excellent stabilization of the fracture fragments; however, concerns about iatrogenic ulnar nerve injury with a medial pin have led to more frequent use of two to three lateral pins for most fractures. Many studies have evaluated the various pin configurations, both from a biomechanical standpoint and with clinical outcome measures. Although crossed pins have more torsional stability, lateral entry pins appear to have appropriate stability for most fractures[26,27] (Figure 6). Typically, 0.062-inch wires are used, but in children younger than 2 years or older patients, different wire sizes may be necessary. Divergence of the pins increases stability, with one pin traversing the lateral column and the other passing through the medial column.[19] Stability can be checked under fluoroscopy after two pins are inserted, and, if necessary, a third pin can be placed to enhance stability. If a medial pin is used, it should be inserted with the elbow extended because the ulnar nerve has been shown to subluxate anteriorly as the elbow is flexed.[28] The surgeon's thumb can be placed over the nerve to displace it posteriorly; if swelling is a concern, a small incision can be made medially to identify the nerve. Increased wire size, increased pin divergence, and/or the use of a Steinmann pin have been shown to enhance stability.[29-31]

A newer technique developed for the fixation of supracondylar humeral fractures is antegrade nailing, which was reported to obtain clinical outcomes similar to those of crossed pins with a low rate (0.4%) of ulnar nerve injury.[32] In 2010, a lateral cross-pinning technique was described consisting of distal and proximal lateral entry sites. In a study of 43 patients, it resulted in no major loss of reduction, return to function, and no ulnar nerve injuries.[33]

In 2011, the American Academy of Orthopaedic Surgeons (AAOS) proposed a clinical practice guideline for the treatment of pediatric supracondylar humeral fractures.[34] Two of the recommendations were based on a consensus, although without reliable evidence: (1) immediate closed reduction of displaced pediatric supracondylar humeral fractures should be performed in patients with decreased perfusion of the hand, and (2) open exploration of the antecubital fossa should be performed in patients who have absent wrist pulses and are underperfused after reduction and pinning of displaced pediatric supracondylar humeral fractures. Two more recommendations, immobilization of the injured limb for acute fractures and closed reduction with pin fixation for type II and III fractures, were graded as having moderate evidence.

Most supracondylar humeral fractures can be treated on a semiemergent basis, provided there is min-

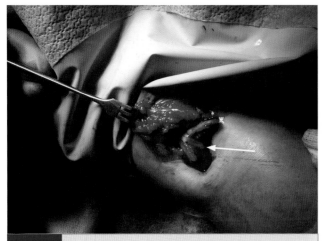

Figure 5 Photograph of an open supracondylar humeral fracture with an anterior wound. Note the median nerve draped over the metaphyseal fragment (arrow).

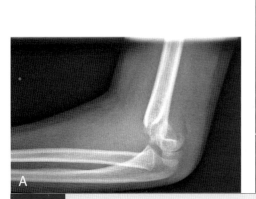
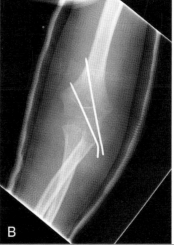
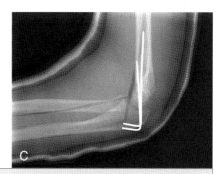

Figure 6 A, Lateral radiograph of a type III supracondylar humeral fracture. AP (B) and lateral (C) radiographs show fixation with two lateral divergent pins.

imal concern about vascular or neurologic compromise.[35] The elbow should be splinted in relative extension (20° to 40°), and hyperflexion or hyperextension should be avoided. Excessive swelling and/or ecchymosis, puckering of the skin at the fracture site, and poor pain control often indicate the need for more urgent treatment. Increased time from injury to surgery has not specifically been shown to increase surgical time or the rate of open reduction.[36-38]

Postoperative Care

Patients often are seen in the office 7 to 10 days after surgery for radiographic monitoring of the fracture and overwrapping of the cast or splint. In general, pins are left in place 3 to 4 weeks, with instructions on range-of-motion activities and gradual return to activities. In older children, pins may be left in place slightly longer if needed for healing. Range of motion often returns without the need for formal physical therapy, although it may take 4 to 6 weeks to regain functional range of motion.[39] By 6 months after surgery, range of motion was found to return to 94% of that of the contralateral elbow, with improvement to 98% at 1 year.[40]

Flexion-type supracondylar humeral fractures are much less common and often are more challenging to treat. Open reduction is often needed, and patients have a higher frequency of preoperative nerve symptoms.[41] Flexion-type supracondylar humeral fractures are reduced and then pinned in the same manner as extension-type fractures.

Complications

Overall, a low complication rate has been reported for closed reduction and percutaneous pinning.[14-16,19,20] Pin migration and infection are the most commonly reported complications.[14] More severe complications, such as malunion (often cubitus varus), compartment syndrome, and a pulseless hand, are less common but can be devastating. Cubitus varus, although often not a functional deformity, can cause distressing cosmetic problems; treatment is a distal humeral corrective osteotomy.

The treatment of a pulseless, perfused hand has been a consistent topic of research and discussion. A perfused hand is pink and has brisk capillary refill (< 2 seconds), whereas a pale hand indicates nonperfusion. A Doppler signal in lieu of a palpable pulse can be accepted with very close clinical monitoring and intervention if the signal is lost. A supracondylar humeral fracture with a nonperfused hand should be treated with urgent closed reduction and reassessment of perfusion. If pulses do not return, open exploration is indicated.[34] Multiple studies have shown that close observation for 48 hours is acceptable for a perfused hand with absent pulses.[42,43] If the examination shows increasing pain, abnormalities in the neurologic examination, or color changes in the hand, vascular exploration through an anterior approach is warranted. Arteriography is not recommended in acute fractures because the artery is almost assuredly injured at the fracture site.

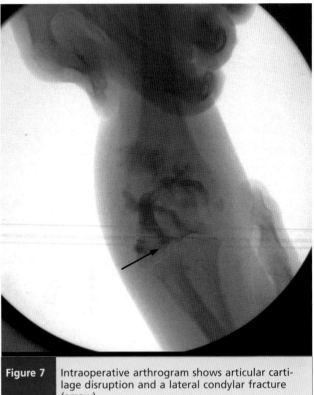

Figure 7 Intraoperative arthrogram shows articular cartilage disruption and a lateral condylar fracture (arrow).

A study from England evaluated two groups of patients with perfused, pulseless hands. The authors concluded that in patients with a concomitant nerve deficit, early exploration of the artery offered better results with no nerve deficits postoperatively.[44]

Compartment syndrome is most often heralded in children by increasing narcotic requirements to relieve pain. A changing neurovascular examination also is a concerning sign. The so-called floating elbow injury, a supracondylar humeral fracture with a concomitant forearm or wrist fracture, has a higher incidence of compartment syndrome.[45]

Fractures of the Lateral Condyle
Classification

Traditionally, lateral humeral condylar fractures had been classified by the Milch system, which defines the fracture based on the location of the fracture line relative to the capitellar ossification center; however, this system is not helpful in guiding treatment. A more modern classification system subdivides fractures based on the amount of displacement and the presence or absence of articular cartilage disruption.[46] Type I fractures have less than 2 mm of displacement and intact articular cartilage, type II fractures have more than 2 mm of displacement with intact articular cartilage, and type III fractures have articular cartilage disruption. The presence or the absence of articular cartilage disruptions can be best assessed by intraoperative arthrography (Figure 7).

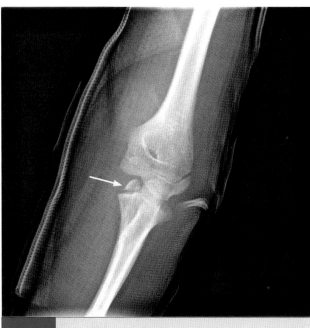

Figure 8 An incarcerated fragment (arrow) can prevent the closed reduction of a medial epicondylar fracture.

Treatment

Nondisplaced fractures can be treated with immobilization in a long arm cast; however, close radiographic follow-up is recommended because early displacement is possible. Oblique radiographs can be helpful in assessing fracture alignment. Displaced fractures with intact articular cartilage (type II) can be treated with closed manipulation and percutaneous pinning. Fractures with disrupted articular cartilage (type III) require open reduction and pinning.

Delayed union and nonunion are much more common with lateral condylar fractures than supracondylar fractures, and longer periods of immobilization are recommended. Five to 6 weeks of cast immobilization often are necessary. Elbow stiffness after a lateral condylar fracture is common. Initial rapid recovery of motion occurs in the first 6 to 12 weeks after removal of the cast and pins, but progressive improvements can be expected for up to 1 year after the injury.[47]

Complications

The most common complication after lateral condylar fractures is lateral spurring or overgrowth, which occurs in 73% of fractures. The amount of spurring seems to be related to the amount of the initial fracture displacement. Despite the appearance, the presence of a spur does not seem to compromise the final functional outcome.[48] Tardy ulnar nerve palsy related to cubitus varus is rare. Causes include nonunion, malunion, and growth disturbance. Cubitus varus and lateral spurring have limited potential for remodeling.[49] Another complication related to the surgical treatment of lateral condylar fractures is osteonecrosis of the capitellum. The risk of osteonecrosis can be minimized by avoiding

aggressive posterior soft-tissue stripping of the lateral condylar fracture during open reduction.

Transphyseal Fractures

Transphyseal fractures are rare and generally occur in children younger than 2 years. The predominantly cartilaginous nature of the distal humerus and the proximal radius makes the diagnosis of this injury challenging. A high index of suspicion is necessary to avoid missing this injury. A normal relationship between the proximal radius and the capitellum can help distinguish this injury from an elbow dislocation. Nonaccidental trauma is the cause of 50% of these injuries. Closed reduction and percutaneous pinning, with or without elbow arthrography, is the preferred treatment to prevent the high rate of cubitus varus that occurs with casting alone.

Fractures of the Medial Epicondyle

In children, medial epicondylar fractures are commonly associated with elbow dislocations. Absolute surgical indications include open injuries, those with incarcerated fragments (Figure 8), and irreducible elbow dislocations. Surgery should be considered for fractures with large displacement or those with associated ulnar nerve palsy. Nondisplaced or minimally displaced fractures (less 5 mm) often can be treated successfully with a brief 2- to 4-week period of immobilization followed by resumption of activity (with or without physical therapy to optimize range of motion).

Precisely measuring the degree of fragment displacement is challenging because of the ovoid shape of the medial epicondyle and the multiple directions of possible displacement. Interobserver and intraobserver reliability of these measurements has been questioned.[50] The degree of displacement often is underestimated on standard AP and lateral radiographs. Internal oblique radiographs often reveal a much larger degree of displacement.[50] The treatment of displaced fractures remains controversial. Surgical fixation of displaced medial epicondylar fractures has been shown to result in higher union rates, but no improvement in pain was demonstrated at intermediate follow-up.[51]

Radial Neck Fractures

Radial neck fractures with minimal displacement (< 5 mm) and minimal angulation (< 30°) can be treated with a short period (2 to 3 weeks) of immobilization and gradual return to activity. Fractures with more displacement or angulation require reduction to maintain the full pronation/supination arc of motion (Figure 9). Direct digital pressure over the fracture, in conjunction with gentle pronation and supination of the forearm under fluoroscopic guidance, can result in successful closed reduction in many fractures. When these methods are unsuccessful, more aggressive techniques must be used. A blunt-tipped pin can be placed percutaneously and used as a joystick to aid in reduction. Alternatively, a flexible intramedullary rod can be placed distally and advanced across the fracture into

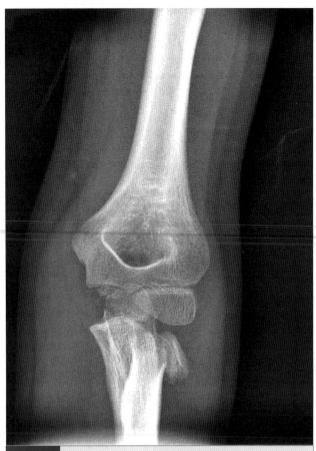

Figure 9 AP radiograph of a severely displaced radial neck fracture.

the radial head; the rod is then rotated to reduce the fragment.[52] Formal open reduction also can be done through a posterolateral approach. Care should be taken to preserve any remaining periosteal attachments. The annular ligament may be transected and repaired to gain further exposure if necessary. Regardless of the method of reduction, unstable fractures should be stabilized with an obliquely placed pin, a small diameter screw, or an intramedullary nail (Metaizeau technique). Radiocapitellar transfixation should be avoided.

Summary

Most upper extremity fractures in children can be treated nonsurgically with good functional and cosmetic results. Some specific fracture types around the elbow, including lateral condylar fractures, fare poorly with nonsurgical treatment.

Key Study Points

- Although the surgical treatment of clavicular fractures in adults has become much more accepted, there is little evidence to suggest that surgical fixation of clavicular fractures in children is superior to nonsurgical treatment.

- The surgical management of supracondylar humeral fractures with the current lateral divergent pinning techniques results in minimal complications and good results. The surgeon should be familiar with the medial pin insertion technique and open approaches for difficult fractures.

- Semiurgent or next-day fixation of supracondylar humeral fractures has not been shown to increase the rate of complications or the need for open reduction, but a nonperfused hand or signs and symptoms of compartment syndrome are indications for immediate surgical reduction.

Annotated References

1. Salter R, Harris WR: Injuries involving the epiphyseal plate. *J Bone Joint Surg Am* 1963;45:587-622.

2. Koch MJ, Wells L: Proximal clavicle physeal fracture with posterior displacement: Diagnosis, treatment, and prevention. *Orthopedics* 2012;35(1):e108-e111.

   The authors provide an algorithm for evaluating and managing proximal clavicular physeal fractures in this case report of undiagnosed posterior clavicular displacement in a 14-year-old boy. Level of evidence: V.

3. Carry PM, Koonce R, Pan Z, Polousky JD: A survey of physician opinion: Adolescent midshaft clavicle fracture treatment preferences among POSNA members. *J Pediatr Orthop* 2011;31(1):44-49.

   Most members of the Pediatric Orthopaedic Society of North America responding to a survey on the treatment of midshaft clavicle fracture in adolescents preferred nonsurgical management of all fracture patterns, with surgical fixation preferred for older adolescents and more severe injuries. Level of evidence: V.

4. Vander Have KL, Perdue AM, Caird MS, Farley FA: Operative versus nonoperative treatment of midshaft clavicle fractures in adolescents. *J Pediatr Orthop* 2010;30(4):307-312.

   In a comparison of two groups of adolescents with closed midshaft clavicular fractures treated surgically or nonsurgically, the authors reported union in all fractures, a faster return to activity in the surgically treated group, and an increase in symptomatic malunions in the nonsurgically treated group. Level of evidence: III.

5. Namdari S, Ganley TJ, Baldwin K, et al: Fixation of displaced midshaft clavicle fractures in skeletally immature

patients. *J Pediatr Orthop* 2011;31(5):507-511.

In 14 skeletally immature patients with displaced diaphyseal clavicular fractures treated with open reduction and internal fixation, scores were high on standardized outcome assessments. Four of the 14 patients required implant removal at or before 24 months. Level of evidence: IV.

6. Neer CS II, Horwitz BS: Fractures of the proximal humeral epiphysial plate. *Clin Orthop Relat Res* 1965;41: 24-31.

7. Bahrs C, Zipplies S, Ochs BG, et al: Proximal humeral fractures in children and adolescents. *J Pediatr Orthop* 2009;29(3):238-242.

8. Hutchinson PH, Bae DS, Waters PM: Intramedullary nailing versus percutaneous pin fixation of pediatric proximal humerus fractures: A comparison of complications and early radiographic results. *J Pediatr Orthop* 2011;31(6):617-622.

    In this study comparing percutaneous pinning and flexible intramedullary nailing in 50 pediatric patients with displaced proximal humeral fractures, the authors reported that those treated with intramedullary nailing had fewer complications, longer surgeries, increased estimated blood loss, and a higher rate of surgical implant removal than those treated with percutaneous pinning. Level of evidence: III.

9. Hwang RW, Bae DS, Waters PM: Brachial plexus palsy following proximal humerus fracture in patients who are skeletally immature. *J Orthop Trauma* 2008;22(4): 286-290.

10. Herman MJ, Boardman MJ, Hoover JR, Chafetz RS: Relationship of the anterior humeral line to the capitellar ossific nucleus: Variability with age. *J Bone Joint Surg Am* 2009;91(9):2188-2193.

11. Omid R, Choi PD, Skaggs DL: Supracondylar humeral fractures in children. *J Bone Joint Surg Am* 2008;90(5): 1121-1132.

12. Skaggs DL, Mirzayan R: The posterior fat pad sign in association with occult fracture of the elbow in children. *J Bone Joint Surg Am* 1999;81(10):1429-1433.

13. Leitch KK, Kay RM, Femino JD, Tolo VT, Storer SK, Skaggs DL: Treatment of multidirectionally unstable supracondylar humeral fractures in children: A modified Gartland type-IV fracture. *J Bone Joint Surg Am* 2006; 88(5):980-985.

14. Bashyal RK, Chu JY, Schoenecker PL, Dobbs MB, Luhmann SJ, Gordon JE: Complications after pinning of supracondylar distal humerus fractures. *J Pediatr Orthop* 2009;29(7):704-708.

15. Iobst CA, Spurdle C, King WF, Lopez M: Percutaneous pinning of pediatric supracondylar humerus fractures with the semisterile technique: The Miami experience. *J Pediatr Orthop* 2007;27(1):17-22.

16. Skaggs DL, Sankar WN, Albrektson J, Vaishnav S, Choi PD, Kay RM: How safe is the operative treatment of Gartland type 2 supracondylar humerus fractures in children? *J Pediatr Orthop* 2008;28(2):139-141.

17. Fitzgibbons PG, Bruce B, Got C, et al: Predictors of failure of nonoperative treatment for type-2 supracondylar humerus fractures. *J Pediatr Orthop* 2011;31(4): 372-376.

    In a retrospective study evaluating risk factors for failure of cast treatment of type II supracondylar humeral fractures, the degree of fracture extension based on the anterior humeral line was significantly related to the failure of cast treatment; the width of the soft-tissue shadow of the upper arm had borderline significance. Level of evidence: III.

18. Camus T, MacLellan B, Cook PC, Leahey JL, Hyndman JC, El-Hawary R: Extension type II pediatric supracondylar humerus fractures: A radiographic outcomes study of closed reduction and cast immobilization. *J Pediatr Orthop* 2011;31(4):366-371.

    Of 155 type II supracondylar humeral fractures treated nonsurgically and evaluated with multiple parameters to assess reduction, 80% had some radiographic extension; however, a determination could not be made regarding the long-term significance of this finding. Level of evidence: IV.

19. Skaggs DL, Cluck MW, Mostofi A, Flynn JM, Kay RM: Lateral-entry pin fixation in the management of supracondylar fractures in children. *J Bone Joint Surg Am* 2004;86(4):702-707.

20. Skaggs DL, Hale JM, Bassett J, Kaminsky C, Kay RM, Tolo VT: Operative treatment of supracondylar fractures of the humerus in children: The consequences of pin placement. *J Bone Joint Surg Am* 2001;83(5): 735-740.

21. Battaglia TC, Armstrong DG, Schwend RM: Factors affecting forearm compartment pressures in children with supracondylar fractures of the humerus. *J Pediatr Orthop* 2002;22(4):431-439.

22. Mapes RC, Hennrikus WL: The effect of elbow position on the radial pulse measured by Doppler ultrasonography after surgical treatment of supracondylar elbow fractures in children. *J Pediatr Orthop* 1998;18(4):441-444.

23. Pretell Mazzini J, Rodriguez Martin J, Andres Esteban EM: Surgical approaches for open reduction and pinning in severely displaced supracondylar humerus fractures in children: A systematic review. *J Child Orthop* 2010;4(2):143-152.

    Based on a meta-analysis of various surgical approaches for the open reduction of supracondylar humeral fractures, the authors concluded that a combined anterior-medial approach allows the best possible functional and cosmetic outcomes.

24. Ersan O, Gonen E, Ilhan RD, Boysan E, Ates Y: Comparison of anterior and lateral approaches in the treat-

6: Pediatrics

ment of extension-type supracondylar humerus fractures in children. *J Pediatr Orthop B* 2012;21(2):121-126.

This comparison study evaluated 46 anterior and 38 lateral approaches for open reduction of supracondylar humeral fractures using the Flynn criteria. The authors reported that both approaches had good to excellent results, but the anterior approach achieved better cosmetic results and had the additional benefit of allowing access to neurovascular structures. Level of evidence: III.

25. Li YA, Lee PC, Chia WT, et al: Prospective analysis of a new minimally invasive technique for paediatric Gartland type III supracondylar fracture of the humerus. *Injury* 2009;40(12):1302-1307.

26. Brauer CA, Lee BM, Bae DS, Waters PM, Kocher MS: A systematic review of medial and lateral entry pinning versus lateral entry pinning for supracondylar fractures of the humerus. *J Pediatr Orthop* 2007;27(2):181-186.

27. Kocher MS, Kasser JR, Waters PM, et al: Lateral entry compared with medial and lateral entry pin fixation for completely displaced supracondylar humeral fractures in children: A randomized clinical trial. *J Bone Joint Surg Am* 2007;89(4):706-712.

28. Zaltz I, Waters PM, Kasser JR: Ulnar nerve instability in children. *J Pediatr Orthop* 1996;16(5):567-569.

29. Hamdi A, Poitras P, Louati H, Dagenais S, Masquijo JJ, Kontio K: Biomechanical analysis of lateral pin placements for pediatric supracondylar humerus fractures. *J Pediatr Orthop* 2010;30(2):135-139.

In the treatment of pediatric supracondylar fractures, a construct consisting of a lateral pin parallel to the lateral metaphysis and a divergent pin crossing at the medial edge of the coronoid was found to be the strongest construct of four lateral entry constructs.

30. Srikumaran U, Tan EW, Belkoff SM, et al: Enhanced biomechanical stiffness with large pins in the operative treatment of pediatric supracondylar humerus fractures. *J Pediatr Orthop* 2012;32(2):201-205.

A comparison of Kirschner wires and Steinmann pins in various constructs found that the most stable construct was crossed pins; however, two large pins (2.8 mm) in any configuration provided more stable fixation than two small wires (1.6 mm) in a lateral divergent fashion.

31. Srikumaran U, Tan EW, Erkula G, Leet AI, Ain MC, Sponseller PD: Pin size influences sagittal alignment in percutaneously pinned pediatric supracondylar humerus fractures. *J Pediatr Orthop* 2010;30(8):792-798.

This retrospective analysis of 159 fractures showed that increased pin diameter improved sagittal alignment without increasing the rate of ulnar nerve injury or infection. Level of evidence: III.

32. Eberl R, Eder C, Smolle E, Weinberg AM, Hoellwarth ME, Singer G: Iatrogenic ulnar nerve injury after pin fixation and after antegrade nailing of supracondylar humeral fractures in children. *Acta Orthop* 2011;82(5):606-609.

In a retrospective review comparing 264 supracondylar humeral fractures treated with antegrade nailing and 176 elbows fixed with crossed pins, ulnar nerve injury occurred in 0.4% of those with antegrade nailing and in 15% of those with crossed pins. The technique for antegrade nailing is described. Level of evidence: III.

33. Queally JM, Paramanathan N, Walsh JC, Moran CJ, Shannon FJ, D'Souza LG: Dorgan's lateral cross-wiring of supracondylar fractures of the humerus in children: A retrospective review. *Injury* 2010;41(6):568-571.

The authors review a technique in which wires were started on the lateral side distal and proximal to a supracondylar humeral fracture to provide cross-wire fixation. In 43 patients, there was no major loss of reduction and no iatrogenic ulnar nerve injuries. Level of evidence: IV.

34. Mulpuri K, Hosalkar H, Howard A: AAOS clinical practice guideline: The treatment of pediatric supracondylar humerus fractures. *J Am Acad Orthop Surg* 2012; 20(5):328-330.

The clinical practice guidelines established by the AAOS for the treatment of pediatric supracondylar humeral fractures are reviewed.

35. Mehlman CT, Strub WM, Roy DR, Wall EJ, Crawford AH: The effect of surgical timing on the perioperative complications of treatment of supracondylar humeral fractures in children. *J Bone Joint Surg Am* 2001;83(3): 323-327.

36. Bales JG, Spencer HT, Wong MA, Fong YJ, Zionts LE, Silva M: The effects of surgical delay on the outcome of pediatric supracondylar humeral fractures. *J Pediatr Orthop* 2010;30(8):785-791.

A comparison of outcomes of 145 supracondylar humeral fractures treated in 21 hours or less after injury or more than 21 hours after injury found no statistical differences between the groups with regard to the need for open reduction (0% in both groups), nerve injuries, vascular complications, surgical time, or compartment syndrome. This study suggests that most of these injuries can be treated in a delayed fashion; however, time to treatment should be determined on an individual basis. Level of evidence: II.

37. Gupta N, Kay RM, Leitch K, Femino JD, Tolo VT, Skaggs DL: Effect of surgical delay on perioperative complications and need for open reduction in supracondylar humerus fractures in children. *J Pediatr Orthop* 2004;24(3):245-248.

38. Murnaghan ML, Slobogean BL, Byrne A, Tredwell SJ, Mulpuri K: The effect of surgical timing on operative duration and quality of reduction in Type III supracondylar humeral fractures in children. *J Child Orthop* 2010;4(2):153-158.

A comparison of 48 type III supracondylar fractures treated less than 8 hours after injury and 39 fractures treated more than 8 hours after injury found no difference in surgical time. No patients in either group had compartment syndromes or conversions to open reduction. The authors caution that this does not necessarily mean that treatment of all supracondylar humeral fractures should be delayed. Level of evidence: II.

39. Wang YL, Chang WN, Hsu CJ, Sun SF, Wang JL, Wong CY: The recovery of elbow range of motion after treatment of supracondylar and lateral condylar fractures of the distal humerus in children. *J Orthop Trauma* 2009; 23(2):120-125.

40. Zionts LE, Woodson CJ, Manjra N, Zalavras C: Time of return of elbow motion after percutaneous pinning of pediatric supracondylar humerus fractures. *Clin Orthop Relat Res* 2009;467(8):2007-2010.

41. Steinman S, Bastrom TP, Newton PO, Mubarak SJ: Beware of ulnar nerve entrapment in flexion-type supracondylar humerus fractures. *J Child Orthop* 2007;1(3): 177-180.

42. Abzug JM, Herman MJ: Management of supracondylar humerus fractures in children: Current concepts. *J Am Acad Orthop Surg* 2012;20(2):69-77.

    This review of treatment and outcomes includes recommendations for nonoperative treatment of type I fractures and surgical intervention for most displaced (types II-IV) injuries.

43. Leet AI, Frisancho J, Ebramzadeh E: Delayed treatment of type 3 supracondylar humerus fractures in children. *J Pediatr Orthop* 2002;22(2):203-207.

44. Mangat KS, Martin AG, Bache CE: The 'pulseless pink' hand after supracondylar fracture of the humerus in children: The predictive value of nerve palsy. *J Bone Joint Surg Br* 2009;91(11):1521-1525.

45. Blakemore LC, Cooperman DR, Thompson GH, Wathey C, Ballock RT: Compartment syndrome in ipsilateral humerus and forearm fractures in children. *Clin Orthop Relat Res* 2000;376:32-38.

46. Weiss JM, Graves S, Yang S, Mendelsohn E, Kay RM, Skaggs DL: A new classification system predictive of complications in surgically treated pediatric humeral lateral condyle fractures. *J Pediatr Orthop* 2009;29(6): 602-605.

47. Bernthal NM, Hoshino CM, Dichter D, Wong M, Silva M: Recovery of elbow motion following pediatric lateral condylar fractures of the humerus. *J Bone Joint Surg Am* 2011;93(9):871-877.

    A prospective evaluation of 141 pediatric patients with lateral humeral condylar fractures found initial rapid recovery in elbow motion up to 1 year after injury regardless of the treatment method. Recovery was slower if the patient was older, had a longer period of elbow immobilization, or had a more severe injury. Level of evidence: II.

48. Pribaz JR, Bernthal NM, Wong TC, Silva M: Lateral spurring (overgrowth) after pediatric lateral condyle fractures. *J Pediatr Orthop* 2012;32(5):456-460.

    In 212 consecutive lateral condylar fractures, a lateral spur developed in 73% of the fractures (43% mild, 38% moderate, and 19% severe). The development of a spur correlated with initial displacement and surgical treatment, and the size of the spur was associated with the amount of initial displacement. Neither the presence nor size of the spur seemed to influence the final outcome. Level of evidence: II.

49. Koh KH, Seo SW, Kim KM, Shim JS: Clinical and radiographic results of lateral condylar fracture of distal humerus in children. *J Pediatr Orthop* 2010;30(5): 425-429.

    In a series of 175 pediatric patients with lateral condylar fractures of the distal humerus followed for more than 1 year, the most common residual deformities were lateral overgrowth and cubitus varus. These deformities had not remodeled at an average of 20 months after injury. Level of evidence: IV.

50. Pappas N, Lawrence JT, Donegan D, Ganley T, Flynn JM: Intraobserver and interobserver agreement in the measurement of displaced humeral medial epicondyle fractures in children. *J Bone Joint Surg Am* 2010;92(2): 322-327.

    In this study, interobserver and intraobserver reliability was poor for measuring the degree of displacement of medial epicondylar fractures.

51. Kamath AF, Baldwin K, Horneff J, Hosalkar HS: Operative versus non-operative management of pediatric medial epicondyle fractures: A systematic review. *J Child Orthop* 2009;3(5):345-357.

52. Metaizeau JP, Lascombes P, Lemelle JL, Finlayson D, Prevot J: Reduction and fixation of displaced radial neck fractures by closed intramedullary pinning. *J Pediatr Orthop* 1993;13(3):355-360.

Video Reference

57.1: Koerner JD, Sabharwal S: Video. *Percutaneous Pinning of Supracondylar Humerus Fractures.* Available at http://orthoportal.aaos.org/emedia/singleVideoPlayer.aspx?resource=EMEDIA_OSVL_13_25. Accessed January 15, 2014.

6: Pediatrics

Chapter 58

Forearm, Wrist, and Hand Trauma: Pediatrics

Christine Ann Ho, MD   Donald S. Bae, MD

Monteggia Fracture-Dislocations

First described by Giovanni Monteggia in 1814, Monteggia fracture-dislocations are fractures of the ulna associated with proximal radioulnar dissociation and radiocapitellar joint dislocation.[1] Although the treatment principles are well established, the diagnosis is frequently missed. Because the reconstruction of chronic Monteggia lesions is fraught with complications, the evaluation of all ulnar fractures should include a careful assessment of the radiocapitellar joint.

Classification and Fracture Patterns

The classic Bado classification of Monteggia fracture-dislocations is still used currently[2] (Table 1). In this scheme, Monteggia lesions are classified by the direction of the radial head dislocation and the apex of the ulnar fracture angulation. This classification system is helpful because it provides insight into both the mechanism of injury and the methods for closed reduction. Bado type I injuries are the most common and are characterized by anterior radial head dislocations and apex anterior ulnar fractures. The mechanism of injury is typically a direct blow to the posterior forearm and/or hyperextension with pronation. Bado type III injuries, which are characterized by lateral radial head dislocation and typically a proximal ulnar fracture, are the second most common Monteggia injury in children. Bado type III lesions are believed to result from either an axial load with forearm supination or an axial load on a partially flexed elbow.

Monteggia fracture-dislocations also have been classified according to the pattern of ulnar fracture: plastic deformation, greenstick, complete anterior, complete

posterior, or lateral.[3] This classification system is particularly useful in guiding surgical treatment.

Assessment

Patients will typically present with pain, swelling, and deformity after a fall onto an outstretched hand. The dislocated radial head may be in close proximity to the median or radial nerve. A thorough neurologic examination is necessary to evaluate for nerve palsies, particularly of the posterior interosseous nerve. In high-energy injuries, it is essential to evaluate the patient for possible compartment syndrome or open fractures.

Radiographic Studies

In general, imaging of forearm injuries should always include an assessment of the wrist and elbow joints. Without exception, all patients with isolated ulnar fractures, whether complete or incomplete, should be evaluated for possible Monteggia lesions. The longitudinal axis of the radius should bisect the capitellar ossification center on all radiographic views.

Occasionally, a congenital radial head dislocation with an acute ulnar fracture may be mistaken for a Monteggia fracture-dislocation. In these instances, the presence of a hypoplastic capitellum, convex or dome-shaped radial head, and bowing of the proximal ulna should alert the examiner to a possible congenital dislocation.

Treatment

Treatment principles for acute Monteggia fracture-dislocations include restoring the length and alignment of the ulnar fracture and obtaining a congruent radiocapitellar reduction. Traditionally, closed reduction and cast immobilization have been advocated. Serial radiography should be performed to assess for subsequent loss of reduction. Given the high risk of late displacement and the challenges associated with the reconstruction of chronic injuries, surgical treatment of acute Monteggia lesions has been advocated.[4] Although closed reduction is recommended for incomplete plastic deformation or greenstick fractures, surgical stabilization is performed for complete ulnar fractures. Transverse or short oblique fractures may be effectively stabilized with intramedullary nailing of the ulna, whereas

---

6: Pediatrics

Table 1

Bado Classification of Monteggia Fracture-Dislocations

Classification	Direction of Radial Head Displacement
Type I	Anterior dislocation
Type II	Posterior dislocation
Type III	Lateral/anterolateral dislocation
Type IV	Anterior dislocation with fractures of both the radius and ulna

long oblique or comminuted fractures require open reduction and plate fixation.

Chronic Monteggia fractures present additional treatment challenges. Although the natural history of these lesions is not well characterized and some patients with neglected Monteggia lesions may have no functional limitations, chronic Monteggia fracture-dislocations can lead to pain, a loss of elbow or forearm motion, deformity, and late neuropathy. The reconstruction of chronic Monteggia lesions consists of restoring ulnar length and alignment, along with open reduction of the radiocapitellar joint, with or without annular ligament reconstruction. A host of techniques ranging from single-stage osteotomy and joint reduction to gradual distraction lengthening of the ulna have been advocated.[5-7] Although the long-term results of chronic fracture-dislocation reconstruction are good in children younger than 12 years or when performed within 3 years of the initial injury, the risk of persistent instability and loss of forearm rotation remains.[7]

Forearm Diaphyseal Fractures

Fractures of the radial and ulnar diaphysis are among the most common skeletal injuries in children, representing up to 50% of all pediatric fractures and having an annual incidence of approximately 1 in 100 children.[8,9] The forearm segment remains one of the most common locations for open fractures and refractures. Recent literature suggests that the incidence of these fractures may be increasing because of changes in the activity patterns and the physical characteristics of children.[10,11] Despite policy statements from the American Academy of Pediatrics (AAP) and the American Academy of Orthopaedic Surgeons (AAOS), recreational trampoline use continues to cause substantial injuries in children, with 55% of injuries occurring as fractures in the upper extremity (34% elbow fractures and 21% forearm fractures); 48% of the injuries require a sedated procedure or surgery for treatment.[12] Although most forearm injuries may be effectively treated nonsurgically, careful clinical and radiographic evaluation, attention to the principles of skeletal remodeling, and

appropriate surgical techniques are critical to optimize clinical results and functional outcomes.

Classification and Fracture Patterns

In general, forearm fractures are described according to anatomic features and the fracture pattern. Injuries may occur in the distal, middle, or proximal diaphysis; may have varying degrees of angulation, displacement, and rotation; and may involve one or both bones. These combinations of fracture characteristics present unique challenges and should guide individualized care. Several characteristic fracture patterns are seen in skeletally immature patients.

Plastic deformation (traumatic bowing) injuries are commonly seen in young patients during the first decade of life. Injuries in which the bones are bent but not broken occur when the applied loads exceed the elastic limits of the radius and ulna but do not surpass the ultimate strength of the bones. Clinically, patients may present with minimal pain, aesthetic deformity, or edema. Forearm rotation is typically limited, and radiographs will demonstrate bowing and a narrowed interosseous space[13] (Figure 1).

Greenstick fractures denote incomplete fractures in which one cortex is disrupted and the other is intact or plastically deformed. In younger patients, these fractures typically result from torsional mechanisms. Radiographs can confirm the diagnosis and guide reduction maneuvers.

Complete fractures of the forearm diaphysis are common. Patients will present with pain, swelling, ecchymosis, and limited forearm motion. Radiographs can confirm the diagnosis.

Remodeling Potential

As with other skeletal injuries in growing children, fractures of the radial and ulnar diaphyses have robust remodeling potential; however, the remodeling capacity is dependent on the proximity of the fracture to the adjacent growth plate, the magnitude and direction of fracture displacement, and the amount of remaining growth. In younger children, fractures closer to the distal physes with deformity in the plane of adjacent joint motion have the greatest remodeling potential. In general, fractures with up to 20° of angulation, complete bayonet apposition, and up to 1 cm of shortening (particularly in the middle and distal thirds of the radius and ulna) can remodel in children younger than 8 years.[14,15] In children older than 10 years with greater than 10° of diaphyseal angulation, remodeling may not occur spontaneously.

Although these general guidelines are helpful in determining how much radiographic deformity will remodel, clinical forearm rotation does not directly correlate with radiographic alignment. Studies suggest that up to 10° of angulation, bayonet apposition, and 45° of malrotation may be tolerated with little functional compromise.[15] Other authors have proposed the use of the axis deviation to predict ultimate forearm motion at the completion of bony healing and skeletal remod-

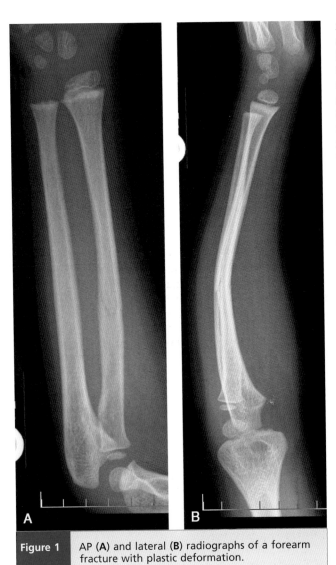

Figure 1 AP (**A**) and lateral (**B**) radiographs of a forearm fracture with plastic deformation.

minimize the risk of complications. To this end, several anatomic considerations guide both injury pattern and fracture treatment in children. The periosteum of the radius and ulna is thick and often incompletely disrupted in forearm fractures. Although the periosteum contributes to rapid healing, promotes remodeling, and may confer mechanical stability, understanding the fracture pattern and the pattern of periosteal disruption is essential to effectuate appropriate reduction maneuvers. The effect of the adjacent muscles and joints on fracture displacement also must be considered. For example, although the biceps and the supinator exert a supinatory force on the proximal third of the radius, a pronation moment to the distal radius is imparted by the pronator teres, the pronator quadratus, and the brachioradialis. These deforming forces must be neutralized during reduction maneuvers and cast immobilization. Pediatric forearm fractures often result from rotational mechanisms of injury, particularly when the radial and ulnar fractures lie at different levels. Correction of rotational malalignment is needed to prevent loss of forearm pronation-supination. In these situations, the so-called rule of thumbs has been advocated. For example, in the typical apex-volar forearm fracture resulting from a supination mechanism, pronation of the distal forearm segment (pointing the thumb to the apex of the deformity) is recommended to correct the malrotation. As was previously discussed in this chapter, the capacity for remodeling further influences fracture management and decision making.

In plastic deformation injuries, closed reduction is advised for injuries with greater than 20° of angulation in patients older than 4 years because of the relatively limited remodeling potential of this particular fracture pattern.[18] It has been shown that up to 30 kg of force sustained over several minutes may be required to correct traumatic bowing; for this reason, reduction is typically performed with the patient under conscious sedation or general anesthesia, with an emphasis on appropriate cast the application to maintain alignment.

In greenstick fractures with unacceptable deformity, closed reduction and the application of a well-molded cast are recommended. Reduction maneuvers involve rotation following the rule of thumbs when the radial and ulnar fractures lie at different levels. Conversely, when the radius and ulna are fractured at the same level, the injury is likely caused by bending mechanisms; reduction can be attained by reversing the deformity with simple three-point molding of the subsequent cast application. Controversy continues regarding whether greenstick fractures should be completed by breaking the "intact" cortex. Although fracture completion may allow for easier manipulation, lower the risk of lost reduction, and lower the subsequent refracture rate, it results in greater fracture instability at the time of the reduction.[19]

Complete nondisplaced fractures can be treated with simple immobilization, whereas patients with unacceptable alignment are treated with closed reduction and casting. In general, closed reduction maneuvers involve first exaggerating the deformity to relax the intact peri-

eling.[16,17] These historical guidelines for acceptable deformity must be carefully balanced against changing patient and family expectations and evolving functional demands.

Assessment

The clinical evaluation should include a careful patient history and physical examination that focuses on the mechanism of injury, the presence or absence of traumatic wounds, and the neurovascular status. Appropriate radiographs should be obtained of the entire forearm segment, including visualization of both the elbow and wrist to rule out concomitant injury (such as a Monteggia or a Galeazzi fracture). Careful evaluation of the entire upper limb is recommended to rule out an ipsilateral fracture (the so-called pediatric floating elbow).

Treatment

The goals of pediatric forearm fracture care are to promote fracture healing, maximize forearm function (particularly forearm rotation), preserve aesthetics, and

6: Pediatrics

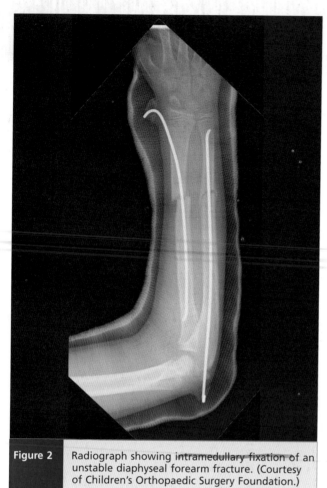

Figure 2 Radiograph showing intramedullary fixation of an unstable diaphyseal forearm fracture. (Courtesy of Children's Orthopaedic Surgery Foundation.)

osteum, applying longitudinal traction to gain length, correcting the rotational alignment, and subsequently reversing the angular deformity. Applying a well-fitting, appropriately molded long-arm cast is important in maintaining alignment after fracture manipulation.

After initial reduction and casting, serial radiographs should be obtained to identify early loss of reduction, which may occur in up to 30% of patients. Risk factors for loss of reduction include older age, more proximal injuries, and greater initial displacement.[20] Six weeks of cast immobilization are typically recommended, followed by a gradual resumption of activities. Recent published information suggests that the risk of refracture is approximately 4% to 7% in the first 12 months after a forearm diaphyseal fracture.[21] Fractures of the middle or proximal third of the radius in which the fracture line is still apparent at the time of cast removal have been shown to have the highest risk of refracture.

Indications for the surgical treatment of diaphyseal forearm fractures include open fractures, fractures with soft-tissue edema or neurovascular compromise precluding circumferential cast immobilization, floating elbow injuries, and unstable or irreducible fractures that fail initial attempts at closed reduction. In these situations, closed or open reduction may be performed followed by internal stabilization. Fixation options in chil-

dren and adolescents generally include intramedullary nailing versus standard plate-and-screw constructs.

Intramedullary nailing is the most common fixation choice for pediatric diaphyseal forearm fractures[22-26] (Figure 2). Although a host of implants are available for use, the treatment principles remain the same. Intramedullary implants are prebent to restore the radial bow and interosseous space and impart rotational stability. Nails are placed via small incisions, which avoid the physes, and are carefully inserted into the intramedullary canals of the affected radius and ulna. After reduction is achieved, these implants are placed across the fracture site and into the medullary canal of the other fracture fragment. In up to 30% of patients, open reduction via small incisions is needed to achieve bony realignment, facilitate nail passage, and avoid excessive manipulation or complications.[22] In select situations, particularly in younger children with closed fractures, single-bone fixation may be sufficient.[27,28] Typically, implants are cut and left beneath the skin; the refracture risk is believed to be lower if implants are not removed until 6 to 12 weeks postoperatively.

Compression plate-and-screw fixation also can be performed using techniques similar to those used in adult forearm fractures, particularly in older adolescents with less remaining growth and remodeling potential. The need for routine implant removal after plate fixation of forearm fractures in children remains controversial.[29-31]

Although the treatment of open forearm fractures adheres to the principles outlined in this chapter, several additional factors should be considered. Open fractures are caused by higher-energy mechanisms of injury and result in greater soft-tissue disruption and fracture instability. There is a higher risk of compartment syndrome in open fractures, particularly after intramedullary fixation.[32] As with all open skeletal injuries, judicious antibiotic coverage and appropriate irrigation and débridement of open fracture sites are needed to avoid infection.

Complications

Although adhering to established treatment principles results in bony healing and functional restoration in most patients, forearm malunions do occur. Etiologies include false assumptions regarding a patient's skeletal remodeling potential, suboptimal reduction and/or casting techniques, a failure to monitor alignment with serial radiography, or incomplete surgical correction. In patients in whom malunion results in a functionally limiting loss of forearm rotation, corrective osteotomy may be indicated. Meticulous surgical technique, typically using closing wedge osteotomies and rigid internal fixation, and careful angular and rotational realignment can provide safe and reliable improvements in forearm rotation.[33,34]

Compartment syndrome is an important and potentially devastating complication of pediatric forearm fracture treatment and can occur in both nonsurgical and surgically treated injuries.[35] Timely diagnosis and appropriate decompressive fasciotomies are critical to avoid permanent neurovascular and functional compromise. The diagnosis of compartment syndrome can be challenging in young, anxious, or nonverbal children. Increasing anxiety, agitation, and analgesic requirements may be signs of an impending compartment syndrome.

Refracture of a diaphyseal forearm fracture occurs in approximately 4% to 7% of patients and is a relative indication for surgical reduction and stabilization.

Fractures of the Distal Radius and Ulna

Fractures of the distal forearm are extremely common in children. Most patients can be managed with cast immobilization and manipulation as needed. Complications can be avoided with close follow-up and careful attention to detail.

Epidemiology and Classification

Although common in all pediatric patients, distal forearm fractures have a predilection for adolescents; this is explained by the decrease of cortical bone in proportion to trabecular bone and the increased porosity of cortical bone during mid to late puberty.[36] A fall onto an outstretched hand while the wrist is extended leads to the more common dorsally displaced distal forearm fracture, whereas a fall onto a flexed wrist results in volar displacement of the fracture fragment.

Fractures can be classified as torus (or buckle), greenstick, metaphyseal, physeal, or Galeazzi (a pattern in which the distal radial fracture is accompanied by dislocation of the distal radioulnar joint [DRUJ]). Metaphyseal fractures are further described as displaced or nondisplaced, and physeal fractures are commonly classified using the Salter-Harris classification system.

Remodeling Capacity

The remodeling capacity of displaced fractures is great because these fractures are in close proximity to the physis in patients with considerable remaining growth, and the deformity is typically in the plane of wrist motion. Translation and complete bayonet apposition almost always remodel, although careful monitoring is required to limit malangulation. Up to 35° of angulation in the sagittal plane can be accepted in patients 10 years and younger. An aspect of the "art of orthopaedics" involves taking into account the skeletal maturity of the patient, the plane and magnitude of the deformity, and the inherent instability of the fracture pattern when deciding on the limits of acceptable angulation for these fractures.

Assessment

Distal radial and ulnar fractures usually result from a fall onto an outstretched hand. Although the classic dinner fork deformity is often present in displaced fractures, minimally displaced fractures can be easily missed, especially in younger children. It is not uncommon for a child with a torus fracture to present for treatment more than 1 week after the initial injury because an assumed sprain has not resolved. Concomitant ipsilateral upper extremity fractures are also easily missed, and careful palpation of the snuffbox for scaphoid tenderness and the elbow for supracondylar humeral fractures should be a routine part of the examination. As with any fracture, assessments of skin integrity and neurovascular status must be performed and documented.

AP and lateral radiographs of the forearm should be obtained, with a low threshold to include dedicated views of the elbow and wrist if only one bone is fractured or if tenderness in the wrist or elbow is present on examination.

Treatment

Torus (or buckle) fractures are inherently stable and are adequately treated with 3 to 4 weeks of immobilization. Care must be taken during radiographic review to ensure that a subtle greenstick fracture, which is at risk for angulation, is not mistaken for a torus fracture. Multiple studies have reported similar outcomes but higher patient and parent satisfaction with the use of a removable splint compared with a short-arm cast,[37,38] although one study found increased pain duration and time to return to full activities in patients immobilized with a volar fiberglass splint compared with those treated with a short-arm plaster cast.[39] Although removable splints may be more convenient for the family and allow unrestricted bathing and water activities, short-arm casts may offer better pain control and more protection during vigorous activities for patients who may be noncompliant with activity restrictions.

Greenstick Fractures

Greenstick fractures in the distal forearm are generally treated with closed manipulation and casting. Adequate analgesia for reduction, especially in the emergency department, may require conscious sedation. The application of a well-molded cast is imperative to prevent redisplacement. These fractures should be monitored with weekly radiographs taken with the arm in the cast for the first 2 to 3 weeks after manipulation, with a low threshold for changing the cast if unacceptable fracture angulation is noted.

Metaphyseal Fractures

Two randomized controlled trials established that treating metaphyseal fractures in a well-molded short-arm cast is as effective as treatment in a long-arm cast.[40,41] Risk factors for redisplacement include complete initial fracture displacement, a higher degree of obliquity of the fracture line, and poor quality of the cast molding.[42] Many quantitative measures of cast molding have been proposed, including the padding index, the Canterbury index, the gap index, the cast index, and the three-point index; all have been variably validated and invalidated in various studies. The cast index, defined as the ratio of the internal diameter of the cast on the

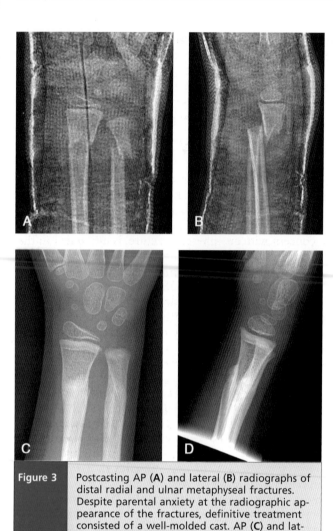

Figure 3 Postcasting AP (**A**) and lateral (**B**) radiographs of distal radial and ulnar metaphyseal fractures. Despite parental anxiety at the radiographic appearance of the fractures, definitive treatment consisted of a well-molded cast. AP (**C**) and lateral (**D**) radiographs taken 4 months after the injury show substantial remodeling. The patient recovered with full range of motion without clinical deformity.

Surgical treatment is generally reserved for fractures that are open, associated with compartment or carpal tunnel syndromes, those with severe swelling that precludes well-molded cast immobilization, ipsilateral fractures that require surgical stabilization, and fractures in which an acceptable reduction cannot be maintained. Closed reduction with percutaneous fixation has been shown to decrease the risk of redisplacement, and it may be considered the primary treatment for an older child with a displaced metaphyseal fracture because these patients have decreased remodeling potential.[45] Although physeal arrest has been associated with pin fixation, it is unclear whether the arrest is caused by the pin or the initial fracture. Despite best efforts, it may not always be possible to avoid crossing the physis during pin fixation; in these instances, the use of a smooth transphyseal pin may minimize the risk of physeal arrest. External fixation of these fractures is generally reserved for patients with extensive soft-tissue injuries.

Physeal Fractures

Most distal radial physeal fractures can be managed in a similar manner to metaphyseal fractures, and the remodeling potential is even greater than that of metaphyseal fractures. These fractures heal fairly rapidly because of the location in the physis; radiographic callus is often visible at 7 to 10 days after injury. Because of this rapid healing, manipulation of these fractures should not be delayed more than 7 days after injury to minimize the risk of further injury to the physis that could result in growth arrest. Patients with physeal fractures who present for treatment more than 7 days after injury should not be treated with manipulation but instead should be placed in a well-molded cast to prevent further displacement. These fractures should be followed for fracture remodeling, which can be profound in patients younger than 11 years. Subsequent corrective osteotomy for symptomatic deformity is rarely needed.

A Salter-Harris type III or IV fracture of the distal radius is an intra-articular fracture. Surgical treatment, generally with small-caliber smooth pins, is usually necessary to achieve anatomic reduction of the articular surface and the physis.

Distal ulnar physeal fractures are uncommon and appear to be associated with a high risk of growth arrest, with one series reporting a 50% arrest rate.[47-49] Open anatomic reduction does not appear to decrease the risk of growth arrest in these fractures. However, the true risk of physeal arrest in these fractures is unknown, and it is unclear if distal ulnar physeal fractures are underreported, underrecognized, and/or inadequately treated. Fortunately, clinically symptomatic ulnar physeal arrest is an infrequent occurrence.

Distal ulnar styloid fractures generally require no treatment despite their low rate of union. One series reported an 80% nonunion rate, with symptomatic nonunions attributable to pathology in the triangular fibrocartilage complex.[50]

sagittal radiograph to the internal diameter on the coronal view, is most commonly used because of its simplicity. The ideal cast index had traditionally been accepted as 0.7, with lower values representing a higher quality molding,[43] although recent literature has suggested that 0.8 may be acceptable.[44]

Considerable controversy surrounds the treatment of displaced distal metaphyseal fractures. Traditionally, closed reduction with some form of sedation or block is followed by immobilization until the fracture has healed. Although some physicians advocate Kirschner wire fixation to decrease the risk of redisplacement,[45] a recent prospective study proved that closed treatment of shortened, displaced, distal radius fractures in well-molded casts without formal manipulation in patients younger than 11 years resulted in full wrist motion, with both clinical and radiographic union[46] (Figure 3). Despite this recent report, the mainstay of emergency department treatment of closed, displaced, metaphyseal fractures continues to be closed reduction and casting, with the patient under conscious sedation.

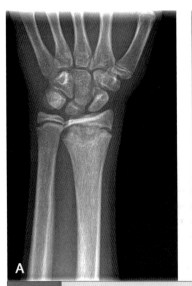
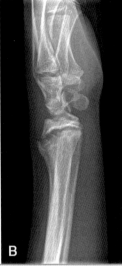

Figure 4 **A,** AP radiograph of the wrist of a 14-year-old adolescent girl who is a level 10 gymnast and spends 32 hours per week in gymnastic training. The patient presented with a report of insidious wrist pain during the prior 3-month period. Fraying and irregularity of the distal radial metaphysis is evident, and ulnar positive deformity is present from the chronic stress to the distal radial physis. **B,** Lateral radiograph shows asymmetric physeal growth with dorsal angulation of the distal radius.

Galeazzi Fractures

Unlike in adults, many Galeazzi fracture patterns in children are amenable to closed manipulation and casting. These fractures should be closely followed to ensure that anatomic reduction of the DRUJ is maintained. Surgical stabilization with either smooth pins or a rigid plate may be required in patients who cannot be managed in a cast. If the DRUJ remains unstable after anatomic reduction and fixation of the radius, a transverse smooth pin across the reduced DRUJ can be used to stabilize the joint. A pseudo-Galeazzi injury or Galeazzi equivalent lesion in children has been described when there is a fracture of the distal ulna physis rather than a DRUJ dislocation. Poorer results with this injury may be caused by the inherent risk of physeal arrest of the distal ulna or the need for open reduction of the distal ulna because of the interposition of soft tissue.[51-53]

Chronic Radial Physeal Injuries

Gymnast's wrist, a stress-related distal radius physeal injury in pediatric patients who are gymnasts, has been well described. These competitive athletes present with chronic pain in the area of the distal radial physis. Radiographically, the distal radial physis appears wide and irregular, with metaphyseal fraying and flaring (Figure 4). On MRI, edema is present on both the metaphyseal and epiphyseal sides of the physis. Distal radial physeal arrest with subsequent ulnar positive deformity will result from continued overuse and stress. Treatment of gymnast's wrist is strict rest and cessation

of any load-bearing activities on that extremity until the pain resolves and the physis shows radiographic recovery. Despite extensive counseling with families regarding the consequences of continued training, it can be difficult to convince these high-level athletes to modify or cease their gymnastic participation.

Complications of Distal Radius and Ulna Fractures

Complications of distal forearm fractures include those common to other pediatric upper extremity fractures: malunion, refracture, tendon or peripheral nerve injury, and compartment syndrome. Resultant physeal arrest, a concern with any physeal fracture, is infrequent in the distal radius, with an estimated incidence of 1% to 7%.[54] This relatively low complication rate (especially when the frequency of distal radial physeal fractures is considered) may be attributed to the fact that most of these fractures result from low-energy injuries (such as a fall from ground level) and the distal radius has significant growth velocity (9 to 10 mm/year after the age of 7 years).[55] Families should be counseled on the risk of physeal arrest, and serial radiography should be recommended for at least 1 year after injury to monitor for continued physeal growth.

After physeal arrest has been identified, surgical intervention should be considered, even in asymptomatic patients, to avoid the risk of future pain, deformity, and functional disability with continued asymmetric growth.[54] Distal radial physeal arrest that is detected early can be treated with complete distal radius epiphysiodesis with concomitant distal ulna epiphysiodesis before the occurrence of substantial ulnar positive variance. Resection of a central distal radial bar, with the placement of interposition material, may be considered in girls younger than 10 years and boys younger than 12 years if the bone bridge involves less than one half of the physis.[56]

When detected late, correction of deformity and pain from distal radial growth arrest requires treatment of all components, including ulnocarpal impaction syndrome, loss of radial inclination and tilt, lunotriquetral injury, triangular fibrocartilage complex injury, and DRUJ instability. Purely ulnar positive variance without distal radial deformity can be treated with an ulnar shortening osteotomy with distal ulnar epiphysiodesis (if the distal ulnar physis is still open) and triangular fibrocartilage complex repair/débridement, as needed. The correction of a distal radial deformity may require distal radial osteotomy to restore radial height and tilt. Good success in correcting severe deformities has been reported with distraction osteogenesis, although this treatment is not commonly used.[57,58]

Scaphoid Fractures

Ossification in the pediatric carpus begins in infancy (Table 2), and all of the carpal bones continue to be

6: Pediatrics

Table 2

Ossification of the Pediatric Carpus

Carpal Bone	Age of Ossification
Capitate	2-3 months
Hamate	3-4 months
Triquetrum	2 years
Lunate	3-4 years
Scaphoid	5 years
Trapezoid	6 years
Trapezium	6 years
Pisiform	8-9 years

mostly cartilaginous in nature until later in adolescence.

As in adults, scaphoid fractures are the most common carpal fracture in children. However, these fractures are rare in children of elementary school age and are often associated with other ipsilateral wrist or forearm fractures from massive trauma when seen in this patient population. Scaphoid fractures in pediatric patients are most commonly seen in adolescent boys, with fracture patterns and incidences similar to those of adults.[59] Pediatric scaphoid waist fractures are the most common type (71%), followed by distal pole fractures (23%), and proximal pole fractures (6%). If a scaphoid injury is suspected, the fracture should be immobilized in a thumb spica cast, with repeated radiography and reexamination in 2 to 3 weeks because 30% of clinically suspected pediatric scaphoid fractures with initial negative radiographic findings have radiographic evidence of a scaphoid fracture at follow-up.[60]

Acute, nondisplaced fractures can be treated in either a long- or short-arm thumb spica cast, although cast immobilization may be required for 3 months or more in proximal pole injuries.[59] As in adults, displaced and unstable fractures are treated with open reduction and internal fixation or, possibly, percutaneous fixation. A recent study reported that one third of contemporary pediatric scaphoid fractures present as chronic nonunions.[59] These fractures should be managed similarly to adult scaphoid nonunions.

Hand Fractures

Most pediatric hand fractures can be treated with splinting or casting. The role of surgical stabilization is dictated by the inherent instability of certain fracture patterns, the need for anatomic reduction in articular fractures, and a failure to maintain fracture reduction. Smooth pin stabilization with small-caliber Kirschner wires (0.028- or 0.035-inch diameter) is the mainstay of fixation in these young patients.

Most Salter-Harris type I and II fractures in the hand occur in the proximal and middle phalanges. They are generally amenable to closed manipulation, buddy taping, and casting, with careful clinical assessment of rotation and malangulation correction (especially with a full-composite fist). Angulation in the sagittal plane has remodeling potential; there is less remodeling potential in coronal plane angulation and minimal to no remodeling in a rotational deformity. Rarely, interposition of tendons or periosteum will necessitate open reduction to remove the offending tissue and pin fixation to maintain the reduction.

Salter-Harris type III and IV fractures with intra-articular step-off or gapping must be reduced and stabilized with pin fixation. In the proximal phalanx of the thumb, the ulnar-sided Salter Harris type III fracture is the equivalent of an ulnar collateral ligament avulsion injury (gamekeeper's thumb) and can result in nonunion and instability if not anatomically reduced and fixed. Salter-Harris type III fractures of the dorsal distal phalanx represent mallet fractures and generally occur in adolescent patients. In fractures with joint involvement greater than 50%, joint incongruity, and joint subluxation, surgical stabilization is required.

A Seymour fracture is a Salter-Harris type I or II fracture of the distal phalanx with an associated germinal matrix nail bed laceration.[61] These open fractures are often underrecognized and undertreated, which can lead to osteomyelitis[62] (Figure 5). Seymour fractures should be treated with antibiotics, nail plate removal, gentle extrication of the interposed germinal matrix, fracture irrigation, fracture reduction, and matrix repair using fine absorbable sutures. The use of 2-octylcyanoacrylate (Dermabond, Ethicon) may also be considered for repair of the nail bed; this repair has been shown to be faster than suture repair, with comparable cosmetic results and patient satisfaction.[63,64] The nail plate may be used as a stent/external splint. Factures that remain unstable after this treatment may require pinning to prevent mallet deformity.

Proximal and middle phalangeal neck (subcondylar) fractures are often undertreated because of a misleading benign radiographic appearance. Clinical rotation and angulation must be carefully assessed, and pin fixation is required to maintain reduction of the small fracture fragments. Dorsal displacement of a subcondylar fracture is an indication for reduction and pin fixation because the volar metaphyseal spike of bone will obliterate the subcondylar fossa and block flexion of the joint. Percutaneous pin osteoclasis is recommended for incipient malunions because open reduction of late-presenting fractures is fraught with complications, including osteonecrosis and loss of motion.[65,66] Despite the traditional belief that there is little remodeling potential in the distal portion of the phalanx, a recent study of eight children with open physes and phalangeal neck fracture malunions reported full remodeling in the sagittal plane but not in the coronal plane.[67] Although the acutely presenting displaced fracture is still best treated with reduction and pin fixation, observation or percutaneous osteoclasis may be considered as a

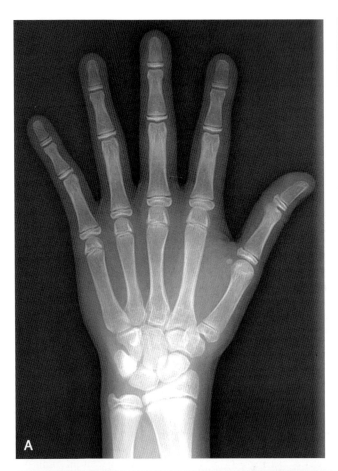
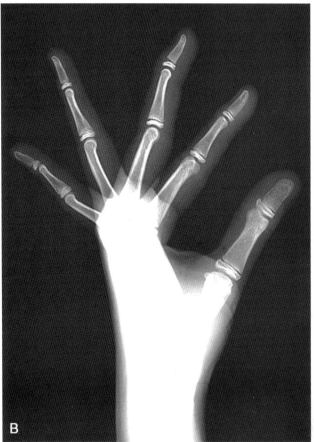
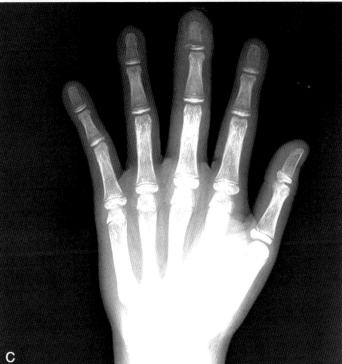
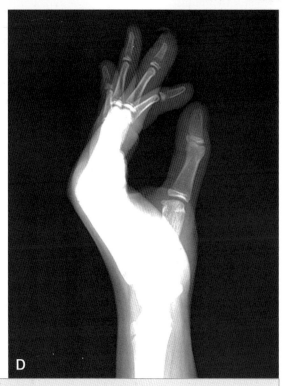

Figure 5   AP (**A**) and lateral (**B**) radiographs of a 12-year-old boy with a Seymour fracture after a hit to his long finger while playing football 4 days prior. The severity of the injury was underappreciated. AP (**C**) and lateral (**D**) radiographs taken 3 weeks later when the boy subsequently presented with frank osteomyelitis of the distal phalanx caused by the untreated open distal phalanx fracture.

treatment for incipient malunion, and observation with subcondylar fossa reconstruction should be the treatment of choice for late presenting healed fractures, especially those with only sagittal plane deformity.

Summary

Although most pediatric upper extremity fractures can be managed nonsurgically because of the high potential for remodeling, careful attention to detail and close follow-up are required to prevent complications. Fracture location and pattern, degree of angulation and displacement, Salter-Harris classification, family beliefs and expectations, and patient age must all be taken into account when determining the best management. A recognition of certain high-risk fracture patterns that dictate surgical management is mandatory for optimal outcomes.

Key Study Points

- Minimally angulated pediatric distal radius fractures can be treated in either a prefabricated wrist splint or short-arm cast with equivalent radiographic and clinical outcomes.

- Although closed manipulation with casting is still the mainstay of emergency department treatment of displaced, closed, metaphyseal distal radius fractures, good clinical and radiographic results can be achieved in patients younger than 11 years with shortened and displaced fractures treated in a well-molded cast to decrease angulation.

- Pediatric scaphoid fracture patterns are similar to patterns in adults. Although 90% of acute, nondisplaced pediatric scaphoid fractures heal uneventfully with cast treatment, union is less certain in chronic, displaced fractures involving the proximal pole.

Annotated References

1. Monteggia GB: *Istituzioni Chirurgiche*, ed 2. Milan, Italy, Giuseppe Maspero, 1814, vol 5, p 130.

2. Bado JL: The Monteggia lesion. *Clin Orthop Relat Res* 1967;50:71-86.

3. Letts M, Locht R, Wiens J: Monteggia fracture-dislocations in children. *J Bone Joint Surg Br* 1985;67(5):724-727.

4. Ring D, Waters PM: Operative fixation of Monteggia fractures in children. *J Bone Joint Surg Br* 1996;78(5):734-739.

5. Gyr BM, Stevens PM, Smith JT: Chronic Monteggia fractures in children: Outcome after treatment with the Bell-Tawse procedure. *J Pediatr Orthop B* 2004;13(6):402-406.

6. Hui JH, Sulaiman AR, Lee HC, Lam KS, Lee EH: Open reduction and annular ligament reconstruction with fascia of the forearm in chronic monteggia lesions in children. *J Pediatr Orthop* 2005;25(4):501-506.

7. Nakamura K, Hirachi K, Uchiyama S, et al: Long-term clinical and radiographic outcomes after open reduction for missed Monteggia fracture-dislocations in children. *J Bone Joint Surg Am* 2009;91(6):1394-1404.

8. Cheng JC, Ng BK, Ying SY, Lam PK: A 10-year study of the changes in the pattern and treatment of 6,493 fractures. *J Pediatr Orthop* 1999;19(3):344-350.

9. Chung KC, Spilson SV: The frequency and epidemiology of hand and forearm fractures in the United States. *J Hand Surg Am* 2001;26(5):908-915.

10. Ryan LM, Brandoli C, Freishtat RJ, Wright JL, Tosi L, Chamberlain JM: Prevalence of vitamin D insufficiency in African American children with forearm fractures: A preliminary study. *J Pediatr Orthop* 2010;30(2):106-109.

    In this study, 10 of 17 African American children with forearm fractures (59%) were found to have vitamin D insufficiency. Level of evidence: IV.

11. Sinikumpu JJ, Lautamo A, Pokka T, Serlo W: The increasing incidence of paediatric diaphyseal both-bone forearm fractures and their internal fixation during the last decade. *Injury* 2012;43(3):362-366.

    The authors reviewed 168 patients younger than 16 years who were treated at a single Finnish institution. A fourfold increase in the number of diaphyseal forearm fractures was seen from 2000 to 2009, and the rate of surgical treatment of pediatric forearm fractures similarly increased. The authors cite changing activity patterns (such as trampoline use) as a reason for the rising incidence of diaphyseal forearm fractures. Level of evidence: IV.

12. Phelps JR, Ho CA, Evans N, Okada P, Wilson PW: Paper No 236: Does following the AAOS and AAP guidelines for trampoline use decrease the severity of injuries? A prospective study. *AAOS 2012 Annual Meeting Proceedings*. CD-ROM. Rosemont, IL, American Academy of Orthopaedic Surgeons, 2012, p 807.

    The authors prospectively evaluated 299 consecutive patients injured during trampoline use and found that following the AAOS and AAP guidelines for trampoline use did not decrease the severity of injuries sustained by children. Ninety-one percent of the injuries were fractures, and 49% of the patients required either an operation or a procedure with conscious sedation to treat the fracture.

13. Firl M, Wünsch L: Measurement of bowing of the radius. *J Bone Joint Surg Br* 2004;86(7):1047-1049.

14. Do TT, Strub WM, Foad SL, Mehlman CT, Crawford AH: Reduction versus remodeling in pediatric distal forearm fractures: A preliminary cost analysis. *J Pediatr Orthop B* 2003;12(2):109-115.

15. Price CT, Scott DS, Kurzner ME, Flynn JC: Malunited forearm fractures in children. *J Pediatr Orthop* 1990; 10(6):705-712.

16. Younger AS, Tredwell SJ, Mackenzie WG: Factors affecting fracture position at cast removal after pediatric forearm fracture. *J Pediatr Orthop* 1997;17(3):332-336.

17. Younger AS, Tredwell SJ, Mackenzie WG, Orr JD, King PM, Tennant W: Accurate prediction of outcome after pediatric forearm fracture. *J Pediatr Orthop* 1994; 14(2):200-206.

18. Vorlat P, De Boeck H: Bowing fractures of the forearm in children: A long-term followup. *Clin Orthop Relat Res* 2003;413:233-237.

19. Schmuck T, Altermatt S, Büchler P, et al: Greenstick fractures of the middle third of the forearm: A prospective multi-centre study. *Eur J Pediatr Surg* 2010;20(5): 316-320.

    An analysis of 103 greenstick fractures showed that completion of a greenstick fracture does not prevent refracture, but the rate of residual malalignment is lower. Level of evidence: IV.

20. Bowman EN, Mehlman CT, Lindsell CJ, Tamai J: Nonoperative treatment of both-bone forearm shaft fractures in children: Predictors of early radiographic failure. *J Pediatr Orthop* 2011;31(1):23-32.

    A multivariate logistical regression analysis of 282 fractures showed that patients older than 10 years, those with proximal-third radial fractures, and fractures with ulnar angulation greater than 15° were at highest risk of failure with closed reduction and casting. Level of evidence: II.

21. Baitner AC, Perry A, Lalonde FD, Bastrom TP, Pawelek J, Newton PO: The healing forearm fracture: A matched comparison of forearm refractures. *J Pediatr Orthop* 2007;27(7):743-747.

22. Flynn JM, Jones KJ, Garner MR, Goebel J: Eleven years experience in the operative management of pediatric forearm fractures. *J Pediatr Orthop* 2010;30(4): 313-319.

    In a review of 2,297 fractures treated over an 11-year period, the authors reported a surgical rate of 6.7%, of which more than two thirds of the patients were treated with intramedullary fixation. Twenty-nine percent of the patients required open reduction to assist nail passage. The overall complication rate was 14.6%, including compartment syndrome and delayed union. Level of evidence: III.

23. Garg NK, Ballal MS, Malek IA, Webster RA, Bruce CE: Use of elastic stable intramedullary nailing for treating unstable forearm fractures in children. *J Trauma* 2008; 65(1):109-115.

24. Kang SN, Mangwani J, Ramachandran M, Paterson JM, Barry M: Elastic intramedullary nailing of paediatric fractures of the forearm: A decade of experience in a teaching hospital in the United Kingdom. *J Bone Joint Surg Br* 2011;93(2):262-265.

    Ninety consecutive children with displaced forearm fractures were treated with intramedullary nailing. The mean time to union was 2.9 months, and 44% of the patients required limited open reduction. Level of evidence: IV.

25. Luhmann SJ, Gordon JE, Schoenecker PL: Intramedullary fixation of unstable both-bone forearm fractures in children. *J Pediatr Orthop* 1998;18(4):451-456.

26. Reinhardt KR, Feldman DS, Green DW, Sala DA, Widmann RF, Scher DM: Comparison of intramedullary nailing to plating for both-bone forearm fractures in older children. *J Pediatr Orthop* 2008;28(4):403-409.

27. Alnaib M, Taranu R, Lakkol S, Aldlyami E, Alcelik I, Tulloch C: Radius-only intramedullary nailing for both-bones diaphyseal forearm fractures in children. *Acta Orthop Belg* 2011;77(4):458-463.

    In this study, 29 children with both-bone diaphyseal forearm fractures were treated with radius-only single-bone intramedullary fixation, with excellent functional outcomes and union rates. Level of evidence: IV.

28. Dietz JF, Bae DS, Reiff E, Zurakowski D, Waters PM: Single bone intramedullary fixation of the ulna in pediatric both bone forearm fractures: Analysis of short-term clinical and radiographic results. *J Pediatr Orthop* 2010;30(5):420-424.

    Single-bone ulnar intramedullary fixation is safe and effective, particularly in younger children with closed injuries. Level of evidence: IV.

29. Clement ND, Yousif F, Duckworth AD, Teoh KH, Porter DE: Retention of forearm plates: Risks and benefits in a paediatric population. *J Bone Joint Surg Br* 2012; 94(1):134-137.

    The authors present a prospective study of 82 patients treated with plating for forearm fractures. Approximately 15% of the plates were removed because of pain, stiffness, or implant-related fractures. Regression analysis of implant-related fracture detected an odds ratio of 4.4 for radial plates and 3.2 for dynamic compression plating. Although complications occurred, the authors concluded that the complications were not more frequent than seen with routine implant removal in children. Level of evidence: IV.

30. Kim WY, Zenios M, Kumar A, Abdulkadir U: The removal of forearm plates in children. *Injury* 2005; 36(12):1427-1430.

31. Peterson HA: Metallic implant removal in children.

6: Pediatrics

J Pediatr Orthop 2005;25(1):107-115.

32. Luhmann SJ, Schootman M, Schoenecker PL, Dobbs MB, Gordon JE: Complications and outcomes of open pediatric forearm fractures. *J Pediatr Orthop* 2004; 24(1):1-6.

33. Price CT, Knapp DR: Osteotomy for malunited forearm shaft fractures in children. *J Pediatr Orthop* 2006;26(2): 193-196.

34. van Geenen RC, Besselaar PP: Outcome after corrective osteotomy for malunited fractures of the forearm sustained in childhood. *J Bone Joint Surg Br* 2007;89(2): 236-239.

35. Yuan PS, Pring ME, Gaynor TP, Mubarak SJ, Newton PO: Compartment syndrome following intramedullary fixation of pediatric forearm fractures. *J Pediatr Orthop* 2004;24(4):370-375.

36. Kirmani S, Christen D, van Lenthe GH, et al: Bone structure at the distal radius during adolescent growth. *J Bone Miner Res* 2009;24(6):1033-1042.

37. Boutis K, Willan A, Babyn P, Goeree R, Howard A: Cast versus splint in children with minimally angulated fractures of the distal radius: A randomized controlled trial. *CMAJ* 2010;182(14):1507-1512.

    The authors randomly assigned 46 children to a prefabricated removable splint and 50 children to a short-arm cast for 4 weeks to treat an angulated fracture of the distal radius. Angulation at 4 weeks, motion, and the Activities Scale for Kids score was not significantly different between the two groups. Level of evidence: I.

38. Abraham A, Handoll HH, Khan T: Interventions for treating wrist fractures in children. *Cochrane Database Syst Rev* 2008;2:CD004576.

39. Oakley EA, Ooi KS, Barnett PL: A randomized controlled trial of 2 methods of immobilizing torus fractures of the distal forearm. *Pediatr Emerg Care* 2008; 24(2):65-70.

40. Bohm ER, Bubbar V, Yong Hing K, Dzus A: Above and below-the-elbow plaster casts for distal forearm fractures in children: A randomized controlled trial. *J Bone Joint Surg Am* 2006;88(1):1-8.

41. Webb GR, Galpin RD, Armstrong DG: Comparison of short and long arm plaster casts for displaced fractures in the distal third of the forearm in children. *J Bone Joint Surg Am* 2006;88(1):9-17.

42. Alemdaroğlu KB, Iltar S, Cimen O, Uysal M, Alagöz E, Atlihan D: Risk factors in redisplacement of distal radial fractures in children. *J Bone Joint Surg Am* 2008; 90(6):1224-1230.

43. Chess DG, Hyndman JC, Leahey JL, Brown DC, Sinclair AM: Short arm plaster cast for distal pediatric forearm fractures. *J Pediatr Orthop* 1994;14(2):

211-213.

44. Kamat AS, Pierse N, Devane P, Mutimer J, Horne G: Redefining the cast index: The optimum technique to reduce redisplacement in pediatric distal forearm fractures. *J Pediatr Orthop* 2012;32(8):787-791.

    This retrospective study of 1,001 children who underwent closed manipulation of a distal forearm fracture found 10.6% fracture redisplacement at 2-week follow-up. The rate of displacement was 5.6% in patients with a cast index less than or equal to 0.80 but 26% in patients with a cast index equal or greater than 0.81. Level of evidence: III.

45. McLauchlan GJ, Cowan B, Annan IH, Robb JE: Management of completely displaced metaphyseal fractures of the distal radius in children: A prospective, randomised controlled trial. *J Bone Joint Surg Br* 2002; 84(3):413-417.

46. Crawford SN, Lee LS, Izuka BH: Closed treatment of overriding distal radial fractures without reduction in children. *J Bone Joint Surg Am* 2012;94(3):246-252.

    In this study, 51 children (aged 3 to 10 years) with closed overriding distal radial fractures were treated with a gently molded fiberglass short-arm cast; no sedation, analgesia, or reduction was used. Clinical and radiographic union with full motion was achieved in all of the patients. Level of evidence: IV.

47. Nelson OA, Buchanan JR, Harrison CS: Distal ulnar growth arrest. *J Hand Surg Am* 1984;9(2):164-170.

48. Golz RJ, Grogan DP, Greene TL, Belsole RJ, Ogden JA: Distal ulnar physeal injury. *J Pediatr Orthop* 1991; 11(3):318-326.

49. Cannata G, De Maio F, Mancini F, Ippolito E: Physeal fractures of the distal radius and ulna: Long-term prognosis. *J Orthop Trauma* 2003;17(3):172-180.

50. Abid A, Accadbled F, Kany J, de Gauzy JS, Darodes P, Cahuzac JP: Ulnar styloid fracture in children: A retrospective study of 46 cases. *J Pediatr Orthop B* 2008; 17(1):15-19.

51. Letts M, Rowhani N: Galeazzi-equivalent injuries of the wrist in children. *J Pediatr Orthop* 1993;13(5):561-566.

52. Imatani J, Hashizume H, Nishida K, Morito Y, Inoue H: The Galeazzi-equivalent lesion in children revisited. *J Hand Surg Br* 1996;21(4):455-457.

53. Kamano M, Ko H, Kazuki K: Paediatric Galeazzi-equivalent fracture: Two case reports. *Hand Surg* 2005; 10(2-3):249-254.

54. Waters PM, Bae DS, Montgomery KD: Surgical management of posttraumatic distal radial growth arrest in adolescents. *J Pediatr Orthop* 2002;22(6):717-724.

55. Pritchett JW: Growth and predictions of growth in the

upper extremity. *J Bone Joint Surg Am* 1988;70(4): 520-525.

56. Lonjon G, Barthel PY, Ilharreborde B, Journeau P, Lascombes P, Fitoussi F: Bone bridge resection for correction of distal radial deformities after partial growth plate arrest: Two cases and surgical technique. *J Hand Surg Eur Vol* 2012;37(2):170-175.

   The authors present two cases of bony bridge resection in the distal radial physis, with a description of surgical technique.

57. Murase T, Oka K, Moritomo H, Goto A, Sugamoto K, Yoshikawa H: Correction of severe wrist deformity following physeal arrest of the distal radius with the aid of a three-dimensional computer simulation. *Arch Orthop Trauma Surg* 2009;129(11):1465-1471.

58. Page WT, Szabo RM: Distraction osteogenesis for correction of distal radius deformity after physeal arrest. *J Hand Surg Am* 2009;34(4):617-626.

59. Gholson JJ, Bae DS, Zurakowski D, Waters PM: Scaphoid fractures in children and adolescents: Contemporary injury patterns and factors influencing time to union. *J Bone Joint Surg Am* 2011;93(13):1210-1219.

   An analysis of 351 pediatric and adolescent scaphoid fractures showed that current patterns and distributions are similar to those of adults. Ninety percent of acute displaced fractures healed with nonsurgical treatment, but lower union rates were seen in chronic, displaced, and proximal fractures. Level of evidence: III.

60. Evenski AJ, Adamczyk MJ, Steiner RP, Morscher MA, Riley PM: Clinically suspected scaphoid fractures in children. *J Pediatr Orthop* 2009;29(4):352-355.

61. Seymour N: Juxta-epiphysial fracture of the terminal phalanx of the finger. *J Bone Joint Surg Br* 1966;48(2): 347-349.

62. Al-Qattan MM: Extra-articular transverse fractures of the base of the distal phalanx (Seymour's fracture) in children and adults. *J Hand Surg Br* 2001;26(3): 201-206.

63. Langlois J, Thevenin-Lemoine C, Rogier A, Elkaim M, Abelin-Genevois K, Vialle R: The use of 2-octylcyanoacrylate (Dermabond(®)) for the treatment of nail bed injuries in children: Results of a prospective series of 30 patients. *J Child Orthop* 2010;4(1):61-65.

   Dermabond instead of suture repair was used to close nail bed injuries not associated with displaced distal phalanx fractures in 30 pediatric patients. The cosmetic results were excellent in all but one patient. Level of evidence: IV.

64. Strauss EJ, Weil WM, Jordan C, Paksima N: A prospective, randomized, controlled trial of 2-octylcyanoacrylate versus suture repair for nail bed injuries. *J Hand Surg Am* 2008;33(2):250-253.

65. Waters PM, Taylor BA, Kuo AY: Percutaneous reduction of incipient malunion of phalangeal neck fractures in children. *J Hand Surg Am* 2004;29(4):707-711.

66. Yousif NJ, Cunningham MW, Sanger JR, Gingrass RP, Matloub HS: The vascular supply to the proximal interphalangeal joint. *J Hand Surg Am* 1985;10(6, pt 1): 852-861.

67. Puckett BN, Gaston RG, Peljovich AE, Lourie GM, Floyd WE III: Remodeling potential of phalangeal distal condylar malunions in children. *J Hand Surg Am* 2012; 37(1):34-41.

   Eight skeletally immature patients with malunions of the distal condyle of the proximal or middle phalanx were followed for a minimum of 1 year. All malunions remodeled completely in the sagittal plane, and functional final range of motion was obtained. Level of evidence: IV.

6: Pediatrics

Chapter 59
Pediatric Upper Extremity Disorders

Scott A. Riley, MD   Ronald C. Burgess, MD

Introduction

Congenital anomalies of the upper extremity represent anatomic differences occurring with a frequency of approximately 1 in 600 live births.[1,2] These congenital differences can present as either an isolated deformity or as part of a multisystem or syndromic condition. Most of these anomalies are believed to develop spontaneously; however, some anomalies follow established genetic patterns. These conditions have varying degrees of clinical expression and often present with a spectrum of involvement from mild to severe (or simple to complex) specific anatomic manifestations.

Embryology

The hand and the upper extremity develop from a limb bud off the lateral body wall at day 26 of gestation, progress in a proximal to distal fashion, and are fully formed by the eighth week[2,3] (Figure 1). Limb deformities that occur as a result of failure of formation are believed to occur during weeks 4 through 8 after gestation. The timing of the appearance of anatomic structures has been well described[3] (Table 1). Anomalies that arise as a result of failures in differentiation occur later in the fetal growth period.

Longitudinal (or proximal to distal) growth is controlled by tissue found at the tip of the limb bud. This collection of cells, known as the apical ectodermal ridge, influences the growth of the somatic and lateral plate mesoderm. The apical ectodermal ridge is mediated by several fibroblastic growth factors and is also influenced by the wingless-type (WNT) signaling center. The interaction between the apical ectodermal ridge and specific fibroblastic growth factors seems to be both time and dose dependent. Inappropriate fibroblastic growth factor signaling is likely a key factor in the development of limb malformations.[4]

The zone of polarizing activity consists of mesodermal cells found on the posterior border of the limb bud that control anteroposterior (radioulnar) development. The activity of these cells is mediated through the sonic hedgehog pathway, which is also dose dependent. A loss of sonic hedgehog pathway expression results in ulnar longitudinal dysplasia, whereas the implantation of additional zone of polarizing activity cells to the anterior limb bud (or higher sonic hedgehog pathway doses) results in ulnar dimelia or mirror hand.[4]

The third center is the non–apical ectodermal ridge ventral ectoderm. This tissue controls limb development along the dorsoventral axis. The key protein involved in this process is WNT-7a. The ventral ectodermal cells express Engrailed-1, which restricts the expression of the WNT-7a protein and allows ventral limb development. In the dorsal non–apical ectodermal ridge ectoderm, WNT-7a induces the *homobox* gene (*Lmx1b*) to regulate dorsal patterning.[2]

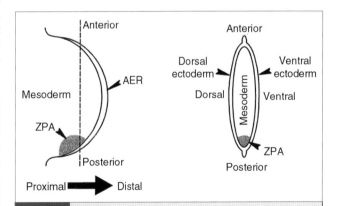

Figure 1 Schematic drawings showing the development of the limb bud in a proximal-to-distal direction coordinated by the apical ectodermal ridge (AER). The zone of polarizing activity (ZPA) signals the differentiation of radius- and ulna-side structures. **A,** The limb bud in the frontal plane. **B,** A cross section of the limb bud at the dashed line shown in A. (Adapted with permission from Daluiski A, Yi SE, Lyons KM: The molecular control of upper extremity development: Implications for congenital hand anomalies. *J Hand Surg Am* 2001;26[1]:8-22.)

Table 1

Timing of the Appearance of Anatomic Structures

Embryonic Age (Days)	Anatomic Findings
26	Limb bud appears
30	Arterial tree present
33	Hand paddle appears
36	Nerve trunks enter arm; chondrification of humerus, radius, and ulna
41	Digital rays present
54	Digital separation complete

(Adapted with permission from Al-Qattan MM, Yang Y, Kozin SH: Embryology of the upper limb. *J Hand Surg Am* 2009;34[7]:1340-1350.)

Table 2

Proposed Modifications to the IFSSH Classification

I. Failure of axis formation and/or differentiation
   Radial longitudinal deficiency
   Radial-ulnar synostosis
   Ulnar longitudinal deficiency
   Transverse deficiency (including symbrachydactyly)
   Dorsal ventral deficiency

II. Failure of hand-plate formation and/or differentiation
   Syndactyly
   Apert syndrome
   Central deficiency (cleft hand)
   Camptodactyly
   Clinodactyly
   Clasped thumb
   Hand-plate synostoses
   Metacarpal synostosis
   Carpal synostosis

III. Duplication
   Radial polydactyly (including triphalangeal thumb)
   Ulnar dimelia
   Ulnar polydactyly

IV. Overgrowth

V. Amniotic band sequence

VI. Generalized skeletal abnormalities

IFSSH = International Federation of Societies for Surgery of the Hand
(Reproduced with permission from Manske PR, Oberg KC: Classification and developmental biology of congenital anomalies of the hand and upper extremity. *J Bone Joint Surg Am* 2009;91[4, suppl 4]:3-18.)

Although each signaling center plays a specific role in limb growth, research has shown that there are also interactions among these three centers that control limb development. By altering the expression of certain mediators, investigators have been able to produce characteristic limb deformities in animal models.[2,3]

Classification of Upper Extremity Anomalies

The precise categorization of limb anomalies in the upper extremity is challenging. The most widely accepted classification system was developed by the International Federation of Societies for Surgery of the Hand and published in the initial volume of the *Journal of Hand Surgery* in 1976.[5] Recent work has attempted to make this system more comprehensive by incorporating newer concepts of developmental biology into the original classification scheme[6] (Table 2).

Failure of Formation

Radial Deficiency

Radial deficiency, which is also known as radial longitudinal deficiency, radial dysplasia, or radial clubhand, is an anomaly characterized by hypoplasia and/or loss of the radial-sided structures of the upper extremity. The classification of the condition depends on the degree of deficiency involving the thumb, the radial-sided carpals, and the radius. The most common type of presentation involves complete absence of the radius (Table 3). The incidence of radial deficiency occurs in approximately 1 in 30,000 live births; these cases are usually sporadic in nature. Both arms are affected in 50% of the patients with radial deficiency, and two thirds of these patients are seen in association with other syndromes that can affect the heart, the kidney, bone marrow, or the gastrointestinal tract.[7] Fetal ultra-

sonography has been able to identify these deficiencies as early as 20 weeks of gestation.[8]

The characteristics and clinical findings seen in specific radial deficient conditions, including thrombocytopenia-absent radius syndrome,[9] Fanconi anemia,[10] VACTERL (defects of vertebral, anal, cardiac, trachea-esophageal, renal, and/or limb systems) association,[11,12] and Holt-Oram syndrome,[12] are summarized in Table 4.

Hypoplastic Thumb

The thumb may be absent or hypoplastic as a part of a radial deficiency.[13] Table 5 describes the five types of hypoplastic thumbs and the recommended treatment options for each type. The most important characteristic of a hypoplastic thumb is whether the child will use the thumb during activities.[14] If the carpometacarpal joint of a hypoplastic thumb is stable, function can be improved by tendon transfers, flap reconstruction, and bone lengthening.[15,16] If the carpometacarpal joint is unstable and the thumb is not used for pinch, the child will come to ignore the thumb during hand use. In these cases, removal of the inefficient thumb is advised, and index finger pollicization may be considered to improve function (Figure 2).

The Global Classification of Radial Longitudinal Deficiencies

Type	Thumb	Carpus[a]	Distal Radius	Proximal Radius
N	Absence or hypoplasia	Normal	Normal	Normal
O	Absence or hypoplasia	Absence, hypoplasia, or coalition	Normal	Normal, radioulnar synostosis, or radial head dislocation
1	Absence or hypoplasia	Absence, hypoplasia, or coalition	> 2 mm shorter than ulna	Normal, radioulnar synostosis, or radial head dislocation
2	Absence or hypoplasia	Absence, hypoplasia, or coalition	Hypoplasia	Hypoplasia
3	Absence or hypoplasia	Absence, hypoplasia, or coalition	Physis absence	Variable hypoplasia
4	Absence or hypoplasia	Absence, hypoplasia, or coalition	Absence	Absence

[a]A carpal anomaly implies hypoplasia, coalition, absence, or bipartite carpal bones. Hypoplasia and absence are more common on the radial side of the carpus, and coalitions are more frequent on the ulnar side. Radiographic findings are valid only if the child is older than 8 years, to allow for ossification of the carpal bones.
(Reproduced from Zlotolow DA, Kozin SH: Upper extremity disorders: Pediatrics, in Flynn JM, ed: *Orthopaedic Knowledge Update*, ed 10. Rosemont, IL, American Academy of Orthopaedic Surgeons, 2011, pp 697-713.)

Findings in Syndromes With Radial Deficiencies

Syndrome	Musculoskeletal Features	Other Body System Features	Additional Findings
Thrombocytopenia-absent radius (TAR syndrome)	Complete bilateral absence of the radii Preservation of the thumbs Short humeri	Hypomegakaryotic thrombocytopenia is present at birth Knee abnormalities	Inheritance: predominantly autosomal recessive
Fanconi anemia	Radial longitudinal deficiency of any type	Pancytopenia: appears at age 3-12 years Can be associated with solid tumors, as well as skin and kidney anomalies	Diagnosis: can be made by chromosome fragility challenge test Treatment: bone marrow transplantation
VACTERL association	Upper limb defects can vary from thumb hypoplasia to severe radial dysplasia	At least three of the following: cardiac malformation, disorders of the vertebral column, anal atresia, tracheoesophageal fistula with esophageal atresia, and renal anomalies	Syndactyly and polydactyly may also be seen
Holt-Oram syndrome	Typical finding in the upper extremity is thumb hypoplasia	Most commonly seen condition affecting both the heart and the upper limb	Autosomal dominant with varying phenotypic expression 35% of patients have a mutation in the *TBX5* transcription factor gene

Treatment Considerations

Except in instances of mild thumb hypoplasia, most children who present with a radial deficiency will have tight radial-sided structures. Early on, the caregivers should be instructed on how to perform gentle passive stretching of a deviated wrist. Ideally, these stretching maneuvers should be done several times each day. Bracing of the limb is begun when the limb is large enough to fit properly and maintain correction inside a fabricated splint. If the forearm does not respond to these conservative treatment modalities, the radial deviation deformity and shortened forearm may remain problematic. Surgical procedures have been attempted to address these concerns. For a persistent radial deviation deformity, repositioning (centralizing) the hand and the wrist on the distal ulna may be clinically appealing. Soft-tissue distraction of the tight radial structures before definitive centralization procedures has been used to aid in correcting the deformity.[17] The typically shortened forearm segment can be gradually lengthened, usually by using ex-

Table 5

The Classification of Thumb Deficiency

Type	Clinical Findings	Treatment
I	Minor generalized hypoplasia	Augmentation
II	Absence of intrinsic thenar muscles Narrowing of first web space Ulnar collateral ligament insufficiency	Opponensplasty First web release Ulnar collateral ligament reconstruction
III	Absence of intrinsic thenar muscles Narrowing of first web space Ulnar collateral ligament insufficiency Extrinsic muscle and tendon abnormalities Skeletal deficiency IIIA: Stable carpometacarpal joint IIIR: Unstable carpometacarpal joint	IIIA: Reconstruction IIIB: Pollicization
IV	Floating thumb	Pollicization
V	Absence of thumb	Pollicization

(Reproduced from Zlotolow DA, Kozin SH: Upper extremity disorders: Pediatrics, in Flynn JM, ed: *Orthopaedic Knowledge Update*, ed 10. Rosemont, IL, American Academy of Orthopaedic Surgeons, 2011, pp 697-713.)

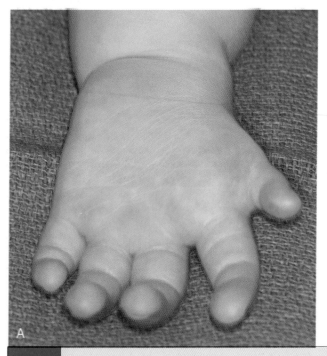 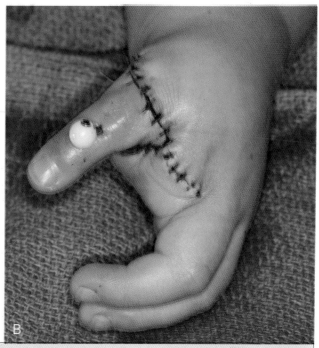

Figure 2 Type IIIB thumb hypoplasia before (**A**) and after (**B**) thumb ablation and index pollicization. It can be difficult for parents to understand the need for surgery, particularly if the thumb is of adequate size. However, the function and appearance of the hand can be dramatically improved through a well-done pollicization. (Courtesy of Shriners Hospital for Children, Philadelphia, PA.)

ternal fixators to achieve distraction osteogenesis of the ulna.[18] In another treatment alternative, the wrist joint is re-created by performing a microvascular transfer of a toe metatarsophalangeal joint.[19] Although these various surgical techniques may allow for improved function and/or appearance, treatment-related complications and unpredictable clinical results are often encountered.[20] Recurrence of the deformity is commonly seen after surgical procedures to centralize the wrist. Because of the uncertain outcomes and potential surgical treatment complications, there remains a lack of consensus regarding treatment recommendations for radial deficiencies.

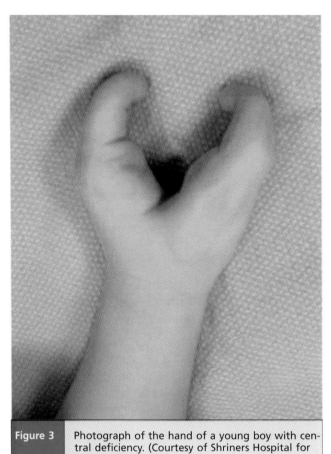

| Figure 3 | Photograph of the hand of a young boy with central deficiency. (Courtesy of Shriners Hospital for Children, Lexington, KY.) |

Ulnar Deficiency

Ulnar deficiency is the underdevelopment or the absence of ulnar-sided structures in the upper extremity. This deformity is usually sporadic in nature, and most patients present with unilateral involvement. This condition occurs much less commonly than radial deficiency and rarely occurs with other organ system anomalies. However, ulnar deficiency can be associated with other skeletal deformities, specifically fibular hemimelia and proximal femoral focal deficiency.[21] The classification system for ulnar deficiency is based on two anatomic components: (1) the degree of elbow and forearm involvement and (2) abnormalities of the thumb and first web space. A typical patient with ulnar deficiency has a loss of some ulnar digits, mild ulnar deviation of the wrist, a shortened forearm, and limited elbow mobility. Syndactyly of some of the remaining digits can be seen as well.

Despite the deformity, most patients with ulnar deficiency are able to achieve a satisfactory level of function. Because a loss of elbow motion can be a challenging to treat surgically, most interventions are designed to improve hand use. As in the case of radial deficiency, early conservative care via passive stretching and splinting is advised. As the child gets older, reliable surgical procedures include syndactyly releases and deepening the first web space to improve grasp and overall hand function.

Central Deficiency

Central deficiency, also known as cleft hand, is believed to develop secondary to failure of formation of the distal and central portion of the limb. The typical patient with central deficiency has bilateral hand and foot involvement, and there is usually a strong family history of similar anomalies. Unilateral central deficits are believed to result from sporadic mutations.[22] The clinical presentation of cleft hand is extremely variable.[23] Along with hypoplastic or missing central digits, unusual positioning of the central phalanges and metacarpals as well as syndactyly and synostosis have been described (Figure 3). Patients may also have clefting of the lip and palate, and tibial hemimelia may be present in the lower extremities.

Many patients with central deficiencies function remarkably well despite the obvious cosmetic deformity. The appearance of the hand with a mild central anomaly may be improved by closing the cleft. More severe deformities are surgically challenging to reconstruct.[24] Families can be advised that reasonable functional goals may be achieved with a hand that has two digits of adequate length that are able to perform a pinching motion.

Symbrachydactyly

The term symbrachydactyly is used to various describe anomalies, ranging from small hypoplastic central digits to complete transverse deficiencies. The condition differs from the classic central deficiency (cleft hand) in that only one limb is usually affected. Although it is believed that the disorder represents a terminal-type deficiency, some patients can present with tiny skin projections (nubbins) on the end of the truncated limb. If these small terminal nubbins are present, the diagnosis may be confused with constriction band syndrome; however, closer examination of the patient will reveal no signs of banding or skin creasing on the other extremities. The disorder may be associated with other conditions, such as Poland syndrome, which is characterized by an ipsilateral loss of the sternal head of the pectoralis major and a concomitant chest wall deformity.

Surgical treatments are designed to give the hand at least two digits of adequate length for grasping and releasing tasks. To gain additional length for small fingers, transferring nonvascularized toe phalanges into the soft tissue at the end of the digits has shown promising results.[25] These phalanges can continue to manifest growth if the transfer is done at a young age and the periosteum is included with the transferred phalanx.[26] If the hand has only one digit, a vascularized toe transfer to the hand may be considered. Although this procedure can be technically difficult, it offers the possibility of providing an additional finger for pinch-related tasks. Distraction osteogenesis also can be used to gain length. Substantial gains in metacarpal and/or phalangeal length have been reported;[27] however, there are complications with this treatment method. Other procedures, such as releasing syndactylized digits, may allow improved hand function.

Prosthesis use in a child with an upper extremity transverse deficiency continues to be unpredictable. Although patients with bilateral transverse deficiencies may benefit from a prosthesis at a young age to assist with sitting and balance, many young children with a unilateral deficiency will not use a passive prosthesis.

Phocomelia

Phocomelia is characterized by significantly shortened or absent long bones of the upper extremity. The hands are small and usually have limited function. Although this anomaly is uncommon (representing less than 1% of all upper extremity congenital deformities), it is fairly well known because of its association with the use of thalidomide, a medication that was used to treat nausea occurring with pregnancy. Recent work has proposed that patients with phocomelia may actually represent a spectrum of severe longitudinal dysplasia.[28] Although upper extremity surgery is rarely recommended for these patients, prosthetic limbs can improve function.

Failure of Differentiation

Syndactyly

Syndactyly is defined as the failure of digital separation with persistence of the skin web between fingers. If there is a family history of syndactyly, it is transmitted in an autosomal dominant pattern with variable penetrance. The genetic defect is located on chromosome 2, and the incidence is approximately 1 in 3,000 live births.[29] Syndactyly is usually an isolated anomaly, but it can be seen in conjunction with Apert syndrome, symbrachydactyly, central deficiency, and ulnar deficiency. The disorder is classified into four types according to both clinical and radiographic features. In complex syndactyly, there is a synostosis between adjacent digits, whereas a syndactyly between two digits without synostosis is classified as simple syndactyly. A complete syndactyly extends to the tips of the fingers, but an incomplete syndactyly does not. The nail plate between two digits that is shared or fused is termed synonychia. Acrosyndactyly is a specific type of digital webbing that describes fingertips that are conjoined distally, but the skin bridging between the fingers is open or incomplete. It can be seen as part of constriction band syndrome.

The primary goal of digital separation in syndactyly is to achieve and maintain an adequate and functional web space. Although there is controversy regarding the timing of surgical treatment, it is generally accepted that early separation should be considered for a syndactyly involving the thumb-index and the ring-little fingers because, as the hand develops, the shorter digits on the border of the hand will tether the longer neighboring digit as it grows and will cause potential angulation and/or rotational deformities. Separating the thumb relatively early (at approximately 6 months of age) allows for pinch activities to develop. Because there is less of a size difference between the central hand digits, these fingers can be separated later. When syndactyly occurs among multiple fingers in the hand, separation between adjacent digits should be delayed approximately 3 months.[30]

The most functional and aesthetically pleasing web spaces are those that have been reconstructed so that no skin grafts or suture lines are found within the web commissure. By paying attention to this detail, interdigital scarring and contracture (also known as web creep) can be minimized.[31,32] Families should be educated that in most instances there is not enough skin available to completely close the incisions of both fingers after separation. Most syndactyly release procedures require skin grafts to cover the remaining defects. These full-thickness grafts can be harvested from the volar wrist crease, the antecubital fossa, or the groin region. It is important to note that as the complexity of the syndactyly becomes more involved, there is greater variability in the neurovascular structures supplying the digits.

Clinodactyly

Radioulnar deformity of a finger at the level of the middle phalanx or the proximal interphalangeal (PIP) joint is called clinodactyly. This deformity occurs in approximately 1% of the population and is most common in the small finger (Figure 4). In some patients, trauma can lead to a physeal injury that then manifests as an angulation deformity of the finger. However, most cases of clinodactyly are inherited and caused by a bracketed or C-shaped physis that causes the development of an abnormally shaped (delta) phalanx. The anomaly is primarily cosmetic, but hand function may be affected if the angulation is severe. Surgical procedures, such as a wedge osteotomy of the middle phalanx or physiolysis of the abnormal bracketed physis, have been described as treatment of the deformity.[33]

Camptodactyly

Finger deformity occurring at the level of the PIP joint in the anteroposterior plane is referred to as camptodactyly. Although many PIP joint contractures are secondary to tendon or joint trauma, true developmental camptodactyly occurs in approximately 1% of the population. It is inherited in an autosomal dominant pattern. The etiology of the contracture is believed to be caused by soft-tissue abnormalities around the PIP joint and commonly involves the flexor digitorum superficialis and the lumbrical. The degree of PIP joint contracture typically worsens during periods of rapid growth. If the condition is left untreated, bone deformity around the PIP joint can occur as a child ages. The disorder can be associated with other conditions, such as arthrogryposis.[34] Surgical treatment of camptodactyly is generally indicated when the PIP joint contracture is greater than 60° and does not respond to passive stretching and splinting. Surgical procedures, including contracture release, tendon transfers, and phalangeal osteotomy, have been described as potential interventions for camptodactyly.[34,35] Regardless of the type of

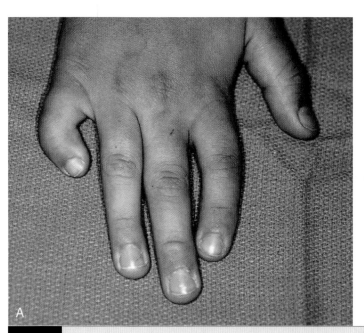
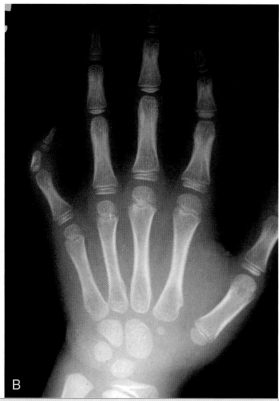

Figure 4 Photograph (**A**) and PA radiograph (**B**) showing the hand of a child with bilateral clinodactyly. (Courtesy of Shriners Hospital for Children, Philadelphia, PA.)

surgical treatment, the family should be advised that complete correction is almost never achieved, and PIP joint motion will likely remain abnormal.

Kirner Deformity

Kirner deformity is a digital anomaly that is characterized by flexion and mild radial deviation of the distal phalanx in the small finger. Although the finger may appear to have a volar curve at the distal interphalangeal joint, the joint is usually normal, and the angulation is within the distal phalanx. Inheritance has been described as autosomal dominant with variable penetrance, yet many cases are sporadic.[36] The condition can be confused with premature physeal growth arrest caused by exposure to cold temperatures (frostbite); however, many fingers are usually affected in Kirner deformity. Because there is minimal or no functional deficit with this condition, surgical correction is rarely needed.

Congenital Synostosis

In the upper extremity, congenital synostosis occurs in two important regions. The first area involves humeroradial synostosis across the elbow, where there are two types based on the morphology of the ulna. Type I is characterized by ulnar hypoplasia, and the elbow is fused in a more extended position. In the more common type II, the elbow is usually fixed in a more flexed position, and the ulna has a more normal appearance.

Because this condition can occur with a variety of syndromes, it is recommended that the patient be referred to a geneticist for a complete evaluation. A child with type II synostosis and a flexed elbow often functions well when performing most activities. A patient with extension or hyperextension posture of the elbow may need a flexion-type osteotomy to change the position of the extremity for improved function.

The second area of synostosis is between the radius and the ulna. It commonly occurs in the proximal one third of the forearm, with the forearm usually in a pronated position[37] (**Figure 5**). This anomaly is inherited in an autosomal dominant fashion with variable expressivity and can also be seen in patients with multiple sex chromosomes.[38] The disorder can occur in association with other conditions, such as Apert syndrome and arthrogryposis. Children with radioulnar synostosis typically have normal flexion and extension of the elbow and can often compensate for loss of forearm rotation by increasing radiocarpal joint flexibility. Because of this, the condition may not be recognized early in life. Most patients with unilateral forearm pronation deformities less than 60° can function well in performing daily activities; however, bilateral hyperpronation deformities can cause limitations, particularly with toileting-related tasks.

Surgical procedures to separate the synostosis have not proven successful. The most reliable method for treating the abnormal forearm position is a derota-

6: Pediatrics

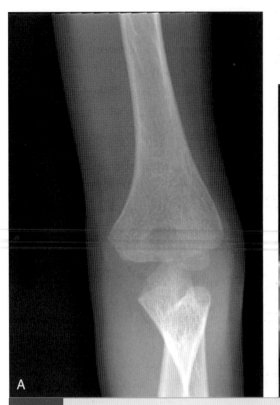
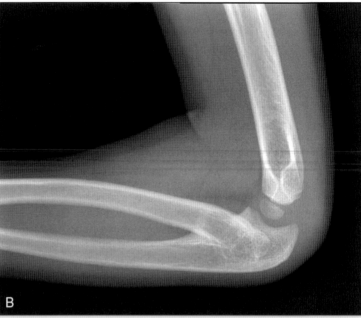

Figure 5 AP (**A**) and lateral (**B**) radiographs showing a radioulnar synostosis. (Courtesy of Shriners Hospital for Children, Philadelphia, PA.)

tional osteotomy through the radioulnar synostosis. Although there may be disagreement regarding what forearm position is ideal in children with unilateral involvement, placing the forearm in mild pronation (30° to 40°) is good for tabletop and keyboarding tasks.[39] In patients with bilateral radioulnar synostosis, having one hand in mild pronation and the other in slight supination can allow for improved self-feeding and personal hygiene.

Sprengel Deformity

Sprengel deformity is characterized by a congenital elevation of the scapula. The condition is usually unilateral and caused by a failure of the scapula to descend to its normal position during weeks 3 to 6 of embryonic growth.[40] A tethering structure called the omovertebral band can be identified along with other abnormal anatomic structures present in patients with the disorder.[41] Sprengel deformity often occurs sporadically, but it can be associated with other conditions, such as congenital scoliosis or Klippel-Feil syndrome (congenital fusions in the cervical spine). Surgical treatment is considered for patients with a severe deformity or a functional deficit. Procedures include resection of the superomedial angle of the scapula, soft-tissue releases, and scapular osteotomy.[40,42]

Duplication

Preaxial Thumb Polydactyly

When polydactyly of the thumb occurs, it is usually a sporadic anomaly that affects one extremity. The incidence is approximately 1 in 10,000 live births, and the condition is more common in males. Because the patient with preaxial polydactyly does not present with two complete and normal sized thumbs, it is inaccurate to consider the condition a true duplication. More likely, the anomaly arises from a delayed involution of the apical ectodermal ridge, which leads to cleaving of the preaxial mesenchymal cells responsible for thumb growth.[43] Usually, the ulnar-sided thumb is larger than its radial counterpart. The thumb deformity can be categorized with the Wassel classification based on the number of abnormal bones[44] (Figure 6). For example, the most common presentation is a Wassel type IV thumb, which has two distal and two proximal phalanges or four abnormal bones. Patients with a Wassel type VII thumb can present with concomitant cardiovascular or musculoskeletal anomalies.[45]

Surgical reconstruction, performed at approximately 1 year of age, is almost always advised. To achieve satisfactory functional and cosmetic results, tissue elements from the excised thumb are often used to supplement the retained digit.[46] A mobile and stable thumb unit is the desired outcome after surgery. Common complications after surgery are angulation deformities and dysfunction of the tendon mechanisms.

Postaxial Polydactyly

Postaxial (or ulnar) polydactyly is a more common condition than radial-sided duplication. The anomaly occurs with relatively common frequency in the black population, affecting 1 in 143 live births. The inheritance pattern is autosomal dominant with variable expression. When the condition presents in a child of European descent, other disorders may be present, so genetic counseling is advised.

There are two basic patterns in the presentation of postaxial polydactyly. Type A is characterized by a digit that appears fairly normal and articulates with the head of the fifth metacarpal or may even have its own (duplicated) metacarpal. In these patients, excision and reconstruction to preserve the stability of the metacarpophalangeal joint may be required. Type B postaxial polydactyly describes a hypoplastic digit that is often attached to the ulnar side of the proximal phalanx by a very small skin bridge.

Two treatment methods exist for this disorder. The anomalous digit can be ligated in the newborn and will eventually become necrotic. This procedure can leave a child with an ulnar-sided skin bump, which is occasionally painful. A recent study reported on a procedure using a topical anesthetic cream followed by surgical excision of the anomalous digit while the patient is in the newborn nursery.[47] The authors found good clinical and cosmetic outcomes with this procedure. Alternatively, the family may elect to have the amputation done electively in the operating room. However, this method will require general anesthesia when the child is older.

Central Polydactyly

Central polydactyly is the least common type of polydactyly. It is characterized by a duplication of a central digit. The condition is caused by a mutation in the *homeobox* gene.[48] The clinical presentation of the duplication can vary from a completely functional finger to a syndactylized partially formed digit (Figure 7). Some patients can adapt quite well to the condition. Although surgical treatment is directed at maximizing hand function, in some patients, digital excision and reconstruction may not offer additional benefits.

Ulnar Dimelia

Ulnar dimelia, often referred to as mirror hand, is a rare condition caused by a duplication of the zone of polarizing activity that forms a limb with two ulnar halves. These hands characteristically have multiple digits, but lack a thumb (Figure 8). A duplicated ulna also may be present and can limit forearm and elbow mobility.

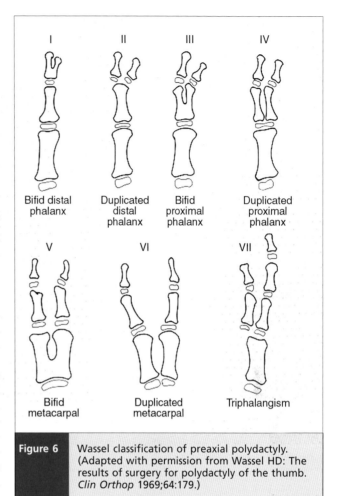

Figure 6 Wassel classification of preaxial polydactyly. (Adapted with permission from Wassel HD: The results of surgery for polydactyly of the thumb. *Clin Orthop* 1969;64:179.)

Developmental Disorders

Trigger Thumb

Originally called congenital trigger thumb, the condition actually develops over time, and its true etiology remains uncertain. The reported incidence among children at age 1 year is 3 per 1,000.[49] A patient commonly presents with the thumb interphalangeal joint in a flexed posture, and a bump (Notta nodule) may be palpated on the flexor pollicis longus tendon at the level of the A1 pulley. Observation, stretching, and splinting have been described as conservative treatment measures, but there remains a large variation in the reported rates of functional recovery.[50,51] Surgical release of the A1 pulley is an effective treatment, but care must be taken to avoid injury to the radial digital nerve of the thumb.

Trigger Finger

In the pediatric population, trigger fingers are quite uncommon and behave differently from those seen in adults. Anatomic abnormalities implicated in the cause of pediatric trigger finger include structural abnormalities of the tendons (such as nodules or aberrant attachments) and thickening of the pulley system. Metabolic

6: Pediatrics

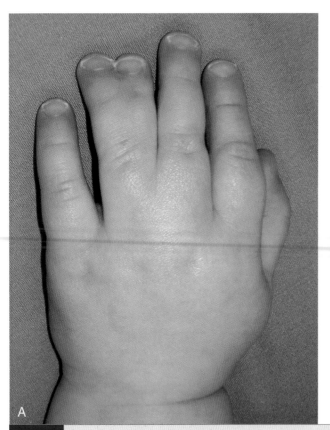
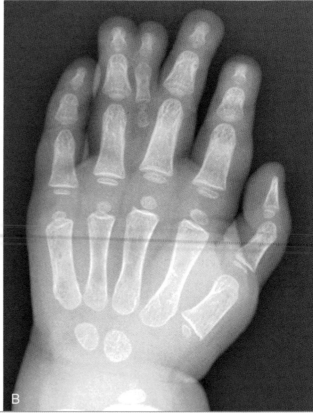

Figure 7 **A,** Photograph of the hand of a child with central polydactyly. **B,** AP radiograph of a hand with central polydactyly. (Courtesy of Shriners Hospital for Children, Lexington, KY.)

diseases (such as Hurler syndrome) and inflammatory conditions (such as juvenile inflammatory arthritis) have been found in association with this disorder. Trigger fingers do not respond well to conservative care. When surgery is needed, treatment of the identified pathology may require an extensive exposure of the flexor tendon mechanism and resection of one slip of the flexor digitorum superficialis tendon.[52]

Madelung Deformity

The developmental disorder known as Madelung deformity becomes apparent in early adolescence and is recognized clinically by a prominent ulnar styloid and a progressive volar posturing of the wrist. Radiographically, the distal radius has an abnormal appearance to the volar-ulnar physis, and the diagnosis can be confused with a physeal growth arrest. An abnormal volar ligamentous tether (Vickers ligament) connecting the lunate and the triangular fibrocartilage complex to the volar-ulnar radial epiphysis has been implicated in the progression of the deformity.[53] The condition usually presents as an isolated disorder, but there are cases that occur as a part of a syndrome (such as Leri-Weill dyschondrosteosis). This disorder occurs more commonly in females.

Despite the clinical appearance, patients with Madelung deformity often function quite well. Early release of the abnormal ligament and physiolysis to help pre-

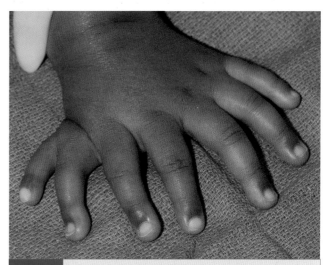

Figure 8 Photograph showing the classic appearance of ulnar dimelia (mirror hand). The ulna-side structures are duplicated, and the thumb is absent. (Courtesy of Shriners Hospital for Children, Philadelphia, PA.)

vent progression of the radial deformity has been recommended.[54] Surgical correction in the symptomatic older child often involves osteotomy of the radius and addressing the distal ulna prominence. A recent study combining release of the Vickers ligament and a radial dome-shaped osteotomy showed promising cosmetic and functional results.[55]

Macrodactyly

Macrodactyly refers to enlargement or overgrowth of either a single digit or multiple digits in the hand (Figure 9). This disorder can occur sporadically or as a clinical finding in other conditions, such as neurofibromatosis, vascular malformations (such as Klippel-Trenaunay-Weber syndrome), osteochondromatosis, and Proteus syndrome. Although neurofibromatosis is inherited as an autosomal dominant condition, the other associated disorders occur sporadically and are rare. In most patients, all anatomic structures in the digit are enlarged, and digital function can be compromised by stiff joints.

One classification of macrodactyly is based on the etiology of the digital enlargement.[56] Type I is caused by a progressive increase in the size of a peripheral nerve secondary to fatty infiltration (lipofibromatosis). The index finger (median nerve distribution) is most commonly involved. Type II macrodactyly is secondary to neurofibromatosis. Type III (polyostotic) is identified by hyperostosis of the digit and stiffness caused by osteochondromas near the joints. Type IV is found in association with hemihypertrophy of the limb.

Surgical treatment of these fingers is challenging because it is difficult to achieve a normal appearance. Simple debulking of the soft-tissue elements is rarely successful because of the accompanying bony enlargement, so osteotomies and physeal arrest techniques are useful.[57] Ultimately, if the finger remains stiff and inhibits its hand function, digital ray amputation may be the best treatment alternative.

Other Disorders

Constriction Band Syndrome

Constriction band syndrome, which is referred to by other names such as Streeter dysplasia, constriction ring syndrome, and amniotic band syndrome,[58] describes the clinical results when detached strands of the amniotic membrane surround portions of the growing fetus. In the extremities, these bands can cause clefting and acrosyndactyly and can lead to amputation. Although the cause of the condition is disputed, it affects between 1 in 1,200 to 15,000 live births, with a slightly increased frequency in females.[59]

Because of the extreme variability of the effects of constriction band syndrome on an extremity, surgical treatment is specifically designed for each patient. However, some general treatment principles exist. Amputated segments may require stump revision for cosmesis or prosthesis fitting. Syndactylized digits are treated in much the same manner as in other patients with a complicated syndactyly (Figure 10). Incomplete or minor bands may be adequately treated by excising the band and incorporating flap elevation and Z-plasty

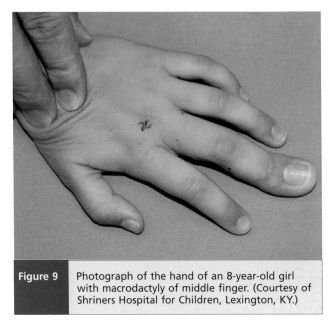

Figure 9 Photograph of the hand of an 8-year-old girl with macrodactyly of middle finger. (Courtesy of Shriners Hospital for Children, Lexington, KY.)

or triangular flap closure techniques.[60,61] In the neonatal setting, emergent release of a band causing venous constriction may prevent an amputation. A recent experimental animal study performing in utero releases of simulated amniotic bands has been reported.[62]

Brachial Plexus Birth Palsy

A traction injury to one or more of the nerves in a neonate's brachial plexus is commonly referred to as brachial plexus birth palsy. Typical injury patterns are shown in Table 6. A thorough knowledge of these patterns is essential to help families understand the treatment alternatives and the expected outcomes. In general, an upper trunk injury at C5-C6 is most common (Erb palsy), whereas an isolated lower plexus injury (Klumpke palsy) is rare. Most infants with brachial plexus birth palsy have mild nerve injuries (neurapraxic type) that can show clinical improvement within a few months. However, in patients with a more substantial nerve injury, spontaneous recovery is less likely. Horner syndrome (ptosis, miosis, enophthalmos, and anhidrosis) is seen with nerve root avulsions and lower plexus injuries.

A complete discussion of brachial plexus birth palsy is beyond the scope of this chapter, but information on current concepts in evaluating and treating this condition can be found in recently published studies.[63,64] The incidence of brachial plexus birth palsy is decreasing in the United States, with a current incidence of 1.5 in 1,000 live births.[65] Although shoulder dystocia is associated with the greatest risk for the disorder, the birth of twins (or multiple birth siblings) and cesarean section delivery were associated with a protective effect against injury. Most children born with brachial plexus birth palsy did not have identifiable risk factors.

6: Pediatrics

Microsurgery

Even though microsurgical procedures are becoming more accepted in the treatment of brachial plexus birth palsy, questions still remain regarding the management of an infant who is not demonstrating timely recovery.[63] It is now believed that simple neurolysis of the involved nerves is not effective as a definitive treatment modality.[66] Nerve transfers and methods for restoring

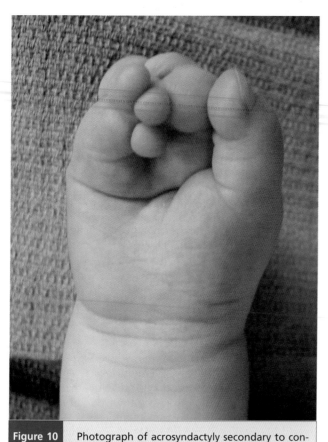

Figure 10 Photograph of acrosyndactyly secondary to constriction band syndrome. (Courtesy of Shriners Hospital for Children, Lexington, KY.)

shoulder motion and elbow flexion have been reported.[67] In one study, at least M3 grade bicep strength was achieved in 92% of the patients treated with an intercostal nerve to musculocutaneous nerve transfer.[68]

Shoulder Evaluation and Management

Obtaining imaging studies of the shoulder of an infant is challenging. Plain radiographs, although easily obtainable, offer limited information about the glenohumeral joint. MRI studies provide the best anatomic detail, but an adequate study requires general anesthesia in the infant.[69] In the hands of an experienced practitioner, ultrasonography is recognized as a good screening tool to diagnose glenohumeral subluxation.[70] Because a glenohumeral joint deformity can occur early in a patient with a persistent internal rotation contracture of the shoulder, treatments involving injections of botulinum toxin type A to the internal rotators, arthroscopic anterior releases, and open surgical release with tendon transfers offer promising results for limiting or reversing the process of glenohumeral dysplasia.[71-74]

Elbow Contracture

Many children with brachial plexus birth palsy have an elbow flexion contracture, and some contractures are severe enough to limit function. A recent study identified a flexion contracture in 48% of the patients with brachial plexus birth palsy.[75] Before treatment, these contractures progressed at a rate of 4.4% per year. Another research study has proposed that the etiology of elbow flexion contracture in brachial plexus birth palsy may be caused by overactivity of the long head of the bicep brachii muscle.[76]

Intrauterine Compartment Syndrome

Intrauterine compartment syndrome is a rare condition that is also known as congenital Volkmann ischemic contracture. In the early stages, the upper extremity of the neonate is typically ischemic, is edematous, and may show some necrosis of the fingertips. The classic

Table 6

Patterns of Brachial Plexus Injuries

Pattern	Involved Nerve Roots	Primary Deficiency
Erb-Duchenne lesion Upper brachial plexus	C5-C6	Shoulder abduction and external rotation Elbow flexion
Extended Erb lesion Upper and middle plexus	C5-C7	Shoulder abduction and external rotation Elbow flexion Elbow and finger extension
Dejerine-Klumpke lesion Lower brachial plexus	C8-T1	Hand intrinsic muscles Finger flexors
Total or global lesion Entire brachial plexus	C5-T1	Entire extremity

(Reproduced from Zlotolow DA, Kozin SH: Upper extremity disorders: Pediatrics, in Flynn JM, ed: *Orthopaedic Knowledge Update*, ed 10. Rosemont, IL, American Academy of Orthopaedic Surgeons, 2011, pp 697-713.)

physical examination finding is a sentinel skin lesion, which has been described as a bluish colored plaque (Figure 11). The true etiology of this condition is unknown, but reported associated factors include prematurity, excessive maternal weight gain, and gestational diabetes.[77] The physical findings can be confused with constriction band syndrome; however, in intrauterine compartment syndrome, there is no banding found proximally on the arm. When recognized early, emergent release of the affected compartments may allow for salvage of the affected limb before tissue loss occurs. In patients where obvious tissue necrosis has occurred in utero, late treatment involves débridement, neurolysis, and muscle reconstruction.[78]

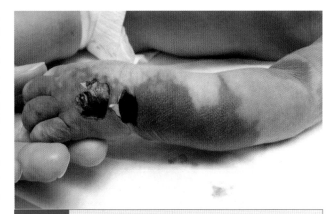

| Figure 11 | Photograph showing neonatal compartment syndrome, with the pathognomonic skin lesion and peripheral ischemia. (Courtesy of Shriners Hospital for Children, Philadelphia, PA.) |

Summary

It is believed that congenital deformities involving the upper extremity represent approximately 10% of all congenital anomalies that are seen. Most of these disorders occur spontaneously or can be found as part of a syndromic condition. Ongoing research that focuses on cell signaling in the developing embryo has improved the understanding of how these anomalies may arise. Care for the child with an upper limb congenital anomaly centers on understanding the unique anatomy of the disorder, identifying potential associated conditions, and designing treatments that allow optimal function

Key Study Points

- New research studying cell-signaling biology has identified certain errors in embryologic development that are thought to be the basis for some congenital upper extremity anomalies.

- Although categorizing these conditions is challenging, a new classification system for congenital upper limb disorders based on recent research in development biology has been proposed. It may eventually supplant the commonly used International Federation of Societies for Surgery of the Hand congenital classifications, which tend to be more descriptive and based on anatomic findings.

- For the young child with brachial plexus birth palsy, treatments such as injections of botulinum toxin type A to the shoulder internal rotator muscles, arthroscopic anterior releases, and open surgical release with tendon transfers offer promising results for limiting or reversing the process of glenohumeral dysplasia.

Annotated References

1. Oberg KC, Feenstra JM, Manske PR, Tonkin MA: Developmental biology and classification of congenital anomalies of the hand and upper extremity. *J Hand Surg Am* 2010;35(12):2066-2076.

   This article presents a new classification system for upper limb anomalies that incorporates the current understandings of molecular biology and how it affects upper limb development. Three broad categories—malformations, deformations, and dysplasias—along with individual subcategories are discussed.

2. Waters PM, Bae DS: Embryology and development, in *Pediatric Hand and Upper Limb Surgery: A Practical Guide*. Philadelphia, PA, Lippincott Williams & Wilkins, 2012, pp 1-9.

   The textbook is an excellent resource that covers most of the anomalies and disorders seen in pediatric upper extremity patients. Each condition is introduced by a case study, which is followed by an in-depth discussion of the clinical findings and treatment algorithms.

3. Al-Qattan MM, Yang Y, Kozin SH: Embryology of the upper limb. *J Hand Surg Am* 2009;34(7):1340-1350.

4. Yang Y, Kozin SH: Cell signaling regulation of vertebrate limb growth and patterning. *J Bone Joint Surg Am* 2009;91(4, suppl 4):76-80.

5. Swanson AB: A classification for congenital limb malformations. *J Hand Surg Am* 1976;1(1):8-22.

6. Manske PR, Oberg KC: Classification and developmental biology of congenital anomalies of the hand and upper extremity. *J Bone Joint Surg Am* 2009;91(4, suppl 4):3-18.

7. Goldfarb CA, Wall L, Manske PR: Radial longitudinal deficiency: The incidence of associated medical and musculoskeletal conditions. *J Hand Surg Am* 2006; 31(7):1176-1182.

6: Pediatrics

8. Mancuso A, Giacobbe A, De Vivo A, Fanara G, Cocivera G: Prenatal identification of isolated bilateral radial dysplasia. *J Clin Ultrasound* 2009;37(3):175-178.

9. Houeijeh A, Andrieux J, Saugier-Veber P, et al: Thrombocytopenia-absent radius (TAR) syndrome: A clinical genetic series of 14 further cases. Impact of the associated 1q21.1 deletion on the genetic counselling. *Eur J Med Genet* 2011;54(5):e471-e477.

   This is a French multicenter clinical study that confirmed the phenotypes of TAR syndrome associated with 1q21.1 deletion. The finding is important in atypical cases and helps guide genetic counseling.

10. Rosenberg PS, Tamary H, Alter BP: How high are carrier frequencies of rare recessive syndromes? Contemporary estimates for Fanconi anemia in the United States and Israel. *Am J Med Genet A* 2011;155A(8):1877-1883.

    Even though Fanconi anemia is a rare condition, this study found that the carrier frequency may be higher than previously determined—about 1 in 181.

11. Holden ST, Cox JJ, Kesterton I, Thomas NS, Carr C, Woods CG: Fanconi anaemia complementation group B presenting as X linked VACTERL with hydrocephalus syndrome. *J Med Genet* 2006;43(9):750-754.

12. de Graaff E, Kozin SH: Genetics of radial deficiencies. *J Bone Joint Surg Am* 2009;91(suppl 4):81-86.

13. Tay SC, Moran SL, Shin AY, Cooney WP III: The hypoplastic thumb. *J Am Acad Orthop Surg* 2006;14(6):354-366.

14. Riley SA, Burgess RC: Thumb hypoplasia. *J Hand Surg Am* 2009;34(8):1564-1573.

15. Kozin SH, Ezaki M: Flexor digitorum superficialis opponensplasty with ulnar collateral ligament reconstruction for thumb deficiency. *Tech Hand Up Extrem Surg* 2010;14(1):46-50.

    This article outlines a treatment plan for type II thumb hypoplasia which is characterized by a narrow web space, the absence of intrinsic thenar muscles, and an insufficient ulnar collateral ligament. The authors describe using the flexor digitorum superficialis tendon for both the opponesplasty and ligament reconstruction.

16. Morisawa Y, Takayama S, Seki A, Nakamura T, Ikegami H: Reconstruction of the first web in congenital thumb anomalies. *Hand Surg* 2011;16(1):63-67.

    This study compared the results of two different skin flaps (Spinner and five-flap Z-plasty) used for thumb web space reconstruction. The authors found that the Spinner flap shows better outcomes in the older child and in those with more severe contractures.

17. Goldfarb CA, Murtha YM, Gordon JE, Manske PR: Soft-tissue distraction with a ring external fixator before centralization for radial longitudinal deficiency. *J Hand Surg Am* 2006;31(6):952-959.

18. Pickford MA, Scheker LR: Distraction lengthening of the ulna in radial club hand using the Ilizarov technique. *J Hand Surg Br* 1998;23(2):186-191.

19. de Jong JP, Moran SL, Vilkki SK: Changing paradigms in the treatment of radial club hand: Microvascular joint transfer for correction of radial deviation and preservation of long-term growth. *Clin Orthop Surg* 2012;4(1):36-44.

    This is a long-term follow-up study of work done originally by Vilkki in 1992. The authors discuss the surgical techniques and outcomes in patients having a vascularized toe metatarsophalangeal joint transfer for treating specific radial deficiencies.

20. Riley SA: An overview of radial longitudinal deficiency. *Curr Orthop Pract* 2008;9:655-659.

21. Flatt AE: *The Care of Congenital Hand Anomalies*, ed 2. St. Louis, MO, Quality Medical Publishing, 1994, pp 411-424.

22. Kozin SH: Upper-extremity congenital anomalies. *J Bone Joint Surg Am* 2003;85(8):1564-1576.

23. Falliner AA: Analysis of anatomic variations in cleft hands. *J Hand Surg Am* 2004;29(6):994-1001.

24. Oberlin C, Korchi A, Belkheyar Z, Touam C, Macquillan A: Digitalization of the second finger in type 2 central longitudinal deficiencies (clefting) of the hand. *Tech Hand Up Extrem Surg* 2009;13(2):110-112.

25. Radocha RF, Netscher D, Kleinert HE: Toe phalangeal grafts in congenital hand anomalies. *J Hand Surg Am* 1993;18(5):833-841.

26. Netscher DT, Lewis EV: Technique of nonvascularized toe phalangeal transfer and distraction lengthening in the treatment of multiple digit symbrachydactyly. *Tech Hand Up Extrem Surg* 2008;12(2):114-120.

27. Dhalla R, Strecker W, Manske PR: A comparison of two techniques for digital distraction lengthening in skeletally immature patients. *J Hand Surg Am* 2001;26(4):603-610.

28. Goldfarb CA, Manske PR, Busa R, Mills J, Carter P, Ezaki M: Upper-extremity phocomelia reexamined: A longitudinal dysplasia. *J Bone Joint Surg Am* 2005;87(12):2639-2648.

29. Kozin SH: Syndactyly. *J Am Soc Surg Hand* 2001;1:1-13.

30. Hutchinson DT, Frenzen SW: Digital syndactyly release. *Tech Hand Up Extrem Surg* 2010;14(1):33-37.

    The authors provide an excellent discussion regarding the different methodologies for syndactyly reconstruction. In addition, updated information on surgical technique, as well as a discussion of postoperative care for these patients, is presented.

31. Vekris MD, Lykissas MG, Soucacos PN, Korompilias AV, Beris AE: Congenital syndactyly: Outcome of surgical treatment in 131 webs. *Tech Hand Up Extrem Surg* 2010;14(1):2-7.

    The authors review syndactyly cases and offer technical advice regarding the management of the more difficult problems, such as the treatment of multiple digit syndactyly.

32. Miyamoto J, Nagasao T, Miyamoto S: Biomechanical analysis of surgical correction of syndactyly. *Plast Reconstr Surg* 2010;125(3):963-968.

    The authors discuss their analysis of the different flaps use for reconstructing the web. They found that the dorsal rectangular flap may be more prone to developing web creep.

33. Strauss NL, Goldfarb CA: Surgical correction of clinodactyly: Two straightforward techniques. *Tech Hand Up Extrem Surg* 2010;14(1):54-57.

    This article shows two methods of surgical correction for addressing a functionally limiting angulation deformity found in patients with clinodactyly.

34. Waters PM, Bae DS: Clinodactyly and camptodactyly, in *Pediatric Hand and Upper Limb Surgery: A Practical Guide*. Philadelphia, PA, Lippincott Williams & Wilkins, 2012, pp 49-58.

35. Goldfarb CA: Congenital hand differences. *J Hand Surg Am* 2009;34(7):1351-1356.

36. Lee J, Ahn JK, Choi S-H, Koh E-M, Cha H-S: MRI findings in Kirner deformity: Normal insertion of the flexor digitorum profundus tendon without soft-tissue enhancement. *Pediatr Radiol* 2010;40(9):1572-1575.

    Although there are many proposed causes, the true etiology of Kirner deformity is unknown. The authors used an MRI of a finger with Kirner deformity and found that there was no inflammation or abnormalities of the flexor tendon insertion on the distal phalanx.

37. Cleary JE, Omer GE Jr: Congenital proximal radioulnar synostosis: Natural history and functional assessment. *J Bone Joint Surg Am* 1985;67(4):539-545.

38. De Smet L, Fryns JP: Unilateral radio-ulnar synostosis and idic-Y chromosome. *Genet Couns* 2008;19(4):425-427.

39. Kasten P, Rettig O, Loew M, Wolf S, Raiss P: Three-dimensional motion analysis of compensatory movements in patients with radioulnar synostosis performing activities of daily living. *J Orthop Sci* 2009;14(3):307-312.

40. Harvey EJ, Bernstein M, Desy NM, Saran N, Ouellet JA: Sprengel deformity: Pathogenesis and management. *J Am Acad Orthop Surg* 2012;20(3):177-186.

    This article is an excellent review of etiology, clinical findings, and proposed treatments of Sprengel deformity. The most common surgical procedures are pre-sented, along with the expected outcomes and potential complications.

41. Mooney JF III, White DR, Glazier S: Previously unreported structure associated with Sprengel deformity. *J Pediatr Orthop* 2009;29(1):26-28.

42. Ahmad AA: Surgical correction of severe Sprengel deformity to allow greater postoperative range of shoulder abduction. *J Pediatr Orthop* 2010;30(6):575-581.

    In patients manifesting severe Sprengel deformity, the author reports on a surgical procedure designed to inferiorly displace and then position the scapula on the rib cage to allow for maximum postoperative shoulder abduction.

43. Waters PM, Bae DS: Preaxial polydactyly, in *Pediatric Hand and Upper Limb Surgery: A Practical Guide*. Philadelphia, PA, Lippincott Williams & Wilkins, 2012, pp 32-42.

    This chapter presents current understanding of the diagnosis and treatment of radial-sided polydactyly.

44. Wassel HD: The results of surgery for polydactyly of the thumb: A review. *Clin Orthop Relat Res* 1969;64:175-193.

45. Ezaki M: Radial polydactyly. *Hand Clin* 1990;6(4):577-588.

46. Baek GH, Gong HS, Chung MS, Oh JH, Lee YH, Lee SK: Modified Bilhaut-Cloquet procedure for Wassel type-II and III polydactyly of the thumb: Surgical technique. *J Bone Joint Surg Am* 2008;90(suppl 2, pt 1):74-86.

47. Katz K, Linder N: Postaxial type B polydactyly treated by excision in the neonatal nursery. *J Pediatr Orthop* 2011;31(4):448-449.

    The authors report on their experience of performing a surgical excision of the rudimentary digit in type B ulnar polydactyly. The families of every patient treated with this method were satisfied with the functional and cosmetic results.

48. Goodman FR: Limb malformations and the human HOX genes. *Am J Med Genet* 2002;112(3):256-265.

49. Kikuchi N, Ogino T: Incidence and development of trigger thumb in children. *J Hand Surg Am* 2006;31(4):541-543.

50. Bae DS: Pediatric trigger thumb. *J Hand Surg Am* 2008;33(7):1189-1191.

51. Ogino T: Trigger thumb in children: Current recommendations for treatment. *J Hand Surg Am* 2008;33(6):982-984.

52. Bae DS, Sodha S, Waters PM: Surgical treatment of the pediatric trigger finger. *J Hand Surg Am* 2007;32(7):1043-1047.

6: Pediatrics

53. Duncan ST, Riley SA: An overview of Madelung's deformity. *Curr Orthop Pract* 2009;20:648-654.

54. Vickers D, Nielsen G: Madelung deformity: Surgical prophylaxis (physiolysis) during the late growth period by resection of the dyschondrosteosis lesion. *J Hand Surg Br* 1992;17(4):401-407.

55. Harley BJ, Brown C, Cummings K, Carter PR, Ezaki M: Volar ligament release and distal radius dome osteotomy for correction of Madelung's deformity. *J Hand Surg Am* 2006;31(9):1499-1506.

56. Flatt AE: *The Care of Congenital Hand Anomalies*, ed 2. St. Louis, MO, Quality Medical Publishing, 1994, pp 317-333.

57. Kakinoki R, Ikeguchi R, Duncan SF: Transverse and longitudinal osteotomy for the treatment of macrodactyly simplex congenita: A case report. *Hand Surg* 2008; 13(2):121-128.

58. Moran SL, Jensen M, Bravo C: Amniotic band syndrome of the upper extremity: Diagnosis and management. *J Am Acad Orthop Surg* 2007;15(7):397-407.

59. Goldfarb CA, Sathienkijkanchai A, Robin NH: Amniotic constriction band: A multidisciplinary assessment of etiology and clinical presentation. *J Bone Joint Surg Am* 2009;91(4, suppl 4):68-75.

60. Upton J, Tan C: Correction of constriction rings. *J Hand Surg Am* 1991;16(5):947-953.

61. Tan P-L, Chiang Y-C: Triangular flaps: A modified technique for the correction of congenital constriction ring syndrome. *Hand Surg* 2011;16(3):387-393.

    The authors present an alternative to the usual resection and Z-plasty flap transposition technique of reconstructing a constriction ring deformity in an extremity.

62. Soldado F, Aguirre M, Peiró JL, et al: Fetal surgery of extremity amniotic bands: An experimental model of in utero limb salvage in fetal lamb. *J Pediatr Orthop* 2009; 29(1):98-102.

63. Hale HB, Bae DS, Waters PM: Current concepts in the management of brachial plexus birth palsy. *J Hand Surg Am* 2010;35(2):322-331.

    This article presents highlights from the recent literature discussing the pathoanatomy and natural history of the injury along with surgical indications, expected outcomes, and complications of treatment modalities.

64. Kozin SH: The evaluation and treatment of children with brachial plexus birth palsy. *J Hand Surg Am* 2011; 36(8):1360-1369.

    The author presents his research involving treatment methods for adolescents and children impaired by nerve injury. As a result of this body of work, Dr. Kozin was presented the 2010 Andrew J. Weiland Medal by the American Society for Surgery of the Hand.

65. Foad SL, Mehlman CT, Ying J: The epidemiology of neonatal brachial plexus palsy in the United States. *J Bone Joint Surg Am* 2008;90(6):1258-1264.

66. Clarke HM, Al-Qattan MM, Curtis CG, Zuker RM: Obstetrical brachial plexus palsy: Results following neurolysis of conducting neuromas-in-continuity. *Plast Reconstr Surg* 1996;97(5):974-984.

67. Kozin SH: Nerve transfers in brachial plexus birth palsies: Indications, techniques, and outcomes. *Hand Clin* 2008;24(4):363-376, v.

68. Luo PB, Chen L, Zhou C-H, Hu S-N, Gu Y-D: Results of intercostal nerve transfer to the musculocutaneous nerve in brachial plexus birth palsy. *J Pediatr Orthop* 2011;31(8):884-888.

    Twenty-four cases of intercostal nerve transfers are presented, and significant gains in bicep strength (of greater than M3) were reported in most of the treated patients.

69. Pearl ML: Shoulder problems in children with brachial plexus birth palsy: Evaluation and management. *J Am Acad Orthop Surg* 2009;17(4):242-254.

70. Pöyhiä TH, Lamminen AE, Peltonen JI, Kirjavainen MO, Willamo PJ, Nietosvaara Y: Brachial plexus birth injury: US screening for glenohumeral joint instability. *Radiology* 2010;254(1):253-260.

    The authors recommend the use of shoulder ultrasonography as a modality for diagnosing glenohumeral subluxation in infants with brachial plexus birth palsy. Interestingly, in 16% of the patients who had posterior subluxation of the humeral head seen on ultrasound, the abnormality was not noted on clinical examination.

71. Waters PM, Bae DS: The early effects of tendon transfers and open capsulorrhaphy on glenohumeral deformity in brachial plexus birth palsy. *J Bone Joint Surg Am* 2008;90(10):2171-2179.

72. Ezaki M, Malungpaishrope K, Harrison RJ, et al: Onabotulinum toxin A injection as an adjunct in the treatment of posterior shoulder subluxation in neonatal brachial plexus palsy. *J Bone Joint Surg Am* 2010;92(12): 2171-2177.

    This article reports on the use of Botox A to treat contractures of the shoulder by temporarily weakening the tight internal rotators that lead to posterior subluxation of the glenohumeral joint. The average age of the patient receiving this treatment was 5.7 months.

73. Kozin SH, Boardman MJ, Chafetz RS, Williams GR, Hanlon A: Arthroscopic treatment of internal rotation contracture and glenohumeral dysplasia in children with brachial plexus birth palsy. *J Shoulder Elbow Surg* 2010;19(1):102-110.

    In children with brachial plexus birth palsy, arthroscopic release of a shoulder contracture combined with tendon transfers showed improved clinical function, as well as improved MRI appearance of the glenohumeral dysplasia compared with preoperative findings. Significant gains in shoulder external rotation and elevation were also noted.

74. Van Heest A, Glisson C, Ma H: Glenohumeral dysplasia changes after tendon transfer surgery in children with birth brachial plexus injuries. *J Pediatr Orthop* 2010; 30(4):371-378.

An important finding in this study was that in children with brachial plexus birth palsy, tendon transfers for decreased external rotation showed greater improvement in glenohumeral dysplasia if the surgery is performed before 2 years of age.

75. Sheffler LC, Lattanza L, Hagar Y, Bagley A, James MA: The prevalence, rate of progression, and treatment of elbow flexion contracture in children with brachial plexus birth palsy. *J Bone Joint Surg Am* 2012;94(5):403-409.

The authors found that the incidence of elbow flexion contracture in brachial plexus birth palsy may be more than previously identified. The contractures were found to increase at a rate of 4.4% per year. Patients with severe contractures showed initial improvement with serial casting. Those children with mild elbow contractures were managed with night splints to help prevent progression.

76. Sheffler LC, Lattanza L, Sison-Williamson M, James MA: Biceps brachii long head overactivity associated with elbow flexion contracture in brachial plexus birth palsy. *J Bone Joint Surg Am* 2012;94(4):289-297.

This article proposes that overactivity of the long head of the bicep tendon, as opposed to an elbow flexor-extensor muscle imbalance, may be the main cause of elbow flexion contracture in brachial plexus birth palsy. Increased activity of this muscle was documented in hand-to-head and high-reach tasks.

77. Raimer L, McCarthy RA, Raimer D, Colome-Grimmer M: Congenital Volkmann ischemic contracture: A case report. *Pediatr Dermatol* 2008;25(3):352-354.

78. Ragland R III, Moukoko D, Ezaki M, Carter PR, Mills J: Forearm compartment syndrome in the newborn: Report of 24 cases. *J Hand Surg Am* 2005;30(5):997-1003.

6: Pediatrics

Chapter 60

Pediatric Spine Disorders and Spine Trauma

Amy L. McIntosh, MD   Patrick Bosch, MD

Torticollis

Congenital Muscular Torticollis

Torticollis means twisted neck. Although there are many causes of torticollis, one of the most common is congenital muscular torticollis (CMT). The etiology of CMT is not established but is likely the result of a compartment syndrome of the sternocleidomastoid muscle secondary to obstruction of venous outflow.[1] In the neonatal period, it presents as a hard mass in the affected sternocleidomastoid muscle that gradually subsides and becomes a tight band as the child ages.[2] The most common position of the head in children with CMT is tilting toward and rotating away from the side of the involved sternocleidomastoid muscle.[2-4]

Children with CMT often have plagiocephaly (asymmetric flattening of the skull). This condition is commonly characterized by a lower than normal position of the eye on the involved side, deviation of the eye and the nose to the affected side, and flattening of the occiput on the opposite side.[2] Most infants will respond to stretching exercises, and there is little justification for surgical release before 12 to 18 months of age.[5] The results of surgical release are good, even in older children (older than 4 to 8 years), although remodeling of plagiocephaly is slower in older children.[2,3] Bipolar release of the sternocleidomastoid muscle is presently favored, but good results are also attainable with unipolar release. Endoscopic release also has been reported.[6]

Atlantoaxial Rotatory Subluxation

Another cause of torticollis in children is atlantoaxial rotatory subluxation. The condition is characterized by excessive movement at the junction between the atlas (C1) and the axis (C2) resulting from either a bony or a ligamentous abnormality. The causes are varied. The condition can result from trauma or can present after an upper respiratory infection or a postoperative infection

---

Dr. McIntosh or an immediate family member serves as a paid consultant to or is an employee of Synthes. Dr. Bosch or an immediate family member serves as a board member, owner, officer, or committee member of the Pediatric Orthopaedic Society of North America.

after head and neck surgery (Grisel syndrome). Other causes include rheumatoid arthritis, congenital anomalies, syndromes, or metabolic diseases. Patients present with torticollis, but the spasm of the sternocleidomastoid muscle is often opposite that seen with CMT, with the head tilting away and rotating toward the involved sternocleidomastoid muscle. Because of pain, the child will resist any attempt to correct the position of the head. Radiography often does not help in establishing the diagnosis. A CT scan of the base of the skull and the cervical spine is the imaging modality of choice (Figure 1).

In 1977, Fielding and Hawkins[7] described four types of atlantoaxial rotatory subluxation. Treatment is based on the degree of displacement and the duration of the symptoms. For a subluxation of a few days, duration, a soft cervical collar and oral NSAIDs may successfully treat the condition. For patients who do not respond to conservative treatment, hospital admission is required. Halter traction is applied, and a muscle relaxant (such as valium) and anti-inflammatory medications are administered. If this treatment is unsuccessful, halo gravity traction and/or surgical stabilization may be necessary to reduce and prevent resubluxation. In a patient with Grisel syndrome, the involvement of an ear, nose, and throat surgeon is essential, and antibiotics are often given in addition to muscle relaxants and anti-inflammatory medications.[8]

Klippel-Feil Syndrome

A patient with Klippel-Feil syndrome has congenital cervical vertebral anomalies (congenital cervical fusions) associated with the characteristic clinical triad of a short neck, a low hairline, and restricted neck mobility. This condition may be erroneously diagnosed as CMT because of the associated head tilt and limited cervical range of motion. Abnormalities in other organ systems are common. Most patients have hearing deficits.[9] Urinary tract anomalies are also common, and renal ultrasonography is indicated in all children with Klippel-Feil syndrome.[10] Because cardiac anomalies are common, an evaluation by a pediatric cardiologist and echocardiography are essential. Patients often have an associated Sprengel deformity (elevated scapula), which presents with limited abduction and forward flexion of

6: Pediatrics

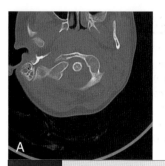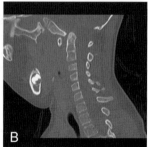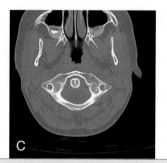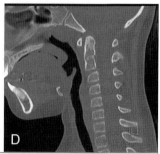

Figure 1 A 6-year-old girl with atraumatic atlantoaxial rotatory instability was unsuccessfully treated with hospitalization, muscle relaxants, NSAIDs, and halter traction. Halo-gravity traction followed by immobilization in a halo vest for 3 months resulted in normal cervical alignment. **A,** Axial CT of C1-C2 rotation before treatment. **B,** Sagittal CT showing a widened atlantodens interval and basilar invagination before treatment. **C,** Axial CT of normal C1-C2 alignment after treatment. **D,** Sagittal CT showing normalization of the atlantodens interval and basilar invagination after treatment.

the involved shoulder. The abnormal position of the scapula is also visible on spinal radiographs. Many children also have associated intradural anomalies; MRI of the brain stem and the spinal cord are essential in the diagnosis of anomalies.

Surgical treatment for orthopaedic problems is often not required for patients with Klippel-Feil syndrome. Radiographic observation with AP, lateral, flexion, and extension views of the cervical spine can be used to determine if progressive instability or degenerative changes at the spinal segments above and below the congenitally fused vertebra have occurred.[11] Patients and their families should be counseled to avoid activities (such as football, hockey, lacrosse, gymnastics, and trampoline use) that place the cervical spine at higher risk for traumatic injury.

Os Odontoideum

Os odontoideum represents a failure of fusion of the dens to the remainder of the axis (C2 body). The etiology of this condition is difficult to determine, but it is believed to be related to either a congenital anomaly or an unrecognized fracture and nonunion of the odontoid synchondrosis before its closure at age 5 to 6 years.[12-14] A child with a symptomatic os odontoideum usually presents with neck pain, headache, transient paresthesias, or myelopathy. The symptoms are attributed to instability of the C1-C2 junction, which leads to spinal cord impingement and/or vertebral artery compression.

Radiographs of the cervical spine (AP, lateral, flexion, and extension views), CT scans, and MRIs are often necessary to thoroughly evaluate these patients. Treatment consists of surgical stabilization and fusion of the C1-C2 junction.

Back Pain

Back pain is uncommon in toddlers and young children; however, the incidence increases dramatically in adolescents, with 24% of adolescents seen annually by a physician because of reported low back pain.[15] As many as 37% of teenage athletes have low back pain, which is associated with the increasing emphasis on participation in competitive athletic competition.[15] The most common identifiable etiologies for low back pain in children and adolescents are spondylolysis, spondylolisthesis, Scheuermann kyphosis, infection, and neoplastic disorders. Most instances of back pain, however, are diagnosed as nonspecific back pain.[15]

Back pain has been positively associated with the female sex, a positive finding on a scoliosis screening examination, and the use of a heavy backpack. It is negatively associated with the use of a light backpack and the availability of a school locker for storing supplies.[16]

It is helpful to use an algorithmic approach in diagnosing back pain. Evaluation should include a thorough history and physical examination, with emphasis on the neurologic examination, and radiographic studies. The use of this approach resulted in a diagnosis in 24% of patients in a recent study.[17] If chronic and constant pain, night pain, radicular pain, or other neurologic signs and symptoms are present, MRI studies should be obtained. The addition of MRI led to a diagnosis in an additional 12% of the patients.[17] If the patient primarily reports lumbosacral low back pain that is reproduced with hyperextension activities, CT and single-photon emission computed tomography (SPECT) should be used to evaluate for spondylosis. If an osteoid osteoma is suspected, CT is the best diagnostic modality. If an infectious, neoplastic, inflammatory, or rheumatologic etiology is suspected, laboratory studies should be obtained, including a complete blood count with differential, erythrocyte sedimentation rate, C-reactive protein level, antinuclear antibody test, rheumatoid factor test, and human leukocyte antigen B27 test. Episodic nonspecific musculoskeletal back pain that is benign in origin develops in many children. These patients are best treated with reassurance, rest, NSAIDs, and physical therapy.[17]

Spondylolysis

Spondylolysis is a term that refers to a stress reaction or a true fracture (cortical disruption) in the pars interarticularis (or posterior elements [lamina/pedicle]). It commonly occurs in athletes who participate in high-risk sports such as gymnastics, diving, football, volleyball, tennis, and rowing. These injuries result from repetitive loading of the lumbar spine in extension and rotation, can be unilateral or bilateral, and occur most commonly at L5.[18] The child or the adolescent typically presents with low back pain or, occasionally, pain that radiates to the buttock or the posterior thigh. Although acute injury may precipitate the onset of pain, insidious onset is more common. Radicular symptoms and disturbance of bowel or bladder function rarely occur with spondylolysis.

Standing PA and lateral radiography of the thoracolumbar spine is the best primary diagnostic test. If the radiographic findings are negative but clinical suspicion remains high, SPECT of the lumbosacral spine is the most effective method for detecting spondylolysis. Thin-section CT, performed with a reverse gantry angle, is the best modality for determining the degree of cortical disruption, lysis, and sclerosis at the pars, the lamina, or the pedicle. Progressive healing of stress reactions can be documented by serial CT evaluations. MRI is indicated when neurologic symptoms and signs are present in conjunction with spondylolysis. The role of MRI as a primary diagnostic tool in young patients with stress reactions or symptomatic spondylolytic defects is not well defined. A high rate of false-positive studies and a low positive predictive value suggest that other modalities may be more effective in diagnosing spondylolysis.[18]

Stress fractures and reactions of the pars interarticularis without cortical disruption (hot areas on SPECT without cortical disruption on CT) have the potential to heal. Osseous healing potential is greater in unilateral than bilateral lesions, and prompt treatment as a result of early detection may improve clinical outcomes. Full-time immobilization in a thoracolumbosacral orthosis, with or without thigh extension for a period of 6 to 12 weeks, is indicated for a child or an adolescent with a stress reaction of the pars interarticularis. Immobilization may be discontinued after pain-free lumbar extension and rotation are achieved; follow-up evaluation with repeat CT imaging should be used to document progressive bony healing. After discontinuation of immobilization and a period of physiotherapy, activities are gradually reintroduced. Surgery is indicated in patients who do not have a positive clinical response after a minimum of 6 months of nonsurgical treatment. In situ L5-S1 posterolateral fusion is the standard treatment in children and adolescents with L5 spondylolysis. Repair of the pars defect is indicated for L1 through L4 spondylolytic defects or spondylolytic defects at multiple vertebral levels.[19]

Spondylolisthesis

Spondylolisthesis describes the forward translation of one vertebra relative to the next lower vertebral segment. In children and adolescents, spondylolisthesis most commonly occurs at the L5-S1 motion segment. The Wiltse classification is most commonly used to help determine the etiology of spondylolisthesis. Of the five types, only types I and II commonly occur in children and adolescents.

Type I, the dysplastic type, defines spondylolisthesis secondary to congenital abnormalities. In dysplastic spondylolisthesis, the pars interarticularis is poorly developed, which allows for elongation or elongation with eventual separation leading to forward slippage of L5 on S1 with repetitive loading over time. This elongated dysplastic pars may cause lumbar stenosis. Patients may present with L5 nerve radiculopathy as well as bowel and bladder dysfunction caused by compression of the sacral nerve roots. Children and adolescents with dysplastic spondylolisthesis are at greater risk for the development of neurologic injury and progressive deformity than patients with isthmic spondylolisthesis.

Type II, the isthmic type, results from osseous disruption of the pars interarticularis. It is hypothesized that isthmic defects are the result of chronic loading of a pars interarticularis that is genetically predisposed to failure. Isthmic spondylolisthesis is the most common type of this disorder in children and adolescents. It has an incidence of 4.4% in children at age 6 years, which increases to 6% by age 18 years.[18] Progressive symptomatic isthmic spondylolisthesis is more likely to develop in children in whom the condition is diagnosed before their adolescent growth spurt, girls, and those presenting with slips greater than 50%. Hamstring spasm is the most frequently associated neurologic abnormality. Lumbar radiculopathy and bowel or bladder symptoms are rare but may occur in children with severe, high-grade, isthmic spondylolisthesis.

Radiography is the primary diagnostic tool when spondylolisthesis is suspected. The Meyerding classification quantifies the amount of forward translation based on a standing lateral radiograph. Spondylolisthesis is considered low grade if the slip is less than 50% (Meyerding classification is grade II or less) and high grade (Meyerding grades III and IV) if the slip is greater than 50% (Figure 2). Measurement of the slip angle quantifies the degree of lumbosacral kyphosis that has occurred in association with anterior translation. MRI is indicated when neurologic signs and symptoms are present. CT is also helpful in defining the bony anatomy to assist with preoperative planning.

Children with symptomatic, low-grade, isthmic spondylolisthesis respond to nonsurgical measures, including NSAIDs, physical therapy, and brace treatment. When pain and other symptoms have resolved, the patient may return to unrestricted athletic activities. Low-grade isthmic spondylolisthesis rarely progresses, regardless of a patient's age or activity level, and it has a benign clinical course in most patients.[18]

© 2014 American Academy of Orthopaedic Surgeons

6: Pediatrics

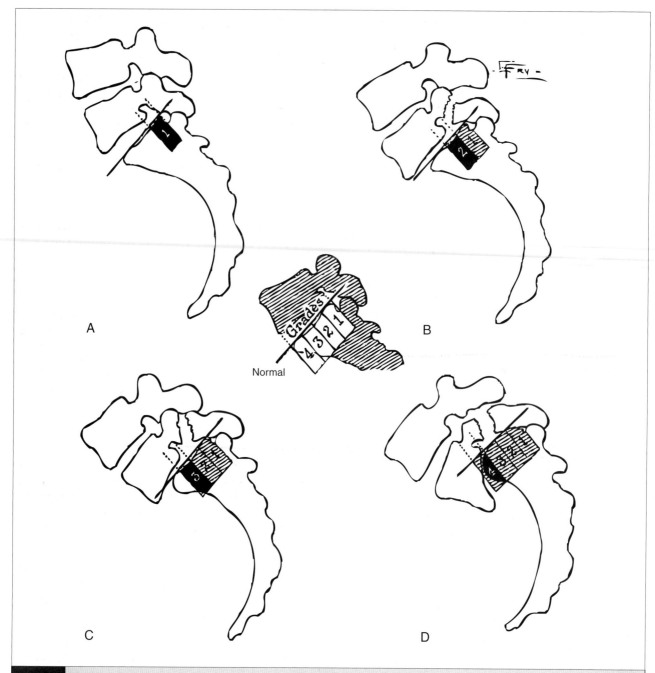

Figure 2   Illustrations of the Meyerding grade for spondylolisthesis. **A**, 25% slippage of L5 on S1 (grade1). **B**, 50% slippage of L5 on S1 (grade 2). **C**, 75% slippage of L5 on S1 (grade 3). **D** 100% slippage of L5 on S1 (grade 4). **E**, All of the representative grades.

In contrast, patients with low-grade dysplastic spondylolisthesis are at greatest risk for progression, the development of a neurologic deficit, and the need for surgical intervention. For these patients, serial physical examinations and radiographic studies are recommended at 6- to 9-month intervals through skeletal maturity.[18]

Children and adolescents with symptomatic high-grade spondylolisthesis, regardless of the type, respond less reliably to nonsurgical measures. Symptomatic re-

lief can be expected in less than 10% of patients. Consequently, surgical management is recommended for children and adolescents with symptomatic high-grade spondylolisthesis.[18]

Surgical treatment of low-grade isthmic spondylolisthesis is indicated for children and adolescents with persistent pain or neurologic dysfunction despite a minimum of 6 to 12 months of nonsurgical treatment. In situ L5-S1 posterolateral fusion is the standard treatment of L5 isthmic defects.[19]

The ideal surgical treatment of patients with high-grade isthmic and dysplastic spondylolisthesis is controversial and determined by the presence or the absence of neurologic symptoms and the amount of localized kyphosis (slip angle). In situ instrumented fusion versus instrumented fusion with partial reduction are the most common surgical treatment strategies.

Scheuermann Kyphosis

Increased kyphosis, or humpbacked deformity, refers to posterior rounding of the spine when viewed from the side. Normal thoracic kyphosis from T5 to T12 ranges from 20° to 45° (Cobb angle). Scheuermann kyphosis is a condition characterized by increased posterior rounding of the thoracic spine in association with structural deformity of the vertebral elements.[20] A lateral radiograph of the spine will show a thoracic kyphosis of more than 40°, along with radiographic findings of more than 5° of anterior wedging of three consecutive adjacent vertebral bodies at the apex of the kyphosis; irregular vertebral apophyseal lines, combined with flattening and wedging; narrowing of the intervertebral disk spaces; and a variable presence of Schmorl nodes.[21]

Patients usually present for evaluation because of increased rounding of the thoracic spine and occasional back pain. When pain is present, it is commonly localized to the interscapular area (apex of the deformity) or the lumbar area and is most likely caused by excessive lordosis and the resultant facet joint stresses. Parental concerns usually are related to cosmesis and the progressive nature of the deformity. On physical examination, the erect patient will demonstrate increased thoracic kyphosis with sloping shoulders. Forward posturing of the head and the neck is secondary to increased cervical lordosis. Increased lumbar lordosis will also be seen in concert with weakened abdominal muscles, which lead to a mildly protuberant abdomen. The Adams forward bending test may demonstrate slight truncal asymmetry associated with mild scoliosis. When viewed from the side, the Adams test will show an abrupt posterior angulation of the thoracic spine. This deformity is not easily corrected with postural changes or passive manipulation. Lumbar lordosis is usually reversible, but cervical lordosis may become fixed. Although the neurologic examination is normal, tight or contracted hamstrings are seen in these patients.

Surgical treatment of Scheuermann kyphosis is reserved for patients with pain, a rigid deformity, a curve of more than 70° to 75° and progressive deformity, and an unacceptable cosmetic appearance. Newer technologies, such as third generation segmental instrumentation in combination with compression rod techniques, have nearly eliminated the need for combined anterior-posterior procedures. When an anterior procedure is deemed to be necessary, prone thoracoscopic anterior release and fusion is an attractive alternative to formal open anterior release.[20]

Bertolotti Syndrome

Bertolotti syndrome is characterized by anomalous enlargement of the transverse process(es) of the lowest lumbar vertebra, which may articulate or fuse with the sacrum or the ilium and cause isolated L4-L5 disk disease. The condition is also described as partial sacralized lumbar vertebra. In a 2006 study, Bertolotti syndrome was found in 11.4% of patients younger than 30 years who underwent MRI evaluation for low back pain.[22] There is no consensus on treatment. Guided injection of steroid and local anesthetic into the anomalous lumbosacral articulation for severe chronic low back pain can lead to immediate but temporary pain relief for most patients.[22] If anomalous lumbosacral articulation is unilateral, a resection of the anomaly can be performed; for bilateral cases, an L5-S1 posterolateral in situ fusion can be attempted.

Scoliosis

The definition of scoliosis is a lateral deviation of the spine of more than 10°; however, it is understood to be a three-dimensional deformity with relative sagittal lordosis and axial rotation. Scoliosis is best considered a clinical finding associated with many and usually unknown etiologies (Table 1).

Congenital Scoliosis

Congenital scoliosis is a spinal deformity caused by structural abnormalities of the spinal column. These abnormalities are the result of unknown embryologic insults, genetic causes, or a combination of factors that occur between the fourth and eighth week of gestation.[23] Other organ systems developing during this time, such as the cardiac and genitourinary systems, may have associated defects. Rates of associated abnormalities as high as 50% justify systemic screening (renal ultrasonography and echocardiography) of patients at the time of diagnosis.[24,25] Abnormalities in the neural axis are present in approximately 40% of patients. MRI to rule out conditions requiring neurosurgical attention (Chiari malformation, tethered or split cord defects) is also often considered part of the initial workup and is strongly recommended before surgical intervention.[24-26] Chest wall deformities, Sprengel deformity or rib fusions, cranial nerve defects, imperforate anus, clubfeet, radial hypoplasia, hemifacial microsomia, and groupings such as oculoauriculovertebral dysplasia (Goldenhar syndrome),VACTERL (vertebral, anal, cardiac, tracheal, esophageal, renal, and limb abnormalities) association, and VATER (vertebral defects, imperforate anus, tracheoesophageal fistula, and radial and renal dysplasia) complex are also associated with congenital scoliosis.[23]

Curve progression is unpredictable in congenital scoliosis;[27] however, large kyphotic and scoliotic deformities can result from congenital abnormalities. Asymmetry in growth of the spinal column causes deformity

6: Pediatrics

Table 1				

Scoliosis Overview

	Presentation	Prognosis	Initial Treatment (25° to 45°)	Definitive Treatment (> 45° and Symptomatic Curve)
Congenital	MRI of spine and check genitourinary and cardiac systems	Variable; higher risk assigned to fully segmented hemivertebrae and unilateral bars	Definitive fusion or excision if curve is progressive and can limit fusion length	Fusion with or without excision or osteotomy
Infantile (younger than 3 years)	MRI of spine (if progressive)	Spontaneous correction possible	Casting	Nonfusion, growing techniques, especially if failed casting
Juvenile (3 to 10 years)	MRI of spine	High risk of progression	Bracing	Nonfusion techniques or definitive fusion
Adolescent (older than 10 years)	MRI if neurologic findings present	Variable	Watchful waiting or bracing	Definitive fusion
Neuromuscular		Generally progressive	Bracing for postural control only. Fusion if symptomatic and progression assured (for example, Duchenne muscular dystrophy)	Fusion, include pelvis if pelvic obliquity. Benign neglect if not symptomatic

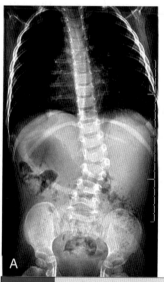
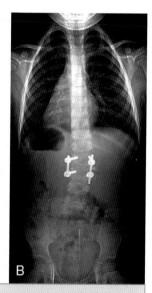

Figure 3   **A,** Radiograph of the spine of a 3-year-old girl with spinal imbalance from a fully segmented hemivertebra. **B,** Standing AP radiograph taken after posterior hemivertebra resection and instrumented fusion. After hemivertebra excision, the patient has improved coronal balance and no clinically apparent asymmetry.

progression. Unbalanced growth because of a hemivertebra or an unsegmented bar typically leads to the most pronounced deformity. A child is at particularly high risk for deformity progression during the major growth period of the spine before 2 years of age and during the pubertal growth spurt.[28]

Children with congenital scoliosis typically should be evaluated every 6 to 12 months with plain radiography. In children with a deformity identified in infancy, the presenting radiographs will be supine. Although these radiographs are often best to delineate the deformity, they are not optimal for monitoring progression. Until standing radiographs can be reliably obtained, patient positioning during radiography must be accounted for when monitoring spinal deformity in younger children. In addition to MRI, CT provides the best detailed representation of the anatomy and is useful for surgical planning.

If progression of deformity occurs, treatment is essentially surgical. Bracing may delay progression of compensatory curves but has no effect on anomalous vertebral growth. Traditional treatment remains in situ stabilization, a prophylactic approach to prevent further deformity with little or no correction. Although good results are possible, long-term follow-up studies have raised concerns about the pulmonary consequences of early fusion.[29] More aggressive correction of the deformity can require osteotomies or vertebral resection,[30] with the resection of isolated segmental hemivertebra proving beneficial[31] (Figure 3). These procedures carry an increased risk of neurologic injury; therefore, monitoring (somatosensory-evoked and transcranial motor-evoked potentials) should be considered mandatory.[32] Attempts at maintaining growth of the spinal column through the deformity with hemiepiphysiodesis of the convexity, growing rod constructs,

6: Pediatrics

and vertical expandable prosthetic titanium rib (VEPTR) devices are described in the literature.[33]

Neuromuscular Scoliosis

Spinal deformity cause by neurologic abnormalities defines a subset of scoliosis patients. Lower motor lesions leading to spinal deformity include myelomeningocele, spinal dysraphism, tumor, muscular dystrophy, or traumatic injury. Upper motor lesions, such as cerebral palsy, often lead to long sweeping curves over the whole spine with pelvic obliquity. The likelihood of deformity is greater with more severe neurologic involvement and loss of ambulation. These curves tend to be progressive. Indications for treatment include gait disturbance, seating imbalance, and quality-of-life disruption.

There is less specific treatment guidance based on the curve magnitude. Although bracing may maintain postural control, surgical stabilization is a definitive treatment. Correction and fixation of pelvic obliquity is particularly challenging. Options for caudal fixation include sacral S-rods, unit rods into the pelvis, iliac bolts, and a newer technique using long screws through the sacroiliac joint.[34] Comorbidities and osteopenia have implications for spinal fixation in patients with neuromuscular scoliosis. Traditionally, sublaminar wires were believed to be more stable in the relatively osteopenic bone, although the use of pedicle screws (off-label) has been supported in the literature.[35]

Idiopathic Scoliosis

Scoliosis in most patients (approximately 80%) has no defined etiology and is called idiopathic scoliosis. Potential causes of scoliosis, including congenital abnormalities, neurologic disorders, tumors, and underlying syndromes (such as Marfan syndrome or neurofibromatosis) should be excluded. A careful history and physical examination will exclude most alternative primary etiologies for spinal deformity, but MRI may be used to rule out intracanal abnormalities, such as Chiari malformation, syringomyelia, or a tethered cord. Certain factors, such as young age, hyperkyphosis, severe rotation, male sex, or an atypical curve pattern, increase the likelihood of a neurologic finding[36-40] (Table 2). Research into the etiology of idiopathic scoliosis suggests a multifactorial, hctcrogenetic disorder. Genome-wide association studies of single nucleotide polymorphisms in families with idiopathic scoliosis are identifying candidate genes, but the pathophysiology of the disorder remains unknown.[41]

Idiopathic scoliosis can be categorized based on a patient's age at onset: infantile (younger than 3 years), juvenile (3 to 10 years), and adolescent (10 to 18 years). Infantile scoliosis is unique in that the deformity can resolve spontaneously over months of observation. It more commonly affects males, and curve patterns tend to have less rotation and are left-sided thoracic curves. Progressive infantile curves, however, represent a very challenging treatment dilemma. Prognostic factors that indicate risk of progression are a rib

Table 2
Relative MRI Indications in Patients With Scoliosis
Congenital abnormality
Younger than 10 years at onset
Male sex
Neurologic finding
Asymmetric reflexes, including abdominal
Atypical curve pattern
Leftward main thoracic curve
Relative kyphosis

vertebral angle difference greater than 20° or the presence of rotation at the apex of the deformity (phase 2 deformity with the rib head overlying the edge of the vertebra on a coronal radiograph).[42] Although the reliability of the rib vertebral angle difference measurement has recently been confirmed, the authors of that analysis cautioned that decision making for infantile scoliosis should include the synthesis of objective and clinical subjective data.[43]

Patients with progressive infantile scoliosis are treated with derotation casting. Diligent and persistent casting techniques can lead to resolution of the deformity. Casts are applied in the operating room with the patient under general anesthesia, often with the aid of specially designed tables to assist in positioning and cast application. The cast is changed at 2- to 4-month intervals, and patients are expected to demonstrate serial improvement in curve magnitude. Casting is more often successful when started before 20 months of age in children with curves of less than 60° and with no underlying syndrome.[44,45] If a curve progresses despite cast and brace treatment, surgery is indicated. Definitive fusion is not desired because it will prevent adequate trunk growth. Growth-preserving techniques include single- and dual-rod growing constructs and VEPTR.[46-48]

Juvenile scoliosis is phenotypically similar to adolescent scoliosis, with a female preponderance of progressive curves, curve patterns that are most commonly right thoracic or double major, and remaining growth as the primary factor in progression. Because patients with juvenile scoliosis are younger than 10 years and are generally ahead of their peak growth spurt, they are believed to be at greater risk for substantial curve progression compared with older patients. This relatively worse prognosis slightly alters decision making from adolescent patients. In most instances, an MRI (whole spine) is obtained to rule out a reversible intracanal abnormality before commencing with brace treatment for curves greater than 25°.[37,39]

Adolescent idiopathic scoliosis is the most common type of spinal deformity. Minor curves of 10° to 20° are present in up to 3% of the population and occur

6: Pediatrics

equally in males and females. However, only 1 in 10 such curves progress to greater than 30°; progression is nearly sevenfold more common in females than in males.

Diagnosis and Curve Morphology

The diagnosis of scoliosis is usually first made by clinical examination. Deformity is often found at the time of well-child or sports physical examinations. Physical findings include asymmetric shoulder levels, waist creases, and rotational prominence detected by the Adams forward bending test. Most curves greater than 20° will be detectable, but certain curve patterns (double major), obesity, and patient modesty in this age group can delay curve detection. Long-cassette or full-length thoracolumbar radiographs are the preferred screening test. Observation with repeat radiography (every 6 to 12 months) is advisable for curves in patients with remaining growth.

Stratifying the risk of curve progression in patients with idiopathic scoliosis remains difficult. The growth remaining, the presenting curve magnitude, the curve pattern, and family history are considered in the risk evaluation.[49] The growth remaining is evaluated by menarche, secondary sexual characteristics (Tanner staging), closure of triradiate cartilage, and the Risser sign. Recently, a simplified skeletal maturity scoring system based on a radiograph of the hand has been shown to better correlate with the behavior of curves in patients with idiopathic scoliosis. Capping (widening of the epiphyses beyond the metaphyses) in phalanges coincides with the stage of maximal height velocity (stage 3 of 8) described in the Tanner-Whitehouse-III classification scheme.[50] Alternatively, a gene-based prognostic test has been developed to predict curve behavior. The use of proprietary gene markers to predict the risk of curve progression (reported as a score from 1 to 200) has yet to be independently validated, and its utility remains unknown.[51]

Adolescent idiopathic scoliosis is further subdivided based on curve morphology and curve magnitude. The direction and the location of perceived structural curves can be described as right thoracic, double major, or left thoracolumbar, which are the most common. Earlier classifications were concerned with specific recommendations for fusion levels in thoracic-based curve patterns.[52] To more comprehensively describe known curve patterns, a new classification scheme was introduced in 2001.[53] This system, known as the Lenke classification, is the main system used to describe adolescent idiopathic scoliosis curves. The Lenke classification includes information about sagittal deformity, allows comparisons for research, and guides surgical treatment (Figure 4).

Bracing

In patients with idiopathic scoliosis, bracing to prevent curve progression during growth remains the only commonly used method of nonsurgical management. There are no data to support the benefits of exercise or manipulative treatment in managing spinal deformity. Bracing is indicated for curves between 25° and 40° in patients with growth remaining (Risser grade 2 or less and less than 1 year postmenarchal). Bracing regimens include full-time wear (typically 16 to 20 hours daily) with removal for sporting activities or nighttime wear of correction braces. The literature supporting brace efficacy is limited.[54,55] A recent prospective study used heat sensors to objectively measure and quantify brace wear. The authors reported less curve progression among patients who wore the brace more than 12 hours per day compared with those who wore it for fewer hours.[56] More rigorous data are being sought in a multicenter, prospective study (Bracing in Adolescent Idiopathic Scoliosis Trial) that has completed patient recruitment and is designed to evaluate the efficacy of bracing. It should be noted that continued regular observation of a patient with scoliosis, so called watchful waiting, remains an accepted treatment alternative.

Surgical Treatment

Surgical treatment of idiopathic scoliosis is indicated for curves that cause spinal imbalance, functional or cosmetic symptoms, or are at risk for continued progression beyond skeletal maturity. Patients with curve magnitudes of more than 50° have been reported to be at risk for continued curve progression throughout life. Continued progression can lead to pain, impaired pulmonary function, and poor body image in adulthood.[57,58] Symptoms can be particularly magnified by different curve patterns. Lumbar curves can lead to imbalance and pain, whereas thoracic curves can lead to pulmonary problems.[59] Despite popular criteria to justify surgical treatment of scoliosis, the data to describe the untreated natural history of this disorder are lacking. The treatment decisions about spinal deformity should be made on an individual patient basis, taking into consideration the curve magnitude, the likelihood of curve progression, other symptoms, and the risks associated with treatment.[60]

The surgical principles for the treatment of spinal deformity are unchanged: loosen the spine to improve alignment, stabilize the correction with implants, and generate fusion mass over deformed segments. Approaches to spinal surgery include posterior, anterior, and thoracoscopic. Instrumentation for spinal surgery has evolved over the years. Pedicle screws, although currently still an off-label use, are the primary form of spinal fixation in scoliosis surgery (Figure 5). Pedicle screws have been shown to be safe; provide superior control of the spinal column, resulting in slightly better coronal and axial correction; and diminish the likelihood of pseudarthrosis compared with all-hook or hybrid constructs.[61-63] The use of pedicle screws has dramatically diminished the role of anterior surgery for even large, stiff deformities.[64,65] Nevertheless, surgical outcomes, based on patient responses have yet to demonstrate any improvement with improved radiographic correction.[66]

Curve Type

Type	Proximal Thoracic	Main Thoracic	Thoracolumbar/ Lumbar	Curve Type
1	Nonstructural	Structural (major*)	Nonstructural	Main thoracic (MT)
2	Structural	Structural (major*)	Nonstructural	Double thoracic (DT)
3	Nonstructural	Structural (major*)	Structural	Double major (DM)
4	Structural	Structural (major*)	Structural	Triple major (TM)
5	Nonstructural	Nonstructural	Structural (major*)	Thoracolumbar/lumbar (TL/L)
6	Nonstructural	Structural	Structural (major*)	Thoracolumbar/lumbar-Main thoracic (TL/L - MT)

Structural Criteria
(Minor Curves)

*Major = largest Cobb measurement, always structural
Minor = all other curves with structural criteria applied

Proximal Thoracic: - Side bending Cobb ≥ 25°
- T2-T5 kyphosis ≥ +20°

Main Thoracic: - Side bending Cobb ≥ 25°
- T10-L2 kyphosis ≥ +20°

Thoracolumbar/Lumbar: - Side bending Cobb ≥ 25°
- T10-L2 kyphosis ≥ +20°

Location of Apex
(SRS definition)

Curve	Apex
Thoracic	T2-T11-12 disk
Thoracolumbar	T12-L1
Lumbar	L1-2 disk - L4

Modifiers

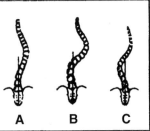

Lumbar Spine Modifier	CSVL to Lumbar Apex
A	CSVL between pedicles
B	CSVL touches apical body(ies)
C	CSVL completely medial

Thoracic Sagittal Profile T5 - T12		
—	(Hypo)	< 10°
N	(Normal)	10°- 40°
+	(Hyper)	> 40°

Curve type (1-6) + lumbar spine modifier (A, B, C) + thoracic sagittal modifier (-, N, or +)

Classification (eg, 1B+): _____

Figure 4 The Lenke classification for adolescent idiopathic scoliosis. SRS = Scoliosis Research Society, CSVL = central sacral vertical line. (Reproduced with permission from Lenke LG, Betz RR, Harms J, et al: Adolescent idiopathic scoliosis: A new classification to determine extent of spinal arthrodesis. *J Bone Joint Surg Am* 2001;83[8]:1169-1181.)

Complications

Reporting from the Scoliosis Research Society's mortality and morbidity database, an overall complication rate for spinal surgery in children is estimated to be approximatley 8.5%. The specific risks of complications were infection, 2.7%; implant-related complications, 1.6%; and new neurologic deficits, 1.4%. The risks were higher among patients undergoing revision surgery, kyphosis correction, or osteotomies. More than one half of the neurologic deficits resolved; however, permanent neurologic injury from scoliosis surgery is recorded.[67] Infection rates were further analyzed in a recent study encompassing 30 years of experience in treating 1,571 pediatric patients at a single institution. The infection rates varied by diagnosis: idiopathic, 0.5%; myelomeningocele, 19.2%; myopathies, 4.3%; and cerebral palsy, 11.2%.[68]

Early-Onset Scoliosis

Early-onset scoliosis is a more recently defined subset in the classification of scoliosis. Children diagnosed with substantial deformity before 5 years of age are at risk for compromised pulmonary development. Underlying diagnoses of early onset scoliosis include progressive infantile scoliosis, congenital scoliosis, or iatrogenic deformity after early fusion. The term thoracic insufficiency syndrome was used to describe conditions of the spine and the chest wall that preclude adequate lung function.[69] From an orthopaedic perspective, the treatment dilemma in these patients is controlling the spinal deformity while maintaining growth of the spinal column to permit lung growth.[48] Traditional treatment included anterior and posterior spinal fusion, which was performed in the belief that no growth was better than further deformity. Unfortunately, early definitive fusion generally failed to control deformity and led to pulmonary morbidity associated with preventing thoracic growth in young children.[70]

6: Pediatrics

Casting has reemerged as an effective growth preserving strategy for the treatment of some patients with early onset scoliosis. Serial casting regimens have been shown to be successful in reversing idiopathic curves in some patients. The technique emphasizes derotation over three-point correction. Casts are typically changed every 2 to 4 months, may require years for full correction, and can include intervals when the patient is out of the cast.[44,45] Even when curves are not corrected, curve progression is often effectively delayed to prevent

significant progression or decompensation. If a curve persists or decompensates, surgical intervention is considered (Figure 6). Efforts should emphasize the maintenance of chest volume and thoracic height. Growing spine constructs with single- or double-rod systems are the most common approach. Spinal implants are placed caudal and cephalad to the segment of spinal deformity. The intervening area is spanned by rods typically placed submuscularly but with care to avoid exposure (and fusion) of the vertebral tissue. Serial lengthening procedures of the rod system to gain spinal column "growth" and maintain deformity correction are undertaken over defined time periods (typically 6 months).[46-48] High rates of complications caused by repeated surgical exposures and diminished lengthening, presumed to be the result of autofusion, have been reported.[71,72]

Externally controlled (magnet-controlled) growing rod implants to address the limitations of traditional growing rods are being developed and tested.[73] The VEPTR device is recommended for deformities with significant rib abnormality or primary chest wall disease.[46-48] Guided growth systems, such as a Luque trolley with sublaminar wires along a smooth rod or the Shilla technique, which uses unlocked pedicle screws, have been described. Despite improved understanding and new technologies and implants, the management of these life-threatening spinal deformities remains difficult.[74] A multidisciplinary approach to these patients should be emphasized.[75]

Pediatric Spine Trauma

Traumatic spinal injuries in children are rare. The most common causes are motor vehicle crashes, falls, sports injuries, and child abuse. The cervical spine is the most

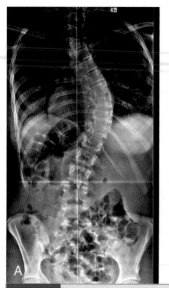
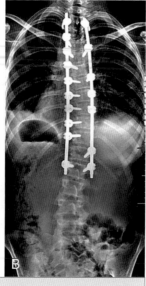

Figure 5 **A,** Radiograph of the spine of a 15-year-old girl with adolescent idiopathic scoliosis, with right thoracic rib prominence and moderate trunk shift. **B,** Postoperative radiograph after posterior spinal fusion with pedicle screw instrumentation.

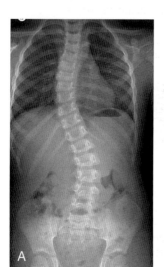
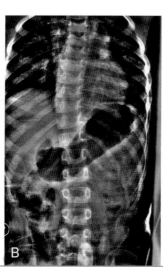
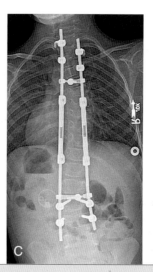
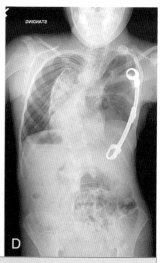

Figure 6 **A,** Standing PA radiograph of a progressive spinal curve in a 3-year-old boy with early-onset scoliosis. **B,** Intraoperative AP radiograph of the same curve during application of the first derotation cast. **C,** PA radiograph of a spine of a child with early onset scoliosis treated with dual growing rods. **D,** PA radiograph of the spine of a child with early-onset scoliosis treated with a VEPTR device.

6: Pediatrics

Table 3

Cervical Spine Fractures

Name/Type of Fracture	Involved Level	Signs and Symptoms	Treatment
Atlanto-occipital dislocation	Occiput/C1	Often fatal Quadriparesis and ventilator dependence if patient survives	Halo stabilization without traction followed by occiput to C1 versus C2 fusion
Jefferson (burst) fracture	C1	Axial load to the head with energy transmitted through the occipital condyles to C1 lateral masses Neurologic injury unlikely	Halo vest immobilization
Odontoid fracture	C2	Younger than 7 years: fixation occurs at the synchondrosis Neck pain and limited range of motion Rare reurologic symptoms	Rigid collar or halo vest immobilization
Hangman's fracture	C2	Bilateral pedicle fractures leading to spondylolisthesis	Rigid collar or halo vest immobilization
Subaxial	C3-C7	Older than 9 years Compression fracture with facet dislocation	Traction followed by rigid collar or halo vest

Table 4

Thoracolumbar Spine Fractures

Name/Type of Fracture	Column Involvement	Signs and Symptoms	Treatment
Compression fracture	Anterior column	Can occur at multiple levels Flexion mechanism	If less than 50% loss of height and stable, 6 weeks in a brace If significant kyphosis, then posterior spinal fusion
Burst fracture	Anterior and middle columns	Axial load Adolescent patient Neurologic involvement from retropulsed fragments	MRI and CT for surgical planning Anterior decompression and column reconstruction followed by posterior spinal fusion with instrumentation (two levels above and below the fracture site)
Flexion-distraction (Chance fracture)	Compression fracture of anterior column and distraction of the middle and posterior columns	Seat belt injury Younger than 10 years Accompanied by major abdominal injuries (including aortic dissection)	More than 15° of segmental kyphosis, then use of an extension brace or cast Posterior spinal fusion with instrumentation if significant kyphosis or ligamentous injury exists
Fracture-dislocation	Anterior, middle, and posterior columns	Thoracolumbar junction Neurologic injury common	Surgery almost always necessary Reduction, decompression, and fusion

frequently injured region of the spine in children because of their larger head size and the greater elasticity and horizontal facet orientation of this spinal region compared with the adult spine (Table 3). The thoracic and lumbar areas of the spine are more commonly involved as a child becomes an adolescent[76] (Table 4).

In contrast with adults, in whom cervical spine injuries account for 30% to 40% of spine trauma, up to 80% of pediatric vertebral injuries and fractures occur within the cervical spine The level of injury correlates with the age of the patient; injuries in the upper cervical spine (occiput to C3) tend to occur in children younger than 8 years. Spinal cord injury is also more common in younger children than older children, but younger children have a better prognosis for recovery. The mortality rate of pediatric patients with cervical spine trauma ranges from 16% to 18%; the rate is higher in patients with upper cervical spine injuries and is highest in children with atlanto-occipital dislocation.[76] The high mortality rate is likely related to the increased rate

6: Pediatrics

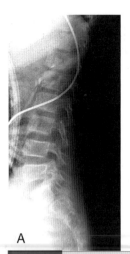
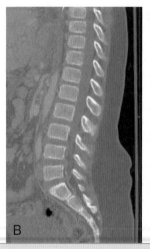
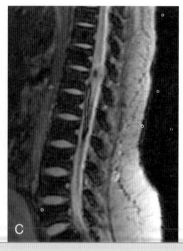
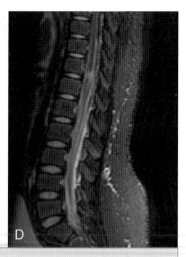

| **Figure 7** | An 8-year-old boy was an unrestrained passenger in a rollover motor vehicle crash. The child presented with dense paraplegia and intact sensation throughout his lower extremities. The patient was treated with bed rest and a thoracolumbar orthosis as he was mobilized. He has regained some motor strength and remains a household ambulator. **A,** Cross-table plain radiograph of the thoracolumbar spine taken after injury. **B,** Sagittal CT reconstruction through the thoracolumbar region shows demonstrable injury. **C,** T-2 weighted MRI shows cord signal change and hematoma. **D,** Short tau inversion recovery image confirms the cord changes but without any appreciable column signal change. |

of concomitant head injury that is associated with a more cephalad location of a cervical spine injury.

Patient Evaluation

Because the head of a child is disproportionately larger than the body, a child with a suspected spinal injury should be immobilized using either a backboard with a recess for the occiput or a standard backboard with pads placed under the torso to accommodate the size of the head. A team approach with coordination of a pediatric general or trauma surgeon is essential. A thorough examination is necessary, with primary and secondary surveys to identify any associated extremity or pelvic injuries and/or noncontiguous spinal trauma.

The radiographic evaluation of a child with a suspected spine injury begins with AP and lateral radiographs of the spine. If the child is older than 5 years, an open-mouth odontoid view also can be obtained. CT may be used conservatively to assess bony anatomy at specific levels, but it cannot be used to clear the cervical spine in pediatric trauma patients who have the potential for instability secondary to soft-tissue injury. Plain radiographs and CT have limited benefit in identifying soft-tissue injuries in the pediatric cervical spine. The use of flexion and extension radiographs is inappropriate to assess for instability in the obtunded or intubated patient or in a patient with a head injury. MRI can be used to evaluate the soft tissues and may aid clinicians in clearing the cervical spine.[76]

Spinal Cord Injury Without Radiographic Abnormality

Spinal cord injury without radiographic abnormality (SCIWORA) is the presence of myelopathy resulting from trauma, without evidence of fracture or ligamentous injury on plain radiographs or CT scans. The term was coined in 1982, before the use of MRI became common.[77] Although MRI has fundamentally changed the meaning of SCIWORA, the concept of spinal cord injury without demonstrable spinal column injury remains valid.[78] MRI typically shows the column injury that was missed on plain radiographs or CT scans; however, there have been extremely rare reports of absent soft-tissue injury on MRI when significant cord injury existed[79] (**Figure 7**).

Recent biomechanical evidence reinforces the epidemiology of SCIWORA. The cervical spine in younger children has greater spinal column plasticity than in older patients, making these children more prone to this type of injury.[80] The overall incidence of SCIWORA is controversial, with reported rates ranging from 5% to 72% of pediatric spinal cord injuries.[76,78,81] Diagnostic criteria, patient demographics (especially the age of patients), and the variable use of imaging technology in different studies account for these differences.

The need for caution should be emphasized in proceeding with acute treatment, with management determined on a case-by-case basis, especially MRI or dynamic studies. Uniform bracing protocols have not been substantiated.[82] A complete recovery occurs in approximately 40% of children with SCIWORA, a partial recovery in 20%, and the remaining 40% do not recover any neurologic function.[83] Secondary spinal deformity as a consequence of persistent neuromuscular weakness can require spinal fusion in patients with SCIWORA.

Summary

Pediatric spinal conditions are common reasons for patients to seek orthopaedic care. Important differences in children compared with adults are ongoing growth and anatomic variants with respect to trauma. Most of these conditions, including back pain, can be managed with the physical examination and history to reassure patients and their families. Spinal deformity and spinal trauma, however, can be major life-changing events for patients.

Key Study Points

- Early-onset scoliosis represents a far more dangerous type of deformity because of its effect on the developing lungs.

- Pediatric spinal trauma demands attention to the anatomic variants of children, including ligamentous laxity, larger head size, and a greater risk of cervical involvement.

- Back pain is a common complaint among adolescent patients, and, most often, the etiology is not apparent; a careful, systematic evaluation should be encouraged.

Annotated References

1. Davids JR Jr, Wenger DR, Mubarak SJ: Congenital muscular torticollis: Sequela of intrauterine or perinatal compartment syndrome. *J Pediatr Orthop* 1993;13(2): 141-147.

2. Lee JK, Moon HJ, Park MS, Yoo WJ, Choi IH, Cho TJ: Change of craniofacial deformity after sternocleidomastoid muscle release in pediatric patients with congenital muscular torticollis. *J Bone Joint Surg Am* 2012;94(13): e93.

   Surgical release of the sternocleidomastoid muscle was performed in 80 patients with CMT. Preoperative and postoperative cephalometric examinations of craniofacial deformity were performed to evaluate curvature and asymmetry. Two groups were identified. Group 1 consisted of patients who had surgery before age 5 years, and group 2 consisted of patients who had surgery after age 5 years. All patients showed improvements in the craniofacial deformity after surgical release of the sternocleidomastoid muscle. Better results were achieved when surgery was performed before age 5 years. Improvements were larger in the first postoperative year than in the second postoperative year.

3. Shim JS, Noh KC, Park SJ: Treatment of congenital muscular torticollis in patients older than 8 years. *J Pediatr Orthop* 2004;24(6):683-688.

4. Shim JS, Jang HP: Operative treatment of congenital torticollis. *J Bone Joint Surg Br* 2008;90(7):934-939.

5. Cheng JC, Au AW: Infantile torticollis: A review of 624 cases. *J Pediatr Orthop* 1994;14(6):802-808.

6. Tang ST, Yang Y, Mao YZ, et al: Endoscopic transaxillary approach for congenital muscular torticollis. *J Pediatr Surg* 2010;45(11):2191-2194.

   The authors present a case report of the endoscopic transaxillary approach for release of the sternocleidomastoid muscle for the treatment of CMT.

7. Fielding JW, Hawkins RJ: Atlanto-axial rotatory fixation: Fixed rotatory subluxation of the atlanto-axial joint. *J Bone Joint Surg Am* 1977;59(1):37-44.

8. Subach BR, McLaughlin MR, Albright AL, Pollack IF: Current management of pediatric atlantoaxial rotatory subluxation. *Spine (Phila Pa 1976)* 1998;23(20):2174-2179.

9. McGaughran JM, Kuna P, Das V: Audiological abnormalities in the Klippel-Feil syndrome. *Arch Dis Child* 1998;79(4):352-355.

10. Moore WB, Matthews TJ, Rabinowitz R: Genitourinary anomalies associated with Klippel-Feil syndrome. *J Bone Joint Surg Am* 1975;57(3):355-357.

11. Baba HM, Maezawa Y, Furusawa N, Chen Q, Imura S, Tomita K: The cervical spine in the Klippel-Feil syndrome: A report of 57 cases. *Int Orthop* 1995;19(4): 204-208.

12. Wang S, Wang C: Familial dystopic os odontoideum: A report of three cases. *J Bone Joint Surg Am* 2011;93(9): e44.

   A case report of three family members with a dystopic type os odontoideum is presented. The patients had progressive neurologic symptoms and were treated with posterior spinal fusion. None of the three family members had trauma or other causative events.

13. Wada E, Matsuoka T, Kawai H: Os odontoideum as a consequence of a posttraumatic displaced ossiculum terminale: A case report. *J Bone Joint Surg Am* 2009; 91(7):1750-1754.

14. Sankar WN, Wills BP, Dormans JP, Drummond DS: Os odontoideum revisited: The case for a multifactorial etiology. *Spine (Phila Pa 1976)* 2006;31(9):979-984.

15. Bhatia NN, Chow G, Timon SJ, Watts HG: Diagnostic modalities for the evaluation of pediatric back pain: A prospective study. *J Pediatr Orthop* 2008;28(2): 230-233.

16. Skaggs DL, Early SD, D'Ambra P, Tolo VT, Kay RM: Back pain and backpacks in school children. *J Pediatr Orthop* 2006;26(3):358-363.

17. Feldman DS, Straight JJ, Badra MI, Mohaideen A, Madan SS: Evaluation of an algorithmic approach to pediatric back pain. *J Pediatr Orthop* 2006;26(3): 353-357.

18. Cavalier R, Herman MJ, Cheung EV, Pizzutillo PD: Spondylolysis and spondylolisthesis in children and adolescents: I. Diagnosis, natural history, and nonsurgical management. *J Am Acad Orthop Surg* 2006;14(7): 417-424.

19. Cheung EV, Herman MJ, Cavalier R, Pizzutillo PD: Spondylolysis and spondylolisthesis in children and adolescents: II. Surgical management. *J Am Acad Orthop Surg* 2006;14(8):488-498.

20. McIntosh AL: Scheuermann's kyphosis. *Curr Opin Orthop* 2007;18(6):536-543.

21. Scheuermann HR: *Juvenile Kyphosis.* Copenhagen, Denmark, Munksgaard, 1964.

22. Quinlan JF, Duke D, Eustace S: Bertolotti's syndrome: A cause of back pain in young people. *J Bone Joint Surg Br* 2006;88(9):1183-1186.

23. Hensinger RN: Congenital scoliosis: Etiology and associations. *Spine (Phila Pa 1976)* 2009;34(17):1745-1750.

24. Shen J, Wang Z, Liu J, Xue X, Qiu G: Abnormalities associated with congenital scoliosis: A retrospective study of 226 Chinese surgical cases. *Spine (Phila Pa 1976)* 2013;38(10):814-818.

    In this retrospective review of 226 patients who were surgically treated for congenital scoliosis, all of the patients were evaluated with whole-spine MRI, echocardiography, and renal ultrasonography. Intraspinal abnormalities were found in 43% of the patients, and other organ defects were found in 40% of the patients.

25. Basu PS, Elsebaie H, Noordeen MH: Congenital spinal deformity: A comprehensive assessment at presentation. *Spine (Phila Pa 1976)* 2002;27(20):2255-2259.

26. Belmont PJ Jr, Kuklo TR, Taylor KF, Freedman BA, Prahinski JR, Kruse RW: Intraspinal anomalies associated with isolated congenital hemivertebra: The role of routine magnetic resonance imaging. *J Bone Joint Surg Am* 2004;86(8):1704-1710.

27. Winter RB, Lonstein JE: Scoliosis secondary to a hemivertebra: Seven patients with gradual improvement without treatment. *Spine (Phila Pa 1976)* 2010;35(2): E49-E52.

    Seven patients from a database of 1,250 patients with congenital scoliosis were identified with a hemivertebra that demonstrated spontaneous improvement over a mean follow-up period of 9 years. This observation highlights the unpredictable nature of deformity progression in congenital scoliosis.

28. Herring JA: *Tachdjian's Pediatric Orthopaedics,* ed 4. Philadelphia, PA, Saunders Elsevier, 2008, p 343.

29. Vitale MG, Matsumoto H, Bye MR, et al: A retrospective cohort study of pulmonary function, radiographic measures, and quality of life in children with congenital scoliosis: An evaluation of patient outcomes after early spinal fusion. *Spine (Phila Pa 1976)* 2008;33(11):1242-1249.

30. Hedequist DJ: Surgical treatment of congenital scoliosis. *Orthop Clin North Am* 2007;38(4):497-509, vi.

31. Ruf M, Jensen R, Letko L, Harms J: Hemivertebra resection and osteotomies in congenital spine deformity. *Spine (Phila Pa 1976)* 2009;34(17):1791-1799.

32. Schwartz DM, Auerbach JD, Dormans JP, et al: Neurophysiological detection of impending spinal cord injury during scoliosis surgery. *J Bone Joint Surg Am* 2007; 89(11):2440-2449.

33. Campbell RM Jr, Hell-Vocke AK: Growth of the thoracic spine in congenital scoliosis after expansion thoracoplasty. *J Bone Joint Surg Am* 2003;85(3):409-420.

34. Sponseller PD, Zimmerman RM, Ko PS, et al: Low profile pelvic fixation with the sacral alar iliac technique in the pediatric population improves results at two-year minimum follow-up. *Spine (Phila Pa 1976)* 2010; 35(20):1887-1892.

    The authors' technique of pelvic fixation was used in 32 consecutive patients and compared with 27 prior patients treated with other techniques. Improved correction of pelvic obliquity was noted, as was radiographic and clinical stability of the sacral alar iliac screws.

35. Modi HN, Hong J-Y, Mehta SS, et al: Surgical correction and fusion using posterior-only pedicle screw construct for neuropathic scoliosis in patients with cerebral palsy: A three-year follow-up study. *Spine (Phila Pa 1976)* 2009;34(11):1167-1175.

36. Dobbs MB, Lenke LG, Szymanski DA, et al: Prevalence of neural axis abnormalities in patients with infantile idiopathic scoliosis. *J Bone Joint Surg Am* 2002;84(12): 2230-2234.

37. Diab M, Landman Z, Lubicky J, et al: Use and outcome of MRI in the surgical treatment of adolescent idiopathic scoliosis. *Spine (Phila Pa 1976)* 2011;36(8): 667-671.

    The authors present a review of a multicenter study group to assess the use of MRI in evaluating patients with idiopathic scoliosis. MRI evaluation was performed in 923 of 2,206 patients, and intracanal abnormalities were identified in 4.2% of those 923 patients. Thoracic hyperkyphosis and juvenile onset scoliosis were risk factors for positive MRI findings.

38. Richards BS, Sucato DJ, Johnston CE, et al: Right thoracic curves in presumed adolescent idiopathic scoliosis: Which clinical and radiographic findings correlate with a preoperative abnormal magnetic resonance image? *Spine (Phila Pa 1976)* 2010;35(20):1855-1860.

    A multicenter review of preoperative MRI evaluation in

scoliosis patients found neural abnormalities in 36 of 529 patients. Those with hyperkyphosis and increased rotation demonstrated higher comparative risk for neural findings.

39. Nakahara D, Yonezawa I, Kobanawa K, et al: Magnetic resonance imaging evaluation of patients with idiopathic scoliosis: A prospective study of four hundred seventy-two outpatients. *Spine (Phila Pa 1976)* 2011; 36(7):E482-E485.

   In this prospective study, 472 patients with presumed idiopathic scoliosis were examined with MRI. Neural axis abnormalities were found in 18 patients (3.8%). Male sex, an age younger than 11 years, and abnormal abdominal reflexes were significantly associated with MRI abnormality.

40. Wu LW, Qiu Y, Wang B, Zhu ZZ, Ma WW: The left thoracic curve pattern: A strong predictor for neural axis abnormalities in patients with "idiopathic" scoliosis. *Spine (Phila Pa 1976)* 2010;35(2):182-185.

   Neural axis abnormalities were found in 37 of 68 (54%) patients with left main thoracic curves. The study cohort was culled over 10 years and was derived from consecutive patients presenting with left thoracic curve patterns who were presumed to have idiopathic scoliosis.

41. Sharma S, Gao X, Londono D, et al: Genome-wide association studies of adolescent idiopathic scoliosis suggest candidate susceptibility genes. *Hum Mol Genet* 2011;20(7):1456-1466.

   One hundred single nucleotide polymorphisms were identified by genome-wide association studies in 419 families with adolescent idiopathic scoliosis. The authors describe some of the identified candidate genes and provide a glimpse into the work of explaining the pathophysiology of scoliosis.

42. Mehta MH: The rib-vertebra angle in the early diagnosis between resolving and progressive infantile scoliosis. *J Bone Joint Surg Br* 1972;54(2):230-243.

43. Corona J, Sanders JO, Luhmann SJ, Diab M, Vitale MG: Reliability of radiographic measures for infantile idiopathic scoliosis. *J Bone Joint Surg Am* 2012;94(12): e86.

   Pediatric orthopaedists and fellows reviewed the radiographs of patients with infantile scoliosis to analyze the radiographic markers. The rib vertebral angle difference and the Cobb angle had high interobserver and intraobserver reliability. Some variability in measurements was noted. The authors cautioned that decision making should not rely on radiographic measurements alone.

44. Mehta MH: Growth as a corrective force in the early treatment of progressive infantile scoliosis. *J Bone Joint Surg Br* 2005;87(9):1237-1247.

45. Sanders JO, D'Astous J, Fitzgerald M, Khoury JG, Kishan S, Sturm PF: Derotational casting for progressive infantile scoliosis. *J Pediatr Orthop* 2009;29(6): 581-587.

46. Thompson GH, Akbarnia BA, Kostial P, et al: Comparison of single and dual growing rod techniques followed through definitive surgery: A preliminary study. *Spine (Phila Pa 1976)* 2005;30(18):2039-2044.

47. Thompson GH, Akbarnia BA, Campbell RM Jr: Growing rod techniques in early-onset scoliosis. *J Pediatr Orthop* 2007;27(3):354-361.

48. Gomez JA, Lee JK, Kim PD, Roye DP, Vitale MG: "Growth friendly" spine surgery: Management options for the young child with scoliosis. *J Am Acad Orthop Surg* 2011;19(12):722-727.

   The authors reviewed the treatment options for early onset scoliosis and the justification for their use in this challenging subset of patients.

49. Lonstein JE, Carlson JM: The prediction of curve progression in untreated idiopathic scoliosis during growth. *J Bone Joint Surg Am* 1984;66(7):1061-1071.

50. Sanders JO, Khoury JG, Kishan S, et al: Predicting scoliosis progression from skeletal maturity: A simplified classification during adolescence. *J Bone Joint Surg Am* 2008;90(3):540-553.

51. Roye BD, Wright ML, Williams BA, et al: Does ScoliScore provide more information than traditional clinical estimates of curve progression? *Spine (Phila Pa 1976)* 2012;37(25):2099-2103.

   The authors compared the use of ScoliScore (Transgenomic) in their clinical practice to traditional predictors of scoliosis curve behavior. Preliminary data are presented. The authors provide an excellent discussion on the limitations and potentials of evolving technologies for predicting curve behavior.

52. King HA, Moe JH, Bradford DS, Winter RB: The selection of fusion levels in thoracic idiopathic scoliosis. *J Bone Joint Surg Am* 1983;65(9):1302-1313.

53. Lenke LG, Betz RR, Harms J, et al: Adolescent idiopathic scoliosis: A new classification to determine extent of spinal arthrodesis. *J Bone Joint Surg Am* 2001;83(8): 1169-1181.

54. Nachemson AL, Peterson LE: Effectiveness of treatment with a brace in girls who have adolescent idiopathic scoliosis: A prospective, controlled study based on data from the Brace Study of the Scoliosis Research Society. *J Bone Joint Surg Am* 1995;77(6):815-822.

55. Danielsson AJ, Hasserius R, Ohlin A, Nachemson AL: A prospective study of brace treatment versus observation alone in adolescent idiopathic scoliosis: A follow-up mean of 16 years after maturity. *Spine (Phila Pa 1976)* 2007;32(20):2198-2207.

56. Katz DE, Herring JA, Browne RH, Kelly DM, Birch JG: Brace wear control of curve progression in adolescent idiopathic scoliosis. *J Bone Joint Surg Am* 2010;92(6): 1343-1352.

   This study was one of the first to use new brace compli-

6: Pediatrics

ance technology. A heat sensor in each brace allowed the researchers to record objective brace use. A dose-response curve supporting brace use was demonstrated.

57. Weinstein SL, Ponseti IV: Curve progression in idiopathic scoliosis. *J Bone Joint Surg Am* 1983;289: 559-567.

58. Weinstein SL, Dolan LA, Spratt KF, Peterson KK, Spoonamore MJ, Ponseti IV: Health and function of patients with untreated idiopathic scoliosis: A 50-year natural history study. *JAMA* 2003;289(5):559-567.

59. Johnston CE, Richards BS, Sucato DJ, et al: Correlation of preoperative deformity magnitude and pulmonary function tests in adolescent idiopathic scoliosis. *Spine (Phila Pa 1976)* 2011;36(14):1096-1102.

This retrospective review of results of pulmonary function tests culled from a large multicenter database showed substantial pulmonary impairment (forced expiratory volume in 1 second and forced vital capacity < 65% predicted) in 19% of the patients with preoperative adolescent idiopathic scoliosis. The risk factors included larger main thoracic curves, more relative lordosis, and greater axial rotation.

60. Weinstein SL: Natural history. *Spine (Phila Pa 1976)* 1999;24(24):2592-2600.

61. Ledonio CG, Polly DW Jr, Vitale MG, Wang Q, Richards BS: Pediatric pedicle screws: Comparative effectiveness and safety. A systematic literature review from the Scoliosis Research Society and the Pediatric Orthopaedic Society of North America task force. *J Bone Joint Surg Am* 2011;93(13):1227-1234.

The authors present a systematic review of the literature emphasizing coronal plane correction and the accuracy of pedicle screw placement. An overall accuracy rate of 94.9% reported in pediatric literature exceeded the safety results reported in adult literature.

62. Suk SI, Kim JH, Kim S-S, Lim D-J: Pedicle screw instrumentation in adolescent idiopathic scoliosis (AIS). *Eur Spine J* 2012;21(1):13-22.

The rationale, the technique, and the results of using thoracic pedicle screws for adolescent scoliosis surgery are presented.

63. Luhmann SJ, Lenke LG, Erickson M, Bridwell KH, Richards BS: Correction of moderate (< 70 degrees) Lenke 1A and 2A curve patterns: Comparison of hybrid and all-pedicle screw systems at 2-year follow-up. *J Pediatr Orthop* 2012;32(3):253-258.

A multicenter, prospective database was culled for scoliosis curve patterns where maximal curve correction could be achieved. The radiographic outcomes were statistically superior among all-pedicle screw constructs.

64. Dobbs MB, Lenke LG, Kim YJ, Luhmann SJ, Bridwell KH: Anterior/posterior spinal instrumentation versus posterior instrumentation alone for the treatment of adolescent idiopathic scoliotic curves more than 90 degrees. *Spine (Phila Pa 1976)* 2006;31(20):2386-2391.

65. Hwang SW, Samdani AF, Wormser B, et al: Comparison of 5-year outcomes between pedicle screw and hybrid constructs in adolescent idiopathic scoliosis. *J Neurosurg Spine* 2012;17(3):212-219.

In a retrospective review of a multicenter database comparing hybrid and all-pedicle screw constructs for idiopathic scoliosis, similar outcomes were achieved with both techniques; however, substantially more anterior releases and thoracoplasties were performed in the hybrid cohort. Slightly larger and stiffer curves were noted among the hybrid cohort preoperatively.

66. Imrie M, Yaszay B, Bastrom TP, Wenger DR, Newton PO: Adolescent idiopathic scoliosis: Should 100% correction be the goal? *J Pediatr Orthop* 2011;31(1, suppl): S9-S13.

A prospective database of Lenke type 1 curves (n = 385) was analyzed in this study. The top 15% of corrections based on the Cobb correction (n = 39, high correction) and bottom 15% (n = 40, low correction) were compared. Although the high correction group had significantly better radiographic outcomes, these outcomes were achieved without achieving higher Scoliosis Research Society scores and possibly at the expense of more loss of kyphosis.

67. Fu KM, Smith JS, Polly DW, et al: Morbidity and mortality associated with spinal surgery in children: A review of the Scoliosis Research Society morbidity and mortality database. *J Neurosurg Pediatr* 2011;7(1):37-41.

This review presents data from the Scoliosis Research Society morbidity and mortality database relevant to pediatric spinal deformity. These data should serve as the benchmark for complication rates in patients treated with surgery for scoliosis and spinal deformity.

68. Cahill PJ, Warnick DE, Lee MJ, et al: Infection after spinal fusion for pediatric spinal deformity: Thirty years of experience at a single institution. *Spine (Phila Pa 1976)* 2010;35(12):1211-1217.

Extensive experience from a single institution was used to establish guidelines for infection risk based on a patient's diagnosis. The treatment of infection is also analyzed and highlights multiple surgical débridements (mean = 2) and implant removal (50% of the cases).

69. Campbell RM Jr, Smith MD, Mayes TC, et al: The characteristics of thoracic insufficiency syndrome associated with fused ribs and congenital scoliosis. *J Bone Joint Surg Am* 2003;85(3):399-408.

70. Karol LA: Early definitive spinal fusion in young children: What we have learned. *Clin Orthop Relat Res* 2011;469(5):1323-1329.

The author provides a clear synopsis of the literature, including her own work, on spinal fusion. The traditional approach of using definitive fusion to treat early spinal deformity was shown to be ineffectual and harmful.

71. Mineiro J, Weinstein SL: Subcutaneous rodding for progressive spinal curvatures: early results. *J Pediatr Orthop* 2002;22(3):290-295.

72. Sankar WN, Skaggs DL, Yazici M, et al: Lengthening of dual growing rods and the law of diminishing returns. *Spine (Phila Pa 1976)* 2011;36(10):806-809.

The authors present a multicenter review of 38 patients treated with growing rod lengthening procedures for early onset scoliosis. The authors reported decreased length gain from each subsequent lengthening procedure.

73. Cheung KM, Cheung JP, Samartzis D, et al: Magnetically controlled growing rods for severe spinal curvature in young children: A prospective case series. *Lancet* 2012;379(9830):1967-1974.

Preliminary data on the first patients treated with magnetically controlled growing rods for spinal curvature are presented. The potential for noninvasive outpatient rod distraction may represent an evolution in instrumentation for early onset scoliosis.

74. Akbarnia BA, Campbell RM, Dimeglio A, et al: Fusionless procedures for the management of early-onset spine deformities in 2011: What do we know? *J Child Orthop* 2011;5(3):159-172.

This review article presents expert opinions from many experienced spine surgeons on the topic of fusionless procedures for treating early onset scoliosis.

75. Sucato DJ: Management of severe spinal deformity: Scoliosis and kyphosis. *Spine (Phila Pa 1976)* 2010;35(25): 2186-2192.

The author reported on his personal experience along with a literature review on the treatment of complex spinal deformity. The article highlights the many concerns involved in treating patients with severe spinal deformity who frequently have many comorbid conditions.

76. Jones TM, Anderson PA, Noonan KJ: Pediatric cervical spine trauma. *J Am Acad Orthop Surg* 2011;19(10): 600-611.

The authors present an excellent review article on the evaluation and the management of pediatric cervical spine trauma.

77. Pang D, Wilberger JE Jr: Spinal cord injury without radiographic abnormalities in children. *J Neurosurg* 1982; 57(1):114-129.

78. Pang D: Spinal cord injury without radiographic abnormality in children: 2 decades later. *Neurosurgery* 2004; 55(6):1325-1343.

79. Mortazavi MM, Mariwalla NR, Horn EM, Tubbs RS, Theodore N: Absence of MRI soft tissue abnormalities in severe spinal cord injury in children: Case-based update. *Childs Nerv Syst* 2011;27(9):1369-1373.

A case report of a 22-month-old child with a profound lower thoracic cord injury is presented. Only ligamentous injury was seen on the MRI scan of the cervical spine. The authors raised concern that undetected spinal column instability can still exist despite MRI evaluation.

80. Luck JF, Nightingale RW, Song Y, et al: Tensile failure properties of perinatal, neonatal and pediatric cadaver cervical spine. *Spine (Phila Pa 1976)* 2013;38(1):E1-12.

The tensile failure properties of the cervical spine are presented, along with data for validating pediatric spine models.

81. Schottler J, Vogel LC, Sturm P: Spinal cord injuries in young children: A review of children injured at 5 years of age and younger. *Dev Med Child Neurol* 2012; 54(12):1138-1143.

In a retrospective review of 159 children 5 years and younger with spinal injury seen at the Shriners Hospital for children in Chicago, the authors reported a 72% incidence of SCIWORA.

82. Bosch PP, Vogt MT, Ward WT: Pediatric spinal cord injury without radiographic abnormality (SCIWORA): The absence of occult instability and lack of indication for bracing. *Spine (Phila Pa 1976)* 2002;27(24):2788-2800.

83. Yalcin N, Dede O, Alanay A, Yazici M: Surgical management of post-SCIWORA spinal deformities in children. *J Child Orthop* 2011;5(1):27-33.

A retrospective review is presented of four patients in whom significant neuromuscular scoliosis developed after a SCIWORA injury. A sweeping curve pattern with pelvic obliquity developed in these patients within 2 years of the spinal cord injury.

6: Pediatrics

Chapter 61

Trauma to the Pelvis, Hip, and Femur: Pediatrics

Jeffrey R. Sawyer, MD   Richard E. Bowen, MD

Introduction

Fractures and dislocations of the pelvis, hip, and femur in a child are usually caused by high-energy trauma; associated injuries are common. Therefore, it is important that all children who sustain these injuries undergo a thorough trauma evaluation. The unique physiologic characteristics of the immature skeleton, such as increased elasticity, the presence of open physes, and the unique blood supply to the pediatric hip, help determine the injury patterns, guide treatment, and predict complications. Nonaccidental trauma should always be included in the differential diagnosis in patients younger than 3 years.

Pelvic Fracture

Characteristics

Pelvic fractures include pelvic ring injuries, acetabular fractures, and avulsions of the various apophyses of the immature pelvis. Pelvic ring fractures are usually sustained by children involved in motor vehicle accidents, either as a passenger or as a pedestrian struck by a vehicle; falls are the second most frequent cause.[1,2] More than one half of children who sustain a pelvic fracture also have an associated fracture or visceral injury,[1] and the mortality rate is 3% to 5%.[1,2] Because children sustain more lateral compression injuries (involving reduction of pelvic volume) and have vascular structures with more elasticity compared with adults, they rarely die of a fracture-related hemorrhage, which can occur

in adults.[3] The increased elasticity of the pediatric pelvis allows isolated injuries to the pelvic ring to occur, especially in children younger than 6 years.[4] Injuries to the pubic rami and symphysis are the most common.[2] Although urogenital injuries are rare, children with significantly displaced or unstable pelvic fractures should undergo a thorough urogenital examination.[5]

Treatment

Most pelvic ring fractures in children are lateral compression injuries[2] and are therefore stable. Stable fractures can be treated with protected weight bearing and, in rare cases, a spica cast. Surgical treatment is required more frequently in skeletally mature adolescent patients.[4] The indications for surgery include fractures with hemodynamic instability, fractures with more than 2 cm of vertical displacement, a displaced acetabular fracture, and fractures with more than 2 mm of triradiate cartilage displacement.[6] The outcomes of surgically treated pelvic fractures are good and similar to those in adult patients,[7,8] except for fractures that involve the triradiate cartilage, which are uncommon.

Complications

Most pediatric pelvic ring fractures heal well and without long-term complications despite the fact that the remodeling potential of the pelvis is limited. Nonunion and residual ligamentous laxity are rare. The final outcome often is determined by any associated injuries, such as head and abdominal injuries, as well as other fractures. Mortality is rare in children with pelvic fractures and usually is the result of associated injuries rather than hemorrhage. The exception is an adolescent patient with either unilateral or bilateral anterior and posterior injuries, which may reflect more of an "adult-type" fracture pattern.[1] Fractures that involve the triradiate cartilage, especially in patients younger than 10 years, can lead to premature closure of the physis and disruption of normal acetabular growth. This may not be readily apparent on initial radiographic studies, and patients should be followed long term for arrested growth that can result in acetabular dysplasia, hip subluxation, and degenerative arthritis.[9]

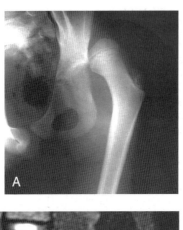
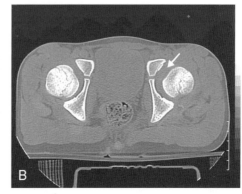
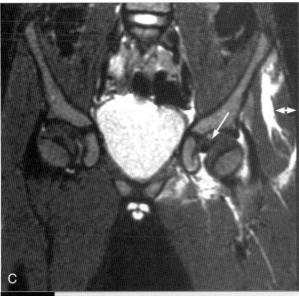
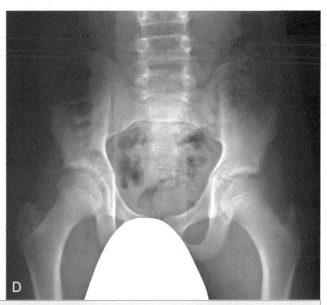

Figure 1 Images of a posterior dislocation of a child's left hip. **A,** AP radiograph showing the dislocation. **B,** Axial CT showing nonconcentric reduction of left hip (arrow). No entrapped osteocartilaginous fragments are present. **C,** Coronal MRI showing an enfolded ligamentum teres or capsule (arrow) causing the nonconcentric hip reduction. **D,** AP pelvic radiograph showing mild coxa magna and subtle femoral neck deformity 4 years after open reduction and removal of the entrapped capsule and ligamentum.

Hip Dislocation

Characteristics

Traumatic hip dislocations in children are rare; 95% of these dislocations are posterior.[10-12] In young children, these dislocations may be caused by low-energy trauma combined with increased periacetabular laxity.[10] This laxity also may account for the lower incidence of associated proximal femoral fractures in children compared with adults.[11] This laxity often causes dislocated hips to reduce spontaneously; the rarity of proximal femoral fractures often causes them to be missed. A spontaneously reduced hip with an eccentric reduction caused by entrapped tissues can result in severe hip pathology.[13] Associated injuries may include ipsilateral femoral epiphyseal fractures, injury to the peroneal branch of the sciatic nerve, and ipsilateral knee injuries.[10,11]

Treatment

Because most traumatic hip dislocations in children are low energy in nature, they can be reduced easily with gentle manipulation.[12] Proper sedation and relaxation along with fluoroscopy are recommended in adolescent patients to prevent iatrogenic fracture of the proximal femoral physis. Urgent reduction is essential to reduce the risk of osteonecrosis.[10] Postreduction imaging, including CT or MRI, is essential to rule out associated injury such as an acetabular or osteochondral fracture and to ensure that the reduction is concentric.[11,14] In children, the interposed tissue usually is capsular or labral, can be attached to an acetabular epiphyseal fragment,[15] and may not appear on radiographs as an osteochondral fragment, as seen in adolescents or adults (**Figure 1**). Immobilization and protected weight bearing are used for 6 to 12 weeks for older patients. Spica casting or abduction splinting can be used for younger and/or noncompliant patients.[11]

The indications for open reduction are nonconcentric reduction or irreducible dislocation. The surgical approach used is most often in the same direction as the dislocation, usually posteriorly. All interposed tissue should be removed, and a capsular, labral, and/or osteochondral repair should be performed when possible. Patients should be followed closely for redislocation. Open reduction may be beneficial for missed or neglected dislocations, which occur most commonly in the developing world.[16,17]

Complications

Common complications of hip dislocations in children are associated nerve injury and osteonecrosis. Approximately 5% of children with a dislocated hip also have an associated nerve injury, usually to the peroneal branch of the sciatic nerve, which usually resolves spontaneously.[11] In one study, osteonecrosis was reported in 12% of children who sustained a hip dislocation.[10] Rapid recognition and reduction of the dislocated hip in children has been shown to reduce the risk of osteonecrosis;[10,16] a 6-hour delay in reduction increases the risk of osteonecrosis by a factor of 20.[10] MRI may help detect osteonecrosis in the postoperative/postreduction period. Although rare, redislocation is not related to the progression of weight bearing and should be treated with capsulorrhaphy.[11]

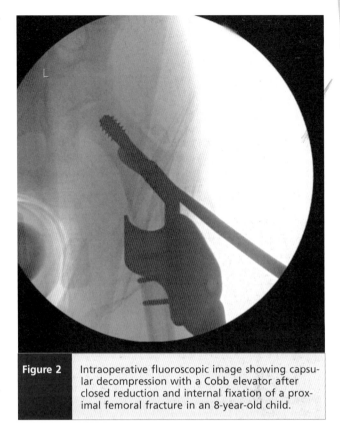

Figure 2 Intraoperative fluoroscopic image showing capsular decompression with a Cobb elevator after closed reduction and internal fixation of a proximal femoral fracture in an 8-year-old child.

Femoral Neck Fractures

Characteristics

Femoral neck fractures account for 1% of pediatric fractures. These fractures are classified using the Delbet system, which not only describes them anatomically but is predictive of the development of osteonecrosis: Type I is a transphyseal separation; type II, transcervical; type III, basicervical; and type IV, intertrochanteric. Because of the absence of transphyseal collateral circulation in the pediatric hip, injuries that are more proximal have a higher risk of damaging the circumflex vessels, resulting in osteonecrosis.[18] A femoral neck fracture in the absence of high-energy trauma may be caused by a neoplastic (either benign or malignant) or metabolic process, as well as by nonaccidental trauma in young children.[19-21]

Treatment

A displaced femoral physeal separation in an infant can be caused by birth trauma.[22] Completely nondisplaced fractures in young children can be treated with a spica cast; however, attentive follow-up is necessary to ensure that late displacement, which can result in deformity and osteonecrosis, does not occur.[23,24] Weight bearing should be advanced slowly to prevent late displacement.[25]

Displaced femoral neck fractures in children should be treated immediately to help decrease the risk of osteonecrosis.[26,27] Anatomic reduction, whether open or closed, is essential for the prevention of osteonecrosis and late deformity.[26,28] Internal fixation should be used, and fracture stability is more important than preservation of the proximal femoral physis.[23,25] Although most Delbet type I, II, and III fractures are treated with cannulated screws, an interlocking implant may be needed for highly unstable vertical and/or comminuted fractures.[29] Because of the relatively small contribution of the proximal femoral physis to overall leg length, iatrogenic growth arrest of the proximal femoral physis usually can be treated with contralateral epiphysiodesis. Capsular decompression also may help decrease the risk of osteonecrosis[18,30] (**Figure 2**). If fixation stability and/or patient compliance is a concern, supplemental spica cast immobilization should be used to prevent excessive forces on the fracture and implants as well as to prevent weight bearing.[24]

Complications

Osteonecrosis is the most common and most serious complication of femoral neck fractures in children. The development of osteonecrosis depends on the location (Delbet classification) and the amount of displacement of the initial fracture, the age of the patient, and the timing and quality of the reduction attained. A large meta-analysis showed that the rate of osteonecrosis was related to the Delbet fracture type: type I, 38%; type II, 28%; type III, 18%; and type IV, 5%.[31] The study also showed that increased age was a risk factor for the development of osteonecrosis. Most authors think that immediate treatment may decrease the risk of osteonecrosis.[26,27] This idea is supported by the fact that

6: Pediatrics

34. Neto PF, Dos Reis FB, Filho JL, et al: Nonunion of fractures of the femoral neck in children. *J Child Orthop* 2008;2(2):97-103.

35. Kanlic E, Cruz M: Current concepts in pediatric femur fracture treatment. *Orthopedics* 2007;30(12):1015-1019.

36. Kanlic EM, Anglen JO, Smith DG, Morgan SJ, Pesántez RF: Advantages of submuscular bridge plating for complex pediatric femur fractures. *Clin Orthop Relat Res* 2004;426:244-251.

37. Sanders S, Egol KA: Adult periarticular locking plates for the treatment of pediatric and adolescent subtrochanteric hip fractures. *Bull NYU Hosp Jt Dis* 2009;67(4):370-373.

38. Ireland DC, Fisher RL: Subtrochanteric fractures of the femur in children. *Clin Orthop Relat Res* 1975;110:157-166.

39. Jeng C, Sponseller PD, Yates A, Paletta G: Subtrochanteric femoral fractures in children: Alignment after 90 degrees-90 degrees traction and cast application. *Clin Orthop Relat Res* 1997;341:170-174.

40. Pombo MW, Shilt JS: The definition and treatment of pediatric subtrochanteric femur fractures with titanium elastic nails. *J Pediatr Orthop* 2006;26(3):364-370.

41. Theologis TN, Cole WG: Management of subtrochanteric fractures of the femur in children. *J Pediatr Orthop* 1998;18(1):22-25.

42. Flynn JM, Garner MR, Jones KJ, et al: The treatment of low-energy femoral shaft fractures: A prospective study comparing the "walking spica" with the traditional spica cast. *J Bone Joint Surg Am* 2011;93(23):2196-2202.

   This prospective study compared walking spica casts with traditional double-leg spica casts for the treatment of femoral shaft fractures and showed a reduced burden on the caregiver and more patient mobility with the walking spica cast. However, more patients had fracture displacement that required cast wedging. Level of evidence: II.

43. Hinton RY, Lincoln A, Crockett MM, Sponseller P, Smith G: Fractures of the femoral shaft in children: Incidence, mechanisms, and sociodemographic risk factors. *J Bone Joint Surg Am* 1999;81(4):500-509.

44. Shrader MW, Bernat NM, Segal LS: Suspected nonaccidental trauma and femoral shaft fractures in children. *Orthopedics* 2011;34(5):360.

   Of 137 children younger than 4 years who presented with a femoral shaft fracture at a trauma center, 43 (mean age, 1.8 years) had injuries suggestive of nonaccidental trauma. Age less than 1 year was a highly significant risk factor for suspected nonaccidental trauma, with 18 of 20 children younger than 1 year referred to child protective services. Level of evidence: IV.

45. Leu D, Sargent MC, Ain MC, Leet AI, Tis JE, Sponseller PD: Spica casting for pediatric femoral fractures: A prospective, randomized controlled study of single-leg versus double-leg spica casts. *J Bone Joint Surg Am* 2012;94(14):1259-1264.

   This study compared 24 patients with single-leg spica casts with 28 patients with double-leg casts and found that all limbs healed in a satisfactory alignment. Children with single-leg spica casts were more likely to fit into car seats and fit more comfortably into chairs; the caregivers of patients with single-leg casts took less time off work. Level of evidence: I.

46. Mansour AA III, Wilmoth JC, Mansour AS, Lovejoy SA, Mencio GA, Martus JE: Immediate spica casting of pediatric femoral fractures in the operating room versus the emergency department: Comparison of reduction, complications, and hospital charges. *J Pediatr Orthop* 2010;30(8):813-817.

   This retrospective comparison of 79 patients treated in the emergency department and 21 patients treated in the operating room found similar results in reduction and complications, with lower costs and shorter hospital stays with spica casting in the emergency department. Level of evidence: III.

47. Lascombes P, Haumont T, Journeau P: Use and abuse of flexible intramedullary nailing in children and adolescents. *J Pediatr Orthop* 2006;26(6):827-834.

48. Altay MA, Erturk C, Cece H, Isikan UE: Mini-open versus closed reduction in titanium elastic nailing of paediatric femoral shaft fractures: A comparative study. *Acta Orthop Belg* 2011;77(2):211-217.

   In this study comparing closed reduction (45 patients) and mini-open reduction (42 patients) for the treatment of femoral shaft fractures fixed with flexible intramedullary nails, patients in the the mini-open group had shorter surgery times, less radiation exposure, and equivalent outcomes to those of the closed reduction group. Level of evidence: III.

49. Rathjen KE, Riccio AI, De La Garza D: Stainless steel flexible intramedullary fixation of unstable femoral shaft fractures in children. *J Pediatr Orthop* 2007;27(4):432-441.

50. Luhmann SJ, Schootman M, Schoenecker PL, Dobbs MB, Gordon JE: Complications of titanium elastic nails for pediatric femoral shaft fractures. *J Pediatr Orthop* 2003;23(4):443-447.

51. Miller DJ, Kelly DM, Spence DD, Beaty JH, Warner WC Jr, Sawyer JR: Locked intramedullary nailing in the treatment of femoral shaft fractures in children younger than 12 years of age: Indications and preliminary report of outcomes. *J Pediatr Orthop* 2012;32(8):777-780.

   Of 17 patients (mean age, 10 years) with femoral shaft fractures who were not candidates for flexible elastic nailing and were treated with small-diameter locked nails using a trochanteric entry, all fractures healed (mean, 13 weeks) with no osteonecrosis. Level of evidence: IV.

6: Pediatrics

52. Jencikova-Celerin L, Phillips JH, Werk LN, Wiltrout SA, Nathanson I: Flexible interlocked nailing of pediatric femoral fractures: Experience with a new flexible interlocking intramedullary nail compared with other fixation procedures. *J Pediatr Orthop* 2008;28(8):864-873.

53. Keeler KA, Dart B, Luhmann SJ, et al: Antegrade intramedullary nailing of pediatric femoral fractures using an interlocking pediatric femoral nail and a lateral trochanteric entry point. *J Pediatr Orthop* 2009;29(4): 345-351.

54. Sink EL, Hedequist D, Morgan SJ, Hresko T: Results and technique of unstable pediatric femoral fractures treated with submuscular bridge plating. *J Pediatr Orthop* 2006;26(2):177-181.

55. Ramseier LE, Janicki JA, Weir S, Narayanan UG: Femoral fractures in adolescents: A comparison of four methods of fixation. *J Bone Joint Surg Am* 2010;92(5): 1122-1129.

    This retrospective study compared elastic stable intramedullary nailing, external fixation, rigid intramedullary nailing, and plate fixation for the management of 194 diaphyseal femoral fractures in 189 children and adolescents (mean age, 13 years). External fixation had the highest rate of complications; the other three methods produced comparable outcomes. Level of evidence: III.

56. Eichinger JK, McKenzie CS, Devine JG: Evaluation of pediatric lower extremity fractures managed with external fixation: Outcomes in a deployed environment. *Am J Orthop (Belle Mead NJ)* 2012;41(1):15-19.

    In 12 femoral shaft fractures, 4 tibial fractures, and 1 subtrochanteric fracture in 17 patients (mean age, 7 years) in a deployed environment, uniplanar external fixation produced good results. Level of evidence: IV.

57. Frech-Dörfler M, Hasler CC, Häcker FM: Immediate hip spica for unstable femoral shaft fractures in preschool children: Still an efficient and effective option. *Eur J Pediatr Surg* 2010;20(1):18-23.

    In 22 preschool children with femoral shaft fracture with up to 2.5 cm of shortening, only 1 developed a clinically significant limb-length discrepancy after immediate spica casting. Level of evidence: IV.

58. Akşahin E, Celebi L, Yüksel HY, et al: Immediate incorporated hip spica casting in pediatric femoral fractures: Comparison of efficacy between normal and high-risk groups. *J Pediatr Orthop* 2009;29(1):39-43.

59. Owen J, Stephens D, Wright JG: Reliability of hip range of motion using goniometry in pediatric femur shaft fractures. *Can J Surg* 2007;50(4):251-255.

60. DiFazio R, Vessey J, Zurakowski D, Hresko MT, Matheny T: Incidence of skin complications and associated charges in children treated with hip spica casts for femur fractures. *J Pediatr Orthop* 2011;31(1):17-22.

    Of 297 patients with 300 spica casts for femoral shaft fractures, the authors reported a 28% frequency of skin complications. Treatment often entailed local skin care, spica cast change in the operating room, or modification of the spica cast in the outpatient setting. Predictors of skin complications included child abuse as the mechanism of injury, younger age, and immobilization with cast more than 40 days. Level of evidence: III.

61. Ellis HB, Ho CA, Podeszwa DA, Wilson PL: A comparison of locked versus nonlocked Enders rods for length unstable pediatric femoral shaft fractures. *J Pediatr Orthop* 2011;31(8):825-833.

    In this retrospective review of 107 femoral shaft fractures treated with Enders rods (37 locked, 70 unlocked), the authors found no statistical differences in demographic data, surgical variables, fracture pattern or location, time to union, femoral alignment, or major complications when compared with fixation with nonlocked rods. However, the patients in the locked-rod group experienced less shortening and fewer distal rod hardware complications. Level of evidence: III.

62. Moroz LA, Launay F, Kocher MS, et al: Titanium elastic nailing of fractures of the femur in children: Predictors of complications and poor outcome. *J Bone Joint Surg Br* 2006;88(10):1361-1366.

63. Sagan ML, Datta JC, Olney BW, Lansford TJ, McIff TE: Residual deformity after treatment of pediatric femur fractures with flexible titanium nails. *J Pediatr Orthop* 2010;30(7):638-643.

    In this combined clinical and biomechanical study, the authors found that recurvatum malunion was common after treatment of midshaft transverse femoral fractures with flexible intramedullary nailing, but turning the proximal tip of at least one nail anteriorly greatly reduced this tendency. Level of evidence: III.

64. Saseendar S, Menon J, Patro DK: Treatment of femoral fractures in children: Is titanium elastic nailing an improvement over hip spica casting? *J Child Orthop* 2010; 4(3):245-251.

    This case-control study demonstrated better radiographic and functional outcomes, as well as shorter rehabilitation times, in 16 patients treated with flexible intramedullary nailing compared with 16 age-matched patients treated with spica casting. Level of evidence: III.

65. MacNeil JA, Francis A, El-Hawary R: A systematic review of rigid, locked, intramedullary nail insertion sites and avascular necrosis of the femoral head in the skeletally immature. *J Pediatr Orthop* 2011;31(4):377-380.

    In this systematic literature review, 19 articles described osteonecrosis rates in patients with femoral shaft fractures treated with antegrade rigid intramedullary nails. Three nail entry sites and their rates of osteonecrosis were identified: the piriformis fossa (2% rate of osteonecrosis); the tip of the greater trochanter (1.4%), and the area lateral to the tip of the greater trochanter (0%).

66. Pate O, Hedequist D, Leong N, Hresko T: Implant removal after submuscular plating for pediatric femur fractures. *J Pediatr Orthop* 2009;29(7):709-712.

6: Pediatrics

67. Butcher CC, Hoffman EB: Supracondylar fractures of the femur in children: Closed reduction and percutaneous pinning of displaced fractures. *J Pediatr Orthop* 2005;25(2):145-148.

68. Fujak A, Kopschina C, Forst R, Gras F, Mueller LA, Forst J: Fractures in proximal spinal muscular atrophy. *Arch Orthop Trauma Surg* 2010;130(6):775-780.

    Of 94 fractures in 60 patients with proximal spinal muscular atrophy, femoral fractures were the most frequent (50 fractures). Most were successfully treated nonsurgically; only 2 femoral shaft fractures were treated surgically. Level of evidence: IV.

69. Marreiros H, Monteiro L, Loff C, Calado E: Fractures in children and adolescents with spina bifida: The experience of a Portuguese tertiary-care hospital. *Dev Med Child Neurol* 2010;52(8):754-759.

    Of 45 fractures reported in 113 children with spina bifida, the most common were fractures of the distal femur. Level of evidence: IV.

70. Arkader A, Friedman JE, Warner WC Jr, Wells L: Complete distal femoral metaphyseal fractures: A harbinger of child abuse before walking age. *J Pediatr Orthop* 2007;27(7):751-753.

71. Kao FC, Tu YK, Hsu KY, Su JY, Yen CY, Chou MC: Floating knee injuries: A high complication rate. *Orthopedics* 2010;33(1):14.

    Of 419 patients with floating knee injuries, 104 (25%) had complications. The lowest complication rate was in the group of patients age 10 to 19 years. Level of evidence: IV.

72. Volpon JB, Perina MM, Okubo R, Maranho DA: Biomechanical performance of flexible intramedullary nails with end caps tested in distal segmental defects of pediatric femur models. *J Pediatr Orthop* 2012;32(5):461-466.

    In a model of distal femur fractures fixed with flexible intramedullary nails with and without threaded end caps, the end-cap nails were 8.75% stiffer in bending and 14.0% stiffer in torsion than nails without end caps.

73. Goodwin R, Mahar AT, Oka R, Steinman S, Newton PO: Biomechanical evaluation of retrograde intramedullary stabilization for femoral fractures: The effect of fracture level. *J Pediatr Orthop* 2007;27(8):873-876.

Chapter 62

Pediatric Hip Disorders

Jonathan G. Schoenecker, MD, PhD   David A. Podeszwa, MD

Developmental Dysplasia of the Hip

Epidemiology and Etiology

Developmental dysplasia of the hip (DDH) encompasses a spectrum of abnormalities of the developing hip, ranging from subtle conditions that can be observed only on imaging studies to subluxation and frank dislocation of the hip joint. Hip dysplasia is the most common orthopaedic defect in newborns, with an incidence ranging from 1 to more than 35 per 1,000 live births. Discrepancies in reports of the incidence of this disorder are believed to result from detection methods (clinical or ultrasound examinations) as well as cultural differences in subpopulations, such as swaddling the hip in extension and adduction. Native Americans and Laplanders have the highest rate of DDH, whereas it is rarely diagnosed in children of African descent. Without any risk factors or family history, the risk of a child being born with DDH is 0.2%, whereas children of parents with DDH have a 12% risk, siblings of children with DDH have a 6% risk, and children whose parents and siblings have DDH have a 36% risk. Through enhanced gene sequencing technology, it is becoming clear that some cases of DDH are, at least in part, a result of specific genetic polymorphisms.[1]

Epidemiologic studies show that first-born progeny of the female sex are at greatest risk for DDH. Approximately 80% of affected infants are girls, and 80% of DDH disorders involve the left hip (60% left alone, 20% right alone, and 20% bilateral). Therefore, the current hypothesis to explain these epidemiologic findings is the DDH is caused by (1) intrauterine positioning, either with the left hip adducted against the mother's lumbosacral spine in the left occiput anterior position (particularly during a first pregnancy) or breech position in the third trimester; (2) change in intrauterine volume (either oligohydramnios or increased birth weight); and (3) response to sex hormones, such as relaxin.

Dr. Schoenecker or an immediate family member has received research or institutional support from ISIS Pharmaceuticals. Dr. Podeszwa or an immediate family member serves as a board member, owner, officer, or committee member of the Pediatric Orthopaedic Society of North America.

Diagnosis and Physical Examination

The objective of examining an infant's hip is to determine the stability of the hip (subluxation or frank dislocation), reduce the hip if it is dislocated or dislocatable, and differentiate instability from normal variations found in a dynamic examination. The examination is most often conducted dynamically, with the infant supine and the hips in flexion. The first aspect of the examination is to determine where the hip(s) are located at rest. This is often done by first bringing the legs into an adducted position. In an infant with a unilateral dislocation at rest, there is an apparent shortening of the thigh (Galeazzi sign), although this sign may be absent with bilateral dislocations. If the hip(s) are believed to be reduced at rest, the examiner then tests whether or not each hip can be dislocated. This is done by gently pressing posteriorly on the flexed, adducted thigh (Barlow test or stress maneuver). If the hip(s) is dislocated at rest or dislocates with posterior stress, the examiner then must determine if the hip is reducible. This is most often accomplished by moving the flexed hip into abduction while gently pressing the greater trochanter toward the acetabulum (Ortolani test or reduction maneuver).

Hips that are dislocated at rest are often reducible before 3 months of age (Ortolani positive sign); however, by 3 to 6 months, soft-tissue contractures often make reduction impossible (Ortolani negative sign). Features of a unilateral fixed dislocation typically include reduced abduction in flexion, walking with a limp because of gluteus medius insufficiency, and toe-walking to compensate for the relative shortening. Bilateral dislocations can cause a hip flexion contracture that is compensated by increased lumbar lordosis. Dysplasia without dislocation can be clinically silent in children and may present in adolescence or adulthood with hip pain and/or degenerative disease.

Imaging

Ultrasonography is the current gold standard for imaging the hip in infants younger than 6 months (Figure 1). Ultrasonography allows changes in hip position to be observed with movement, and real-time ultrasonography permits multiplanar examinations that can clearly determine the position of the femoral head with respect to the acetabulum. Currently, the most common ultrasonographic technique is the dynamic standard minimum examination. This method provides information similar to the physical examination, including assess-

Table 1

Stages of Legg-Calvé-Perthes Disease

Stage	Name	Radiographic Findings	Duration
I	Osteosclerosis	Normal appearing radiographs or epiphyseal sclerosis with or without widening of the joint	Up to 6 months
II	Fragmentation	Maximal sclerosis with areas of progressive radiographic resorption of the epiphysis	6 months to 2 years
III	Reossification	Recognizable new bone formation	1-3 years
IV	Healing/remodeling	Epiphyseal bone density normalizes and trabecular patterns appear; secondary deformities may appear, and focal physeal arrest may be apparent.	Until skeletal maturity

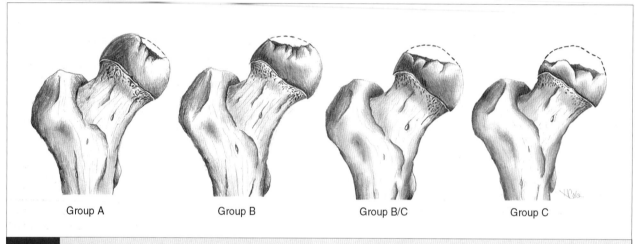

Group A   Group B   Group B/C   Group C

Figure 4   Illustrations of the Herring lateral pillar classification system. The lateral one third of the epiphysis, usually located lateral to the central sequestrum, is compared with the contralateral hip and measured for grading. The epiphysis is considered group A if the height is equal to the contralateral epiphysis, group B if there is partial collapse but the height is greater than 50% of the contralateral epiphysis, and group C if there is greater collapse and the height is less than 50% of the contralateral epiphysis. A fourth type, called B/C, is a borderline group that is included to categorize hips with a thin or poorly ossified lateral pillar and loss of exactly 50% of the original height of the lateral pillar. (Courtesy of Heather A. Cole, Children's Hospital Vanderbilt, Nashville, TN.)

poorly ossified lateral pillar with loss of exactly 50% of the original height of the lateral pillar. This classification system has been proven to have good intraobserver and interobserver reliability and correlation with the prognosis. Approximately 30% of hips may progress in their lateral pillar classification during fragmentation, with changes more frequent in extensively involved hips.

Other radiographic signs associated with poor outcomes are lateral subluxation, hinge abduction, and the presence of a metaphyseal cyst and a physeal bar. Common residual deformities after Legg-Calvé-Perthes disease include head widening (coxa magna) and flattening (coxa plana). If the capital femoral physis is significantly involved, these findings are accentuated by and typically may include femoral neck shortening (coxa breva) and relative overgrowth of the greater trochanter. Accommodative secondary remodeling in acetabular depth and orientation occur throughout the course of Legg-Calvé-Perthes disease and may result in

paradoxic DDH and femoral acetabular impingement (FAI). Although MRI, CT, and bone scans have been investigated as a means of better defining the pathology of Legg-Calvé-Perthes disease, their clinical value in classifying or predicting disease outcomes has yet to be validated.

Treatment and Outcomes

The goal of treatment is to obtain and maintain containment of the involved femoral head within the acetabulum. Ideally, it would be beneficial to decrease the duration of the disease; however, there are few conclusive scientific data supporting the ability to alter the time course of Legg-Calvé-Perthes disease. Early femoral head containment (defined as acetabular coverage of the anterolateral femoral epiphysis) protects the femoral head from deforming stresses. Treatment to achieve effective containment maximizes subsequent joint congruity. Containment must be radiographically

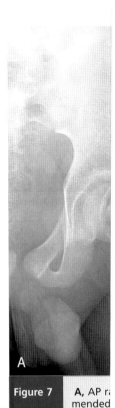

Figure 7 A, AP ra[...]
mended [...]
result of [...]

All patients wit[...]
sidual proximal fe[...]
been recognized a[...]
stantial intra-artic[...]
articular cartilage[...]
alignment osteoto[...]
correct alignment[...]
and improving fur[...]
location approach[...]
oral osteotomy, l[...]
chronic deformity[...]
ogy.[54] Despite ear[...]
dications for thi[...]
lished.[46,55]

Summary

Hip dysplasia, L[...]
can each present[...]
radiographic find[...]
cal characteristics[...]
recognition and t[...]
ing potential co[...]
long-term outcon[...]
individual patien[...]
presentation. Lor[...]
being diagnosed i[...]
tions that can aff[...]
tient's function th[...]

confirmed. Nonsurgical therapies include activity modification, non–weight-bearing or partial weight-bearing restrictions, NSAIDs, abduction bracing, or physical therapy. The inability to maintain femoral head containment with nonsurgical therapy may be an indication for surgical intervention. Surgical treatment options include adductor tenotomy followed by abduction casting/bracing, proximal femoral varus osteotomy, acetabular redirectional osteotomy (single or triple innominate), or acetabular augmentation (shelf procedure).

Nonsurgical techniques have a higher success rate in patients younger than 6 years and those with less involvement of the epiphysis (lateral pillar A). There is little controversy regarding initiating nonsurgical therapy in these patients because approximately 80% will have a favorable prognosis without surgery. It is essential to continuously monitor these patients for loss of motion and/or containment and to switch to a surgical treatment algorithm if changes occur. Patients older than 6 years with a more involved epiphysis (greater than lateral pillar A) should be treated surgically. A systematic review of the literature suggests that a proximal femoral varus osteotomy or a Salter innominate osteotomy in patients 6 years or older before or in the early fragmentation phase results in improved femoral head sphericity compared with nonsurgical treatment.[22] The Norwegian experience paralleled those findings by demonstrating improved femoral head sphericity in patients between 6 and 10 years of age with whole femoral head involvement who were treated with a femoral varus osteotomy at an average of 5.6 months after diagnosis.[23] A proximal femoral varus osteotomy also has been shown to be superior to nonsurgical treatment in certain patients with lateral pillar classifications of B or B/C but not C.[24] Although some valgus remodeling of the femoral neck is expected with growth, too much varus can lead to a poor outcome; 10° to 15° of varus is the recommended correction.[25]

A 2013 study reported that patients with a lateral pillar classification of B or B/C treated with an adductor tenotomy followed by an A-frame orthosis and physical therapy have outcomes equivalent to those treated with proximal femoral osteotomy.[26] Their outcomes are superior to those with a lateral pillar classification of C who are treated with a varus osteotomy. The authors concluded that the combination of the tenotomy (to regain abduction and containment), followed by an orthosis (to maintain motion), and physical therapy takes advantage of the biologic plasticity of epiphyseal cartilage and uses the femoroacetabular articulation as an environment for dynamic, physiologic containment and remodeling. In support of the need for an adductor tenotomy and physical therapy in this protocol, a recent literature review found that abduction bracing alone does not result in substantial improvement in containment, femoral head sphericity, or range of motion after brace wear.[27] In hips that present late with severe deformity, passive hip abduction may be very limited because the lateral epiphysis engages the acetabulum even when the patient is asleep (referred to as hinge abduction). Containment-type procedures are contraindicated for hinge abduction, which can be treated with a proximal femoral valgus osteotomy, with or without a shelf arthroplasty.

The proximal femoral and acetabular residual deformity in the symptomatic skeletally mature patient is frequently complex and challenging to treat. Clinically, these patients commonly present with signs and symptoms of FAI, such as activity-related groin pain and a positive impingement sign. Relative to normal hips and those with idiopathic FAI, hips with residual deformity from Legg-Calvé-Perthes disease demonstrate decreased range of motion, different locations of impingement zones, and a higher prevalence of intra- and extra-articular impingement.[28] Plain radiography and gadolinium-enhanced magnetic resonance arthrography with radial sequencing are useful for evaluating extra- and intra-articular pathology. An evaluation of intraoperative findings in skeletally mature patients with Perthes or Perthes-like deformities reported labral, acetabular, and femoral cartilage abnormalities in 76%, 59%, and 81% of cases, respectively. Male sex, a high trochanter, and joint incongruity were associated with more advanced intra-articular disease.[29]

The advent of surgical hip dislocation has created a safe and efficacious approach for dynamically evaluating the hip for FAI and treating intra-articular, acetabular, and proximal femoral pathology (**Figure 5**). In a study of 29 symptomatic patients with residual Legg-Calvé-Perthes disease who were treated with a surgical hip dislocation at an average age of 17 years and followed for a minimum of 1 year, there was substantial improvement in self-reported function and a low complication rate.[30] Femoral head-neck osteochondroplasty and a variety of concomitant procedures were performed without difficulty. Similarly, another study reported an 86% survival rate for symptomatic Perthes hips treated through a surgical hip dislocation approach, with specific procedures based on the femoral and acetabular pathomorphology.[31] Absolute indications and long-term efficacy of joint preservation surgery in this patient population are not yet defined.

The long-term outcomes of the mature hip with residual deformity of Legg-Calvé-Perthes disease initially treated nonsurgically are generally related to the sphericity of the femoral head and the congruity of the hip joint. A recent prospective study reported that pain, arthritis, and ongoing hip dysfunction were common in patients with Legg-Calvé-Perthes disease who were treated nonsurgically.[32] Fifty-eight hips were examined at a mean of 20.4 years after enrollment in the study; 76% of the patients reported at least occasional hip pain, and 39% reported daily pain or pain several times weekly (most commonly groin pain). Only 26% of the patients had no radiographic evidence of arthritis, whereas 44% had moderate or severe arthritic changes. Clinically, a positive impingement sign (pain with flexion, adduction, and internal rotation of the hip) was associated with an increased frequency of hip pain and a lower Iowa Hip Score and Nonarthritic Hip Score (NAHS). The lateral pillar classification was as-

6: Pediatrics

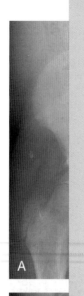

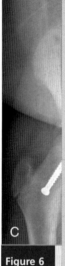

Figure 6

warrant st[
The modifi[
Oxford bo[
predict the[
the overall[
open trirad[
best predic[
The sho[
for mild sl[
sults may [
a 12% rat[
16 years a[
undergoing[
patients w[
One third [
but did no[
limitation.[
Osteone[
most seriou[

2. Harcke HT, Kumar SJ: The role of ultrasound in the diagnosis and management of congenital dislocation and dysplasia of the hip. *J Bone Joint Surg Am* 1991;73(4): 622-628.

3. Mahan ST, Katz JN, Kim YJ: To screen or not to screen? A decision analysis of the utility of screening for developmental dysplasia of the hip. *J Bone Joint Surg Am* 2009;91(7):1705-1719.

4. Roposch A, Liu LQ, Hefti F, Clarke NM, Wedge JH: Standardized diagnostic criteria for developmental dysplasia of the hip in early infancy. *Clin Orthop Relat Res* 2011;469(12):3451-3461.

   Among pediatric orthopaedic surgeons worldwide, the most relevant clinical criteria for making the diagnosis of DDH in infants younger than 9 weeks include the Ortolani and Barlow tests, hip asymmetry in abduction of 20° or greater, breech presentation, limb-length discrepancy, and a first-degree relative treated for DDH. Level of evidence: V.

5. Murnaghan ML, Browne RH, Sucato DJ, Birch J: Femoral nerve palsy in Pavlik harness treatment for developmental dysplasia of the hip. *J Bone Joint Surg Am* 2011; 93(5):493-499.

   Femoral nerve palsy is an uncommon yet clinically important complication of Pavlik harness treatment of DDH. It is strongly predictive of treatment failure, and its effect is greatest when DDH is more severe. Level of evidence: IV.

6. Gould SW, Grissom LE, Niedzielski A, Kecskemethy HH, Bowen JR, Harcke HT: Protocol for MRI of the hips after spica cast placement. *J Pediatr Orthop* 2012; 32(5):504-509.

   The authors reviewed 34 consecutive MRIs performed without sedation after spica cast placement in patients with DDH. They concluded that two sequences accurately assessed the concentric reduction, with a potential study time of 15 minutes. These findings obviate the need for sedation. Level of evidence: II.

7. Gholve PA, Flynn JM, Garner MR, Millis MB, Kim YJ: Predictors for secondary procedures in walking DDH. *J Pediatr Orthop* 2012;32(3):282-289.

   The authors tried to identify predictors for secondary procedures after open reduction of the hip in walking children with DDH. They found that an open reduction without concurrent femoral osteotomy strongly predicted the need for a secondary procedure. Level of evidence: IV.

8. Sankar WN, Schoenecker JG, Mayfield ME, Kim YJ, Millis MB: Acetabular retroversion in Down syndrome. *J Pediatr Orthop* 2012;32(3):277-281.

   The morphology of DDH in patients with Down syndrome and idiopathic DDH were studied. The authors found that the anterolateral acetabulum was most often deficient in patients with idiopathic DDH. Level of evidence: III.

9. Salter RB: Innominate osteotomy in the treatment of congenital dislocation and subluxation of the hip. *J Bone Joint Surg Br* 1961;43:518-539.

10. Pemberton PA: Pericapsular osteotomy of the ilium for treatment of congenital subluxation and dislocation of the hip. *J Bone Joint Surg Am* 1965;47:65-86.

11. Holman J, Carroll KL, Murray KA, Macleod LM, Roach JW: Long-term follow-up of open reduction surgery for developmental dislocation of the hip. *J Pediatr Orthop* 2012;32(2):121-124.

    The long-term results of open reduction surgery in DDH were studied. The authors found that the results deteriorate with the increasing age of patients at the time of surgery. Osteonecrosis and redislocation predict a poor functional and radiographic result. Level of evidence: IV.

12. Firth GB, Robertson AJ, Schepers A, Fatti L: Developmental dysplasia of the hip: Open reduction as a risk factor for substantial osteonecrosis. *Clin Orthop Relat Res* 2010;468(9):2485-2494.

    The authors determined that the type of reduction (closed with traction versus open without femoral shortening) but not age influenced the risk of osteonecrosis. Level of evidence: IV.

13. Wu KW, Wang TM, Huang SC, Kuo KN, Chen CW: Analysis of osteonecrosis following Pemberton acetabuloplasty in developmental dysplasia of the hip: Long-term results. *J Bone Joint Surg Am* 2010;92(11):2083-2094.

    The authors propose that the lateral epiphyseal branch of the medial circumflex artery is vulnerable to compression with increased inferior reduction/displacement of the femoral head, thus increasing the risk of osteonecrosis. Level of evidence: III.

14. Pospischill R, Weninger J, Ganger R, Altenhuber J, Grill F: Does open reduction of the developmental dislocated hip increase the risk of osteonecrosis? *Clin Orthop Relat Res* 2012;470(1):250-260.

    Early reduction of a dislocated hip (within the first year of life) is advocated to avoid the need for concomitant osteotomies combined with open reduction.

15. Roposch A, Odeh O, Doria AS, Wedge JH: The presence of an ossific nucleus does not protect against osteonecrosis after treatment of developmental dysplasia of the hip. *Clin Orthop Relat Res* 2011;469(10):2838-2845.

    Thirty-five percent (37/105) hips treated for DDH before 18 months of age developed osteonecrosis. When considering only grade II or greater changes (Bucholz-Ogden classification), there was no difference in the risk of osteonecrosis with or without an ossific nucleus present at initial treatment.

16. Roposch A, Liu LQ, Offiah AC, Wedge JH: Functional outcomes in children with osteonecrosis secondary to treatment of developmental dysplasia of the hip. *J Bone Joint Surg Am* 2011;93(24):e145.

    The authors determined that patients with an ossific nu-

6: Pediatrics

6: Pediatrics

cleus at the time of hip reduction showed a slight tendency toward better outcomes, but the ossific nucleus did not protect against osteonecrosis. Level of evidence: III.

17. Kobayashi D, Satsuma S, Kuroda R, Kurosaka M: Acetabular development in the contralateral hip in patients with unilateral developmental dysplasia of the hip. *J Bone Joint Surg Am* 2010;92(6):1390-1397.

After 6 years of age, a difference in acetabular growth develops in patients with and without primary acetabular dysplasia. A final prognosis for acetabular development appears to be difficult to determine until the age of 12 years. Level of evidence: IV.

18. Herrera-Soto JA, Price CT: Core decompression and labral support for the treatment of juvenile osteonecrosis. *J Pediatr Orthop* 2011;31(2, suppl):S212-S216.

Juvenile osteonecrosis responds differently in younger patients in whom Legg-Calvé-Perthes develops, and it is similar to adult osteonecrosis. The treatment rationale should be tailored to address these differences. Level of evidence: IV.

19. Hailer YD, Montgomery SM, Ekbom A, Nilsson OS, Bahmanyar S: Legg-Calve-Perthes disease and risks for cardiovascular diseases and blood diseases. *Pediatrics* 2010;125(6):e1308-e1315.

Patients with Legg-Calvé-Perthes disease had a hazard ratio of 1.70 (95% confidence interval: 1.39-2.09) for cardiovascular diseases compared with individuals without the disease. There was a statistically significant higher risk for blood diseases, including anemias, coagulation defects, and hypertensive disease. Level of evidence: III.

20. Daniel AB, Shah H, Kamath A, Guddettu V, Joseph B: Environmental tobacco and wood smoke increase the risk of Legg-Calvé-Perthes disease. *Clin Orthop Relat Res* 2012;470(9):2369-2375.

The authors attempted to confirm an association between environmental tobacco smoke, firewood smoke, and socioeconomic status with the risk of Legg-Calvé-Perthes disease. Level of evidence: III.

21. Vosmaer A, Pereira RR, Koenderman JS, Rosendaal FR, Cannegieter SC: Coagulation abnormalities in Legg-Calvé-Perthes disease. *J Bone Joint Surg Am* 2010; 92(1):121-128.

The risk of Legg-Calvé-Perthes disease increases with an increasing number of coagulation abnormalities in males but not in females. Level of evidence: III.

22. Saran N, Varghese R, Mulpuri K: Do femoral or salter innominate osteotomies improve femoral head sphericity in Legg-Calvé-Perthes disease? A meta-analysis. *Clin Orthop Relat Res* 2012;470(9):2383-2393.

Children 6 years or older during or before the fragmentation phase of Legg-Calvé-Perthes disease are more likely to have better femoral head sphericity with surgical treatment (femoral or innominate osteotomies) than with nonsurgical treatment.

23. Terjesen T, Wiig O, Svenningsen S: Varus femoral osteotomy improves sphericity of the femoral head in

older children with severe form of Legg-Calvé-Perthes disease. *Clin Orthop Relat Res* 2012;470(9):2394-2401.

In children 6 to 10 years of age in whom the whole femoral head is affected, femoral head sphericity 5 years after a femoral varus osteotomy was better than the sphericity after physical therapy.

24. Herring JA, Kim HT, Browne R: Legg-Calve-Perthes disease: Part II. Prospective multicenter study of the effect of treatment on outcome. *J Bone Joint Surg Am* 2004;86(10):2121-2134.

25. Kim HK, da Cunha AM, Browne R, Kim HT, Herring JA: How much varus is optimal with proximal femoral osteotomy to preserve the femoral head in Legg-Calvé-Perthes disease? *J Bone Joint Surg Am* 2011;93(4): 341-347.

The authors report that 10° to 15° of varus correction is recommended when performing proximal femoral varus osteotomy on hips in the early stages of Legg-Calvé-Perthes disease.

26. Rich MM, Schoenecker PL: Management of Legg-Calvé-Perthes disease using an A-frame orthosis and hip range of motion: A 25-year experience. *J Pediatr Orthop* 2013;33(2):112-119.

Treatment of 240 hips in 213 patients resulted in spherically concentric hips in 101 of 113 (89%) lateral pillar B hips and 77 of 115 (67%) of lateral pillar C hips. Patient age did not affect the outcome.

27. Hardesty CK, Liu RW, Thompson GH: The role of bracing in Legg-Calve-Perthes disease. *J Pediatr Orthop* 2011;31(2, suppl):S178-S181.

A comprehensive literature review of abduction bracing suggests bracing alone has no effect on containment, femoral head shape, or hip range of motion. Petrie casts still have a limited role in short-term treatment before complete reossification.

28. Tannast M, Hanke M, Ecker TM, Murphy SB, Albers CE, Puls M: LCPD: Reduced range of motion resulting from extra- and intraarticular impingement. *Clin Orthop Relat Res* 2012;470(9):2431-2440.

Hips with Legg-Calvé-Perthes disease show decreased range of motion, differences in the location of impingement zones, and a higher prevalence of intra- and extra-articular impingement compared with normal hips and hips in patients with idiopathic FAI. Level of evidence: III.

29. Ross JR, Nepple JJ, Baca G, Schoenecker PL, Clohisy JC: Intraarticular abnormalities in residual Perthes and Perthes-like hip deformities. *Clin Orthop Relat Res* 2012;470(11):2968-2977.

Chondral lesions and labral tears are common in symptomatic patients with Perthes or Perthes-like deformities. Male sex, a high trochanter, and joint incongruity are associated with more advanced intra-articular disease. Level of evidence: IV.

30. Shore BJ, Novais EN, Millis MB, Kim YJ: Low early failure rates using a surgical dislocation approach in

6: Pediatrics

healed Legg-Calvé-Perthes disease. *Clin Orthop Relat Res* 2012;470(9):2441-2449.

The surgical hip dislocation approach allowed evaluation and treatment of all intra-articular and proximal femoral deformities of healed Legg-Calvé-Perthes disease. There was a low complication rate and improved postoperative Western Ontario and McMaster Universities Osteoarthritis Index scores. Level of evidence: IV.

31. Albers CE, Steppacher SD, Ganz R, Siebenrock KA, Tannast M: Joint-preserving surgery improves pain, range of motion, and abductor strength after Legg-Calvé-Perthes disease. *Clin Orthop Relat Res* 2012; 470(9):2450-2461.

The authors reported on 50 patients (age range, 7 to 47 years) treated with a variety of joint-preserving procedures based on the authors' treatment algorithm. Postoperative improvement in hip pain and function were reported. The hip survival rate at 5 years after surgery was 86%. Level of evidence: IV.

32. Larson AN, Sucato DJ, Herring JA, et al: A prospective multicenter study of Legg-Calvé-Perthes disease: Functional and radiographic outcomes of nonoperative treatment at a mean follow-up of twenty years. *J Bone Joint Surg Am* 2012;94(7):584-592.

The Stulberg classification was significantly associated with impingement on physical examination, increased NAHS, and higher Tönnis grade. Hips rated as Stulberg type III or IV more frequently had poor or fair outcomes based on the Iowa Hip Score and NAHS. Level of evidence: III.

33. Traina F, De Fine M, Sudanese A, Calderoni PP, Tassinari E, Toni A: Long-term results of total hip replacement in patients with Legg-Calvé-Perthes disease. *J Bone Joint Surg Am* 2011;93(7):e25.

In the 32 hip replacements in this study, there was a 96.9% cumulative survival rate at 15 years, with an overall complication rate of 12.5%. Harris hip scores were significantly improved postoperatively.

34. Lehmann CL, Arons RR, Loder RT, Vitale MG: The epidemiology of slipped capital femoral epiphysis: An update. *J Pediatr Orthop* 2006;26(3):286-290.

35. Zupanc O, Krizancic M, Daniel M, et al: Shear stress in epiphyseal growth plate is a risk factor for slipped capital femoral epiphysis. *J Pediatr Orthop* 2008;28(4): 444-451.

36. Loder RT, Richards BS, Shapiro PS, Reznick LR, Aronson DD: Acute slipped capital femoral epiphysis: The importance of physeal stability. *J Bone Joint Surg Am* 1993;75(8):1134-1140.

37. Ziebarth K, Domayer S, Slongo T, Kim YJ, Ganz R: Clinical stability of slipped capital femoral epiphysis does not correlate with intraoperative stability. *Clin Orthop Relat Res* 2012;470(8):2274-2279.

The Loder classification of unstable SCFE had poor specificity (39%) and limited sensitivity (76%) for identifying complete physeal disruption, which was confirmed intraoperatively. Using the chronologic classification system (acute, acute-on-chronic, and chronic) did not improve results (specificity 44%, sensitivity 82%). Level of evidence: III.

38. Mamisch TC, Kim YJ, Richolt JA, Millis MB, Kordelle J: Femoral morphology due to impingement influences the range of motion in slipped capital femoral epiphysis. *Clin Orthop Relat Res* 2009;467(3):692-698.

39. Goodwin RC, Mahar AT, Oswald TS, Wenger DR: Screw head impingement after in situ fixation in moderate and severe slipped capital femoral epiphysis. *J Pediatr Orthop* 2007;27(3):319-325.

40. Loder RT, Dietz FR: What is the best evidence for the treatment of slipped capital femoral epiphysis? *J Pediatr Orthop* 2012;32(suppl 2):S158-S165.

A systematic review of the literature with treatment recommendations for stable and unstable SCFE and the role of surgical dislocation in the treatment of SCFE are presented. Level of evidence: IV.

41. Dragoni M, Heiner AD, Costa S, Gabrielli A, Weinstein SL: Biomechanical study of 16-mm threaded, 32-mm threaded, and fully threaded SCFE screw fixation. *J Pediatr Orthop* 2012;32(1):70-74.

When comparing 16-mm, 32-mm, and fully threaded screws in an immature porcine model, the 16-mm threaded screws had the highest rate of femoral neck failure. Fully threaded or 32-mm threaded screws may confer additional femoral neck strength. Level of evidence: IV.

42. Mooney JF III, Sanders JO, Browne RH, et al: Management of unstable/acute slipped capital femoral epiphysis: Results of a survey of the POSNA membership. *J Pediatr Orthop* 2005;25(2):162-166.

43. Sonnega RJ, van der Sluijs JA, Wainwright AM, Roposch A, Hefti F: Management of slipped capital femoral epiphysis: Results of a survey of the members of the European Paediatric Orthopaedic Society. *J Child Orthop* 2011;5(6):433-438.

Seventy percent of the survey respondents from the European Paediatric Orthopaedic Society use a single screw for fixation of stable or mild unstable SCFE. There is no consensus regarding the treatment of moderate or severe unstable SCFE and the treatment of the contralateral hip.

44. Segal LS, Jacobson JA, Saunders MM: Biomechanical analysis of in situ single versus double screw fixation in a nonreduced slipped capital femoral epiphysis model. *J Pediatr Orthop* 2006;26(4):479-485.

45. Huber H, Dora C, Ramseier LE, Buck F, Dierauer S: Adolescent slipped capital femoral epiphysis treated by a modified Dunn osteotomy with surgical hip dislocation. *J Bone Joint Surg Br* 2011;93(6):833-838.

Short-term follow-up (mean, 3.8 years) of 30 hips demonstrated an excellent outcome in 28 hips, with anatomic or near anatomic reduction and osteonecrosis in

1 hip (3.3%). Four hips (13.3%) required revision of failed implants. Level of evidence: IV.

46. Slongo T, Kakaty D, Krause F, Ziebarth K: Treatment of slipped capital femoral epiphysis with a modified Dunn procedure. *J Bone Joint Surg Am* 2010;92(18): 2898-2908.

   The authors report excellent short-term clinical and radiographic outcomes in 21 of 23 patients treated for severe SCFE (stable and unstable) with the modified Dunn procedure. Two poor outcomes (8.7%) were reported, including the development of osteonecrosis and severe osteoarthritis. Level of evidence: IV.

47. Yildirim Y, Bautista S, Davidson RS: Chondrolysis, osteonecrosis, and slip severity in patients with subsequent contralateral slipped capital femoral epiphysis. *J Bone Joint Surg Am* 2008;90(3):485-492.

48. Zide JR, Popejoy D, Birch JG: Revised modified Oxford bone score: A simpler system for prediction of contralateral involvement in slipped capital femoral epiphysis. *J Pediatr Orthop* 2011;31(2):159-164.

   The modified Oxford bone score had excellent intraobserver and very good interobserver reliability and is easier to apply than the original Oxford bone score. Level of evidence: II.

49. Popejoy D, Emara K, Birch J: Prediction of contralateral slipped capital femoral epiphysis using the modified Oxford bone age score. *J Pediatr Orthop* 2012;32(3): 290-294.

   The modified Oxford bone age score and a triradiate score of 1 were found to be significant predictors (*P* < 0.0001) of the development of contralateral SCFE in patients presenting with a unilateral slip, with the modified Oxford bone age score a better overall predictor. Level of evidence: IV.

50. Larson AN, Sierra RJ, Yu EM, Trousdale RT, Stans AA: Outcomes of slipped capital femoral epiphysis treated with in situ pinning. *J Pediatr Orthop* 2012;32(2): 125-130.

   At a mean follow-up of 16 years, one third of patients with SCFE treated with in situ pinning reported residual pain. Approximately 10% required some form of reconstructive surgery within 10 years of in situ pinning, with 5% undergoing hip replacement within 20 years. Level of evidence: IV.

51. Sankar WN, McPartland TG, Millis MB, Kim YJ: The unstable slipped capital femoral epiphysis: Risk factors for osteonecrosis. *J Pediatr Orthop* 2010;30(6): 544-548.

   Osteonecrosis developed in 14 of 70 patients (20%) with unstable SCFE. Younger age and shorter duration of prodromal symptoms were the only risk factors identified. Level of evidence: IV.

52. Sink EL, Zaltz I, Heare T, Dayton M: Acetabular cartilage and labral damage observed during surgical hip dislocation for stable slipped capital femoral epiphysis. *J Pediatr Orthop* 2010;30(1):26-30.

   Acetabular cartilage injury was present in 33 of 39 (84.6%) and labral injury in 34 of 39 (87.1%) hips treated for pain associated with residual SCFE deformity using a surgical hip dislocation approach. There was no correlation between the severity of damage and the severity of SCFE. Level of evidence: IV.

53. Leunig M, Casillas MM, Hamlet M, et al: Slipped capital femoral epiphysis: Early mechanical damage to the acetabular cartilage by a prominent femoral metaphysis. *Acta Orthop Scand* 2000;71(4):370-375.

54. Ganz R, Gill TJ, Gautier E, Ganz K, Krügel N, Berlemann U: Surgical dislocation of the adult hip: A technique with full access to the femoral head and acetabulum without the risk of avascular necrosis. *J Bone Joint Surg Br* 2001;83(8):1119-1124.

55. Rebello G, Spencer S, Millis MB, Kim YJ: Surgical dislocation in the management of pediatric and adolescent hip deformity. *Clin Orthop Relat Res* 2009;467(3): 724-731.

6: Pediatrics

Chapter 63

Knee, Leg, Ankle, and Foot Trauma: Pediatrics

M. Lucas Murnaghan, MD, MEd, FRCSC   Debra Popejoy, MD

Introduction

Injuries to the lower extremity are common in children and can occur from a variety of mechanisms. Athletic participation by children and adolescents is an increasing cause of lower extremity fractures. The implications of growth disturbance caused by these fractures are magnified by the growth potential of the lower extremity and its intolerance of substantial angular and rotational deformities. Many of the fractures discussed in this chapter are classified using the Salter-Harris classification system, which is outlined in chapter 57, Shoulder, Upper Arm, and Elbow Trauma: Pediatrics, in *Orthopaedic Knowledge Update 11*. In this chapter, additional information is also provided on the previously discussed diaphyseal and metaphyseal femoral fractures described in chapter 61, Pelvis, Hip, and Femur Trauma: Pediatrics, in *Orthopaedic Knowledge Update 11*.

Distal Femoral Physeal Fractures

The physis of the distal femur contributes 40% of the growth of the lower extremity. Fractures that involve this physis can have substantial effects on subsequent growth, including partial or complete premature growth arrest. Partial growth arrest can lead to angular deformity, whereas complete growth arrest can lead to limb-length discrepancy. The physis is also at particular risk for growth disturbance because of the morphology of the distal femoral physis and the proximity to the uniplanar knee joint.

After obtaining a complete patient history and physical examination, AP and lateral radiographs of the

knee should be obtained. Based on these radiographs, the fracture can be classified and the amount of displacement assessed. Nondisplaced Salter-Harris type I fractures can be difficult to diagnose from plain radiographs and may require further investigation. Although the addition of stress radiographs was previously recommended, the advent and availability of MRI makes this imaging modality a more favored diagnostic approach. Nondisplaced fractures or fractures with displacement of less than 2 mm can be treated in a well-molded cast.

Displaced Salter-Harris type I and II fractures are at higher risk for further displacement and growth arrest. Salter-Harris type I fractures and type II fractures with a small metaphyseal (Thurston Holland) fragment can be fixed with crossed Kirschner wires. The wires can be placed in either an antegrade or a retrograde fashion. Kirschner wires are removed at 6 weeks in the outpatient clinic. Salter-Harris type II fractures with a large metaphyseal fragment can be treated with screw fixation placed from the side of the fragment, fixing the distal fragment to the intact metaphysis. After clinical and radiographic union is achieved, physiotherapy may be required to regain knee range of motion.

Because Salter-Harris type III and IV fractures traverse the articular surface, close attention must be paid to the degree of displacement. Advanced imaging studies (CT or MRI) may be required to accurately assess the amount of displacement. Intra-articular fractures with more than 2 mm of step or gap require reduction and fixation. Described techniques include closed reduction with fluoroscopic assistance, arthroscopically assisted reduction, and open reduction and internal fixation. At the time of stabilization or after fracture union, the treating physician should carefully assess for concomitant ligamentous injuries about the knee.[1] The likelihood of growth arrest is associated with the degree of initial displacement and has been reported in up to 50% of patients regardless of an anatomic reduction. The implications of partial or complete growth arrest are determined by the years of remaining growth in the patient. In patients with the potential for growth arrest, the treating physician may consider surgical resection of the physeal bar, completion of the epiphysiodesis, and/or contralateral epiphysiodesis.

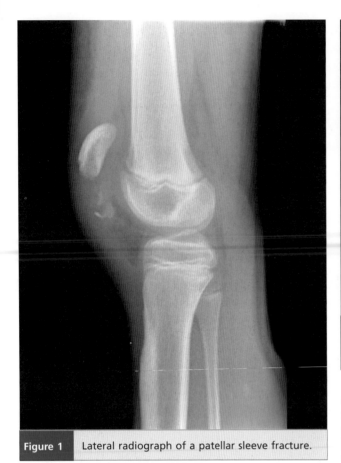

Figure 1   Lateral radiograph of a patellar sleeve fracture.

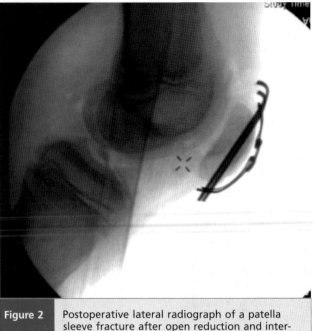

Figure 2   Postoperative lateral radiograph of a patella sleeve fracture after open reduction and internal fixation with a tension-band technique.

Patella Fractures

Patella fractures are relatively rare injuries in children, representing less than 1% of all pediatric fractures.[2] The mechanism of injury in a patella fracture is variable, including a direct blow, sudden forceful contraction of the extensor mechanism, and patellar dislocation. The physical examination must focus on the integrity of the extensor mechanism because this will dictate management. The radiographic examination should include AP, lateral, and skyline views. Nondisplaced fractures with an intact extensor mechanism can be treated nonsurgically with a long leg cast. Immobilization for 4 to 6 weeks, followed by progressive weight bearing and range of motion, are then instituted. Displaced fractures require surgical stabilization to restore knee extension and articular congruity. A variety of techniques have been described, including tension-band wiring, nonabsorbable sutures, and cannulated screws.

Patella sleeve fractures represent a uniquely pediatric type of patella fracture.[3] The mechanism of injury is commonly a sudden deceleration or eccentric contraction of the quadriceps mechanism. The patella in patients in this age group has a thick layer of unossified cartilage. The radiographic finding of a small rim of bone substantially underestimates the cartilaginous portion of this injury. The nonossified portion consists of articular cartilage on the deep surface and periosteum and cartilage on the superficial surface. Displaced

sleeve fractures should be treated with open reduction and internal fixation (Figures 1 and 2). Described fixation methods include transosseous sutures, tension-band wires, or suture anchors.[4,5] Similar to the more common distal fracture, a superior pole sleeve fracture has been described.[6]

Patellar dislocations are often associated with osteochondral fracture or chondral injury. The most common locations for these injuries are the lateral femoral condyle and the medial patellar facet. Careful examination of postreduction plain radiographs is required to look for evidence of fracture. A skyline radiograph is particularly helpful in diagnosing injuries that may otherwise be missed on AP and lateral radiographic views. Any evidence of fracture on early radiographs or the persistence of an effusion more than 6 weeks after injury warrants advanced imaging studies (CT or MRI). Knee arthroscopy is helpful to determine the size, location, and status of the fragment. Primary fixation of the osteochondral fragment can be performed arthroscopically or through an arthrotomy. A variety of fixation methods have been described, including bioabsorbable implants and headless metal screws.

Tibial Fractures

Tibial Tuberosity Fracture

Tibial tuberosity fractures are relatively uncommon injuries that most often occur in the adolescent years and result from eccentric quadriceps contraction.[7]

The Ogden classification system describes the relative displacement, propagation, and comminution of these fractures.[8] Further additions to this classification system include type IV fractures, with near complete in-

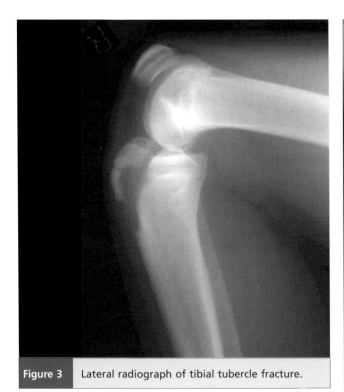

Figure 3 Lateral radiograph of tibial tubercle fracture.

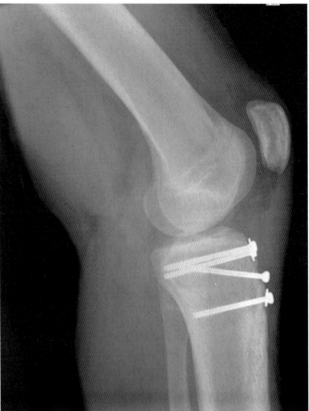

Figure 4 Postoperative lateral radiograph of a tibial tubercle fracture after open reduction and internal fixation.

volvement of the epiphysis, and type V fractures, which are a combination of type IIIB and type IV fractures.[7] Posterior metaphyseal involvement should be carefully evaluated because such involvement can be associated with compartment syndrome and refracture.[9]

Ogden type IA (nondisplaced) fractures are best treated with immobilization in a long leg cast for 6 weeks. Displaced fractures require open reduction and internal fixation. Fluoroscopic guidance and an arthrotomy will assist the surgeon in obtaining an anatomic reduction (Figures 3 and 4). A recent case series described the use of suture anchors to assist in maintaining the meniscal-articular relationship and providing additional fixation for smaller fragments.[10]

The most important acute complication of a tibial tuberosity fracture is recurrent anterior tibial artery laceration and associated compartment syndrome. Late complications include anterior growth arrest and associated recurvatum deformity.

Proximal Tibial Physeal Fractures

Proximal tibial physeal fractures typically result from a high-energy traumatic injury. These fractures can cause devastating vascular injuries resulting from tethering of the popliteal artery at the trifurcation. Vascular compromise occurs in 5% to 7% of these injuries. Prompt reduction typically restores blood flow; however, patients must be monitored closely after initial treatment.

Salter-Harris type II fractures are the most common. Nondisplaced type I and II fractures can be treated with long leg casting; careful follow-up is needed to ensure that reduction is maintained. Displaced type I and II fractures can be treated with closed reduction and per-

cutaneous fixation under fluoroscopic guidance. A recently described flexion-type physeal separation can be managed by closed means with cast immobilization.[11] Type III and IV fractures are by definition intra-articular, and they require anatomic reduction to minimize the risk of physeal bar formation and optimize the long-term outcomes of the knee. When internal fixation for type III and IV fractures is required, intraepiphyseal screws oriented parallel to the physis are used.

Compartment syndrome is a feared complication of proximal tibial physeal fractures. Angular deformity and limb-length discrepancy also have been well documented. Patients should be followed for 2 to 3 years after injury to allow for early detection and treatment, if necessary, of potential problems.

Proximal Tibial Metaphyseal Fractures

Proximal metaphyseal fractures of the tibia typically occur in children age 3 to 6 years. Posttraumatic valgus deformity resulting from these fractures is a concern, along with the Cozen phenomenon, which can occur regardless of treatment.[12] Posttraumatic deformity peaks at 1 year after injury and will often spontaneously resolve over the next 3 to 4 years. In the rare instances in which the deformity does not resolve, guided growth through hemiepiphysiodesis has been advocated.[13]

6: Pediatrics

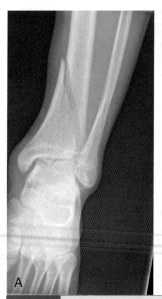
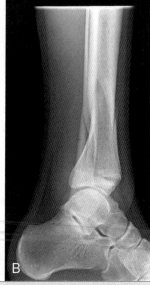

Figure 5   AP (**A**) and lateral (**B**) radiographs of a triplane fracture. On the AP view, the fracture resembles a Salter-Harris type III injury. On the lateral view, the fracture resembles a Salter-Harris type II injury.

Tibial Diaphyseal Fractures

Tibial shaft fractures are a common pediatric fracture and typically result from indirect forces. Most pediatric tibial shaft fractures can be treated by long leg casting or with closed manipulation and casting. A recent report summarized the absolute and relative indications for the surgical treatment of tibial shaft fractures in children.[14] The indications for surgical intervention include an open fracture, tibial fractures complicated by compartment syndrome, injury to multiple systems, a fracture that cannot be adequately reduced by closed means, and a floating knee. Relative indications include comminuted fractures and displaced fractures with an intact fibula. Acceptable alignment is influenced by the skeletal maturity of the patient, with treatment guidelines resembling those applicable to adult tibial fractures as the potential for remodeling decreases.

When surgical treatment is indicated, options for fixation include external fixation, elastic intramedullary nailing, and plating. The implant choice is tailored to the fracture pattern, the age of the child, and the associated soft-tissue injuries. As with adults, the development of compartment syndrome after a tibial fracture is an important concern. Making the diagnosis of compartment syndrome in children can be a challenging. Specific attention should be paid to the presence of anxiety, agitation, and an increased need for analgesics (the three A's) to alert the physician of possible compartment syndrome.[15] Confirmation of the diagnosis can be made by measuring intracompartmental pressures. Definitive treatment of compartment syndrome requires emergent decompression of the affected compartments.

Distal Tibial Physeal Fractures

Salter-Harris type I and II fractures make up more than 50% of all distal tibial physeal fractures. Closed treatment of these injuries is typical, except in the rare instances in which soft-tissue interposition blocks adequate reduction. The mechanism of injury and the initial fracture displacement have been shown to affect the rate of premature physeal closure. High-energy mechanisms, such as motor vehicle crashes, result in a significantly higher rate of physeal closure versus low-energy mechanisms, such as sports injuries or falls. For every 1 mm of initial fracture displacement, there is a 15% increased risk for physeal arrest compared with a nondisplaced fracture.[16]

Salter-Harris type III and IV injuries involving the medial malleolus present the challenging combination of both physeal and intra-articular injuries. These injuries carry a substantial risk (20%) of subsequent growth problems regardless of the type of appropriate treatment used. Surgical intervention is indicated for displaced fractures and is best performed through an open reduction with visualization of the joint surface, with the use of intraepiphyseal cannulated screws placed parallel to the physis and the joint to transfix the fragment to the intact epiphysis. Transphyseal fixation should be avoided, but, when necessary, it should consist of temporary, smooth Kirschner wires.

Extensor retinaculum syndrome has been described in patients with distal tibial physeal fractures. The extensor tendons and neurovascular bundle are compressed under the extensor retinaculum. This condition is treated by releasing the extensor retinaculum.[17]

Transitional Fractures of the Distal Tibia

Tillaux and triplane fractures occur during the transition to skeletal maturity. The distal tibial physis closes in a predictable manner (centrally first, then medially, and then laterally) over an 18-month period. The order of closure of the distal tibial physis is responsible for the fracture patterns seen during this period of adolescence.

Tillaux fractures are Salter-Harris type III injuries that occur from an external rotation injury when only the anterolateral portion of the distal tibial physis remains open. Because these fractures occur when the growth plate is almost closed, premature growth arrest has minimal implications. Nondisplaced fractures can be treated nonsurgically with cast immobilization. Fractures with more than 2 mm of displacement are treated surgically, with attention to restoring the articular surface. The fragment can be reduced and transfixed with a single screw. Careful attention must be paid to avoid intra-articular penetration; crossing the physis is less concerning because of the closing growth plate.

Triplane fractures are Salter-Harris type IV injuries and occur in slightly younger patients than Tillaux fractures. On the AP and mortise views, they appear like Salter-Harris type III injuries and on lateral films resemble Salter-Harris type II injuries (Figure 5). Triplane fractures have components in the sagittal, coronal, and

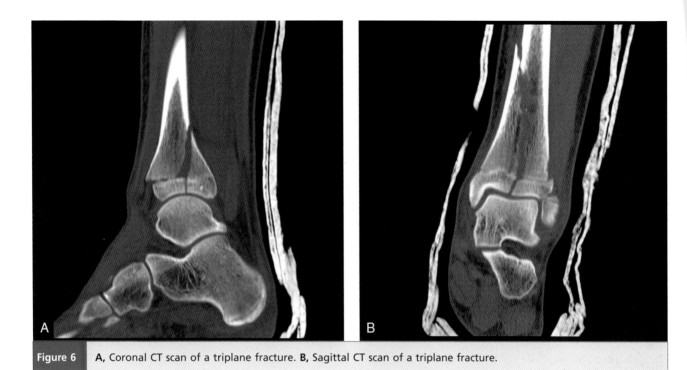

Figure 6 **A,** Coronal CT scan of a triplane fracture. **B,** Sagittal CT scan of a triplane fracture.

transverse planes. CT is useful in determining the number of fragments and the amount of displacement (Figure 6). A recent study reported that the use of CT changed the diagnosis from a Tillaux to a triplane fracture in 5% of cases.[18]

Fractures with more than 2 mm of displacement may be associated with posttraumatic arthritis and warrant special attention. These fractures may be treated with closed manipulation, closed manipulation and percutaneous fixation (most successful for a two-part fracture), or open reduction and internal fixation. Open reduction is typically performed through an anterior approach, which can be biased medially or laterally depending on the fracture pattern. The posteromedial fragment is reduced first, followed by the Tillaux component. A recent report suggests the need to clinically and radiographically examine the patient for an associated high fibular fracture.[19]

Distal Fibular Fractures

Distal fibular fractures are commonly seen in children and typically represent Salter-Harris type I or II fractures. Children with a distal fibular fracture present with pain and swelling over the distal fibular physis. Radiographs may not show any bony injury, but soft-tissue swelling over the distal fibula is the hallmark sign. In a recent comparison, the Ottawa Ankle Rules were found to be the most sensitive in the pediatric population for predicting ankle fracture.[20] Nondisplaced fractures can be treated with casting or bracing. In children with nondisplaced fractures, functional bracing has been shown to be more effective in achieving recovery of physical function, a faster return to baseline activities, and a higher patient satisfaction rate compared with casting.[21] Complications from distal fibular fractures are rare but can include growth arrest and nonunion. A recent study in which children with suspected distal fibular physeal injuries were evaluated with MRI suggested that lateral ligament sprains in children may be more common than previously believed.[22]

Foot Fractures

Talus Fractures

Talus fractures are quite rare and can result from forced dorsiflexion or supination. Nondisplaced fractures can be safely managed with non–weight-bearing immobilization.[23] Open reduction is indicated with displacement of more than 5 mm or 10° of malalignment. Because there is a risk of osteonecrosis in displaced talar neck fractures, every attempt should be made at anatomic alignment and rigid fixation.[24] With the increasing popularity of snowboarding and skateboarding, lateral process fractures present a specific subset of talus fractures that can be treated nonsurgically or with fixation or excision if symptomatic.[25]

Calcaneus Fractures

Fractures of the calcaneus are not often seen in the pediatric population. Along with the distal first and fifth metatarsals, the calcaneus serves as one of the three major weight-bearing centers of the foot. Excessive pressure on the heel of the foot is a typical mechanism of injury, as is jumping from a height and landing forcefully on a hard surface. Lawnmower injuries can also cause damage to the posterior calcaneus and disrupt the attachment of the Achilles tendon.

6: Pediatrics

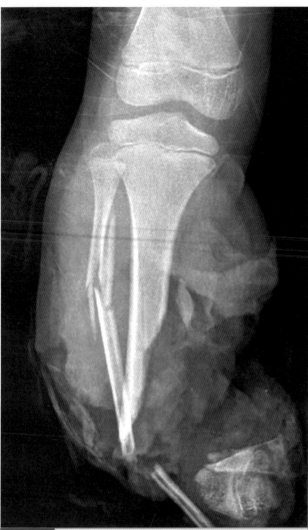

Figure 7	AP radiograph of the lower extremity following a lawnmower injury. The patient sustained an open comminuted fracture of the tibia with near-complete amputation of the foot.

Calcaneal fractures can be classified as extra- or intra-articular. Different classification schemes have been developed, such as the Essex-Lopresti or Sanders systems. Determination of the fracture pattern may be challenging with plain radiographs and can be further elucidated with CT. A hybridized classification system suggested by Schmidt and Weiner[26] includes the loss of insertion of the Achilles tendon and substantial soft-tissue damage, which can result from a lawnmower injury. Generally, calcaneal fractures can be treated nonsurgically, with cast immobilization and protected weight bearing for a period of 4 to 6 weeks.[27] Certain scenarios, however, necessitate surgical intervention, including avulsion fractures of the tuberosity of the calcaneus in which closed reduction is recommended,[28] and displaced intra-articular fractures, in which good to excellent results have been achieved with open reduction and internal fixation.[29] Fracture of the sustentaculum tali has been reported in pediatric patients. Treatment

of this fracture includes fragment excision and reconstruction of the deltoid ligament.[30]

Midfoot Fractures

Midfoot fractures range from relatively benign compression-type fractures requiring immobilization to severe fracture-dislocations (Lisfranc) injuries requiring open reduction and internal fixation. The nutcracker fracture of the cuboid results from forceful abduction and axial loading on the cuboid; this injury often occurs during participation in an equestrian sport.[31]

Metatarsal Fractures

The first and fifth metatarsals are the most commonly fractured. The first metatarsal is more likely injured in a fall from a height, whereas the fifth metatarsal is more commonly injured during athletic participation.[32] Nonsurgical management is the mainstay of treatment of most metatarsal fractures, although severely displaced fractures or fractures with delayed union may require surgical fixation. It has been shown that surgical treatment of proximal fractures of the fifth metatarsal may allow for more rapid return to activity.[33]

Phalangeal Fractures

For the most part, phalangeal fractures can be managed with a stiff-soled shoe or buddy taping. Open Salter-Harris fractures can occur in the distal phalanx with associated nail bed lacerations. These fractures warrant débridement and antibiotic administration, although internal fixation of the fracture itself may not be required.

Lawnmower Injuries and Traumatic Amputations

Lawnmower injuries are a devastating traumatic event, which can result in partial or complete amputation of the lower extremity (Figure 7). Management in the trauma room includes ensuring hemodynamic stability and early treatment with broad-spectrum antibiotics, tetanus vaccine, and sterile dressings. Urgent surgical treatment with formal irrigation and débridement, treatment of vascular injury, and osseous stabilization should follow. Vacuum-assisted closure therapy can be a helpful strategy in managing these injuries.[34] Amputation may be required as well as consultation with a plastic surgeon for reconstructive planning of soft-tissue coverage. Early mobilization and a prosthesis fitting should be encouraged to optimize return to aid-free ambulation.

Summary

Fractures of the lower extremity are less common than those of the upper extremity. Many of these fractures can be managed nonsurgically, but special surgical consideration is required in some cases. Malalignment (coronal, sagittal, or rotational) can result from the malunion of diaphyseal fractures or partial growth arrest of physeal injuries and is less well tolerated in these weight-bearing limbs. An understanding of the potential acute and long-term complications of these fractures is crucial to their overall management.

Key Study Points

- Injuries to the distal femoral or proximal tibial physis require careful consideration with regard to possible partial or complete growth arrest.

- Transitional fractures of the distal tibia may require cross-sectional imaging to fully appreciate the anatomy of the injury and optimal treatment.

- Although most fractures of the foot in the pediatric population can be treated nonsurgically, certain displaced fractures (talus, calcaneus, Lisfranc) require special surgical consideration.

Annotated References

1. Bertin KC, Goble EM: Ligament injuries associated with physeal fractures about the knee. *Clin Orthop Relat Res* 1983;177:188-195.

2. Ray JM, Hendrix J: Incidence, mechanism of injury, and treatment of fractures of the patella in children. *J Trauma* 1992;32(4):464-467.

3. Hunt DM, Somashekar N: A review of sleeve fractures of the patella in children. *Knee* 2005;12(1):3-7.

4. Kaar TK, Murray P, Cashman WF: Transosseous suturing for sleeve fracture of the patella: Case report. *Ir J Med Sci* 1993;162(4):148-149.

5. Houghton GR, Ackroyd CE: Sleeve fractures of the patella in children: A report of three cases. *J Bone Joint Surg Br* 1979;61-B(2):165-168.

6. Gettys FK, Morgan RJ, Fleischli JE: Superior pole sleeve fracture of the patella: A case report and review of the literature. *Am J Sports Med* 2010;38(11):2331-2336.

   The authors present a case report of a superior pole sleeve fracture in a healthy 10-year-old boy. The surgical treatment is described as well as the 3-year follow-up results. A summary of previous cases from the literature is also provided.

7. Frey S, Hosalkar H, Cameron DB, Heath A, David Horn B, Ganley TJ: Tibial tuberosity fractures in adolescents. *J Child Orthop* 2008;2(6):469-474.

8. Ogden JA, Tross RB, Murphy MJ: Fractures of the tibial tuberosity in adolescents. *J Bone Joint Surg Am* 1980;62(2):205-215.

9. Brey JM, Conoley J, Canale ST, et al: Tibial tuberosity fractures in adolescents: Is a posterior metaphyseal fracture component a predictor of complications? *J Pediatr Orthop* 2012;32(6):561-566.

   This study reported that the presence of a posterior metaphyseal fracture associated with a tibial tuberosity fracture was a marker for potential complications, including refracture.

10. Howarth WR, Gottschalk HP, Hosalkar HS: Tibial tubercle fractures in children with intra-articular involvement: Surgical tips for technical ease. *J Child Orthop* 2011;5(6):465-470.

    A retrospective review of six tibial tubercle fractures over a 2.5-year period was performed. The authors highlight technical considerations for fixation, with an emphasis on clinical and radiographic outcomes.

11. Vyas S, Ebramzadeh E, Behrend C, Silva M, Zionts LE: Flexion-type fractures of the proximal tibial physis: A report of five cases and review of the literature. *J Pediatr Orthop B* 2010;19(6):492-496.

    The authors report on five patients who sustained a rare flexion-type fracture separation of the proximal tibial epiphysis. All of the patients were treated with closed reduction and immobilization; no complications were reported.

12. Jackson DW, Cozen L: Genu valgum as a complication of proximal tibial metaphyseal fractures in children. *J Bone Joint Surg Am* 1971;53(8):1571-1578.

13. Stevens PM, Pease F: Hemiepiphysiodesis for posttraumatic tibial valgus. *J Pediatr Orthop* 2006;26(3):385-392.

14. Gordon JE, O'Donnell JC: Tibia fractures: What should be fixed? *J Pediatr Orthop* 2012;32(suppl 1):S52-S61.

    A literature review of nonsurgical and surgical management of tibial shaft fractures is presented. The authors describe indications and relative indications for surgical fixation, although they recognize that most of these fractures can be treated with closed reduction and casting.

15. Bae DS, Kadiyala RK, Waters PM: Acute compartment syndrome in children: Contemporary diagnosis, treatment, and outcome. *J Pediatr Orthop* 2001;21(5):680-688.

16. Leary JT, Handling M, Talerico M, Yong L, Bowe JA: Physeal fractures of the distal tibia: Predictive factors of premature physeal closure and growth arrest. *J Pediatr Orthop* 2009;29(4):356-361.

17. Mubarak SJ: Extensor retinaculum syndrome of the ankle after injury to the distal tibial physis. *J Bone Joint Surg Br* 2002;84(1):11-14.

18. Liporace FA, Yoon RS, Kubiak EN, et al: Does adding computed tomography change the diagnosis and treatment of Tillaux and triplane pediatric ankle fractures? *Orthopedics* 2012;35(2):e208-e212.

A retrospective review by blinded reviewers was performed on 24 pediatric Tillaux or triplane fractures. Intraobserver and interobserver agreements about primary treatment plans did not differ substantially between radiographs and radiographs plus CT scans (0.4 and 0.5, respectively). The authors also reported that the diagnosis was changed from a Tillaux fracture to a triplane fracture in seven cases.

19. Singleton TJ, Cobb M: High fibular fracture in association with triplane fracture: Reexamining this unique pediatric fracture pattern. *J Foot Ankle Surg* 2010;49(5): 491-494.

The authors present a case report of a 12-year-old boy with a triplane fracture with an associated high fibular fracture. The rarity of this type of fracture is discussed, and the importance of making the diagnosis with an adequate physical examination and appropriate imaging is highlighted.

20. Gravel J, Hedrei P, Grimard G, Gouin S: Prospective validation and head-to-head comparison of 3 ankle rules in a pediatric population. *Ann Emerg Med* 2009; 54(4):534-540, e1.

21. Boutis K, Willan AR, Babyn P, Narayanan UG, Alman B, Schuh S: A randomized, controlled trial of a removable brace versus casting in children with low-risk ankle fractures. *Pediatrics* 2007;119(6):e1256-e1263.

22. Boutis K, Narayanan UG, Dong FF, et al: Magnetic resonance imaging of clinically suspected Salter-Harris I fracture of the distal fibula. *Injury* 2010;41(8):852-856.

A prospective cohort study of 18 patients investigated the role of MRI in the diagnosis of suspected Salter-Harris type I fractures of the distal fibula. The authors reported that suspected Salter-Harris type I fractures of the distal fibula are frequently misdiagnosed clinically and more likely represent ligamentous sprains or bony contusions.

23. Eberl R, Singer G, Schalamon J, Hausbrandt P, Hoellwarth ME: Fractures of the talus—differences between children and adolescents. *J Trauma* 2010;68(1): 126-130.

A retrospective review of 25 talar fractures in children and adolescents is presented. The study reported a higher rate of surgical treatment in the adolescent group; no cases of osteonecrosis were reported in patients younger than 12 years.

24. Fernandez ML, Wade AM, Dabbah M, Juliano PJ: Talar neck fractures treated with closed reduction and percutaneous screw fixation: A case series. *Am J Orthop (Belle Mead NJ)* 2011;40(2):72-77.

The authors performed a retrospective review of fractures of the talar neck that were treated with closed reduction and percutaneous fixation.

25. von Knoch F, Reckord U, von Knoch M, Sommer C: Fracture of the lateral process of the talus in snowboarders. *J Bone Joint Surg Br* 2007;89(6):772-777.

26. Schmidt TL, Weiner DS: Calcaneal fractures in children: An evaluation of the nature of the injury in 56 children. *Clin Orthop Relat Res* 1982;171:150-155.

27. Yu GR, Zhao HM, Yang YF, Zhou JQ, Li HF: Open reduction and internal fixation of intra-articular calcaneal fractures in children. *Orthopedics* 2012;35(6):e874-e879.

The authors report on a retrospective review of nine intra-articular calcaneal fractures in eight children treated with open reduction and internal fixation. Clinical and radiographic outcomes are reported based on functional outcome scores.

28. Cole RJ, Brown HP, Stein RE, Pearce RG: Avulsion fracture of the tuberosity of the calcaneus in children: A report of four cases and review of the literature. *J Bone Joint Surg Am* 1995;77(10):1568-1571.

29. Ceccarelli F, Faldini C, Piras F, Giannini S: Surgical versus non-surgical treatment of calcaneal fractures in children: A long-term results comparative study. *Foot Ankle Int* 2000;21(10):825-832.

30. Huri G, Atay AO, Leblebicioğlu GA, Doral MN: Fracture of the sustentaculum tali of the calcaneus in pediatric age: A case report. *J Pediatr Orthop B* 2009;18(6): 354-356.

31. Ceroni D, De Rosa V, De Coulon G, Kaelin A: Cuboid nutcracker fracture due to horseback riding in children: Case series and review of the literature. *J Pediatr Orthop* 2007;27(5):557-561.

32. Singer G, Cichocki M, Schalamon J, Eberl R, Höllwarth ME: A study of metatarsal fractures in children. *J Bone Joint Surg Am* 2008;90(4):772-776.

33. Herrera-Soto JA, Scherb M, Duffy MF, Albright JC: Fractures of the fifth metatarsal in children and adolescents. *J Pediatr Orthop* 2007;27(4):427-431.

34. Halvorson J, Jinnah R, Kulp B, Frino J: Use of vacuum-assisted closure in pediatric open fractures with a focus on the rate of infection. *Orthopedics* 2011;34(7):e256-e260.

A retrospective review was performed on 37 open pediatric fractures treated with vacuum-assisted closure. The specific outcome measure being investigated was the rate of surgical infection (both superficial and deep). The authors concluded that, when compared with historical controls, the use of vacuum-assisted closure therapy was effective and safe.

Chapter 64

Lower Extremity and Foot Disorders: Pediatrics

Vishwas R. Talwalkar, MD   Theresa A. Hennessey, MD

Lower Extremity Disorders

Normal alignment of the lower extremities is dynamic, changing with growth and development. These changes occur simultaneously and three-dimensionally in the transverse, coronal, and sagittal planes. The evolution of normal alignment has been well described. Knowledge of age-appropriate values is essential when evaluating, identifying, and treating patients with limb deformities.[1-3]

Limb deformities are assessed both clinically and radiographically. When possible, observation of walking, with attention paid to the foot progression angle and any gait disturbance, is an essential component of the examination. The AP radiograph of the legs with the patella forward is the primary image used for assessing frontal plane alignment.[4] Identification of the mechanical axis and any deviation from normal should be noted. A range of normal values for joint alignment and a systematic approach to assessing deformity has been thoroughly described (Figure 1). After the nature and location of the deformity have been identified, the physician must decide on management options, including reassurance, continued observation, or treatment. Familiarity with the multiple conditions that can lead to limb deformity will allow for the formulation of an informed and rational management plan. Techniques available for treatment continue to evolve and now include but are not limited to accommodation with a shoe lift; guided growth; hemiepiphysiodesis; epiphysiodesis; osteotomy, with gradual or acute angular correction; limb lengthening; limb shortening; internal, external, or intramedullary fixation; amputation with prosthetic management; or some combination of these treatment options.

Conditions that can cause limb deformity can be divided into developmental (idiopathic tibia vara, idiopathic genu valgum, and rotational anomalies), acquired (posttraumatic and postinfectious conditions,

renal failure, and vitamin D deficient rickets), and congenital (femoral, fibular, or tibial deficiency; congenital tibial pseudarthrosis; posteromedial bowing; hypophosphatemic rickets; hemihypertrophy; bony dysplasias; and congenital joint dislocation) groups. The con-

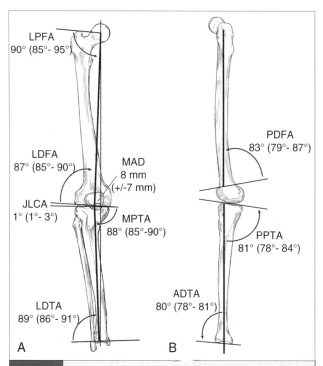

Figure 1   **A,** Illustration showing the measurement of the mechanical axis deviation (MAD), lateral proximal femoral angle (LPFA), lateral distal femoral angle (LDFA), medial proximal tibial angle (MPTA), and lateral distal tibial angle (LDTA) and their normal values and ranges. JLCA = joint line congruity angle. **B,** The measurement of the posterior distal femoral angle (PDFA), posterior proximal tibial angle (PPTA), and anterior distal tibial angle (ADTA) and their normal values and ranges. (Reproduced from Gordon JE, Dobbs MB: Lower extremity and foot disorders: Pediatrics, in Flynn JM, ed: *Orthopaedic Knowledge Update*, ed 10. Rosemont, IL, American Academy of Orthopaedic Surgeons, 2011, pp 763-782.)

6: Pediatrics

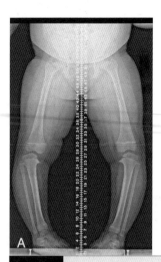
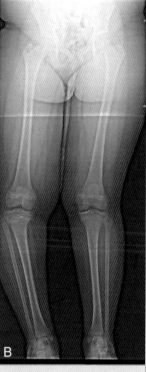

Figure 2 **A,** Standing AP radiograph of the lower extremities of a 3-year-old child with progressive infantile tibia vara shows proximal medial metaphyseal beaking and tibial torsion. **B,** Standing AP radiograph of the lower extremities of an 11-year-old child with unilateral adolescent tibia vara showing the deformity is at the level of the physis, with a normal proximal tibial epiphysis.

common, typically occurs bilaterally, and displays concomitant distal femoral varus.

The stages of proximal tibial epiphyseal deformity have been classified by Langenskiöld. Stages IV through VI represent physeal bar formation that can result in severe deformity with tibial plateau depression. Treatment of mild (Langenskiöld stages I and II) deformity with bracing may be attempted; some success has been reported. Spontaneous resolution of mild deformity in some patients with these changes also has been reported. Progressive deformity is most often treated with proximal tibial and fibular osteotomy. Osteotomy before 4 years of age with overcorrection of the deformity usually yields good results, but patients should be followed closely for signs of recurrence (**Figure 2, A**). Guided growth implants have recently been used for primary treatment and managing recurrence.[5] Medial proximal tibial epiphysiolysis in conjunction with osteotomy may be necessary in patients with Langenskiöld stages IV to VI deformities.[6]

Adolescent tibia vara does not present with epiphyseal deformity and tends to be less severe than the infantile form. As is the case with the infantile form, many patients are obese. Many patients have associated medical comorbidities, including insulin resistance, hypertension, and obstructive sleep apnea.[7] Early identification and treatment of these patients with guided growth methods is preferable to osteotomy, but these methods may be challenging to use in obese patients[8] (**Figure 2, B**). Distal femoral varus is also a component of the deformity in many patients.[9] If an osteotomy is necessary, both the tibia and the femur frequently require treatment. In rare instances, tibial plateau elevation is necessary to achieve full correction.[10]

Genu Valgus

Excessive valgus about the knee is much less common than pathologic varus. Physiologic valgus is typically most noticeable at approximately age 4 years, with a tibiofemoral angle of 10° to 15°. This angle gradually normalizes to the adult physiologic alignment of 5° to 7° valgus by age 8 years. A careful evaluation for some underlying etiology is crucial because the deformity may be caused by conditions that require treatment, including chronic renal failure, metabolic bone disease, bone dysplasia, congenital limb deficiency, or mucopolysaccharidosis. The most common cause is valgus deformity after a proximal tibial metaphyseal fracture (Cozen phenomenon). Valgus deformity occurs in approximately 50% of these injuries and tends to worsen until 18 months after the injury, with gradual correction for several years afterward. Observation for several years after a proximal tibial metaphyseal fracture is recommended. Regardless of the etiology, treatment by guided growth is the preferred method to restore alignment in patients with open physes[11-13] (**Figure 3**). A varus-producing osteotomy of either the distal femur or proximal tibia carries a potential risk of peroneal nerve injury and should be reserved for symptomatic, skeletally mature patients.

ditions also can be grouped by deformity (varus, valgus, or rotational). However, no system of classification is perfect because many of the causes and the descriptions of the deformities are complex, with crossover characteristics between the groups.

Specific Conditions

Tibia Vara

Idiopathic tibia vara (Blount disease) occurs as either infantile, juvenile, or adolescent forms. Infantile tibia vara typically is detected before aged 3 years. The juvenile form occurs in children age 4 to 10 years, and the adolescent form in children older than 10 years. Although the primary deformity is in the proximal tibia, patients may display varying degrees of distal femoral deformity, distal tibial valgus, procurvatum of the tibia, and limb-length discrepancy.

Pathologic infantile tibia vara is characterized by progressive varus deformity of the proximal tibia along with internal tibial torsion. This condition can be differentiated from physiologic genu varum by its progressive nature and the presence of radiographic changes in the proximal tibia. Physiologic bowing is much more

Metabolic Bone Disease

Metabolic bone disease can cause complex deformities, depending on the type of disease and the patient's age at onset. Normal physeal function is disturbed, affecting growth and remodeling. Although the orthopaedist may play an important role in correcting the limb deformities in these patients, consistent management of the underlying metabolic disturbance is essential for successful outcomes. Rickets, a classic example of a metabolic bone disease, may have early onset in the case of the X-linked hypophosphatemic form, leading to varus, or later onset in the case of dietary deficiency or renal failure, leading to valgus. Weight bearing tends to exacerbate preexisting alignment so that varus, valgus, anterior bowing, and/or recurvatum all tend to get progressively worse. Because there is frequently three-dimensional distortion of the entire limb, osteotomy planning can be challenging. Slight overcorrection may lead to deformity in the opposite direction, and slight undercorrection may lead to recurrence. Many patients require multiple corrective procedures.[14]

Rotational Deformities

Severe rotational deformities that interfere with functional activities are rare. The deformities are usually persistent femoral anteversion and/or tibial internal/external rotation. Many of these patients will present with reports of nonspecific anterior knee pain or difficulty with running. Remodeling of limb rotation with growth ceases by age 10 years, and rotational alignment at this age will persist for many decades. Treatment should be reserved for children in whom limb rotation remodeling has ceased. Children who have persistent deformities that interfere with running or patients with symptomatic deformities may be candidates for acute correction by open, percutaneous, or intramedullary osteotomy. Nonsurgical treatment is ineffective at any age for bony rotational deformities. Fixation methods include plates, pins, screws, or intramedullary devices.

The combination of femoral anteversion and external tibial torsion is called miserable malalignment syndrome and may be a source of patellofemoral maltracking and anterior knee pain. Initial treatment with physical therapy for extensor (particularly vastus medialis obliquus) and hamstring strengthening is the first step in treatment. Patients with persistent symptoms may be candidates for concurrent or staged derotational osteotomies of both the femur and the tibia.[15]

Tibial Bowing

Congenital bowing deformities of the diaphysis of the tibia and the fibula can occur. Posteromedial bowing is associated with calcaneovalgus foot deformity and usually resolves spontaneously by age 4 years, but it may result in clinically important limb-length discrepancy requiring a shoe lift, contralateral epiphysiodesis, or lengthening. Persistent ankle valgus deformity may also occur.[16]

Anterolateral bowing is associated with congenital tibial pseudarthrosis; 50% of the cases are also associ-

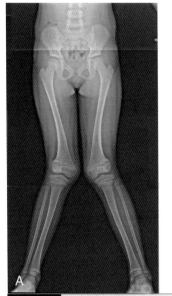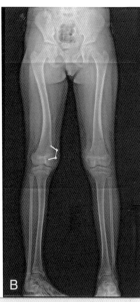

Figure 3 **A,** Standing AP radiograph of the lower extremities of a 7-year-old child with progressive genu valgum in association with X-linked hypophosphatemic rickets and congenital patellar dislocations shows characteristic physeal widening and cupping along with valgus deformity. **B,** Standing AP radiograph shows correction of the valgus deformity bilaterally with guided growth. The left patella underwent extensor realignment and is now reduced. The right knee was addressed at the time of plate removal. The physeal widening normalized after restoration of normal forces and medical therapy.

ated with neurofibromatosis type I. Bowing without fracture is managed with protective clamshell bracing to avoid fracture until skeletal maturity and occasionally even into adulthood. True tibial pseudarthrosis is challenging to treat. Obtaining and maintaining union has not been universally achieved with any technique. Surgical treatment is recommended if the pseudarthrosis is atrophic or persists for more than 3 months. Techniques have been described using bone transport via an external fixator, vascularized fibular transfer, resection with autogenous grafting and intramedullary fixation, and the use of additional biologic stimulation such as bone morphogenetic protein.[6]

Limb-Length Discrepancy

Limb-length discrepancy may be an acquired condition, as seen in patients with postinfectious or posttraumatic physeal arrest, or a congenital condition, as seen in patients with femoral, tibial, or fibular deficiency or hemihypertrophy. Management of the limb-length discrepancy depends on the magnitude of the deformity, the location of the deformity, the function of the involved limb, and the associated findings in each patient.

Treatment of idiopathic, posttraumatic, or postinfectious growth arrest with normal joint function is based primarily on the magnitude of the deformity and the

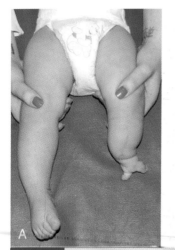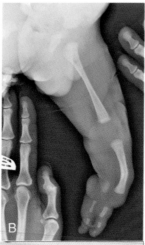

Figure 4 **A,** Photograph of the lower extremities of a 3-month-old child with left fibular deficiency shows shortening and anterior bowing of the tibia as well as severe foot deformity. **B,** AP radiograph of the same patient at age 1 month shows complete absence of the fibula, anterior tibial bowing, and foot deformity.

Congenital Limb Deficiency and Deformity

Congenital limb deficiency includes the problem of limb-length discrepancy in addition to abnormal joint formation. Fibular deficiency is the most common presentation and is often associated with femoral deficiency. Associated conditions include hip dysplasia, acetabular retroversion, femoral deficiency, lateral femoral condyle hypoplasia, patellar instability, and ligamentous insufficiency of the knee, tibial bowing, lateral ray deficiency, ankle valgus, and tarsal coalition. Each patient with a congenital limb deficiency represents a complex clinical situation. The management of these patients is usually dictated by the magnitude of the discrepancy and the stability of the foot and ankle. Children with a stable foot and ankle can be managed with all of the previously mentioned methods to equalize limb lengths. Children with an unstable foot and ankle are usually best managed with Symes or modified Boyd amputation and a prosthesis, which is fitted at walking age (Figure 4). Occasionally, cultural and social factors as well as access to prosthetic care play a large role in decision making. The functional status of the upper limbs is also an important point to consider because many of these patients use their feet for grasping and fine motor tasks.

Femoral Deficiency

Femoral deficiency includes a broad spectrum of pathology, ranging from a mild congenital short femur to frank absence of the femur except for a small residual tuft. The presence of a stable hip joint is the variable that dictates the quality of a patient's gait regardless of whether the patient has been treated with reconstruction, lengthening, or amputation. Approximately 50% of patients will have an associated fibular deficiency. As is the case with other forms of congenital limb deficiency, the treatment necessary depends on the projected discrepancy and the stability of the joints in the limb (Figure 5). Patients with moderate limb-length discrepancy and joint function are managed with length equalization by some combination of a shoe lift, epiphysiodesis, and lengthening, depending on the clinical scenario. Patients with a large projected discrepancy (> 20 cm), severe joint deformity and/or instability, or a nonfunctional foot are usually candidates for knee fusion and distal amputation at a relatively young age to appropriately manage growth of the limb. Van Ness rotationplasty is also an option for a selected patient with a stable and relatively normal foot and ankle but severe shortening.

Tibial Deficiency

Tibial deficiency is rare compared with fibular or femoral deficiency, is more often familial, and is associated with ulnar hypoplasia. Treatment is usually dictated by the presence or absence of a stable knee joint and extensor mechanism. If a functioning extensor mechanism exists, it should be preserved (Figure 6). The limb distal to the knee is managed according to the particular deformity in each patient. Knee disarticulation is usually necessary if no functional extensor mechanism exists.

predicted discrepancy at maturity. Multiple methods have been used to predict the extent of the discrepancy at maturity, including the Moseley graph, the growth-remaining method, and the multiplier method. It is recommended that at least two different techniques be used to analyze a patient's growth pattern and predict the limb-length discrepancy before any surgical intervention. Differences of up to 2.5 cm are well tolerated and may be managed with a shoe lift or observation. Differences from 2.5 to 5 cm are usually treated with an external shoe lift, contralateral epiphysiodesis, a shortening osteotomy, or limb lengthening. Differences of more than 5 cm may be similarly managed. However, a femoral shortening osteotomy greater than 4 cm may lead to permanent weakness, and epiphysiodesis may result in a disproportionate limb appearance. If a shoe lift is used for this magnitude of difference, it can be heavy and difficult to manage; therefore, a prosthesis may be considered. In patients with limb shortening of more than 20% to 30%, reconstruction usually requires multiple lengthening procedures, with or without contralateral epiphysiodesis. Patients with a postseptic physeal injury are particularly difficult to manage and require long-term evaluation because of their unpredictable growth patterns.[17] Limb lengthening is most commonly performed with external fixators, either uniplanar or multiplanar, but intramedullary motorized nails are also being used. Their efficacy and cost-effectiveness are still being studied.[18,19] The addition of a flexible intramedullary rod to lengthening procedures using an external fixator has been shown to decrease the healing index and time in a frame.[20] Transarticular amputation and prosthetic fitting is also an option that should be discussed in patients with a large predicted discrepancy.

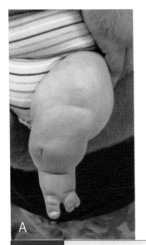
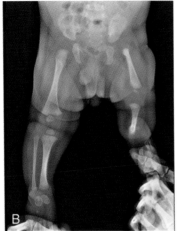

Figure 5 **A,** Clinical photograph of 4-month-old child with left proximal focal femoral deficiency shows an anterior tibial dimple, ray deficiency of the foot, and a funnel-shaped thigh. **B,** Supine radiographic view of the same child showing the proximal femoral deformity, small distal femoral epiphysis, complete fibular deficiency, and foot deformity.

Hemihypertrophy

Hemihypertrophy (anisomelia) is a condition in which a limb, limbs, or the entire side of the body is enlarged. The girth of the limb and its length are enlarged. It can be syndromic (for example, Beckwith Wiedemann syndrome) or idiopathic and related to retroperitoneal or abdominal tumors, such as a Wilms tumor, a hepatoblastoma, or a neuroblastoma. Interval screening for these tumors has been recommended, but specific protocols are evolving.[21] The limb-length difference is managed with shoe lifts and, in some cases, epiphysiodesis.

Congenital Patellar Dislocation

Congenital patellar dislocation is a condition in which the patella is laterally dislocated and irreducible. It differs from traumatic patellar instability or habitual dislocation because the deformity is present at birth and the patella is not mobile. It is usually detected before age 5 years and is associated with valgus and flexion deformity of the knee and external rotation of the tibia. Trochlear hypoplasia is present in all cases, but stability can be achieved with careful soft-tissue balancing. Treatment consists of extensive realignment of the extensor mechanism, sometimes involving medial transfer of the entire patellar tendon insertion, and release of the contracted lateral structures. Additional lengthening of the extensor mechanism by quadriceps tendon lengthening or femoral shortening may also be necessary for adequate knee range of motion and patellar stability. The valgus deformity of the knee may need to be addressed before soft-tissue realignment.

Congenital Dislocation of the Knee

Congenital dislocation of the knee is another relatively rare condition that presents as a spectrum of deformi-

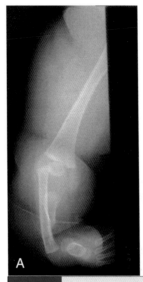
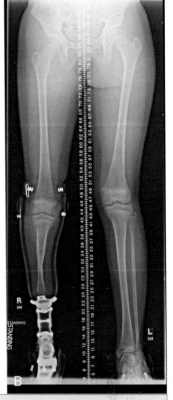

Figure 6 **A,** AP radiograph showing tibial deficiency with absence of the distal portion of the tibia, proximal fibular migration, and severe equinovarus foot deformity in a 6-month-old child. **B,** AP radiograph of the lower extremities of same child at age 13 years after proximal tibiofibular synostosis and a distal modified Boyd amputation.

ties ranging from mild subluxation to fixed dislocation. The dislocation is anterior and associated with hip dislocation in approximately 50% of patients. Children should be assessed for neuromuscular or syndromic causes. Treatment is with initial serial casting or splinting. If the associated hip dislocation is reducible in a Pavlik harness and the knee can be flexed to 90°, this is an excellent method to treat both hip and knee deformities. Irreducible dislocations can be treated with reduction and quadriceps lengthening or, in some cases, a femoral shortening osteotomy.[22,23]

Foot Disorders

Clubfoot

Clubfoot deformity, or congenital talipes equinovarus, is one of the most common musculoskeletal deformities, occurring in approximately 1 to 2 individuals in 1,000 live births worldwide. Approximately 80% of affected individuals are believed to have an isolated, idiopathic deformity. The remaining 20% of patients with clubfoot have associated neuromuscular conditions and genetic syndromes. There is strong evidence of genetic

6: Pediatrics

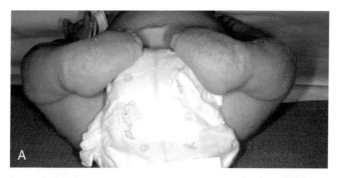

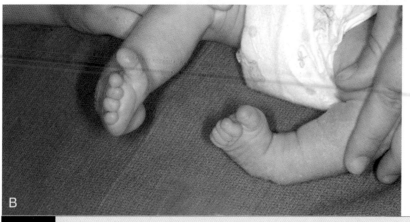

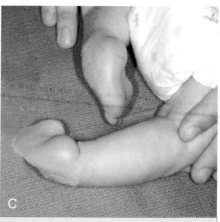

Figure 7 Clinical photographs of bilateral clubfeet in a 2-week-old infant. The deformities include hindfoot varus and equinus, midfoot cavus, and adduction. **A,** Inferior view. **B,** Frontal view. **C,** Posterior view.

causation; however, clubfoot is not caused by a single gene disorder, but it is a heterogeneous condition that is likely caused by multiple genes and epigenetic factors, most of which are not yet understood.[22] The primary goal of clubfoot treatment is to correct the deformity and obtain a functional, pain-free, plantigrade foot with good mobility and without calluses requiring shoe modifications.

Clubfoot is a complex congenital deformity that can be difficult to treat. It is characterized by midfoot cavus, forefoot adduction, hindfoot varus, and hindfoot equinus (**Figure 7**). At presentation, the deformity has a wide spectrum of severity. The long-term outcomes of treatment are not easily predictable.

Historically, clubfoot was treated with casting and extensive soft-tissue surgery. Long-term studies have reported the development of pain, arthritis, stiffness, and ambulation difficulties in adulthood in many patients treated in this manner. In North America and many countries in the world, the current standard of care for treating clubfoot is the Ponseti method, which consists of an initial correction phase of serial casting placed at weekly intervals to correct the various deformities in sequence: cavus, adductus, varus, and equinus. Because the cavus deformity is further accentuated by pronation of the forefoot, the forefoot must be supinated to unlock the foot and allow for abduction and simultaneous correction of the cavus, adductus, and varus deformities.[23] The casts are traditionally placed at 1-week intervals, with several minutes of stretching the foot before casting. In most patients, a percutaneous Achilles tenotomy is performed to correct the residual equinus after hyperabduction of the foot is achieved. After casting is complete, a prolonged bracing regimen is prescribed, consisting of 3 months of full-time wear followed by 3 to 4 years of nighttime and naptime wear.

The initial correction rates are reported at nearly 100% in most studies, with relapse rates varying from 10% to 56%.[24-26] Long-term studies have reported a high recurrence rate associated with the failure of the family to maintain the postcasting brace protocol.[27] It has been shown that relapses occur in only 6% of compliant families and in more than 80% of noncompliant families. Noncompliance with the bracing protocol increases the relative risk of recurrence 5 to 17 times.[28,29] Attempts have been made at modifying the brace, although no modification has resulted in a brace as consistently effective as the original foot abduction orthosis (boots and a bar) designed and used by Ponseti.

A recurrent deformity is one that has been previously well corrected and maintained in a foot abduction orthosis but recurs after a period of several months to years. A rapid recurrence may be related to a neurologic cause, and the possibility of a tethered cord should be investigated. In all cases, it is recommended that the elements of the recurrence be determined: equinus, midfoot adduction, supination, cavus, dynamic intoeing, rocker-bottom foot, or a major recurrence with multiple elements. Treatment should be directed to the specific deformity. Soft-tissue stretching with physical therapy and repeat casting are often very successful, followed by return to treatment with a foot abduction orthosis. Surgical treatment may include plantar release, abductor hallucis lengthening, midfoot capsulotomies, midfoot osteotomies, posterior tibialis tendon recession, tibialis anterior tendon transfer, and tibial osteotomy. Most importantly, if surgical treatment is undertaken, it should be implemented using a stepwise approach after stretching and casting have failed to provide further correction. Tibialis anterior tendon transfer for a dynamic supination gait in an otherwise corrected foot is an accepted part of the Ponseti method. It was reported in 51% of patients treated by the Ponseti method.

The upper age limit of children who can be treated with the Ponseti method is yet to be defined, with reports of correction obtained in children 10 years and older at the initiation of treatment. The method also has been used successfully in patients with nonidiopathic clubfeet, including clubfeet in patients with arthrogryposis, myelomeningocele, and other syndromes.[30,31] The Ponseti method also has been used in feet that had been previously treated with extensive surgery. As a result, there is no type of clubfoot or situation for which the Ponseti method should not be initially applied. Even in the most difficult cases of clubfoot, the method allows partial correction and can limit the amount of surgery needed.

Metatarsus Adductus

Metatarsus adductus is a common foot deformity characterized by adduction of the forefoot with respect to the hindfoot. The lateral border of the foot is curved, the heel is neutral, and the sole has a characteristic bean shape. The ankle and the subtalar joints are normal and have full range of motion. This disorder is very common, occurring in as many as 1 in 100 live births, and is believed to be a molding deformity related to intrauterine positioning. It is often associated with late pregnancy, first pregnancies, twin pregnancies, and oligohydramnios.

The treatment of metatarsus adductus is generally conservative, with 90% to 95% of patients having spontaneous resolution with no treatment. Parents can be taught gentle stretching exercises for the child's foot, which are performed a few times each day. The foot is stretched by gently abducting the forefoot while placing the thumb on the cuboid to use as the fulcrum. The stretch is held a few seconds and repeated 10 to 20 times. For a rigid foot, or a foot that is not showing improvement after 6 months of age, gentle stretching and serial casting can be performed. For a foot that requires additional treatment, a foot abduction orthosis (as is used for clubfoot) may be warranted at night for 1 year.

Congenital Vertical Talus/Oblique Talus

Congenital vertical talus is a rare deformity that is present at birth. This deformity is associated with neuromuscular (myelomeningocele, arthrogryposis, sacral

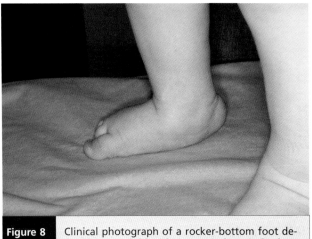

Figure 8 Clinical photograph of a rocker-bottom foot deformity in a child with congenital vertical talus.

agenesis, and diastematomyelia) and genetic disorders (trisomy 13-15, 18) in more than 50% of patients. Children with this deformity should undergo a careful neurologic examination, and MRI of the spine should be considered. Specific gene mutations with autosomal dominant inheritance have been identified.[32]

Congenital vertical talus is a rigid deformity characterized by a hindfoot in equinus, a dorsiflexed forefoot, and a convex rocker-bottom deformity created by the dorsally dislocated talonavicular joint (**Figure 8**). AP and lateral radiographs along with a maximum plantar flexion lateral radiograph will assist in the diagnosis (**Figure 9**). In an oblique talus or a flatfoot deformity, persistent dislocation of the talonavicular joint on the plantar-flexion lateral view will not be seen.

Treatment has traditionally consisted of an open release and reduction, with pinning of the talonavicular joint between the ages of 6 and 12 months. More recently, a technique has been described consisting of serial manipulation and casting, percutaneous pin fixation of the talonavicular joint after reduction is obtained, and a percutaneous Achilles tenotomy.[33,34] This technique has resulted in excellent short-term results in both idiopathic and nonisolated congenital vertical talus.

Positional Calcaneovalgus Foot Deformity

Positional calcaneovalgus foot deformity is a common deformity noted at birth and is characterized by a foot that is hyperdorsiflexed to the point that the dorsum of the foot may rest on the anterior surface of the lower leg. It is believed to be a positional deformity and is more common in firstborn children and females. No congenital deformity or dislocation is present. It is not associated with a posteromedial bow of the tibia and must be differentiated from congenital vertical talus and paralytic deformities. Spontaneous improvement is expected. The parents may be instructed on the use of gentle foot stretching exercises to aid in improvement.

6: Pediatrics

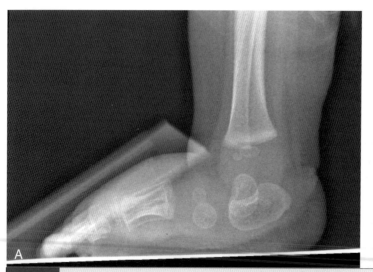
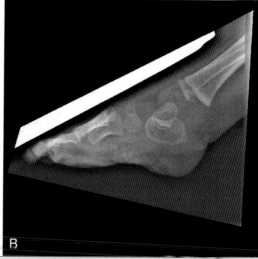

Figure 9 Standing lateral (**A**) and maximum plantar flexion lateral radiograph (**B**) of the foot of a child with congenital vertical talus deformity. Note the persistent dorsal dislocation of the navicular on the talus in the plantar flexion view.

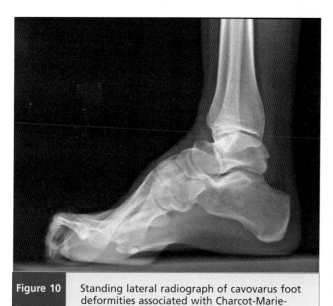

Figure 10 Standing lateral radiograph of cavovarus foot deformities associated with Charcot-Marie-Tooth disease.

Cavus Foot Deformity

In the simplest terms, a cavus foot is a foot with an elevated longitudinal arch. More specifically, this deformity results from a forefoot that is plantar flexed in relationship to the hindfoot. It may be secondary to plantar flexion of the forefoot, dorsiflexion of the calcaneus, or both. In general, the hindfoot is in varus (a cavovarus foot), but it may be neutral or in valgus (Figure 10). Patients will present with a report of frequent ankle sprains or pain related to the calluses on the bottom of the feet.

In more than two thirds of patients with a cavus foot deformity, an underlying neurologic disorder is the cause. Cerebral palsy, poliomyelitis, myelomeningocele, spinal cord abnormality, and Friedreich ataxia are fre-

quently associated with a cavus foot deformity. The most common neurologic disorder resulting in this deformity is a hereditary sensory motor neuropathy, usually Charcot-Marie-Tooth disease type I or II. A residual deformity related to clubfoot or a recurrence of clubfoot may also have a cavus component. An idiopathic cavus foot deformity should be made by a diagnosis of exclusion.

At presentation, the patient and family history should be obtained and a thorough examination should be performed because many neurologic conditions are hereditary. A thorough neurologic examination is critical. Sensory disturbances in light touch, pain, vibratory sense (often in a stocking glove distribution) are commonly found in patients with peripheral neuropathies. Deep tendon reflexes are often diminished in a patient with a hereditary sensory motor neuropathy or Friedreich ataxia. Spinal cord pathology may be associated with clonus. Often, a patient with a neurologic disease presents with bilateral deformities. Unilateral deformities can result from traumatic spinal cord injuries, sequelae of lower extremity compartment syndrome, spinal cord tumor, syringomyelia, lipomeningocele, diastematomyelia, and a tethered spinal cord. Electromyography and nerve conduction velocity studies may help delineate the cause. MRI of the neural axis is important to rule out spinal cord pathology. Referral to a neurologist and a geneticist may be appropriate.

Radiographic evaluation of the cavus foot should include AP and lateral images of the feet with the patient in the standing position. The cavus foot will demonstrate plantar flexion of the metatarsals. The spine also should be imaged with PA and lateral views to evaluate for congenital malformations, interpedicular widening, or atypical scoliosis.

After the appropriate workup has been completed, treatment may include stretching exercises if there is true equinus associated with the cavus deformity.

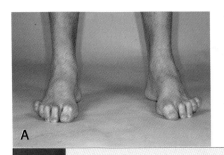
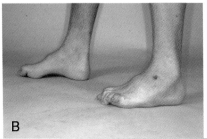
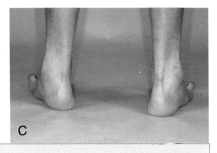

Figure 11 Frontal (**A**), lateral (**B**), and posterior (**C**) clinical photographs of cavovarus foot deformities related to Charcot-Marie-Tooth disease. Note the hindfoot varus, midfoot cavus, and clawing of the toes.

Stretching and the use of orthotics have not been shown to prevent or effectively treat the cavus deformity. In planning treatment, it is important to understand the pathogenesis of the condition. In all settings, the cavus (and associated varus or valgus) results from a muscle imbalance. In Charcot-Marie-Tooth disease, for example, there is weakness and contracture of the intrinsic musculature of the foot (**Figure 11**). Although the posterior tibialis and peroneus longus remain strong, the anterior tibialis and peroneus brevis are weak. This results in hindfoot varus, forefoot equinus and pronation, and a contracted arch. Flexibility of the varus hindfoot can be evaluated with the Coleman block test.

Video 64.1: Coleman Block Test. Vishwas R. Talwalkar, MD (0.19 min)

Surgical treatment is indicated for progressive deformity, ankle instability, and painful calluses. The principles of surgery are to initially correct the deformity and then balance the soft tissues to maintain the correction. Surgery may involve the release of soft-tissue structures and selective osteotomies. Rebalancing depends on tendon transfers such as the peroneus longus to brevis transfer to remove the deforming force of the longus and strengthen the pull of the brevis. Transfer of the posterior tibialis to the dorsum of the foot may be helpful in patients with a weak anterior tibialis.

Flatfoot

Flexible flatfoot is an extremely common condition characterized by decreased medial arch height and valgus in the hindfoot. The degree of flexibility defines the condition as a variation of normal. A rigid flatfoot is indicative of an underlying pathologic state, such as a tarsal coalition. The incidence of flatfoot is very high in infants and young children and decreases with age; approximately 20% of adults have a flatfoot deformity.

The flexible flatfoot seen in children is often termed hypermobile, which refers to the mobility of the subtalar joint. In these feet, the arch is decreased in standing, but reconstitutes nicely with toe standing or hyperextension of the great toe (the toe-raise test and the Jack test, respectively). A normal-appearing arch is usually

Video 64.2: Tip-Toe Test. Vishwas R. Talwalkar, MD (0.27 min)

Video 64.3: Jack's Test. Vishwas R. Talwakar, MD (0.17 min)

present when not standing. Approximately 25% of flexible flatfeet are associated with a tight Achilles tendon.

Treatment is not necessary for an asymptomatic flexible flatfoot. If there is a tight heel cord in an asymptomatic foot, stretching should be recommended because the tight heel cord may lead to symptoms in the future. For a flatfoot with a tight heel cord and pain, stretching often alleviates symptoms. If pain persists, soft orthotics seem to relieve symptoms in many patients. Surgery, although rarely indicated, should be considered only when conservative management has failed. Surgical options include soft-tissue reconstruction, gastrocnemius/heel cord lengthening, osteotomy, and arthrodesis.

Skewfoot

Skewfoot, also called serpentine or z-foot, is a rare and complex foot deformity that includes malalignment of the hindfoot, the midfoot, and the forefoot. The etiology, pathogenesis, and natural history of this disorder are not clear. The deformity is characterized by forefoot adduction, midfoot abduction, hindfoot valgus, and a tight Achilles tendon (**Figure 12**).

In the infant, it is sometimes difficult to differentiate skewfoot from simple metatarsus adductus. Lack of spontaneous improvement, excessive hindfoot valgus, and a tight Achilles tendon sometimes make the diagnosis more clear. After ossification has progressed, this deformity can be diagnosed radiographically, as previously described (**Figure 13**). In some instances, skewfoot is believed to be related to improper casting tech-

6: Pediatrics

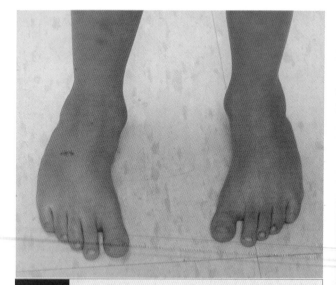

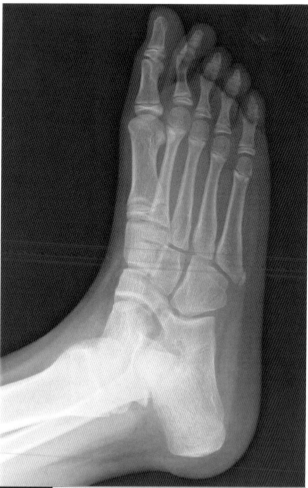

Figure 12 Clinical photograph of bilateral skewfoot deformity in an 8-year-old boy showing forefoot adduction, midfoot abduction, and hindfoot valgus. (Reproduced from Gordon JE, Dobbs MB: Lower extremity and foot disorders: Pediatrics, in Flynn JM, ed: *Orthopaedic Knowledge Update*, ed 10. Rosemont, IL, American Academy of Orthopaedic Surgeons, 2011, pp 763-782.)

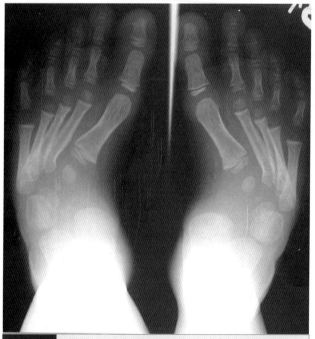

Figure 13 AP radiograph of the patient in Figure 12 with bilateral skewfeet, showing lateral translation of the midfoot on the hindfoot. (Reproduced from Gordon JE, Dobbs MB: Lower extremity and foot disorders: Pediatrics, in Flynn JM, ed: *Orthopaedic Knowledge Update*, ed 10. Rosemont, IL, American Academy of Orthopaedic Surgeons, 2011, pp 763-782.)

Figure 14 Internal oblique radiograph of the right foot of a patient with a bony and cartilaginous calcaneonavicular coalition.

niques in the treatment of clubfoot or metatarsus adductus.

Treatment is generally nonsurgical, with stretching for the tight Achilles tendon and the use of custom soft orthotics. The goal of the orthotics is to pad and support the midfoot with weight bearing. Surgery, which is extensive and includes soft-tissue release, medial reefing, and osteotomies, is rarely indicated. Surgery should be performed only if the patient has substantial pain that does not respond to stretching and the use of orthotics.

Tarsal Coalition

A tarsal coalition is a fibrous, cartilaginous, or bony union between two or more tarsal bones of the midfoot or hindfoot. It is believed to occur in 3% to 6% of the general population and is twice as common in males. The most common coalitions (90%) are calcaneonavicular or at the middle facet of the talocalcaneal articulation (**Figure 14**). Coalitions are found bilaterally in

50% to 60% of patients, tend to be familial, and 20% of patients with one coalition have a second coalition.

Coalitions may become symptomatic, with activity-related pain and increasing deformity, as the coalition changes from a cartilaginous to a bony union. This occurs at age 8 to 12 years for calcaneonavicular coalitions and age 12 to 16 years for talocalcaneal coalitions.[35] The patient often reports repeated ankle sprains.

The physical examination shows a rigid flatfoot deformity with minimal subtalar motion. When the patient is asked to stand on his or her toes, the hindfoot does not invert into varus. Occasionally, the patient presents with a rigid foot and painful peroneal spasm.[36] In a calcaneonavicular coalition, an internal oblique radiograph will show frank, bony bridging or blunting and fibrous union. A standing lateral radiograph may show beaking of the talus dorsally, resulting from restricted movement. Making a diagnosis of talocalcaneal coalition is more difficult using plain radiographs; CT or MRI may be necessary.

The treatment of a tarsal coalition varies based on the location of the coalition and the severity of the symptoms. Nonsurgical therapy, which includes rest, orthotic wear, and anti-inflammatory medication, is usually the initial treatment in symptomatic coalitions.[36-38] A limited trial of cast immobilization (3 to 6 weeks) also has been reported to be beneficial.[38]

Surgical treatment is indicated if conservative management has failed. The recommended surgical treatment in calcaneonavicular coalitions is resection and interposition of the extensor digitorum brevis, fat, bone wax, or other material.[38,39] The optimal surgical management of talocalcaneal coalitions is less clearly defined. The options are resection, isolated subtalar fusion, or triple arthrodesis. Poor results with resection have been associated with valgus of the heel of more than 16° or coalition greater than 50% of the posterior facet.[40,41] There is agreement that younger age at the time of resection likely leads to better outcomes.[42]

Osteochondroses

An osteochondrosis is a disturbance in endochondral ossification in a previously normal growth center. In general, osteochondroses are considered to be idiopathic, although some cases may be associated with repetitive trauma.

Kohler disease is an osteochondrosis that affects the tarsal navicular. In general, it occurs in children 4 to 7 years of age; 80% of the cases occur in boys. The patient presents with a limp, sometimes walking on the lateral border of the foot. Patients also present with pain, swelling, erythema, and tenderness at the medial midfoot over the navicular. On radiographs, the navicular will appear flattened and sclerotic (**Figure 15**). This condition is self-limiting, and no long-term sequelae have been noted. Treatment is based on the symptoms. In mild cases, an over-the-counter arch support may relieve symptoms. If the patient has severe or prolonged pain, a short-leg walking cast can be used for 4 to 8 weeks.

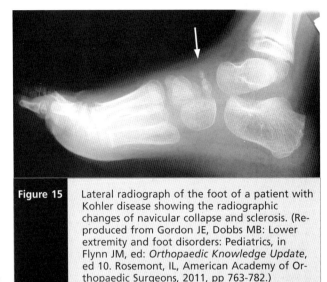

Figure 15 Lateral radiograph of the foot of a patient with Kohler disease showing the radiographic changes of navicular collapse and sclerosis. (Reproduced from Gordon JE, Dobbs MB: Lower extremity and foot disorders: Pediatrics, in Flynn JM, ed: *Orthopaedic Knowledge Update*, ed 10. Rosemont, IL, American Academy of Orthopaedic Surgeons, 2011, pp 763-782.)

Freiberg infraction affects the head of the metatarsal, most frequently the second metatarsal. This type of osteochondrosis may present early with swelling, pain, and an absence of radiographic changes. As the condition progresses, osteonecrosis becomes visible radiographically, and the necrotic bone is gradually replaced as healing occurs. Freiberg infraction is more frequent in girls than boys and occurs during adolescence. For most patients, treatment consists of activity modification and metatarsal padding. In severe, prolonged cases, surgery may be indicated. Surgical treatment may include débridement of the joint or a dorsiflexion osteotomy of the metatarsal neck.

Juvenile Hallux Valgus

Hallux valgus or bunion deformity is an abnormal prominence on the medial side of the foot at the first metatarsophalangeal joint. The juvenile bunion appears in the preteen or teen years when the physes are still open. There is a female predilection and a strong genetic component to juvenile hallux valgus. In the teenage years, the deformity is best treated conservatively with shoe modifications of a wide toe box and a low heel. Splinting helps alleviate symptoms in some patients but has no long-term effect. Surgery is considered if long-term conservative management is unsuccessful. There is believed to be a high risk for recurrence of deformities treated while the physes are still open. The natural history in juvenile hallux valgus is not clear.

The deformity is evaluated with standing AP and lateral radiographs of the feet. The common measurements are the intermetatarsal angle, the hallux valgus angle (first metatarsal-proximal phalanx angle), the distal metatarsal articular angle, the proximal metatarsal articular angle, and the metatarsophalangeal joint congruity. The treatment, as is the case with adult deformities, is determined based on the magnitude of the deformity. A chevron osteotomy or McBride procedure is often used for mild deformities, a distal soft-tissue pro-

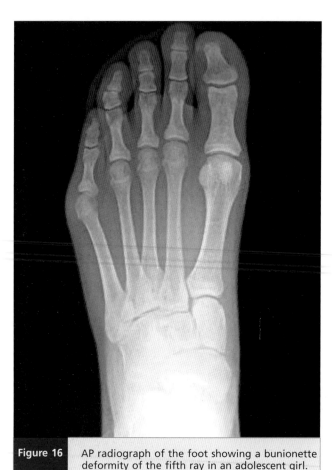

Figure 16 AP radiograph of the foot showing a bunionette deformity of the fifth ray in an adolescent girl. (Reproduced from Gordon JE, Dobbs MB: Lower extremity and foot disorders: Pediatrics, in Flynn JM, ed: *Orthopaedic Knowledge Update*, ed 10. Rosemont, IL, American Academy of Orthopaedic Surgeons, 2011, pp 763-782.)

cedure with a proximal osteotomy is used for moderate to severe deformities with subluxation, and a double osteotomy is used for moderate to severe deformities with an increased distal metatarsal articular angle.[43]

Lateral hemiepiphysiodesis of the first metatarsal has been proposed as an alternative treatment in the growing patient. With this procedure, correction occurs slowly with continued growth. The only published study of lateral hemiepiphysiodesis reported significant deformity correction in 50% of patients.[44] The appropriate timing and technique for this procedure requires further investigation. The procedure is appealing because the surgery is substantially less invasive and has the potential for permanent correction, whereas the risk of recurrence in other surgical procedures is high.

Lesser Toe Deformities

Deformities of the lesser toes are concerning to parents. In curly toe deformity, the interphalangeal joint of a lesser toe (or toes) is flexed and medially deviated so that it underlaps the adjacent toe. This deformity, which is caused by congenital tightening of the toe flexors, most commonly occurs in the third and fourth toes

but may be present in all four toes. In most patients, the deformity is asymptomatic; approximately 25% of patients have spontaneous resolution. Treatment is indicated for patients with pain and difficulty with shoe wear. A surgical release of the toe flexor at the level of the distal interphalangeal joint usually results in substantial improvement in toe positioning and relief of symptoms.

Congenital overriding fifth toe is a genetic disorder in which the fifth toe appears shortened, dorsiflexed, adducted, and overlaps the fourth toe. It often occurs bilaterally. This disorder is a rigid deformity, and 50% of patients have persistent symptoms of pain with shoe wear and are affected enough to require treatment. Conservative treatments are ineffective because of the rigidity of the deformity. Surgical treatment consists of release of the contracted metacarpophalangeal joint capsule, extensor tendon lengthening, and pinning the toe in the corrected position. A racquet-type incision is used, and some soft-tissue rearrangement is often required.

The most common congenital toe deformity is polydactyly. It is often a familial disorder and is bilateral in 50% of patients. The fifth toe is the most commonly duplicated digit. Duplications on the lateral side of the foot are called postaxial polydactyly, and those on the medial side of the foot are called preaxial polydactyly. Preaxial polydactyly is most often seen with tibial hemimelia, whereas postaxial polydactyly is usually an isolated and familial disorder. Polydactyly usually is treated surgically because the forefoot is widened by the extra toes and obtaining properly fitting shoe wear is challenging. The best age for treatment has not been determined. Some physicians prefer to treat patients between 9 to 12 months of age, whereas others wait until the patient is 2 to 3 years of age. The condition requires radiologic evaluation to determine the extent of the duplication and which digit to excise.

Bunionette deformity is a painful osseous deformity on the lateral aspect of the head of the fifth metatarsal (**Figure 16**). It is less common than bunion deformity (hallux valgus). Patients present secondary to pain and swelling in the area of the deformity. The initial treatment is shoe modifications, which are usually successful. If pain is persistent, a variety of surgical osteotomy procedures have been described for bunionette deformity. Metatarsal osteotomies narrow the forefoot, maintain the length of the metatarsal, and preserve function of the metatarsophalangeal joint. Distal metatarsal osteotomies produce less correction and reduce postoperative disability; however, they pose a risk of inadequate correction because of the small width of the fifth metatarsal head and transfer lesions if shortened or dorsiflexed excessively. The sliding oblique metaphyseal osteotomy, described by Smith and Weil (without fixation) and later by Steinke (with fixation), is easy to perform, provides good cancellous bone contact, and is safe and effective.[45]

Idiopathic Toe Walking

Idiopathic toe walking is a diagnosis of exclusion. Toe walking is quite normal and is frequently seen in children who are starting to walk. Persistent toe walking after the age of 2 years merits investigation because it may be a sign of an underlying neuromuscular or developmental abnormality. A recent investigation in Sweden reported the prevalence of idiopathic toe walking at 4.9% in 5-year-old children.[46] Other causes (neurologic, neuromuscular, developmental, psychological, and anatomic disorders) must be ruled out before a diagnosis is made.

If toe walking develops in a child who previously had a normal gait, it is necessary to rule out primary muscle or neurologic diseases, including muscular dystrophy, myotonic dystrophy, dystonia, tethered cord, and central or peripheral nervous system disorders. Unilateral toe walking should also incite a workup for an underlying etiology.

The physical examination of the child with idiopathic toe walking demonstrates loss of passive ankle dorsiflexion. The neurologic examination will be normal. Depending on the severity of the contracture of the triceps surae, treatment can begin with stretching and dorsiflexion strengthening exercises, nighttime bracing, or (in more severe cases) serial casting followed by exercise therapy and possibly bracing. Children who do not respond to serial casting and exercises can be treated with gastrocnemius and soleus myofascial lengthening or formal lengthening of the Achilles tendon.

Purely voluntary toe walking is often the most difficult form of the disorder to treat because the physical examination is completely normal (no evidence of contracture). The child simply prefers to walk on his or her toes. Bracing to encourage behavior change has been used to treat these patients.

Summary

Orthopaedic issues in the lower extremity of the pediatric patient are diverse. In the pediatric patient, secondary to the tremendous growth potential and remodeling capability, treatments exist that are not possible in the adult patient.

Key Study Points

- Guided growth is an effective treatment for patients with growth deformities. In larger patients with large deformities, multiple implants or implants that accommodate multiple screws may be necessary. A variety of methods, including single transphyseal screws as well as various tension band plate-screw constructs have been described.

- Distraction osteogenesis (limb lengthening) via an external fixator is augmented by intramedullary devices. The healing index can be accelerated and time in frame can be reduced with the addition of an intramedullary device. Increased risk of infection in this setting continues to be an evolving issue. The efficacy and cost of isolated intramedullary lengthening devices also requires continued study.

- Manipulative treatment of congenital vertical talus is effective for syndromic and nonsyndromic feet. Manipulation and serial casting followed by percutaneous or mini-open reduction and pinning have been shown to achieve good short-term results in children with idiopathic and non-idiopathic deformities.

Annotated References

1. Staheli LT, Corbett M, Wyss C, King H: Lower-extremity rotational problems in children: Normal values to guide management. *J Bone Joint Surg Am* 1985; 67(1):39-47.

2. Vankka E, Salenius P: Spontaneous correction of severe tibiofemoral deformity in growing children. *Acta Orthop Scand* 1982;53(4):567-570.

3. Jacquemier M, Glard Y, Pomero V, Viehweger E, Jouve JL, Bollini G: Rotational profile of the lower limb in 1319 healthy children. *Gait Posture* 2008;28(2):187-193.

4. Sabharwal S, Zhao C, Edgar M: Lower limb alignment in children: Reference values based on a full-length standing radiograph. *J Pediatr Orthop* 2008;28(7):740-746.

5. McIntosh AL, Hanson CM, Rathjen KE: Treatment of adolescent tibia vara with hemiepiphysiodesis: Risk factors for failure. *J Bone Joint Surg Am* 2009;91(12): 2873-2879.

6. Johnston CE II: Congenital pseudarthrosis of the tibia: Results of technical variations in the charnley-williams procedure. *J Bone Joint Surg Am* 2002;84-A(10):1799-1810.

7. Gordon JE, Hughes MS, Shepherd K, et al: Obstructive sleep apnoea syndrome in morbidly obese children with tibia vara. *J Bone Joint Surg Br* 2006;88(1):100-103.

6: Pediatrics

8. Park SS, Gordon JE, Luhmann SJ, Dobbs MB, Schoenecker PL: Outcome of hemiepiphyseal stapling for late-onset tibia vara. *J Bone Joint Surg Am* 2005;87(10): 2259-2266.

9. Gordon JE, King DJ, Luhmann SJ, Dobbs MB, Schoenecker PL: Femoral deformity in tibia vara. *J Bone Joint Surg Am* 2006;88(2):380-386.

10. Gordon JE, Heidenreich FP, Carpenter CJ, Kelly-Hahn J, Schoenecker PL: Comprehensive treatment of late-onset tibia vara. *J Bone Joint Surg Am* 2005;87(7): 1561-1570.

11. Mesa PA, Yamhure FH: Percutaneous hemiepiphysiodesis using transphyseal cannulated screws for genu valgum in adolescents. *J Child Orthop* 2009;3(5): 397-403.

12. Guzman H, Yaszay B, Scott VP, Bastrom TP, Mubarak SJ: Early experience with medial femoral tension band plating in idiopathic genu valgum. *J Child Orthop* 2011;5(1):11-17.

    The authors of this retrospective radiographic study of 47 knees in 25 patients with idiopathic genu valgum reported good correction with lateral tension band plating, with more rapid correction using multiple plates and in younger patients.

13. Stevens PM, Maguire M, Dales MD, Robins AJ: Physeal stapling for idiopathic genu valgum. *J Pediatr Orthop* 1999;19(5):645-649.

14. Saran N, Rathjen KE: Guided growth for the correction of pediatric lower limb angular deformity. *J Am Acad Orthop Surg* 2010;18(9):528-536.

    This comprehensive review article outlines the multiple methods of temporary and permanent growth modulation and indications for their use.

15. Bruce WD, Stevens PM: Surgical correction of miserable malalignment syndrome. *J Pediatr Orthop* 2004;24(4): 392-396.

16. Shah HH, Doddabasappa SN, Joseph B: Congenital posteromedial bowing of the tibia: A retrospective analysis of growth abnormalities in the leg. *J Pediatr Orthop B* 2009;18(3):120-128.

17. Park DH, Bradish CF: The management of the orthopaedic sequelae of meningococcal septicaemia: Patients treated to skeletal maturity. *J Bone Joint Surg Br* 2011; 93(7):984-989.

    This review of 10 patients with limb deformity after meningococcal septicemia treated over a 12-year period and followed to maturity discusses the complexity of this patient population. Most patients required multiple procedures to treat angular and length deformities.

18. Mahboubian S, Seah M, Fragomen AT, Rozbruch SR: Femoral lengthening with lengthening over a nail has fewer complications than intramedullary skeletal kinetic distraction. *Clin Orthop Relat Res* 2012;470(4):1221-1231.

    A comparison of functional outcomes and complications in patients treated with femoral lengthening with an external fixator over a nail versus an intramedullary device showed equivalent lengthening but a higher rate of unanticipated interventions in the group treated with the intramedullary device.

19. Krieg AH, Speth BM, Foster BK: Leg lengthening with a motorized nail in adolescents: An alternative to external fixators? *Clin Orthop Relat Res* 2008;466(1):189-197.

20. Popkov D, Popkov A, Haumont T, Journeau P, Lascombes P: Flexible intramedullary nail use in limb lengthening. *J Pediatr Orthop* 2010;30(8):910-918.

    This study compared two groups of patients treated with upper and lower limb lengthening for congenital and noncongenital deformities. In one group, a flexible intramedullary rod was also placed to facilitate alignment and provide stability. The group treated with the intramedullary rod healed more rapidly and required less time in the external fixator for all diagnoses.

21. Dempsey-Robertson M, Wilkes D, Stall A, Bush P: Incidence of abdominal tumors in syndromic and idiopathic hemihypertrophy/isolated hemihyperplasia. *J Pediatr Orthop* 2012;32(3):322-326.

    The authors report on a 10-year review of abdominal imaging studies performed on patients with isolated and syndromic anisomelia. Intra-abdominal tumors developed in 1 of 10 patients with syndromic hemihypertrophy and 3 of 250 patients with idiopathic hemihypertrophy. The authors recommend taking advantage of molecular screening to focus screening protocols.

22. Oetgen ME, Walick KS, Tulchin K, Karol LA, Johnston CE: Functional results after surgical treatment for congenital knee dislocation. *J Pediatr Orthop* 2010;30(3): 216-223.

    At an average follow-up of 12 years, seven patients who were surgically treated for congenital knee dislocation had good functional outcomes despite knee instability and a stiff-knee gait pattern. No difference was observed between those treated with femoral shortening versus quadricepsplasty.

23. Johnston CE II: Simultaneous open reduction of ipsilateral congenital dislocation of the hip and knee assisted by femoral diaphyseal shortening. *J Pediatr Orthop* 2011;31(7):732-740.

    A 5-year review of patients treated with concomitant hip and knee reductions showed superior results in knee function and equivalent results in hip outcomes when compared with traditional staged treatment.

24. Staheli L, Ponseti I: *Clubfoot: Ponseti Management*, ed 3. Seattle, WA, Global Help Organization, 2009. http://www.global-help.org/publications/books/ book_cfponseti.html.

    This book describing the Ponseti method for treating clubfoot is an indispensable guide. It is now published in 30 languages by the Global Help Organization and is also available electronically.

25. Morcuende JA, Dolan LA, Dietz FR, Ponseti IV: Radical reduction in the rate of extensive corrective surgery for clubfoot using the Ponseti method. *Pediatrics* 2004; 113(2):376-380.

26. Laaveg SJ, Ponseti IV: Long-term results of treatment of congenital club foot. *J Bone Joint Surg Am* 1980;62(1): 23-31.

27. Ponseti IV, Smoley EN: Congenital club foot: The results of treatment. *J Bone Joint Surg Am* 1963;45:261-275.

28. Morcuende JA, Egbert M, Ponseti IV: The effect of the internet in the treatment of congenital idiopathic clubfoot. *Iowa Orthop J* 2003;23:83-86.

29. Haft GF, Walker CG, Crawford HA: Early clubfoot recurrence after use of the Ponseti method in a New Zealand population. *J Bone Joint Surg Am* 2007;89(3): 487-493.

30. Boehm S, Limpaphayom N, Alaee F, Sinclair MF, Dobbs MB: Early results of the Ponseti method for the treatment of clubfoot in distal arthrogryposis. *J Bone Joint Surg Am* 2008;90(7):1501-1507.

31. Gerlach DJ, Gurnett CA, Limpaphayom N, et al: Early results of the Ponseti method for the treatment of clubfoot associated with myelomeningocele. *J Bone Joint Surg Am* 2009;91(6):1350-1359.

32. Merrill LJ, Gurnett CA, Connolly AM, Pestronk A, Dobbs MB: Skeletal muscle abnormalities and genetic factors related to vertical talus. *Clin Orthop Relat Res* 2011;469(4):1167-1174.

    The authors reviewed muscle biopsies performed in patients with congenital vertical talus. They concluded that abnormal skeletal muscle biopsies are common in patients with vertical talus, although it is unclear whether this is primary or secondary to the joint deformity. Associated anomalies are present in 62% of all patients.

33. Alaee F, Boehm S, Dobbs MB: A new approach to the treatment of congenital vertical talus. *J Child Orthop* 2007;1(3):165-174.

34. Chalayon O, Adams A, Dobbs MB: Minimally invasive approach for the treatment of non-isolated congenital vertical talus. *J Bone Joint Surg Am* 2012;94(11, e73): 1-7.

    Fifteen consecutive patients (25 feet) with nonisolated congenital vertical talus were retrospectively reviewed at a minimum of 2 years after treatment with serial casting followed by limited surgery. Initial correction was obtained in all patients. All radiographic parameters measured at the time of the latest follow-up had improved significantly (*P* < 0.0001) compared with the values before treatment. The mean values of the measured angles did not differ significantly from age-matched normal values.

35. Cowell HR, Elener V: Rigid painful flatfoot secondary to tarsal coalition. *Clin Orthop Relat Res* 1983;177:54-60.

36. Harris RI, Beath T: Etiology of peroneal spastic flat foot. *J Bone Joint Surg Br* 1948;30(4):624-634.

37. Morgan RC Jr, Crawford AH: Surgical management of tarsal coalition in adolescent athletes. *Foot Ankle* 1986; 7(3):183-193.

38. Zaw H, Calder JD: Tarsal coalitions. *Foot Ankle Clin* 2010;15(2):349-364.

    The authors present a comprehensive review of the history, etiology, incidence, pathophysiology, diagnosis, and treatment of tarsal coalition. A succinct discussion of the evidence-based literature on the current management of tarsal coalition is presented.

39. Badgely CE: Coalition of the calcaneus and the navicular. *Arch Surg* 1927;15:75-88.

40. Wilde PH, Torode IP, Dickens DR, Cole WG: Resection for symptomatic talocalcaneal coalition. *J Bone Joint Surg Br* 1994;76(5):797-801.

41. Luhmann SJ, Schoenecker PL: Symptomatic talocalcaneal coalition resection: indications and results. *J Pediatr Orthop* 1998;18(6):748-754.

42. Giannini S, Ceccarelli F, Vannini F, Baldi E: Operative treatment of flatfoot with talocalcaneal coalition. *Orthop Clin Relat Res* 2003;411:178-187.

43. Coughlin MJ: Roger A. Mann Award. Juvenile hallux valgus: Etiology and treatment. *Foot Ankle Int* 1995; 16(11):682-697.

44. Davids JR, McBrayer D, Blackhurst DW: Juvenile hallux valgus deformity: Surgical management by lateral hemiepiphyseodesis of the great toe metatarsal. *J Pediatr Orthop* 2007;27(7):826-830.

45. Weil L Jr, Weil LS Sr: Osteotomies for bunionette deformity. *Foot Ankle Clin* 2011;16(4):689-712.

    A comprehensive review of the multiple described osteotomies for bunionette deformity is presented.

46. Engström P, Tedroff K: The prevalence and course of idiopathic toe-walking in 5-year-old children. *Pediatrics* 2012;130(2):279-284.

    A cross-sectional prevalence study of idiopathic toe walking in 5.5-year-old children in Sweden is presented. The authors found a 4.9% prevalence of idiopathic toe walking in this patient population. A 41.2% prevalence of toe walking was found in children with neuropsychiatric diagnoses and developmental delays.

Video References

64.1: Talwalkar VR: Video. *Coleman Block Test*. Lexington, KY, 2013.

64.2: Talwalkar VR: Video. *Tip Toe Test*. Lexington, KY, 2013.

64.3: Talwalkar VR: Video: *Jack's Test*. Lexington, KY, 2013.

6: Pediatrics

Chapter 65

Injuries and Conditions of the Pediatric and Adolescent Athlete

Cordelia W. Carter, MD   Jennifer Weiss, MD

Introduction

The number of children and adolescents participating in sports in the United States continues to increase. For the 2009 to 2010 academic year, it was estimated that more than 7 million adolescents participated in high school athletics. An estimated 30 million youths participate annually in sports outside the academic setting.[1] Increased participation in sports has resulted in a concomitant increase in the number of sports-related injuries. It has been estimated that more than 4 million visits annually to the emergency department can be attributed to sports-related injuries, with an even larger number of outpatient visits attributed to injuries sustained during athletic participation.[1] Because of the possible short- and long-term consequences associated with sports-related injuries, there is an understandable need to improve the diagnosis, treatment, and prevention of these injuries in young athletes.

Upper Extremity

Shoulder

Anterior Shoulder Instability

Traumatic anterior shoulder dislocation is a common upper extremity injury in young athletes. Patients with anterior shoulder instability are typically young males who participate in high-demand contact sports. The primary mechanism of injury in this population is a collision or a contact event with the arm in abduction and external rotation. The physical examination in the acute setting may reveal loss of the normal shoulder contour, associated pain, and limited shoulder motion. The patient is initially treated with prompt reduction under conscious sedation, followed by sling immobili-

zation. The radiographic evaluation of a patient with a suspected shoulder dislocation typically includes AP, axillary lateral, and scapular Y views. Radiography is essential for determining the direction of dislocation; confirming adequate reduction; and identifying bony injuries associated with the dislocation, including compression fractures of the humeral head (such as Hill-Sachs lesions) or anterior glenoid rim fractures (such as bony Bankart lesions). MRI arthrography may better delineate associated intra-articular pathology, including tears of the glenoid labrum or the rotator cuff.

Traumatic anterior shoulder instability is associated with a high risk of recurrence, with young age and male sex being primary factors in the increased risk of reinjury. In young patients, the reported risk of shoulder redislocation has ranged from 75% to 100% after immobilization, rehabilitation, and gradual return to sports.[2] In the young adult population, research has documented improved functional outcomes of the shoulder with primary surgical stabilization, usually consisting of arthroscopic Bankart repair.[3] Recently, this approach has been used in the pediatric and adolescent populations (age 11 to 18 years), with reports of dramatically decreased recurrence rates, improved patient satisfaction, and good functional outcomes after primary arthroscopic repair.[4,5] Although surgical repair for patients with first-time dislocations has gained in popularity and has scientific support, not every patient should be treated surgically. Recent data suggest that primary surgical repair for very young patients (age 10 to 13 years at the time of injury) may not be as beneficial as had been originally reported.[6]

After the decision to proceed with surgical repair, it is imperative that all associated injuries be identified and appropriately addressed. These include soft-tissue injuries that may be underestimated by conventional imaging modalities and osseous defects affecting the humeral head, the anterior glenoid, or both.[7,8]

Clavicle Fractures

Traumatic fractures of the clavicle are common in young athletes and represent more than 15% of all fractures in this population.[9,10] The usual mechanisms of injury are falls onto the affected upper extremity or a direct blow to the collarbone itself. Midshaft fractures of the clavicle are the most common fracture pattern in

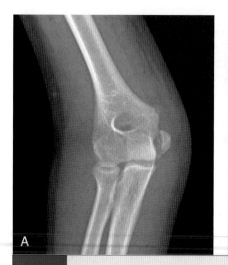
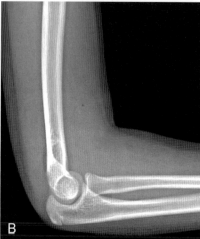
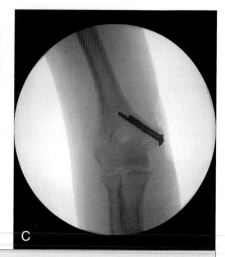

Figure 1   AP (**A**) and lateral (**B**) views of a widely displaced medial epicondyle fracture in the elbow of an 11-year-old girl who is a gymnast. **C,** Intraoperative fluoroscopic view of the same elbow after open reduction and internal fixation of the fracture.

children, although injuries to the proximal and distal clavicle may also occur. The physeal injury pattern is unique to children and adolescents. Physeal injury can occur through the distal or proximal clavicular growth plate and can mimic dislocation of the acromioclavicular and sternoclavicular joints, respectively.[11,12]

Patients with clavicular fractures typically present with deformity, swelling, ecchymosis, and localized tenderness. Radiographic evaluation includes AP and 30° cephalic tilt views of the clavicles to assess fracture displacement, comminution, and shortening. Traditionally, clavicular fractures in pediatric and adolescent patients have been treated nonsurgically with immobilization in a sling or figure-of-8 bandage, followed by early mobilization. Because of the excellent capacity of the clavicle to heal and remodel in this population, nonsurgical treatment of clavicular fractures remains the gold standard for most young patients.[13]

Because the clinical and functional outcomes of adult patients seem to be improved with open reduction and internal fixation of displaced fractures,[14] this finding has been extrapolated to adolescent patients. It has recently been shown that surgical fixation of shortened, displaced, and comminuted midshaft clavicular fractures in adolescents can be performed safely, with faster bony healing and return to sports compared with nonsurgical management. Because hardware prominence and hardware-related discomfort are common complications in adolescents, return to the operating room for hardware removal is frequently required.[9,10,15,16] The successful use of alternative fixation devices, including intramedullary clavicle pins and absorbable implants, recently has been reported.[15] Indications for the surgical treatment of adolescents with shortened or comminuted clavicular fractures continue to evolve.

Elbow
Medial Epicondyle Fractures
Medial epicondyle fractures are common injuries in the pediatric and adolescent populations, representing approximately 10% of all elbow fractures. Three primary mechanisms of injury have been identified for medial epicondylar fractures: (1) a direct blow to the elbow; (2) an elbow dislocation; and (3) an avulsion-type injury, with overwhelming traction forces applied to the apophysis through the musculotendinous attachment of the flexor-pronator mass and/or the origin of the ulnar collateral ligament. Gymnasts and throwing athletes are especially susceptible to isolated fractures of the medial epicondylar apophysis; symptomatic apophysitis may precede acute apophyseal failure.[17]

Typical findings in patients with apophyseal avulsions include localized swelling, crepitation, ecchymosis, and tenderness to palpation. Valgus elbow instability and ulnar nerve symptoms may also be present. Traditionally, AP, lateral, and oblique radiographs of the elbow have been used to evaluate these injuries. Some recent studies have questioned the ability of physicians to accurately and reliably assess the degree of fracture displacement using plain radiographs. Anterior displacement of the fracture fragment is frequently underestimated.[18,19]

Treatment of medial epicondyle fractures has traditionally been guided by the degree of fracture displacement. Displacement of less than 2 mm is generally accepted as a clear indication for nonsurgical management, with immobilization in a long-arm cast for 3 to 4 weeks. Incarceration of the fracture fragment in the joint, open fracture, ulnar nerve dysfunction with suspected nerve entrapment, and frank valgus instability of the elbow are widely accepted indications for surgical treatment, which generally consists of open reduction and internal fixation of the fracture[20-22] (Figure 1). The amount of fracture displacement that requires surgical reduction and fixation remains controversial.

Some authors have reported good long-term functional outcomes in patients with fracture displacement up to 15 mm who were managed nonsurgically.[20,21] In contrast, other authors have suggested that nonsurgical treatment of widely displaced medial epicondyle fractures can result in nonunion and is associated with elbow instability, pain, and impaired elbow function.[22] These authors recommend open reduction and internal fixation for fractures with displacement greater than 5 mm. Patients who rely heavily on the stabilizers of the elbow joint for their athletic activities (such as gymnasts, baseball players, quarterbacks, and wrestlers) may benefit from a solid, anatomic bony union of the fracture, which is more reliably achieved with surgical treatment. Symptomatic nonunion, when present, is a challenging clinical complication. A recent study reported improved outcomes after delayed open reduction and internal fixation in patients with symptomatic nonunions.[23]

Osteochondritis Dissecans of the Capitellum

Juvenile osteochondritis dissecans (OCD) of the humeral capitellum is a disorder that primarily affects adolescent athletes (age 11 to 21 years). It is characterized radiographically by fragmentation of the subchondral bone of the capitellum, which may progress over time to separation of the overlying articular cartilage and ultimately to loosening of the osteochondral fragment. The presence of intra-articular loose bodies, osteochondral defects, and osteophytic changes of the radiocapitellar joint represent the most advanced stages of the disease. The etiology of OCD is poorly understood, although it is generally accepted that repetitive microtrauma to the lateral side of the elbow (as seen in throwing athletes, such as baseball pitchers, or in upper extremity weight-bearing athletes, such as gymnasts and cheerleaders) in the setting of a tenuous osseous blood supply results in the characteristic subchondral fragmentation.[24,25] Importantly, capitellar OCD should be distinguished from Panner disease, which is a self-limited osteochondrosis of the capitellum that occurs in children younger than 10 years, is usually not activity related, and routinely resolves with time and supportive care.

Patients with OCD typically report activity-related elbow pain, which is frequently accompanied by swelling, loss of motion, and in the later stages of the disease, mechanical symptoms such as locking, clicking, or catching. The physical examination may reveal swelling, flexion contracture, crepitation, and tenderness over the anterolateral capitellum. Radiographic evaluation (AP, lateral, 45° flexion AP, and/or oblique views) frequently shows a focal lesion in the capitellum with associated irregularity of the joint surface. Additional evaluation usually consists of MRI, which helps to determine the integrity of the articular cartilage.[24,25]

There are many systems for staging capitellar OCD, but the simplest system tries to determine if the lesion is stable (open capitellar growth plate, localized radiolucency of the subchondral bone, and preserved elbow range of motion) or unstable (closed capitellar physis, fragmentation of the lesion, and loss of elbow motion of more than 20°).[26] This staging system is useful both prognostically and therapeutically because stable lesions are more likely to heal without surgical intervention, whereas unstable lesions fare better with surgical treatment.

The treatment of capitellar OCD lesions is typically guided by the stage of the lesion and the appearance of the articular cartilage. Patients with small, stable, intact lesions often improve with a course of activity modification (such as sports cessation) followed by gentle physical therapy to improve motion and strength. Patients with large unstable lesions, loss of articular cartilage integrity, and intra-articular loose bodies, and those in whom nonsurgical management has been unsuccessful may benefit from surgical intervention. The first-line surgical treatment usually consists of elbow arthroscopy with débridement and drilling of the lesion, with removal of loose bodes and microfracture performed as necessary (Figure 2). Unstable lesions may be fixed in situ using either an arthroscopic or an open approach. Several recent studies have reported good clinical outcomes with these methods in the pediatric and adolescent populations.[27-30] Data also support autologous osteochondral mosaicplasty for the treatment of very large, advanced OCD lesions.[31] Uncontained lesions, which extend beyond the lateral cartilaginous margin of the capitellum, may be associated with greater postoperative flexion contractures. Failure to adequately restore the lateral margin of the capitellum has been associated with radial head deformity and/or radiohumeral arthrosis.[27-30]

Lower Extremity

Pelvis and Hip
Apophyseal Avulsion Fractures

Avulsion fractures of the apophyses of the pelvis and the hip are injuries unique to young athletes (age 11 to 25 years), with adolescents being primarily affected. These injuries commonly occur as the result of a sudden, forceful contraction of the musculotendinous unit, with failure occurring through the growth plate itself.[32,33] The ischial tuberosity is the most common site of injury, followed by the anterior inferior iliac spine and the anterior superior iliac spine.[33] Injuries to the other apophyses around the pelvis are rare.[32-34]

Typically, the patient with an apophyseal avulsion fracture describes the acute onset of well-localized pain during participation in athletics, especially during sprinting or jumping activities. Apophyseal avulsion injuries are frequently associated with participation in soccer and gymnastics. Often, patients will hear a popping sound before the onset of hip pain. Occasionally, patients may report a prodrome of symptoms consistent with apophysitis (such as less intense pain or discomfort associated with activities) in the days or weeks before the acute avulsion event. The physical

6: Pediatrics

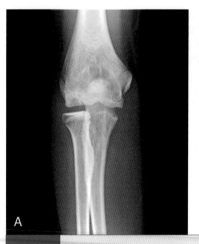
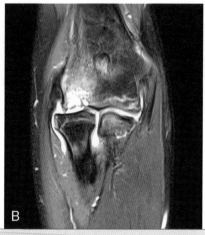
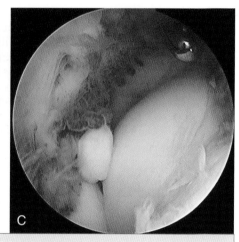

Figure 2   **A,** AP radiograph of the elbow of a 12-year-old boy who is a basketball player shows a large osteochondritis dissecans lesion of the capitellum. **B,** A coronal fat-suppressed MRI scan shows the cystic nature of the lesion, with thinning of the articular cartilage. **C,** An arthroscopic image shows extensive synovitis and intra-articular loose bodies.

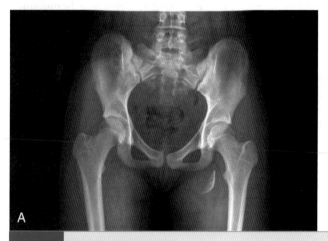
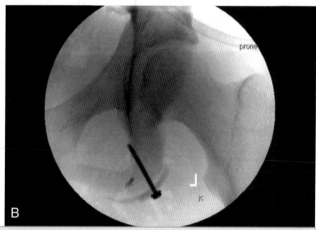

Figure 3   **A,** AP radiograph of the pelvis of a 14-year-old girl who is a sprinter shows a widely displaced apophyseal avulsion fracture of the ischial tuberosity. Sciatic nerve irritation subsequently developed in this patient, and she was treated with open reduction and internal fixation of the fracture. **B,** Intraoperative fluoroscopic view after fracture fixation.

examination will reveal localized swelling, ecchymosis, and tenderness to palpation of the affected site; the pain symptoms can be re-created with passive stretching and/or active contraction of the involved muscle. Muscle weakness may be noted. Plain radiographs of the pelvis, in conjunction with a good history and physical examination, usually can confirm the diagnosis.

The initial treatment of these injuries usually involves a combination of protected weight bearing, activity modification, the application of ice, and the administration of oral anti-inflammatory medications followed by physical therapy for regaining strength and motion and then a gradual return to sports participation. In rare instances, widely displaced fractures may require surgical treatment to avoid late sequelae of the injury, including symptomatic fibrous nonunion, persistent muscle weakness or dysfunction, sciatic nerve irritation (with ischial tuberosity avulsions; Figure 3), and

painful bony impingement (with anterior superior iliac spine avulsions).[35,36]

Overuse Injuries of the Hip

Many chronic hip injuries affect pediatric and adolescent athletes, including extra-articular conditions such as muscle strains, ligament sprains, and bursitis of the bony prominences around the hip (the greater trochanter, the ischial tuberosity, and the iliopectineal eminence). Coxa saltans interna (internal snapping hip) occurs when the iliopsoas tendon anteriorly snaps over the pelvic brim and/or the femoral head. Coxa saltans externa (external snapping hip) occurs when the posterior aspect of the iliotibial band snaps over the greater trochanter laterally. Most of these soft-tissue injuries occur in the setting of improper training regimens (overtraining, poor periodization, and poor techniques) and respond well to a prescribed course of activity modification, physical therapy, and oral anti-inflammatory medications. In recalcitrant cases, more aggressive treatments may be warranted, including corticosteroid injection, surgical lengthening, and débridement and/or the release of the involved structures.[37]

Intra-articular hip pathology may also occur in the young athlete. For example, stress fractures of the femoral neck have been reported in skeletally immature patients. Osteochondral defects of the femoral head and/or acetabulum can result from trauma, such as a hip dislocation.[37] Intra-articular snapping hip syndrome can occur as a result of loose bodies within the joint or injury to the labrum or the ligamentum teres. Slipped capital femoral epiphysis should always be considered in a young patient with hip pain regardless of sports participation.

Femoroacetabular Impingement

No discussion of hip pathology in the young athletic population is complete without discussing femoroacetabular impingement, which can be defined as the anomalous physical contact that occurs between the proximal femur and the acetabular rim. This disorder is characterized by a reproducible pattern of abnormal bony abutment that occurs secondary to morphologic abnormalities of the proximal femur (the cam lesion), the acetabulum (the pincer lesion), or a combination of both (mixed impingement).[38,39] The cam-type deformity is typified by the aspheric extension of the articular surface at the anterosuperior head-neck junction of the proximal femur. With hip motion, especially in the maximal ranges of flexion and internal rotation, the irregularly shaped proximal femur abuts or jams into the anterosuperior acetabulum. In pincer impingement, excessive coverage of the femoral head, which results from acetabular retroversion, coxa profunda, or posttraumatic osteophyte formation, effectively pinches the labrum between the adjacent bony structures. Over time, the abnormal bony contact results in recurrent microtrauma to the articular cartilage and labrum, with premature degenerative joint disease of the hip representing the final end point in the disease process.

Patients with femoroacetabular impingement typically report activity-related groin pain, which is occasionally associated with mechanical symptoms of clicking or popping. Common physical examination

Video 65.1: Physical Evaluation of Hip Pain in Non/Prearthritic Patient and Athlete. Allston J. Stubbs, MD; Adam William Anz, MD; Benjamin L. Long, MD; John Frino, MD; Stephanie Cheetham, MD (18.05 min)

findings include decreased internal rotation of the hip and reproducible pain with flexion, adduction, and internal rotation of the affected hip (the impingement test). Associated inflammation of the adjacent soft tissues (iliopsoas, piriformis, and sacroiliac joint) is common. Diagnostic imaging studies may show the presence of a pistol-grip deformity and/or decreased head-neck offset (α angle > 55°) in cam impingement. Pincer impingement is associated with a positive crossover sign, coxa profunda, and/or an increased center-edge angle. MRI arthrography of the affected hip is commonly used to detect associated labral pathology.[38,39] The treatment of femoroacetabular impingement is discussed in detail in *Orthopaedic Knowledge Update 11*, chapter 35, Hip and Pelvic Reconstruction and Arthroplasty).

Knee
Anterior Cruciate Ligament Tears

The management and treatment of anterior cruciate ligament (ACL) injuries in skeletally immature patients is controversial. Because most studies on this topic have been retrospective, prospective studies with a large number of patients are needed to achieve a better understanding of ACL injuries.[40]

ACL deficiency in the skeletally immature knee has been shown to lead to poor outcomes, including instability, meniscal tears, and cartilage damage. A 2011 study examined the effect of delayed surgical treatment of ACL tears in skeletally immature athletes. The authors found that patients who underwent surgical treatment more than 12 weeks after injury had a higher incidence of irreparable meniscal tears and chondral injuries, with an even stronger association when the knee was subjectively unstable.[41]

Treatment options vary depending on the patient's age and stage of skeletal maturity. There are many techniques available to treat ACL tears in prepubescent patients or those with Tanner stage 1 or 2 disease. A retrospective review of 16 prepubescent patients treated with transphyseal reconstruction using soft-tissue grafts found that all of the patients were able to return to sports participation, and no growth disturbances were reported.[42]

At a mean follow-up of 3.6 years, a 3% failure rate with no angular deformities or limb-length discrepancies was reported in patients with Tanner stage 3 disease who were treated with transphyseal reconstruction with quadrupled hamstring autograft and metaphyseal fixation.[43] No reported growth disturbance occurred in 16 children and adolescents with Tanner stage 3 and 4 disease who underwent ACL reconstruction with patellar tendon autograft. The authors cautioned that meticulous surgical technique was used for placing the bone plugs proximal to the physes, and the graft was not overtensioned.[44]

Complications after ACL reconstruction in young athletes include retears and arthrofibrosis. The prevalence of arthrofibrosis in children and adolescents after ACL reconstruction has been reported to be 8.3%. Surgical manipulation can be used to restore motion, but functional outcome may be affected. Vigilance is important in monitoring postoperative range of motion in young patients after ACL reconstruction.[45]

6. Pediatrics

Partial ACL Tears

Partial tearing of the ACL is difficult to diagnose with MRI, with an accuracy as low as 25% to 53%.[46] Patients are often unable to return to their preinjury level of sports participation, and full rupture of the ACL will occur in many patients.[46] An adolescent patient with a partial ACL tear can be considered for nonsurgical treatment if the patient's skeletal age is younger than 14 years. If the patient has a positive pivot shift test result or the tear is greater than 50% of the ACL or predominantly involves the posterolateral corner, reconstruction is more likely required to achieve stability.[47] A prospective study found that the best predictor of the need for reconstruction of a partially torn ACL was a positive finding in the pivot shift test performed in an awake patient at least 3 months after injury. The authors suggested that a negative pivot shift test result at the approximate 3-month follow-up examination is predictive of knee stability.[48]

Discoid Meniscus

The incidence of symptomatic discoid meniscus of the knee is not known. An asymptomatic discoid meniscus may be diagnosed as an incidental finding. The discoid meniscus is more prone to tears than the normal C-shaped meniscus. It was proposed that discoid menisci should be classified first by whether the meniscus is complete or incomplete and then by the location of the instability.[49] In a study of 30 knees, it was reported that 77% of surgically treated discoid menisci were unstable. The location of instability was anterior in 53% of the knees, posterior in 16%, and a combination of anterior and posterior in 6%.[49] A 2004 study reported that peripheral rim instability was more common in complete discoid menisci. The authors reported that instability was located anteriorly in 47% of the knees, posteriorly in 38%, and less commonly at the middle third peripheral attachment (11.1%).[50] Instability is thought to be the etiology of knee flexion contracture (the inability to fully extend the knee). It has been proposed that knee flexion contracture is caused by a redundant anterior segment of the meniscus in combination with posterior rim instability.[51]

A patient with symptomatic discoid meniscus will present with knee pain, catching, clunking, and, in some instances, the onset of knee flexion contracture. Treatment is indicated if the patient is symptomatic. When symptoms are present, arthroscopy should be performed. If a discoid meniscus is identified as an incidental finding on MRI or with arthroscopy, treatment is not warranted. When instability is identified, stabilization of the meniscus is recommended, but long-term outcomes after repair are not yet known. Reoperation rates after arthroscopy for discoid meniscus are high, and the long-term outcomes for stabilization procedures are not well understood.

Traumatic Patellar Dislocations

Patellar dislocations are thought to occur most frequently among young patients (age 10 to 17 years). Patients with recurrent episodes of patellar instability are more likely to be female, and patients with a history of a prior patellar dislocation are seven times more likely to have recurrent patellar dislocation than first-time dislocators.[52] A 2011 study reported that in patients younger than 18 years, the location of the tear of the medial patellofemoral ligament (MPFL) was at the patellar attachment in 61% of patients and at the femoral attachment in 12%. An additional 12% of patients had injury to both attachments, 6% had no identifiable MPFL tear, and 9% had combination midsubstance and attachment injuries.[53] In contrast, a 2009 study of older patients reported that the location of the MPFL rupture was at the femoral attachment in 66% of patients, the patellar attachment in 13%, and the midsubstance in 21%.[54] Patients with MPFL rupture at the femoral attachment were less likely to return to their preinjury level of activity.

Valgus malalignment can pose a risk for patellar instability. Valgus alignment can be measured using the Q angle, the angle formed by a line drawn from the anterior superior iliac spine to the central patella and a second line drawn from the patella to the tibial tubercle. A normal Q angle is up to 14° in males and 17° in females. The distance between the tibial tuberosity and the trochlear groove may also play a role in susceptibility to patellar instability. This distance has been reported to be significantly greater in patients with a patellar dislocation.[55]

The management of an initial traumatic patellar dislocation is also controversial. A prospective randomized study of surgical treatment for a first-time traumatic patellar dislocation correlated with a lower rate of redislocation.[56] However, a randomized clinical trial examining the outcomes of children after surgical medial imbrications did not confirm improvement in long-term outcomes for surgically treated patients compared with those treated nonsurgically.[57]

Nonsurgical treatment remains the initial approach to managing patellar instability. Physical therapy to address core and hip abductor strengthening, bracing with patellar stabilizing braces, and patellar taping are strategies that should be pursued before surgery is considered. The distinction between traumatic patellar dislocation and atraumatic recurrent instability is an important one, and patients with atraumatic recurrent instability are rarely indicated for surgical treatment.

Tibial Spine Fractures

Avulsion fractures of the tibial spine or the tibial eminence are far more common in children than in skeletally mature individuals. Patients older than 18 years may have worse outcomes than children after treatment of tibial spine fractures.[58]

Tibial spine fractures have been classified into four types[59] (Figure 4). Displaced fractures require surgical reduction and fixation using open or arthroscopic techniques. Although arthroscopic techniques have become popular, to date no data support the benefit of arthroscopic over open techniques. The intermeniscal ligament

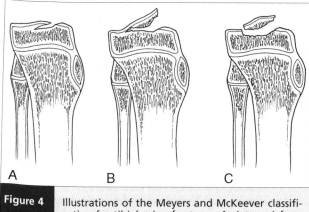

Figure 4 Illustrations of the Meyers and McKeever classification for tibial spine fractures. **A,** A type 1 fracture is not displaced and can be treated in a cast, either in full extension or in 25° of flexion. **B,** A type 2 fracture is hinged out of place and can often be treated with closed reduction and casting. **C,** A type 3 fracture is completely displaced. A type 4 fracture (not illustrated) is displaced and rotated. Type 3 and 4 fractures require surgical reduction and stabilization.

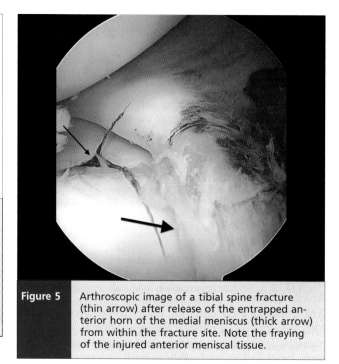

Figure 5 Arthroscopic image of a tibial spine fracture (thin arrow) after release of the entrapped anterior horn of the medial meniscus (thick arrow) from within the fracture site. Note the fraying of the injured anterior meniscal tissue.

is frequently a block to reduction, and care should be taken to retract the ligament out of the way when reducing the fracture (**Figure 5**). Fixation options include screws and sutures. Screw fixation has been shown to have a higher reoperation rate because of symptoms caused by the hardware.[58] Different suture techniques have been studied with regard to biomechanical strength. No suture configuration has been proven to provide a biomechanical advantage over the others.[60]

Postoperative care of tibial eminence fractures can be complicated by arthrofibrosis. Early motion after surgical fixation has been shown to correlate with an earlier return to sports and activities.[58,61]

OCD of the Knee

OCD of the knee is an idiopathic pathologic finding that involves the bone and the overlying cartilage of the knee. The cause of this disorder may be repetitive trauma, inflammation, or ischemia. The patient may provide a nonspecific report of knee pain and swelling, possibly with popping, clicking, and locking. OCD of the knee is frequently an incidental diagnosis. Workup includes radiography, with care to obtain a notch view to visualize the posterior aspect of the femoral condyles. MRI is appropriate to further clarify the stability of the lesion. The most common location for OCD of the knee is the lateral aspect of the medial femoral condyle. Nonsurgical treatment (activity modification, possible protected weight bearing, and possible bracing or casting of the involved leg) is appropriate for a skeletally immature patient with a stable lesion. If a patient is near skeletal maturity or the lesion is unstable, surgical options can be considered. If the lesion is stable, transarticular or extra-articular drilling is appropriate. For unstable lesions, fixation of the lesion should be performed.[62,63] For completely unattached lesions, fixation is still preferred.[64] If this is not possible, then mar-

Table 1

Recommendations From the AAOS Clinical Practice Guideline for the Diagnosis and the Treatment of Osteochondritis Dissecans of the Knee

In a patient with knee symptoms and/or signs, radiographs are an option.

In a patient with a known OCD lesion on radiographs, MRI of the knee is an option to characterize the OCD lesion.

Symptomatic, skeletally immature patients with salvageable unstable or displaced OCD lesions can be offered the option of surgery.

Patients who remain symptomatic after treatment of OCD may have a history, physical examination, radiography, and/or MRI to assess healing.

Patients who have been surgically treated for OCD may be offered postoperative physical therapy.

OCD = osteochondritis dissecans.

row stimulation, osteoarticular transfer, or autologous chondrocyte implantation can be considered.[65] Guidelines from a workgroup of the American Academy of Orthopaedic Surgeons have addressed the diagnosis and treatment of OCD of the knee[66] (**Table 1**). Further research is under way to guide orthopaedic surgeons in the diagnosis and treatment of this challenging condition.

6: Pediatrics

74. Perumal V, Wall E, Babekir N: Juvenile osteochondritis dissecans of the talus. *J Pediatr Orthop* 2007;27(7): 821-825.

75. Letts M, Davidson D, Ahmer A: Osteochondritis dissecans of the talus in children. *J Pediatr Orthop* 2003; 23(5):617-625.

76. Weiss JM, Jordan SS, Andersen JS, Lee BM, Kocher M: Surgical treatment of unresolved Osgood-Schlatter disease: Ossicle resection with tibial tubercleplasty. *J Pediatr Orthop* 2007;27(7):844-847.

Video Reference

65.1: Stubbs AJ, MD; Anz AW, MD; Long BL, MD; Frino J, MD; Cheetham SG, MD: Video. *Physical Evaluation of Hip Pain in Non/Pre-Arthritic Patient and Athlete*. Available at http://orthoportal.aaos.org/emedia/ singleVideoPlayer.aspx?resource=EMEDIA_OSVL_10_04. Accessed January 15, 2014.

Chapter 66

Skeletal Dysplasias, Connective Tissue Diseases, and Other Genetic Disorders

Klane K. White, MD   William G. Mackenzie, MD

Introduction

The human genome codes for a variety of proteins that play an important role in the structure and function of the tissues of the musculoskeletal system. Genetic mutations can therefore result in an array of cytokine, enzyme, and structural malfunctions of the tissues in which they are expressed. As a rule, germline mutations are expressed throughout the body, resulting in a generalized phenotype, as opposed to postmeiotic mutations, which generally are expressed in a mosaic or localized fashion, such as found in conditions such as fibular hemimelia or proximal femoral focal deficiency. There are a wide variety of genetically mediated conditions with significant orthopaedic manifestations. Deformities of the spine, forearms, hips, and lower extremities can result in substantial functional impairment. The skeletal dysplasias, or osteochondrodystrophies, are a subset of these conditions in which the genetic abnormality primarily affects endochondral bone formation. These conditions are typified by generalized skeletal involvement that evolves with development, generally resulting in a disproportionate short stature.

Historically, genetic disorders of the skeleton have been defined by their radiologic manifestations. With an evolving understanding of the molecular origins of these disorders, they now can be classified accordingly. This chapter presents a review of genetically mediated disorders.

Disorders Caused by Defects in Genes of Structural Elements

Differential gene expression among the various structural tissues (such as bone, cartilage, and ligaments) does occur, resulting in variations of disease effects within these tissues (Table 1). If the structural abnormality involves cartilage, a growth abnormality may be caused by physeal failure, resulting in a failure of bone growth and deformity, and articular cartilage failure, resulting in degenerative joint disease, such as in spondyloepiphyseal dysplasia congenita. If the affected protein is important for ligament or tendon strength, joint subluxation may occur, such as in Marfan syndrome or Ehlers-Danlos syndrome. In osteogenesis imperfecta, the structural abnormality is caused by a type I collagen mutation, resulting in bone fragility. In addition, the phenotype may evolve with time and growth as the abnormal structural deficiencies progressively accumulate, and tissue damage associated with these deficiencies can also progress. Furthermore, deformities may recur after corrective surgery because the structural components are abnormal.

Marfan Syndrome

Marfan syndrome results from a mutation in the gene encoding for the fibrillin protein. Fibrillin plays a key role in maintaining the normal mechanical properties of soft tissues, especially in resisting the cyclic stresses of the cardiovascular, ocular, and skeletal systems.[1,2] Fibrillin mutations cause some extracellular growth factors, such as transforming growth factor–β and the bone morphogenetic proteins (BMPs), to become more readily accessible to cell receptors.[3,4] The increased availability of these growth factors likely increases cellular growth, leading to the development of tall stature and long, thin fingers and toes. The increased availability of growth factors also is likely responsible for many of the changes in the mechanical properties of the soft tissues. Consequently, future therapies for this disorder may be tailored to growth factor activity modulation.[3]

The revised Ghent nosology (2010) emphasizes the

6: Pediatrics

Table 1

Disorders Caused by Defects in Genes of Structural Elements

Disorder	Gene Defect		Orthopaedic Phenotype/Inheritance Pattern
Marfan syndrome	FBN1 15q21.1		Scoliosis, aortic root aneurysm, protrusion acetabuli, ectopia lentis, hand joint laxity, chest deformity, pes planovalgus, and loss of elbow extension
Osteogenesis imperfecta	COL1A1 17q21.33 or COL1A2 7q22.1		Variable, short stature; extensive bone fragility; and multiple fractures
		Type I, autosomal dominant	Normal or low-normal height and blue sclerae, multiple bone fractures occur during childhood, and 50% deaf
		Type II, autosomal dominant	Short, crumpled-appearing femurs and ribs; hypoplastic lungs; and central nervous system malformations and hemorrhage common
		Type III, autosomal recessive	The most severe type: large skull, with triangular appearance of the facial bones; pale blue sclerae (normal at puberty); multiple long-bone and vertebral fractures; kyphosis, and severe scoliosis
		Type IV, autosomal dominant	Short stature, bowed bones, and vertebral fractures; sclerae typically are white
		Type V, autosomal recessive	Hypertrophic callus after fracture and ossification of the interosseous membrane between the tibia and fibula and between the radius and ulna
		Type VI, autosomal recessive	Similar to type IV; abnormalities of mineralization rather than collagen
		Type VII, autosomal recessive	Rhizomelia and coxa vara
		Type VIII, autosomal recessive	White sclerae, severe undermineralization of skeleton
Type II collagen disorders	COL2A1 12q13.11	Achondrogenesis type II, autosomal dominant	Short trunk with prominent abdomen, striking micromelia, flat midface, micrognathia, cleft patella, hydropic appearance, absence of ossification of the sacrum, and barrel-shaped thorax with short ribs
		Stickler syndrome, autosomal dominant	Scoliosis and a mild epiphyseal dysplasia, osteochondritis dissecans–type lesions (multiple) and precocious arthritis, joint hypermobility, and midface hypoplasia Type I often present with Pierre-Robin sequence at birth
		Kniest dysplasia, autosomal dominant	Short stature; a round, flat face with central depression; prominent eyes; enlargement and stiffness of joints; scoliosis; contractures of fingers; bell-shaped chest; coxa vara; genu valga; and dumbbell metaphyses on extremity radiographs
		Spondyloepiphyseal dysplasia congenita, autosomal dominant	Disproportionate short stature (short trunk), abnormal epiphyses, flattened vertebral bodies (platyspondyly), odontoid hypoplasia or os odontoideum common, atlantoaxial instability, scoliosis, lumbar lordosis, coxa vara, hip flexion contractures, and genu valgum

importance of family history, aortic root aneurysm, and ectopia lentis as the cardinal diagnostic features of this disorder.[5] Other key musculoskeletal findings are a part of the systemic score, including laxity of the wrist and thumb, chest deformity, pes planovalgus, protrusio acetabuli, scoliosis, and loss of elbow extension. In a pa-

tient with Marfan syndrome, scoliosis is sometimes diagnosed first. It is important for the orthopaedist to recognize the underlying condition, because referral for appropriate prophylactic management of the cardiovascular abnormities can be a lifesaving intervention. The clinical findings of laxity and subluxation of the joints and weakening of arterial walls with resultant aortic root dilatation are easily understood based on the function of fibrillin. The tall stature and arachnodactyly associated with the syndrome are likely caused by the growth factor activity modulation previously discussed.[4]

Hyperlaxity is responsible for many of the orthopaedic aspects of Marfan syndrome, including joint subluxation, scoliosis, and a predisposition to sprains. Scoliosis in Marfan syndrome is treated in a manner similar to idiopathic scoliosis, although bracing appears to be less effective[6] (Figure 1). Management of scoliosis in these patients differs in several ways. First, the incidence of dural ectasia is higher in these patients, and appropriate imaging (MRI) is recommended for all patients indicated for surgical intervention. Second, the complication rate in scoliosis surgery is higher for patients with Marfan syndrome compared with those with idiopathic scoliosis. Infection, instrumentation failure, pseudarthrosis, or coronal and sagittal curve decompensation are reported to occur in 10% to 20% of patients,[7] whereas overcorrection can cause cardiovascular complications.[8] Traction should be used with caution; subluxation of vertebrae can occur and worsen, especially in the presence of associated kyphosis.[9] Infection often is associated with a dural tear (increased risk with dural ectasia), and perioperative death from valvular insufficiency has been reported.

Osteopenia is commonly found in patients with Marfan syndrome; however, this is not associated with an increased risk of fractures.[10,11] Protrusio acetabuli may be treated with prophylactic fusion of the triradiate cartilage with mixed results, and therefore is not warranted in most patients.[12]

Osteogenesis Imperfecta

Osteogenesis imperfecta (OI) occurs in about 1 in 20,000 children and is most commonly the result of a mutation in the genes that code for type I collagen strands (COL1A1 and COL1A2) or the genes that encode for the processing of these strands. Type I collagen is composed of three tightly packed procollagen chains in the form of a triple helix. Defects in type I collagen can be qualitative or quantitative in nature. A substitution of glycine by another amino acid, leading to structural abnormalities, prevents proper triple helix formation of the collagen molecule and subsequent qualitative deficiencies of the bone matrix. Meanwhile, mutations that result in a premature stop codon lead to abnormal messenger RNA production and, therefore, less collagen production. Bone in patients affected by OI shows a decreased number of trabeculae and decreased cortical thickness. There is an increased number of osteoblasts and osteoclasts, which are biologically hypermetabolic. Despite an increase in the frequency of fractures during childhood in patients with OI bone healing occurs at a normal rate but with abnormal bone.

The phenotype of OI is quite variable, with some individuals only mildly affected and having no skeletal deformity. Others have short stature, extensive bone

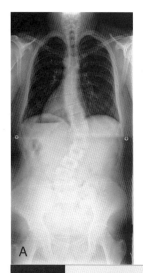
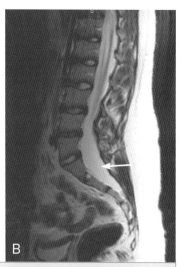

Figure 1 **A,** Radiograph of the spine of a 15-year-old adolescent with Marfan syndrome shows thoracolumbar scoliosis. The neurologic examination was normal, but the patient reported back pain. **B,** MRI showing dural ectasia (arrow) and a Tarloff cyst.

fragility, and multiple fractures. The most severe forms of OI are fatal during the perinatal period. The Sillence classification was established in 1979 as a clinical classification with four types of OI and has been subsequently modified to include eight forms based on clinical, radiographic, biochemical, and genetic information.[13,14] Types I, II, III, and IV are autosomal dominant, whereas the other types are autosomal recessive. Type I is a mild disorder characterized by a deficient quantity of type I collagen. Clinically, type I OI is characterized by normal or below-normal stature, blue sclerae, and multiple fractures. Fractures occur with greater frequency during early childhood but are less common after puberty. Deafness is common, and audiology screening is recommended.

Type II OI is the lethal perinatal form of OI. Respiratory failure is the most common cause of death as a result of a restrictive chest wall further compromised by pain associated with multiple rib fractures. Radiographically, these children are found to have short, crumpled-appearing (accordion-like) femurs.

Type III OI presents with the most severe of the survivable phenotypes, typically presenting with multiple fractures and severe deformities at birth. Skull films reveal wormian bone (irregular isolated intrasutural bones that appear in addition to the usual centers of ossification in the cranium). Facial characteristics include an underdeveloped triangular appearance of the facial bones and pale blue sclerae. Multiple vertebral compression fractures, which have a so-called codfish appearance on radiographs, commonly lead to kyphosis and severe scoliosis. Ultimately, most patients with type III OI are relegated to a wheelchair for mobility.

Patients with type IV OI have a variable fracture incidence. Characteristics include short stature, bowed

6: Pediatrics

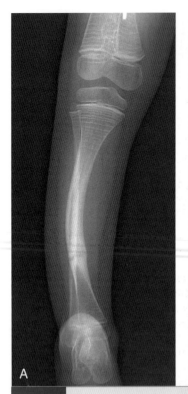
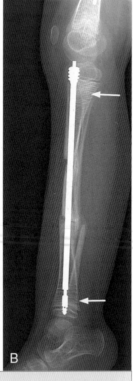

Figure 2	**A,** Radiograph of the leg of a 6-year-old child with OI shows a tibial deformity and pseudarthrosis. Note the metaphyseal lines secondary to pamidronate therapy. **B,** Postoperative lateral radiograph of the tibia after realignment osteotomies and intramedullary fixation with an expansile telescoping rod. Arrows indicate metaphyseal lines.

monly with telescoping rods) are the standard treatment in children with bone deformities that interfere with function (**Figure 2**).

Pharmacologic treatment of OI with bisphosphonates is not FDA approved but is now commonly used in the care for children sustaining two or more long-bone fractures per year.[18] Cyclical treatment with intravenous pamidronate results in improved bone mineral density, a reduction in fracture incidence, a reduction in pain, and improved remodeling of vertebral body compression fractures.[18] Data supporting the use of other forms of bisphosphonates exist in the treatment of low bone mineral density in children and in children with OI, but pamidronate remains the standard in bisphosphonate therapy. Because animal data suggest that impaired bone healing may occur in the presence of bisphosphonate therapy, elective osteotomies should be timed accordingly (infusions should be delayed approximately 3 months after surgical intervention).

Type II Collagen Disorders

Defects in the formation of type II collagen result in an array of physical manifestations and disabilities. Nonmusculoskeletal manifestations that are common to these disorders include myopia and cleft palate anomalies. Achondrogenesis type II represents a type II collagen disorder in its most severe form and is lethal. The primary musculoskeletal manifestations of Stickler syndrome are scoliosis and a mild epiphyseal dysplasia, with osteochondritis dissecans–type lesions and precocious arthritis. Infants with type I Stickler syndrome often present with Pierre-Robin sequence at birth. Kniest dysplasia is typified by significant short stature; a round, flat face with central depression; prominent eyes; enlargement and stiffness of joints; contractures of fingers; normal head circumference; a bell-shaped chest; and dumbbell-like metaphyses on extremity radiographs.

Spondyloepiphyseal dysplasia congenita is an autosomal dominant disorder characterized by a disproportionate short stature (short trunk), abnormal epiphyses, and flattened vertebral bodies (platyspondyly). Odontoid hypoplasia is essentially universal in individuals with spondyloepiphyseal dysplasia congenita, and os odontoideum is common. Atlantoaxial instability presents a technically difficult challenge for the spine surgeon. In a study of 21 patients with spondyloepiphyseal dysplasia congenita, the authors found a significant correlation between stature of less than seven SDs below the mean, coxa vara, and a decreased posterior atlantodens interval.[19] Myelopathy may develop during childhood, but often does not present until adulthood, and is more common when os odontoideum is present. Occipitocervical fusion to C2 with decompression should be recommended for instability and cord compression.

Thoracolumbar kyphosis can be associated with scoliosis in spondyloepiphyseal dysplasia congenita.[20] An apparent lumbar lordosis is also quite common and is related to the presence of coxa vara.[20] Lower extremity

bones, and vertebral fractures, but these patients generally are less severely affected than those with type III OI. Most patients with type IV OI are ambulatory, but the phenotype is variable.

Type V OI is characterized radiographically by hypertrophic callus after fracture. Ossification of the interosseous membrane between the tibia and fibula and between the radius and ulna is also seen.[15] Patients with type VI OI sustain fractures more often than patients with type IV OI. Sclerae are white or faintly blue, and dentinogenesis imperfecta is uniformly absent.[16] In type VII OI, the phenotype is moderate to severe and is characterized by fractures at birth, bluish sclerae, early deformity of the lower extremities, coxa vara, osteopenia, and rhizomelia.[17] Type VIII OI results from a mutation in the *LEPRE1* gene, and represents a very severe form of OI that is often lethal. It is characterized by white sclerae, severe growth deficiency, extreme skeletal undermineralization, and bulbous metaphyses.

Managing fractures and orthopaedic deformities (such as scoliosis) in OI can be exceedingly challenging. Nonsurgical management of fractures consists of a short course of splinting to minimize the effects of disuse osteoporosis and prevent cyclic fracturing. Realignment osteotomies with intramedullary fixation (com-

Table 2

Disorders Caused by Tumor-Related Genes and Overgrowth Syndromes

Disorder	Gene Defect	Orthopaedic Phenotype/Inheritance Pattern	
Neurofibromatosis	NF1 17q11.2	Autosomal dominant	Scoliosis: idiopathic or dystrophic; overgrowth of the limbs; pseudarthrosis of long bones (usually tibia); benign subcutaneous fibromas; plexiform neurofibromas; dumbbell intraforaminal tumors; dural ectasia
Proteus syndrome	AKT1 14q32.32	Does not run in families	Hemihypertrophy; macrodactyly; superficial soft-tissue tumors; partial gigantism of the hands, feet, or both; plantar surface of the feet with gyriform creases; focal and regional gigantism; scoliosis and kyphosis; large vertebral bodies; angular malformations of the lower extremities (especially genu valgum)

Table 3

The Cardinal Clinical Findings for the Diagnosis of Neurofibromatosis

Six or more café-au-lait spots (larger than 5 mm in diameter in a child or 15 mm in an adult)

Two neurofibromas or a single plexiform neurofibroma

Freckling in the axilla or inguinal region

An optic glioma

Two or more Lisch nodules (hamartoma of the iris)

A distinctive osseous lesion, such as vertebral scalloping or cortical thinning

A first-degree relative with neurofibromatosis type 1

findings include coxa vara, hip flexion contractures, and genu valgum. Proximal femoral extension osteotomies have been described to treat the associated hip flexion contractures and indirectly increase lumbar lordosis.[21] Substantial epiphyseal dysplasia can lead to early arthrosis of the hips and knees.

Disorders Caused by Tumor-Related Genes and Overgrowth Syndromes

Mutations of genes coding for growth and cell proliferation are commonly implicated in neoplastic disorders and syndromes associated with limb overgrowth (Table 2). Overgrowth disorders, unlike other genetically mediated orthopaedic syndromes, often present with asymmetry. Leg length discrepancies and scoliosis are therefore a common aspect of these disorders.

Neurofibromatosis

Neurofibromatosis (NF) is the most common single-gene disorder in humans. This disorder has several forms, of which NF type 1 (NF1) is relevant to orthopaedic surgeons. These children appear normal at birth, with the disease progressing with age. Diagnosis is made based on the presence of at least two of the seven cardinal clinical findings (Table 3).

NF1 results from a mutation in the NF1 gene, coding for neurofibromin, which is a tumor suppressor protein that stimulates the conversion of Ras-GTP to Ras-GDP, which in turn activates the Rat sarcoma (Ras) signaling system. Mutations in the NF1 gene lead to the production of a nonfunctional version of neurofibromin that cannot regulate cell growth and division. As a result, tumors such as neurofibromas can form along nerves throughout the body. Medical therapies such as the farnesyl transferase inhibitors, which block the downstream effects of Ras signaling activation, and the statin inhibitors, which regulate Ras signaling by interfering with its membrane binding, are currently under investigation.[22,23]

In addition to scoliosis and limb overgrowth, pseudarthrosis of the long bones may develop in patients with NF. Scoliosis in NF is categorized as idiopathic or dystrophic. Dystrophic curves have short, sharp, single curves that are kyphotic and typically involve a short segment. These curves are typically early in onset and aggressively progressive. Brace treatment is largely ineffective in dystrophic curves. Surgical intervention can be complicated by the presence of severe dural ectasia and rib head dislocation into the spinal canal. As such, preoperative imaging with MRI is mandatory for patients with dystrophic curves. The risk of paraplegia is high in patients with dystrophic curves, particularly those with severe kyphosis. Nondystrophic curves are managed using standard techniques applicable to idiopathic scoliosis.

Pseudarthrosis of the long bones, most commonly the tibia, is common in NF (Figure 3). Pseudarthrosis of the tibia presents with a characteristic anterolateral bow that is obvious in infancy. The pseudarthrosis site is composed of a hamartoma of undifferentiated mesenchymal cells.[24,25] Early tibial management should be directed at preventing fractures with a clamshell orthosis. Surgical intervention in not warranted until a fracture is established. Although many approaches have been proposed, the common elements leading to suc-

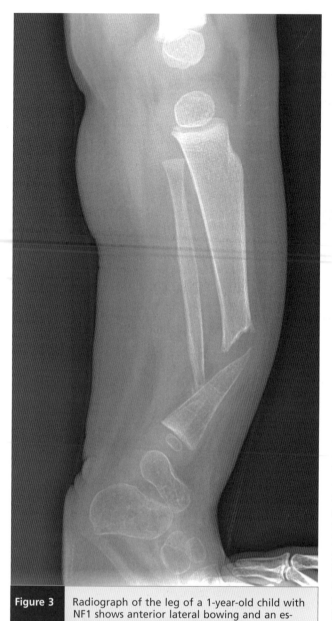

Figure 3   Radiograph of the leg of a 1-year-old child with NF1 shows anterior lateral bowing and an established congenital pseudarthrosis of the tibia. The pseudarthrosis consists of hamartomatous tissue, which require aggressive resection at the time of treatment.

of positron emission tomography holds promise for identifying a malignancy. There is a propensity for the development of other malignancies, such as Wilms' tumor or rhabdomyosarcoma, in children with a neurofibroma.

Proteus Syndrome

Proteus syndrome is a rare condition characterized by overgrowth of the bones, skin, and other tissues and is thought to be the result of an activating mutation in AKT1 kinase in a mosaic pattern (post germline). A characteristic appearance of Proteus syndrome is gyriform creases of the plantar surface of the feet. Symptoms worsen over time. Unlike other overgrowth syndromes, malignancies are not thought to be a part of this disorder. Regional gigantism, scoliosis, and kyphosis are typical. Angular malformations of the lower extremities, especially genu valgum, may be managed by guided growth;[32] however, recurrence of deformities after surgical intervention is common. Scoliosis is likely the result of asymmetric overgrowth, and resultant spinal cord compression can be difficult to treat because of vertebral overgrowth.

Disorders Caused by Defects in Developmentally Important Signaling Pathways

Axial and appendicular skeletal growth occurs through a discrete and tightly regulated series of programmed cell growth, differentiation, and apoptosis. Systemic hormonal regulation (endocrine) and local cytokine regulation (paracrine) can be affected by both intrinsic and extrinsic (environmental) factors. Dysregulation of these processes through either mutations in germline DNA or postfertilization can manifest at any point in this process, either through upregulation or downregulation of cellular activity (Table 4). When genetically mediated, the effects of these processes are generally intrinsic to all growth centers throughout the body and therefore result in generalized growth retardation, with deformities that can continue to evolve with growth.

Achondroplasia and Related Disorders

Mutations in the gene coding for fibroblast growth factor receptor-3 (*FGFR-3*) gene result in upregulation of *FGFR-3* receptor activity and consequently impaired differentiation of physeal cartilage with impaired growth of the proliferative and hypertrophic zones.[33-35]

Depending on the location of the mutation the severity of the skeletal dysplasia can vary, resulting in the conditions of achondroplasia, hypochondroplasia, and thanatophoric dysplasia. These disorders are inherited in an autosomal dominant manner, with sporadic mutations accounting for at least 80% of patients.

Rhizomelic shortening with normal trunk length (the proximal bones are most affected), macrocephaly, frontal bossing, and trident hands are the hallmark of achondroplasia. Hypotonia and gross motor development are delayed in early life but quickly normalize

cessful treatment include aggressive débridement of the hamartoma and adequate stabilization of the tibia and fibula. Intramedullary fixation, free vascularized bone graft, and Ilizarov bone transport have been described.[26-29] Studies using BMPs at the pseudarthrosis site suggest that this modality may help in achieving union.[30] The results of BMP use have demonstrated variable success. Concerns about the use of BMPs in patients with an inherited premalignant condition still exist.[31]

The risk of malignant degeneration of a neurofibroma into a neurofibrosarcoma has been reported to be between 1% and 20%.[7] Distinguishing a malignant lesion from a benign lesion can be difficult, and the use

Table 4

Disorders Caused by Defects in Developmentally Important Signaling Pathways

Disorder	Gene Defect	Orthopaedic Phenotype/Inheritance Pattern	
Achondroplasia and related disorders	*FGFR-3* 4p16.3	Achondroplasia, autosomal dominant, 80% sporadic mutation	Rhizomelic limb shortening with normal trunk length, macrocephaly, frontal bossing, trident hands, foramen magnum and upper cervical stenosis, lumbar spinal stenosis, genu varum with internal tibial torsion, ligamentous laxity at the knee and ankles, flexion contractures of the elbows, and subluxation of the radial heads
		Hypochondroplasia, autosomal dominant	Similar to those of achondroplasia but are less severe
		Thanatophoric dysplasia, autosomal dominant	Severe and almost always fatal before age 2 years; severe rhizomelic shortening, platyspondylysis, protuberant abdomen, small thoracic cavity, and cardiorespiratory failure
Pseudoachondroplasia	*COMP* 19p13.1	Autosomal dominant	Radiographically detectable delays in epiphyseal ossification; rhizomelic short stature and ligamentous laxity with normal facial features; scoliosis and thoracolumbar kyphosis common; high prevalence of C1-C2 instability and varus or valgus knees.
Camptomelic dysplasia	*SOX9* 17q23	Autosomal dominant	Severe short-limbed dwarfism; sometimes fatal; bowing of the long bones, primarily the tibia and femur; laryngotracheomalacia and restricted chest size; kyphosis and scoliosis; plagiocephaly; a cleft palate; micrognathia; renal and cardiac defects; and sex reversal (phenotypic females have an XY karyotype)
Cleidocranial dysplasia	*RUNX2* 6p21	Autosomal dominant	Intramembranous ossification (clavicles, cranium, pelvis), hypoplasia or absence of the clavicles, mild short stature, a high palate, abnormal permanent tooth development, widening of the symphysis pubis, coxa vara, short femoral neck, and lumbar spondylolysis

through childhood. Foramen magnum stenosis with cervicomedullary spinal cord compression, is common in infancy, with progressive enlargement of the foramen magnum with age. Severe foramen magnum stenosis is believed to result in central sleep apnea, which combined with upper airway obstruction and mild restrictive lung disease can result in sudden death during infancy. Screening polysomnography and MRI of the occipital cervical junction are essential in avoiding this complication. Thoracolumbar junction kyphosis generally resolves with the attainment of independent ambulation, but a small percentage of patients with residual vertebral body wedging and delayed development ultimately require surgical treatment. Lumbar spinal stenosis is also common, typically becoming symptomatic in the third to fourth decade of life, but it can be symptomatic in a skeletally immature patient. Children with residual kyphosis also can manifest symptoms of spinal stenosis. Surgical decompression should be accompanied by instrumentation and fusion in these patients because progressive sagittal deformity ensues with continued growth after a laminectomy.[36]

The lower extremity malalignment in achondroplasia is genu varum with associated internal tibial torsion (Figure 4), as well as ligamentous laxity at the knees, which is accentuated in slight knee flexion. With few exceptions, genu varum in achondroplasia is asymptomatic and does not lead to precocious arthritis. Genu varum in achondroplasia rarely requires treatment; however, an osteotomy may be required with reduced function caused by lateral leg or foot pain (which must be differentiated from pain of spinal or radicular origin). In the upper extremities, flexion contractures of the elbows and subluxation of the radial heads are present. Humeral lengthening is indicated for children lacking the ability to independently engage in personal

6: Pediatrics

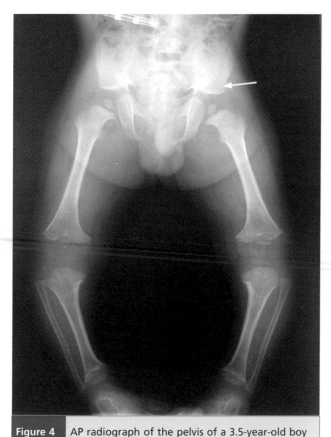

Figure 4   AP radiograph of the pelvis of a 3.5-year-old boy with achondroplasia. Note the genu varum and typical champagne glass pelvis (arrow).

hygiene because of rhizomelic shortening. Nonorthopaedic manifestations of achondroplasia include difficulty with weight control, sleep apnea, recurrent otitis media, and hydrocephalus. These patients have normal intelligence, and life expectancy is not significantly diminished.

The mutation for hypochondroplasia resides in a different location within the *FGFR-3* gene than in achondroplasia, resulting in the differing phenotype. Hypochondroplasia presents with findings similar to those of achondroplasia but presents later because they are less severe. These include short stature, small hands, lumbar stenosis, and genu varum.[37] Thanatophoric dysplasia is severe and almost always is fatal before the patient reaches 2 years of age. It is characterized by severe rhizomelic shortening, platyspondyly, a protuberant abdomen, and a small thoracic cavity that is responsible for cardiorespiratory failure.

Pseudoachondroplasia

Pseudoachondroplasia is an autosomal dominant disorder resulting from a defect in the cartilage oligomeric matrix protein, which disrupts normal physeal extracellular matrix formation.[38] This disruption results in radiographically detectable delays in epiphyseal ossifica-

tion. The hallmarks of pseudoachondroplasia, like achondroplasia, are rhizomelic short stature and ligamentous laxity but with normal facial features. Scoliosis and thoracolumbar kyphosis are common in this condition.[39] The high prevalence of C1-C2 instability is of primary importance in pseudoachondroplasia.[21,40] Substantial C1-C2 instability is common in pseudoachondroplasia. Screening flexion and extension lateral C-spine radiographs are recommended in this patient population. As is the case with other skeletal dysplasias, routine radiographic examination is warranted, and occipitocervical fusion is indicated when radiographic evidence of instability or myelopathy is present.

Lower extremity deformities can manifest as either varus or valgus (or both) malalignment of the knees. Maintaining deformity correction in skeletally immature patients can be exceedingly difficult and often requires revision surgeries. Given the propensity for precocious arthritis in this group, correction of malalignment is believed to be important to preserve long-term function.

Camptomelic Dysplasia

Diaphyseal bowing of the long bones, primarily the tibia and femur, are the hallmarks of camptomelic dysplasia, whereas the absence of thoracic pedicles on plain radiographs is diagnostic. Plagiocephaly, cleft palate, micrognathia, renal and cardiac defects, and sex reversal (phenotypic females have an XY karyotype) are common in this disorder. Camptomelic dysplasia is the result of a mutation in the *SOX9* gene, which is critical to the ossification of long-bone cartilage anlagen during fetal development. Endochondral ossification is normal. Defective tracheal cartilage and restricted chest size often result in respiratory failure and death during the neonatal period. Progressive spinal deformity (kyphosis and scoliosis) is common and further compromises pulmonary function.[41] For those children who survive past infancy, aggressive management of spinal deformities has been recommended.[42] Treatment of spinal deformities may be complicated by the presence of hydromyelia and diastematomyelia. Neurologic complications and pseudarthrosis may also make the treatment of these complicated patients difficult.[43]

Cleidocranial Dysplasia

The gene mutation in cleidocranial dysplasia is in runt-related transcription factor 2 (RUNX2) and is inherited in an autosomal dominant fashion. RUNX2 is an osteoblast-specific transcription factor that regulates osteoblast differentiation.[44] A failure of the development of membranous bones is manifested as a deficiency of the clavicles and pelvis as well as delayed closure of the cranial fontanels. As a result, the shoulders appear narrow and sloping and can be brought close together in front of the body. Mild short stature, coxa vara, a high palate, and abnormal permanent tooth development also are present, with lumbar spondylolysis occurring in 24% of patients.[45]

Table 5

Disorders Caused by Multiple Genes and Chromosome Abnormalities

Disorder	Gene Defect	Inheritance Pattern	Orthopaedic Phenotype
Multiple epiphyseal dysplasia	COMP 19p13.1 COL9A1 6q12-q14 COL9A2 1p33-p32 COL9A3 20q13.3 MATN3 2p24-p23	Autosomal dominant	Mild short stature, genu valgum, and precocious arthritis (hips and knees); delayed ossification of the epiphyses or osteochondritis dissecans– type lesions (multiple)
	SLC26A2 5q31-q34	Autosomal recessive	Clubfoot, cleft palate, clinodactyly, and characteristics of diastrophic dysplasia; double layer patella on lateral views
Down syndrome	Trisomy 21		Hypotonia, joint hyperlaxity, atlantoaxial and occipitoatlantal instability, short stature, a flat face, mental retardation, short and broad hands, hip dysplasia, patellofemoral instability, flatfoot, and hallux valgus; congenital heart defect and thyroid dysfunction
Turner syndrome	Partial absence of one of the X chromosomes		Short stature; wide and webbed neck; low-set ears and hairline; cubitus and genu valgum; swollen hands and feet; scoliosis; chest that is broad, flat, and shield shaped; diabetes; weight gain; osteoporosis; a high incidence of fractures; congenital heart disease; kidney abnormalities; cognitive deficits related to memory, mathematics, and visuospatial discrimination; inadequate production of estrogen
Noonan syndrome	PTPN11 12q24 SOS1 2p21 KRAS 12p12.1 NRAS 1p13.2 RAF1 3p25 BRAF 7q34 SHOC2 10q25		Short stature, congenital cervical spine defects, low-set ears and hairline, scoliosis, and pectus carinatum or excavatum type I; Arnold-Chiari malformation in some patients
Prader-Willi syndrome	Deletion of 5q11-q13 of paternal origin		Obesity, somnolence, increased appetite, scoliosis (90%), small hands and feet
Angelman syndrome	Deletion of 5q11-q13 of maternal origin		Mental deficiency, puppet-like gait, paroxysms of laughter, and scoliosis

Disorders Caused by Multiple Genes or Chromosome Abnormalities

Many genetically mediated disorders exist in which a single gene mutation does not account for an ascribed phenotype. These disorders may result from deletion, addition, or translocation of large chromosomal fragments (Table 5). Historically, these disorders have been diagnosed by karyotype analysis or fluorescent in situ hybridization techniques. More recently, microarray comparative genomic hybridization has been effectively used to detect and localize the presence or absence of specific DNA sequences on chromosomes. For smaller and yet undiscovered genetically mediated defects (which may involve more than one gene mutation), the development of exome and full genome sequencing may soon offer clinicians extremely powerful tools to diagnose and ultimately understand the molecular basis of many disorders.

Multiple Epiphyseal Dysplasias

Multiple epiphyseal dysplasias manifest as both autosomal dominant and autosomal recessive forms. The dominant forms appear to result from five different possible gene mutations (COMP, COL9A1, COL9A2, COL9A3, and MATN3). Clinically, these patients present with mild short stature (often presenting in late childhood); genu valgum; and precocious arthritis, which is most pronounced in the hips and knees. Radiographically, there is delayed ossification of the epiphyses or the presence of osteochondritis dissecans– type lesions. When multiple sites of osteochondritis dissecans are present, Stickler syndrome also should be considered in the differential diagnosis. The recessive

6: Pediatrics

form of multiple epiphyseal dysplasia has been attributed to mutations in the *SLC26A2* gene. Compared with the dominant forms, up to 50% of affected individuals with the recessive form have an abnormal finding at birth (such as clubfoot, cleft palate, or clinodactyly) and have characteristics of diastrophic dysplasia. Radiographically, this form of multiple epiphyseal dysplasia is typified by a double-layer patella on lateral views.

Down Syndrome

Down syndrome occurs in the presence of part or all of a third copy of chromosome 21 (trisomy 21). Down syndrome is the most common chromosomal disorder, occurring in approximately 1 in 700 births. Hypotonia and joint hyperlaxity, particularly involving the upper cervical spine (atlantoaxial and occipitoatlantal instability), the hips, and the patellofemoral joint constitute most of the orthopaedic manifestations of this disorder. Other clinical concerns for these children include short stature, flatfoot and hallux valgus, congenital heart defects, and thyroid dysfunction.

Acetabular dysplasia or hip dislocation occurs between the ages of 2 and 10 years and is found in approximately 5% of patients. Treatment of hip dislocation in Down syndrome should include capsulorrhaphy, with pelvic and femoral varus osteotomies. Slipped capital femoral epiphysis and osteonecrosis also can occur. A patient with Down syndrome and slipped capital femoral epiphysis should undergo pinning of both the symptomatic and the contralateral hip.

Orthopaedic surgeons are often asked to provide an evaluation for clearance to participate in the Special Olympics.[46,47] Activities that put the cervical spine at risk for injury are to be avoided, including gymnastics, diving, and any tumbling activities. Radiographic evaluation for cervical spine instability should be interpreted with caution. Motion up to 10 mm between flexion and extension lateral radiographs of the cervical spine is considered normal in these children. Surgical intervention should be reserved for children with neurologic symptoms rather than based on radiographic criteria because of the high rate of surgical complications.

Turner Syndrome

Turner syndrome occurs with a complete or partial absence of an X chromosome (monosomy X). It often presents with a mosaic distribution of cells.[48] Orthopaedic abnormalities include elbow and knee deformities, Madelung deformity of the wrist, and short stature. Other physical findings include a wide, webbed neck; low-set ears and hairline; and a shield-shaped (broad) chest.[49] Osteoporosis and a high incidence of fractures have also been reported. Girls with Turner syndrome typically experience gonadal dysfunction with amenorrhea and sterility. Further clinical concerns for these patients include diabetes, weight gain, congenital heart disease, and kidney abnormalities. Learning difficulties are common in Turner syndrome, specifi-

cally with regard to memory, mathematics, and visuospatial discrimination.

Noonan Syndrome

Noonan syndrome, historically known as the "male version of Turner syndrome," is a relatively common congenital disorder that affects girls and boys equally and is clinically and genetically distinct from Turner syndrome. The following genes are known to cause Noonan syndrome: *PTPN11* (50%), *RAF1* (3-17%) *SOS1* (10%), *KRAS* (1%), *NRAS* (unknown), or *BRAF* (unknown).[50] Orthopaedic manifestations of Noonan syndrome include short stature, congenital cervical spine fusions, scoliosis, joint laxity or contractures, and scapular winging. Congenital heart defects, impaired blood clotting, hypotonia, and learning disabilities are also part of Noonan syndrome. Joint or muscle pain, often with no identifiable cause, is typical. Type I Arnold-Chiari malformation in Noonan syndrome has been described.[51,52]

Prader-Willi Syndrome and Angelman Syndrome

Partial deletion of chromosome 15, which includes a series of seven genes, is the cause of Prader-Willi syndrome (PWS). Paternal expression is ensured by the process of imprinting (an epigenetic process that involves DNA methylation and histone modifications to achieve monoallelic gene expression without altering the genetic sequence). The maternal copy is imprinted and thus silenced, whereas the mutated paternal copy is expressed and not functional. In Angelman syndrome, affected maternal genes are expressed, whereas the paternal genes are silenced in the same region. The orthopaedic manifestations include scoliosis, often early in onset; hip dysplasia; and joint hyperlaxity.[53,54] Individuals with PWS have short stature, are obese with abnormal body composition, have reduced fat free mass, lean body mass, and total energy expenditure. Patients with PWS are at increased perioperative risk because of hypercapnia and hypoxia, obstructive sleep apnea, thick secretions, and a exaggerated response to sedatives. Growth hormone therapy has been shown to improve weight and behavioral issues, and increases bone mineral density.[55] The effect of growth hormone therapy on scoliosis is unclear, but it does not appear to adversely affect the development of scoliosis.[56]

Disorders Caused by Defects in Processing Proteins (Enzymes)

Enzymes catalyze the physiologic molecular processes required for normal cellular and tissue function. Mutations to the genes encoding enzymes required for glycoprotein degradation and transport result in the accumulation of these substances, cytokine dysregulation, cell dysfunction, and ultimately cell death (Table 6). These mutations can have a wide variety of effects on cells, resulting in a broad range of abnormalities in cell func-

Table 6

Disorders Caused by Defects in Processing Proteins (Enzymes)

Disorder	Gene Defect	Syndrome	Orthopaedic Phenotype/Inheritance Pattern	
Mucopolysaccharidoses	*IDUA* 4p16.3	Hurler	Type I, autosomal recessive	Thoracolumbar kyphosis, scoliosis, progressive hip subluxation and genu valgum, finger triggering, and carpal tunnel syndrome
		Scheie		Joint stiffness, thoracolumbar kyphosis, scoliosis, progressive hip subluxation, genu valgum, finger triggering, and carpal tunnel syndrome
	IDS Xq28	Hunter	Type II	Spinal deformities, carpal tunnel syndrome, ankle equinus contractures, and hip dysplasia
	GNS 12q14 *HGSNAT* 8p11.1 *NAGLU* 17q21 *SGSH* 17q25.3	Sanfilippo	Type III, autosomal recessive	Ankle equinus contractures, hip dysplasia, and scoliosis
	GALNS 16q24.3 *GLB1* 3p21.33	Morquio	Type IV, A and B autosomal recessive	Short trunk and ligamentous laxity, significant genu valgum, progressive acetabular dysplasia, odontoid hypoplasia or aplasia, C1-C2 instability, platyspondylysis, and thoracic kyphosis
	ARSB 5q14.1	Maroteaux-Lamy	Type VI, autosomal recessive	Stenosis at the occipitocervical junction, hypoplasia of the C1 arch posteriorly, thoracolumbar kyphosis, osteonecrosis, and femoral head resorption
Diastrophic dysplasia	*SLC26A2* 5q31-q34	Autosomal recessive		Rhizomelic dwarfism, multiple joint contractures, severe clubfeet, patellar dislocation, joint instability, hitchhiker's thumb, cervical kyphosis, severe kyphoscoliosis, hypoplastic vertebrae, and quadriplegia spina bifida occulta (75%)

tion and a wide range of clinical findings. Medical treatments have been developed to replace the defective enzyme in many of these disorders. Such treatments often can arrest but not reverse the skeletal manifestations of the disorder. Orthopaedists are treating an increasing number of patients with these disorders. Because of early diagnoses, appropriate medical treatments can be applied, with increased life expectancies as a result.

Mucopolysaccharidoses

The mucopolysaccharidoses (MPSs) are a family of autosomal recessive disorders characterized by single gene defects resulting in abnormal degradation and accumulation of glycosaminoglycans (GAGs) within the lysosome[57] (Table 7). Ten distinct enzyme deficiencies are described for the six commonly recognized MPS syndromes (MPS type VIII has been reported in only one individual). For each enzyme deficiency, there is a spectrum of clinical severity, which depends on the relative dysfunction caused by the gene mutation. All forms of MPS result in progressive disability. The more severe forms of MPS are typified by relentless multiorgan dysfunction and early death. For those forms with heparan

sulfate accumulation (MPS types I, II, and III) this may include variable neurocognitive decline. The classic clinical findings for patients with MPS include spinal instability and stenosis, hepatosplenomegaly, recurrent otitis media, hearing loss, obstructive sleep apnea, cardiac valve dysfunction, umbilical and inguinal hernias, recurrent respiratory infections, and clouding of the corneas. Treatment by hematopoietic stem cell transplantation and enzyme replacement therapy has resulted in substantial improvements in cardiac, respiratory, and neurologic function and has subsequently improved overall function and longevity.[58,59]

Mucopolysaccharidosis Type I

Hurler syndrome represents the most severe form of MPS type 1, whereas Scheie syndrome represents the mild end of the clinical spectrum. Hurler-Scheie is the intermediate form. Children with Hurler syndrome suffer from progressive cognitive decline, diffuse skeletal disease (dysostosis multiplex), organomegaly, cardiopulmonary disease, and joint contractures. The average life expectancy is less then 10 years when the condition is not treated. The Scheie form is characterized by joint stiffness and normal cognition. The diagnosis usually is

6: Pediatrics

Table 7

The Mucopolysaccharidoses

Designation	Syndrome	Enzyme Defect	Substance Stored	Inheritance Pattern
MPS IH MPS 1HS MPS 1S	Hurler Hurler-Scheie Scheie	α-l-iduronidase	DS, HS	Autosomal recessive
MPS II	Hunter	Iduronidase-2-sulfatase	DS, HS	X-linked recessive
MPS IIIA	Sanfilippo A	Heparin-sulfatase (sulfamidase)	HS	Autosomal recessive
MPS IIIB	Sanfilippo B	α-N-acetylglucosamidase	HS	Autosomal recessive
MPS IIIC	Sanfilippo C	Acetyl-CoA: α-glucosaminide- N-acetyltransferase	HS	Autosomal recessive
MPS IIID	Sanfilippo D	Glucosamine 6-sulfatase	HS	Autosomal recessive
MPS IVA	Morquio A	N-acetyl galactosamine-6-sulfate sulfatase	KS, CS	Autosomal recessive
MPS IVB	Morquio B	β-d-galactosidase	KS, CS	Autosomal recessive
MPS VI	Maroteaux-Lamy	Arylsulfatase B, N-acetylgalactosamine- 4-sulfatase	DS	Autosomal recessive
MPS VII	Sly	β-d-glucuronidase	CS, HS, DS	Autosomal recessive
MPS VIII		Glucosamine-6-sulfatase	CS, HS	Autosomal recessive

CS = chondroitin sulfate, DS = dermatan sulfate, HS = heparan sulfate, KS = keratan sulfate, MPS = mucopolysaccharidosis.

made during the teenage years, and patients have a normal life expectancy. Hematopoietic stem cell transplantation is used to treat the Hurler form, but its effect on skeletal manifestations is limited.[60] Musculoskeletal deformities, including thoracolumbar kyphosis, scoliosis, progressive hip subluxation, and genu valgum, develop after stem cell transplantation and often require surgical treatment.[61] The accumulation of GAGs in flexor tendon tenosynovium can cause finger triggering and carpal tunnel syndrome.

Mucopolysaccharidosis Types II and III

Skeletal manifestations tend to be milder in Hunter syndrome (MPS type II) and Sanfilippo syndrome (MPS type III). Although all patients with Sanfilippo syndrome suffer from persistent and pervasive neurocognitive decline, Hunter syndrome patients may present anywhere along the spectrum; those with no cognitive involvement to extremely severe involvement. Spinal deformities may warrant surgical intervention. Carpal tunnel syndrome is almost universal in Hunter syndrome. Ankle equinus contractures are also common in both syndromes, with treatment being guided by the expected functional benefits. Hip dysplasia is mild in these disorders and typically does not require surgical intervention.[62,63]

Mucopolysaccharidosis Type IV

There are two known types of Morquio syndrome (MPS IVA and IVB). Both types are caused by enzyme defects involved in the degradation of keratan sulfate. An affected child has a short trunk and ligamentous laxity. There is substantial genu valgum, which is aggravated by the ligamentous laxity. Guided growth is an attractive treatment option for lower extremity deformities, but there is a high risk for deformity recurrence after implant removal. Femoral head collapse and cartilage delamination results in precocious arthrosis. The hips develop progressive acetabular dysplasia and subluxation. In young patients, radiographs demonstrate a small femoral ossific nucleus. but MRI or arthrography reveal a normally sized cartilaginous femoral head. Total joint arthroplasty is effective but technically challenging in these patients.[64] Radiographs of the cervical spine demonstrate odontoid hypoplasia, with C1-C2 instability commonly seen on flexion-extension films. An extradural, fibrocartilaginous mass behind the odontoid process can contribute to spinal cord compression. Prophylactic C1-C2 fusion has been suggested by some authors; however, many patients with Morquio syndrome never develop instability.[7] Platyspondyly is found throughout the spine, typically resulting in a gentle thoracic kyphosis (**Figure 5**). Progressive, angular deformities at the cord level should be surgically stabilized. Longevity is typically into the fourth or fifth decade in the classic form of the disease and much later in the less severe, or nonclassic, disease. Death is usually the result of cardiorespiratory disease, but disease of the upper cervical spine accounts for most of the disability experienced by these patients.

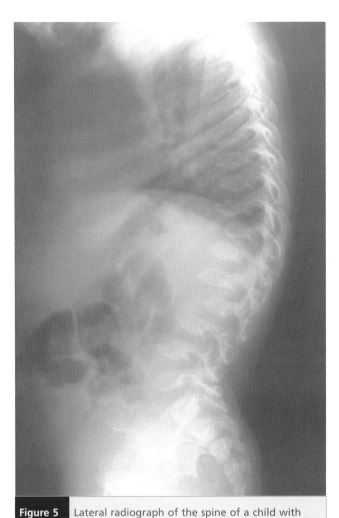

Figure 5 Lateral radiograph of the spine of a child with Morquio syndrome. Note the generalized platy-spondylysis with anterior beaking. More focal hypoplasia at the thoracolumbar junction is seen in other forms of MPS.

Mucopolysaccharidosis Type VI

Maroteaux-Lamy syndrome presents with a spectrum of musculoskeletal involvement. Cognitive function is normal. Stenosis at the occipitocervical junction is common and is usually caused by hypoplasia of the C1 arch posteriorly. In addition, the dura in MPS type VI can become extremely thickened and the intervertebral disks become prominent, further contributing to spinal cord compression. Thoracolumbar kyphosis occurs, but it typically does not require surgery. The hips commonly subluxate, such as in Morquio syndrome, and can deteriorate secondary to inflammatory osteonecrosis and femoral head resorption.

Diastrophic Dysplasia

Diastrophic dysplasia is an autosomal recessive, rhizomelic dwarfism associated with multiple severe and, at times, life-threatening spinal deformities.[65,66] Although diastrophic dysplasia is not a true enzyme deficiency, this disorder is the result of a sulfate transporter protein defect, localized to the *SLC26A2* (solute carrier

family 26, member 2) gene.[39] The result is similar to the storage effects seen in MPS. Clinically, these patients present with multiple joint contractures, severe clubfeet, patellar dislocation, and joint instability; the presence of the classic hitchhiker's thumb and cauliflower ears are pathognomonic for the condition.[21] Normal intelligence is associated with diastrophic dwarfism.

Cervical kyphosis occurs in 25% to 40% of children with diastrophic dysplasia, is present in early infancy, and tends to resolve spontaneously in most children by 6 years of age.[65-67] Severe kyphosis (> 60°) associated with hypoplastic vertebrae often progresses. Bracing has been recommended in young children for kyphosis; however, good outcomes likely represent the benign natural history of this condition in some children. Severe complications can be expected with surgical treatment, with multiple reports of quadriplegia and cardiopulmonary failure. Traditionally, anterior stabilization and posterior stabilization have been recommended; however, no reports of long-term follow-up exist. When planning their surgical approach, treating surgeons should be aware of the high incidence (up to 75%) of spina bifida occulta within the cervical spine;[68] good preoperative imaging, including multiplanar CT and MRI, is warranted.

Scoliosis is the hallmark deformity of diastrophic dysplasia, with a reported incidence of the disorder in 37% to 88% of affected individuals.[65,66,68,69] The most common curve pattern is a double thoracic scoliosis with hyperkyphosis. Curves often present early, before age 5 years; are prone to severe progression; become extremely rigid; and adversely affect pulmonary function. After age 10 years, trunk height usually does not develop in children with diastrophic dwarfism. Early intervention for curves greater 50° is recommended regardless of the patient's age.[69]

Contracture-Related Syndromes

Contractures are common in a variety of orthopaedic conditions and are the most prominent phenotypic feature of several syndromes (**Table 8**). These syndromes have a wide variety of etiologies, including mutations that cause developmental problems, mutations that dysregulate muscle function, and fetal environmental causes. Many of these syndromes are associated with muscle dysfunction. For example, distal arthrogryposis is caused by mutations that disrupt fast-twitch muscle fiber activity. There is some overlap in phenotype between these conditions and some of the myopathies. Despite their different etiologies, these disorders have similar management guidelines. Arthrogryposis is a physical finding, not a diagnosis, in a large group of disorders characterized by joint contractures present at birth. These disorders can be considered as contracture syndromes and grouped into three general categories, each of which can be represented by a prototypic disease.

6: Pediatrics

Table 8

Contracture-Related Syndromes

Disorder	Gene Defect	Orthopaedic Phenotype/Inheritance Pattern	
Arthrogryposis multiplex congenita	*CHRNG* 2q37.1	Autosomal recessive	Shoulders adducted and internally rotated; elbow more often extended than flexed; wrist severely flexed with ulnar deviation; hips are flexed, abducted, and externally rotated; knees are typically in extension, although flexion is possible; clubfeet; scoliosis; and hip dislocation
Larsen syndrome	*FLNB* 3p14.3	Autosomal dominant / Autosomal recessive	Multiple congenital dislocations of large joints; flat face; ligamentous laxity; kyphosis and abnormal cervical spine segmentation, with instability; and structural abnormality in the cervical spine
Distal arthrogryposis	*MYBPC1* 12q23.2 *TPM2* 9p13	Type I autosomal dominant	Fixed hand contractures and foot deformities; good overall function
	MYH3 17p13.1	Type II, Freeman-Sheldon	Fixed hand contractures and foot deformities
Pterygia syndromes	*CHRNG* 2q37.1	Multiple pterygium syndrome, autosomal recessive	Web across every flexion crease in the extremities, most prominently across the popliteal space, the elbow, and the axilla; webbing across the neck; webbed fingers; vertical talus; and significant spinal deformity
	IRF6 1q32.3-q41	Popliteal pterygium syndrome, autosomal dominant	Born with webs of skin on the backs of the legs across the knee joint, syndactyly, and triangular folds of skin over the nails of the large toes

Arthrogryposis Multiplex Congenita

Arthrogryposis is defined as the presence of contractures involving more than two joints at more than two levels. Arthrogryposis multiplex congenita (AMC) or amyoplasia is the best known and most involved form of arthrogryposis. Although the etiology of AMC is unknown, studies have shown that some mothers of children with AMC have serum antibodies that inhibit fetal acetylcholine receptor function, and the number of anterior horn cells in the spinal cord is decreased. The appearance of the neonate's upper extremities is similar to that found in brachial plexus palsy and spinal muscular atrophy (shoulders adducted and internally rotated, with the elbow extended, and the wrist is severely flexed, with ulnar deviation). In the lower extremities, the hips are flexed, abducted, and externally rotated, with the knees typically in extension, (although flexion is possible). Clubfeet are common. Unlike paralytic disorders, however, joint motion is restricted as a result of contractures. Ambulatory potential is limited in patients with AMC. The presence of knee flexion deformities results in decreased ambulatory potential compared with those with extension deformities.[70] Up to 25% of affected patients are nonambulatory, and many others are household ambulators.

The goals of managing AMC are to optimize lower limb alignment and stability for ambulation and upper extremity motion for independent self-care. Outcomes appear to be improved if surgery is performed at ages younger than 4 to 6 years, when adaptive intra-articular changes can occur. Hip dislocation is common, but treatment is controversial. Although range of motion of the hips is important for normal gait, it is unclear whether hip reduction significantly improves motion and, therefore, ambulatory ability. Closed reduction is rarely, if ever, successful. A medial approach to open reduction has yielded excellent results, and, as a result, at least one early attempt at surgical reduction of bilaterally dislocated hips may be worthwhile.

Flexion and extension deformities of the knee are commonly present in AMC, with flexion deformities being more common. As mentioned previously, waling ability, as measured by gait analysis, is significantly better in children born with extension deformities compared with those with flexion deformities, particularly when knee flexion exceeds 30°. Posterior soft-tissue releases initially improve range of motion, but the flexion contractures typically recur, with loss of motion and function.[70-72] Posterior release may be repeated later, and often supracondylar extension osteotomies of the femur can be helpful to correct residual deformity. Femoral shortening is often required in addition to soft-tissue releases or extension osteotomies to facilitate safe and effective correction. Anterior growth modulation plates of the distal femur may also be used to correct milder, residual flexion deformities of the knee.

Like other joints, clubfoot deformities in AMC are extremely rigid, traditionally requiring extensive surgical release. Ponseti casting, however, has demonstrated good results in several studies and should be considered

6: Pediatrics

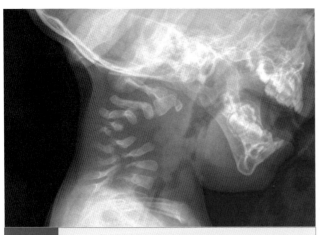

Figure 6 Severe cervical kyphosis is seen in a child with Larsen syndrome. Early posterior stabilization is recommended to prevent progression and associated neurologic compromise.

as the first line of treatment.[73-75] More recalcitrant deformities may still require limited surgical release, osteotomies, or treatment with external frame fixators.

Splinting may be useful to treat hand deformities in young children with AMC. Surgical releases of the upper extremities are typically not warranted. It has been suggested that 90° of elbow flexion is the minimum desired, such that if both elbows are involved, surgery to address inadequate flexion should be done on one side with augmentation of elbow flexion by triceps tendon transfer.[76]

Complex and rigid spinal deformities develop in approximately one third of patients with AMC. C-shaped neuromuscular patterns are the most common, but double and triple major curves associated with significant kyphosis can also occur. Like other neuromuscular disorders, surgery is indicated for progressive curves that interfere with balance or function. For severe deformities, a course of gravity halo traction may be considered. Because some patients have regained ambulatory function after surgical correction of their spinal deformity, the loss of walking ability associated with progressive scoliosis has also been suggested as an indication for surgical intervention.[7]

Larsen Syndrome

Mutations in the *FLNB* gene, which codes for the filamin B protein, is the most common cause of Larsen syndrome as well as the more severe atelosteogenesis type 3. These disorders are inherited in an autosomal dominant manner. Autosomal recessive Larsen syndrome results from a deficiency of carbohydrate sulfotransferase 3.[77] A mosaic phenotype also has been reported, which results in asymmetric disease.[78] The common features of Larsen syndrome are multiple congenital dislocations of large joints, a characteristic flat face, and ligamentous laxity, with the autosomal dominant form typically presenting with a milder phenotype than the autosomal recessive form. A duplicate os calcis

on a lateral radiograph of the foot is highly suggestive of the diagnosis, whereas a double-layer patella can be found on lateral radiographs of the knee in the autosomal recessive form.

Knee extension deformities are common in Larsen syndrome. The associated ligamentous laxity may mean that the knee remains unstable after reduction. Bracing or extra-articular reconstruction of the anterior cruciate ligament may be beneficial in patients with residual knee laxity.[79] Hip dislocations are also common in Larsen syndrome, despite a relatively normal-appearing acetabulum. There is typically good range of motion and little functional loss associated with hip dislocation in Larsen syndrome. The hips are usually irreducible by nonsurgical management and often have poor results (redislocation) with surgical reduction. Consequently, any treatment of hip dislocations in Larsen syndrome is controversial.

Cervical instability, anterolisthesis, and kyphosis are common in Larsen syndrome and are often recognizable during infancy. Kyphosis results from hypoplasia of the vertebral bodies, with dissociation between the vertebral bodies and the posterior arch (Figure 6). Screening of the cervical spine by serial radiographs and careful neurologic examination are critical during the first year of life. Myelopathy is common, and quadriplegia, including death, has been reported as a result of these deformities. Posterior stabilization is warranted in the presence of myelopathy and may allow the kyphotic deformity to correct with growth. With severe kyphosis, anterior and posterior decompression and fusion may be required.[80,81]

Distal Arthrogryposis

In contrast with other forms of arthrogryposis, distal arthrogryposis is characterized by involvement of the hands and the feet; the more proximal joints are not involved. There are two main types of distal arthrogryposis. Type I is characterized by isolated hand and foot anomalies, and patients with type II, or Freeman Shelton syndrome, present with facial abnormalities and cognitive delay. Type I can be caused by mutations in the *TPM2* gene. These mutations result in abnormal levels of β-tropomyosin, a protein important for fast-twitch muscle fibers. Type II is caused by mutations in an isoform of troponin I that is involved in the troponin-tropomyosin complex of fast-twitch myofibers. These disorders cause abnormal activity of fast-twitch muscle fibers and are thought to result in distal arthrogryposis.

Children with distal arthrogryposis have much less severe deformities than those with classic arthrogryposis. The hands usually function quite well despite the contractures. Hand surgery can improve function and usually involves lengthening of the flexor pollicis longus and rebalancing of the thumb extensor. Foot deformity can be quite severe; clubfoot deformities are typical. These deformities can be treated with the Ponseti technique, including serial manipulation and casting. Surgical releases and foot osteotomies are often re-

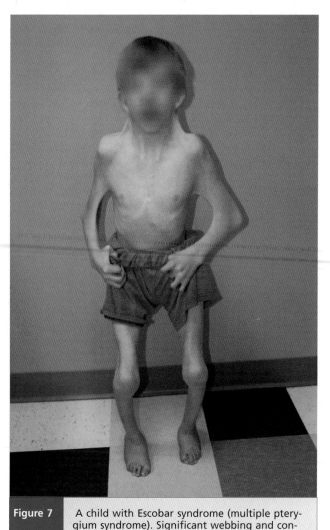

Figure 7   A child with Escobar syndrome (multiple pterygium syndrome). Significant webbing and contractures at multiple joints are seen.

quired. The outcome of treatment is better in the distal arthrogrypotic than the classic arthrogrypotic syndromes.

Pterygia Syndromes
The most common pterygia syndromes are multiple pterygia syndrome, or Escobar syndrome, and popliteal pterygia syndrome.

Multiple pterygia syndrome is characterized by webbing at all flexion creases in the extremities, most prominent in the popliteal space, the elbow, and the axilla (Figure 7). Webbing can be seen extending from the ear to the shoulders and across the neck laterally. Despite webbing, function is usually very good. The patient's independence and mobility depends on the magnitude of the lower extremity webbing and joint motion. Spinal deformity resulting in restrictive and obstructive pulmonary problems can be severe. A common associated foot deformity is vertical talus.

Popliteal pterygium syndrome is the result of mutations in the gene encoding interferon regulatory factor-6. Patients can have cleft lip and palate, intraoral

adhesions, and occasionally fibrous bands that cross the perineum and can distort the genitalia. The popliteal web can be extensive, running from the ischium to the calcaneus and causing a severe knee flexion deformity. Knee flexion contractures can be treated surgically, but it is extremely important to understand the web anatomy. A superficial fibrous band with an overlying muscle runs from the ischium to the calcaneus and is called the calcaneoischiadicus muscle. The sciatic nerve is extremely superficial just under the fibrous band, with the popliteal artery and vein lying deeper. Early surgery is recommended to avoid vascular shortening and adaptive changes in the joint. Lengthening of the skin using plastic surgical procedures and femoral shortening, extension osteotomies can improve knee flexion contractures. Care must be taken to avoid injury to the sciatic nerve. Gradual elongation of the web using fixators has been attempted, but recurrence is common.

Summary

This chapter reviews skeletal dysplasias, connective tissue abnormalities, and other genetic disorders. There is a wide variety of these genetically mediated conditions, with significant orthopaedic manifestations involving the spine and extremities that can reduce function and cause early mortality.

Key Study Points

- Organization of the extensive information available on these disorders is difficult; patterns of involvement can help organize the content. For example, the *FGFR-3* disorders (thanatophoric dysplasia, severe achondroplasia with acanthosis nigricans, achondroplasia, and hypochondroplasia) share similar genotypic and phenotypic characteristics and can be arranged in order of lessening severity.

- Identification of the severe skeletal abnormalities that can result in catastrophic injury that may result in significant loss of function is important. These abnormalities typically occur as a result of spine instability with or without stenosis. All children with a skeletal dysplasia, with the exception of achondroplasia, require flexion/extension upper cervical spine radiographs to assess for instability.

- The clinician should focus on treatments that improve function and reduce pain rather than those that result solely in improvement of a deformity.

Annotated References

1. Pyeritz RE, McKusick VA: The Marfan syndrome: Diagnosis and management. *N Engl J Med* 1979;300(14): 772-777.

2. Doman I, Kövér F, Illés T, Dóczi T: Subluxation of a lumbar vertebra in a patient with Marfan syndrome: Case report. *J Neurosurg* 2001;94(1, suppl):154-157.

3. Pearson GD, Devereux R, Loeys B, et al: Report of the National Heart, Lung, and Blood Institute and National Marfan Foundation Working Group on research in Marfan syndrome and related disorders. *Circulation* 2008;118(7):785-791.

4. Rifkin DB, Todorovic V: Bone matrix to growth factors: Location, location, location. *J Cell Biol* 2010;190(6): 949-951.

    A review of the role of fibrillin-1 mutations in transforming growth factor-β bioavailability/signaling in Marfan syndrome and the downstream effects on osteoblast maturation is presented. Level of evidence: V.

5. Loeys BL, Dietz HC, Braverman AC, et al: The revised Ghent nosology for the Marfan syndrome. *J Med Genet* 2010;47(7):476-485.

    The authors present a revision of the diagnostic criteria for Marfan syndrome composed by an international panel of experts. Level of evidence: V.

6. Ahn NU, Sponseller PD, Ahn UM, Nallamshetty L, Kuszyk BS, Zinreich SJ: Dural ectasia is associated with back pain in Marfan syndrome. *Spine (Phila Pa 1976)* 2000;25(12):1562-1568.

7. Alman BA, Goldberg MJ: *Lovell and Winter's Pediatric Orthopaedics*, ed 6. Philadelphia, PA, Lippincott Williams and Wilkins, 2006, pp 251-313.

8. Skaggs DL, Bushman G, Grunander T, Wong PC, Sankar WN, Tolo VT: Shortening of growing-rod spinal instrumentation reverses cardiac failure in child with Marfan syndrome and scoliosis: A case report. *J Bone Joint Surg Am* 2008;90(12):2745-2750.

9. Yang JS, Sponseller PD: Severe cervical kyphosis complicating halo traction in a patient with Marfan syndrome. *Spine (Phila Pa 1976)* 2009;34(1):E66-E69.

10. Beighton P, De Paepe A, Steinmann B, Tsipouras P, Wenstrup RJ; Ehlers-Danlos National Foundation (USA) and Ehlers-Danlos Support Group (UK): Ehlers-Danlos syndromes: Revised nosology, Villefranche, 1997. *Am J Med Genet* 1998;77(1):31-37.

11. Burrows NP, Nicholls AC, Yates JR, et al: The gene encoding collagen alpha1(V) (COL5A1) is linked to mixed Ehlers-Danlos syndrome type I/II. *J Invest Dermatol* 1996;106(6):1273-1276.

12. Wenstrup RJ, Langland GT, Willing MC, D'Souza VN,

    Cole WG: A splice-junction mutation in the region of COL5A1 that codes for the carboxyl propeptide of pro alpha 1(V) chains results in the gravis form of the Ehlers-Danlos syndrome (type I). *Hum Mol Genet* 1996;5(11):1733-1736.

13. Sillence DO, Senn A, Danks DM: Genetic heterogeneity in osteogenesis imperfecta. *J Med Genet* 1979;16(2): 101-116.

14. Cole WG: The molecular pathology of osteogenesis imperfecta. *Clin Orthop Relat Res* 1997;343:235-248.

15. Glorieux FH, Rauch F, Plotkin H, et al: Type V osteogenesis imperfecta: A new form of brittle bone disease. *J Bone Miner Res* 2000;15(9):1650-1658.

16. Glorieux FH, Ward LM, Rauch F, Lalic L, Roughley PJ, Travers R: Osteogenesis imperfecta type VI: A form of brittle bone disease with a mineralization defect. *J Bone Miner Res* 2002;17(1):30-38.

17. Ward LM, Rauch F, Travers R, et al: Osteogenesis imperfecta type VII: An autosomal recessive form of brittle bone disease. *Bone* 2002;31(1):12-18.

18. Glorieux FH: Bisphosphonate therapy for severe osteogenesis imperfecta. *J Pediatr Endocrinol Metab* 2000; 13(suppl 2):989-992.

19. Miyoshi K, Nakamura K, Haga N, Mikami Y: Surgical treatment for atlantoaxial subluxation with myelopathy in spondyloepiphyseal dysplasia congenita. *Spine (Phila Pa 1976)* 2004;29(21):E488-E491.

20. Bethem D, Winter RB, Lutter L, et al: Spinal disorders of dwarfism: Review of the literature and report of eighty cases. *J Bone Joint Surg Am* 1981;63(9):1412-1425.

21. Herring JA: *Tachdjian's Pediatric Orthopaedics*, ed 3. Philadelphia, PA, WB Saunders, 2002, pp 213-322.

22. Kolanczyk M, Kühnisch J, Kossler N, et al: Modelling neurofibromatosis type 1 tibial dysplasia and its treatment with lovastatin. *BMC Med* 2008;6:21.

23. Korf BR: Statins, bone, and neurofibromatosis type 1. *BMC Med* 2008;6:22.

24. Cho TJ, Seo JB, Lee HR, Yoo WJ, Chung CY, Choi IH: Biologic characteristics of fibrous hamartoma from congenital pseudarthrosis of the tibia associated with neurofibromatosis type 1. *J Bone Joint Surg Am* 2008; 90(12):2735-2744.

25. Stevenson DA, Moyer-Mileur LJ, Murray M, et al: Bone mineral density in children and adolescents with neurofibromatosis type 1. *J Pediatr* 2007;150(1):83-88.

26. Grill F, Bollini G, Dungl P, et al: Treatment approaches for congenital pseudarthrosis of tibia: Results of the

6: Pediatrics

EPOS multicenter study. *J Pediatr Orthop B* 2000;9(2): 75-89.

27. Dobbs MB, Rich MM, Gordon JE, Szymanski DA, Schoenecker PL: Use of an intramedullary rod for treatment of congenital pseudarthrosis of the tibia: A long-term follow-up study. *J Bone Joint Surg Am* 2004;86(6): 1186-1197.

28. Romanus B, Bollini G, Dungl P, et al: Free vascular fibular transfer in congenital pseudoarthrosis of the tibia: Results of the EPOS multicenter study. *J Pediatr Orthop B* 2000;9(2):90-93.

29. Paley D, Catagni M, Argnani F, Prevot J, Bell D, Armstrong P: Treatment of congenital pseudoarthrosis of the tibia using the Ilizarov technique. *Clin Orthop Relat Res* 1992;280:81-93.

30. Richards BS, Oetgen ME, Johnston CE: The use of rhBMP-2 for the treatment of congenital pseudarthrosis of the tibia: A case series. *J Bone Joint Surg Am* 2010; 92(1):177-185.

   A single institution's retrospective review of patients treated surgically for congenital pseudoarthrosis of the tibia to include rhBMP-2 in addition to the Williams intramedullary rod technique is presented. Level of evidence: IV.

31. Senta H, Park H, Bergeron E, et al: Cell responses to bone morphogenetic proteins and peptides derived from them: Biomedical applications and limitations. *Cytokine Growth Factor Rev* 2009;20(3):213-222.

32. Stevens PM, Klatt JB: Guided growth for pathological physes: Radiographic improvement during realignment. *J Pediatr Orthop* 2008;28(6):632-639.

33. Hall JG: The natural history of achondroplasia. *Basic Life Sci* 1988;48:3-9.

34. Horton WA: Fibroblast growth factor receptor 3 and the human chondrodysplasias. *Curr Opin Pediatr* 1997; 9(4):437-442.

35. Maynard JA, Ippolito EG, Ponseti IV, Mickelson MR: Histochemistry and ultrastructure of the growth plate in achondroplasia. *J Bone Joint Surg Am* 1981;63(6): 969-979.

36. Baca KE, Abdullah MA, Ting BL, et al: Surgical decompression for lumbar stenosis in pediatric achondroplasia. *J Pediatr Orthop* 2010;30(5):449-454.

   The authors reviewed pediatric patients with achondroplasia treated for lumbar stenosis. Higher revision rates were reported in patients who did not have concomitant fusion and instrumentation. Level of evidence: IV.

37. Yamanaka Y, Ueda K, Seino Y, Tanaka H: Molecular basis for the treatment of achondroplasia. *Horm Res* 2003;60(suppl 3):60-64.

38. Rousseau F, Bonaventure J, Legeai-Mallet L, et al: Clinical and genetic heterogeneity of hypochondroplasia. *J Med Genet* 1996;33(9):749-752.

39. Online Mendelian Inheritance in Man. National Center for Biotechnology: US National Library of Medicine website. http://omim.org/entry/134934. Accessed September 20, 2013.

   An updated review of disorders associated with FGFR3 gene mutations is presented. Level of evidence: V.

40. Tolo VT: *The Pediatric Spine: Principles and Practice.* New York, NY, Raven Press Ltd, 1994, pp 369-393.

41. Svensson O, Aaro S: Cervical instability in skeletal dysplasia: Report of 6 surgically fused cases. *Acta Orthop Scand* 1988;59(1):66-70.

42. Thomas S, Winter RB, Lonstein JE: The treatment of progressive kyphoscoliosis in camptomelic dysplasia. *Spine (Phila Pa 1976)* 1997;22(12):1330-1337.

43. Coscia MF, Bassett GS, Bowen JR, Ogilvie JW, Winter RB, Simonton SC: Spinal abnormalities in camptomelic dysplasia. *J Pediatr Orthop* 1989;9(1):6-14.

44. Lee B, Thirunavukkarasu K, Zhou L, et al: Missense mutations abolishing DNA binding of the osteoblast-specific transcription factor OSF2/CBFA1 in cleidocranial dysplasia. *Nat Genet* 1997;16(3):307-310.

45. Richie MF, Johnston CE II: Management of developmental coxa vara in cleidocranial dysostosis. *Orthopedics* 1989;12(7):1001-1004.

46. Winell J, Burke SW: Sports participation of children with Down syndrome. *Orthop Clin North Am* 2003; 34(3):439-443.

47. Doyle JS, Lauerman WC, Wood KB, Krause DR: Complications and long-term outcome of upper cervical spine arthrodesis in patients with Down syndrome. *Spine (Phila Pa 1976)* 1996;21(10):1223-1231.

48. Gicquel C, Cabrol S, Schneid H, Girard F, Le Bouc Y: Molecular diagnosis of Turner's syndrome. *J Med Genet* 1992;29(8):547-551.

49. Kim JY, Rosenfeld SR, Keyak JH: Increased prevalence of scoliosis in Turner syndrome. *J Pediatr Orthop* 2001; 21(6):765-766.

50. Tartaglia M, Kalidas K, Shaw A, et al: PTPN11 mutations in Noonan syndrome: Molecular spectrum, genotype-phenotype correlation, and phenotypic heterogeneity. *Am J Hum Genet* 2002;70(6):1555-1563.

51. Wedge JH, Khalifa MM, Shokeir MH: Skeletal anomalies in 40 patients with Noonan's syndrome. *Orthop Trans* 1987;11:40-41.

52. Lee CK, Chang BS, Hong YM, Yang SW, Lee CS, Seo

JB: Spinal deformities in Noonan syndrome: A clinical review of sixty cases. *J Bone Joint Surg Am* 2001; 83(10):1495-1502.

53. Holm VA, Cassidy SB, Butler MG, et al: Prader-Willi syndrome: Consensus diagnostic criteria. *Pediatrics* 1993;91(2):398-402.

54. Rees D, Jones MW, Owen R, Dorgan JC: Scoliosis surgery in the Prader-Willi syndrome. *J Bone Joint Surg Br* 1989;71(4):685-688.

55. Festen DA, de Lind van Wijngaarden R, van Eekelen M, et al: Randomized controlled GH trial: Effects on anthropometry, body composition and body proportions in a large group of children with Prader-Willi syndrome. *Clin Endocrinol (Oxf)* 2008;69(3):443-451.

56. de Lind van Wijngaarden RF, de Klerk LW, Festen DA, Duivenvoorden HJ, Otten BJ, Hokken-Koelega AC: Randomized controlled trial to investigate the effects of growth hormone treatment on scoliosis in children with Prader-Willi syndrome. *J Clin Endocrinol Metab* 2009; 94(4):1274-1280.

57. Kircher S, Bajbouj M, Beck M: *Mucopolysaccharidoses: A Guide for Physicians and Parents.* Bremen, Germany, Uni-Med Verlag AG, 2007.

58. Vellodi A, Young EP, Cooper A, et al: Bone marrow transplantation for mucopolysaccharidosis type I: Experience of two British centres. *Arch Dis Child* 1997; 76(2):92-99.

59. Giugliani R, Federhen A, Rojas MV, et al: Mucopolysaccharidosis I, II, and VI: Brief review and guidelines for treatment. *Genet Mol Biol* 2010;33(4):589-604.

The authors reviewed MPS disorders currently amenable to enzyme replacement therapy. Level of evidence: V.

60. Taylor C, Brady P, O'Meara A, Moore D, Dowling F, Fogarty E: Mobility in Hurler syndrome. *J Pediatr Orthop* 2008;28(2):163-168.

61. Malm G, Gustafsson B, Berglund G, et al: Outcome in six children with mucopolysaccharidosis type IH, Hurler syndrome, after haematopoietic stem cell transplantation (HSCT). *Acta Paediatr* 2008;97(8):1108-1112.

62. White KK, Hale S, Goldberg MJ: Musculoskeletal health in Hunter disease (MPS II): ERT improves functional outcomes. *J Pediatr Rehabil Med* 2010;3(2): 101-107.

The authors retrospectively reviewed musculoskeletal findings and functional outcomes as measured using the Pediatric Outcomes Data Collection Instrument in MPS type II after enzyme replacement therapy. Level of evidence: IV.

63. White KK, Karol LA, White DR, Hale S: Musculoskeletal manifestations of Sanfilippo Syndrome (mucopolysaccharidosis type III). *J Pediatr Orthop* 2011;31(5): 594-598.

The authors provided a two-institution review of the orthopedic manifestations of Sanfilippo syndrome. Level of evidence: IV.

64. Tassinari E, Boriani L, Traina F, Dallari D, Toni A, Giunti A: Bilateral total hip arthroplasty in Morquio-Brailsford's syndrome: A report of two cases. *Chir Organi Mov* 2008;92(2):123-126.

65. Bethem D, Winter RB, Lutter L: Disorders of the spine in diastrophic dwarfism. *J Bone Joint Surg Am* 1980; 62(4):529-536.

66. Poussa M, Merikanto J, Ryöppy S, Marttinen E, Kaitila I: The spine in diastrophic dysplasia. *Spine (Phila Pa 1976)* 1991;16(8):881-887.

67. Remes V, Marttinen E, Poussa M, Kaitila I, Peltonen J: Cervical kyphosis in diastrophic dysplasia. *Spine (Phila Pa 1976)* 1999;24(19):1990-1995.

68. Herring JA: The spinal disorders in diastrophic dwarfism. *J Bone Joint Surg Am* 1978;60(2):177-182.

69. Matsuyama Y, Winter RB, Lonstein JE: The spine in diastrophic dysplasia: The surgical arthrodesis of thoracic and lumbar deformities in 21 patients. *Spine (Phila Pa 1976)* 1999;24(22):2325-2331.

70. Ho CA, Karol LA: The utility of knee releases in arthrogryposis. *J Pediatr Orthop* 2008;28(3):307-313.

71. Devalia KL, Fernandes JA, Moras P, Pagdin J, Jones S, Bell MJ: Joint distraction and reconstruction in complex knee contractures. *J Pediatr Orthop* 2007;27(4):402-407.

72. van Bosse HJ, Feldman DS, Anavian J, Sala DA: Treatment of knee flexion contractures in patients with arthrogryposis. *J Pediatr Orthop* 2007;27(8):930-937.

73. Boehm S, Limpaphayom N, Alaee F, Sinclair MF, Dobbs MB: Early results of the Ponseti method for the treatment of clubfoot in distal arthrogryposis. *J Bone Joint Surg Am* 2008;90(7):1501-1507.

74. van Bosse HJ, Marangoz S, Lehman WB, Sala DA: Correction of arthrogrypotic clubfoot with a modified Ponseti technique. *Clin Orthop Relat Res* 2009;467(5): 1283-1293.

75. Morcuende JA, Dobbs MB, Frick SL: Results of the Ponseti method in patients with clubfoot associated with arthrogryposis. *Iowa Orthop J* 2008;28:22-26.

76. Van Heest A, James MA, Lewica A, Anderson KA: Posterior elbow capsulotomy with triceps lengthening for treatment of elbow extension contracture in children with arthrogryposis. *J Bone Joint Surg Am* 2008;90(7): 1517-1523.

77. Hermanns P, Unger S, Rossi A, et al: Congenital joint

6: Pediatrics

dislocations caused by carbohydrate sulfotransferase 3 deficiency in recessive Larsen syndrome and humerospinal dysostosis. *Am J Hum Genet* 2008;82(6):1368-1374.

78. Debeer P, De Borre L, De Smet L, Fryns JP: Asymmetrical Larsen syndrome in a young girl: A second example of somatic mosaicism in this syndrome. *Genet Couns* 2003;14(1):95-100.

79. Johnston CE II, Birch JG, Daniels JL: Cervical kyphosis in patients who have Larsen syndrome. *J Bone Joint Surg Am* 1996;78(4):538-545.

80. Madera M, Crawford A, Mangano FT: Management of severe cervical kyphosis in a patient with Larsen syndrome: Case report. *J Neurosurg Pediatr* 2008;1(4):320-324.

81. Sakaura H, Matsuoka T, Iwasaki M, Yonenobu K, Yoshikawa H: Surgical treatment of cervical kyphosis in Larsen syndrome: Report of 3 cases and review of the literature. *Spine (Phila Pa 1976)* 2007;32(1):E39-E44.

Chapter 67

Neuromuscular Disorders in Children

Unni G. Narayanan, MBBS, MSc, FRCSC   Michelle S. Caird, MD

Introduction

This chapter is an updated review of some of the more common childhood onset neuromuscular disorders that are associated with significant musculoskeletal consequences. The disorders arise from a wide range of etiologies (congenital, developmental, genetic, or chromosomal or acquired disorders) at the level of the brain, the spine, the peripheral nervous system, or muscle. Although basic science and epidemiologic research continues to evolve, an understanding of these conditions will possibly lead to prevention or cure. Orthopaedic surgery plays an important role in the management of children with these disorders, within the context of a multidisciplinary approach involving numerous healthcare disciplines.

Cerebral Palsy

Definitions, Etiology, and Pathophysiology

Cerebral palsy (CP) comprises a heterogeneous group of disorders of the development of movement and posture, which arise from permanent but nonprogressive disturbances in the developing brain of the fetus or infant. The motor disorders are often accompanied by disturbances in sensation, perception, cognition, communication, and behavior; epilepsy; and secondary musculoskeletal problems.[1] Collectively, CP is the most common cause of chronic disability in children, with a prevalence of 2 to 3 instances per 1,000 live births.[2]

The etiology of CP is diverse, with most cases being related to prenatal and neonatal causes; premature

Dr. Narayanan or an immediate family member serves as a board member, owner, officer, or committee member of the American Academy for Cerebral Palsy and Developmental Medicine and the Pediatric Orthopaedic Society of North America. Dr. Caird or an immediate family member serves as a board member, owner, officer, or committee member of the Pediatric Orthopaedic Society of North America, the Scoliosis Research Society, the Orthopaedic Research and Education Foundation, and the University of Michigan Medical School Alumni Society.

birth is the most common risk factor. The premature brain is particularly vulnerable because of its fragile vasculature and the immature autonomic nervous system that regulates cerebral blood flow. Periventricular leukomalacia is the most common lesion associated with prematurity. Other prenatal causes include intrauterine infections (toxoplasmosis, other intrauterine infection, rubella, cytomegalovirus, and herpes simplex virus, commonly referred to as the TORCH group), placental malformations, intrauterine hemorrhages, and prenatal and neonatal strokes. Congenital cerebral malformations such as encephaloceles, segmental defects, microcephaly, and cortical dysgenesis account for approximately 15% of all CP cases. Hypoxic encephalopathy at birth in full-term infants accounts for only 10% of cases. Postnatal causes include hyperbilirubinemias, metabolic abnormalities, postnatal trauma (shaken baby syndrome), infections, and toxicities.

The primary disturbance in the brain results in an upper motor neuron disorder that is associated with abnormal muscle tone (most often hypertonia) and is accompanied by a loss of selective motor control, muscle weakness, impaired balance, and a delay in the development of motor milestones. The location and the extent of the brain disturbance determine regional involvement as well as the severity of the disorder, which can vary from subtle physical findings and minimal limitations to severe functional disability. Motor disorders contribute to secondary musculoskeletal problems, including muscle contractures, because muscles around a joint are not equally affected. Muscles grow in response to stretch that occurs from typical physical activities associated with normal motor developmental milestones, such as rolling over, sitting, crawling, pulling up to stand, walking, running, and jumping. In patients with CP, the abnormal muscle tone initially results in dynamic contractures, where the muscle is taut (because of hypertonia) but of normal length. As motor development is delayed or fails to progress, muscle growth fails to keep pace with skeletal growth, so tight muscles gradually become short relative to the length of the bones that they traverse. Dynamic contractures become more fixed or static. Delayed developmental milestones and the forces associated with contractures result in altered development of the growing skeleton. Infantile morphology (increased femoral anteversion)

6: Pediatrics

Table 1

Cerebral Palsy Classifications Based on the Predominant Type of Tone and Movement Disorder

	Characteristics	Other Features
Spastic CP	Spasticity Velocity dependent hypertonia	Most common
Dystonic CP	Hypertonia Involuntary muscle contractions Slow repetitive movements or abnormal postures	Lesions of the basal ganglia
Athetoid CP	Involuntary twisting, writhing movements of limbs, trunk, and neck	Associated with neonatal kernicterus
Ataxic CP	Balance difficulties Sometimes hypotonia	Cerebellar lesions
Mixed movement CP	Combinations of spasticity and dystonic movements	

CP = cerebral palsy.

fails to remodel naturally and results in secondary bony deformities and joint instability that contribute to lever arm dysfunction,[3] which in turn affects the quality and the efficiency of gait and other aspects of physical function in children who are ambulatory or results in deformities of the trunk and limbs that can affect the health-related quality of life of those who are nonambulatory.

Classification

CP has been classified based on the predominant type of tone and movement disorder (Table 1); by anatomic distribution (hemiplegia, diplegia, or quadriplegia); and by the severity of the motor disability according to the Gross Motor Functional Classification System (GMFCS)[4] (Table 2). The five-level GMFCS has been shown to be stable and prognostically useful and is the current gold standard method for classifying CP.

Natural History

Motor function improves in all children with CP, leveling off between 6 and 7 years of age. Functional levels typically remain stable until early adolescence.[5] During adolescence, many ambulatory children will experience some decline in function associated with worsening musculoskeletal pathology that accompanies the adolescent growth spurt and is compounded by an increase in body weight.[6] Understanding this natural history is critical to put in context the perceived or real benefits of any treatments that these children receive. Improvements after treatment in a younger child must be greater than the expected improvements in gross motor function that occur naturally prior to age 7 years. Interventions in older children who show little change in outcomes might still be effective in preventing functional deterioration associated with growth.[7] The true benefits of different treatments can be inferred only from studies that include natural history controls for comparison. Longer-term studies are needed because the growing child is at risk for recurrent deformity and deteriorating function over time.

Goals of Treatment and Measurement of Outcomes

Optimization of gait function and improvement of gait appearance are the main goals of treatment of ambulatory children with CP. Better gait should be associated with an increase in speed and endurance, improved balance, fewer falls, reduced reliance on walking aids, reduced fatigue, and pain relief. Ideally, optimizing gait function should lead to increased independence and participation in sports and other physical activities. Outcome measures currently used for children with ambulatory CP include gait analysis and derived gait analysis-derived indices (Gait Deviation Index,[8] Gait Profile Score,[9] and Movement Analysis Profile[10]), which are summary measures of the overall patterns of gait; the Gross Motor Function Measure (GMFM-66),[11] the Pediatric Outcomes Data Collection Instrument,[12] the Gillette Functional Assessment Questionnaire,[13] and the Functional Mobility Scale.[14]

Nonambulatory children with CP (GMFCS levels IV and V) often experience several comorbidities such as seizures; cognitive, visual, and hearing impairments; communication difficulties; swallowing difficulties; drooling; aspiration; gastroesophageal reflux; constipation; and incontinence. Many of these children are at risk for aspiration pneumonias or malnutrition requiring insertion of gastrostomy or gastrojejunostomy tubes for safe feeding. They are also at high risk for developing contractures of the upper and lower limbs, progressive hip displacement, and scoliosis, which can be associated with pain and difficulties with positioning, seating, and caregiving. These children rely on caregivers for much of their activities of daily living. The goals of treatment for nonambulatory children include prevention or relief of pain, facilitation of caregiving, and preservation or improvement of health and quality of life. The Caregiver Priorities and Child Health Index of Life with Disability is the only validated condition-specific outcome measure for children with nonambulatory CP.[15]

Table 2

The Gross Motor Functional Classification System is a five-level ordinal rating system that has become the international standard for categorizing individuals based on the severity of their motor disability. The following definitions are for children age 6 to 12 years.

Level	Descriptors	
I	Can perform all the activities of their age-matched peers, albeit with some difficulties with their speed, balance, and coordination	
II	Similar functional abilities on flat and familiar surfaces as level I but require support when negotiating uneven surfaces or stairs	
III	Independent walkers but require a walking aid such as one or two canes, crutches, or a walker and may use wheelchairs for longer distances	
IV	Nonambulatory but able to functionally bear weight for transfers and use a walker for exercise purposes only	
V	Nonambulatory; poor head control and sitting balance; unable to do any functional weight bearing and are usually totally dependent on caregivers	

Treatment Strategies for Ambulatory CP

Physical therapy (stretching and strengthening), orthotics (braces), and serial casting are early treatment strategies for some of the musculoskeletal consequences of CP. Dynamic contractures secondary to increased muscle tone are treated with targeted injections of botulinum toxin or phenol into specific muscles or more systemically by neurosurgical methods, such as selective dorsal rhizotomy or intrathecal baclofen. These are believed to prevent or delay the onset of static contractures and bony deformities, which are best addressed with orthopaedic surgery. The current evidence for the effectiveness of these interventions for children with ambulatory CP is well summarized in systematic reviews on the subject.[16]

Botulinum toxin A (BTX-A) injections are effective in reducing calf muscle spasticity and increasing ankle dorsiflexion in the short term but are not superior to serial casting. Contradictory evidence exists regarding

6: Pediatrics

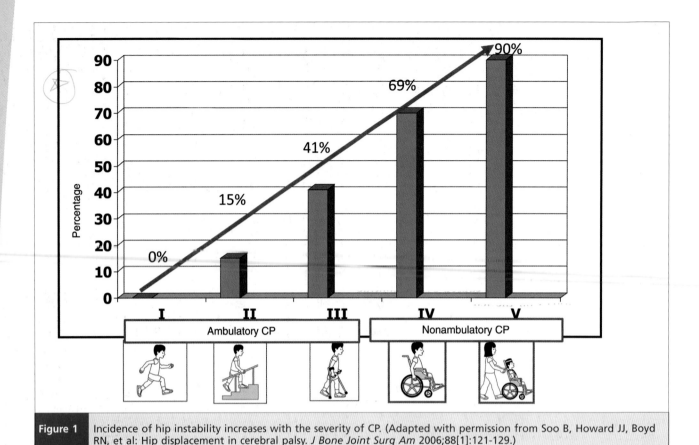

Figure 1 Incidence of hip instability increases with the severity of CP. (Adapted with permission from Soo B, Howard JJ, Boyd RN, et al: Hip displacement in cerebral palsy. *J Bone Joint Surg Am* 2006;88[1]:121-129.)

the effectiveness of combining BTX-A with serial casting. Limited evidence exists that the reduction in spasticity brought on by BTX-A potentiates the effect of physical therapy interventions to reduce hypertonicity, and these interventions result in measurable functional benefits. Furthermore, the long-term effects or benefits of BTX-A remain unknown.[17]

Selective dorsal rhizotomy followed by physiotherapy, when compared with physiotherapy alone, has been effective in reducing spasticity in the lower extremities of children age 4 to 8 years with spastic CP, but this reduction in spasticity was associated with a modest improvement in gross motor function.[18] Furthermore, selective dorsal rhizotomy may not reduce the need for subsequent orthopaedic surgery, and evidence regarding long-term benefits is sparse.[19,20]

Baclofen, a γ-aminobutyric acid agonist, can reduce generalized spasticity. However, oral baclofen is poorly absorbed, and the large doses required for any significant clinical effect are associated with undesirable side effects. Intrathecal administration of baclofen with an implantable pump allows for very small doses (μg) to directly reach the target tissue and is an effective way to control severe generalized hypertonia, but it is usually reserved for children with severe symptoms (GMFCS level V) because it is expensive and can be associated with several complications.[21,22]

Fixed contractures and bony deformities are best treated with musculotendinous lengthening or tendon transfers and corrective osteotomies using the strategy of single-event multilevel surgery (SEMLS) compared with staged single-level procedures.[23,24] In one small prospective trial, 11 children with spastic diplegia who underwent SEMLS demonstrated a substantial improvement in gait as measured by the Gait Profile Score and the Gillette Gait Index, compared with a control group of 8 children who underwent progressive resistance strength training. Functional outcomes were neither clinically nor statistically different between the two groups at 12 months. At 24-month follow-up, significant functional differences (five points on the GMFM-66) compared with baseline were detectable in the SEMLS group.[25] There are few published studies of the durability of outcomes or the long-term effects of multilevel orthopaedic surgery.[26]

Treatment Strategies in Nonambulatory CP
Hip Instability
Children with CP have normal hips at birth. Progressive hip displacement arises from spasticity of the hip adductors and hip flexors in combination with abnormal proximal femoral morphology (increased anteversion and coxa valga). The risk of hip instability is strongly correlated with increasing severity of CP, occurring in up to 90% of children at GMFCS level V[27] (Figure 1).

Dislocated hips are associated with contractures; the dislocations reduce mobility and interfere with dressing

© 2014 American Academy of Orthopaedic Surgeons

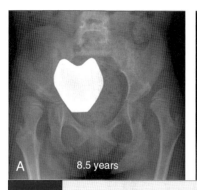
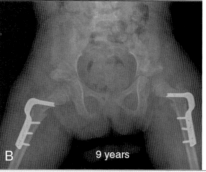
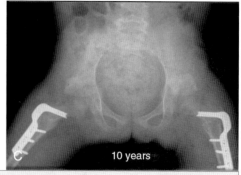

Figure 2   Radiographic views showing lateral reconstructive surgery for progressive hip subluxation. **A,** Preoperative AP radiograph of the pelvis shows significant bilateral hip subluxation. **B,** Postoperative AP radiograph following bilateral femoral and acetabular osteotomies shows reduced hips. **C,** One year postoperative radiograph of the pelvis shows healed osteotomies and maintenance of hip reductions bilaterally.

and perineal care. Pain may be caused by the contracture, abnormal forces on the femoral head or the acetabulum, or degenerative arthritis, which is present in 50% of adults with severe CP. Untreated hip dislocations in adults with CP have been associated with increased risk of sitting discomfort, pressure sores, and femoral fractures.[28,29] These symptoms can have a significant effect on health-related quality of life, and interventions to prevent these consequences in general are thought to be worthwhile. Clinical and radiographic surveillance is recommended, particularly for children with severe CP.[30]

In children with hips at risk of dislocation, the use of BTX-A injections along with abduction bracing does not prevent hips from further displacement but does reduce the rate of this displacement by one half, reduces the adduction contracture, and delays surgery until the child is older.[31] Although surgery may still be required, when performed in an older child, the risk of recurrence and the need for repeated reconstructive surgery may be reduced.

Some controversy exists regarding whether the strategy of early prophylactic surgery is superior to an early reactive surgical procedure performed at the first signs of symptoms (contracture interfering with caregiving or pain). Early prophylactic surgery (when the migration percentage has increased 30% to 40% without symptoms) has the theoretic benefit of less surgery[32] but at the greater risk of repeat surgery, which might include the same operations done if primary surgery was performed later. Early prophylactic adductor releases alone are associated with high recurrence rates, with up to 67% of patients requiring additional reconstructive procedures.[33] The rate of recurrence is highest for children in GMFCS levels IV and V.[34] Hip reconstructive procedures include adductor and psoas lengthening combined with proximal femoral varus derotational osteotomy to contain the hip. An open reduction of the femoral head generally is not required. A periacetabular pelvic osteotomy is added if there is significant acetabular dysplasia in children older than 6 years (Figure 2). In children with severe bilateral CP (diplegia and quadriplegia), bilateral reconstructive surgery is recommended, even when the hip instability is unilat-

eral, because the risk of dislocation of the contralateral side after unilateral surgery is high.[35,36]

Hip salvage surgery is reserved for symptomatic, long-standing, untreated hip dislocations where the femoral head is severely deformed, thereby precluding a congruent reconstruction. One effective salvage procedure is a proximal femoral head resection at the base of the neck, along with a subtrochanteric valgus osteotomy of the femur, in addition to adductor and psoas lengthening.[37] This combination effectively provides sufficient abduction for perineal hygiene, provides pain relief from the previous dislocation, and permits weight bearing in a stander. This procedure is seldom associated with heterotopic ossification or proximal migration noted with other more extensive proximal femoral resections.

Spinal Deformities in CP

Spinal deformity is common in children with severe motor disability (GMFCS levels IV and V).[38] Spinal deformity has been classified into three types: type 1, predominantly thoracic or thoracolumbar scoliosis with no pelvic obliquity; type 2, long C-shaped curves extending to the sacropelvis; and type 3, collapsing type of kyphosis with no coronal plane deformity.[39] Thoracolumbar curves tend to progress more than thoracic or lumbar curves, and the larger a curve at presentation, the more likely it is to get worse. Many spinal deformities remain flexible, allowing a child to be positioned comfortably in a wheelchair with appropriate lateral supports and back tilt to keep the child upright. External bracing sometimes is not tolerated because these children are often fed by gastrostomy tubes. There is also little evidence that braces prevent progression of the deformity. Rigid curves causing discomfort and pressure-related problems may require custom seating with molded backs to accommodate and support the child in an upright position.

Instrumented spinal fusion may be performed prophylactically while the curve is still relatively small (< 70°) and flexible or reactively at the onset of difficulties associated with the deformity. There is little evidence that a prophylactic surgical approach is neces-

Table 3

Orthopaedic Manifestations by Defect Level in Myelomeningocele

Level	Motor Examination	Orthopaedic Manifestations	Functional Manifestations
Thoracic	Flaccid lower extremities	Scoliosis (neuromuscular, congenital) Kyphosis Possible clubfeet, hip dislocations	Household ambulation with HKAFO bracing when small Wheelchair when bigger
Upper lumbar	Hip flexion/adduction partially intact Knee flexion/extension, ankle power, hip extension/abduction absent	Hip dislocation from unbalanced muscles common	Ambulation with HKAFO bracing when small Often wheelchair when bigger
Lower lumbar	Knee extension intact (L4— quadriceps) Ankle dorsiflexion possible (L5— tibialis anterior)	Clubfeet Calcaneus (L5) Hip dislocation or subluxation sometimes	Ambulation with KAFO bracing
Sacral	Hip flexion/adduction, knee flexion/extension, ankle power present Hip extension/abduction partially intact Gastrocnemius-soleus complex and foot weakness	Cavovarus foot deformity Hip dislocation much less common Ulcers may lead to osteomyelitis	Very good ambulation with AFO bracing

HKAFO = hip-knee-ankle-foot orthosis; KAFO = knee-ankle-foot orthosis; AFO = ankle-foot orthosis.

sary. A reactive approach may be just as effective when seating modifications are not effective. The standard surgical intervention is a long instrumented posterior spinal fusion to include the upper thoracic levels to the pelvis. This can be accomplished with unit rods and sublaminar wires or with more modern and stronger but more expensive pedicle screw constructs. The latter in combination with intraoperative traction obviates the need for anterior releases for larger curves.[40] The surgical objectives are to level the pelvis, improve the truncal balance to improve sitting comfort and endurance, and prevent pulmonary problems associated with a large curve.

Myelomeningocele

Defects of the neural tube occur in approximately 2 to 9 per 1,000 births and are the third most common birth defect in the United States. Bowel and bladder control are affected, and the lower extremities and the trunk are involved to varying extents, depending on the level of the defect. The goals of orthopaedic care for patients with myelomeningocele are correcting and preventing the deformity to maximize mobility and function. The orthopaedic surgeon is one member of the multidisciplinary team, which also includes neurosurgeons, urologists, rehabilitation specialists, physical and occupational therapists, nutritionists, neuropsychologists, orthotists, and social workers. Table 3 shows the orthopaedic and functional manifestations associated with the level of the lesion.

Several advances have been made in fetal surgery for myelomeningocele. The Management of Myelomeningocele Study (MOMS) randomized prenatal versus postnatal repair of myelomeningocele. It was stopped for efficacy of prenatal treatment at 183 of 200 patients because prenatal treatment reduced death and the need for shunting and improved motor function, but it was associated with increased preterm delivery and uterine dehiscence.[41] Improved motor function was measured as the difference between the neuromotor function level and the anatomic lesion level. The prenatal group was also more likely to be able to walk independently compared with the postnatal group, even though the prenatal group had higher lesion levels. Other outcomes of interest to orthopaedists require longer follow-up periods.

Spinal deformities may develop, including neuromuscular scoliosis, congenital scoliosis, or kyphosis. Scoliosis occurs in 50% to 90% of patients with myelomeningocele and may progress depending on the level of the lesion, patient maturity, and curve size.[42] Scoliosis treatment may include bracing to offer support and delay fusion but ultimately will not control curve progression. Surgery should achieve good sitting balance, maximize function, and halt curve progression.[43] Spinal fusion may be performed, but the risk of complications in this patient group is very high compared with other types of scoliosis. Patients with poor preoperative nutrition status and positive urine cultures have a high risk for perioperative wound infection and should be treated before fusion.[44] In patients with a thoracic-level lesion and kyphosis, several recent studies have shown that radical kyphectomy and long fusion to the pelvis improve sitting and skin ulcers but are associated with a significant risk of complications.[45,46]

Hip subluxation or dislocation is influenced by the level of the lesion. Controversy exists regarding attempts to reconstruct and relocate the hips. A func-

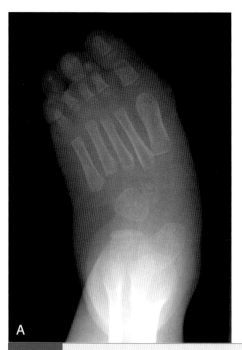
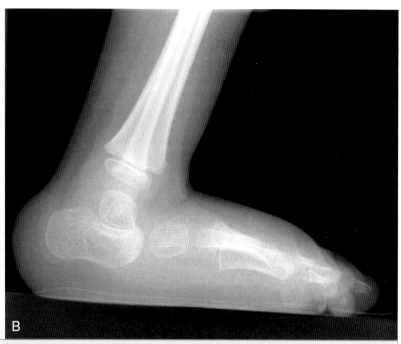

Figure 3 AP and lateral simulated weight-bearing views of a foot in calcaneovalgus in a 3-year-old boy with L5 myelomeningocele. Note the abducted forefoot with divergence of the talus and the calcaneus on the AP view (**A**) and the obliquity of the talus on the lateral view (**B**).

tional approach to the patient in this situation has been advocated. Gait may depend more on hip contractures than on hip location, and complications associated with surgery, including a decline in strength and increased fracture risk, may outweigh the benefits of reduction.[47]

The knees may experience excessive movements that can cause pain or destabilize ambulation. In some cases, bracing the knee with knee-ankle-foot orthoses offers stabilization. In addition, marked external tibial torsion may play a role in abnormal knee movement, which may require a derotational osteotomy. Patients with low lumbar or sacral myelomeningocele and knee flexion contractures who undergo radial posterior knee capsulectomy have improved contracture, dynamic sagittal kinematics, and walking velocity.[48] Knee extension is also important for standing in patients with higher level lesions, and flexion contractures may require treatment even in nonambulatory patients.

Common foot deformities in myelomeningocele include equinus, equinovarus, and calcaneus deformity, as shown in Figure 3. The Ponseti method for the treatment of equinovarus may be helpful but may not be as successful as in other diagnoses. Preservation of motion throughout the foot while correcting deformity is important to decrease the risks of skin breakdown and the development of adjacent arthritis in a neuropathic foot.[47]

Fractures occur in the lower extremities in patients with myelomeningocele. Low bone mineral density associated with minimal weight bearing may predispose patients to fractures from low-energy trauma. These

fractures present with painless swelling, warmth, and redness in the involved limb and can mimic infection with occasional fever and an elevated erythrocyte sedimentation rate. In this setting, radiographs should be obtained to evaluate for a fracture. Thoracic-level myelomeningocele is associated with a significantly higher fracture rate than at the sacral level.[49] The duration of immobilization should be minimized to decrease the risk of secondary fractures.

Muscular Dystrophies

The most common forms of muscular dystrophy are Duchenne muscular dystrophy (DMD) and Becker muscular dystrophy, which are progressive muscle diseases in which the gene encoding the large cell-membrane protein dystrophin is affected. The cell membrane is destabilized by the abnormal dystrophin, and cells become permeable to creatine kinase (CK), which can be detected in the blood in elevated levels. The muscle fibers degenerate and are replaced by fibroadipose tissue. DMD is inherited in an X-linked recessive manner, and 20% to 30% of cases result from spontaneous mutations. The condition occurs in 2 to 3 of 10,000 male births. Patients with DMD have no dystrophin detectable in muscle cells. Patients typically present between 18 months and 4 years of age with late walking, an abnormal stiff-kneed gait, pseudohypertrophy of the calves, or toe walking; they may have a positive Gower sign. CK levels are highly elevated, and muscle biopsy, if needed, shows an absence of dystrophin. Orthopaedic manifestations include mus-

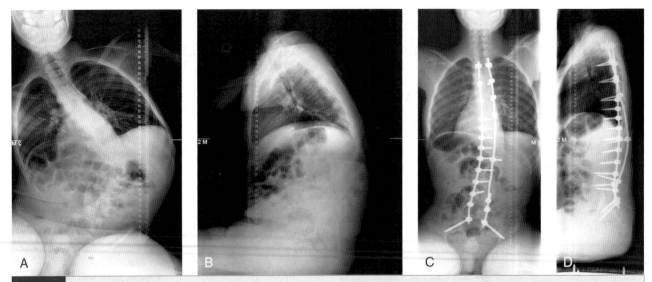

Figure 4   AP (**A**) and lateral (**B**) preoperative views of the spine of a 12-year-old boy with Duchenne muscular dystrophy showing an 82° curvature. AP (**C**) and lateral (**D**) views following posterior spinal fusion with instrumentation to the pelvis show improvement in both scoliosis and sitting position.

cle weakness that is greater proximally than distally, lumbar lordosis, scoliosis, and joint contractures. Becker muscular dystrophy may present with more mild weakness than with DMD, elevated levels of CK (but not as high as with DMD), and abnormal dystrophin on muscle biopsy.

Historically, patients with DMD generally stopped ambulating in their early teens and often died in their 20s from respiratory compromise or cardiac disease. However, corticosteroid treatment has been shown to slow the decrease in muscle strength and the progression of scoliosis.[50] Other studies have reported delayed loss of muscle strength, preservation of function, and extension of independent ambulation but increased vertebral compression fractures and long bone fractures with steroid treatment.[51] Questions remain regarding whether corticosteroids prevent scoliosis or merely delay its onset and whether the delayed onset of scoliosis increases the cardiac and respiratory risks associated with posterior spinal fusion and instrumentation.

The onset of scoliosis in DMD typically occurs when patients stop ambulating, and the general agreement is that spinal fusion should be performed early when the curve magnitude reaches 35°.[52] Some studies have shown that spinal fusion delays the rate of respiratory decline,[53] whereas others have shown no difference in respiratory change.[54] In addition, families of high-risk patients express satisfaction with posterior spinal fusion and believe surgery improved function and quality of life.[53] Studies of instrumentation constructs show that pedicle screw constructs, like those shown in Figure 4, compare well in curve correction and have lower blood loss and surgical times than Luque-Galveston techniques.[55] Preoperative assessment should include cardiac and pulmonary function tests to optimize patient condition before surgery.

Joint contractures can be addressed nonsurgically or

surgically to maintain function, assist with seating, and improve comfort. There is a wide variety of treatments depending on the patient's level of function and walking ability, from bracing and stretching to tendon lengthening.

Spinal Muscular Atrophy

Spinal muscular atrophy (SMA) is an autosomal recessive disorder caused by a deletion in the *SMN1* gene that results in the loss of the α motor neurons in the anterior horn of the spinal cord. This manifests as motor weakness with preserved sensation. Patients present with hypotonia, delayed milestones, and proximal greater than distal muscle weakness. Orthopaedic manifestations include scoliosis and hip dysplasia. Confirmation of the diagnosis includes screening for *SMN1* deletion. CK levels are normal in these patients, and an electromyogram (EMG) shows a motor nerve disorder with normal nerve conduction velocity studies.[56]

SMA is classified by age of onset and function. Type 1 (Werdnig-Hoffman) presents before 6 months of age with hypotonia, swallowing difficulty, and absent deep tendon reflexes. These patients never sit and have significant respiratory difficulty. Type 2 patients have symptom onset between 6 and 18 months with delayed motor milestones and muscle fasciculations. They gain the ability to sit and have variable walking ability. Type 3 (Kugelberg-Welander) patients present after 18 months of age, are generally ambulatory, and have Trendelenburg gait and muscle fasciculations.

Scoliosis occurs in nearly all patients with severe SMA types 1 and 2 and in about one half of the patients with type 3. It usually develops by the age of 10 years, and long, C-shaped neuromuscular type curves or thoracolumbar curves are most common. In SMA

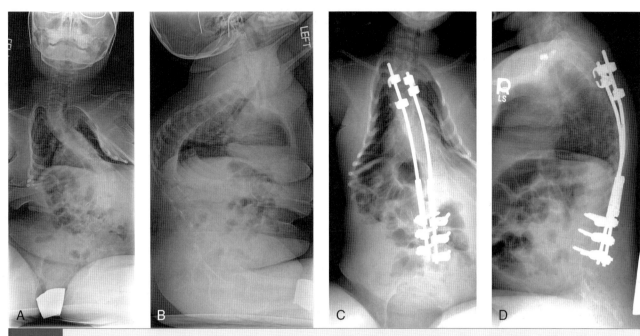

Figure 5 AP (**A**) and lateral (**B**) preoperative views of the spine of an 8-year-old boy with spinal muscular atrophy type II showing an 84° curvature with significant kyphosis. AP (**C**) and lateral (**D**) views following growing rod instrumentation shows improvement in both scoliosis and sitting position but persistence in rib collapse of the thorax.

types 1 and 2, bracing is ineffective and may result in respiratory compromise. Surgery for scoliosis results in improved sitting balance and endurance. In older children and adolescents, posterior spinal fusion is recommended. In juveniles, posterior spinal fusion to the pelvis may be considered based on a recent study,[57] which found that only 36% had major curve progression with Luque-Galveston fixation. In young children with large curves, a growing rod construct controlled the curves and pelvic obliquity well and promoted thoracic growth with little effect on other thoracic dimensions. Patients have longer hospital stays but fewer complications compared with patients with other diagnoses treated with growing rods[58,59] (Figure 5). Hip dislocation is common, especially in severe SMA, and observation is widely recommended. In a study of 41 patients with severe SMA, 17 of 82 hips (21%) were dislocated, and 20 hips were subluxated. Two patients had pain, and one had difficulty sitting, prompting the authors to recommend observation only.[60] In one study, hip reconstruction is not recommended in patients with severe SMA because no pain and no problems with perineal care were found in the study group, and because all four of the operated patients had recurrent dislocation.[61]

Hereditary Motor Sensory Neuropathy

Hereditary motor sensory neuropathy (HMSN) is the most common hereditary neuropathy and occurs about 1 in 5000 people. Multiple forms are described, but the most common is HMSN type 1, which is the autosomal dominant demyelinating type. HMSN types 1 and 2 are more commonly known as Charcot-Marie-Tooth disease types 1 and 2, respectively. The gene resides on chromosome 22 and encodes peripheral myelin protein.[62]

Diagnosis is made by family history, examination findings, EMG and nerve conduction velocity studies, and genetic testing. Patients present with intrinsic weakness, foot deformities, ankle sprains, and tripping. Orthopaedic manifestations include cavovarus foot deformity, scoliosis, and hip dysplasia.

Deformities of the foot and the ankle are progressive and begin with selective motor weakness of the foot intrinsic muscles. This is followed by weakness of the peroneus brevis and then the tibialis anterior, whereas the peroneus longus and tibialis posterior muscles are spared. This pattern of weakness results in cavus, claw toes, and hindfoot varus. Abnormal stress during ambulation may result in stress fractures, especially along the lateral foot. For skeletally immature feet with early weakness, bracing, night splints, physical therapy, and possibly BTX-A injections may temporarily maintain good foot position. As deformities continue and cavus progresses, the Coleman block test can be used to evaluate flexibility of the hindfoot. A block placed under the lateral border of the foot removes the influence of the fixed, plantar-flexed first ray. A plantar fascia release can be performed in young children. In older children an osteotomy along the first ray is added to treat the plantar flexion deformity. A calcaneal osteotomy can be added to treat rigid hindfoot varus. Transfers of the tibialis anterior or posterior, possible medial cuneiform osteotomies, and Achilles lengthening may also be

6: Pediatrics

needed to correct the deformity. Triple arthrodesis is reserved for salvage because arthritis of the ankle and the foot may develop.[63]

Spine deformity develops most commonly in adolescence, but unlike adolescent idiopathic scoliosis, curves are noted to be left sided in one third of the cases; kyphoscoliosis is present in almost one half of these patients.[64] Patients with various types of HMSN were studied; scoliosis developed in one fourth of the patients and three fourths of those with scoliosis had HMSN type 1. In addition, the deformity rates varied by genotype.[65] Bracing was found to be less successful than in adolescent idiopathic scoliosis.[64] The surgical indications are similar to those for idiopathic scoliosis, but curve progression may occur if selective short fusion is performed. Intraoperative spinal cord monitoring is not possible in most patients, but neurologic injury is uncommon.[64]

Hip dysplasia in HMSN is often asymptomatic until adolescence.[66] It is more commonly noted with HMSN type 1, and radiographs show a shallow acetabulum combined with a proximal femur abnormality.[67] Radiograph evaluation of the hips is recommended on an annual basis. Surgical procedures include osteotomies of the acetabulum and the proximal femur. Postoperative nerve palsy is more common because patients with HMSN may be more susceptible to subtle injury. Rigid internal fixation is recommended to minimize immobilization, which may cause severe debilitation.[66]

Friedreich Ataxia

Friedreich ataxia is an autosomal recessive disorder that occurs in approximately 1 in 50,000 live births. A defect in the responsible gene on chromosome 9 results in the loss of the mitochondrial protein frataxin. Iron accumulates in the mitochondria. Patients present at an average age of 11 or 12 years with areflexia, ataxic gait, weakness, and speech difficulties. Orthopaedic manifestations include cavovarus foot deformity, ataxic gait, and scoliosis. Other features include cardiomyopathy and respiratory insufficiency. The disease itself is progressive, with death occurring in the third or fourth decade of life.

Scoliosis occurs in 60% to 80% of patients, and progression is common. Left-sided curves and kyphoscoliosis are noted more frequently than in idiopathic scoliosis.[68,69] Bracing is poorly tolerated because it may interfere with walking, and its benefit is questionable. Outcomes with posterior spinal fusion are excellent,[68] but selective short fusion should be avoided to prevent postoperative progression. Intraoperative spinal cord monitoring may be difficult.[68,69]

Cavovarus feet that are supple or have significant growth left may require soft-tissue surgery, including Achilles lengthening or transfers of the tibialis anterior or tibialis posterior tendons, to achieve good foot position. Triple arthrodesis may be needed in the skeletally mature but stiff foot.[70,71]

Summary

Neuromuscular disorders in the growing child can result in a wide variety of musculoskeletal pathology. Patients are most effectively managed using a multidisciplinary disorder-based approach that involves therapists, orthotists, developmental pediatricians, physiatrists, and orthopaedic and neurosurgeons. Although orthopaedic surgery plays an important role in the management of children with these disorders, the evidence-based outcomes of the effectiveness of these interventions remain to be established. Continued clinical and basic science research is still needed to reverse musculoskeletal effects, halt progression, and improve treatment.

Key Study Points

- The GMFCS is the gold standard classification for CP.

- The goals of orthopaedic interventions for ambulatory CP are to improve gait-related function and gait appearance; prevent or relieve pain; promote independence; and increase physical activities, including sports and recreation.

- The MOMS study, which randomized patients to undergo prenatal myelomeningocele repair or postnatal repair, was stopped for efficacy of prenatal treatment at 183 of 200 patients. Prenatal repair reduced the need for shunting and improved motor function but was associated with increased preterm delivery and uterine dehiscence.

- Good curve control and few postoperative complications were shown in patients with SMA treated with growing rods from the thoracic spine to the pelvis for scoliosis.

Annotated References

1. Rosenbaum P, Paneth N, Leviton A, et al: A report: The definition and classification of cerebral palsy. *Dev Med Child Neurol Suppl* 2007;109:8-14.

2. Stanley F, Alberman ED, Blair E: *Cerebral Palsies: Epidemiology and Causal Pathways*. London, United Kingdom, Mac Keith Press, 2000.

3. Gage JR, Schwartz M: Pathologic gait and lever arm dysfunction, in Gage JR, ed: *The Treatment of Gait Problems in Cerebral Palsy*. London, United Kingdom, Mac Keith Press, 2004, pp 180-204.

4. Palisano R, Rosenbaum P, Walter S, Russell D, Wood E, Galuppi B: Development and reliability of a system to

classify gross motor function in children with cerebral palsy. *Dev Med Child Neurol* 1997;39(4):214-223.

5. Rosenbaum PL, Walter SD, Hanna SE, et al: Prognosis for gross motor function in cerebral palsy: Creation of motor development curves. *JAMA* 2002;288(11):1357-1363.

6. Hanna SE, Rosenbaum PL, Bartlett DJ, et al: Stability and decline in gross motor function among children and youth with cerebral palsy aged 2 to 21 years. *Dev Med Child Neurol* 2009;51(4):295-302; and Palisano R, Rosenbaum P, Walter S, Russel D, Wood E, Galuppi B: Development and reliability of a system to classify gross motor function in children with cerebral palsy. *Dev Med Child Neurol* 1997:39(4):214-223; and Can Child, www.canchild.ca; and Graham K, Reid B, Harvey A, The Royal Children's Hospital, Melbourne.

7. Gough M, Eve LC, Robinson RO, Shortland AP: Short-term outcome of multilevel surgical intervention in spastic diplegic cerebral palsy compared with the natural history. *Dev Med Child Neurol* 2004;46(2):91-97.

8. Schwartz MH, Rozumalski A: The Gait Deviation Index: A new comprehensive index of gait pathology. *Gait Posture* 2008;28(3):351-357.

9. Baker R, McGinley JL, Schwartz MH, et al: The gait profile score and movement analysis profile. *Gait Posture* 2009;30(3):265-269.

10. Beynon S, McGinley JL, Dobson F, Baker R: Correlations of the Gait Profile Score and the Movement Analysis Profile relative to clinical judgments. *Gait Posture* 2010;32(1):129-132.

    The authors investigated the validity of the Gait Profile Score and the Movement Analysis Profile related to clinical judgments. It appears that both measures may be helpful in clinical practice and education in addition to the traditional presentation of kinematic data.

11. Russell DJ, Avery LM, Rosenbaum PL, Raina PS, Walter SD, Palisano RJ: Improved scaling of the Gross Motor Function Measure for children with cerebral palsy: Evidence of reliability and validity. *Phys Ther* 2000; 80(9):873-885.

12. Daltroy LH, Liang MH, Fossel AH, Goldberg MJ; Pediatric Outcomes Instrument Development Group. Pediatric Orthopaedic Society of North America: The POSNA pediatric musculoskeletal functional health questionnaire: Report on reliability, validity, and sensitivity to change. *J Pediatr Orthop* 1998;18(5):561-571.

13. Novacheck TF, Stout JL, Tervo R: Reliability and validity of the Gillette Functional Assessment Questionnaire as an outcome measure in children with walking disabilities. *J Pediatr Orthop* 2000;20(1):75-81.

14. Graham HK, Harvey A, Rodda J, Nattrass GR, Pirpiris M: The Functional Mobility Scale (FMS). *J Pediatr Orthop* 2004;24(5):514-520.

15. Narayanan UG, Fehlings D, Weir S, Knights S, Kiran S, Campbell K: Initial development and validation of the Caregiver Priorities and Child Health Index of Life with Disabilities (CPCHILD). *Dev Med Child Neurol* 2006; 48(10):804-812.

16. Narayanan UG: Management of children with ambulatory cerebral palsy: An evidence-based review. *J Pediatr Orthop* 2012;32(suppl 2):S172-S181.

    Current evidence of the effectiveness for specific interventions in children with ambulatory CP, including BTX-A injections, selective dorsal rhizotomy, multilevel orthopaedic surgery, and the role of gait analysis for surgical decision making before surgery are reviewed.

17. Bjornson K, Hays R, Graubert C, et al: Botulinum toxin for spasticity in children with cerebral palsy: A comprehensive evaluation. *Pediatrics* 2007;120(1):49-58

18. McLaughlin J, Bjornson K, Temkin N, et al: Selective dorsal rhizotomy: Meta-analysis of three randomized controlled trials. *Dev Med Child Neurol* 2002;44(1):17-25.

19. Langerak NG, Tam N, Vaughan CL, Fieggen AG, Schwartz MH: Gait status 17-26 years after selective dorsal rhizotomy. *Gait Posture* 2012;35(2):244-249.

    Thirty-one adults were assessed an average of 21 years after selective dorsal rhizotomy: 58% showed improvements in gross motor function, whereas none deteriorated. Sixty-one percent required additional orthopaedic surgery.

20. Grunt S, Becher JG, Vermeulen RJ: Long-term outcome and adverse effects of selective dorsal rhizotomy in children with cerebral palsy: A systematic review. *Dev Med Child Neurol* 2011;53(6):490-498.

    This systematic review found moderate evidence for the long-term effects of selective dorsal rhizotomy on spasticity reduction but little evidence that this resulted in meaningful functional benefits. Level of evidence: II.

21. Butler C, Campbell S; AACPDM Treatment Outcomes Committee Review Panel: Evidence of the effects of intrathecal baclofen for spastic and dystonic cerebral palsy. *Dev Med Child Neurol* 2000;42(9):634-645.

22. Campbell WM, Ferrel A, McLaughlin JF, et al: Long-term safety and efficacy of continuous intrathecal baclofen. *Dev Med Child Neurol* 2002;44(10):660-665.

23. McGinley JL, Dobson F, Ganeshalingam R, Shore BJ, Rutz E, Graham HK: Single-event multilevel surgery for children with cerebral palsy: A systematic review. *Dev Med Child Neurol* 2012;54(2):117-128.

    A systematic review of 31 studies of SEMLS highlights that current evidence stems from small, uncontrolled case series with short-term outcomes and few controlled studies or clinical trials.

24. Fabry G, Liu XC, Molenaers G: Gait pattern in patients with spastic diplegic cerebral palsy who underwent staged operations. *J Pediatr Orthop B* 1999;8(1):33-38.

6: Pediatrics

25. Thomason P, Baker R, Dodd K, et al: Single-event multilevel surgery in children with spastic diplegia: A pilot randomized controlled trial. *J Bone Joint Surg Am* 2011;93(5):451-460.

   In this small trial, gait outcomes improved at 12 months in children who underwent SEMLS compared with a control group that received only strengthening. In the SEMLS group, functional outcomes (based on GMFM-66) improved 24 months from baseline. Level of evidence: II.

26. Saraph V, Zwick EB, Auner C, Schneider F, Steinwender G, Linhart W: Gait improvement surgery in diplegic children: How long do the improvements last? *J Pediatr Orthop* 2005;25(3):263-267.

27. Soo B, Howard JJ, Boyd RN, et al: Hip displacement in cerebral palsy. *J Bone Joint Surg Am* 2006;88(1):121-129.

28. Cooperman DR, Bartucci E, Dietrick E, Millar EA: Hip dislocation in spastic cerebral palsy: Long-term consequences. *J Pediatr Orthop* 1987;7(3):268-276.

29. Noonan KJ, Jones J, Pierson J, Honkamp NJ, Leverson G: Hip function in adults with severe cerebral palsy. *J Bone Joint Surg Am* 2004;86(12):2607-2613.

30. Gordon GS, Simkiss DE: A systematic review of the evidence for hip surveillance in children with cerebral palsy. *J Bone Joint Surg Br* 2006;88(11):1492-1496.

31. Graham HK, Boyd R, Carlin JB, et al: Does botulinum toxin A combined with bracing prevent hip displacement in children with cerebral palsy and "hips at risk"? A randomized, controlled trial. *J Bone Joint Surg Am* 2008;90(1):23-33.

32. Hägglund G, Andersson S, Düppe H, Lauge-Pedersen H, Nordmark E, Westbom L: Prevention of dislocation of the hip in children with cerebral palsy: The first ten years of a population-based prevention programme. *J Bone Joint Surg Br* 2005;87-B(1):95-101.

33. Stott NS, Piedrahita L; AACPDM: Effects of surgical adductor releases for hip subluxation in cerebral palsy: An AACPDM evidence report. *Dev Med Child Neurol* 2004;46(9):628-645.

34. Shore BJ, Yu X, Desai S, Selber P, Wolfe R, Graham HK: Adductor surgery to prevent hip displacement in children with cerebral palsy: The predictive role of the Gross Motor Function Classification System. *J Bone Joint Surg Am* 2012;94(4):326-334.

   In 330 children who underwent adductor surgery to prevent progressive hip displacement, this was successful only 32% of the time. In nonambulatory children (GMFCS IV and V), the success rate dropped to less than 20%. Level of evidence: II.

35. Canavese F, Emara K, Sembrano JN, Bialik V, Aiona MD, Sussman MD: Varus derotation osteotomy for the treatment of hip subluxation and dislocation in GMFCS level III to V patients with unilateral hip involvement:

   Follow-up at skeletal maturity. *J Pediatr Orthop* 2010; 30(4):357-364.

   Twenty-seven children with bilateral CP (GMFCS levels III to V) underwent unilateral hip reconstructive surgery. Twelve of the 27 (44%) developed contralateral hip displacement requiring surgery by skeletal maturity. Level of evidence: IV.

36. Park MS, Chung CY, Kwon DG, Sung KH, Choi IH, Lee KM: Prophylactic femoral varization osteotomy for contralateral stable hips in non-ambulant individuals with cerebral palsy undergoing hip surgery: Decision analysis. *Dev Med Child Neurol* 2012;54(3):231-239.

   Using decision analysis, this study suggests that nonambulatory children (10 years or younger) with bilateral CP (GMFCS levels IV and V) and unilateral hip displacement would benefit from a prophylactic proximal femoral osteotomy of the contralateral hip concurrently with reconstruction for the affected side.

37. McHale KA, Bagg M, Nason SS: Treatment of the chronically dislocated hip in adolescents with cerebral palsy with femoral head resection and subtrochanteric valgus osteotomy. *J Pediatr Orthop* 1990;10(4):504-509.

38. Persson-Bunke M, Hägglund G, Lauge-Pedersen H, Wagner P, Westbom L: Scoliosis in a total population of children with cerebral palsy. *Spine (Phila Pa 1976)* 2012;37(12):E708-E713.

   Data from the CP registry in southern Sweden show that GMFCS level IV or V had a 50% risk of having moderate or severe scoliosis by 18 years of age, whereas children in GMFCS level I or II had almost no risk. Level of evidence: II.

39. Lonstein JE, Akbarnia A: Operative treatment of spinal deformities in patients with cerebral palsy or mental retardation: An analysis of one hundred and seven cases. *J Bone Joint Surg Am* 1983;65(1):43-55.

40. Keeler KA, Lenke LG, Good CR, Bridwell KH, Sides B, Luhmann SJ: Spinal fusion for spastic neuromuscular scoliosis: Is anterior releasing necessary when intraoperative halo-femoral traction is used? *Spine (Phila Pa 1976)* 2010;35(10):E427-E433.

   In this retrospective study, intraoperative halo-femoral traction with posterior spinal fusion was associated with equivalent curve correction and spinal balance but shorter operating room times, lower blood loss, fewer postoperative intubations, and fewer cases of pneumonias when compared with anterior releases combined with posterior spinal fusions. Level of evidence: III.

41. Adzick NS, Thom EA, Spong CY, et al: A randomized trial of prenatal versus postnatal repair of myelomeningocele. *N Engl J Med* 2011;364(11):993-1004.

   This study randomized patients to undergo prenatal myelomeningocele repair or postnatal repair and was stopped for efficacy of prenatal treatment at 183 of 200 patients. Prenatal repair reduced the need for shunting and improved motor function, but it was associated with increased preterm delivery and uterine dehiscence. Level of evidence: I.

42. Müller EB, Nordwall A, Odén A: Progression of scoliosis in children with myelomeningocele. *Spine (Phila Pa 1976)* 1994;19(2):147-150.

43. Guille JT, Sarwark JF, Sherk HH, Kumar SJ: Congenital and developmental deformities of the spine in children with myelomeningocele. *J Am Acad Orthop Surg* 2006; 14(5):294-302.

44. Hatlen T, Song K, Shurtleff D, Duguay S: Contributory factors to postoperative spinal fusion complications for children with myelomeningocele. *Spine (Phila Pa 1976)* 2010;35(13):1294-1299.

    This retrospective review of 59 patients with myelomeningocele who underwent spinal fusion found that positive preoperative urine cultures and poor nutrition status significantly increased the risk for a postoperative wound infection. Level of evidence: III.

45. Altiok H, Finlayson C, Hassani S, Sturm P: Kyphectomy in children with myelomeningocele. *Clin Orthop Relat Res* 2011;469(5):1272-1278.

    This retrospective review of 33 patients with myelomeningocele who underwent kyphectomy and posterior spinal fusion with instrumentation to the pelvis showed good correction and maintenance of alignment but a risk for complications; 11 secondary surgeries were required. Level of evidence: IV.

46. Garg S, Oetgen M, Rathjen K, Richards BS: Kyphectomy improves sitting and skin problems in patients with myelomeningocele. *Clin Orthop Relat Res* 2011; 469(5):1279-1285.

    This retrospective review of 18 patients with thoracic myelomeningocele who underwent kyphectomy and spinal fusion found frequent complications, with 7 patients requiring multiple procedures, but improved sitting balance and resolved skin problems in 17 of 18 patients. Level of evidence: IV.

47. Thomson JD, Segal LS: Orthopedic management of spina bifida. *Dev Disabil Res Rev* 2010;16(1):96-103.

    The authors present a review of the changes over the past 10 years in diagnosis, functional assessment, and orthopaedic management of myelomeningocele with emphasis on gait, scoliosis, and kyphosis.

48. Moen TC, Dias L, Swaroop VT, Gryfakis N, Kelp-Lenane C: Radical posterior capsulectomy improves sagittal knee motion in crouch gait. *Clin Orthop Relat Res* 2011;469(5):1286-1290.

    This retrospective review of 11 patients with low lumbar or sacral myelomeningocele and knee flexion contractures found that radial posterior knee capsulectomy improved the contracture, dynamic sagittal kinematics, and walking velocity. Level of evidence: IV.

49. Akbar M, Bresch B, Raiss P, et al: Fractures in myelomeningocele. *J Orthop Traumatol* 2010;11(3):175-182.

    This retrospective study of 862 patients with myelomeningocele found that 11% of the patients had one or more fractures, and those with thoracic level paralysis were at highest risk. Level of evidence: IV.

50. Alman BA, Raza SN, Biggar WD: Steroid treatment and the development of scoliosis in males with Duchenne muscular dystrophy. *J Bone Joint Surg Am* 2004;86(3): 519-524.

51. King WM, Ruttencutter R, Nagaraja HN, et al: Orthopedic outcomes of long-term daily corticosteroid treatment in Duchenne muscular dystrophy. *Neurology* 2007;68(19):1607-1613.

52. Karol LA: Scoliosis in patients with Duchenne muscular dystrophy. *J Bone Joint Surg Am* 2007;89(suppl 1):155-162.

53. Takaso M, Nakazawa T, Imura T, et al: Surgical management of severe scoliosis with high risk pulmonary dysfunction in Duchenne muscular dystrophy: Patient function, quality of life and satisfaction. *Int Orthop* 2010;34(5):695-702.

    This study identified 14 patients with DMD and severe pulmonary dysfunction who underwent posterior spinal fusion for scoliosis and found good long-term deformity correction, no major complications with surgery, and high family satisfaction and improved quality of life after surgery. Level of evidence: IV.

54. Roberto R, Fritz A, Hagar Y, et al: The natural history of cardiac and pulmonary function decline in patients with duchenne muscular dystrophy. *Spine (Phila Pa 1976)* 2011;36(15):E1009-E1017.

    This retrospective review of 174 patients with DMD tracked the decline in pulmonary and cardiac function and found no difference in those patients treated with posterior spinal fusion and those whose scoliosis was followed nonsurgically. Level of evidence: III.

55. Arun R, Srinivas S, Mehdian SM: Scoliosis in Duchenne's muscular dystrophy: A changing trend in surgical management. A historical surgical outcome study comparing sublaminar, hybrid and pedicle screw instrumentation systems. *Eur Spine J* 2010;19(3): 376-383.

    This retrospective study compares surgical correction of scoliosis in DMD using different types of instrumentation and found similar good maintenance of correction at long-term follow-up but lower blood loss and surgical time with pedicle screw constructs. Level of evidence: IV.

56. Mesfin A, Sponseller PD, Leet AI: Spinal muscular atrophy: Manifestations and management. *J Am Acad Orthop Surg* 2012;20(6):393-401.

    The authors reviewed the genetics, presentation, diagnosis, and management of SMA with emphasis on the orthopaedic aspects.

57. Zebala LP, Bridwell KH, Baldus C, et al: Minimum 5-year radiographic results of long scoliosis fusion in juvenile spinal muscular atrophy patients: Major curve progression after instrumented fusion. *J Pediatr Orthop* 2011;31(5):480-488.

    This retrospective multicenter review of 22 SMA patients who had undergone posterior spinal fusion with

6: Pediatrics

Index

titanium, 69
TKA applications of, 69
Metaphyseal fractures
distal radius and ulna, 801–802, 802*f*
proximal tibial, 877
Metastatic disease
skeletal
biology of, 278–279
bisphosphonate role in, 279–280
epidemiology of, 278
fracture risk prediction in, 280
treatment of, 280–282, 281*f*
spinal
radiation for, 770–771
surgical decision making for, 769–770, 770*t*
Metatarsal fractures, 639
pediatric, 880
Metatarsus adductus, 889
Methadone, postoperative pain management with, 311
Methicillin-resistant *Staphylococcus aureus* (MRSA)
in athletes, 121
in orthopaedic infections, 288
in osteomyelitis, 292–293
in septic arthritis, 293–294
Methotrexate (Rheumatrex)
for psoriatic arthritis, 217
for RA, 214*t*
Methylprednisolone
for cervical SCI, 680–681
during lumbar disk herniation surgery, 720
for UBCs, 269–270
Meyerding classification, of spondylolisthesis, 831, 832*f*
Microbiology, of orthopaedic infections, 288
Microfracture, for cartilage repair, 545*f*, 546
Micromechanics, 54–55
Micronutrient recommendations, for athletes, 116, 116*t*
Microsurgery, for brachial plexus birth palsy, 821–822
Middle third tibia, soft-tissue coverage about, 569–571, 570*f*, 571*f*
Midfoot amputation, 662, 662*t*
Midfoot fractures
pediatric, 880
tarsal navicular, 635–636, 635*f*, 636*f*, 637*f*
Midfoot reconstruction, 647
Midshaft clavicular fractures, 325, 326*f*
Mirror hand, 819, 820*f*
Mitochondriopathies, metabolic, 243, 244*t*
MMN. *See* Multifocal motor neuropathy
MMP-9. *See* Matrix metalloproteinase 9
MMP-13. *See* Matrix metalloproteinase 13

Mobile-bearing TKAs, 587
Modified Gibson approach, for acetabular fractures, 460–461
Modified Stoppa approach, for acetabular fractures, 461
Modularity, in TKA, 587
Molecular markers. *See* Biomarkers
Molecular therapy, for low back pain, 733
MOMS. *See* Management of Myelomeningocele Study
MoM surfaces. *See* Metal-on-metal surfaces
Monoclonal antibodies, for RA, 213, 214*t*
Mononucleosis, in athletes, 121
Monteggia injuries, 394
pediatric, 797–798, 798*t*
Morality, medical ethics and, 6–7
Morphine
for lower extremity amputations, 664
postoperative pain management with, 312–313, 312*t*
Morquio syndrome, 923*t*, 924, 924*t*, 925*f*
Moving valgus stress test, for MCL injury, 377, 377*f*
MPFL reconstruction. *See* Medial patellofemoral ligament reconstruction
MPSs. *See* Mucopolysaccharidoses
MRI. *See* Magnetic resonance imaging
MRSA. *See* Methicillin-resistant *Staphylococcus aureus*
MSTS. *See* Musculoskeletal Tumor Society
MTM. *See* Myotubular myopathy
Mucopolysaccharidoses (MPSs), 11–13, 923*t*, 924*t*, 925*f*
Multidirectional instability (MDI), 361
Multifocal motor neuropathy (MMN), 259–260
Multiple epiphyseal dysplasias, 921, 921*t*
Multiple myeloma, 275
Multiple pterygia syndrome, 926*t*, 927–928, 928*f*
Mupirocin, for skin infections, 121
Muscle
architecture of, 237
in human arm, 36–37, 37*f*
in human leg, 37–38
fiber types in, 38
functional anatomy of, 35, 35*f*
function of, 237
passive biomechanical properties of, 36*f*, 38
regeneration of, 39
sarcomeres of, 35–36, 35*f*, 36*f*
tendon interactions with, 40, 41*t*
Muscle disorders, 237
congenital structural myopathies, 241–242, 243*t*

diagnosis of, 245–248, 247*f*, 248*f*
fibromyalgia, 243–245
genetic counseling for, 245–248, 247*f*, 248*f*
inflammatory myopathies, 238–239, 238*t*
metabolic myopathies–mitochondriopathies, 243, 244*t*
muscular dystrophies, 239–240, 239*t*, 939–940, 940*f*
myasthenia gravis and myasthenic syndromes, 240–241
myotonias/channelopathies, 242–243, 244*t*
neuropathic disorders, 241, 242*t*
paraneoplastic myopathy, 245
rhabdomyolysis, 245, 246*t*
Muscle relaxants, for low back pain, 730
Muscular dystrophies, 239–240, 239*t*, 939–940, 940*f*
Musculoskeletal biomechanics
of articular cartilage, 49–50
of bone, 49
clinical applications from
mechanical testing for fracture treatment insight, 55
optimal implant positioning, 55–56, 56*f*
patient-specific treatment, 56–57
of knee extensor mechanism, 528
of ligaments, 42, 50–51, 51*f*
after injury, 43, 43*f*
new and developing focus areas in
locked plating and related concepts, 53–54, 53*f*
micromechanics, 54–55
noninvasive mechanical assessment, 54
patient-specific treatment, 51–53, 52*f*, 53*f*
of pelvic ring, 449
in rotator cuff disease, 362–363
in shoulder instability, 357–358, 358*f*
of skeletal muscle
active properties, 35–38, 36*f*, 37*f*
passive properties, 36*f*, 38
of tendons, 39, 50–51, 51*f*
aging and injury effects on, 40–41
terminology used in, 50*t*
Musculoskeletal tumors
biopsy of, 268
clinical presentation of, 265
epidemiology of, 265
imaging of
bone scintigraphy, 267, 267*f*
MRI, 266
PET, 267–268, 268*f*
plain film radiography, 265, 266*f*
ultrasonography, 265–266
initial workup of, 265
metastatic skeletal disease
biology of, 278–279